ISBN 978-1-332-19690-6
PIBN 10296854

FB &c Ltd, Dalton House, 60 Windsor Avenue, London, SW19 2RR.
Company number 08720141. Registered in England and Wales.

For support please visit www.forgottenbooks.com

SMITHSONIAN

CONTRIBUTIONS TO KNOWLEDGE.

VOL. XII.

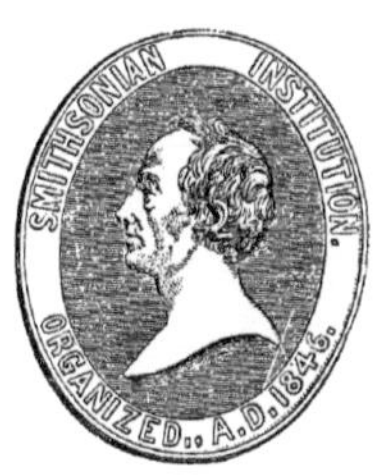

EVERY MAN IS A VALUABLE MEMBER OF SOCIETY, WHO, BY HIS OBSERVATIONS, RESEARCHES, AND EXPERIMENTS, PROCURES KNOWLEDGE FOR MEN.—SMITHSON.

CITY OF WASHINGTON:
PUBLISHED BY THE SMITHSONIAN INSTITUTION.
MDCCCLX.

ADVERTISEMENT.

This volume forms the twelfth of a series, composed of original memoirs on different branches of knowledge, published at the expense, and under the direction, of the Smithsonian Institution. The publication of this series forms part of a general plan adopted for carrying into effect the benevolent intentions of James Smithson, Esq., of England. This gentleman left his property in trust to the United States of America, to found, at Washington, an institution which should bear his own name, and have for its objects the "*increase* and *diffusion* of knowledge among men." This trust was accepted by the Government of the United States, and an Act of Congress was passed August 10, 1846, constituting the President and the other principal executive officers of the general government, the Chief Justice of the Supreme Court, the Mayor of Washington, and such other persons as they might elect honorary members, an establishment under the name of the "Smithsonian Institution for the increase and diffusion of knowledge among men." The members and honorary members of this establishment are to hold stated and special meetings for the supervision of the affairs of the Institution, and for the advice and instruction of a Board of Regents, to whom the financial and other affairs are intrusted.

The Board of Regents consists of three members *ex officio* of the establishment, namely, the Vice-President of the United States, the Chief Justice of the Supreme Court, and the Mayor of Washington, together with twelve other members, three of whom are appointed by the Senate from its own body, three by the House of Representatives from its members, and six persons appointed by a joint resolution of both houses. To this Board is given the power of electing a Secretary and other officers, for conducting the active operations of the Institution.

To carry into effect the purposes of the testator, the plan of organization should evidently embrace two objects: one, the increase of knowledge by the addition of new truths to the existing stock; the other, the diffusion of knowledge, thus increased, among men. No restriction is made in favor of any kind of knowledge; and, hence, each branch is entitled to, and should receive, a share of attention.

The Act of Congress, establishing the Institution, directs, as a part of the plan of organization, the formation of a Library, a Museum, and a Gallery of Art, together with provisions for physical research and popular lectures, while it leaves to the Regents the power of adopting such other parts of an organization as they may deem best suited to promote the objects of the bequest.

After much deliberation, the Regents resolved to divide the annual income into two equal parts—one part to be devoted to the increase and diffusion of knowledge by means of original research and publications—the other half of the income to be applied in accordance with the requirements of the Act of Congress, to the gradual formation of a Library, a Museum, and a Gallery of Art.

The following are the details of the parts of the general plan of organization provisionally adopted at the meeting of the Regents, Dec. 8, 1847.

DETAILS OF THE FIRST PART OF THE PLAN.

I. To INCREASE KNOWLEDGE.—*It is proposed to stimulate research, by offering rewards for original memoirs on all subjects of investigation.*

1. The memoirs thus obtained, to be published in a series of volumes, in a quarto form, and entitled "Smithsonian Contributions to Knowledge."

2. No memoir, on subjects of physical science, to be accepted for publication, which does not furnish a positive addition to human knowledge, resting on original research; and all unverified speculations to be rejected.

3. Each memoir presented to the Institution, to be submitted for examination to a commission of persons of reputation for learning in the branch to which the memoir pertains; and to be accepted for publication only in case the report of this commission is favorable.

4. The commission to be chosen by the officers of the Institution, and the name of the author, as far as practicable, concealed, unless a favorable decision be made.

5. The volumes of the memoirs to be exchanged for the Transactions of literary and scientific societies, and copies to be given to all the colleges, and principal libraries, in this country. One part of the remaining copies may be offered for sale; and the other carefully preserved, to form complete sets of the work, to supply the demand from new institutions.

6. An abstract, or popular account, of the contents of these memoirs to be given to the public, through the annual report of the Regents to Congress.

II. TO INCREASE KNOWLEDGE.—*It is also proposed to appropriate a portion of the income, annually, to special objects of research, under the direction of suitable persons.*

1. The objects, and the amount appropriated, to be recommended by counsellors of the Institution.

2. Appropriations in different years to different objects; so that, in course of time, each branch of knowledge may receive a share.

3. The results obtained from these appropriations to be published, with the memoirs before mentioned, in the volumes of the Smithsonian Contributions to Knowledge.

4. Examples of objects for which appropriations may be made:—

(1.) System of extended meteorological observations for solving the problem of American storms.

(2.) Explorations in descriptive natural history, and geological, mathematical, and topographical surveys, to collect material for the formation of a Physical Atlas of the United States.

(3.) Solution of experimental problems, such as a new determination of the weight of the earth, of the velocity of electricity, and of light; chemical analyses of soils and plants; collection and publication of articles of science, accumulated in the offices of Government.

(4.) Institution of statistical inquiries with reference to physical, moral, and political subjects.

(5.) Historical researches, and accurate surveys of places celebrated in American history.

(6.) Ethnological researches, particularly with reference to the different races of men in North America; also explorations, and accurate surveys, of the mounds and other remains of the ancient people of our country.

I. TO DIFFUSE KNOWLEDGE.—*It is proposed to publish a series of reports, giving an account of the new discoveries in science, and of the changes made from year to year in all branches of knowledge not strictly professional.*

1. Some of these reports may be published annually, others at longer intervals, as the income of the Institution or the changes in the branches of knowledge may indicate.

2. The reports are to be prepared by collaborators, eminent in the different branches of knowledge.

3. Each collaborator to be furnished with the journals and publications, domestic and foreign, necessary to the compilation of his report; to be paid a certain sum for his labors, and to be named on the title-page of the report.

4. The reports to be published in separate parts, so that persons interested in a particular branch, can procure the parts relating to it, without purchasing the whole.

5. These reports may be presented to Congress, for partial distribution, the remaining copies to be given to literary and scientific institutions, and sold to individuals for a moderate price.

The following are some of the subjects which may be embraced in the reports:—

I. PHYSICAL CLASS.

1. Physics, including astronomy, natural philosophy, chemistry, and meteorology.
2. Natural history, including botany, zoology, geology, &c.
3. Agriculture.
4. Application of science to arts.

II. MORAL AND POLITICAL CLASS.

5. Ethnology, including particular history, comparative philology, antiquities, &c.
6. Statistics and political economy.
7. Mental and moral philosophy.
8. A survey of the political events of the world; penal reform, &c.

III. LITERATURE AND THE FINE ARTS.

9. Modern literature.
10. The fine arts, and their application to the useful arts.
11. Bibliography.
12. Obituary notices of distinguished individuals.

II. To DIFFUSE KNOWLEDGE.—*It is proposed to publish occasionally separate treatises on subjects of general interest.*

1. These treatises may occasionally consist of valuable memoirs translated from foreign languages, or of articles prepared under the direction of the Institution, or procured by offering premiums for the best exposition of a given subject.

2. The treatises to be submitted to a commission of competent judges, previous to their publication.

DETAILS OF THE SECOND PART OF THE PLAN OF ORGANIZATION.

This part contemplates the formation of a Library, a Museum, and a Gallery of Art.

1. To carry out the plan before described, a library will be required, consisting, 1st, of a complete collection of the transactions and proceedings of all the learned societies in the world; 2d, of the more important current periodical publications, and other works necessary in preparing the periodical reports.

2. The Institution should make special collections, particularly of objects to verify its own publications. Also a collection of instruments of research in all branches of experimental science.

3. With reference to the collection of books, other than those mentioned above, catalogues of all the different libraries in the United States should be procured, in order that the valuable books first purchased may be such as are not to be found elsewhere in the United States.

4. Also catalogues of memoirs, and of books in foreign libraries, and other materials, should be collected, for rendering the Institution a centre of bibliographical knowledge, whence the student may be directed to any work which he may require.

5. It is believed that the collections in natural history will increase by donation, as rapidly as the income of the Institution can make provision for their reception; and, therefore, it will seldom be necessary to purchase any article of this kind.

6. Attempts should be made to procure for the gallery of art, casts of the most celebrated articles of ancient and modern sculpture.

7. The arts may be encouraged by providing a room, free of expense, for the exhibition of the objects of the Art-Union, and other similar societies.

8. A small appropriation should annually be made for models of antiquity, such as those of the remains of ancient temples, &c.

9. The Secretary and his assistants, during the session of Congress, will be required to illustrate new discoveries in science, and to exhibit new objects of art; distinguished individuals should also be invited to give lectures on subjects of general interest.

In accordance with the rules adopted in the programme of organization, each memoir in this volume has been favorably reported on by a Commission appointed for its examination. It is however impossible, in most cases, to verify the statements of an author; and, therefore, neither the Commission nor the Institution can be responsible for more than the general character of a memoir.

The following rules have been adopted for the distribution of the quarto volumes of the Smithsonian Contributions:—

1. They are to be presented to all learned societies which publish Transactions, and give copies of these, in exchange, to the Institution.

2. Also, to all foreign libraries of the first class, provided they give in exchange their catalogues or other publications, or an equivalent from their duplicate volumes.

3. To all the colleges in actual operation in this country, provided they furnish, in return, meteorological observations, catalogues of their libraries and of their students, and all other publications issued by them relative to their organization and history.

4. To all States and Territories, provided there be given, in return, copies of all documents published under their authority.

5. To all incorporated public libraries in this country, not included in any of the foregoing classes, now containing more than 10,000 volumes; and to smaller libraries, where a whole State or large district would be otherwise unsupplied.

OFFICERS

OF THE

SMITHSONIAN INSTITUTION.

THE PRESIDENT OF THE UNITED STATES,
Ex-officio PRESIDING OFFICER OF THE INSTITUTION.

THE VICE-PRESIDENT OF THE UNITED STATES,
Ex-officio SECOND PRESIDING OFFICER.

ROGER B. TANEY,
CHANCELLOR OF THE INSTITUTION.

JOSEPH HENRY,
SECRETARY OF THE INSTITUTION.

SPENCER F. BAIRD,
ASSISTANT SECRETARY.

W. W. SEATON, TREASURER.

JAMES A. PEARCE,
ALEXANDER D. BACHE, } EXECUTIVE COMMITTEE.
JOSEPH G. TOTTEN,

REGENTS.

JOHN C. BRECKENRIDGE, ...	*Vice-President of the United States.*
ROGER B. TANEY, ...	*Chief Justice of the United States.*
JAMES G. BERRET, ...	*Mayor of the City of Washington.*
JAMES A. PEARCE, ...	*Member of the Senate of the United States.*
JAMES M. MASON, ...	" " " " " "
STEPHEN A. DOUGLAS, ...	" " " " " "
WILLIAM H. ENGLISH, ...	*Member of the House of Representatives U. S.*
L. J. GARTRELL, ...	" " " " " "
BENJAMIN STANTON, ...	" " " " " "
GIDEON HAWLEY, ...	*Citizen of New York.*
——— ———	———
GEORGE E. BADGER, ...	" *of North Carolina.*
CORNELIUS C. FELTON, ...	" *of Massachusetts.*
ALEXANDER D. BACHE, ...	" *of the District of Columbia.*
JOSEPH G. TOTTEN, ...	" " "

MEMBERS EX-OFFICIO OF THE INSTITUTION.

JAMES BUCHANAN, ...	*President of the United States.*
JOHN C. BRECKENRIDGE, ...	*Vice-President of the United States.*
LEWIS CASS, ...	*Secretary of State.*
HOWELL COBB, ...	*Secretary of the Treasury.*
JOHN B. FLOYD, ...	*Secretary of War.*
ISAAC TOUCEY, ...	*Secretary of the Navy.*
JOSEPH HOLT, ...	*Postmaster-General.*
JEREMIAH S. BLACK, ...	*Attorney-General.*
ROGER B. TANEY, ...	*Chief Justice of the United States.*
P. F. THOMAS, ...	*Commissioner of Patents.*
JAMES G. BERRET, ...	*Mayor of the City of Washington.*

HONORARY MEMBERS.

Robert Hare,*	Albert Gallatin,*
Washington Irving,*	Parker Cleaveland,*
Benjamin Silliman,	A. B. Longstreet,

Hon. Jacob Thompson, *Secretary of the Interior.*

(* Deceased.)

TABLE OF CONTENTS.[1]

---

[1] Each memoir is separately paged and indexed.

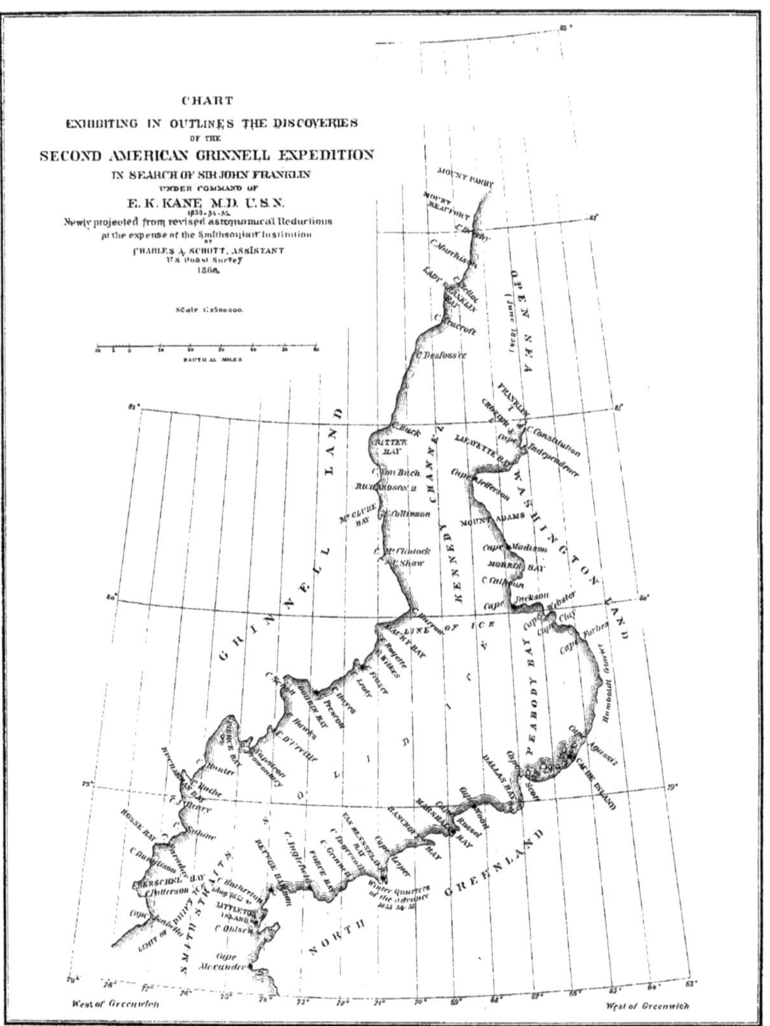

Lith. of J. Bien, 60 Fulton Street N.Y.

SMITHSONIAN CONTRIBUTIONS TO KNOWLEDGE.

ASTRONOMICAL OBSERVATIONS

IN THE

ARCTIC SEAS.

BY

ELISHA KENT KANE, M.D., U.S.N.

MADE DURING THE SECOND GRINNELL EXPEDITION IN SEARCH OF SIR JOHN FRANKLIN, IN 1853, 1854, AND 1855, AT VAN RENSSELAER HARBOR, AND OTHER POINTS IN THE VICINITY OF THE NORTHWEST COAST OF GREENLAND.

REDUCED AND DISCUSSED,

BY

CHARLES A. SCHOTT,
ASSISTANT U. S. COAST SURVEY.

[ACCEPTED FOR PUBLICATION, MARCH, 1860.]

COLLINS, PRINTER,
PHILADELPHIA.

CONTENTS.

INTRODUCTORY LETTER.

WASHINGTON, March 7, 1860.

PROFESSOR JOSEPH HENRY, LL.D.,

Secretary of the Smithsonian Institution:

DEAR SIR: The records of the astronomical observations made under the direction of Dr. Kane, in the second expedition to the Arctic regions, were placed in my hands by his late lamented father, Judge Kane, in December, 1857.

Dr. Kane had selected Assistant Charles A. Schott, of the Coast Survey, for the reduction of a considerable portion of the observations made in that expedition; and I, therefore, placed these in Mr. Schott's possession for reduction and discussion. The work has been faithfully performed, and I recommend it for publication in the "Smithsonian Contributions to Knowledge." It is proper to state that the instruments were furnished in part by the U. S. Coast Survey, and that the computations have been made at the expense of the Smithsonian Institution.

Very respectfully, yours,

A. D. BACHE.

ASTRONOMICAL OBSERVATIONS AND REDUCTIONS.

OF the astronomical observations made by the second Grinnell Expedition, under command of Dr. Kane, those for the longitude of Van Rensselaer Harbor, the winter quarters during 1853–'54 and 1854–'55, were most numerous and most carefully attended to. The geographical location of the shore line, traced by the expedition, depends for its longitude on that of Van Rensselaer Harbor, as the central meridian. The latitude of Van Rensselaer Harbor, or Fern Rock Observatory, was likewise carefully determined, as far as the instrumental means of the expedition permitted. The astronomical and geodetic material collected by the various travelling parties, and required for the geographical position of their tracks, is given in Appendix No. 6, to the second volume of the Narrative of the Expedition. Part of this material was collated with the manuscript, and the revised results will be given, in the present paper, after the discussion of the latitude and longitude of Van Rensselaer Harbor. The record of the observations discussed is taken from the original log-book, or other manuscript documents, belonging to the expedition. The astronomical observations were under the special care of Mr. Augustus Sonntag. The principal instruments for the determination of the geographical positions, were sextants, a Gambey theodolite, a transit instrument, and five mean time chronometers.

Fern Rock Observatory was established on the northernmost of the rocky group of islets in Van Rensselaer Harbor: the highest point of Observatory Island is twenty-nine feet above mean tidal level. For directions to sites of Van Rensselaer Harbor, it will be sufficient to refer to note 56, page 430, of the first volume of the Narrative.[1]

On the 25th of August, 1853, a general survey of the harbor was made, and on the 12th of September following, the site of the Observatory was selected. This observatory consisted of four walls of granite blocks, cemented together with moss and water, and the aid of frost. These walls were covered in with a substantial wooden roof, with openings in the direction of the meridian and prime vertical. The transit and theodolite were mounted on piers, formed by a conglomerate of gravel and ice, well rammed down, in iron-hooped pemmican casks, and cemented by freezing water. These piers were found as firm as the rock on which they rested.[2]

[1] For a copy see appendix (No. 1) to this paper.

[2] See page 116, vol. I, of the Narrative.

Observations for Latitude of Van Rensselaer Harbor Observatory, and the Winter Quarters of the Brig Advance.

The first observation for latitude was made on September 12, 1853, with the theodolite. Later observations were obtained by means of a sextant and artificial horizon. The Gambey theodolite[1] was furnished with repeating circles; the diameter of the horizontal circle was six inches, with the limb divided from five to five seconds, and provided with two verniers; the vertical circle has four verniers, and is of the same size and graduation as the horizontal circle. The following observations were made by Mr. Sonntag, at Washington, D. C., for the angular value of a division of the large level belonging to the instrument.

Level readings.	Difference.	Value of 10″.	Level readings.	Difference.	Value of 10″.	Level readings.	Difference.	Value of 10″.
32.5 —0.5	33.0	15d.6	8.2 25.2	—17.0	9d.7	32.1 2.0	30.1	9d.6
24.7 7.3	17.4	7.7	13.0 20.3	— 7.3	8.9	27.2 6.7	20.5	9.3
21.0 11.3	9.7	7.8	17.8 16.2	+ 1.6	6.7	23.2 11.0	11.2	7.1
17.0 15.1	1.9	8.3	21.0 12.7	+ 8.3	10.0	19.2 15.1	4.1	8.6
13.0 19.4	— 6.4	9.7	26.2 7.9	+18.3	8.6	15.0 19.5	— 4.5	10.7
9.0 25.1	—16.1	5.4	30.2 3.3	+26.9	8.3	9.8 25.0	—15.2	7.6
5.7 27.2	—21.5		34.3 —0.9	+35.2		6.0 28.8	—22.8	
		9.08			8.70			8.82

One division of level from set 1 . . . . 1.″10
" " " 2 . . . . 1.15
" " " 3 . . . . 1.13

Resulting value 1.13

(The length of the bubble was 16d.3, 16d.7, and 17d.1 in the three sets respectively.) The level is connected with the Y supporting the vertical circles.

This instrument was much injured by a fall in the water, and rendered unfit for use, by a second accident, two months later, in November, 1853, when it fell from the pier at the observatory. It may be remarked, here, that Mr. Sonntag has deduced approximate results from his observations with this instrument, and with the sextant, insufficient refraction tables not permitting him to deduce final results.

Observations of September 12, 1853. (A. M.)
Observations of the sun's zenith distance for time.

Circle east.	Chronometer time.	Level.	Reading of circle.		Circle west.	Chronometer time.	Level.	Reading of circle	
$\underline{\odot}$	3h 04m 42s	9d.5	195° 02′ 25″	45″	$\underline{\odot}$	3h 14m 44s	11d.0	76° 18′ 35″	30″
		14.7	35	45			14.3	35	30
$\overline{\odot}$	3 09 25	16.0	195 40 25	15	$\overline{\odot}$	3 17 42	10.5	75 43 30	20
		8.0	25	30			14.2	25	25

[1] This instrument, marked United States Coast Survey, No. 34, was kindly lent by the Superintendent of the Survey, Prof. A. D. Bache.

The north end of the level was always read first; the temperature of the air, and the barometer and attached thermometer readings, are taken from the meteorological record, and discussed by me in 1859 (see Smithsonian Contributions to Knowledge, vol. XI, Parts I and III, of the Meteorological paper).

Thermometer + 22°.6 Fahr.	Approximate latitude + 78° 37′ 12″.
Barometer 29.70 inch.	Approximate longitude 4h 43m 28s west of Greenwich.
Attached thermometer 66°.	From a preliminary discussion of the moon culminations.

Time is noted by the pocket chronometer.

We find: Reading of ⊙'s centre, corrected for level	195°	21′	29″.9	Circle east.
" " " "	76	00	56.8	" west.
⊙'s apparent zenith distance	75	19	43.4	
Correction for refraction	+	3	50.3	
" for parallax	—		8.2	
⊙'s corrected zenith distance	75	23	25.5	

Hence, by the usual formula:—

Apparent time of observation	22h	32m	00s.7
Equation of time		3	48.4
Mean time of observation	22	28	12.3
Chronometer time of observation	27	11	38.2
Pocket chronometer fast of Fern Rock mean time	4	43	25.9

(Hence this chronometer indicates very nearly Greenwich mean time.)

Observations of circum-meridian altitudes of the sun, for latitude.

Circle east.	Chronometer.	Level.	Reading of circle.		Circle east.	Chronometer.	Level.	Reading of circle.	
$\underline{\odot}$	4h 27m 40s	13d.0	195° 58′ 50″	45″	$\underline{\odot}$	4h 45m 12s	14d.0	195° 58′ 60″	35″
		10.6	55	60			11.0	50	65
$\overline{\odot}$	4 30 40	12.0	196 30 40	30	$\overline{\odot}$	4 47 32	13.3	196 30 25	05
		12.0	40	55			11.4	10	35
Circle west.					Circle west.				
$\underline{\odot}$	4 35 45	10.3	75 33 25	15	$\underline{\odot}$	4 53 54	10.8	75 35 30	25
		14.0	10	15			13.4	25	30
$\overline{\odot}$	4 38 10	10.8	75 01 30	30	$\overline{\odot}$	4 56 30	11.2	75 03 65	55
		14.0	35	25			14.0	60	70

Thermometer + 20°.1.			
Barometer 29.71 inch.	We find: Reading of ⊙, corr'd for level,	196° 14′ 45″ Cir. E.	196° 14′ 34″
Attached thermometer 68°.	" " "	75 17 21 " W.	75 19 43
Approx. rate of pocket chron.	⊙'s apparent zenith distance	74 31 18	74 32 34
2 .5 gaining on mean time.	Corr'n for refraction.—paral.	+ 3 31	3 31
	Corrected zenith distances	74 34 49	74 36 05
	Chronometer time of observation	4h 33m 03s.8	4h 50 47s.0
	Chronometer fast	4 43 25.9	4 43 25.9
	Mean time of observation	23 49 37.9	0 07 21.1
	Equation of time	+ 3 55.2	3 55.4
	Apparent time	23 53 33.1	0 11 16.5

Hence, by the usual formula, reduction to meridian 16″.8 and 51″.2.

Meridional zenith distance	74° 34′ 32″	74° 35′ 14″
⊙'s declination	+ 4 03 00	+ 4 02 43
Resulting latitude of Fern Rock	78 37 32	78 37 57
Mean	78 37 44	

The following observations were made with the Gambey sextant and artificial mercurial horizon. The mercury was covered with a glass roof, the sides of which were reversed during the observations, in order to eliminate any error arising from a want of parallelism in the surfaces of the glass. The zero-point of the sextant was examined, and its index determined for each set of observations. The positive sign of the index error indicates that the zero-point is on the large arc, and that the correction to the observed altitude is subtractive. The long astronomical telescope belonging to the sextant was always used.[1] In Appendix, No. X, of the second volume of the Narrative,[2] Dr. Kane remarks, that the sextants used were made by Gambey, and divided to ten seconds; he believed that an error of ten seconds, depending on the want of parallelism in the glass cover of the horizon, could not exist in the results.

The time observations, with the transit instrument, made between November 18, 1853, and January 10, 1854, will be found recorded and discussed after the completion of the latitude observations; the following record, and result for time on February 20, 1854, however, is here inserted, as made with the Gambey sextant, and in order to follow the date as near as may be convenient.

February 20, 1854. Observation of the altitude of Saturn, for time.
(With Gambey sextant and artificial horizon.) Time noted by pocket chronometer.

Chronometer time.	Double altitude.	Chronometer time.	Double altitude.
12h 35m 11s	53° 7′ 20″	12h 40m 17s	52° 49′ 50″
36 22	3 30	42 16	43 00
38 37.5	52 56 30	43 21.5	38 00

Approx. long. + 4h 43m 28s. Approx. lat. 78° 37′ 12″. Index error + 8′ 22″.5.
$t = -28°.6$ F. $b = 29.27$ in. $\tau = +33°$.

Apparent altitude of Saturn	26° 27′ 00″.4	26° 17′ 37″.1
Correction for refraction and parallax	— 2 15.8	— 2 16.7
Corrected altitude	26 24 44.6	26 15 20.4
Saturn's declination	+17 17 28.1	+17 17 28.4
From which data we find the hour angle	2h 21m 51s.7	2h 26m 55s.2
AR of Saturn	3 34 33.0	3 34 33.0
Sidereal time of observation	5 56 24.7	6 01 28.2
" " mean noon	22 01 08.7	22 01 08.7
Whence mean time of observation	7 53 58.1	7 59 00.8
And chronometer time	12 36 43.5	12 41 58.2
Pocket chronometer fast of Fern Rock mean time	4 42 45.4	4 42 57.4
Chronometer error (mean)	— 4 42 51.4	

[1] Extracted from a Report of Mr. Sonntag's to the Commander, dated "Brig Mariane, Godhavn, September 12, 1855."

[2] See Appendix containing extracts.

May 14, 1854. Observations of circum-meridian altitudes of the sun, for latitude.
Gambey sextant; on the floe near the brig.

	Pocket chronometer.	Double altitude.		Pocket chronometer.	Double altitude.
$\underline{\odot}$	4h 33m 16s	59° 35′ 55″	$\underline{\odot}$	4h 40m 56s	59° 36′ 00″
	34 31	35 40		41 47	35 50
	35 35	35 50		42 35	35 40
$\overline{\odot}$	4 36 35	60 39 00	$\overline{\odot}$	4 43 40	60 38 45
	37 24	38 50		44 40	38 20
	38 58	39 40		45 34	37 50

Index error — 1′ 10″. $t = +7°.4$ F. $b = 29.84$ in. $\tau = +51°$.
For chronometer error and rate, see observations for time, May 16, 17, 19.

⊙'s corrected alt. (for index, refraction, and parallax)	30° 02′ 38″	30° 02′ 25″
Chronometer time of observation	4h 36m 03s	4h 43m 12s
Chronometer fast of Fern Rock mean time	4 39 27[1]	4 39 27
Mean time of observation	23 56 36	0 03 45
Hour angle	+ 0 0 30	+ 0 07 40
Hence reduction to meridian	+ 0″.2 and	+ 24″.9
⊙'s declination	+18° 39′ 53″	18° 39′ 57″
Resulting latitude	78 37 15	78 37 07
Mean	78 37 11	

May 15, 1854. Observations of circum-meridian altitudes of the sun, for latitude.
Gambey sextant; on the floe near the brig.

	Pocket chronometer.	Double altitude.		Pocket chronometer.	Double altitude.
$\underline{\odot}$	4h 28m 38s	59° 51′ 10″	$\underline{\odot}$	4h 35m 25s	59° 52′ 40″
	29 12	51 45		36 22	52 40
	30 15	51 30		37 12	52 30
$\overline{\odot}$	4 31 37	60 55 10	$\overline{\odot}$	4 38 07	60 55 10
	32 30	55 10		39 14	55 10
	34 23	55 30		39 53	54 30

Index error — 14′ 1″. $t = +8°.4$ F. $b = 29.93$ in. $\tau = +46°$.

⊙'s corrected alt. (for index, refraction, and parallax)	30° 17′ 01″	30° 17′ 13″
Chronometer time of observation	4h 31m 06s	4h 37m 42s
Chronometer fast of Fern Rock mean time	4 32 26[2]	4 39 26
Mean time of observation	23 51 40	23 58 16
Hour angle	— 0 04 26	+ 0 02 10
Reduction to meridian	+ 8″.3	+ 2″.0
⊙'s declination	+18° 54′ 09″	+18° 54′ 10″
Resulting latitude	78 37 00	78 36 55
Mean	78 36 58	

[1] For chronometer error and rate see subsequent observations.
[2] For chronometer error and rate see further on.

May 16, 1854. Observations of circum-meridian altitudes of the sun, for latitude.
Gambey sextant; on the floe near the brig.

	Pocket chronometer.	Double altitude.		Pocket chronometer.	Double altitude.
$\underline{\odot}$	4h 29m 15s	60° 33′ 20″	$\overline{\odot}$	4h 39m 05s	61° 37′ 30″
	32 56	33 40		39 39	37 10
	34 05	33 40		40 47	37 05
$\overline{\odot}$	4 35 36	61 37 05	$\underline{\odot}$	4 42 08	60 33 40
	36 35	37 30		43 00	33 45
	37 41	36 50		44 09	33 20

Index error + 0′ 16″. $t = +12°.5$ F. $b = 30.07$ in. $\tau = +39°$.

⊙'s corrected alt. (for index, refraction, and parallax)	30° 30′ 56″		30° 30′ 58″
Chronometer time of observation	4h 34m 21s		4h 41m 28s
Chronometer error	— 4 39 25[1]		4 39 25
Mean time of observation	23 54 56		0 02 03
Hour angle	— 1 10		+ 5 58
Reduction to meridian	+ 0″.5	and	+ 15″.1
⊙'s declination	+19° 08′ 08″		+19° 08′ 12″
Resulting latitude	78 37 12		78 36 59
Mean	78 37 06		

May 16, 1854. Observations of equal altitudes of the sun, for time.
Gambey sextant; on the floe near the brig.

Pocket chronometer. A. M.	Double altitude.		Pocket chronometer. P. M.	Pocket chronometer. A. M.	Double altitude.		Pocket chronometer. P. M.
0h 46m 18s	$\underline{\odot}$	49° 30′	8h 25m 21s.5	0h 53m 16s.5	$\underline{\odot}$	50° 05′	8h 18m 31s.5
47 24		35	24 21	54 15		10	17 36
48 17.5		40	23 29	55 16.5		15	16 33.5
0 49 33	$\overline{\odot}$	50 50	8 22 0.5	0 56 22.5	$\overline{\odot}$	51 25	8 15 20.5
50 35.5		55	21 11	57 33.5		30	14 19.5
51 31		51 00	20 10.5	58 32.5		35	13 8.5

A. M. Index error + 0′ 26″. $t = +11°.2$ F. $b = 30.06$ in. $\tau = +46°$.
P. M. Index error + 0′ 24″. $t = +15°.0$ F. $b = 30.07$ in. $\tau = +53°$.

The reductions of observations of equal altitudes are made according to the method given in the American Ephemeris and Nautical Almanac, for 1856.

On reducing the observations, it was found that the chronometer error came out too small by 24s.5; and, after working each set separately, the discrepancy was traced to the morning observations. The following reductions, therefore, are based on the two sets taken in the afternoon. It is probable that there was either an

[1] For chronometer error see following observation.

unusual amount of refraction in the morning, or else the rate of the chronometer has changed in the interval.

Afternoon altitudes of the sun.	1st set.	2d set.
☉'s corrected altitude (for index, refraction, and parallax)	25° 05′ 11″	25° 22′ 44″
☉'s declination	19 10 18	19 10 26
And the hour angle	3h 47m 12s.5	3h 40m 24s.9
Equation of time	— 3 53.4	3 53.4
Mean time of observation	3 43 19.1	3 36 31.5
Chronometer time of observation	8 22 45.5	8 15 55.0
Chronometer error on Fern Rock mean time . . .	— 4 39 26.4	— 4 39 23.5
Mean	— 4 39 24.9	

May 17, 1854. Observations of equal altitudes of the sun, for time.
Gambey sextant; on the floe near the brig.

Pocket chronometer. A. M.	Double altitude.	Pocket chronometer. P. M.	Pocket chronometer. A. M.	Double altitude.	Pocket chronometer. P. M.
0h 16m 45s	☉̄ 48° 10′	8h 55m 39s.5	0h 23m 32s	☉̄ 48° 45′	8h 49m 14s.2
17 37	15	54 36	24 20	50	48 22.5
18 36	20	53 48.5	25 22	55	47 21.5
0 20 23	☉̲ 47 25	8 52 18	0 26 48	☉̲ 48 0	8 46 26
21 13	30	51 23	27 44	5	45 35
22 15	35	50 24.5	28 34	10	44 41

For A. M. observations, index error — 7′ 46″. $t = +9°.3$ F. $b = 30.00$ in. $\tau = +53°$.
For P. M. observations, index error — 7′ 28″. $t = +14°.1$ F. $b = 29.95$ in. $\tau = +56°$.

A. M. Chronometer time 0h 19m 28s.1	P. M. Chronometer time 8h 53m 01s.5 set 1.	
A. M. Chronometer time 0 26 03.4	P. M. Chronometer time 8 46 56.7 set 2.	
Equation of equal altitudes	— 50s.8 (set 1.)	— 50s.2 (set 2.)
Middle chronometer time	4h 36m 14.8	4h 36m 30.0
Chronometer time of apparent noon. . .	4 35 24.0	4 35 39.8
Equation of time	+ 3 52.5	+ 3 52.5
Chronometer time of mean noon . . .	4 39 16.5	4 39 32.3
Chronometer error on Fern Rock mean time		—4 39 24.4

May 17, 1854. Observations of circum-meridian altitudes of the sun, for latitude.
Gambey sextant; on the floe near the brig.

	Pocket chronometer.	Double altitude.		Pocket chronometer.	Double altitude.
$\overline{\odot}$	4h 29m 46s.5	61° 56′ 0″	$\overline{\odot}$	4h 37m 05s.5	61° 56′ 20″
	30 39.5	56 30		37 49	56 30
	31 32.0	56 25		38 27	56 30
$\underline{\odot}$	4 33 02	60 53 30	$\underline{\odot}$	4 39 25	60 53 45
	34 12	54 00		40 01.5	53 30
	35 55	53 40		40 58.5	53 25

Index error —7′ 40″. $t = +10°.5$ F. $b = 29.95$ in. $\tau = +53°$.

☉'s corrected altitude (for index, refraction, and parallax)	80° 44′ 31″	80° 44′ 31″
Chronometer time of observation	4h 32m 31s.2	4h 38m 57s.8
Chronometer error	— 4 39 24.4	— 4 39 24.4
Mean time of observation	23 53 07	23 59 33
Hour angle	— 8 01	+ 3 26
Reduction to meridian	3″.9 and	5″.0
☉'s declination	+19° 21′ 45″	+19° 21′ 49″
Resulting latitude	78 37 10	78 37 13
Mean	78 37 12	

May 19, 1854. Observations of equal altitudes of the sun, for time.
Gambey sextant; on the floe near the brig.

Pocket chronometer. A. M.	Double altitude.	Pocket chronometer. A. M.	Pocket chronometer. P. M.	Double altitude.	Pocket chronometer. P. M.
0h 33m 29s	$\overline{\odot}$ 50° 30′	8h 39m 9s.5	0h 37m 09s	$\underline{\odot}$ 49° 45′	8h 35m 34s
34 37	35	38 4	37 57	50	34 41
35 28	40	37 16.5	38 54	55	33 43.5

A. M. Index error — 8′ 44″. P. M. Index error — 9′ 22″.
$t = +13°.5$ F. $b = 30.05$ in. $\tau = +52°$. $t = +19°.3$ F. $b = 30.20$ in. $\tau = +53°$.
Observation not very exact, the mercury being in motion.

A. M. Chronometer time 0h 36m 15s.6 P. M. Chronometer time 8h 36m 24s.7

Equation of equal altitudes	— 46s.7
Middle chronometer time	4h 36m 20.1
Chronometer time of apparent noon	4 35 33.4
Equation of time	+ 3 48.4
Chronometer time of mean noon	4 39 21.8

RECAPITULATION OF CHRONOMETER ERRORS DETERMINED IN MAY, 1854.

May 16.	Pocket chronometer fast of Fern Rock mean time	4h 39m 24s.9
" 17.	" " " " "	4 39 24.4
" 19.	" " " " "	4 39 21.8

Approximate rate 1s losing per day.

The pocket chronometer was made to indicate Greenwich mean time within a few minutes; between October 5 and October 10, 1853, it ran down; October 29, it was carried about for nine hours; again, November 4, it was carried on a journey for three days; on the 22d of November it ran down, and on December 21 it was exposed for four hours to a temperature of —38° F. Its rate, as indicated by the other chronometers, 2143, 370, 2721, and 264 (all mean time chronometers), was tolerably uniform, and varying between 3ˢ.6 and 0ˢ.0.

May 20, 1854. Observations of circum-meridian altitudes of the sun, for latitude. Gambey sextant; on the floe near the brig.

Pocket chronometer.	Double altitude.	Pocket chronometer.	Double altitude.
$\overline{\odot}$ 4ʰ 31ᵐ 09ˢ.5	63° 14′ 5″	$\overline{\odot}$ 4ʰ 36ᵐ 44ˢ.5	63° 14′ 5″
32 09.5	13 50	37 28	14 5
33 02	14 5	38 23.5	13 55
$\underline{\odot}$ 4 33 59	62 11 20	4 40 07	62 10 45
34 41	11 00	40 49	10 40
35 30.5	11 10	41 40	10 45

Index error — 8′ 17″.5. $t = +12°.9$ F. $b = 39.25$ in. $\tau = +53°$.

☉'s corrected altitude (for index, refraction, and parallax)	31° 23′ 49″	31° 23′ 43″
Chronometer time of observation	4ʰ 33ᵐ 25ˢ.2	4ʰ 39ᵐ 12ˢ.0
Chronometer error	— 4 39 21.0	4 39 21.0
Mean time of observation	23 54 04	23 59 51
Hour angle	— 2 11	+ 3 37
Reduction to meridian	— 2″.0 and	5.″6
☉'s declination	+20° 00′ 43″	+20° 00′ 46″
Resulting latitude	78 36 52	78 36 57
Mean	78 36 55	

RECAPITULATION OF RESULTS FOR LATITUDES OF VAN RENSSELAER HARBOR.

September 12, 1853. From two sets of Z. D.'s of the sun at the Fern Rock Observatory 78° 37′ 44″.

This result will be used for the reduction of the transit observations at the observatory. This observatory was some distance (as we learn from pages 108, 116, 167, and 168, of vol. I, of the Narrative) to the northward of the position of the brig. The following results for latitude refer to the position of the Brig Advance in the winter quarters:—

May 14, 1854.	From two sets of altitudes	78° 37′ 11″[1]
" 15,	" " " "	36 58
" 16,	" " " "	37 06
" 17,	" " " "	37 12
" 20,	" " " "	36 55
	Mean	78 37 04 ± 3″

[1] The recapitulation of the approximate values for latitude of the brig, on p. 387, appendix No. VI, vol. II of the Narrative, has two additional values between May 14 and 15, for which I could not find any record.

which result is to be used for the reduction of astronomical observations taken on or near the brig; it gives also the position of the meteorological observatory on the floe.

In the above reductions, Ivory's refraction tables have been used, as given in the convenient form for logarithmic computation (and extended if required) in Lee's Collection of Tables and Formulæ. All observed altitudes were greater than 14½°.

Observations for Longitude of Van Rensselaer Harbor Observatory, and the Winter Quarters of the Brig Advance.

Observations of Transit for Time and of the Moon and Moon Culminating Stars for Longitude of Fern Rock Observatory.

The transit observations commence November 18, 1853, and end January 10, 1854. The time was noted by the pocket chronometer, showing within a few minutes Greenwich mean time. The transit instrument was supplied with five wires, and the observations are recorded, from I to V, in the order in which the star (or moon) passes them at the upper culmination, the circle being east of the telescope. The letter R, attached to the name of the object observed, indicates that its transit was observed reflected from a mercurial horizon; this method of observing became necessary for the measure of the inclination of the axis, in consequence of the intense cold affecting the length of the bubble of the level to such a degree that it became useless. At temperatures below —40°, no use could be made of the instrument. The instrument was properly adjusted, an operation somewhat troublesome in so high a latitude, and at so low temperatures. For the azimuthal adjustment there remained but an arc of 11⅓° between the pole and the zenith; Dr. Kane remarks,[1] "Some of our instruments, in consequence of the cold, became difficult to manage in consequence of the unequal contraction of brass and iron."

Appendix No. VIII, of vol. II of the Narrative, contains the record of the transit observations, as made by Mr. Sonntag. The following pages contain the same extracted from the manuscript.

In the reduction, I have adopted the latitude 78° 37½', and the longitude 4^h 43^m 28^s W. of Greenwich (an approximate result from the moon culminations). The reduction was made by application of the method of least squares; to know the instrumental deviations with the greatest accuracy is not of so much importance for the moon culminations, since the result for longitude depends more on the differences of time between the transit of the moon and stars, but it is otherwise with the occultations, where the chronometer error must be known with the greatest precision.

A peculiarity in the construction of the instrument requires to be noticed, viz: it does not permit direct observation of a star elevated more than about 50° above the horizon, hence all observations upon the pole star, and others near the zenith, had to be taken reflected.

---

[1] Page 154, vol. I, of the Narrative.

OBSERVATIONS OF THE TRANSIT OF THE STARS AND THE MOON AT FERN ROCK OBSERVATORY.

Transit instrument. A. SONNTAG, Observer.

Object.		Wire I.	Wire II.	Wire III.	Wire IV.	Wire V.
		November 18, 1853. Circle West. Time by pocket chronometer.				
☾ II.	s. p.[1]	6^h 49^m 16^s	49^m 37^s	50^m $01^s.5$	50^m 24^s	50^m $45^s.5$
μ Geminor.	s. p.	7 05 39.5	06 01.5	06 23	06 44.5	07 06.5
ι Geminor.	s. p.	7 26 24	26 45.5	27 07	27 29.5	27 51.5
		Changed azimuth and inclination.				
Polaris	R.	14 16 44	02 39	49 21	36 50	13 22 55
η Ursæ maj.	s. p.	14 32 12	32 41.5	.. ..	33 42.5	34 15
α Arietis		50 26.5	50 05	49 44	49 23.0	14 .. ..
α Bootis	s. p.	14 59 19	59 39	00 00.5	00 21.0	15 00 42.5
γ Ceti		27 14	26 54	26 34.5	26 14.5	15 25 54
		Circle East.				
β Ursæ min.	R. s. p.	15 45 17	44 01.5	42 47	41 31.5	15 40 14
		November 21, 1853. Circle East. Pocket chronometer.				
51 Cephei	R. s. p.	7	16 42.5	09 18.5	02 45	6 .. ..
β Lyræ		7 23 08	23 29	23 53.5	24 14.5	24 37.5
ε Aquilæ		7 37 14.5	37 34.5	37 54.0	38 16.0	38 37.0
δ Geminor.	s. p.	51 32.5	51 12.0	50 50.0	50 29.5	7 50 07.0
δ Aquilæ		7 56 41.5	57 02.0	57 19.5	57 43.0	58 02.5
γ Cancri	s. p.	9 14 44.0	14 24.0	14 02.5	13 42.5	9 .. ..
☾ II.	s. p.	20 01.0	.. ..	19 15	18 52.5	9 18 28.5
ι Ursæ maj.	s. p.	29 35	29 06.5	28 37	28 07.5	9 27 35
ζ Cygni		9 44 46.5	45 09	45 30.5	45 53.5	46 17
α Cephei	R.	9 52 49	53 30	54 13.5	54 55	55 38.5
λ Leonis	s. p.	03 11	02 50.5	02 28.5	02 07	10 01 44
		November 23, 1853. Circle East. Pocket chronometer.				
η Draconis	R.	4 53 44	54 27	55 06.5	55 50	56 32.5
α Tauri	s. p.	5 01 11	00 51	00 29.5	00 09	4 59 47
α Aurigae	s. p.	40 01	39 33	39 04.5	38 35	5 38 06.5
γ Draconis	R.	6 24 56.5	25 31	26 02	26 33	27 07
α Lyræ		7 03 12.5	03 39	04 04	04 30	04 56
β Lyræ		7 15 02	15 25	15 47	16 12	16^m 35^s + 1^m
ζ Aquilæ		7 30 16.5	30 36.5	30 57	31 17	31^m $37^s.5$
δ Geminor.	s. p.	44 40	44 21	43 59	43 36	7 43 14.5
α Leonis		22 29 44.5	30 04	30 25.5	30 45	31 05.5
γ Leonis		22 40 56	41 16	41 37	41 59	42 23
☾ II.		23 18 25	18 45	19 07	19 29	19 49.5
χ Leonis		23 26 30	26 50	.. ..	27 31	27 52
		December 8, 1853. Circle East. Pocket chronometer.				
ι Piscium		11 03 55	04 15	04 35	04 54	05 15
α Andromedæ		11 31 46	32 08	32 31	32 54	33 16.5
γ Pegasi		11 36 57	37 17	37 37	37 57.5	38 19
☾ I.		11 54 49	55 11.5	55 31	55 53.5	56 13
δ Piscium		12 12 23	12 41	13 03.5	13 22	13 42.5

[1] Sub polo.

Object.		Wire I.	Wire II.	Wire III.	Wire IV.	Wire V.
		December 9, 1853. Circle East. Pocket chronometer.				
α Andromedæ		11^h 27^m 52^s	28^m 15^s	28^m 36^s	29^m 00^s	29^m $21^s.5$
γ Pegasi		11 33 02	33 22.5	33 42	34 03.5	34 24
☾ I.		12 36 57.5	37 17	37 38	37 58.5	38 20[1]
		December 12, 1853. Circle East. Pocket chronometer.				
δ Arietis		2	18 41	19 03.5	19 25	19 44
☾ I.		2 44 30	44 53.5	45 15	45 36.5	45 58
η Tauri		2 53 38.5	54 00	54 23.5	54 44.5	55 07
27 Tauri[2]		2 55 20	55 41	56 04	56 25.5	56 48
A′ Tauri		3 10 55.5	11 17	11 38.5	12 00	12 22
		December 13, 1853. Circle East. Pocket chronometer.				
Polaris	R.	11 51 56	04 10	17 39.5		
		Circle West.				
Polaris	R.	12 41 37	28 36.5			
α Arietis	R.	11 27	11 06	10 44.5	10 23.5	1 10 04
α Bootis	s. p.	1 20 04.5	20 26	20 46.5	21 08	21 29.5
γ Ceti		48 10.0	47 51	47 30	47 11	1 46 49.5
β Ursæ min.	R. s. p.	2	01 38	02 56.5	04 13	05 28
α Coronæ	s. p.	2 39 20	39 42	40 03.5	40 25	40 48
η Tauri		2 51 05.5	50 43.5	50 22.5	50 02.0	2 49 38
27 Tauri[2]		52 45	52 25	52 03	51 39	2 51 20
A′ Tauri		08 18.5	07 57	07 30.5	07 12	3 06 50.5
☾ I.		31 20.5	30 59.5	30 38	30 17	3 29 52.5
		December 14, 1853. Circle West. Pocket chronometer.				
ι Ursæ min.[3]	R. s. p.	4 03 52.5	06 27	09 21.5	.. ..	.. .. ..
☾ I.		19 01	18 41.5	18 16.5	17 56	4 17 35.5
☾ II.		21 15	20 52.5	20 31	20 07.5	4 19 44.5
ο Tauri		26 56	26 34.5	26 13	25 50.5	4 25 30
δ Orionis		32 36.5	32 16.5	31 57	31 36.5	4 31 16.5
ζ Tauri		36 58	36 35.5	36 15.5	35 53.5	4 35 31.5
α Orionis		55 15.5	54 54	54 35	54 14	4 53 53.5
μ Geminor		22 05.5	21 43.5	21 23	21 01	5 20 39.5[4]
		December 15, 1853. Circle West. Pocket chronometer.				
Polaris	R.	12 33 22	20 13.5	07 32.5	54 18.5	11 41 27
η Ursæ maj.	s. p.	12 44 55.5	45 27.5	45 57	46 29	46 58.5
η Bootis	s. p.	12 51 05.5	51 26.5	51 47.5	52 09	52 31
α Arietis	R.	03 40	03 18.5	02 58	02 35.5	1 02 13
α Bootis	s. p.	1 12 19.5	12 40.5	13 01	13 23.0	13 43
γ Ceti		40 18.5	39 59	39 39	39 19	1 38 59.5
β Ursæ min.	R. s. p.	1 52 49	54 06	55 20	56 35	57 52.5
ο Tauri		23 02	22 39	22 19.5	21 57.5	4 21 35.5
ζ Tauri		33 02.5	32 41.5	32 20.0	31 58.5	4 31 37
α Orionis		51 17	50 57.5	50 37	50 17.5	4 49 58
γ Draconis	s. p.	4 55 38	56 10.5	56 42.5	57 15	57 47.5
☾ II.		10 42.0	10 19.0	09 56.5	09 34	5 09 11
μ Geminor.		18 07.5	17 46.5	17 25.5	17 03.5	5 16 41

[1] Through clouds. [2] In original Plj. [3] The original has τ. [4] The record has 5^h 20^m $29^s.5$.

Object.		Wire I.	Wire II.	Wire III.	Wire IV.	Wire V.
January 8, 1854. Circle West. Pocket chronometer.						
α Bootis	s. p.	11^h ..^{m} ..^{s}	37^m 34^s	37^m 55^s	38^m $16^s.5$	11^h 38^m $37^s.5$
845 B. A. C.		06 34.5	06 14	05 54.5	05 33.5	12 05 12.5
π Arietis		10 39.5	10 18.5	09 58.5	09 38	12 09 15.5
α Ceti		24 06.5	23 45.5	23 27	23 06.5	12 22 45.5
☾ I.		42 42.5	42 20.5	41 57	41 37.5	12 41 15
Saturn (centre)		02 41.5	02 20.5	01 59	01 39.5	1 01 18
17 Tauri		05 36.5	05 15	04 53	04 31	1 04 08.5
η Tauri		08 12.5	07 50.5	07 29	07 07.5	1 06 45
27 Tauri		09 53.5	09 31.5	09 09.5	08 47.5	1 08 26
January 9, 1854. Circle West. Pocket chronometer.						
γ Pegasi		9 31 42.5	31 23	31 02.5	30 40	9 30 19
α Cassiopeæ	R.	59 08.5	58 34	57 58.5	57 23	9 56 46.5
Polaris	R.	11 09 00	56 12	43 10	30 09.5	10 17 54.5
η Ursæ maj.	s. p.	11 05 45	06 17.5	06 46	07 18	07 49.5
α Arietis		24 39.5	24 18.5	23 58	23 36.5	11 23 13
January 10, 1854. Circle West. Pocket chronometer.						
γ Pegasi		9 27 48.5	27 28	27 07	26 47.5	9 26 27
α Cassiopeæ	R.	55 15	54 41.5	54 05.5	53 30	9 52 52.5
Polaris	R.	11 06 09.5	53 06	39 30	26 11	10 13 22
α Bootis	s. p.	11 29 20.5	29 42	30 02.5	30 24	30 46

Reduction of Preceding Transits.

There being no level readings, the amount of inclination of the transit axis has to be found from the transit observations themselves; the number of unknown quantities in the normal equations, however, could be reduced to three, since the collimation error could be deduced independently. The instrument was adjusted for collimation on November 18, and on December 13, Polaris was observed, reflected, circle east and circle west, from which observation the collimation has been deduced; the result was, however, satisfactorily checked in those sets of observations, including stars above and below the pole. A preliminary reduction was made in order to ascertain an approximate value for the rate of the chronometer; this instrument was considered as a sidereal chronometer with a large rate.

The following notation has been used in the reduction.

a = azimuthal deviation, in seconds of time $\left\{\begin{matrix}+\\-\end{matrix}\right\}$, when instrument is $\left\{\begin{matrix}\text{east}\\\text{west}\end{matrix}\right\}$ of south.

A = azimuthal factor; correction for azimuthal deviation Aa.

b = inclination of axis, in seconds of time $\left\{\begin{matrix}+\\-\end{matrix}\right\}$, when $\left\{\begin{matrix}\text{west}\\\text{east}\end{matrix}\right\}$ end is high.

B = level factor; correction for level Bb.

c = collimation error, in seconds of time; for upper culmination $\left\{\begin{matrix}+\\-\end{matrix}\right\}$ when mean of wires is $\left\{\begin{matrix}\text{east}\\\text{west}\end{matrix}\right\}$ of line of collimation.

C = collimation factor; correction for collimation Cc.

E = error of chronometer $\left\{\begin{matrix}+\\-\end{matrix}\right\}$ when $\left\{\begin{matrix}\text{slow}\\\text{fast}\end{matrix}\right\}$ of sidereal time at an assumed time T.

E_0 = an assumed chronometer error and ϵ its correction; $E = E_0 + \epsilon$.

$t_1\ t_2\ t_3 \ldots$ = the observed times of transits of a group of stars, already corrected for rate of chronometer and collimation.

$AR_1 - t_1 = e_1 \quad AR_2 - t_2 = e_2 \quad AR_3 - t_3 = e_3 \ldots\ldots$ and $e_1 - E_0 = n_1 \quad e_2 - E_0 = n_2 \ldots\ldots$

The values a, b and ϵ can be deduced from the normal equations:

$$\Sigma\,\epsilon + \Sigma\,Aa + \Sigma\,Bb = \Sigma\,n$$
$$\Sigma\,A\epsilon + \Sigma\,A^2a + \Sigma\,ABb = \Sigma\,An$$
$$\Sigma\,B\epsilon + \Sigma\,ABa + \Sigma\,B^2b = \Sigma\,Bn.$$

It is essential, however, that the instrument be not disturbed during the time of the transits of the group of stars.

For the reduction of the incomplete transits and for deducing the collimation error, the equatorial intervals of the wires have been deduced from transits of 18 stars, as follows:—

For circle *east* and *upper* culmination.

I	$-39.^s71$
II	-19.82
III	$-\ \ 0.22$
IV	$+19.84$
V	$+39.91$

The probable error of each interval is on the average $\pm\ 0.^s07$. From a preliminary reduction of the observations of December 15 and January 9, the daily rate of the chronometer was found $+\ 3^m\ 56.^s0$, or the rate (losing) per minute $+\ 0.^s164$ approximately.

The observations of Polaris, upper culmination reflected, of Dec. 13, 1853, circle east and circle west, give the collimation error $c = -1.^s40$ (for upper culmination and) circle *east*, the observed chronometer times having been corrected for rate, and the equatorial intervals were multiplied by $\sqrt[3]{sec.\ H}$, where H the hour angle. This value of c has been used for the reduction of transits on and after Dec. 13; for Nov. 18, $c = o$, and between this date and Dec. 13 a gradual change was assumed to have taken place.

The immediate purpose of the following reduction is to obtain values for the level and azimuthal deviation, to apply the required corrections to the observed transits of the moon and moon-culminating stars; it is, however, only the difference of these corrections which affects the resulting longitude.

For the first three observations of Nov. 18, 1853, we have no means of ascertaining the above two instrumental corrections; the level and azimuthal factors, however, for the moon and the two stars are nearly equal. After these observations the level and azimuth were changed.

It was found advisable to omit the observations of Polaris *R.* and 51 Cephei *s. p. R.* in the conditional equations of Nov. 18 and 21, since it is probable that the form of the pivots of the axis is very imperfect, or that the instrument was otherwise disturbed.

November 18, 1853. Circle West.

Object.	Mean of wires.	$R.$	$Cc.$	$t.$	Difference.	$AR.$	Deduced sidereal time of moon's limb.
☾ II. s. p.	$6^h\ 50^m\ 00^s.8$	$0^s.0$	$0^s.0$	$6^h\ 50^m\ 00^s.8$			$17^h\ 57^m\ 43^s.2$
μ Geminor s. p.	7 06 23.0	+2.6	0.0	7 06 25.6	$-0^h\ 16^m\ 24^s.8$	$18^h\ 14^m\ 07^s.1$	17 57 42.3
ϵ Geminor s. p.	7 27 07.5	+6.1	0.0	7 27 13.6	−0 37 12.8	18 34 56.4	17 57 43.6

The result by ϵ Gem. has the weight 2; μ Gem. the weight 1; the former star having very nearly the same level and azimuthal factor.

Object.	Mean of wires.	$R.$	$Cc.$	$t.$	$AR.$	$AR-t=\epsilon.$
Polaris R.	$13^h\ 49^m\ 29^s.8$	$-11^s.6$	$0^s.0$	$13^h\ 49^m\ 18^s.2$	$1^h\ 06^m\ 34^s.7$	
η Urs. maj. s. p.	14 33 12.7	− 4.4	0.0	14 33 08.3	1 41 44.3	$11^h\ 08^m\ 36^s.0$
α Arietis	14 49 44.0	− 1.7	0.0	14 49 42.3	1 58 56.7	11 09 14.4
α Bootis s. p.	15 00 00.4	0.0	0.0	15 00 00.4	2 08 57.6	11 08 57.2
γ Ceti	15 26 34.2	+ 4.4	0.0	15 26 38.6	2 35 44.1	11 09 05.5
Circle East.						
β Urs. min. s. p. R.	15 42 46.2	+ 7.0	0.0	15 42 53.2	2 51 06.7	11 08 13.5

$T = 15^h\ 00^m.0$

$E_0 = +11^h\ 08^m\ 40^s0$

$E = +11\ 10\ 42$

Normal equations.

$$5\,\epsilon + 5.87\,a + 3.0\,b = +46.6 \qquad a = -100^s$$
$$+5.87\,\epsilon + 7.32\,a + 5.2\,b = +23.7 \qquad b = +7.1$$
$$+3.0\,\epsilon + 5.2\,a + 13.0\,b = -63.8 \qquad \epsilon = +122$$

November 21, 1853. Circle East.

Object.	Mean of wires.	$R.$	$Cc.$	$t.$	$AR.$
51 Cephei s. p. R.	$7^h\ 09^m\ 31^s.1$	$-22^s.9$	$+2^s.1$	$7^h\ 09^m\ 10^s.3$	$18^h\ 30^m\ 45^s.4$
β Lyræ	7 23 51.5	−18.9	−0.1	7 23 32.5	18 44 39.0
ζ Aquilæ	7 37 55.2	−16.6	−0.1	7 37 38.5	18 58 39.6
δ Geminor s. p.	7 50 50.2	−14.5	+0.1	7 50 35.8	19 11 23.4
δ Aquilæ	7 57 21.7	−13.4	−0.1	7 57 08.2	19 18 05.8
γ Cancri s. p.	9 14 03.0	− 0.9	+0.1	9 14 02.2	20 34 48.9
☾ II. s. p.	9 19 14.1	0.0	+0.1	9 19 14.2	
ι Urs. maj. s. p.	9 28 36.2	+ 1.5	+0.2	9 28 37.9	20 49 10.2
ζ Cygni R.	9 45 31.3	+ 4.3	−0.1	9 45 35.5	21 06 41.7
α Cephei R.	9 54 13.2	+ 5.7	−0.2	9 54 18 7	21 15 08.8
λ Leonis s. p.	10 02 28.2	+ 7.1	+0.1	10 02 35.4	21 23 21.8

$T = 9^h\ 19^m.2$

$E_0 = +11^h\ 20^m\ 50^s.0$

$E = +11\ 22\ 02.$

Normal equations.

$$+9\,\epsilon + 8.57\,a - 2.6\,b = +19.5 \qquad a = -70^s.4$$
$$+8.57\,\epsilon + 8.2\,a - 2.0\,b = +11.4 \qquad b = +13.6$$
$$-2.6\,\epsilon - 2.0\,a + 6.3\,b = +37.3 \qquad \epsilon = +72.5$$

Object.	Mean+R+$Cc.$	$Bb.$	$Aa.$	$t.$	Difference.	$AR.$	Deduced sidereal time of moon's limb.
δ Geminor s. p.	$7^h\ 50^m\ 35^s.8$	$-2^s.9$	$-73^s.9$	$7^h\ 49^m\ 19^s.0$	$+1^h\ 28^m\ 37^s.0$	$19^h\ 11^m\ 23^s.4$	$20^h\ 40^m\ 00^s.4$
γ Cancri s. p.	9 14 02.2	− 2.7	−75.3	9 12 44.2	+ 5 11.8	20 34 48.9	20 40 00.7
☾ II. s. p.	9 19 14.2	− 2.9	−75.3	9 17 56.0			20 40 00.7
(ζ Cygni R.)	9 45 35.5	−10.2	−60.5	9 44 24.8	− 26 28.8	21 06 41.7	(20 40 12.9)
λ Leonis s. p.	10 02 35.4	− 3.1	−75.3	10 01 17.0	− 43 21.0	21 23 21.8	20 40 00.8

Omitting ζ Cygni, R., the deduced sidereal time of the ☾'s IId limb becomes $20^h\ 40^m\ 00^s.7$.

November 23. Circle East.

Object.	Mean of wires.	R.	Cc.	Mean + R + Cc.	AR.	ε.
η Draconis R.	4h 55m 08s.0	—20s.5	—0s.4	4h 54m 47s.1	16h 21m 58s.6	11h 27m 11s.5
α Tauri s. p.	5 00 29.5	—19.6	+0.2	5 00 10.1	16 27 32.6	11 27 22.5
α Aurig. s. p.	5 39 04.0	—13.3	+0.3	5 38 51.0	17 05 54.4	11 27 03.4
γ Drac. R.	6 26 01.9	— 5.6	—0.3	6 25 56.0	17 53 10.4	11 27 14.4
α Lyræ	7 04 04.3	+ 0.7	—0.3	7 04 04.7	18 31 57.3	11 27 52.6
β Lyræ	7 16 48.2	+ 2.8	—0.2	7 16 50.8	18 44 39.0	11 27 48.2
ζ Aquilæ	7 30 56.9	+ 5.1	—0.2	7 31 01.8	18 58 39.6	11 27 37.8
δ Gemi. s. p.	7 43 58.1	+ 7.2	+0.2	7 44 05.5	19 11 23.5	11 27 18.0

The normal equations give: $a = -34^s.4$

$T = 7^h\ 00^m.0$ $b = +\ 1.2$

$E_0 = +\ 11^h\ 27^m\ 30^s$ $\varepsilon = +\ 27$

Object.	Mean of wires.	R.	Cc.	Bb.	Aa.	t.	Difference.	AR.	Deduced sid. time of moon's limb.
α Leonis	22h 30m 24s.9	—8s.0	—0s.2	+0s.5	—32s.3	22h 29m 44s.9	+48m 50s.5	10h 00m 34s.2	10h 49m 24s.7
γ Leonis	22 41 38.3	—6.2	—0.2	+0.7	—31.0	22 41 01.6	+37 33.8	10 11 53.6	10 49 27.4
☾ II.	23 19 07.1	0.0	—0.2	+0.5	—32.0	23 18 35.4			10 49 25.0
χ Leonis	23 27 10.7	+1.3	—0.2	+0.4	—32.3	23 26 39.9	— 8 04.5	10 57 27.4	10 49 22.9

The mean from the three stars has been adopted.

For the following observations on Dec. 8, Dec. 9, and Dec. 12, the azimuth error has been assumed zero, as it nearly results from the mean found on December 13, 14, and 15; the level error is — 2.8, as found on the 13th and the two following days. The difference in the values of A on Dec. 8, 9, and 12, is in maximo but 0.1.

December 8, 1853. Circle East.

Object.	Mean of wires.	R.	Aa.	Bb.	Cc.	t.	Difference.	AR.	Deduced sid. time of moon's limb.
ι Piscium	11h 04m 34s.8	—8s.3	0s.0	—0s.8	—1s.1	11h 04m 24s.6	+51m 05s.3	23h 32m 25s.4	0h 23m 30s.7
(α Andro.)	11 32 31.1	—3.8	0.0	—2.0	—1.3	11 32 24.0	+23 05.9	0 00 49.9	(0 23 55.8)
(γ Pegasi)	11 37 37.5	—3.0	0.0	—1.4	—1.1	11 37 32.0	+17 57.9	0 05 42.3	(0 23 40.2)
☾ I.	11 55 31.6	0.0	0.0	—0.6	—1.1	11 55 29.9			0 23 31.5
δ Piscium	12 13 02.4	+2.9	0.0	—0.8	—1.1	12 13 03.4	—17 33.5	0 41 05.9	0 23 32.4

Excluding the results from α Androm. and γ Pegasi, the observed AR. of the moon becomes $0^h\ 23^m\ 31^s.5$.

December 9, 1853. Circle East.

Object.	Mean of wires.	R.	Aa.	Bb.	Cc.	t.	Difference.	AR.	Deduced sid. time of moon's limb.
α Andro.	11h 28m 36s.9	—11s.3	0s.0	—2s.0	—1s.3	11h 28m 22s.3	+1h 09m 13s.9	0h 00m 49s.9	1h 09m 63s.8
γ Pegasi	11 33 42.8	—10.5	0.0	—1.4	—1.2	11 33 29.7	+1 04 06.5	0 05 42.3	1 09 48.8
☾ I.	12 37 38.2	0.0	0.0	—0.8	—1.2	12 37 36.2			?(1 09 53.8)

Moon seen through clouds.

Giving the result by γ Pegasi the weight two, the observed AR of the moon results as above; it is, however, preferable to reject the result altogether, on account of the great difference in the results by the two stars.

December 12, 1853. Circle East.

Object.	Mean of wires.	*R.*	*Aa.*	*Bb.*	*Cc.*	*t.*	Difference.	*AR.*	Deduced sid. time of moon's limb.
δ Arietis	$2^h\ 19^m\ 02^s.9$	$-4^s.3$	$0^s.0$	$-1^s.4$	$-1^s.4$	$2^h\ 18^m\ 55^s.8$	$+26^m\ 16^s.1$	$3^h\ 03^m\ 17^s.0$	$3^h\ 29^m\ 33^s.1$
☽ I.	2 45 14.6	0.0	0.0	—1.4	—1.3	2 45 11.9			3 29 35.6
η Tauri	2 54 22.7	+1.5	0.0	—1.7	—1.3	2 54 21.2	—09 09.3	3 38 48.7	3 29 39.4
27 Tauri	2 56 03.7	+1.8	0.0	—1.7	—1.4	2 56 02.4	—10 50.5	3 40 29.1	3 29 38.6
A' Tauri	3 11 38.6	+4.3	0.0	—1.7	—1.4	3 11 39.8	—26 27.9	3 56 04.1	3 29 36.2

δ Arietis is nearer to the moon in reference to declination than any of the other stars, and since they differ considerably in their value for the ☾'s sidereal time, it seemed to be preferable to combine the results from η, 27, and A' Tauri into one, and take the mean between it and that obtained by δ Arietis. $E_{\odot} = +\ 12^h\ 44^m\ 24^s.9.$

December 13, 1853. Circle West.

Object.	Mean of wires.	*R.*	*Cc.*	Mean + *R* + *Cc.*	*AR.*
Polaris R.	$12^h\ 15^m\ 44^s.0$	$-17^s.1$	$+54^s.6$	$12^h\ 16^m\ 21^s.5$	$1^h\ 06^m\ 19^s.7$
α Arietis R.	1 10 45.0	— 8.1	+ 1.5	13 10 38.4	1 58 56.6
α Bootis s. p.	1 20 46.9	— 6.4	— 1.5	13 20 39.0	2 08 58.2
γ Ceti	1 47 30.3	— 2.0	+ 1.4	13 47 29.7	2 35 44.1
β Urs. min. s. p. R.	2 02 56.1	+ 0.5	— 5.3	14 02 51.3	2 51 07.6
α Coron. s. p.	2 40 03.7	+ 6.6	— 1.5	14 40 38.8	3 28 28.1
η Tauri	2 50 22.3	+ 8.3	+ 1.5	14 50 32.1	3 38 48.7
27 Tauri	2 52 02.4	+ 8.5	+ 1.5	14 52 12.4	3 40 29.1
A' Tauri	3 07 33.7	+11.1	+ 1.5	15 07 46.3	3 56 04.1
☾ I.	3 30 37.5	+14.9	+ 1.5	15 30 53.9	

$T = 14^h\ 00^m.0 \qquad E_{\odot} = +\ 12^h\ 48^m\ 20^s$

The above data were used in three different forms: 1st, omitting Polaris; 2d, omitting Polaris and β Urs. min.; and last, taking all the stars. The first hypothesis gave apparently the best results, viz:—

Normal equations:

$$+8\,\epsilon + 8.55\,a + 4.3\,b = -51.5 \qquad a = +26^s.4$$
$$+8.55\,\epsilon + 9.3\,a + 6.5\,b = -55.8 \qquad b = -\ 2.8$$
$$+4.3\,\epsilon + 6.5\,a + 13.3\,b = -\ 8.5 \qquad \epsilon = -33.1$$
$$E = +\ 12^h\ 47^m\ 47^s$$

Object.	*Bb.*	*Aa.*	*t.*	Difference.	*AR.*	Observed sid. time of moon's limb.
η Tauri	$-1^s.7$	$+24^s.0$	$14^h\ 50^m\ 54^s.4$	$+40^m\ 22^s.1$	$3^h\ 38^m\ 48^s.7$	$4^h\ 19^m\ 10^s.8$
27 Tauri	—1.7	+24.0	14 52 34.7	+38 41.8	3 40 29.1	4 19 10.9
A' Tauri	—1.7	+24.3	15 08 08.9	+23 07.6	3 56 04.1	4 19 11.7
☽ I.	—1.7	+24.3	15 31 16.5			4 19 11.1

The mean result from the three stars has been adopted.

December 14, 1853. Circle West.

Object.	Mean of wires.	*R.*	*Cc.*	Mean + *R* + *Cc.*	*AR.*
ε Urs. min. s. p. R.	4^h 09^m $01^s.7$	— $1^s.9$	—$10^s.4$	16^h 08^m $49^s.4$	5^h 00^m $55^s.9$
☾ I.	4 18 17.9	— 0.4	+ 1.5	16 18 19.0	
☾ II.	4 20 30.1	0.0	+ 1.5	16 20 31.6	
ο Tauri	4 26 12.8	+ 0.9	+ 1.5	16 26 15.2	5 18 52.2
δ Orionis	4 31 56.6	+ 1.9	+ 1.4	16 31 59.9	5 24 33.2
ζ Tauri	4 36 14.8	+ 2.6	+ 1.5	16 36 18.9	5 28 55.4
α Orionis	4 54 34.4	+ 5.6	+ 1.4	16 54 41.4	5 47 16.2
μ Geminor	5 21 22.5	+10.0	+ 1.4	17 21 34.0	6 14 07.7

T = 16^h $20^m.5$ $E_0 = + 12^h\ 52^m\ 40^s$

The normal equations: $+\ 6\,\varepsilon + 7.1\,a + 9.3\,b = -\ 58.2$ give $a = -5^s.0$

$+ 7.1\,\varepsilon + 10.2\,a + 18.3\,b = -102.0$ $b = -3.3$

$+ 9.3\,\varepsilon + 18.3\,a + 50.3\,b = -245.1$ $\varepsilon = +1.3$

Object.	*Bb.*	*Aa.*	*t.*	Differences. (Very near full moon.)		*AR.*	Deduced sid. time of moon's limb.	
				I.	II.		I.	II.
☾ I.	—$2^s.0$	—$4^s.5$	16^h 18^m $12^s.5$				5^h 10^m $53^s.8$	
☾ II.	—2.0	—4.5	16 20 25.1					5^h 13^m $06^s.4$
ο Tauri	—2.0	—4.5	16 26 08.7	—0^h 7^m $56^s.2$	—0^h 5^m $43^s.6$	5^h 18^m $52^s.2$	5 10 56.0	5 13 08.6
δ Orionis	—0.7	—5.0	16 31 54.2	—0 13 41.7	—0 11 29.1	5 24 33.2	5 10 51.9	5 13 04.1
ζ Tauri	—2.0	—4.5	16 36 12.4	—0 17 59.9	—0 15 47.3	5 28 55.4	5 10 55.5	5 13 08.1
α Orionis	—1.0	—5.0	16 54 35.4	—0 36 22.9	—0 34 10.3	5 47 16.2	5 10 53.3	5 13 05.9
μ Geminor	—2.0	—4.5	17 21 27.5	—1 03 15.0	—1 01 02.4	6 14 07.7	5 10 52.7	5 13 05.3

December 15, 1853. Circle West.

Object.	Mean of wires.	*R.*	*Cc.*	Mean + *R* + *Cc.*	*AR.*
Polaris R.	12^h 07^m $22^s.7$	—$24^s.7$	+$54^s.6$	12^h 07^m $52^s.6$	1^h 06^m $18^s.4$
η Urs. maj. s. p.	12 45 57 5	—18.3	— 2.2	12 45 37.0	1 41 45.1
η Bootis s. p.	12 51 47.9	—17.5	— 1.4	12 51 29.0	1 47 42.2
α Arietis R.	1 02 57.0	—15.6	+ 1.5	13 02 42.9	1 58 56.6
α Bootis s. p.	1 13 01.4	—13.9	— 1.5	13 12 46.0	2 08 58.3
γ Ceti	1 39 39.0	— 9.6	+ 1.4	13 39 30.8	2 35 44.1
β Urs. min. s. p. R.	1 55 20.5	— 7.0	— 5.3	13 55 08.2	2 51 07.7
ο Tauri	4 22 18.7	+17.1	+ 1.5	16 22 37.3	5 18 52.3
ζ Tauri	4 32 19.9	+18.9	+ 1.5	16 32 40.3	5 28 55.4
α Orionis	4 50 37.4	+21.8	+ 1.4	16 51 00.6	5 47 16.2
γ Draconis s. p.	4 56 42.7	+22.7	— 2.2	16 57 03.2	5 53 10.3
☾ II.	5 09 56.5	+24.9	+ 1.5	17 10 22.9	
μ Geminor	5 17 24.8	+26.1	+ 1.5	17 17 52.4	6 14 07.8

T = 14^h $38^m.0$ $E_0 = + 12^h\ 56^m\ 15^s$

A preliminary discussion showed that the result from Polaris was accordant with the results from the other stars; the whole group gave the following normal equations :—

$+\ 12\,\varepsilon + 10.87\,a - 35.65\,b = +\ 94.1$ $a = -22^s.9$ $E = + 12^h\ 56^m\ 37^s.1$

$+ 10.87\,\varepsilon + 13.9\,a + 38.4\,b = -\ 168.1$ $b = -2.26$

$- 35.65\,\varepsilon + 38.4\,a + 1497.5\,b = -\ 5072.0$ $\varepsilon = + 22.1$

Object.	*Bb.*	*Aa.*	*t.*	Difference.	*AR.*	Deduced sidereal time of moon's limb.
ο Tauri	—1^s.4	—20^s.6	16^h 22^m 15^s.3	+47^m 45^s.4	5^h 18^m 52^s.3	6^h 06^m 37^s.7
ζ Tauri	—1.4	—20.6	16 32 18.3	+37 42.4	5 28 55.4	6 06 37.8
α Orionis	—0.7	—22.9	16 50 37.0	+19 23.7	5 47 16.2	6 06 39.9
(γ Draconis s. p.)	+2.3	—27.5	16 56 38.0	+13 22.7	5 53 10.3	(6 06 33.0)
☾ II.	—1.6	—20.6	17 10 00.7			6 06 38.4
μ Geminor	—1.4	—20.6	17 17 30.4	— 7 29.7	6 14 07.8	6 06 38.1

Excluding γ Draconis, we obtain from the mean of four stars the deduced *AR* of the moon as above.

January 8, 1854. Circle West.

Object.	Mean of wires.	*R.*	*Cc.*	*Aa.*[1]	*M+R+Cc+Aa.*	*AR.*
α Bootis s. p.	11^h 37^m 55^s.2	—10^s.5	—1^s.5	+24^s.9	11^h 38^m 08^s.1	2^h 08^m 58^s.9
845 B. A. C.	12 05 53.8	— 5.9	+1.4	+24.9	12 06 14.2	2 37 02.9
π Arietis	12 09 58.0	— 5.2	+1.4	+22.4	12 10 16.6	2 41 08.6
α Ceti	12 23 26.2	— 3.1	+1.4	+24.9	12 23 49.4	2 54 38.8
☾ I.	12 41 58.5	0.0	+1.4	+24.9	12 42 24.8	
Saturn centre	1 01 59.7	+ 3.3	+1.4	+24.9	13 02 29.3	3 33 19.6
17 Tauri	1 04 52.8	+ 3.8	+1.5	+24.9	13 05 23.0	3 36 12.7
η Tauri	1 07 28.9	+ 4.2	+1.5	+24.9	13 07 59.5	3 38 48.6
27 Tauri	1 09 09.6	+ 4.5	+1.5	+24.9	13 09 40.5	3 40 29.1

T = 12^h 42^m.0 $E_o = + 14^h\ 30^m\ 50^s$

Normal equations: $8\,\epsilon + 3.3\,b = -1.4$ $b = -1.3$

$3.3\,\epsilon + 1.9\,b = -1.27$ $\epsilon = + 0.4$

Object.	*Bb.*	*t.*	Difference.	Deduced sidereal time of moon's limb.
845 B. A. C.	—0^s.5	12^h 06^m 13^s.7	+0^h 36^m 10^s.5	3^h 13^m 13^s.4
π Arietis	—0.6	12 10 16.0	+ 32 08.2	3 13 16.8
α Ceti	—0.4	12 23 49.0	+ 18 35.2	3 13 14.0
☾ I.	—0.6	12 42 24.2		3 13 14.5
Saturn centre	—0.6	13 02 28.7	— 20 04.5	3 13 15.1
17 Tauri	—0.8	13 05 22.2	— 22 58.0	3 13 14.7
η Tauri	—0.8	13 07 58.7	— 25 34.5	3 13 14.1
27 Tauri	—0.8	13 09 39.7	— 27 15.5	3 13 13.6

January 9, 1854. Circle West.

Object.	Mean of wires.	*R.*	*Cc.*	*M+R+Cc.*	*AR.*
γ Pegasi	9^h 31^m 01^s.4	—9^s.7	+ 1^s.4	9^h 30^m 53^s.1	0^h 05^m 42^s.0
α Cassiop. R.	9 57 58.1	—5.2	+ 2.4	9 57 55.3	0 32 13.3
Polaris R.	10 43 17.2	+2.1	+54.6	10 44 13.9	1 05 58.3
η Urs. maj. s. p.	11 06 47.2	+6.0	— 2.2	11 06 51.0	1 41 46.2
α Arietis	11 23 57.1	+8.8	+ 1.5	11 24 07.4	1 58 56.3

T = 10^h 30^m $E_o = + 14^h\ 34^m\ 50^s$ The normal equations give $a = + 38^s.9$

$b = + 20.0$

$\epsilon = - 24.7$

Omitting Polaris, ϵ would be $= - 35.8$

[1] The azimuthal deviation cannot be found from the above observations. The mean *a* has, therefore, been used, as found on the 9th and 10th, viz: $a = + 24''.9$.

January 10, 1854. Circle West.

Object.	Mean of wires.	R.	Co.	M+R+Co.	AR.
γ Pegasi	9h 27m 07s.6	—10s.3	+ 1s.4	9h 26m 58s.7	0h 05m 42s.0
α Cassiop. R.	9 54 04.9	— 5.8	+ 2.4	9 54 01.5	0 32 13.3
Polaris R.	10 39 39.7	+ 1.5	+54.6	10 40 35.8	1 05 57 3
α Bootis s. p.	11 30 03.0	+ 9.8	— 1.5	11 30 11.3	2 08 59.1

T = 10h 30m E$_0$ = + 14h 38m 40s The normal equations give a = + 10s.9

b = + 20.6

c = — 3.5

RECAPITULATION OF THE DEDUCED SIDEREAL TIMES OF THE MOON'S LIMB.

1853. Nov. 18	☾ II. s. p.	17h 57m 43s.2	1853. Dec. 13	☾ I.	4h 19m 11s.1
" 21	☾ II. s. p.	20 40 00.7	" 14	☾ I.	5 10 53.8
" 23	☾ II.	10 49 25.0	" 14	☾ II.	5 13 06.4
Dec. 8	☾ I.	0 23 31.5	" 15	☾ II.	6 06 38.4
" 9	☾ I.	(1 09 53.8)?	1854. Jan. 8	☾ I.	3 13 14.5
" 12	☾ I.	3 29 35.6			

The longitude is deduced from the above values by a method received from Prof. Peirce in 1851, an account of which is given in Coast Survey Report for 1858, Appendix No. 21, p. 186.

From the Greenwich observations[1] we have the following corrections to the tabular places of the moon's right ascension, as given in the Greenwich Nautical Almanac:—

	From transit observations.	From altazimuth observations.	Mean adopted.
1853. November 18	—0s.36	—0s.58	—0s.47
" 21	—0.24		—0.24
" 23	—0.10		—0.10
December 8	—0.70	—0.99	—0.84
" 9	—0.77		—0.77
" 12	—0.22	—0.10	—0.15
" 13		+0.02	+0.02
" 14		—0.64	—0.64
" 15		—0.54	—0.54
1854. January 8	—0.36	—0.78	—0.57

The weights assigned to the moon culminations are approximations; the greater the number and the better the agreement of the results from the moon culminating stars the greater the weight. The result deduced for December 9 is unreliable, and has been rejected; the result for December 8 is not much better, but has been worked up along with the rest.

[1] Astronomical and Magnetic and Meteorological Observations at the Royal Observatory, Greenwich. Volumes for 1853 and 1854. London, 1855 and 1856.

REDUCTION OF THE LONGITUDE OF VAN RENSSELAER HARBOR OBSERVATORY.

From observations of the moon and the moon culminating stars.

	1853. ☾ II. s. p. November 18.	☾ II. s. p. November 21.	☾ II. November 23.	☾ I. December 8.	☾ I. December 12.
Approx. sid. time of obs'n.	17^h 58^m	20^h 40^m	10^h 49^m	0^h 24^m	3^h 30^m
" Greenwich m. t.	6 50	9 20	23 19	11 57	14 46
Moon's declination	+25° 09′.5	+22° 58′.8	+13° 19′.6	—2° 37′.8	+17° 31′.8
" semidiameter	14′ 44″.7	14′ 58″·1	15′ 26″.6	15′ 16″.2	14′ 47″.2
Semidiameter × sec. D.	— 65^s.16	— 65^s.03	— 63^s.48	+61^s.14	+62^s.03
Sid. t. of transit of ☾'s limb	17^h 57^m 43^s.2	20^h 40^m 00^s.7	10^h 49^m 25^s.0	0^h 23^m 31^s.5	3^h 29^m 35^s.6
Observed AR of centre	17 56 38.0	20 38 55.7	10 48 21.5	0 24 32.6	3 30 37.6
Corr'd tab. AR of prec. full hour at Greenwich	17 54 45.4	20 38 11.9	10 47 40.7	0 22 37.2	3 29 02.4
Difference	1 52.6	43.8	40.8	1 55.4	1 35.2
Hourly motion	2 10.06	2 08.64	2 02.45	1 53.65	1 58.02
Greenwich mean time	6 51 58	9 20 25	23 19 59	12 00 53	14 48 26
Corresp'g G. sid. time	22 42 51	25 23 33	15 33 18	5 11 28	8 15 15
Longitude W. of Green'h	4 45 08	4 43 32	4 43 53	4 47 57	4 45 39
Weight	1	3	2	1	1

	1853. ☾ I. December 13.	☾ I. December 14.	☾ II. December 14.	☾ II. December 15.	1854. ☾ I. January 8.
Approx. sid. time of obs'n.	4^h 19^m	5^h 11^m	5^h 13^m	6^h 07^m	3^h 13^m
" Greenwich m. t.	15 31	16 19	16 21	17 11	12 43
Moon's declination	+21° 07′.7	+23° 46′.9	+23° 47′.0	+25° 19′.4	+16° 13′.3
" semidiameter	14′ 44″.6	14′ 43″.7	14′ 43″.7	14′ 44″.4	14′ 50″.6
Semidiameter × sec. D.	+58^s.97	+58^s.91	—58^s.91	—58^s.96	+59^s.37
Sid. t. of transit of ☾'s limb	4^h 19^m 11^s.1	5^h 10^m 53^s.8	5^h 13^m 06^s.4	6^h 06^m 38^s.4	3^h 13^m 14^s.5
Observed AR of centre	4 20 14.3	5 11 58.2	5 12 02.0	6 05 33.2	3 14 16.3
Corr'd tab. AR of prec. full hour at Greenwich	4 19 08.9	5 11 16.6	5 11 16.6	6 05 08.0	3 12 54.5
Difference	1 05.4	41.6	45.4	25.2	1 21.8
Hourly motion	2 02.87	2 07.52	2 07.52	2 10.82	1 56.53
Greenwich mean time	15 31 57	16 19 35	16 21 22	17 11 33	12 42 08
Corresp'g G. sid. time	9 02 50	9 54 32	9 56 20	10 50 36	7 55 04
Longitude W. of Green'h	4 43 39	4 43 38	4 43 14	4 43 58	4 41 50
Weight	3	$\frac{3}{2}$	$\frac{3}{2}$	3	3

RECAPITULATION OF RESULTS, FROM MOON CULMINATIONS, OF THE LONGITUDE OF VAN RENSSELAER HARBOR OBSERVATORY.

	Moon's limb.	Longitude W. of Greenwich.	W.
1853. November 18	☾ II. s. p.	4^h 45^m 08^s	1
" 21	☾ II. s. p.	4 43 32	3
" 23	☾ II.	4 43 53	2
December 8	☾ I.	4 47 57?	1
" 12	☾ I.	4 45 39	1
" 13	☾ I.	4 43 39	3
" 14	☾ I.	4 43 38	1.5
" 14	☾ II.	4 43 14	1.5
" 15	☾ II.	4 43 58	3
1854. January 8	☾ I.	4 41 50	3

The value of December 8 must be rejected on the ground of imperfect transits; it is also thrown out by Peirce's Criterion; if included it would make the final result 13^s greater.

The weighted mean from nine observations is $4^h\ 43^m\ 34^s \pm 13^s$. If we combine the results according to the moon's limb, we find:—

From observations of ☾ I.	. . . . . .	$4^h\ 43^m\ 14^s$	weight 8.5
" " ☾ II.	. . . . . .	4 43 50	" 10.5
Mean	. . . . . .	4 43 32	

which last value I have adopted.

Record and Reduction of the Occultations and Eclipse, observed at Van Rensselaer Harbor.

The observations of occultations and of an eclipse were made at the Winter Quarters in latitude 78° 37′ 04″, and in approximate west longitude $4^h\ 43^m\ 32^s$.

In the following record, the times are given by chronometer, uncorrected for error and rate, in the two accounts of it in Appendix No. IX., second volume of the Narrative, pages 398 and 399, and in No. 1017 of the Astronomische Nachrichten, pages 135 and 136, the time is mean local time, as made out by Mr. Sonntag.

Occultation of Saturn. December 12, 1853.

Immersion at	$7^h\ 03^m\ 11^s.6$	Pocket chronometer.	A. Sonntag, observer.
"	7 28 49.0	Chronometer No. 2143.	Dr. Hayes, "
		1ˢ before the complete disappearance.	
Emersion at	7 36 50	Pocket chronometer.	A. Sonntag, observer.
		Perhaps 10ˢ too late.	

Note.—Moon's limb much undulating. The telescopes were one of English make and one by Fraunhofer, each of thirty-inch focal length. At immersion the time was noted when the last point of Saturn's ring disappeared behind the moon's limb; at the emersion, the time is given when the last point of the ring parted from the moon's limb. Chronometer comparisons:—

Pocket chronometer	$6^h\ 21^m\ 19^s.3$	No. 2143	$6^h\ 47^m$	All mean time chronometers.
	22 36.0	" 370	40	
	24 34.0	" 2721	19	
	26 30.7	" 264	29	

Occultation of Saturn. January 8, 1854.

Immersion at	$10^h\ 10^m\ 30^s$	Pocket chronometer.	A. Sonntag, observer.
		Doubtful, perhaps obscured by a cloud.	
Emersion at	11 07 06.5	Pocket chronometer.	A. Sonntag, observer.

Moment when the last point of Saturn's ring parted from the moon's limb.

For points of contact see note to the occultation of the 12th of December. Chronometer comparison

Pocket chronometer $10^h\ 18^m\ 30^s.0$ No. 2143 $10^h\ 45^m$

Occultation of Saturn. February (4) 5, 1854.

Immersion at	$4^h\ 25^m\ 10^s.5$	Pocket chronometer.	A. Sonntag, observer.
" at	4 52 55.0	No. 2143.	Dr. Kane, "
		Disappearance of last point of ring.	
Emersion at	5 23 09.0	Pocket chronometer.	A. Sonntag, observer.
		Saturn's centre.	
" at	5 51 13.0	No. 2143.	Dr. Kane, observer.
		Last contact of ring.	The moon's limb was much undulating.

Chronometer comparisons :—

Pocket chronometer	4^h 33^m $17^s.2$	No. 2143	5^h	01^m
	34 48.4	" 370	4	58
	36 01.4	" 2721		29
	37 17.9	" 264		40

The sky was very clear. Thermometer at immersion —53° (corrected temp. = —58°.2), at the emersion —52° (corrected temp. = —54°.6).

Occultation of Mars. February 13, 1854.

Immersion, first contact at	1^h 04^m $59^s.0$	Pocket chronometer.	A. Sonntag, observer.
" second " at	1 06 01.5	" "	" "
		(Disappearance.)	
" " " at	1 33 47.0	No. 2143.	Dr. Kane, observer.
		(Disappearance.)	
Emersion, last contact at	1 36 05.5	Pocket chronometer.	A. Sonntag, observer.

Chronometer comparisons :—

Pocket chronometer	1^h 14^m $01^s.2$	No. 2143	1^h	42^m
	15 51.2	" 370		40
	16 20.8	" 2721		9
	17 18.0	" 264		20

Note.—Moon near the horizon, limb much undulating. Immersion reliable, emersion doubtful; perhaps too late. The planet reappeared at a different place than expected.

The observations for time, for the above occultations, were made with the eighteen inch transit instrument.

Observation of the solar eclipse. May 15, 1855.

The original entry of the observations of this eclipse I could not find: the following has been copied from the published account in the Narrative:—

Mean local time of beginning	9^h 13^m 41^s	Dr. Kane, observer.
	38	A. Sonntag, "
" " " ending	10 55 44	Dr. Kane, "
	52	A. Sonntag,

Altitude of the sun at beginning 10° 17′, at ending 8°. The time was obtained from observations of equal altitudes of the sun.

Reduction of the preceding Observations for Longitude.

Converting the chronometer error on sidereal time to its equivalent on mean time, we have, from the preceding transit reductions, the following results:—

1853. December 8	7^h 13^m	$E = -4^h$ 42^m $24^s.8$	} $22^s.2$
9	7 54	—4 42 17.9	}
12	10 02	—4 42 23.9	}
13	9 17	—4 42 48.9	
14	11 38	—4 42 16.6	
15	9 56	—4 42 00.5	
Mean, December 13.5		$E = -4$ 42 22.1 ± 5^s	

The differences in the values of E are due to the imperfect transits arising from the difficulty of obtaining a reliable azimuthal determination, and since the rate of the chronometer has been found by frequent comparisons with the other mean time chronometers to be uniform, I have preferred to use the mean E from the several determinations. The next reliable time observations are on February 20, 1854, which gave $E = -4^h\ 42^m\ 51^s.4$ at $7^h\ 56^m$ (mean time); the daily rate is accordingly $-0^s.42$ (gaining), and the chronometer error on mean time for the several occultations becomes:—

1853.	December 12, 14^h	$E = -4^h\ 42^m\ 21^s.7$	Occultation of Saturn.
1854.	January 8, 18	-4 42 33.3	" "
"	February 4–5, 1	-4 42 44.8	" "
"	" 13, 20	-4 42 48.2	" of Mars.

That the rate of the pocket chronometer during the above times was uniform is proved by the comparisons with the other chronometers; between December 12 and January 8, 2143 had a gaining rate on the pocket chronometer of $1^s.9$, between the latter date and February 5 it was $2^s.3$, and between the last date and February 13 it was $2^s.2$. The true rate of 2143 is, therefore, $-2^s.2 - 0^s.4 = -2^s.6$.

The following table contains the observed times of the several phases of the occultations of Saturn and ring:—

Van Rensselaer mean time.	December 12, 1853.	January 8, 1854.	February 4–5, 1854.
Immersion, contact of last point of ring	$14^h\ 20^m\ 48^s.8$	$17^h\ 27^m\ 56^s.7$	$4^d\ 23^h\ 42^m\ 23^s.2$
Emersion, centre			5 0 40 20.8
" last contact of ring	14 54 18.3	18 24 33.2	0 40 42.0

The method of reduction used is that of finding the time of true conjunction in right ascension, and the notation the same as given in vol. II. of Sawitsch's Treatise on Practical Astronomy (German edition, by Dr. W. C. Goetze, Hamburg, 1851). Hansen's interpolation formula was used. The tabular Nautical Almanac places and data have been corrected, when practicable, from the Greenwich observations.

Longitude from the Observations of the Occultation of Saturn's Ring.

December 12, 1853.

Immersion, last contact of ring	$7^h\ 48^m\ 20^s.0$	Sidereal time	or $19^h\ 04^m\ 20^s.8$	Approx. Green-
Emersion, " "	8 21 55.0	at Van Rensselaer	19 37 50.3	wich mean time.

From the Greenwich Nautical Almanac, as corrected from the Greenwich observations:—

At immersion, α ☾ . . . . $3^h\ 39^m\ 02^s.59$
At emersion 3 40 08.92
(Correction to Nautical Almanac $-0^s.22$)
At immerson, δ ☾ . . . . $+18°\ 12'\ 55''.1$
At emersion 18 18 08.9
(Correction to Nautical Almanac $-5''.0$)
At immersion, horizontal parallax ☾ $54'\ 07''.1$
At emersion 54 06.8
(Correction $+0''.3$ according to Adams.)
At immersion, semidiameter ☾ . . $14'\ 45''.5$
At emersion 14 45.4
(Correction $-1''.1$ according to Oudeman's Astronomische Nachr. No. 1202.)

At immersion, α ♄ . . . $3^h\ 39^m\ 09^s.11$
At emersion 3 39 08.71
(Correction to Nautical Almanac $+0^s.15$.)
At immersion δ ♄ . . . $+17°\ 14'\ 26''.3$
At emersion 17 14 25.2
(Correction to Nautical Almanac $-8''.9$.)

Horizontal parallax ♄ . . . . $1''.0$
Semidiameter ♄ . . . . . $9''.2+1''.0$

Mean time of ☌, Greenwich $19^h\ 07^m\ 39^s.3$

Immersion.				Emersion.			
☾'s horizontal paral. at Van Rensselaer	53′	56″.7		☾'s horizontal paral. at Van Rensselaer	53′	56″.4	
Relative parallax π	53	55.7		Relative parallax π	53	55.4	
$a-s$	—62° 19	21.1		$a-s$	—70° 26	31.5	
$a'-a=p=$	— 10	00.09		$a'-a=p=$	— 10	38.50	
$\delta'-\delta=q=$	— 48	57.19		$\delta'-\delta=q=$	— 49	20.16	
Augmented semidiameter ☾ .		890.9		Augmented semidiameter ☾ .		890.5	

The following quantities were computed for the purpose of plotting the phenomenon to obtain the points of contact on the ring, and the required radial correction to the moon's semidiameter to refer the point on the ring to the centre of Saturn.

Approximate α ☾ at immersion $3^h\ 38^m\ 22^s.58$ At emersion $3^h\ 39^m\ 26^s.35$
" α ♄ " 3 39 09.11 " 3 39 08.71

	At immersion.	At emersion.
Relative approximate difference in AR (reduced to a great circle)	—11′ 06″.3	+ 4′ 12″.5
" " " in declination	+ 9 31.6	+14 23.5

Geocentric elements of Saturn's ring :—

$p=-2°\ 38'$	$a'=\ 30''.3$	From the Greenwich N. A.
$a=\ 45''.6$	$b'=-12.3$	
$b=\ -18.6$	Southern surface visible.	

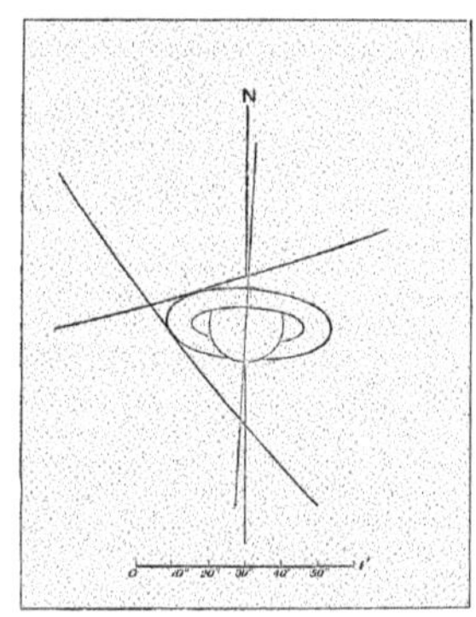

By means of the above numbers, the moon's path relative to Saturn was plotted, and the correction to refer the points of contact to the centre was obtained graphically. See above diagram, showing the position of the planet and ring, and contacts of the moon's limb.

Reduction to centre . .	—17″.5	Reduction to centre . .	+11″.5
$k'=$	873.4	$k'=$	902.0
$k'+b'=$	+1445.0	$k'+b'=$	+1765.5
$k'-b'=$	+ 301.8	$k'-b'=$	+ 88.5
$d'=$	+17° 19′ 12″.1	$d'=$	+17° 21′ 37″.0
$a'+p=a=$	+90.65	$a'+p=a=$	—911.66
$m-n=$	118ˢ.09	$m-n=$	118ˢ.14
Reduction to time of true ☌ .	+3 04.2	Reduction to time of true ☌ .	—30ᵐ 52ˢ.0
t	14 20 48.8	t	14 54 18.3
τ	14ʰ 23ᵐ 53ˢ.0	τ	14ʰ 23ᵐ 26ˢ.3
$\psi'=40°\ 52'.7$		$\psi'=106°\ 48'.0$	

Time of true ☌ in Van Rensselaer mean time 14ʰ 23ᵐ 53ˢ.0 + 1.84 dB from immersion.
14 23 26.3 — 7.05 dB from emersion.

$dB=-3''.0$ Hence longitude of Van Rensselaer Harbor from immersion 4ʰ 43ᵐ 51ˢ.8
from emersion 4 43 51.8

Longitude from the Observations of the Occultation of Saturn's Ring.

January 8, 1854.

Immersion, last contact of ring	12ʰ 42ᵐ 25ˢ.7	Sidereal time at Van Rensselaer	or 22ʰ 11ᵐ 28ˢ.7 Approx. Greenwich mean time.
Emersion, " "	13 39 11 5		23 08 05.2

From the Greenwich Nautical Almanac, as corrected by the Greenwich observations:—

At immersion, α ☾	3ʰ 32ᵐ 49ˢ.40	At immersion, α ♄	3ʰ 33ᵐ 16ˢ.75
At emersion	3 34 40.95	At emersion	3 33 16.45
(Correction to Nautical Almanac—0ˢ.36.)		(Correction to Nautical Almanac +0ˢ.18.)	
At immersion, δ ☾	+17° 47′ 21″.3	At immersion, δ ♄	+17° 00′ 34″.3
At emersion	17 56 22.2	At emersion	17 00 33.9
(Correction to Nautical Almanac—10″.0.)		(Correction to Nautical Almanac —9″.0.)	
At immersion, horizontal parallax ☾	54′ 14″.9		
At emersion	54 14.3	Horizontal parallax ♄	1″.0
(Correction —0″.1 according to Adams.)		Semidiameter ♄	8″.9+1″.0
At immersion, semidiameter ☾ . .	14′ 47″.6		
At emersion	14 47.4	Mean time of ☌, Greenwich .	22ʰ 25ᵐ 18ˢ.9
(Correction —1″.1 according to Oudeman.)			

Immersion.		Emersion.	
☾'s horizontal paral. at Van Rensselaer	54′ 04″.5	☾'s horizontal paral. at Van Rensselaer	54′ 03″.9
Relative parallax $\pi=$ . .	54 03.5	Relative parallax $\pi=$ . .	54 02.9
$\alpha-s=$	—137° 24 04.5	$\alpha-s=$	—151° 07 39
$\alpha'-\alpha=p=$	— 7 36.83	$\alpha'-\alpha=p=$	— 5 25.96
$\delta'-\delta=q=$	— 52 59.54	$\delta'-\delta=q=$	— 53 24.21
Augmented semidiameter ☾ .	889.7	Augmented semidiameter ☾ .	889.2

For the construction of the diagram the following quantities were used:—

Apparent α ☾ at immersion	3ʰ 32ᵐ 18ˢ94	At emersion 3ʰ 34ᵐ 19ˢ.22
Relative apparent difference in AR (reduced) .	—13′ 49″.4	+15′ 00″.0
" " " in declination .	— 6 12.5	+ 2 24.2

Geocentric elements of Saturn's ring:—

$p=-2°\ 26'$	$a'=\ 29''.4$
$a=\ 44''.3$	$b'=-12.0$
$b=-17.9$	Southern surface visible.

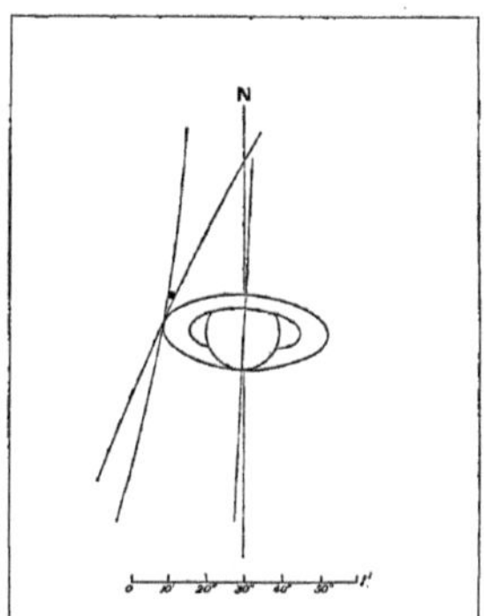

The radial correction, obtained graphically, see diagram, is, therefore,

Reduction to centre . .	$-20''.0$	Reduction to centre . .	$+\ 21''.0$
$k'=$	869.7	k'	910.2
$k'+b'=$	$+\ 497.2$	$k'+b'$	$+1054.3$
$k'-b'=$	$+1242.2$	$k'-b'$	$+\ 766.1$
d'	$+16°\ 57'\ 28.0$	d'	$+17°\ 01'\ 46.0$
$a'+p=a$	$+364.78$	$a'+p=a$	-1265.89
$m-n$	$117^s.78$	$m-n$	$117^s.83$
Reduction to time of true ☌ .	$+12^m\ 23.3$	Reduction to time of true ☌ .	$-42^m\ 58.4$
t	$17^h\ 27\ 56.7$	t	$18^h\ 24\ 33.2$
τ	17 40 20.0	τ	17 41 34.8
$\psi'=334°\ 38'\ 20''$		$\psi'=170°\ 53'\ 02''$	

Time of true ☌ in Van Rensselaer time $17^h\ 40^m\ 20^s.0 - 1.01\ dB$

$17\ \ 41\ \ 34.8\ - 0.34\ dB$ Hence $dB = -112$.

Longitude of Van Rensselaer from immersion and emersion $4^h\ 43^m\ 06^s$; but since the immersion is marked doubtful, I give the weight one-half to the above result, and combine it with the uncorrected result from the emersion, viz: $4^h\ 43^m\ 44^s.1$. The resulting longitude becomes $4^h\ 43^m\ 31^s$.

Longitude from the Observations of the Occultation of Saturn's Ring and Centre.

February 4–5, 1854.

Immersion, last contact of ring	20^h	44^m	$20^s.8$	Sidereal time at Van Rensselaer	or 5^d	4^h	25^m	$55^s.2$	Approximate Greenwich mean time.
Emersion, centre	21	42	27.8			5	23	52.8	
" last contact of ring	21	42	49.1			5	24	14.0	

From the Greenwich Nautical Almanac, as corrected by the Greenwich observations:—

At immersion, α ☾ . . . . $3^h\ 30^m\ 51^s.73$
At emersion (*C*) 3 32 46.79
" (*R*) 3 32 47.50
(Correction to Nautical Almanac $-0^s.35$.)
At immersion, δ ☾ . . . . +17° 51′ 04″.3
At emersion (*C*) 18 00 24.4
" (*R*) 18 00 27.9
(Correction to Nautical Almanac —5″.5.)
At immersion, horizontal parallax ☾ 54′ 34″.4
At emersion (*C*) 54 33.4
" (*R*) 54 33.4
(Correction +1″.0 according to Adams.)
At immersion, semidiameter ☾ . . 14′ 52″.5
At emersion (*C*) 14 52.3
" (*R*) 14 52.3
(Correction —1″.1 according to Oudeman.)

At immersion, α ♄ . . . . $3^h\ 32^m\ 30^s.91$
At emersion (*C*) 3 32 31.09
" (*R*) 3 32 31.09
(Correction to Nautical Almanac $+0^s.25$.)
At immersion, δ ♄ . . . . +17° 05′ 46″.4
At emersion (*C*) 17 05 47.7
" (*R*) 17 05 47.7
(Correction to Nautical Almanac —8″.6.)

Horizontal parallax ♄ . . . . 1.″0
Semidiameter ♄ . . . . . 8.4 + 1.2

Greenwich mean time of ☌ $5^d\ 5^h\ 15^m\ 57^s.5$

	Immersion (*R*).	Emersion (*C*).	Emersion (*R*).
☾'s horizontal paral. at Van Rensselaer	54′ 23″.9	54′ 22″.9	54′ 22″.9
Relative parallax π	54 22.9	54 21.9	54 21.9
α—s	—258° 22 16.5	—272° 25 15	—272° 30 24
α′—α=*p*	+ 11 06.42	+ 11 20.72	+ 11 20.68
δ′—δ=*q*	— 51 36.75	— 50 46.80	— 50 46.56
Augmented semidiameter ☾ . . .	896.1	896.6	896.6

For the construction of the diagram the following quantities were used:—

		At emersion (*C*)	(*R*)
Apparent α ☾ at immersion	$3^h\ 31^m\ 36^s.16$	$3^h\ 33^m\ 32^s.17$	$3^h\ 33^m\ 32^s.88$
Relative app. dif. in AR (red.)	—13′ 05″.1	+14′ 35″.5	+14′ 45″.7
" " in declination	— 6 18.9	+ 3 49.9	+ 3 53.6

Geocentric elements of Saturn's ring:—

p = —2° 24′
a = 42.1
b = —17.1

a′ = 28.0
b′ = —11.5
Southern surface visible.

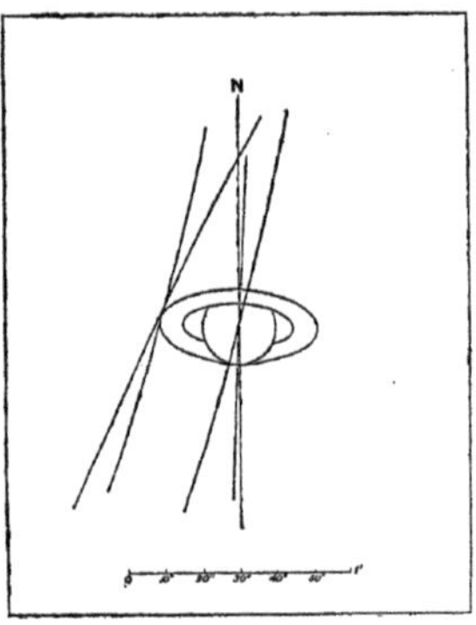

The radial correction, obtained graphically, is as follows:—

Reduction to centre . . .	—19″.5	0″.0	+20″.5
k'	876.6	896.6	917.1
$k'+b'$	497.7	1126.5	1150.7
$k'-b'$	1255.5	666.7	683.5
d'	+17° 02′ 37.0	+17° 07′ 42.6	+17° 07′ 44.5
$a'+p=a$	+1493.21	—226.13	—247.33
$m-n$	118ˢ.91	118ˢ.98	118ˢ.98
Reduced to time of true ☌ .	+50ᵐ 13.8	—7ᵐ 36.2	—8ᵐ 18.9
t	4ᵈ 23ʰ 42 23.2	5ᵈ 0ʰ 40 20.8	5ᵈ 0ʰ 40 42.0
τ	5 0 30 37.0	5 0 32 44.6	5 0 32 23.1
ψ'	334° 23′ 25″	165° 08′ 32″	165° 14′ 32″

Time of true ☌ in Van Rensselaer mean time 5ᵈ 0ʰ 32ᵐ 37ˢ.0 —1.01 dB $dB=+7.1$
0 32 44.6 —0.56 dB }
0 32 23.1 —0.56 dB }

Hence longitude of Van Rensselaer from immersion 4ʰ 43ᵐ 27ˢ.6
emersion (C) 4 43 16.9 } 27ˢ.6
" (R) 4 43 38.4 }

Resulting longitude 4 43 27.6

Longitude from the Observations of the Occultation of Mars.

February 13, 1854.

Immersion, first contact	20ʰ 22ᵐ 10ˢ.8 mean time.	17ʰ 59ᵐ 04ˢ.4 sid. time.	
" second "	20 23 06.6	" 18 00 00.4	"
Emersion, last "	20 53 17.3	" 18 30 16.1	"

Approx. Greenwich mean time, phase (1) 14ᵈ 1 05 42.8
" (2) 1 06 38.6
" (3) 1 36 49.3

From the Greenwich Nautical Almanac, as corrected from the Greenwich observations:—

At immersion (1), α ☾ . . 11ʰ 02ᵐ 21ˢ.84
" (2) . . 11 02 23.65
At emersion (3) . . 11 03 24.21
(Correction to Nautical Almanac —0ˢ.28)
At immersion (1), δ ☾ . . +11° 34′ 05″.8
" (2) . . 11 33 54.4
At emersion (3) . . 11 27 32.9
(Correction to Nautical Almanac +0″.4.)
At immersion (1), horizontal paral. ☾ 56′ 12″.6
" (2) . . . 56 12.7
At emersion (3) . . . 56 13.2
(Adams' correction +0″.5.)
At immersion (1), semidiameter ☾ . 15′ 19″.3
" (2) . . . 15 19.3
At emersion (3) . . . 15 19.4
(Correction to Nautical Almanac —0″.3
+Oudeman's correction —1″.1.)

At immersion (1), α ♂ . . 11ʰ 02ᵐ 32ˢ.24
" (2) . . 11 02 32.20
At emersion (3) . . 11 02 30.65
(Correction to Nautical Almanac +1ˢ.56.)
At immersion (1), δ ♂ . . +10° 47′ 54″.7
" (2) . . 10 47 55.0
At emersion (3) . . 10 48 05.5
(Correction to Nautical Almanac —17″.4.)
Horizontal parallax ♂ . . 12″.3
Semidiameter ♂ . . 6″.4+1″.8=8″.2

Reduction of observation of immersion, first and second contact :—

I.		II.	
I. Horizontal paral. at V. R.	56′ 01″.8	II. Horizontal paral. at V. R.	56′ 01″.9
Relative parallax π	55 49.5	Relative parallax π	55 49.6
$\alpha-s=$	—104° 10 39	$\alpha-s=$	—104° 24 12
$\alpha'-\alpha=p=$	—10 57.8	$\alpha'-\alpha=p=$	—10 57.2
$\delta'-\delta=q=$	—54 16.4	$\delta'-\delta=q=$	—54 16.9
Augmented semidiameter ☾	921.4	Augmented semidiameter ☾	921.4
$k'=$	929.6	$k'=$	913.2
$k'+b'=$	+ 444.3	$k'+b'=$	+ 415.6
$k'-b'=$	+1414.9	$k'-b'=$	+1410.8
$a'+p=a=$	+ 149.13	$a'+p=a=$	+ 122.15
$m-n=$	1759.6	$m-n$	1759.6
Reduction to time of true ☌	$+5^m\ 05^s.1$	Reduction to time of true ☌	$+4^m\ 09^s.9$
$t=$	20^h 22 10.8	t	20^h 23 06.6
$\tau=$	20 27 15.0	τ	20 27 16.5
(ψ'=328° 32′)		(ψ'=326° 59′)	

Reduction of observation of last contact—emersion (marked doubtful) :—

☾'s horizontal par. at Van Rensselaer	56′ 02″.4	$a'+p=a=$	—842″.19
Relative parallax π	55 50.1	$m-n=$	1759.5
$\alpha-s$	—111° 42 55.5	Reduction to time of true ☌	$-28^m\ 43^s.1$
$\alpha'-\alpha=p=$	—10 29.98	$t=$	20^h 53 17.3
$\delta'-\delta=q=$	—54 33.0		
Augmented semidiameter ☾	15 21.1	$\tau=$	20 24 34.2
$k'=$	929.3		
$k'+b'=$	+ 23.7	(ψ'=257° 02′)	
$k'-b'=$	+1834.9	Greenwich time of ☌	$1^h\ 10^m\ 45^s.0$

For the time of the true conjunction in Van Rensselaer time, we have from the mean of the two phases of the immersion and from the emersion—

$$20^h\ 27^m\ 16^s.2 + 2.46\ dr - 0.02\ dR + 1.31\ dB$$
$$20\ \ 24\ \ 34.2\ - 9.28\ dr - 9.28\ dR + 9.04\ dB$$

and omitting dr and dR, we find by subtraction $dB = +\ 21''$, and the resulting longitude—

From immersion	(1)	$+4^h\ 43^m\ 02^s.5$	
" "	(2)	4 43 00.2	Mean $4^h\ 43^m\ 01^s.2$.
" emersion	(3)	4 43 01.0	

LONGITUDE FROM THE OBSERVATIONS OF THE SOLAR ECLIPSE OF MAY 15, 1855.

Observations at Van Rensselaer Harbor :—

Immersion, first contact	$9^h\ 13^m\ 39^s.5$ mean time.	$12^h\ 46^m\ 32^s.7$ sid. time.
Emersion, last contact	10 55 48.0 " "	14 28 58.0 " "
Approximate Greenwich mean time, immersion	13 57 11.5	
" " " emersion	15 39 20.0	

From the Greenwich Nautical Almanac, as corrected from the Greenwich observations:—

At immersion, α ☾	$3^h\ 27^m\ 18^s.79$	At immersion, α ⊙	$3^h\ 28^m\ 59^s.69$
At emersion	3 31 05.89	At emersion	3 29 16.60
(Correction to Nautical Almanac —$0^s.67$)		(Correction to Nautical Almanac $+0^s.23$)	
At immersion, δ ☾ . . .	+19° 56′ 09″.2	At immersion, δ ⊙ . . .	+18° 56′ 19″.5
At emersion	20 14 45.7	At emersion	18 57 19.7
(Correction to Nautical Almanac —0″.1)		(Correction to Nautical Almanac —0″.8)	
At immersion, horizontal parallax ☾	57′ 09″.1	Semidiameter ⊙	15′ 50″.4
At emersion " "	57 06.6	Horizontal parallax ⊙	8″.48
(Adams' correction —3″.8)			
At immersion, semidiameter ☾ . .	15′ 35″.0		
At emersion " . .	15 34.3		
(Oudeman's correction —2″.3)			

Observations at Dorpat, Russia:—
See No. 966 of the Astronomische Nachrichten.

Commencement and middle of eclipse before sunrise, end of the eclipse was observed as follows:—

Mädler, with the great refractor	$20^h\ 01^m\ 19^s.1$	sidereal time.
Clausen, with a five foot telescope . . .	20.6	
Lais, with a two foot telescope . . .	21.9	

Strong undulations of the sun's limb, at 5° altitude, caused a perceptible uncertainty. [M.]

Giving the weights 3, 2, 1, to the above observed times, the adopted sidereal time at Dorpat is $20^h\ 01^m\ 20^s.1$.

Latitude of the Dorpat Observatory	+58° 22′ 47″.1	From Dr. Gould's table
Longitude " "	—26 43 38.4	in the American Eph.
" " "	— $1^h\ 46^m\ 54^s.6$	& Nautical Almanac.

Dorpat mean time of end	$16^h\ 28^m\ 19^s.6$
Approximate Greenwich mean time	14 41 25.0

The corrected data from the Nautical Almanac are:—

α ☾	$3^h\ 28^m\ 57^s.08$	δ ☾	+20° 04′ 15″.2
α ⊙	3 29 07.05	δ ⊙	+18 56 45.7
Horizontal parallax ☾ . .	57′ 08″.0	Horizontal parallax ⊙ . .	8″.48
Semidiameter ☾ . . .	15 34.6	Semidiameter ⊙	15′ 50″.3

Reduction of the observation of the commencement of the eclipse at Van Rensselaer:—

Horizontal par. ☾ at Van Rensselaer	56′ 58″.12		
Relative parallax π = ...	56 49.64		
$\frac{\alpha☾-\alpha⊙}{401}$ = ...	$-0^s.25$	$\frac{\delta☾-\delta⊙}{401} = +9''.0$	
$\alpha-\delta = -9^h\ 19^m\ 14^s.2$	$= -139°\ 48'\ 33''$		
$\alpha'-\alpha=p=-463''.67$		$\eta = 98°\ 48'\ 31''$	
$\delta'-\delta=q=-3328.30$			
Augmented semidiameter ☾ .	$=937''.85$	$k' = r☾ + r⊙ = 1888''.25$	
$\delta'=\delta+q=$	19° 00′ 40″.9		
$\delta'-D=b'=$	4 21.4	$\frac{\delta'+D}{2} = d' = +18°\ 58'\ 30''.2$	
$k'+b'=$	2149.65		
$k'-b'=$	1626.85	ό Greenwich	$14^h\ 46^m\ 17^s.0$
$a'+p=a=$	+1513.85	Hourly motion ☾ . . .	1999″.65
Reduction to true ό . .	$+49^m\ 03^s.6$	" " ⊙ . . .	148.20
t, or observed time . . .	9 13 39.5	$\psi' = 7°\ 57'\ 23''$	
τ , ...	10 02 43.1		

Reduction of the observations of the end of the eclipse at Van Rensselaer :—

Horizontal par. ☾ at Van Rensselaer	$=56' 55''.62$	
Relative parallax $\pi=$	56 47.14	
Correction to α	$+0^s.27$	Correction to δ $+11''.6$
$\alpha - s =$	$=-10^h\ 57^m\ 51^s.8$	
$\alpha' - \alpha = p =$	$-192''.49$	
$\delta' - \delta = q =$	-3367.19	$\eta = 101° 03' 02''$
Augmented semidiameter ☾	$936''.65$	$k' = 1886''.95$
$\delta' = \delta + q =$	$+19° 18' 38''.5$	
$\delta' - D = b' =$	+21 18.8	$\frac{\delta' + D}{2} = d' = + 19° 07' 59.''1$
$k' + b' =$	+3165.75	
$k' - b' =$	+608.15	
$a' + p = a =$	-1661.16	$m - n = 1853''.99$
Reduction to true δ	$-53^m\ 45^s.6$	$\psi' = 137° 20' 6''$
t, or observed time	10^h 55 48.0	
τ	10 02 02.4	

Reduction of the observations of the end of the eclipse at Dorpat :—

$\phi' = 58° 12' 31''.2$		
Horizontal par. ☾ at Dorpat	$=56' 59''.73$	
Relative parallax π	=56 51.25	
Correction to α	$0^s.00$	Correction to δ $+10''.1$
$\alpha - s =$	$-16^h\ 32^m\ 23^s.0$	
$\alpha' - \alpha = p =$	$+1769''.08$	
$\delta' - \delta = q =$	-2960.85	$\eta = 103° 09' 13''$
Augmented semidiameter ☾	$=936''.13$	$k' = 1886''.43$
$\delta' = \delta + q =$	$19° 14' 54''.4$	
$\delta' - D = b' =$	+18 08.7	$\frac{\delta' + D}{2} = d' = + 19° 05' 50''$
$k' + b' =$	+2975.13	
$k' - b' =$	+797.73	
$a' + p = a =$	+138.8	$m - n = 1852''.65$
Reduction to true δ	$+4^m\ 29^s.7$	$\psi' = 144° 45' 8''$
t, or observed time	16^h 28 19.6	
τ	16 22 49.3	

We have, therefore, the following expressions for the time of true conjunction in—

Van Rensselaer mean time	$10^h\ 02^m\ 43^s.1 + 2.08\,dr + 2.08\,dR + 0.29\,dB$	(phase 1)
" "	$10\ 02\ 02.4 - 2.88\,dr - 2.88\,dR - 1.90\,dB$	(" 2)
Dorpat "	$16\ 32\ 49.3 - 2.51\,dr - 2.51\,dR - 1.45\,dB$	(" 2)

Neglecting the smaller terms dr and dR, we find, from the Dorpat observations, $dB = -15''.3$; and substituting this value in the two preceding equations, we obtain the longitude of Van Rensselaer harbor—

From the commencement of the eclipse	$+4^h\ 43^m\ 33^s.9 - 0.29\,dB$	$= + 4^h\ 43^m\ 38^s.3$
" end " "	$+4\ 44\ 14.6 + 1.90\,dB$	$= +4\ 43\ 45.5$
Adopted longitude, mean value		+4 43 41.9

Recapitulation of results for longitude of Van Rensselaer Harbor by occultations of planets and a solar eclipse:—

Occultation of Saturn	December 12, 1853	$4^h\ 43^m\ 51^s.8$
" "	January 8, 1854	4 43 31.0
" "	February 4–5, 1854	4 43 27.6
" of Mars	February 13, 1854	4 43 01.2
Eclipse of the sun	May 15, 1855	4 43 41.9
Mean		4 43 30.7 ± 6^s

Resulting longitude from 9 moon culminations, 1853–54	$4^h\ 43^m\ 32^s.0 \pm 13^s$
" " " 4 occultations and one eclipse, 1853–4–5	4 43 30.7 ± 6
Final longitude of Fern Rock Observatory and Van Rensselaer Harbor winter quarters, adopted	$4^h\ 43^m\ 31^s \pm 7^s$ W. of Greenw.
	$= 70°\ 52'\ 45'' \pm 1\frac{3}{4}'$

The approximate longitude adopted by Mr. Sonntag, as given in the Narrative, page 398, Appendix No. IX, vol. II, is $4^h\ 42^m\ 40^s$, or 70° 40′ 00″; in my reduction of the magnetic observations of the expedition, this approximate result was retained, it should therefore be increased by 51^s, or 12′ 45″; in my reduction of the meteorological observations, I have adopted a value resulting from a preliminary reduction of the moon culminations, viz.: $4^h\ 43^m\ 32^s$, or 70° 53′.

If we compare any of the separate results for longitude with the final value, and, in considering the probable errors, it should be remembered that one degree of longitude in the parallel (78° 37′) of Van Rensselaer is but 11.88 nautical miles, thus the above uncertainty of 7^s, in the final result for longitude, is but half a mile of linear measure.

The following pages contain the record and reduction of some astronomical observations obtained on the coast of Greenland by the expedition, in 1853, when on the way to Van Rensselaer Harbor. The names of these stations are as follows:—

1. Fiskernaes, flagstaff near the Governor's house.
2. " small island, on the northern side of the harbor.
3. Pröven, place near the Governor's house.
4. Upernavik, garden near the Governor's house.
5. Fog Inlet, or Refuge Harbor, southwest end of inner harbor.
6. " " hill to the northward of the harbor.
7. Bedevilled Reach, afterwards called Cape Inglefield.
8. Marshall Bay.

Fiskernaes, June 30, 1853. Station, flagstaff near the Governor's house.

Observations with the sextant of the sun's altitude near the meridian, for latitude.

	Chronometer time.	Double altitude.		Chronometer time.	Double altitude.
$\underline{\odot}$	4h 06m 40s	98° 25′ 40″	$\overline{\odot}$	4h 18m 30s	98° 41′ 40″
	7 40	22 10		20 29	32 55
	9 15	16 30		21 37	27 55
$\overline{\odot}$	4 12 32	99 06 40	$\underline{\odot}$	4 23 49	97 14 30
	13 50	01 20		25 20	7 25
	15 00	98 56 20		26 49	96 59 55

Index error — 1′ 50″. Temperature 41° F. Aneroid barometer 30.15 inches.

REDUCTION.

Chronometer time of observation ⊙	4h 10m 49s.5	4h 22m 45s.6	
[1] Chronometer error	—3 21 45.6	—3 21 45.6	
Mean time of observation	0 49 03.9	1 01 00.0	
Apparent time of observation	0 45 46.6	0 57 42.7	
P	11° 28′ 31″	14° 28′ 03″	
Apparent altitude	49° 21′ 38″.3	48° 56′ 16″.6	
A	49 20 52.5	48 55 30.1	
⊙'s declination	+23 10 22.9	+23 10 20.9	
Meridional arc	66° 24′ 20″	66° 09′ 08″	
Meridional arc + latitude . .	129 29 37	129 14 07	
Latitude	63 05 17	63 04 59	Mean 63° 05′ 08″

Observations of double altitudes of the sun for time.

	Chronometer time.	Double altitude.		Chronometer time.	Double altitude.
$\overline{\odot}$	7h 45m 23s	63° 54′ 40″	$\overline{\odot}$	7h 54m 24s	61° 55′ 10″
	46 22	42 45		55 23	41 20
	47 06	33 00		56 16	30 35
$\underline{\odot}$	7 48 53	62 06 10	$\underline{\odot}$	7 58 53	59 53 25
	49 49	61 53 55		8 00 26	32 10
	51 19	61 34 20		01 39	15 55

Index error of sextant — 7′ 55″. Temperature 45° F. Aneroid barometer 30.10 inches.

REDUCTION.

⊙'s apparent altitude	31° 27′ 41″.6	30° 23′ 00″.4
A	31 26 11.9	30 21 30.8
⊙'s Δ	66 50 11.9	66 50 13.9
Latitude	63 05 (08)	63 05 (08)
Hour angle	4h 23m 04s.3	4h 32m 44s.0
Equation of time	+ 3 19.5	+ 3 19.8
Mean time of observation	4 26 23.8	4 36 03.8
Chronometer time of observation . . .	7 48 08.6	7 57 50.2
Chronometer error	—3 21 44.8	3 21 46 4
Mean	—3 21 45.6	

Chronometer error on Greenwich mean time . + 24.4 bro't up by rate from N. York.
Approximate longitude of Fiskernaes . . 3h 22m 10s = 50° 32½′ W. of Greenwich.

[1] See following observations and reductions.

Fiskernaes, July 1, 1853. Station on small island on the northern side of the harbor.
Observations of double altitudes of the sun with the sextant, for latitude.

Chronometer time.	Double altitude.	Chronometer time.	Double altitude.
$\underline{\odot}$ 5h 18m 15s	91° 59′ 10″	$\underline{\odot}$ 5h 29m 30s	89° 16′ 05″
19 25	49 00	30 31	08 00
20 34	39 25	31 15	01 05
$\overline{\odot}$ 5 23 14	?91 14 35	$\overline{\odot}$ 5 35 47	89 21 15
24 11	04 40	36 29	15 05
25 07	89 56 30	37 07	8 50

Index error of sextant —8′ 45″. Temperature about 43° F. Aneroid barometer 30.05 inches.

Reduction.

⊙'s apparent altitude	45° 32′ 49″	44° 40′ 14″	
A	45 31 56	44 39 20	
Chronometer time	5h 21m 47s.7	5h 33m 26s.5	
Chronometer error	—3 21 45.6	—3 21 45.6	Assumed.
Mean time of observation . .	2 00 02.1	2 11 40.9	
Apparent time	1 56 32.1	2 08 10.8	
Meridional arc	63° 57′ 06″	63° 15′ 45″	
Meridional arc + latitude . .	127 00 06	126 18 25	
Latitude	63 03 00	63 02 40	Mean 63° 02′ 50″

(This result is only approximate.)

Pröven, July 19, 1853. Station near the house of the Governor.
Observations of the sun's altitude for time.

Chronometer time.	Double altitude.	Chronometer time.	Double altitude.
$\underline{\odot}$ 1h 54m 43s	71° 28′ 10″	$\overline{\odot}$ 2h 5m 26s	73° 21′ 50″
56 10	35 45	6 41	28 05
57 31	42 00	7 37	32 05
$\overline{\odot}$ 1 59 33	72 54 55	$\underline{\odot}$ 2 9 56	72 38 50
2 01 00	73 01 40	11 19	45 20
2 43	09 10	12 32	51 00

Index error of sextant —3′ 0″. Approximate temp. 40° F. Approximate bar. 29.5 inches.
Approximate longitude 55° 25′ W. of Greenwich.

Reduction.

⊙'s apparent altitude . . .	36° 10′ 48″.3	36° 34′ 35″.8
A	36 09 34.9	36 33 22.5
Δ	69 10 20	69 10 23
Latitude (approx.) . . .	72 23 00	72 23 00
Hour angle	24h —1h 49m 33s.9	24h —1h 39m 17s.0
Equation of time . . .	5 56.7	5 56.8
Mean time of observation . .	22 16 22.8	22 26 39.8
Chronometer time . . .	25 58 36.6	26 08 55.2
Chronometer error	—3 42 13.8	—3 42 15.4 Mean —3h 42m 14s.6

The longitude is probably greater than the above value, assumed 3h 42m 30s or 55° 37′.5.

? Probably 90° 12′ 35″.

Pröven, July 19, 1853. Place near the Governor's house.
Circum-meridian altitudes of the sun, for latitude.

	Chronometer time.	Double altitude.		Chronometer time.	Double altitude.
$\overline{\odot}$	3h 27m 5s	77° 13′ 5″	$\overline{\odot}$	3h 49m 2s	77° 23′ 30″
	29 5	15 25		52 10	22 55
	30 55	16 25		54 0	22 30
$\underline{\odot}$	3 33 14	76 15 20	$\overline{\odot}$	3 57 38	77 20 50
	34 42	15 50		58 55	20 15
	36 50	16 40		4 01 00	19 10
$\underline{\odot}$	3 40 0	76 18 5	$\underline{\odot}$	4 3 10	76 14 00
	42 40	19 10		4 49	13 5
	44 47	19 30		6 16	11 20

Index error of sextant. —3′ 10″. Approximate temp. 42° F. Approximate bar. 29.6. inches.

Reduction.

⊙'s apparent altitude	38° 24′ 41″	38° 25′ 10″
Chronometer time	3h 38m 52s.0	4h 00m 06s.0
Mean time of observation . .	23 51 37	0 17 51
Apparent time	23 45 41	0 11 55
k	404.2	280.3
x	145.9	101.2
$A+x$	38° 26′ 00″	38° 25′ 44″
⊙'s declination	20 48 55	20 48 44
Latitude	72 22 55	72 23 00 Mean 72° 22′ 58″

Upernavik,[1] July 22, 1853. Station in garden near the Governor's house.
Sextant. Circum-meridian altitudes of the sun, for latitude.

	Chronometer time.	Double altitude.		Chronometer time.	Double altitude.
$\underline{\odot}$	3h 47m 50s	75° 25′ 30″	$\underline{\odot}$	3h 57m 00s	75° 24′ 10″
	49 13	26 10		57 45	24 30
	50 45	25 30		58 25	24 20
$\overline{\odot}$	3 52 10	74 22 10	$\overline{\odot}$	3 59 22	74 20 10
	53 20	22 10		4 0 10	19 30
	54 30	22 50		1 00	19 20

Index error — 3′ 31″. (No record of time observations.)

The observations are uncertain, on account of the imperfect image reflected from the artificial horizon, the molasses being covered with a film. (A set of observations for azimuth of Sanderson's Hope is here omitted for want of time observations.) Approximate temperature 39° Fah., barometer 29.5 inches. Mr. Sonntag

[1] Position according to Capt. Inglefield: Lat. 72° 46′ 51″. Long. 56° 02′ 46″ W. of Greenwich.

obtained the result for latitude 72° 50′; a better observation August 26, 1855, by means of a mercurial horizon, gave 72° 46′.2.

Fog Inlet, or *Refuge Harbor*,[1] August 10, 1853. Station on southwest end of inner harbor.
Approximate latitude 78° 31′. Approximate longitude 73° 50′.
Observations with the sextant of the sun's altitude, for time.

	Chronometer time.	Double altitude.		Chronometer time.	Double altitude.
⨀̄	6h 48m 46s	51° 22′ 40″	⨀̲	6h 58m 11s	49° 45′ 40″
	49 42	16 20		59 28	41 00
	51 37	10 20		7 00 29	37 50
⨀̲	6 53 20	50 01 50	⨀̄	7 01 49	50 37 10
	55 27	49 54 50		3 13	31 50
	56 38	50 50		4 25	27 30

Index error —4′ 50″. Approximate temperature 32° F. Approximate barometer 29.7 inches.

	Chronometer time.	Double altitude.		Chronometer time.	Double altitude.
⨀̄	10h 49m 30s	31° 04′ 20″	⨀̲	10h 54m 25s	29° 32′ 15″
	50 37	30 57 30		55 36	24 15
	51 34	52 20		57 23	15 00

Index error —5′ 5″.

REDUCTION.

Apparent altitude	25° 20′ 27″	25° 05′ 50″	15° 08′ 01″
A	25 18 28	25 03 50	15 04 30
Δ	74 32 38	74 32 42	74 35 35
Latitude approximate	78 31 00	78 31 00	78 31 00
Hour angle	29 55 00	32 08 18	90 04 50
Equation of time	+ 5m 02s.1	+ 5m 02s.1	+ 5m 00s.8
Mean time of observation	2h 04m 42s.1	2h 13m 35s.3	6h 05m 20s.1
Chronometer time	6 52 35.0	7 01 15.8	10 53 10.8
Chronometer error	—4 47 52.9	—4 47 40.5	—4 47 50.7
Mean error		—4 47 48	

[1] Number LXXXII of Dr. Kane's map, vol. I of Narrative.

Fog Inlet, or *Refuge Harbor*, August 11, 1853. Station on hill to the northward of the harbor.

Observations with the theodolite, of circum-meridian altitudes of the sun, for latitude.

Circle west.	Chronometer.	Level.	Vertical circle.	Circle east.	Chronometer.	Level.	Vertical circle.
$\bar{\odot}$	4h 18m 17	N. 12.2	207° 6′ 10″	$\bar{\odot}$	4h 44m 2s	N. 13.9	63° 20′ 50″
		S. 11.0	5 55			S. 8.2	20 55
			5 55				21 10
			6 15				21 5
$\bar{\odot}$	4 21 17	12.0	207 8 00	$\bar{\odot}$	4 47 47	9.2	63 20 35
		11.3	7 40			13.4	55
			7 50				50
			7 55				50
$\underline{\odot}$	4 24 08	11.0	206 37 00	$\bar{\odot}$	4 53 19	11.8	63 21 10
		12.2	36 35			11.0	30
			35				30
			50				20
$\underline{\odot}$	4 27 06	10.8	206 38 15	Circle west. $\bar{\odot}$	4 58 41	12.0	207 14 30
		12.9	37 55			11.0	5
			37 55				5
			38 10				15
Circle east. $\underline{\odot}$	4 35 08	11.2	63 54 0	$\underline{\odot}$	5 01 52	11.8	206 42 25
		11.8	5			12.0	41 55
			10				42 00
			5				42 10
$\underline{\odot}$	4 38 16	9.5	63 53 35	Circle east. $\underline{\odot}$	5 07 6	11.8	63 54 20
		13.2	40			11.0	54 30
			45				35
			50				35

Approximate temperature 35° F. Approximate barometer 29.7 inches.

REDUCTION.

Combining the first four observations with the following four observations, we obtain the readings for ⊙ W. and ⊙ E.; the last four observations furnish similar quantities, but the resulting latitude from the first combination has the weight 2, from the last combination the weight 1.

⊙ W.	4h 22m 42s	206° 52′ 11″	⊙ W.	5h 00m 16s	206° 58′ 10″
⊙ E.	4 41 18	63 37 25	⊙ E.	5 00 12	63 37 56
⊙	4 32 00	63 22 37	⊙	5 00 14	63 19 53

⊙'s apparent altitude .	26° 37′ 23″	26° 40′ 07″	
Chronometer time . .	4h 32m 00s	5h 00m 14s	Chronometer error as before.
Mean time	23 44 12	0 12 26	
Hour angle	20 45	7 34	
x	181″.5	24″.1	
$A + x$	26° 38′ 33″	26° 38′ 40″	
Declination	15 11 22	15 11 00	
Latitude	78 32 49	78 32 20	
Resulting latitude . .	78 32 39		

Bedevilled Reach (station afterwards called Cape Inglefield), August 12, 1853.

Observations with the theodolite, circum-meridian altitudes of the sun, for latitude.

Circle west.	Chronometer.	Level.	Reading.	Circle west.	Chronometer.	Level.	Reading.
$\underline{\odot}$	4h 53m 32s	N. 10.0	206° 45′ 50″	$\underline{\odot}$	5h 10m 52s	10.0	206° 42′ 25″
		S. 11.5	25			11.0	41 50
			30				42 00
			45				42 10
$\overline{\odot}$	4 57 32	12.2	207 17 55	$\overline{\odot}$	5 14 37	10.3	207 13 5
		9.2	45			10.3	12 50
			35				12 30
			50				13 00
Circle east.				Circle east.			
$\overline{\odot}$	5 02 02	6.2	64 05 10	$\overline{\odot}$	5 19 36	15.8	64 10 10
		14.8	30			4.2	30
			30				20
			25				25
$\underline{\odot}$	5 05 24	15.3	64 37 0	$\underline{\odot}$	5 23 07	8.0	64 44 5
		5.0	5			12.4	20
			10				20
			10				20

Approximate long. 72½° W. of Gr. Approximate temp. 33° F. Approximate bar. 29.7 inches.

REDUCTION.

⊙ W.	4h 55m 32s	207° 01′ 44″	⊙ W.	5h 12m 44s	206° 57′ 28″
⊙ E.	5 03 43	64 21 14	⊙ E.	5 21 22	64 27 14

	⊙'s apparent zenith distance.	Apparent altitude.	A
At 4h 59m 37s.5	63° 39′ 45″	26° 20′ 15″	26° 18′ 21″
" 5 17 03.0	63 44 53	26 15 07	26 13 13

Chronometer error	4h 44m 55s. See below.	
Mean time of observation	0 14 42	0h 32m 08s
Hour angle	0 10 00	0 27 29

k	196″	Meridional arc . . .	75° 01′ 06″
x	41.9	Meridional arc + ϕ . .	153 35 17
$A + x$	26° 19′ 03″	Latitude	78 34 11
⊙'s declination	14 52 58		
Latitude	78 33 55	Mean	78 34 03

Bedevilled Reach (Station Cape Inglefield), August 12, 1853. Theodolite observations for time.

Circle east.	Chronometer.	Level.	Reading.	Circle west.	Chronometer.	Level.	Reading.
$\overline{\odot}$	10h 23m 27s	8.0	74° 17′ 55″	$\overline{\odot}$	10h 39m 35s	11.4	195° 45′ 30″
		12.0	18 05			10.4	5
			18 05				0
			17 50				10
$\overline{\odot}$	10 26 57	15.2	74 28 10	$\underline{\odot}$	10 42 32	10.5	195 5 5
		5.0	15			11.2	4 50
			15				4 50
			5				5 0
$\underline{\odot}$	10 30 28	12.2	75 10 15	$\underline{\odot}$	10 46 34	11.8	194 53 5
		8.2	30			10.0	52 40
			25				52 40
			20				52 55
Circle west.				Circle east.			
$\overline{\odot}$	10 35 16	11.2	195 58 5	$\underline{\odot}$	10 50 49	13.0	76 10 30
		10.0	58 0			8.2	40
			57 45				45
			58 5				45

(NOTE.—Between the 13th and 14th there were two more observations taken, for which, however, there is no need.) Atmospheric temperature and pressure as above.

REDUCTION.

Taking means, we find			
$\overline{\odot}$ E.	10h 25m 12s	74° 22′ 56″	
$\underline{\odot}$ E.	10 30 28	75 10 18	
$\overline{\odot}$ W.	10 37 25	195 51 36	
$\underline{\odot}$ W.	10 44 33	194 58 53	Reduction to ⊙ + 15′ 50″
$\underline{\odot}$ E.	10 50 49	76 10 35	" — 15 50

⊙ E.	10h 27m 50s	74° 46′ 37″	⊙ W.	195° 14′ 43″	
⊙ W.	10 40 59	195 25 15	⊙ E.	75 54 45	
Mean	10 34 25	74 40 42		75 20 01	10h 47m 41s
Apparent altitude		15 19 18		14 39 59	
A		15 15 48		14 36 19	
Δ		75 11 17		75 11 26	
L		78 34 30		78 34 30	
m		84 30 48		84 11 07	
p		86 12 14		89 31 06	
Time of observation		5h 49m 30s.3		6h 02m 45s.7	
Time by chronometer		10 34 25.0		10 47 41.0	
Error		—4 44 54.7		4 44 55.3	
Mean		—4 44 55.0 which was used in the reduction for latitude.			

August 23, 1853. Station 3 miles E. S. E. from the brig (either in Force Bay or Van Rensselaer Harbor). Sextant observations of circum-meridian altitudes of the sun.

	Chronometer time.	Double altitude.		Chronometer time.	Double altitude.
$\underline{\odot}$	4h 37m 2s	45° 14′ 30″	$\overline{\odot}$	4h 48m 20s	46° 17′ 40″
	39 17	14 45		49 43	17 30
	40 42	15 00		50 40	17 30
$\overline{\odot}$	4 43 25	46 18 00	$\underline{\odot}$	4 52 0	45 14 10
	44 30	18 10		54 0	13 50
	46 00	18 10		55 12	13 5

Mr. Sonntag deduced the latitude 78° 37′ 9″

Marshall Bay. September 3, 1853. According to p. 390, vol. II. of the Narrative, this station is from bearings 1° 59′ east of the winter quarters, and hence in longitude 68° 54′. Rate of chronometer about $2^s.5$ gaining daily; error, September 12, on Fern Rock mean time $-4^h\ 43^m\ 26^s$.

Theodolite observations. Circum-meridian altitudes of the sun, for latitude.

Circle east.	Chron'r time.	Level.	Reading.	Circle west.	Chron'r time.	Level.	Reading.
$\underline{\odot}$	$4^h\ 13^m\ 27^s$	N. 7.0	199° 7′ 10″	$\overline{\odot}$	$4^h\ 43^m\ 00^s$	N. 10.0	71° 52′ 15″
		S. 15.0	6 45			S. 13.0	52 10
			6 45				51 50
			7 05				52 25
				Circle east.			
$\underline{\odot}$	4 20 25	11.8	199 7 20	$\overline{\odot}$	4 59 50	10.8	199 35 50
		11.7	6 50			12.3	30
			6 40				35
			6 55				50
Circle west.				Circle west.			
$\overline{\odot}$	4 27 22	12.0	71 52 5	$\underline{\odot}$	5 08 09	10.0	72 31 30
		11.3	51 55			13.0	30
			51 50				35
			52 10				40

Temperature 27°.5. Barometer 29.98 inches. The sun seen occasionally through clouds, observed without shade-glass.

Reduction.

$\underline{\odot}$ E.	$4^h\ 16^m\ 56^s$	199° 07′ 00″		$\overline{\odot}$ E.	$4^h\ 59^m\ 50^s$	199° 35′ 43″
$\overline{\odot}$ W.	4 35 11	71 52 03		$\underline{\odot}$ W.	5 08 · 09	72 31 31
$\odot$	4 26 04	71 22 32		$\odot$	5 04 00	71 27 54
Approximate altitude . .		18 37 28				18 32 06

On account of the uncertainty in the chronometer error it was considered safer to use the first combination alone, as being nearest to true noon.

Chronometer error . .	$-\ 4^h\ 35^m\ 9^s$	$x =$	27″
Mean time of observation .	23 50 55	$a + x$	18° 35′ 03
Equation of time . .	+ 0 53	Declination	7 26 11
h	8 13	Latitude	78 51 08

Recapitulation of Results for Latitude and Adopted Longitudes.

	Latitude.	Longitude W. of Greenwich.				
Fiskernaes	63° 02′.8	50° 32′.5 = 3^h	22^m	10^s	Approx. longitude.
Pröven	72 23.0	55 37.5 3	42	30	" "
Upernavik	72 46.2	56 02.8 3	44	11	Long. by Inglefield.
Refuge Harbor	78 32.7	73 50 4	55	20	
Cape Inglefield	78 34.1	72 55 4	51	40	
Winter-quarters, Van Rensselaer Harbor	78 37.1	70 52.8 4	43	31	
Marshall Bay	78 51.1	68 54.0 4	35	36	

6

Determination of the elevation of station on Marshall Bay by means of the depression of the sea horizon. Observations with the theodolite.

	Level.	Reading.		Level.	Reading.
Circle east.	11.8	90° 56′ 5″	Circle west.	13.3	180° 37′ 10″
	11.8	55 50		10.0	5
		55 55			15
		56 5			20
	Mean	90 55 59		Corrected and converted	89 22 44

Apparent zenith distance of horizon 90 09 22

Using 0.08 for the co-efficient of refraction, the corresponding elevation is 27.8 metres or 91 feet.

The following record of determinations of latitudes, by various travelling parties, has been copied from volume II. of the Narrative, Appendix Nos. V. and VI.

Cape John Frazer, position XXIII, May 28, 1854.

This position is determined by an observation with sextant and ice horizon.

Altitude	$\overline{\odot}$	31° 33′.5
	$\underline{\odot}$	32 05.5
	⊙	31 49.5
Correction for dip, refraction, and parallax		—3.0
		31 46.5
Declination		21 29.4
Latitude		79 42.9

Cape Prescott, position XX, May 29, 1854.

Double altitude	$\overline{\odot}$	64° 42′.0
	$\underline{\odot}$	63 38.0
Altitude ⊙'s centre		32 05.0
Correction for refraction and parallax		—1.4
		32 03.6
Declination		21 38.8
Latitude		79 35.2

The determination of the latitude of Cape Hawks, position XV., does not agree with its location on the map, it is therefore here omitted.

Cape William Wood, position LXXI, June 7, 1854.

Double altitude ⊙	$\overline{\odot}$	68° 16′		
" "	$\underline{\odot}$	67 8		
		67 42		
Index error		—3		
		67 39	⊙	33° 50′
Correction for refraction and parallax				—2
				33 48
Declination				22 47
Latitude				78 59

Cache Island, position LXVII, June 14 and 16, 1854.

Double altitude ⊙ . . .	67° 43′.5		67° 54′.0	
	68 47.5		68 57 5	
	68 15.5		68 25.7	
Index error	—3.5		—3.9	
	68 12.0	34 06.0	68 21.8	34 10.9
Correction for refraction and parallax .		—1.4		—1.3
		34 04.6		34 09.6
Declination		23 17.1		23 22.1
Latitude		79 12.5		79 12.5

Cape Andrew Jackson, position LVII, June 21, 1854.
Observations with pocket sextant and artificial horizon. One mile from entering cape of the channel.

Double altitude	⊙̲	66° 21′.5	
	⊙̅	67 27.5	
		66 54.5	33 27.2
Correction for refraction and parallax			—1.3
			33 25.9
Declination			23 27.5
Latitude			80 01.6

Cape Jefferson, position LI, June 24, 1854.

Double altitude	⊙̲	64° 59′.5	
	⊙̅	66 04.0	
		65 31.8	32 45.9
Correction for refraction and parallax			—1.3
Altitude ⊙			32 44.6
Declination			23 25.8
Latitude			80 41.2

Cape Madison, position LIV, June 26, 1854.

Double altitude	⊙̲	65° 35′.0	
	⊙̅	66 40.0	
		66 07.5	33 03.7
Correction for refraction and parallax			—1.3
Altitude ⊙			33 02.4
Declination			23 22.6
Latitude			80 20.2

(The data given on page 383, vol. II. of the Narrative, for longitude of the two last stations, are insufficient; the resulting longitude, as given on the map, must therefore be adopted. The index error of the sextant has been applied to the observations of the preceding three stations.)

Littleton Island, June 12, 1855.

The latitude of Littleton Island is determined by a set of circum-meridian altitudes of the sun, made on the east end of the island; the individual observations give (when corrected for refraction)—

Altitude ⊙'s centre	34° 47′ 27″	
	32	
	25	
	22	Mean. 34 47 29
	38	
	26	
	26	
	35	
Altitude ⊙ corrected for parallax . .	34° 47′ 36″	
Declination	23 9 37	
Latitude	78 22 01	

Cape Alexander, June 17, 1855.

This position is obtained by an observation at a point on the ice five miles distant and N. 7° 26′ E. (true) from the cape.

Double altitude	$\bar{\odot}$	70° 45′	
	$\underline{\odot}$	69 41	
		70 13	
Index error		+8.7	
Corrected double altitude		70 21.7	35 10.8
Correction for refraction and parallax			—1.4
			35 09.4
Declination			23 23.7
Latitude			78 14.3
Latitude Cape Alexander			78 9.3

The map appended to this paper is based upon the preceding astronomical results; the astronomically determined positions (either in latitude or longitude) are indicated by a star; for its longitudes, it depends on the well determined meridian of the winter quarters; the detail of shoreline and the principal names are from Dr. Kane's map, in vol. I. of the Narrative. The projection depends on the following data, derived from Bessel's elements of the figure of the earth.

1° of the meridian in middle latitude . .	80½°	111649m.1
1° of longitude in parallel	78	23216.2
" " "	79	21306.9
" " "	80	19391.0
" " "	81	17469.2
" " "	82	15541.8
" " "	83	13609.7

Examining the original map in the Narrative, I found that the longitude of the Observatory in Van Rensselaer harbor actually adopted was not that given in the text, but a value so nearly agreeing with my final result, that no change in the longitude of that part of the coast was required in the transfer of the shoreline to the new map. By request, Mr. Sonntag marked the exact position of the observatory in reference to the shoreline of the harbor, an important datum, not given before. It will be perceived that the only change of importance made in the present map, is the shifting of the shores of Kennedy Channel to the southward to an amount of about nineteen nautical miles; it is well known that Dr. Kane had adopted the mean positions resulting from astronomical observations and dead reckoning, whereas in my map the astronomical determinations alone have been used. This change I made with the concurrence of Professor Bache, who, in May, 1858, communicated to the Royal Geographical Society, in England, that such a step seemed desirable and proper. The highest point of the shoreline, traced by Morton, on the east side of the Channel, is now placed in latitude 80° 56′, and, on the opposite side, the highest point distinctly seen by him is located in latitude 82° 07′.[1]

The following table contains the geographical positions of stations determined by travelling parties, and the latitudes of which have been given above.

	Latitude.	Long. W. of Gr.
Cape John Frazer	79° 42′.9	71° 30′
Cape Prescott	79 35.2	72 56
Cape William Wood	78 59	68 20
Cache Island	79 12.5	65 30
Cape Andrew Jackson	80 01.6	66 52
Cape Jefferson	80 41.2	67 52
Cape Madison	80 20.2	66 52
Littleton Island	78 22.0	74 10
Cape Alexander	78 09.3	74 20

The following results are taken from a report of Mr. Sonntag's to Dr. Kane, dated September 12, 1855 (at Godhavn).

	Latitude.	Long. W. of Gr.
Fitzclarence rock	76° 55′.0	
Dalrymple rock	76 30.5	70° 23′
Parker snow point	76 04.2	68 44
Cape York	75 56	66 48
Godhavn	69 14.6	

(NOTE.—In my discussion of the magnetic observations of the expedition the latitudes and longitudes of the stations could only be given approximately, and the results now obtained should be substituted instead of them.)

Observations in Connection with Twilight.—The following notes, made by Dr. Kane, has been extracted from his Log-Book. In calculating the sun's depression below the horizon, I have applied a correction for horizontal refraction, taking into account the temperature actually observed on that day.

Oct. 15, 1853.—Last entry of sunlight having been seen. "Astronomically, the upper limb of the sun should disappear at noon, October 25, if the horizon was free, but it is obstructed by a mountain ridge."[2]

---

[1] In a letter (dated Albany, February 29, 1860), Mr. Sonntag expresses himself as follows: "I am very glad to learn that you are going to reconstruct the map, and to reduce the upper portion of it, and I feel confident that, after the reduction is made, it will have claims to as much accuracy as any other map of any parts of the Arctic Regions."

[2] Page 105, vol. I. of the Narrative.

Nov. 2, 1853.—"A star observed at 2 P. M., and on the following day at half past one o'clock; on the 4th the thermometer had to be read by means of a lantern at 3 P. M., and on the following day at 2 P. M."

Nov. 7, 1853.—"Observed the first faint streak of daylight at 6 A. M. On the following day, stars of the 2d magnitude were visible at noonday; on the 2d instant, Capella had been seen at the same hour, and but for the misty haze probably earlier." Polaris was seen at noon on the 16th.

Nov. 22, 1853.—"The darkness is now (nearly) complete, being barely able to read at noonday." Sun's centre below the horizon 8° 09′ (temp. —35°).

Dec. 22, 1853.—Maximum depression of the sun's centre below the horizon at noon 11° 23′; temp. —35°.

Jan. 4, 1854.—"To-day at noon a distinct zone of illumination was seen to the south clearly defining the highest hills. This is the first departure we have had from our uniform darkness. The largest print is illegible at noon." Sun's centre below the horizon 10° 41′ (temp. —11°). On the following day, the first appearance of twilight was noticed at 7 A. M.; on the 7th and 18th, the largest print was not yet readable at noon.

Jan. 19, 1854.—"To-day at noon read the title page of my prayer book by turning the type towards the illuminated sky to the southward." Sun's centre below the horizon 8° 11′ (temp. —51°.)

Jan. 20, 1854.—"A faint appearance of brownish-red appeared above the hills to the southward between 11 A. M. and 1 P. M." On the 22d the standard thermometer could be read at noon without a lantern, and on Feb. 3, at 9 A. M.

Feb. 13, 1854.—"The light at noonday had a decided yellow tinge."

Feb. 20, 1854.—"At noon saw the sun's rays shining on the cliffs on the eastern side of the bay." Astronomically, the sun's upper limb should reappear on the horizon on the 16th. On the 2d and 4th of March twilight appeared at 3 A. M."

March 26, 1854.—"The standard thermometer is read at midnight without artificial light. On the 30th, stars of the 2d magnitude still visible at 1 A. M."

Oct. 29, 1854.—"The red of the graduated zone of sunset is deep cherry-red, running into crimson, which, after being cut by bluish-gray strata, blends with the higher blue by rosy pink."

Nov. 15, 1854.—"Can read type in Parry's Narrative at noon, but with great difficulty." Sun's centre below the horizon 6° 25′ (temp. —35°).

Nov. 19, 1854.—"At noon cannot read Parry's type." Sun's centre below the horizon 7° 26′ (temp. —14°).

Dec. 31, 1854.—"The twilight was remarkably apparent at noon to-day."

For comparison with the above, the following information has been extracted from Gehler's Physical Dictionary: In latitude 51°, Brandes was able to read the largest type, with the book turned toward the light, the sun's centre being 10½° below the horizon; ordinary large type was read with the sun's depression of 8½°. At Van Rensselaer Harbor, in latitude 78½, the limits of legibility, for ordinary large type, were with a depression of 7° 26′ and 8° 11′. It is generally assumed that, in temperate latitudes, complete darkness sets in when the sun's depression reaches 18°; on the 2d of March, the first appearance of twilight was noticed at a depression of 15° 0′ (temp. —37°) in latitude 78½; thus it appears that in this high latitude twilight is more feeble with the same depression of the sun than in lower latitudes. This circumstance is, doubtless, owing to the diminished height of the atmosphere (by contraction, on account of the cold, and by compression) in these high latitudes.

APPENDIX.

Directions to Sites of Rensselaer Harbor.

1. The observatory was placed upon the northernmost of the rocky group of islets that formed our harbor. It is seventy-six English feet from the highest and northernmost salient point of this island, in a direction S. 14° E., or in line with said point and the S. E. projection of the southernmost islet of the group.

2. A natural face of gneiss rock formed the western wall of the observatory. A crevice in this rock has been filled with melted lead, in the centre of which is a copper bolt. Eight feet from this bolt and in the direction indicated by the crevice stood the magnetometer. This direction is given in case of local disturbance from the nature of the surrounding rocks.

3. On the highest point of the island mentioned in paragraph 1 is a deeply chiselled arrow-mark filled with lead. This is twenty-nine feet above the mean tidal plane of our winter quarters for the years 1853–4. The arrow points to a mark on a rocky face denoting the lowest tide of the season; both of these are referred by sextant to known points.

4. In an enlarged crack five feet due west of the above arrow is a glass jar containing documents.

5. A cairn calls attention to these marks: nothing is placed within it.

Extract from Appendix No. X, 2d volume of the Narrative, pp. 400—404, on methods of survey.

"It is proposed in the following sketch to give a general account of the methods used in surveying the coasts of Smith's Straits, and of Greenland as far south as Melville Bay. For a large portion of this labor I am indebted to my assistant Mr. Sonntag.

"It will be seen that the survey conducted by the returning expedition has more claims to accuracy than is attainable by a mere running or flying survey, although the operations were limited by the peculiar condition of the party.

"The means employed were, of course, not new; yet a short and precise account of the methods used to secure as perfect a delineation of the shore line as circumstances would permit may be properly given, with a view to a comparison of results with other surveys of the same region.

"It may be remarked at the outset that the geographical results of the expedition depend altogether for their longitude on the meridian of Rensselaer Harbor. The establishment of this prime meridian was, therefore, an object of great attention.

"As a general rule, the geographical positions were determined on shore whenever practicable; on some occasions on large floes, which afforded a firm basis for the artificial horizon. On several occasions in Smith's Straits, observations for latitude and longitude were made by means of a theodolite. This instrument was provided with a vertical circle of ten inches diameter, and its limb was divided to four seconds: attached to it was a very sensitive level, the value of a scale-division of which had been determined at Washington, and was found to equal 1″.13.

"For latitude a number of measurements of the altitude of the sun's upper and lower limb were taken, commencing about twenty minutes before and ending twenty minutes after the culminations. An equal number of readings of both limbs were taken with the instrument in the direct and reversed position. A screen of pasteboard protected the instrument from the direct action of the sun's rays.

"Observations for time (and longitude) were taken about 9 o'clock A. M. or 3 o'clock P. M.

"The apparent path of the sun in these high latitudes is but slightly inclined to the horizon; and the azimuth of any object was determined from the transit of the sun's first and second limb over the vertical wires of the instrument. The time being known, the azimuth of the zero of the limb is easily calculated, and nothing remained but to measure the horizontal angle between that direction and any object the astronomical bearing of which was desired. The azimuth is reckoned from north by east round to 360°. As objects for azimuthal determination, well defined glaciers, bluffs, islands, prominent capes, and the most distant headlands were selected; and, in order to make sure of the stability of the instrument during the period of observation, a second set of observations of the sun for azimuth of zero of limb was obtained.

"By means of two positions thus determined, a number of objects were located by the intersections of the bearings of the known points, and whenever practicable a third or check azimuth was obtained; in this latter case any discrepancy was properly taken into account according to known principles.

"In observing with the sextant for altitude of the sun, the usual precautions were taken, and in particular the parallelism of the upper and lower surfaces of the covering-glass of the artificial mercurial horizon was tested. An error of ten seconds, it is thought, cannot exist on this account, although another roof gave results differing as much as fifteen minutes (?) in the direct and reversed position, and consequently had to be rejected.

"The sextants used were made by Gambey, and divided to ten seconds. They were provided with an astronomical telescope, which has invariably been made use of in connection with the artificial horizon. When observing for latitude, multiplied observations were generally taken: first, three of the sun's upper limb; next, three of the lower; and finally, again three of the upper limb. These observations were commenced eight or ten minutes before noon. The corresponding index error was always determined.

"Observations for longitude were never made nearer than three hours from noon; and, whenever weather and time permitted, corresponding observations in the forenoon and afternoon were secured. On these occasions twelve observations, divided into four groups, and an equal number for the upper and lower limb, were taken. In observing corresponding altitudes, the index was set to an even five or ten minutes, and the time noted when the contact was perfect. The successive changes of the index were regulated according to the sun's relative changes in altitude. * * *

* * * * * "In working up the observations, index error, refraction, and change of the sun's declination, during the interval, were properly taken into account.

"In a few instances, when the weather or other causes prevented an observation for latitude at noon, two sets of observations were taken, as far distant from one another as practicable, and latitude and longitude deduced accordingly. Such was the case at Fiskernaes and Refuge Inlet. This method proved very accurate, provided one set was not more than two hours from noon, and the other at least two hours distant from the first.

"Time was noted by a pocket-chronometer, which was compared before and after each set of observations with four box-chronometers, the rates of which had been determined at New York before leaving port. At St. John's, Newfoundland, and at different times in our winter quarters the box-chronometers were rated by Mr. Sonntag by means of a transit instrument. The mean rate of the pocket-chronometer as found by comparison with each box-chronometer was adopted. As an approximate longitude of the prime meridian of Rensselaer Harbor, 70° 40′ W. of Greenwich has at present been adopted. A slight change is anticipated from some observed occultations of planets by the moon and a solar eclipse: these observations have not yet been worked up. Any change made hereafter in this longitude will, as has already been remarked, equally affect all the other longitudes.

"For the determination of azimuths by means of a sextant, the angle between the sun's centre and the object was measured and the time noted. For this purpose the smaller telescope was used, and sometimes a pocket-sextant. Whenever the object, the azimuth of which was to be found, was farther removed from 120° than from the sun, the angular distance of an intermediate object, about 90° from the sun, was introduced. At the same time the altitude of the sun was observed, to allow for the reduction of the arc of the horizon; this reduction was always small, since the sun was seldom higher than 30°, and in no case higher than 36°.

"When the azimuth of an object was thus determined, a number of other conspicuous objects were connected with it by horizontal angles. Two determinations of the azimuth of an object, obtained from two astronomically-determined points, seldom differed more than seven minutes.

"The principal points of the coast have thus become known, either by direct observations of latitude and longitude, by latitude and solar bearing, or by the intersection of two azimuths, according to methods explained above.

"The filling in of the minor or secondary points remains yet to be explained. The position was generally obtained by solar or compass bearings and estimated distances. In regard to the solar bearings, it may be remarked that their frequent application rendered the construction of a table of double entry for every degree of altitude of the sun from 5° to 36°, and for every degree of angular distance from 10° to 125°, quite an acceptable improvement in facilitating the reduction. In regard to magnetic bearings, it is to be remarked that they were taken with a pocket-compass, the face of which, divided into degrees, was fastened to the bottom of the box to allow the needle free play. The magnetic declination (variation of compass) observed with this instrument at different times at the same place seldom differed more than three degrees, while on the contrary, other compasses, with the card fastened to the needle, would remain stationary in any position in which they were placed, in consequence of the small horizontal force in the region traversed. Care was taken to keep the compass perfectly level, and in sighting the eye was kept directly over the north end of the needle.

"The estimation of distances of intermediate points was the only thing loosely obtained; but it must be remembered, however, that these distances were always checked by means of astronomically determined positions, and hence, no error of this kind, although they were of frequent occurrence, could be propagated. Distances estimated at the same time have in some instances received a proportionate correction obtained from the check of any single line directly from comparison with astronomical data. At other times, distances paced were found to agree remarkably well with their distance astronomically determined. In this way a journey undertaken in March, 1854, was found correct to within one-thirtieth of the whole distance travelled over in six days.

"The survey of bays and harbors was conducted in the ordinary way, by means of a base-line measured, either with a cord properly stretched or by pacing. Angles were then measured at each extremity, and occasionally another point was determined trigonometrically. The head-lands, prominent bluffs, and islands for these maps generally were determined astronomically. * * * *

* * * "The whole survey, made as explained above, embraces that portion of the coast north of Capes Alexander and Sabine. That portion of it included between Cape Alexander and Upernavik, which was in revision of the work of our English predecessors, as laid down in the Admiralty charts, was made during the escape of the party in boats. For the greater portion of this labor I am indebted to Mr. Sonntag.

E. K. K."

PUBLISHED BY THE SMITHSONIAN INSTITUTION,

WASHINGTON CITY,

MAY, 1860.

SMITHSONIAN CONTRIBUTIONS TO KNOWLEDGE.

ON

FLUCTUATIONS OF LEVEL

IN THE

NORTH AMERICAN LAKES.

BY

CHARLES WHITTLESEY.

[ACCEPTED FOR PUBLICATION, APRIL, 1859.]

COMMISSION

TO WHICH THIS MEMOIR HAS BEEN REFERRED.

Capt. A. A. HUMPHREYS, U. S. A.,
Capt. A. W. WHIPPLE, U. S. A.

JOSEPH HENRY,
Secretary S. I.

COLLINS, PRINTER,
PHILADELPHIA.

FLUCTUATIONS OF LEVEL

IN THE

NORTH AMERICAN LAKES.

In the year 1838 a remarkable rise was observed in all the Lakes, since which date I have neglected no opportunity to collect information concerning the fluctuations of level that occur in these waters. For Lake Erie, by the assistance of various observers to whom I have given credit in the proper place, I am now able to present daily measurements for four entire though not consecutive years, besides registers for parts of several years, and also to give some statistical tables for other Lakes.

The observations show three kinds of fluctuation.

1. A general rise and fall, extending through a period of many years, which may be called the *secular variation* of level, having no regular period of return, and depending upon peculiar combinations in the meteorology of the country drained by the tributaries to the waters of the great Northern Lakes.

2. An annual rise and fall within certain limits, the period of which is completed in about twelve months. This, which is caused by changes of the seasons within the year, and can be predicted with much certainty, may properly be called the *annual variation.* It occurs regularly, without reference to a general height of the waters.

3. A sudden, frequent, but irregular movement, varying from a few inches to several feet. This is of two kinds: one due to obvious causes, such as winds and storms; another resulting from rapid undulations in calm water, the cause of which is not yet satisfactorily explained. Both classes may be styled *transient fluctuations.*

In this paper I shall do little more than classify the statistics which I possess. Meteorological registers for the Lake regions, owing to the recent settlement of the country, are very scarce; and such as are to be found do not extend through many years. The Army Meteorological Reports embrace the greatest length of time, but reach no farther back than the year 1822.

In the reports of the regents of the University of New York there is much valuable information on meteorology in general; a part of which refers to the basin of the great Lakes. Half a century hence, when, by means of the records now established, a good annual abstract of the temperature, rain, and cloudiness of the region can be made out, I have no doubt that there will be found a direct correspondence between the secular fluctuations of the level of the Lakes and the meteorology of the surrounding country.

When a wet, cold, and cloudy year is succeeded by another of the same character, the reservoirs, into which so many rivers, creeks, and streamlets discharge their waters, gradually fill up. A contrary combination, viz: a series of dry, warm, and clear seasons, by diminishing the supply and increasing evaporation, will produce a visible depression of the surface of the Lakes. To discuss thoroughly the phenomena of fluctuation we need daily registers, kept at different and distant places on each Lake, for a period of at least twenty-five years. It is probable that within that length of time the seasons complete a cycle, and return to pass again through a similar course of changes. To establish and continue such registers would, however, require the assistance of the government. The Topographical Bureau has required its agents at the Lake harbors, in some cases, to keep water tables; and these form the most minute and reliable information we possess. This corps, however, is engaged in harbor constructions only at irregular intervals, and consequently leave in their records many blank spaces. Government has, however, through its light-house keepers, the means of procuring perfect registers of water levels on all the Lakes, with the least possible expense; and there would be little difficulty in pointing out numerous practical results that would justify such a system of observations, without regarding the unseen benefits that always follow the acquisition of scientific knowledge. In this case there are important benefits accruing to commerce, not requiring demonstration. The soundings, made in the prosecution of the hydrographical survey of the Lakes, to be reliable marks for knowing the depth, should be referred to a well determined stage of water. Docks, warehouses, and harbor channels derive their value from being at all times accessible to vessels. The tables now presented show extreme changes of level of seven feet; and from the average of entire months, in different years, a difference of five feet three inches.

There are some vessels on the Lakes that draw more than nine feet, and, therefore, a dock constructed at the time of high water, into which a vessel of this draught could enter, would require between five and six feet of dredging, in order to be used during low water.

As a question of science and of utility, the whole subject has engaged the attention of prominent men. De Witt Clinton and General Cass, among others, have bestowed upon it the most careful study. General Henry Whiting, of the army, while residing at Detroit, at and subsequent to the war of 1812, kept the first registers to which we can refer. Dr. Douglass Houghton, the lamented geologist of Michigan, made it one of the objects of his examination during his short but active life.

I have condensed, from all sources within my reach, information respecting the state of the waters since the settlement of the Lake country. This is put into a tabular form; but is in many cases based upon general report, upon tradition, and the memory of living witnesses, but latterly upon measurements. The authorities are given on the same sheet, so that the value of what it contains may be properly estimated.

Since 1838, reliable measurements have greatly increased. That which I have given for Lake Erie is an abstract of the registers at three ports—one at each end of the Lake, and one near the middle or widest part.

At Detroit, Messrs. A. E. Hathan and S. W. Higgins made use of the base of the hydraulic tower connected with the water-works of that city as a bench mark, counting downwards to the surface of the water in the river. At Cleveland the high water line of June, 1838, has been used as zero, also reckoning downwards. This line was two feet below the surface of the east pier, at the south end of the steps leading up the parapet wall. The mitre sill of the guard lock at Black Rock was at first used by the engineers of the State of New York on which to register the depth of water. When the enlargement of the Erie Canal was commenced, Mr. John Lothrop, C. E., transferred the measurements to the bottom of the canal, at Buffalo, which is one foot below the mitre sill of the guard lock. (See Plate I., No. 1.)

As the records at different places are but seldom of the same dates, it is not easy to bring them into comparison with each other. To effect this, in the only manner they admit of, I neglect the descent of the Detroit River from that city to the Lake, and regard the surface of the Lake as level. The longest period of the Detroit tables, which correspond with those at Cleveland, was compared by the mean of both, which gave the elevation of the stone water table of the hydraulic tower above the Cleveland zero at three feet $\frac{43}{100}$ths. By Mr. Hathan's register this mark was, in June, 1838, three feet $\frac{20}{100}$ths above the surface of the river.

During the month of July, 1851, Mr. Lothrop, at Buffalo, and I myself, at Cleveland, kept registers. The fluctuations of this month were small, the weather being very calm. The high water line of June, 1838, by this comparison, corresponds to a depth of water in the enlarged canal of eleven feet $\frac{42}{100}$ths. The base of the hydraulic tower is, therefore, fourteen feet $\frac{85}{100}$ths above the bottom of canal.

TABLE OF WATER LEVELS

All the measurements reduced to one expression, which is the depth

Year.	Monthly Average.												Yearly change of level.
	Jan.	Feb.	March.	April.	May.	June.	July.	Aug.	Sept.	Oct.	Nov.	Dec.	
1788 to 1790	...	...	...	...	...	...	...	...	...	...	...	...	...
1796	...	...	...	...	...	...	...	...	...	...	...	...	...
1797	...	...	...	...	...	...	...	...	...	...	...	...	...
1798	...	...	...	...	...	...	...	...	...	...	...	...	...
1800	...	...	...	...	...	...	...	...	...	...	...	...	...
1801	...	...	...	...	...	...	...	...	...	...	...	...	...
1802	...	...	...	...	...	...	...	...	...	...	...	...	...
1806	...	...	...	...	...	...	...	...	...	...	...	...	...
1809	...	...	...	...	...	...	...	...	...	...	...	...	...
1810	...	...	...	...	...	...	...	...	...	...	...	...	...
1811	...	...	...	...	...	...	...	...	...	...	...	...	...
1812	...	...	...	...	...	...	...	...	...	...	...	...	...
1813	...	...	...	...	...	...	...	...	...	...	...	...	...
1814	...	...	...	...	...	...	...	...	...	...	...	...	...
1815	...	...	...	...	...	...	...	9.40	...	...	...	...	...
1816	...	...	...	...	...	...	...	...	...	...	...	...	...
1819	...	...	...	...	...	6.30	...	...	...	...	...	...	...
"	...	...	...	...	...	...	...	6.30	...	...	...	...	...
1820	...	...	...	...	...	...	...	6.30	...	...	...	...	...
1821	...	...	...	...	...	...	...	...	...	...	...	...	...
1822	...	...	...	...	...	...	...	...	...	...	...	...	...
1823	...	...	...	...	...	...	...	...	...	...	...	...	...
1824	...	...	...	...	...	...	...	...	...	...	...	...	...
1825	...	...	...	...	...	...	...	...	...	...	...	...	...
1826	...	...	...	...	...	...	...	...	...	...	...	...	...
1827	...	...	...	...	...	...	...	...	...	...	...	...	...
1828	...	...	...	...	...	7.30	...	7.80	...	...	...	...	...
1829	...	...	...	...	...	...	...	...	...	...	...	...	...
1830	...	...	...	...	...	...	...	...	...	...	...	...	...
1831	...	...	...	...	...	...	...	...	...	...	...	...	3.00
1832	...	...	...	...	...	...	...	...	...	...	...	...	...
1833	...	...	...	...	...	...	...	...	...	...	...	...	...
1834	...	...	...	...	...	8.82	...	...	...	...	...	...	...
1835	...	...	...	...	...	8.57	...	...	8.07	...	...	...	...
1836	...	...	...	...	...	9.82	...	9.82	...	...	...	...	...
1837	8.30	...	...	...	...	8.82	...	(10.07)	...	...	...	...	...
1838	...	...	...	...	10.39	(11.40)	11.15	10.64	10.10	9.89	...	9.46	1.94
"	...	...	...	...	...	...	...	(11.40)	11.16	10.41	9.31	9.40	2.09
1839	7.74	...	...	...	9.50	9.83	10.08	10.13	9.33	(10.30)	...	...	2.56
1840	6.92	...	...	8.33	8.37	8.42	(8.60)	...	8.11	8.04	7.84	7.61	1.68
"	...	...	...	...	10.33	(10.90)	10.33	10.40	9.30	9.10	...	...	...
1841	6.68	...	6.65	7.04	6.95	7.15	7.57	(7.99)	7.17	6.86	6.85	6.97	1.34
"	...	...	8.65	...	(9.50)	9.24	8.80	8.30	7.75	6.87	...	...	...
1842	8.99	...	...	...	9.50	...	...	...	...	...	...	...	...
1843	...	...	...	...	8.96	...	...	...	...	...	...	...	...
1844	...	...	...	...	9.21	...	...	...	...	...	...	...	...
1845	...	...	...	...	(9.30)	...	...	8.71	8.43	8.27	7.84	7.60	1.34
1846	7.34	6.97	6.91	7.30	8.26	(8.57)	(8.57)	8.34	...	...	...	...	1.66
1847	...	...	...	...	8.80	...	...	...	...	8.50	...	...	...
1848	...	...	...	...	8.46	...	...	...	...	8.94	...	...	...
1849	...	...	8.32	...	8.07	...	8.02	...	...	...	...	...	...
"	...	...	...	...	9.40	...	...	...	...	...	...	...	...
1850	...	...	...	...	8.96	8.49	...	...	...	...	7.71	7.83	...
1851	7.88	7.86	8.40	8.47	8.59	9.34	(9.46)	9.34	9.07	9.13	9.21	...	1.58
"	7.49	...	...	...	...	(9.49)	9.46	(9.49)	9.15	8.99	8.74	8.50	2.00
1852	8.35	8.07	8.42	9.47	10.07	(10.30)	10.20	9.97	9.61	9.35	9.10	9.07	2.23
1853	9.56	9.40	9.49	10.07	10.15	...	...	...	...	...	...	...	...
1856	...	...	...	...	...	...	...	...	...	...	8.30	7.90	...
1857	...	8.15	8.15	8.78	9.65	9.90	(10.15)	9.99	9.60	9.55	9.32	9.32	2.00
Mean	...	...	...	...	...	...	...	...	...	...	...	...	1.85

FOR LAKE ERIE.

of water on the Mitre Sill of the enlarged Erie Canal at Buffalo.

YEAR.	PLACE OF OBSERVATION.	OBSERVERS.	EXPLANATIONS, REMARKS, ETC.
1788 to 1790	E. end of Lake Erie	......	By tradition derived from the early settlers, very high; according to some as high as 1838, but this is doubtful.
1796	W'rn Reserve	......	By the first emigrants and surveyors, reported as very low—five feet below 1838.
1797	Buffalo	......	Rising rapidly; statement of a lake captain to De Witt Clinton.
1798	Cleveland	Alonzo Carter	Water continues to rise, but three feet below June, 1838.
1800	Detroit	......	Very high; old roads flooded; report of old people to Dr. Houghton.
1801	"	......	Still high.
1802	"	......	Very low; reported by old settlers as lower than 1797.
1806	Cleveland	......	Very low; reported by old settlers as lower than 1801-2, and declining regularly to 1809-10, when it reached a level by many regarded as low as that of 1819. Bird Island left bare and dry.
1809	Detroit	......	
1810	Buffalo & Erie	M. Sanford	
1811	Buffalo	A Lake Captain	Rise of six inches in the spring over 1810, by measurement, and a fall of two inches.
1812	"	"	Rise of fourteen inches in spring over 1810, by measurement, and a fall of three inches.
1813	"	"	Rise of two feet two inches in spring over 1810, by measurement.
1814	Erie, Pa.	Capt. Dobbin	Rise of two feet six inches in spring above general level of 1813.
1815	Detroit	Col. Whiting	Rise of three feet above average level of 1814; also M. Sanford and A. Carter.
1816	Cleveland	A. Carter	Water still high but falling, and continued to fall till 1819.
1819	Detroit	Col. Whiting	LOWEST WELL-ASCERTAINED LEVEL OF THE WATER IN LAKE ERIE, though it was reported to have been 1.60 feet lower at Detroit in February, 1819.
"	Black Rock	......	
1820	"	......	Old residents at Buffalo state, in August as low as 1819.
1821	"	Gen. Dearborn	Rising, as reported by Major Lachlan and Mr. McTaggart, of Canada.
1822	Cleveland	A. Carter	Rising; in the spring four feet below June, 1838.
1823	Canada	Mr. McTaggart	Rising; in the spring three feet three inches below June, 1838.
1824	Cleveland	......	Rising gradually.
1825	"	A. Walworth	Rising; lowest level three feet below June, 1838.
1826	"	A. Merchant	Rising; lowest level two feet ten inches below June, 1838.
1827	Canada	McTaggart	About the general level of 1815.
1828	Detroit	A. E. Hathan	
1829	"	Dr. Houghton	Water still rising. See geological report of Michigan for 1839.
1830	"	S. W. Higgins	General level same as 1828. Mr. H. was topographer of Michigan.
1831	"	Col. Whiting	Lower than last year; yearly change at least three feet.
1832	Cleveland	A. Walworth	General average two feet ten inches below June, 1838.
1833	"	"	General average three feet two inches below June, 1838.
1834	"	"	Mr. Wolworth was the first agent of the works at the harbor.
1835	"	"	
1836	Detroit	A. E. Hathan	Mr. Hathan was at the time city engineer.
1837	Buffalo	J. Lothrop	Mr. Lothrop was an engineer upon the Erie Canal.
1838	Cleveland	Geo. C. Davies	From July to October inclusive, measurements several times a day.
"	Detroit	S. W. Higgins	HIGHEST KNOWN LEVEL OF LAKE ERIE, occurring at Cleveland in June, and at Detroit and Buffalo in August of this year.
1839	Black Rock	Com. Advertiser	
1840	Detroit	A. E. Hathan	Occasional measurements.
"	Black Rock	Com. Advertiser	Measurements daily during the summer months by direction of the State Engineer.
1841	Detroit	A. E. Hathan	
"	Black Rock	Com. Advertiser	According to the Detroit register, the water in the Detroit River was comparatively lower, during the whole of the years 1840 and 1841, than at Black Rock. In September and October, 1841, the two records agree.
1842	"	"	
1843	"	"	
1844	"	"	From 1838 to 1852, the Black Rock, Buffalo, and Cleveland figures are the mean of daily measurements.
1845	Cleveland	T. B. W. Stockton	Col. Stockton was the government agent for the works at the harbor, and caused the water level, the barometer, and thermometer, to be noted three times a day.
1846	"	"	
1847	Cleveland	......	The *Buffalo Commercial Advertiser* has occasionally published the results of the observations made at Black Rock, particularly for the month of May, and sometimes all the summer months, but I have not been able to procure the original record.
1848	Buffalo	......	
1849	Detroit	......	
"	Buffalo	......	
1850	"	John Lothrop	Mr. Lothrop was the engineer of the enlarged Erie Canal, western division. His zero is the mitre sill of the guard lock, Buffalo, which is one foot lower than the sill of the old guard lock of Black Rock.
1851	"	"	The agreement between the contemporaneous readings at Buffalo and at Cleveland, in the year 1851, is very close.
"	Cleveland	C. Whittlesey	
1852	"	B. Stanard	At Detroit, the lowest observed month since 1838, was March, 1841, 6.65; at Black Rock, October, 1841, 6.87; and at Cleveland, March, 1846, 6.91.
1853	"	C. Whittlesey	
1856	"	"	Greatest known difference at Detroit, six feet eight inches.
1857	"	"	Greatest known difference at Cleveland (about), six feet.
Mean			Greatest known difference at Buffalo, fifteen feet six inches. Greatest permanent difference of general level, five feet one inch.

Neither general opinion nor tradition can be reduced to feet and inches, and I have, therefore, discarded from the above table whatever depended solely upon the recollection of one person, who had taken no measurements or preserved no memoranda. There are, however, certain objects, such as roads, wharves, and buildings, that serve as points of reference for high and low water, and tend by association vividly to impress upon the memory facts of this character. The old French inhabitants of Detroit have no tradition of a water level below that of the year 1819, although Detroit has been occupied since 1702. At Buffalo the year 1810 is remembered as one of low water, nearly or quite as low as 1819.

In discussing the data here presented, it is apparent that the surface of the Lake is not strictly level, and thus there are discrepancies as to the time of high and low water at different places. The form of the coast at Buffalo is such that the height of water is affected by it in connection with certain winds. Those from the east and northeast keep back the waters, and cause a depression that may be observed for one or two months at a time. The reverse occurs with prevailing winds from the west and southwest. The waters driven eastward between two shores, constantly approaching each other, are raised above the general surface like the tides in the Bay of Fundy. On the 18th of April, 1848, it appears from the register of Mr. Lothrop that a gale from the northeast reduced the level of the Lake to a point fifteen feet six inches below the surface of October 18th, 1849, when a terrible storm occurred from the southwest. At Cleveland the greatest observed local fluctuation was three feet two inches, which took place on the 19th of November, 1845. As the Lake is broad opposite Cleveland, and the place is situated not far from the middle, its surface would be less affected by winds; and here the level during the summer of 1819 is regarded as the lowest.

But if that year did not differ from other years in the period of the annual rise and depression, it must have been still lower in the winter than in the summer months. Dr. Houghton has mentioned one observation, made some time in the winter of 1818 and 1819, by which the water in the Detroit River was six feet eight inches below the flood time of 1838. The winter season, however, has been little noticed, except by those who keep water tables; and at that time a regular register was not known.

For want of better data, the well noted low water in the summer of 1819 is compared with the great rise of the summer of 1838, two of the most remarkable years in the history of the fluctuations. In 1838, on the shores of Lake Erie, grounds were submerged on which old orchards had come to maturity, and on forest lands trees that were centuries old were killed by the overflow of the Lake water. In the month of June I observed small boats passing from house to house in the streets of the village, at the mouth of the Conneaut river, Ohio. The water rose at Cleveland, in the month of July, so as to cover the floor of a warehouse to the depth of one foot. These events served to revive the memory of past times, and to stimulate observation in coming years.

Among the old inhabitants it brought up afresh the popular idea derived from the aborigines, that the rise is periodical, occurring once in seven years. This belief is very generally entertained, and many persons related the several years when the rise occurred. This belief shows the tendency to hasty generalization, and the superstitious proneness to attribute to the number seven a peculiar applicability to the recurrence of natural phenomena.

By examining the table we have given, containing observations that have been made since 1819, there will appear a continual rise until 1838, a period of nineteen years, without any decline. Other tables show an uninterrupted decline from 1838 to 1841, three years; in 1841, a slight rise; from 1842 to 1851, a regular decline of eight years. During a space of thirty-two years, there is no instance of a return of high water in the period of seven years. For the years since 1838, I am able to offer a much more satisfactory exhibit. To simplify the result, I have constructed a diagram of curves whose ordinates are the monthly average of the surface reduced to the Buffalo zero for such months and years as have a good mean. There are four years complete, the means of which are consolidated into one curve, which is placed, to prevent confusion, below the other curves. See Plate I, No. 1.

The regularity of the annual rise and fall is evident from an inspection of the form of the curves. The months of June and July are high as compared with other months, whatever the general level may be. A depression follows immediately, which reaches the lowest points in the months of December and January. This is the law, to which there are exceptions, arising from variations of the seasons. In fourteen of the best ascertained years high water occurred in June and July ten times; in ten years, the annual decline reached the lowest point in the months of December and January six times. There is, therefore, a spring flood and a winter ebb, the same as in the Mississippi and other large rivers or ponds. The surplus water due to melting snows and spring rains causes an accumulation of water. In winter the frost and drought, by diminishing the supply, causes the surface to settle below that of summer. The amount of fluctuation within the year, deduced from sixteen years' observation, is as follows:—

	Feet.	Inches.
Cleveland, greatest average monthly difference of high and low water	1	3
Detroit, " " " "	1	2½
Buffalo, " " " "	0	10½
Mean annual difference of highest and lowest months	1	1½

Lakes Huron and Michigan have not received much attention; but are known to have been high in 1838 and low in 1819. It does not necessarily follow that the highest or lowest level of different Lakes will occur at the same time, nor that the quantity of rise and fall should be the same. There should be, however, in all of them an annual flux and reflux, and also secular fluctuations. As the lower Lakes receive more water from those above during years that are high than they do when there is a depressed surface, there should be a greater range between high and low water in them than in those nearer the source of supply. Lake Superior is the only one of the chain that exhibits the effects of conditions strictly its own.

TABLE OF WATER LEVELS

Reduced to an expression of the depth of water

Year.	Average of the month in feet and inches.												Annual range.
	Jan.	Feb.	March.	April.	May.	June.	July.	Aug.	Sept.	Oct.	Nov.	Dec.	
	ft. in.	ft. in.	ft. in.	ft. in.	ft. in.	ft. in.	ft. in.	ft. in.	ft. in.	ft. in.	ft. in.	ft. in.	ft. in.
1827–8	...	...	...	...	...	...	...	...	...	...	...	...	...
1838	...	...	...	...	...	...	...	...	...	...	...	...	...
1844–5	...	...	...	...	...	...	...	...	...	...	...	...	...
1846	...	...	...	...	...	...	...	...	...	...	...	...	...
1847	...	...	10	...	...	...	...	...	...	...	...	...	...
1851	...	...	...	...	...	...	...	...	(12 3)	...	...	...	...
1852	...	...	...	...	...	11 7	...	...	...	...	...	...	...
1853	...	...	...	...	9 11	10 7	11 0	10 6	(11 4)	11 1	...	10 9	...
1854	...	...	9 9	10 3	10 4½	10 9	11 2	11 4	11 6½	(11 9)	11 7	11 3	2 0
1855	11 1	11 2½	11 3½	11 3½	11 4½	12 1	12 6	12 10	12 10 $\frac{8}{10}$	(13 2 $\frac{9}{10}$)	13 0	...	2 1
1856	...	...	...	...	12 3	12 7	12 9	13 1 $\frac{1}{10}$	(13 4 $\frac{2}{10}$)	13 2 $\frac{2}{10}$	...	...	...

Here the high water month, from the meagre observations hitherto made, is September; and the low water month is March. The streams are numerous, but short and rapid. Their waters soon reach the Lake in the spring, but to counteract this rapidity the season is late. Snow does not entirely disappear from the swamps and gorges of the mountains before the middle of May. The area draining into this Lake is small compared with its extent. There are but three considerable rivers: the St. Louis, Ontonagon, and Michipicoton, the longest of which does not exceed two hundred miles, yet Captain Bayfield states that more than ten times the quantity is received than is discharged at St. Mary's. On account of the small extent of the basin, the spring floods are insufficient to bring the annual rise to its maximum. It requires the additional rains of the summer and the early fall months to effect this. The observations are not sufficient to determine correctly the amount of either the annual or the secular variations. The greatest measured difference is two feet six inches, that is, from the high water of September, 1851, to the low water of March, 1854. The greatest difference of months in the year 1853, is one foot five inches; in 1854 two feet, and in 1855 two feet one inch.

All those who journeyed along the shores of this Lake in 1845–6, observed that the summer months were unusually dry. Fires raged in all parts of the country, not upon the mountains only, but in swamps which had been saturated with water so long that large cedar-trees had grown up and died of old age. In consequence of this the surface of the Lake declined in those years, and in 1847 still more—according to the general estimate three feet.

The position of Sault St. Mary's I am well aware is not a good one for ascertaining the actual changes that occur in the open Lake. For this purpose Copper Harbor, Eagle river, Rock Harbor on Isle Royal, or Ontonagon would be much preferable. Places on the broad parts of the water, and not at the heads of bays and inlets, are much the best points to observe the fluctuations of level. They

FOR LAKE SUPERIOR.

on the Mitre Sill, head of Canal, Sault St. Mary.

YEAR.	PLACE OF OBSERVATION.	OBSERVERS.	REMARKS.
1827–8	Sault St. Mary	Capt. Dearborn, U. S. A.	Reported to be at the lowest level.
1838	......	......	Reported by Major Lachlan as three feet higher than 1828.
1844–5	......	......	Water high in these years, but not measured.
1846	CopperHarbor	W. W. Mather, C. Whittlesey	From two to three feet below general level of 1845.
1847	"	W. W. Mather, Mr. Turrill	Rise from June to September, twelve inches; trees a hundred years old within four feet of the present level.
1851	"	D. D. Brockway	This being at the time the highest then known state of the water, a mark was made on the rocks of Duck Island, near the end of Turrill's dock; this, by a comparison of seven months in 1855–6, corresponds to twelve feet three inches in the canal.
1852	"	Mr. Turrill	
1853	Eagle River	C. Whittlesey	Mean of frequent observations during the month. Copper Harbor mark, or zero, transferred to the Eagle River dock.
1854	"	"	
1855	Sault St. Mary	Wm. Finney	Taken frequently during the summer months, under the direction of John Burt, superintendent of the canal.
1856	"	M. B. Sherwood	Highest water in September three times, in October twice, in five years. High months in parentheses.

are less affected by winds and currents, and the irregularities that arise from indentations of the coast. Whoever undertakes to compare observations made at the Sault St. Mary's, at Detroit, Buffalo, Niagara, and Ogdensburg, which are situated upon straits or outlets, will at once perceive that the range of fluctuation is greater than it is at Eagle river, Cleveland and Oswego, situated on the open water. There is between them a correspondence, but, from causes that are apparent, the changes of level at the same time may be greater or may be less upon the St. Lawrence, the Detroit, or the St. Mary's rivers than upon Lake Ontario, Lake Huron, or Lake Superior.

If the width of the Detroit river at Fort Gratiot is greater than it is at Detroit, a rise of a given number of feet in Lake Huron must result in a greater rise at Detroit, the channel being narrower and more compressed. This is known to be the case in the Niagara river.

Below the falls for many miles is a narrow gorge where the river is compressed into much narrower limits than it has at Black Rock, where Lake Erie discharges itself. While this Lake varies secularly, not to exceed six feet, the rise and fall in the gorge below the suspension bridge is reported to be fifteen and even twenty feet. But on Lake Erie and Lake Superior the best zero or line of reference is furnished by the guard locks of the Erie and the Sault St. Mary's canals, and although the position is not favorable in other respects, the zero is so convenient and well established that I have reduced all the registers for these Lakes to the same expression as those at the canals just named.

In June, 1855, soon after the completion of the canal at the Sault, connecting Lake Huron and Lake Superior, Mr. John Burt, the superintendent, caused his assistants, Messrs. Wm. Finney and M. B. Sherwood, to keep a register of the depth of water at the upper and at the lower locks. These have been kindly furnished me as late as the fall of 1856. They were not made daily but frequently during the month; the course and strength of the wind were recorded, with occasional observations of the barometer.

The mean elevation of Lake Superior above Lake Huron is not yet known, nor the precise difference of elevation at any one time.

It is evident that the mean elevation of Lake Erie, or any of the Lakes above the ocean, cannot be determined till the mean of its fluctuations are known. We call the height of Lake Erie five hundred and sixty-five feet above mean tide at Albany, because it was found to be so at the time when the Erie Canal was surveyed. But without knowing the state of the water at Black Rock or Buffalo at that day, it is evident there may be an error of two and a half to three feet.

The same may be said of all the Lakes. The rise to be overcome by the canal at the Falls of St. Mary's was reported by the engineers to be seventeen and one-half feet; but if there is a change of level in Lake Superior above the falls, it does not follow, as has been just observed, that the same change of level would be noticed below the falls where the river is wider.

Mr. Murray, of the geological survey of Canada, in 1848, examined the other rapids of the St. Mary's river, and made their united descent two feet $\frac{91}{100}$ths, which, added to the above and neglecting the descent of the water between the rapids, the difference is twenty feet $\frac{41}{100}$. As measured barometrically by Captain Bayfield, the elevation of Lake Superior is six hundred and twenty-seven feet above the ocean, and Lake Huron is stated by Mr. Higgins to be five hundred and seventy-eight, making a difference of forty-nine feet.

The elevation of Lake Huron is, however, subject to correction by future levels along the connecting straits. I have not, in this paper, given the details of the water tables, reserving them for publication within their respective States. The results are shown in the proper tables, in the form of a monthly average, with remarks.

The register of Messrs. Finney and Sherwood for the six summer months of 1855 and 1856, show a difference between the depth of water at the lower and at the upper locks of about ten inches during those years, as follows:—

	Feet.	Inches.
Mean depth of water at upper lock six months, 1855	12	9.00
" " " " 1856	12	10.25
lower lock six months, 1855	12	00.38
" " " " 1856	12	1.00

These tables show conclusively the effect of winds in raising and depressing the water in a narrow and crooked strait connecting two Lakes. On the morning of July 16, 1855, the wind was from the northwest, and off Lake Superior. As usual, in that case, the water rose at the upper gate, varying from twelve feet one inch to thirteen feet six inches, or about one and one-half feet.

At noon the wind had changed to the opposite quarter and blew from the southeast. The water fell to eleven feet five inches, and at one P. M. to ten feet nine inches, making a difference of two feet nine inches in less than eight hours.

On the 3d of June, 1856, the observers witnessed a still more remarkable change, because it occurred while the wind was steadily from the same quarter. It blew a continued gale from the southeast during the entire day. At 7½ A. M. the water was low. At 3½ P. M. it was still lower, being at nine feet nine inches, rising in the space of three hours to thirteen feet ten inches, a change of four feet one inch.

The highest monthly average is that of September, 1856, when the mean depth in the canal was thirteen feet four and $\frac{20}{100}$ inches. During the season of navigation the water of Lake Superior is higher than during the winter months, but a fall of four feet in the general surface of the Lake below the highest known state would reduce the canal depth in September to nine feet four inches, and might interfere with the passage of large craft.

At present the shallowest parts of the St. Mary's river are less than nine feet, but the canal was intended to have a depth of water of never less than twelve feet.

This is an instance of the importance of Lake registers to engineers and those engaged in improving navigation.

TABLE OF WATER LEVELS

All the measurements reduced to the zero, or line of reference, at

Year.	Monthly Average.												Yearly change of level.
	Jan.	Feb.	March.	April.	May.	June.	July.	Aug.	Sept.	Oct.	Nov.	Dec.	
	ft. in.	ft. in.	ft. in.	ft. in.	ft. in.	ft. in.	ft. in.	ft. in.	ft. in.	ft. in.	ft. in.	ft. in.	ft. in.
1795	...	...	...	...	...	...	...	...	...	...	...	...	3 0
1815	...	7 4	7 6	...	...	...	(6 8)	...	...	...	...	...	2 8
1816	...	...	6 10	...	...	(4 11)	(5 10)	...	...	...	...	...	1 8
1817	...	...	...	7 4	...	(5 6)	...	...	...	...	...	...	1 11
1818	...	...	8 3	...	...	(5 10)	...	...	...	...	...	...	1 10
1819	...	...	8 9	...	...	...	(6 10)	...	...	...	...	...	2 5
1820	...	...	...	8 4	...	...	(5 2)	...	...	...	...	...	1 11
1821	...	...	8 1	...	...	(5 10)	...	...	...	...	...	...	3 2
1822	...	...	8 0	...	...	(5 6)	...	...	...	...	...	...	2 3
1823	...	...	7 10	...	...	...	(5 4)	...	...	...	...	...	2 6
1824	...	...	9 4	...	...	(7 1)	...	...	...	...	...	...	2 6
1825	...	...	9 4	...	...	...	(6 10)	...	...	...	...	...	2 3
1826	...	...	...	...	...	(5 2)	...	...	...	5 10	...	...	2 6
1827	...	...	...	...	...	...	(2 10)	3 11	...	4 6	...	...	...
1837	...	...	...	...	...	...	4 6	...	...	5 1	...	...	...
1838	...	...	...	...	...	...	(3 0½)	...	3 11¾	4 5	...	...	...
1839	5 5½	...	...	...	...	...	4 5	4 5½	4 10	5 4½	5 9	...	...
1840	...	6 3½	5 8	5 2	4 5¼	(4 1½)	4 2	4 5	4 11⅓	...	5 5 9/10	5 8 1/10	2 3
1841	5 8 2/10	5 9 4/10	5 11½	5 2 7/10	(4 6½)	4 6 8/10	4 8½	5 1½	...	6 3	6 11 7/10	7 0	2 5
1842	6 9	6 5½	6 2	5 10 7/10	...	5 5	(5 2 7/10)	5 7	5 9	6 1 2/10	6 4 1/10	6 6 8/10	1 6
1843	6 5 3/10	...	6 1 2/10	6 6	5 3 1/10	5 0 8/10	(5 1)	5 6 7/10	6 0½	6 1½	6 2½	6 5	1 5
1844	6 7	6 7	6 4 6/10	6 1 6/10	...	5 3	(5 2 8/10)	5 4 0/10	5 6 2/10	6 5½	...	...	1 4
1845	6 7 2/10	6 4½	...	5 1	...	(5 1)	5 5	5 10 6/10	6 6	6 5	6 9½	...	1 8½
1846	7 5½	7 7	7 8 7/10	6 7	6 4	6 4 2/10	(6 1)	6 4	6 8 2/10	7 1½	7 5½	6 7	1 8
1847	6 10	6 4	6 6	5 10	5 3	(5 1)	5 4 7/10	5 11	5 10 7/10	6 1	6 5	6 8	1 9
1848	(5 3)	5 8	6 5	6 0	6 2½	6 2	6 3 7/10	6 5½	6 11½	7 3 8/10	7 8 3/10	6 8	2 5
1849	7 0	7 0	7 2	6 8	5 10	(5 9½)	5 11	6 4½	6 8	6 11½	6 7	6 3	1 2½
1850	6 7	6 2	6 2	6 2	(5 6)	5 6½	5 8	6 3½	6 9	6 10	7 5	6 5	1 11
1851	6 6	7 4	6 4 1/10	6 9	6 6	(5 4)	5 9	5 6	5 10	6 9	7 3	7 1	2 0
1852	7 0	7 1	6 10	6 6	5 0	(4 5)	4 8	4 10	5 4	4 9	6 0	5 8	2 8
1853	5 9	5 6	5 6	4 11	4 6	(3 6)	3 9	4 3	4 8½	5 1	5 4 8/10	5 6	2 3
1854	6 1	6 1	6 0	6 1	4 5½	(4 5)	4 8½	5 1	5 9	6 0½	6 6	6 10	2 5
1855	7 0	6 11	7 0½	6 9	6 0	5 9	5 1½	(5 1)	5 5	5 5	5 8	5 7½	1 11
1856	...	...	...	4 10	4 3	...	4 0½	4 4	5 2	5 5½	5 10½	5 11½	...
1857	...	6 0½	...	5 0½	...	3 8	(3 4)	3 5	...	...	...	...	...

The diagram of monthly variations for Lake Ontario (see Plate I, No. 2) is constructed from the register of H. T. Spencer, Esq., made once a month at the mouth of the Genesee river. A single reading for each month may fail to give a good average, but the regularity of the figures show that care was taken to avoid rough weather.

The table for Rochester is copied from the annual reports of the regents of the university. For a transcript of the registers at Oswego, I am indebted to M. P. Hatch, Esq., the harbor agent at that place. This includes a greater number of years, but except for the last two they are incomplete.

FOR LAKE ONTARIO.

Oswego, N. Y., reckoning downward from top of west pier.

YEAR.	PLACE OF OBSERVATION.	OBSERVERS.	EXPLANATIONS AND GENERAL REMARKS.
1795	Kingston	Mr. Weld	*Weld's Travels in Canada*, quoted by Major Lachlan. The lake reported to be higher than during the previous thirty years, or since 1765; its overflow destroying an orchard planted that year.
1815	F't Niagara	Edw. Giddings	Mr. Giddings kept a register while he resided at Fort Niagara from 1815 to 1827, but has published only the extremes of each year. The lowest water within the year occurred in the month of March nine times out of twelve, and the highest months during fourteen years are June and July, divided in equal numbers between them. The Niagara zero, or line of reference, was five feet below the top of the sill of the dock. To reduce his figures to the Oswego standard, the data are slight, but I have preferred to make the reduction, and thus exhibit all the measurements for this lake at one view. The only months of the Oswego and Niagara registers in common are those of July and October, 1838. By them, Mr. Giddings's line of reference was ten feet below the Oswego zero, and the top of the capsill of the dock five feet. Highest months of the year in parentheses. Mean of yearly fluctuations for twelve years at Niagara two feet three inches. HIGHEST KNOWN RISE.
1816	"		
1817	"		
1818	"		
1819	"		
1820	"		
1821	"		
1822	"		
1823	"		
1824	"		
1825	"		
1826	"		
1827	"		
1837	Oswego	Lieut. R. C.	The Oswego zero, or line of reference, is the top of the coping of the west pier, near its southern end, at the boat-house, counting downwards to the surface of the water. Messrs. Smead, Judson, and Hatch were successively the agents of the government in the construction of the harbor at Oswego. Up to the year 1854, there are months in the Oswego register that are wanting, and these are supplied by reducing the measurements made since 1846 for the Regents of the New York University at Rochester harbor by H. T. Spencer. By a comparison of twenty months, common to both registers, Mr. Spencer's zero, or the top of the Rochester dock, is two feet ten inches below the Oswego zero. Prior to the time of Messrs. Hatch and Malcolm, the readings were made only occasionally in calm weather from one to eight times a month, but those gentlemen observed the water daily. In all cases, the mean of all the measurements is here given. Dr. Guest's observations at Ogdensburg extend from February, 1851, to August, 1857, made from time to time with occasional vacant spaces. By a comparison of eight months, his zero being the top of the railroad dock, is equivalent to eight and seven-tenths inches below the Oswego zero. The range of the fluctuations is about the same, and thus the descent of the river may be neglected for the purposes of this table. Mean of yearly fluctuations at Rochester and Oswego for eighteen years, one foot ten and a half inches. Highest water in the month of June eight times, July six, May twice, August once, January once. Lowest water in November three times, December twice, January three times, February twice, March three times. Greatest absolute height of all observations, July, 1838. Greatest absolute depression of all observations, March, 1824 and 1825. Greatest absolute difference at Niagara, six feet six inches.
1838	"	Smead, U.S.A.	
1839	"	"	
1840	"	"	
1841	"	J. W. Judson	
1842	"	"	
1843	"	"	
1844	"	"	
1845	"		
1846	Oswego &	J. W. Judson &	
1847	Rochester	H. T. Spencer	
1848	"	"	
1849	"	"	
1850	"	"	
1851	"	"	
1852	"	"	
1853	"	M. P. Hatch &	
1854	"	H. T. Spencer	
1855	"	W. S. Malcolm	
1856	Ogdensburg	W. E. Guest	
1857	"	"	

By comparing the records of both places, it is plain that for such periods as are common there is a close correspondence. The two ports are about sixty miles apart, situated on the same shore, and at about the broadest part of the Lake. In the average of the seven last months of 1853 the greatest discrepancy occurs. The difference is six and one-half inches. On both registers the year 1853 is one of high and the year 1848 of low water. The year 1850, which is almost a blank in the Oswego tables, shows the lowest month of the Rochester records.

Mr. Edward Giddings, in a pamphlet published at Lockport, New York, in 1838, explaining his views upon the causes of the rise and fall in the surface of the

Lakes, gives to the public a part of his registers taken at the dock at Fort Niagara. The fluctuations of the Niagara river are not exactly coincident with those in the general surface of either the Lake above or the one below; but those reported by Mr. Giddings vary so little that I have reduced them to the same standard as the others and placed them in my abstract.

From the yearly average 1846 was the lowest, but differed only one-tenth of an inch from 1851. That portion of 1846 which appears in the Oswego tables shows the lowest stage observed there. Like Lake Erie, the spring rise is reached in the months of June and July; but there is more irregularity in the low water months.

According to Mr. Spencer's observations, high water occurred in the months of June and July, seven years in eight; the minimum of the year in the months of November and December, four times; January and February, three; and March, once. The records of nineteen years at Oswego show that the month of July, 1838, was higher than any month since, which corresponds in time with the noted flood on Lake Erie. From the high level of that year, the decline of Lake Ontario was not as rapid as Lake Erie. The lowest state since 1838 on the last named Lake is that of 1842, but on Lake Ontario that of 1848.

The question of the existence of a daily or lunar tide in this and other Lakes, corresponding to that of the ocean, has been, like the idea of a seven year's rise and a seven year's fall, so often brought forward that it deserves notice. In Weld's Travels in Canada, 1790–5, it is stated that "it is believed by many that the waters of Lake Ontario are influenced by a tide that ebbs and flows frequently in the course of twenty-four hours, as in the Bay of Quintè, where it has been observed to rise fourteen inches every four hours."

The same idea had its origin on Lake Michigan, at the head of Green Bay, which, like that of Quintè, is a narrow inlet extending far inland.

Colonel Henry Whiting, of the army, observed the fluctuations at Green Bay, in 1828, during the months of July and August, and states that in no case did they correspond to the passage of the moon over the meridian, and that there are no lunar tides. Mr. George C. Davies, who assisted Mr. Walworth in keeping a daily water table at Cleveland, in 1838, says, "I can say, without fear of contradiction, that there is no lunar tide on Lake Erie."

Captain Jonathan Carver, who passed through the Upper Lakes, in 1766–9, states that "observations made by the French at the Straits of Mackinaw show that there is no diurnal flood and ebb there."

The difficulty of reducing observations made at one port to those made at another, even on the same Lake, is owing to a want of correspondence in the rise and fall of water in the same months at different places. It is also impossible to free the readings from erratic "local oscillations," some of which are due to visible causes, such as winds and the shape of the coast, and others to causes not visible, and not yet well understood. This difficulty is apparent on comparing the means of the same months at different places on Lake Erie, as shown in the table of levels. We have for the years 1838, 1839, 1840, and 1841, pretty fair annual averages at

Detroit and at Buffalo. The mean annual average, however, is quite different, being greatest at the east end of the Lake.

MEAN ANNUAL DIFFERENCE FOR THREE YEARS.

	DETROIT. Feet.	BUFFALO. Feet.
1839 below 1838	1.33	1.25
1840 " 1839	0.99	1.25
1841 " 1840	1.00	1.65
Fall in three years	3.32	4.15

Between the highest and lowest months within the year, the extremes of fluctuation are also quite different at different places.

GREATEST DIFFERENCE OF LEVEL BY MONTHLY AVERAGES WITHIN A YEAR.

DETROIT. Feet.	BUFFALO. Feet.	CLEVELAND. Feet.
2.33	1.27	2.30

There is no way of eliminating such discrepancies, but by a more perfect series of observations, and the rejection of such as are affected by sudden causes. This cannot be done with the imperfect registers hitherto kept.

I now pass to the third class of "fluctuations," namely, transient fluctuations.

I shall here give some extracts from my memoranda upon the pulsations or oscillations that occur on Lake Superior, in calm as well as in stormy weather. Those of the 25th, 26th, and 27th of June, 1854, were very marked and regular.

The Lake for several days was without storms, winds, or waves. The first table is from observations made on the 29th of June.

Time of flood A. M.	Time of ebb A. M.	Period of reflux.	Time from flood to flood.	Extreme change of level.	REMARKS, WEATHER, &c.
11 h. 20 m.	11 h. 28 m.	8 min.	. .	5 inches	Calm; light rain.
11 33	11 38	5	13 min.	4 "	Light breezes off shore.
11 44	11 47	3	11	3 "	" "
11 50	11 55	5	6	Slight	Rain and wind increased.
12 1	12 5	6	11	3 inches	Stationary at ebb three minutes.
12 50	12 20	5	14	7 "	Slight wind off shore.

The same movement continued throughout the day. The place of observation was within the creek called Eagle river, about twenty rods from the Lake.

The flood or influx came into the stream, rapidly carrying boats, logs, and brush violently against the current as far as the rapids. No storms or severe winds occurred for several days before or after the 29th. The prevailing wind for the month of July was from the west. For two weeks in the latter part of June and forepart of July scarcely a day passed without the pulsations.

The next table is from my register for October 11, 1854. The play of the waters began early in the day, with a stiff south-easterly or off-shore breeze; and no waves visible along the shore line. The observations were made in the open Lake, at the pier, in three feet of water, eight rods from shore.

Time of flood A. M.	Time of ebb A. M.	Time elapsed ebb to flood.	Time elapsed flood to flood.	Range of level.	WEATHER, &c.
...	7 h. 35 m.	...	...	10 inches	Water calm.
7 h. 43 m.	7 46	8 min.	...	18 "	A current down the lake one mile per hour.
7 50	7 58	4	7 min.	18 "	
8 00	8 3	2	10	15 "	
8 13	8 19	10	13	Slight	
8 24	8 25	5	11	18 inches	Very sudden.
8 26	8 30	1	2	2 feet	
8 36	8 43	5	10	Slight	
8 46	8 53	3	10	...	
8 58	8 00	5	12	...	

The same southerly breeze and cloudy weather existed at the close as at the commencement.

The coast is visible from the pier each way one-fourth of a mile, over a clear sand beach.

At the moment of each influx a low wave broke on the shore along the whole field of view, and at each depression the water retired from one to three rods on the beach. This occurred everywhere at precisely the same instant. It had the appearance of a succession of undulations too slight and broad to create a visible swell on the surface coming directly upon the shore. The waves must have been parallel to the coast line and not oblique to it, or they would not have arrived at the same moment. If the crest of the undulations made an angle with the shore, the breaking of the water would have been progressive along the beach, as in the case of oblique waves.

Both the flood and ebb occurring as nearly as I could determine along a line of half a mile in length at the same time, the swell must have moved directly toward shore. On the 2d and 3d of this month (October, 1854) a destructive storm occurred, beginning at the east, changing to northeast and north, and finally to northwest, with heavy rain.

On my return to the Lake in the afternoon of the 11th, the movement was as active as in the morning. There had been no cessation during the day.

RECORD OF FLUCTUATIONS. October 11th, 1854.

Ebb P. M.	Flood P. M.	Ebb to flood.	Flood to flood.	Change of level.	REMARKS.
3 h. 25 m.	3 h. 26 m.	1 min.	...	1 ft. 2 in.	Weather calm; cloudy and rain.
3 33	3 35	2	9 min.	0 4½	
3 38	3 39	1	4	0 1	Observers Dr. S. H. Whittlesey and James S. Morgan.
3 41	3 44	3	5	0 10	
3 51	3 55	4	9	1 2	
3 58	3 59	1	4	0 7	
4 4	4 7	3	8	1 2	
4 11	4 17	6	10	0 11½	

This table shows greater rapidity of movement than that for the morning. The readings were made in the creek at the usual place, where the range from high to low level, as might be expected, was somewhat less than in the open Lake at the pier. As a general rule, it will be observed that the pulsation which is longest in its period from high to low, is the greatest in its range; but to this there are exceptions. On the morning of the 12th the water was still in motion, as it was the evening before, the weather being very calm, with a ground swell, coming in from the open Lake. At eleven o'clock A. M. it increased in rapidity, and in the range. About the 14th of the same month, another severe gale set in from the northwest, and continued three days. The remainder of the month was calm.

In the year 1855, the first oscillations of the season were noticed on the 20th of June, at 10 o'clock A. M., the weather being calm and clear.

The same thing occurred in the same kind of weather on the 26th, and again on the 13th of July. Hitherto, since the 22d of April, when the Lake ice broke up, there had been no prolonged gales nor storms, and only a few thunder-gusts. On the 14th, 15th, 16th, 17th, 18th, 19th, the movements were almost continuous. At the Sault, as Mr. Emerson informs me, the water rose three feet three inches on the 18th. The weather was cloudy and rainy, with frequent thunder-storms; but the Lake was calm most of the time. From the 24th to the 31st fluctuations occurred daily, with close, calm, cloudy, and foggy weather, the thermometer at night varying from 55° to 88° F.

From the 1st to the 12th of August, inclusive, there was no cessation of the oscillation, except for parts of two days. During this time there was but one gale, which was from the west, on the 9th instant, and lasted twenty hours. Thunder-storms were frequent, between which the sky was clear and the Lake calm.

I did not notice any more till the 25th of August. In the meantime the autumn winds had set in. During the afternoon of the 25th a violent thunder-storm arose from the northwest, and the oscillations came on as rapidly and as marked as at any period of the summer. Again, on the 30th and 31st the same thing occurred in calm weather, a thunder-storm having taken place during the intervening night. This phenomenon was observed in the month of September on eleven different days, and three times during the first eight days of October; after which, my residence having been changed, the observations ceased.

The month of September on this Lake and on Lake Erie was more stormy than the month of October. Whether these movements occur in the winter season, I am unable to say.

For the purpose of furnishing memoranda covering as wide a space as possible, I insert two more tables of an hour's readings each, one on the 2d, and another on the 3d of August, 1855, in different parts of the day.

OSCILLATIONS. August 2d and 3d, 1855.

Ebb A. M.	Flood A. M.	From ebb to flood.	From flood to flood.	Change of level.	REMARKS.
8 h. 23 m.	8 h. 31 m.	8 min.	. . .	0 ft. 3 in.	Weather calm; sultry, cloudy;
8 36	Wanting	. . .	. . .	0 6	movements continue all day.
8 49	8 53	4	. . .	0 5	
9 2	9 7	5	14 min.	0 4	
9 14	9 17	3	10	0 3	
9 25	9 29	4	12	0 4	
Aug. 3d, P. M.	P. M.				
. . .	1 h. 5 m.	. . .	. . .	. . .	Thunder-storm and rain in the
1 h. 7 m.	1 12	5	7	0 4	morning; wind N. W., chang-
1 16	1 20	4	8	0 2½	ing to S. in the afternoon;
1 30	1 37	7	17	0 4¾	movements all day.
1 44	1 51	7	14	0 4	
1 54	1 56	3	5	0 3½	
2 00	1 4	4	8	0 2½	

Such agitations of the water, in perfectly calm weather, attracted the attention of travellers at an early day. The relations of the Jesuit fathers are replete with accounts of sudden waves and swells, on which their canoes were tossed by some invisible agent. All those who reside on the shores of the Lakes have made the same observations. They have been so frequently noticed, and so often commented upon in the public prints, that the subject has ceased to excite surprise. Even the small Lakes of the interior sometimes exhibit the same mysterious movements, and at times when neither storms nor winds are within view. But notwithstanding the notoriety which they have acquired, there has been little direct observation. I know of only two instances in past time in which registers have been kept.

When General Cass was at Green Bay in 1820, he caused the flux and reflux of water at the mouth of the Fox river to be measured by a gauge set upon the shore. He concluded that the fluctuations of level at that place had no connection with lunar tides, and the observations show that they are not of the class which I have recorded.

The Eagle river tables show a uniformity and rapidity of motion quite different from the Green Bay registers. Without going into details upon the nature and cause of the changes of level at Green Bay, I will remark that a residence of one summer at Fort Howard confirmed me in the correctness of the conclusion of General Cass, in regard to the absence of any apparent effect from lunar attraction. This appears to be the case in an estuary, whose shores terminate at an acute angle, where very slight movements in the bay were made conspicuous at the point of intersection of the shore lines. The general form of Green Bay is such that the winds and currents of the open Lake affect its surface from whatever direction they come. The discharge of water from the Fox river is considerable, and the meeting of a wave of influx from the bay with this current would create an observable rise. Vibrations would follow, which should occur as they are observed to do, at irregular intervals of from half an hour to several hours.

The only records relating purely to "barometrical waves," that I know of, are those of Professor Mather, made at Copper Harbor in July, 1847. He compared, during one day, the fluctuations of his barometer, with those of the level of the water. The opinion has been so often advanced that these oscillatory movements are due to rapid variations of the barometrical pressure, that the term of "barometrical waves" has come to be their received name. It is doubtful whether, if this be the case, a mercurial barometer would show them. The movements of the column are too sluggish, and the apparatus for reading too imperfect to indicate a change of pressure that sometimes occurs in the space of one minute. My tables show that an oscillation may be completed in that time. Some more sensitive instrument is needed to indicate atmospherical changes that occupy at intervals of so short a period.

Professor Mather's observations were taken under circumstances that should be well considered in comparing them with others, made in calm weather and on the open Lake. (See Plate II, No. 3.)

Copper Harbor is a long narrow inlet, within which the movements are augmented, and may also be broken up, by counter waves reflected from the sides. During the time of Prof. M.'s observations, violent storms and winds were raging at the harbor, or were visible in the distance. Such agitations of the atmosphere, although they do not prevent the regular oscillations, would materially interfere with them. His observations were carefully made, and are the earliest exact data of a scientific kind relative to this subject within my reach.

There is to be found, moreover, in the geological reports upon the Upper Peninsula, a comprehensive historical notice of these phenoména.

Whether such movements have been observed upon the ocean, I am not aware. But it would seem probable, that, whatever the cause may be, it should be universal, and produce its effects on all bodies of water.

It is plain, after the barometer recovered from the effects of the tornado in the forenoon, it declined regularly till night, as might have been expected from the stormy condition of the weather.

The pulsations within the harbor continued all day, although there is a break in the readings from 11 A. M. till 2 P. M., with the exception of one at twelve hours eight minutes. So far, therefore, as these observations indicate, there is no apparent connection between the oscillations and the barometrical pressure; at least the movements for twelve hours were very marked, while the barometer was regularly falling, except during the tornado. The day commenced with the barometer at 29.288, and closed with it at 29.150.

In the autumn of 1856 I had the first opportunity of comparing the state of the barometer with the movements of the water. It was done with an aneroid recently compared with a good cistern barometer. I had not assistants to enable me at the same time to note the actual range of the wâve in a vertical direction; but in this respect it was apparently the same as is shown in the preceding tables.

On the 19th of October the Lake was calm, a light breeze blowing off shore from the southeast. The weather was calm and foggy on the 20th, with a gentle breeze from the south, and a hazy, warm atmosphere, like the Indian summer. It rained during a greater part of the night between the 20th and 21st, and on the morning of the last named day the wind was northeast by east, or about parallel with the coast line. During the day rain continued to fall, and the wind, continuing in the same quarter, increased to a gale, raising a heavy swell upon the Lake. The oscillations were visible early in the morning, and continued with unusual rapidity all day. It was not until late in the afternoon that a barometer could be procured.

The readings were made at the moment of the culmination, and also at the lowest ebb of the wave or oscillatory movement. The results agree in general with those of Professor Mather, and show a steady motion of the barometrical column in one direction during the fluctuations of the water level.

REGISTER OF BAROMETRICAL READINGS TAKEN AT THE MOMENT OF THE EBB AND FLOOD.
Eagle River, Lake Superior, October, 1856.

Day and hour.	Reading of the barometer.	State of the pulsation.	STATE OF THE WEATHER—REMARKS.
October 21st	Inches.		
4h. 50m. P. M.	29.440	Ebb	Wind northeasterly, a moderate gale, with a drizzling rain.
4 51	29.445	Flood	
4 55	29.451	Ebb	
4 57	29.453	Flood	Extreme fluctuations, four to twelve inches.
4 58	29.460	Ebb	
4 59	29.470	Flood	Heavy swells, rolling into the creek, interfere with the regularity of the oscillations.
5 1	29.475	Ebb	
5 3	29.480	Flood	
5 4½	29.489	Ebb	
5 6	29.500	Flood	
5 7	29.500	Ebb	
5 8	29.500	Flood	
5 10	29.500	Ebb	
5 11	29.510	Flood	
5 13	29.510	Ebb	
5 13½	29.510	Flood	
5 14	29.510	Ebb	
5 15	29.510	Flood	
5 16½	29.510	Ebb	
5 18	29.520	Flood	
5 19	29.520	Ebb	
5 20½	29.520	Flood	Movements very strong.
5 33	29.535		Darkness sets in; oscillations continue till 9 P. M., and probably all night.
5 40	29.546		
6 00	29.575		
6 10	29.582		
6 20	29.595		
6 30	29.600		
6 40	29.595		
6 50	29.602		
7 00	29.600		
7 10	29.602		
7 20	29.602		
7 30	29.603		
7 40	29.601		
7 50	29.601		
8 00	29.600		
8 30	29.505		
9 00	29.601		Oscillations continue.
October 22d			
6h. 45m. A. M.	29.500		Wind north, light; oscillations going on, but the movements are slight; water calm.
7 15	29.485		
8 15	29.500		
8 45	29.500		Fog on the adjacent mountains.
9 15	29.500		Oscillations languid, but with a great vertical range.
9 45	29.500		

REGISTER OF BAROMETRICAL READINGS—Continued.

Day and hour.	Reading of the barometer.	State of the pulsation.	STATE OF THE WEATHER—REMARKS.
October 22d	Inches.		
11h. 00m. A. M.	29.510		
11 30	29.510		Weather same as in the morning.
12 00 M.	29.525		
1 00 P. M.	29.510		Wind north, increasing; no movement.
2 00	29.490		
3 00	29.480		Oscillations commence.
3 10	29.480		
3 15	29.500	Flood	
3 20	29.495	Ebb	
3 28	29.500	Flood	
3 45	29.500	Ebb	
3 48	29.510	Flood	
4 00	29.512		Movement ceases.
4 30	29.515		Wind north, light.
4 45	29.520		
5 00	29.525		
5 15	29.525		
5 45	29.570		
7 00	29.600		From 4 to 9 P. M., weather clear, cool, and calm, and no movement in oscillation.
8 00	29.600		
9 00	29.600		
October 23d			
7h. 00m. A. M.	29.640		Clear and cool; light breeze from the north; oscillations ranging from four to six inches.
8 00	29.725		
9 00	29.770		
9 33	29.775	Flood	Very full.
9 38	29.775	Ebb	Breeze lulls.
9 42	29.780	Flood	
9 47	29.785	Ebb	
9 53	29.785	Flood	Movement very slight.
9 55	29.785	Ebb	Movement very slight.
9 59	29.790	Flood	Very full.
10 3	29.790	Ebb	Slight.
10 8	29.795	Flood	
10 13	29.796	Ebb	Very low.
10 17	29.797	Flood	
10 20	29.797	Ebb	
10 25	29.797	Flood	Movement dying out.
10 32	29.785	Ebb	Movement dying out.
10 45	29.785		Movement ceases.
11 30	29.790		The general level of the lake is four inches lower than yesterday, but the vertical range of the pulsations is greater.
12 00 M.	29.780		
12 10 P. M.	29.780		
12 15	29.785		
12 20	29.802		
12 23	29.820	Flood	
12 30	29.830	Ebb	
12 35	29.840		No movement.
12 40	29.850	Flood	
12 45	29.855	Ebb	
12 50	29.860		Wind freshening from the north; movements succeed each other rapidly, but with a very slight rise and fall.
1 15			
1 30			
3 00			
3 30			Observations cease.

To the facts here given I propose to add very little in the way of a discussion. During the observations, embracing parts of three days, the barometer was lowest at the commencement, on the 21st. There had been no recent storms. The weather was close, foggy, and warm for the season and the latitude. From 4 o'clock and 50 minutes in the afternoon of the 21st to 9 o'clock in the evening, the rise was from 29.440 to 29.600. After a drizzling, foggy night, and a scarcely perceptible northerly breeze, the column stood about as it did the evening previous, and so remained until 3 P. M. of the 22d. The movements of the water were not marked till about this hour, when the wind, still continuing in the north, increased slightly, and the mercury began to rise.

On the morning of the 23d it was still higher, and the play of the waters very lively, the wind continuing in the north. So long as the observations continued, the movements of the surface were slight in quantity, but rapid in time, with only a slight wind. The barometer was all this time steadily rising. From 7 A. M. to 3 P. M. it rose from 29.640 to 29.870 inches.

For several days following the 23d there were moderate gales on the Lake, and rain. On the 28th of the month the regular autumn winds commenced, with snow. The middle day (the 22d) showed more fluctuation of the barometer and less of the water than either of the others.

It is not easy to conceive of a change in the weight of the atmosphere that shall be completed in an average period of ten minutes, and in some cases much less. Is not the cause therefore still to be sought for?

By my observations there is no apparent connection with storms, except thunder-storms. That season of the year, and the kind of weather when thunder-gusts are most frequent, with intervening calms and fogs, is most prolific of oscillations.

There is a distinct class of movements due to the direct driving force of winds that I shall notice below. For the consideration of those who wish to theorize upon the facts I have presented, I suggest that they turn their attention to the agency of electricity.

In May, 1855, the surface of Seneca Lake, as reported in the Geneva Gazette, rose and fell during two entire days as often as once in ten to thirty minutes, ranging through a vertical distance of five inches to two feet. The presence of storms is not mentioned. Could a difference of barometrical pressure exist on different sides of a narrow inland Lake only a few miles across? If so, can we rely upon the barometer to obtain difference of elevation?

While observing the influx and reflux at Eagle river, in July, 1855, the air was frequently agitated by the usual detonations of lightning. Shocks in the atmosphere which produce thunder, which stunned the ear, and cause walls and floors of buildings to tumble, might also produce agitations of the surface of water. There is physical force sufficient in the electricity of the atmosphere at all times to produce this effect; the difficulty occurs in applying it. Electrical movements may be brought into existence by opposite conditions of the atmosphere which rests upon the water and the surrounding shores, especially if there are adjacent mountains.

Vapor is condensed by winds which meet with peaks or mountain crests, and rain and thunder-storms are produced in this way. A breeze from the water pressing against the side of an abrupt highland chain frequently causes its summits to be enveloped in fogs and clouds of condensed moisture. Fogs excite electrical action like clouds, though with less intensity. Winds and unequally heated bodies of air may produce the same effect, causing rapid undulations in the atmosphere, and these may be transmitted to the water beneath.

Without offering this as a satisfactory explanation, I present it for consideration. To discuss the question rationally, we need observations upon the electrical state of the atmosphere during a period of oscillations.[1]

Upon fluctuations caused by winds it will not be necessary to enlarge, as they are produced by a visible cause, and little is left for speculation. The mechanical power of winds, heaping up water on a lea and depressing it on a windward shore, is generally known. On the North American Lakes the registers show that it is a force worthy of attention where the construction of harbors and piers is concerned. In such cases there must be added to the general stage of water something for the temporary rise due to storms.

Certain winds cause at the same place a greater rise than others. At each port the amount of this kind of fluctuation is shown by the daily registers for each direction of the wind. I select some instances from the tables in my possession, choosing from among those on Lake Erie only such as were registered three times a day, and on Lake Ontario once a day.

Those at Cleveland are from Colonel Stockton's observations; those at Buffalo from Mr. Lathrop's; and at Oswego they are taken from those of Messrs. Hatch and Malcolm.

[[1] The simplest hypothesis for the explanation of these phenomena is, that they are produced by the passage of thunder-storms, and perhaps, in some cases, of water-spouts, across distant parts of the Lake. It is well established, by observations at this Institution, that rapid oscillations of the barometer are produced during the passage of a thunder-storm across the meridian of this city. The mercury suddenly descends, then rises a little, and again falls, and after this regains its former level as the storm passes off to the east. A thunder-storm, therefore, crossing the lake at a distance, would transmit to the place of observation undulations from every point of its path, and these, arriving in succession, would produce effects similar to those described. This hypothesis can be tested by the observations which are now about to be established along the lake.—SEC. SMITHSONIAN INSTITUTION.]

TABLE SHOWING THE GREATEST CHANGE OF SURFACE WITHIN A MONTH ARISING FROM THE EFFECT OF WINDS.

CLEVELAND.		BUFFALO.		OSWEGO.	
Date.	Extreme change.	Date.	Extreme range.	Date.	Extreme range.
1845	Ft. In.	1850	Ft. 1/100.	1854	Ft. 1/100.
August	0 10	November	2.70	June	0.35
September	1 1	December	4.60	July	0.45
October	1 2	1851		August	0.90
November	2 0	January	5.55	September	1.00
December	2 5	February	5.60	October	0.65
1846		March	2.90	November	0.50
January	1 5	April	6.25	December	1.00
February	1 8	May	5.20	1855	
March	1 0	June	1.30	January	0.42
April	1 6	July	1.50	February	0.35
May	1 0			March	0.70
June	0 8			April	1.00
July	0 10			May	0.60
August	2 11			June	0.65
				July	0.20
				August	0 40
				September	0.30
				October	0.35
				November	0.70
				December	0.60
				1856	
				January	0.40

There are at each of these places momentary floods and subsidencies that exceed the recorded range of the surface, of which memoranda are made, and which I have already given.

In water tables, the object of which is to ascertain an average level for each month and for each year, sudden movements are avoided as much as possible. They are noted in the column of remarks, but do not enter the general average.

The table of extreme fluctuations just given represents, therefore, more properly the effect of such winds or storms as prevailed for some hours or days in one direction, rather than the result of sudden gusts producing impulses that pass away as suddenly.

The monthly range is far greater at Buffalo than at Cleveland, for reasons already given.

At Oswego it is less than at any place on Lake Erie, owing, probably, to a greater depth of water, especially near the shore.

For the port of Cleveland, Ohio, in twenty-one cases of high water—the wind was northeasterly, eight; northwest, three; south, three; and the remainder calm. At Buffalo, in six cases out of nine, it occurred under the influence of a southwest or down Lake breeze; and in the same number of instances of lowest water, the wind was from the east, or up the Lake, six times.

At Oswego the effect of winds is equally apparent, but the amount of fluctuation produced is less. In twenty-one cases—the highest water happened with a west wind, fifteen times; northwest, once; southwest, once; and south (or off shore), once. Lowest water occurred under a westerly breeze, four times; and with southerly (or off shore) winds, ten times; northerly, four; and in calm weather, twice.

At Cleveland, therefore, northeast winds pile up the waters more than any other. At Buffalo southwest, and at Oswego the west winds produce the same effect.

REGULARITY OF THE RISE AND FALL.

To show more perfectly the regular progress of the changes of level within the year, I have divided the observations for a few months into weeks, and constructed curves accordingly. For Buffalo I have selected two months in a rising stage of water, and for Cleveland five months in a falling stage. With these remarks the diagram will be understood. (Plate II, number 4.)

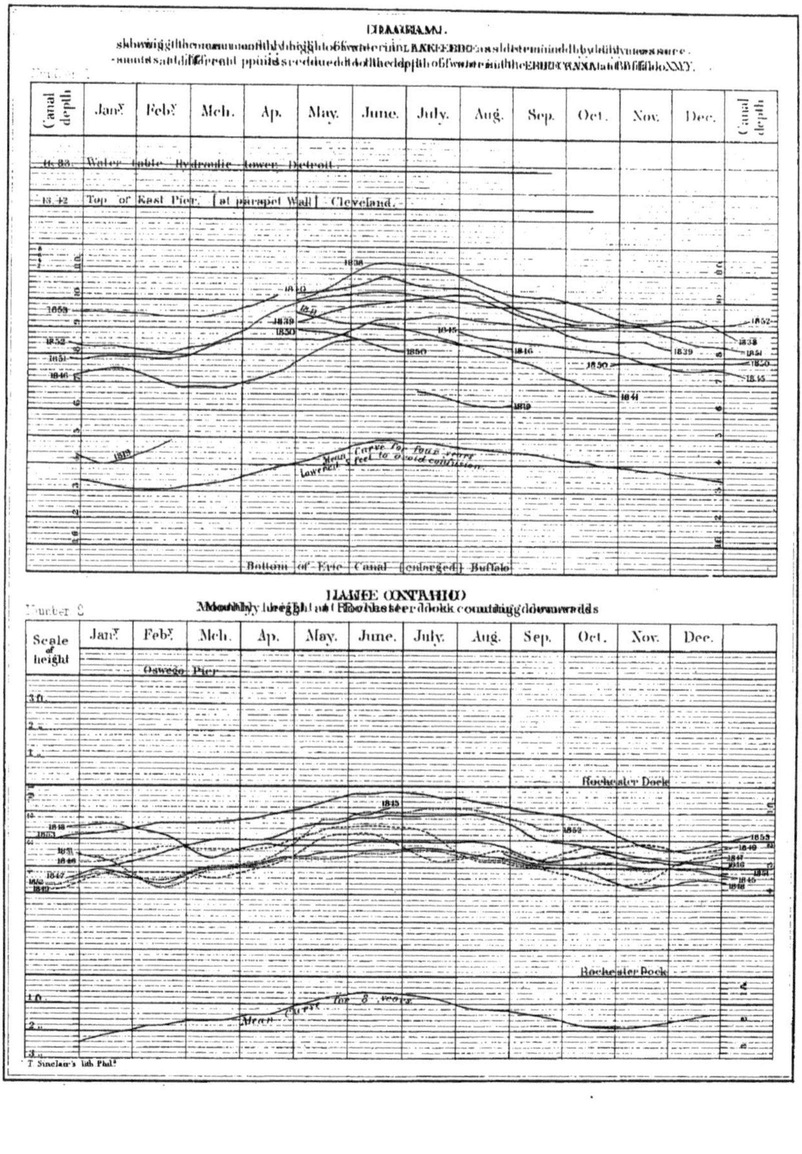

DIAGRAM,

showing the mean monthly height of water in LAKE ERIE as determined by the measurements at different points reduced to the depth of water in the ERIE CANAL at Buffalo N.Y.

Canal depth	Jan.y	Feb.y	Mch.	Ap.	May.	June.	July.	Aug.	Sep.	Oct.	Nov.	Dec.	Canal depth

11.83. Water table Hydraulic tower. Detroit.

13.42 Top of East Pier. [at parapet Wall] Cleveland.

Mean Curve for four years Lowered 3 feet to avoid confusion.

Bottom of Erie Canal (enlarged) Buffalo

LAKE ONTARIO

Number 2

Monthly height at Rochester dock counting downwards

Scale of height	Jan.y	Feb.y	Mch.	Ap.	May.	June.	July.	Aug.	Sep.	Oct.	Nov.	Dec.

Oswego Pier

Rochester Dock

Rochester Dock

Mean Curve for 8 years

T. Sinclair's lith Phil.a

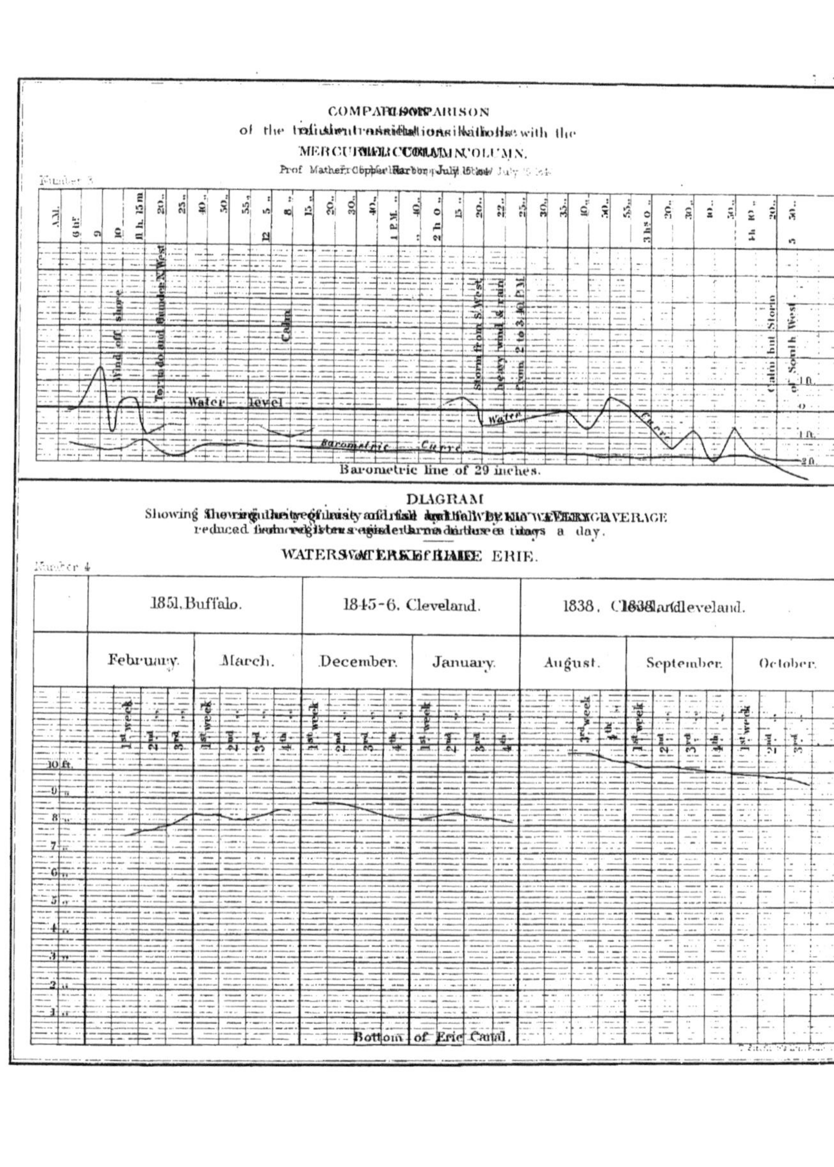

COMPARISON
MERCURIAL COLUMN.
Prof Mather, Copper Harbor, July 15th
Wind off shore
Calm
Storm from S. West
heavy wind & rain
from 2 to 3.40 P.M.
Calm but Storm
of South West
Water level
Water Curve
Barometric Curve
Barometric line of 29 inches.
DIAGRAM
WATERS OF LAKE ERIE.
1851, Buffalo.
1845-6. Cleveland.
1838, Cleveland.
February.
March.
December.
January.
August.
September.
October.
Bottom of Erie Canal.

SMITHSONIAN CONTRIBUTIONS TO KNOWLEDGE.

METEOROLOGICAL OBSERVATIONS

MADE AT

PROVIDENCE, R. I.

EXTENDING OVER A PERIOD OF TWENTY-EIGHT YEARS AND A HALF, FROM DECEMBER 1831 TO MAY 1860.

BY

ALEXIS CASWELL,
PROFESSOR OF NATURAL PHILOSOPHY AND ASTRONOMY IN BROWN UNIVERSITY, PROVIDENCE, RHODE ISLAND.

[ACCEPTED FOR PUBLICATION, AUGUST, 1859.]

ERRATA.

Year 1831,	page	1, December,	Amount of rain	*for*	blank	*read*	1.95 in.
" 1832,	"	1, February,	Mean temp. 1 P. M.	"	34°.2	"	32°.4
" 1832,	"	4, December,	Extreme range temp.	"	48°	"	40°
" 1834,	"	9, Sept. 5,	Daily mean thermometer	"	73°.3	"	73°.5
" 1834,	"	10, December,	Barom. mean of month	"	30.993	"	30.093
" 1835,	"	12, April,	Mean temp. of month	"	41°.1	"	42°.5
" 1835,	"	12, May,	Mean temp. of month	"	54°.9	"	54°.5
" 1835,	"	13, June,	Extreme range temp.	"	30°	"	35°
" 1835,	"	15, October 10,	Daily mean thermometer	"	47°.3	"	49°.3
" 1837,	"	23, March,	Max. temp. 1 P. M.	"	49°	"	51°
" 1837,	"	26, August,	Extreme range temp.	"	35°	"	37°
" 1837,	"	26, September,	Mean temp. for month	"	58°.5	"	58°.1
" 1837,	"	26, September,	Extreme range temp.	"	42°	"	43°
" 1838,	"	32, September,	Mean temp. of month	"	61°.4	"	62°.0
" 1839,	"	35, February,	Barom. mean of month	"	29.390	"	30.043
" 1839,	"	37, June,	Extreme range temp.	"	36°	"	38°
" 1840,	"	40, January,	Max. temp. 1 P. M.	"	38°	"	40°
" 1840,	"	43, June,	Mean temp. of month	"	66°.3	"	66°.6
" 1841,	"	49, July,	Mean temp. of month	"	70°.0	"	70°.3
" 1841,	"	51, October,	Extreme range temp.	"	31°	"	42°
" 1842,	"	58, December,	Barom. mean of month	"	20.980	"	29.980
" 1843,	"	62, September,	Barom. mean of month	"	20.977	"	29.977
" 1844,	"	64, January,	Extreme range temp.	"	45°	"	47°
" 1844,	"	66, April,	Mean temp. 1 P. M.	"	60°.1	"	60°.9
" 1844,	"	67, July,	Extreme range temp.	"	26°	"	28°
" 1844,	"	69, October,	Mean temp. of month	"	49°.8	"	50°.0
" 1845,	"	70, January,	Mean temp. 10 P. M.	"	30°.7	"	29°.0
" 1845,	"	70, January,	Mean temp. 1 P. M.	"	84°.4	"	34°.7
" 1847,	"	83, February,	Max. temp. 1 P. M.	"	57°	"	51°
" 1849,	"	99, October,	Barom. mean at sunrise	"	25.97	"	29.97
" 1853,	"	119, March,	Red. barom. mean 1 P. M.	"	99.80	"	29.80
" 1853,	"	121, June,	Red. barom. mean of month	"	35.027	"	30.027
" 1854,	"	129, October,	Red. barom. mean of month	"	30.030	"	30.090
" 1857,	"	145, July,	Extreme range temp.	"	35°.0	"	39°.0
" 1857,	"	146, August,	Extreme range temp.	"	31°.0	"	32°.0

geographical position of University Hall, as fixed by the determinations of the coast survey, is lat. 41° 50′ 17″ N., long. 71° 23′ 20″ W. from Greenwich.

The barometer used from the commencement of the register till May, 1847, was constructed with a flexible leather bottom. It was a good one of its kind, and gave average results which are probably reliable. In respect to the barometric range and the absolute heights it was probably less accurate than for mean results.

PREFACE.

In presenting the following Meteorological Observations to the public, it is proper to offer a few words of explanation.

They were commenced in December, 1831, with the hope that a careful record of the changes in the weather might be of use to myself and possibly to others in after years. As month after month passed, I found myself gradually extending my range of observation, and daily incorporating in my register a greater and greater number of phenomena. And I at length came to embrace nearly all the points which I supposed would be of special use in future meteorological researches. It was my practice for several years to publish in one of the papers of this city abstracts from my register, giving such general information as was most interesting to the public. In the American Almanac of 1850 I published summaries of the monthly mean height of the barometer, of the monthly and annual mean temperatures, and the monthly and annual quantity of rain, &c. These summaries extended from 1832 to 1848, inclusive. Similar ones have been continued in the same work to the present time.

Dr. Henry, the Secretary of the Smithsonian Institution, learning that my register extended without interruption over a period of nearly thirty years, was favorably impressed with the service which its publication might render to the progress of meteorological science, rightly judging that so long a series of observations made at the same place under the same general circumstances, and by the same person, would have a value in developing the laws of atmospheric changes which would not otherwise belong to them. The subject of their publication having been fully considered, it was determined to place them among the *Smithsonian Contributions to Knowledge.*

For the information of meteorologists who may wish to know the position of my place of observation, and the character of the instruments which I have used, I may state that my residence, where the instruments have been used, is on College Hill, a few hundred feet north of University Hall, Providence, at an elevation of a little more than a hundred and fifty feet above tide-water in the river. The geographical position of University Hall, as fixed by the determinations of the coast survey, is lat. 41° 50′ 17″ N., long. 71° 23′ 20″ W. from Greenwich.

The barometer used from the commencement of the register till May, 1847, was constructed with a flexible leather bottom. It was a good one of its kind, and gave average results which are probably reliable. In respect to the barometric range and the absolute heights it was probably less accurate than for mean results.

In May of 1847, I procured an open cistern barometer, made by Mr. William H. Temple, of Boston, with a micrometer screw for the adjustment of the surface of the mercury in the cup to an ivory point. It was similar to others which he had constructed for the use of the coast survey. The Vernier is moved by rack-work, and reads to the *one-hundredth of an inch.* The interior diameter of the tube is very nearly *three-tenths of an inch.* In the reduction of the barometric observations, no account has been taken of capillarity.

The reductions to the temperature of 32° Fahr. and to the sea-level, with the exception of the last year, were made under the direction of the Smithsonian Institution, by Prof. J. H. Coffin, of Easton, Pa. The reduction to sea-level was based upon the result of direct experiment. The barometer, when standing at or near 30.00 inches, with steady weather, was several times transferred from College Hill to the water-level, and the mean result gave for the reduction +0.18 of an inch. This is the correction which has been employed.

Several different thermometers have been used, but always the most accurate which could be obtained in this country. For the three years (since April of 1857) I have used the thermometers made by Mr. James Green, of New York, and known as the Smithsonian thermometers.

The actual times of observation have sometimes differed a little from the hours indicated at the head of the columns, although as a general practice the observations have been made very nearly at the times specified. The direction and force of the winds, and the degree of cloudiness have been determined without the aid of special instruments. From the nature of the case these observations cannot lay claim to any minute accuracy; yet it was thought desirable, and not without its utility, to make a record of the facts as they would appear in the judgment of a practiced observer.

Besides the deductions which appear on the current pages of the work, an appendix has been added, containing elaborate summaries, which it is hoped will facilitate the researches of scientific meteorologists, and thus repay in some degree the labor which has been bestowed upon them.

I may state, in conclusion, that all due care has been bestowed upon the preparation of the manuscript, and upon the correction of the proof, as the sheets have passed through the press, with a view to prevent and exclude errors. But in so large a mass of figures it is hardly possible to secure entire accuracy; and I can only hope that any errors which may have escaped notice will not be such as to mislead the inquirer.

A. CASWELL.

PROVIDENCE, *June* 6, 1860.

TABLES OF SUMMARIES.

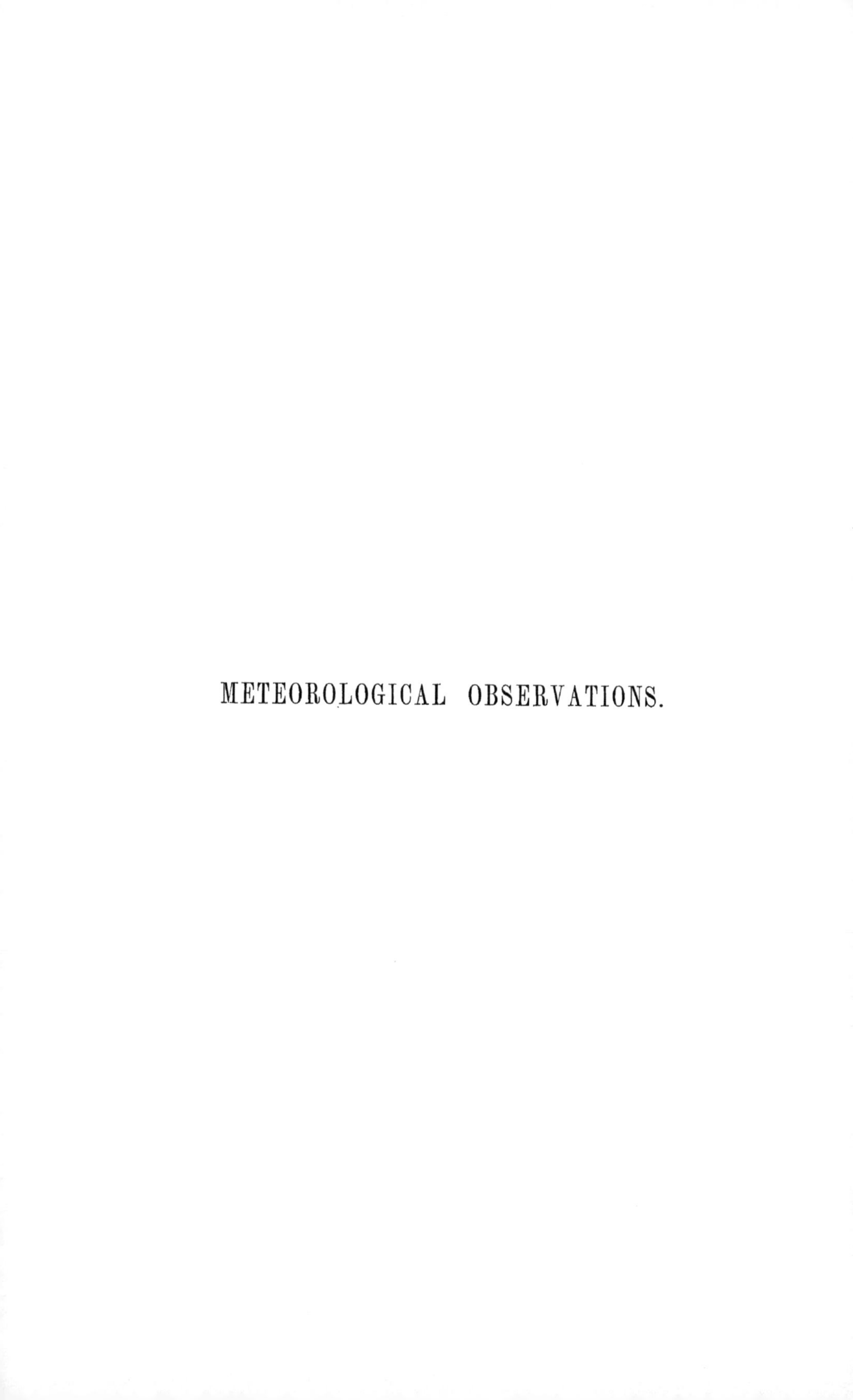

METEOROLOGICAL OBSERVATIONS.

December, 1831.

DAYS.	BAROMETER, REDUCED TO 32° F. At 7 A. M.	At 1 P. M.	At 9 P. M.	THERMOMETER. At 7 A. M.	At 1 P. M.	At 9 P. M.	Daily mean.	WINDS.	WEATHER.	RAIN AND SNOW IN INCHES OF WATER.
1	...	...	...	21	...	15	...	N. E.	Snow 2 in.	0.10
2	...	...	...	13	18	15	15.3	N. W'ly	Clear	
3	...	...	...	14	17	16	15.7	N. E.	Sn. } 3 in.	0.15
4	...	...	...	16	21	20	19.0	N. E.	Sn. }	
5	29.18	29.39	29.60	13	22	18	17.7			
6	29.88	29.83	29.90	10	22	16	16.0	W.	Clear	
7	29.95	29.93	29.92	14	24	20	19.3	W'ly		
8	29.91	29.89	29.93	10	25	15	16.7	W.	Clear	
9	29.95	29.92	30.03	18	32	19	23.0	W'ly	Cloudy	
10	30.12	30.16	30.16	15	25	18	19.3	W.	Clear	
11	30.24	30.13	29.99	13	35	31	26.3	S'ly		
12	29.90	29.92	29.99	22	25	12	19.7	N'ly	Clear	
13	29.91	29.84	29.91	8	20	10	12.7	N. W.	Clear	
14	30.06	30.11	30.20	11	21	...	...	N. W.		
15	30.11	30.04	30.03	11	16	5	10.7	N. E.	Snow 11 in.	0.55
16	30.03	29.74	29.50	4	23	28	18.3			
17	29.11	28.99	...	24	27	12	21.0	W.	Snow 1 in.	0.05
18	...	29.86	30.00	2	11	8	7.0	W.	Clear	
19	29.92	29.70	29.80	13	25	14	17.3	W'ly		
20	29.91	29.84	29.69	13	25	22	20.0	W'ly	Clear	
21	29.42	29.27	29.37	25	35	20	26.7	W.		
22	29.73	29.86	30.10	9	7	0	5.3	W.	Clear	
23	30.18	30.20	30.14	—1	17	13	9.7	S. W.	Clear	
24	29.85	29.34	29.40	23	14	34	23.7	S'ly	Sn. & rain	0.60
25	29.68	29.71	29.69	31	32	25	29.3	W'ly		
26	29.58	29.49	...	20	24	17	20.3	W'ly	Clear	
27	29.48	29.55	29.67	20	23	13	18.7	W'ly	Clear	
28	29.66	29.50	...	11	25	22	19.3	N. E.	Snow 7½ in.	0.40
29	29.47	29.31	29.35	22	28	25	25.0	N. E.	Cloudy	
30	29.48	29.59	29.78	18	19	12	16.3	N. W.	Clear	
31	29.88	29.85	29.66	4	24	30	19.3	N'ly	Snow 2 in.	0.10
Means	29.79	29.74	29.83	14.4	22.7	17.5				
REDUCED TO SEA LEVEL.										
Max.	30.42	30.38	30.38	31	35	34	29.3			
Min.	29.36	29.17	29.53	—1	7	0	5.3			
Mean	29.97	29.92	30.01							
Range	1.06	1.21	0.85	32	28	34	24.0			
Mean of month			29.967	...	...	...	18.20	...	Rain	0.58
Extreme range			1.25	...	...	...	36.00	...	Snow	0.85

January, 1832.

DAYS.	At 7 A. M.	At 1 P. M.	At 9 P. M.	At 7 A. M.	At 1 P. M.	At 9 P. M.	Daily mean.	WINDS.	WEATHER.	RAIN AND SNOW.
1	29.60	...	29.76	17	...	16	...	N. W.	Variable	
2	29.92	29.94	29.97	8	27	17	17.3	W'ly		
3	28.73	29.64	29.83	22	35	24	27.0		Sn. & rain	
4	30.09	30.11	30.08	6	26	15	15.7	W'ly	Variable	
5	29.94	29.83	29.85	22	36	35	31.0	S'ly	Variable	
6	29.87	29.52	29.66	34	43	40	39.0	S. W'ly	Rain	0.50
7	29.90	29.96	30.05	26	28	22	25.3	N'ly	Clear	
8	30.02	29.94	29.56	14	28	33	25.0	S. E'ly	Rain	1.50
9	28.93	29.24	29.48	37	44	34	38.3	W'ly	Clear	
10	29.56	29.53	29.47	26	38	32	32.0	S'ly	Clear	
11	29.36	29.29	29.41	31	33	22	28.7	N'ly	Snow 1 in.	0.05
12	29.63	29.72	29.84	13	20	20	17.7	W'ly	Clear	
13	29.82	29.72	29.85	20	38	34	30.7	W'ly	Clear	
14	30.00	30.06	30.09	26	40	28	31.3	W'ly	Clear	
15	30.07	30.06	30.05	27	50	36	37.7	W'ly	Clear	
16	30.04	30.03	30.04	36	52	29	42.3	W'ly	Clear	
17	30.05	30.04	30.02	32	46	34	37.3	S. W.	Clear	
18	29.86	29.75	29.71	36	49	44	43.0	S. W.	Cloudy	
19	29.55	29.54	29.69	47	54	41	47.3	W'ly	Clear	
20	29.80	29.82	29.84	35	39	35	36.3	W'ly	Cloudy	
21	29.69	29.62	29.83	31	37	26	31.3	W'ly	Snow 1½ in.	0.07
22	29.97	...	30.15	17	...	16	...	N. W.	Clear	
23	30.20	30.17	30.13	11	29	28	22.7	W'ly	Variable	
24	30.01	29.86	29.78	32	41	38	37.0	E'ly	Mist	
25	29.47	29.44	29.60	48	43	17	36.0	S. E'ly	Rain	0.60
26	29.78	29.98	30.17	—1	5	—2	0.7	N. W.	Clear	
27	30.01	30.12	30.17	—7	16	0	3.0	W'ly	Variable	
28	30.21	30.15	30.11	—4	16	16	9.3	S. W'ly	Variable	
29	30.07	30.05	30.05	18	26	22	22.0	N. E.	Snow 3 in.	0.15
30	29.86	29.67	29.47	31	37	36	34.7	E'ly	Rain	1.00
31	29.68	29.76	29.89	32	32	24	29.3	W'ly	Variable	
Means	29.79	29.81	29.84	23.3	34.8	26.5	...	...	...	3.87
REDUCED TO SEA LEVEL.										
Max.	30.39	30.35	30.35	47	54	44	47.3			
Min.	28.91	29.42	29.59	—7	5	—2	0.7			
Mean	29.97	29.99	30.02							
Range	1.48	0.93	0.76	54	49	46	44.3			
Mean of month			29.991	...	...	...	28.2			
Extreme range			1.48	...	...	...	61.0			

February, 1832.

DAYS.	BAROMETER, REDUCED TO 32° F. At 7 A. M.	At 1 P. M.	At 10 P. M.	THERMOMETER. At 7 A. M.	At 1 P. M.	At 10 P. M.	Daily mean.	WINDS.	WEATHER.	RAIN AND SNOW IN INCHES OF WATER.
1	30.03	30.09	30.10	18	28	26	24.0	W'ly	Variable	
2	29.93	29.76	29.71	30	44	41	38.3	W'ly	Variable	
3	29.66	29.68	29.67	42	57	41	46.7	W'ly	Variable	
4	29.68	29.72	29.72	34	36	32	34.0	N. E'ly	Sn. & rain	0.35
5	29.62	...	29.92	27	...	11	...	N. E.	Snow 6½ in.	0.35
6	30.11	30.06	29.85	—1	19	20	12.7	W'ly	Var. snow	
7	29.71	29.82	30.03	27	32	20	26.3	W'ly	Clear	
8	30.13	30.11	30.13	16	22	18	18.7	N. E.	Variable	
9	30.02	29.94	29.68	22	26	17	21.7	N. E.	Snow 7 in.	0.40
10	29.72	29.86	30.04	13	30	16	19.7	W'ly	Clear	
11	30.23	30.19	29.98	14	32	32	26.0	S. E'ly	Variable	
12	29.64	29.54	29.41	42	45	48	45.0	S. W'ly	Rain	0.75
13	29.66	29.92	30.18	36	35	28	33.0	W'ly	Variable	
14	30.29	30.29	30.25	26	33	31	30.0	N. E.	Snow ¼ in.	
15	30.08	30.01	30.09	32	36	32	33.3	N. E'ly	Mist	
16	30.22	30.27	30.32	20	20	9	16.3	N'ly	Variable	
17	30.33	30.19	29.89	3	20	20	14.3	W'ly	Variable	
18	29.55	29.50	29.61	28	42	34	34.7	W'ly	Variable	
19	29.52	29.40	29.46	32	36	34	34.0	N. E.	Rain	0.67
20	29.47	29.43	29.27	32	34	32	32.7	N. E.	Rain	1.03
21	29.47	29.60	30.00	28	23	14	21.7	N. W.	Clear	
22	30.19	30.23	30.23	10	29	27	22.0	S. W'ly	Clear	
23	30.08	29.84	29.81	32	36	31	33.0	S. W.	Rain	0.32
24	30.19	30.34	30.40	6	10	4	6.7	N. W.	Clear	
25	30.33	30.43	29.86	8	25	28	20.3	N. E.	Rain	0.28
26	29.87	29.82	29.85	28	40	30	32.7	W'ly	Variable	
27	29.98	29.98	29.94	22	37	30	29.7	W'ly	Clear	
28	29.87	29.69	29.64	32	36	33	33.7	S. W'ly	Sn. & rain	0.10
29	29.72	29.81	29.97	35	44	31	36.7	W.	Clear	
Means	29.91	29.91	29.90	23.9	34.2	26.5	...	...	...	4.25
REDUCED TO SEA LEVEL.										
Max.	30.51	30.61	30.58	42	57	48	46.7			
Min.	29.65	29.58	29.45	—1	10	4	6.7			
Mean	30.09	30.09	30.18							
Range	0.86	1.03	1.13	43	47	44	40.0			
Mean of month			30.087	...	...	...	27.6			
Extreme range			1.16	...	...	...	58.0			

March, 1832.

DAYS.	At 6 A. M.	At 1 P. M.	At 10 P. M.	At 6 A. M.	At 1 P. M.	At 10 P. M.	Daily mean.	WINDS.	WEATHER.	RAIN AND SNOW.
1	30.15	30.16	30.22	20	33	24	25.7	W.	Clear	
2	30.24	30.21	29.99	17	34	30	27.0	S. W	Variable	
3	29.69	29.61	29.81	36	48	34	39.3	W'ly	Variable	
4	29.86	...	...	29	...	...	...	W.	Clear	
5	29.71	29.54	29.39	34	41	42	39.0	S. E'ly	Rain	1.50
6	29.27	29.24	29.29	40	41	37	39.3	N. W.	Cloudy	
7	29.44	29.50	29.66	30	35	24	29.7	N. W.	Clear	
8	29.91	29.86	29.84	20	41	38	33.0	S. W.	Variable	
9	26.89	29.84	29.80	35	59	44	46.0	S. W.	Variable	
10	29.84	29.90	30.06	45	63	44	50.7	W'ly	Clear	
11	30.10	30.02	29.91	38	52	45	45.0	N. E.	Cloudy	
12	29.68	29.49	29.31	46	56	44	48.7	S'ly	Rain	0.65
13	29.23	29.31	29.30	45	54	39	46.0	N. W.	Clear	
14	29.42	29.55	29.80	21	24	17	20.7	N. W.	Variable	
15	30.04	30.13	30.17	12	31	25	22.7	N. W.	Clear	
16	30.17	30.11	30.06	27	44	31	34.0	N. W.	Clear	
17	29.73	29.36	29.22	35	40	37	37.3	N. E.	Rain	0.40
18	29.24	29.38	29.69	16	14	16	15.3	N. W.	Snow	0.05
19	29.86	29.92	29.98	12	26	20	19.3	N. W.	Clear	
20	29.98	29.87	29.68	16	40	35	30.3	S. W.	Variable	
21	29.36	29.23	29.41	40	42	32	38.0	S. W.	Rain	0.30
22	29.47	29.56	29.74	22	30	22	24.7	N. W.	Variable	
23	29.81	29.87	29.82	19	39	34	30.7	N. W.	Clear	
24	29.78	29.70	29.94	37	62	48	49.0	W.	Clear	
25	29.78	29.77	29.70	40	56	51	48.7	S. W.	Variable	
26	29.65	29.58	29.69	50	57	34	47.0	S. W.	Rain	0.30
27	29.89	29.98	30.05	24	37	28	39.7	N. W.	Clear	
28	30.07	30.04	30.00	24	40	32	32.0	S. W'ly	Clear	
29	29.96	29.97	30.10	38	38	28	34.7	N. E.	Cloudy	
30	30.17	30.13	30.03	22	43	32	32.3	N. W.	Clear	
31	29.86	29.64	29.44	33	59	49	47.0	S. W.	Variable	
Means	29.78	29.75	29.76	29.8	42.6	33.7	...	...	...	3.20
REDUCED TO SEA LEVEL.										
Max.	30.42	30.39	30.40	50	59	51	50.7			
Min.	29.41	29.41	29.40	12	14	16	15.3			
Mean	29.96	29.93	29.94							
Range	1.01	0.98	1.00	38	45	35	35.4			
Mean of month			29.943	...	...	...	35.4			
Extreme range			1.02	...	...	...	47.0			

April, 1832.

DAYS.	BAROMETER, REDUCED TO 32° F. Sun-rise.	At 1 P. M.	At 9 P. M.	THERMOMETER. Sun-rise.	At 1 P. M.	At 9 P. M.	Daily mean.	WINDS.	WEATHER.	RAIN AND SNOW IN INCHES OF WATER.
1	29.45	29.34	29.49	42	57	38	45.7	W'ly	Variable	
2	29.60	29.65	29.71	29	45	36	36.7	W'ly	Clear	
3	29.58	29.26	29.25	38	37	37	37.3	N. E.	R'n & snow	0.55
4	29.53	29.49	29.45	28	44	42	38.0	N. W.	Variable	
5	29.66	29.78	29.92	26	36	28	30.0	N. W.	Clear	
6	30.04	30.06	30.08	22	40	28	30.0	N. W.	Clear	
7	30.03	29.91	29.79	24	46	34	34.7	W.	Clear	
8	29.79	29.83	29.91	30	38	27	31.7	N. E.	Clear	
9	29.99	30.03	30.02	20	37	26	27.7	N.	Clear	
10	29.99	29.88	29.81	29	51	37	39.0	S. W.	Variable	
11	29.69	29.64	29.69	39	59	40	46.0	S. W.	Rain	0.05
12	29.69	29.61	29.53	33	56	54	47.7	S. E'ly	Variable	
13	29.50	29.47	29.42	48	74	59	60.3	W'ly	Clear	
14	29.43	...	29.59	37	...	37	...	N. E.	Variable	
15	29.62	29.75	29.79	36	40	36	37.3	N. E.	Cloudy	
16	29.76	29.69	29.68	36	44	36	38.7	N. E.	Cloudy	
17	29.59	29.56	29.58	38	38	38	38.0	N. E.	Rain	1.75
18	29.58	29.63	29.66	35	34	34	34.3	N. E.	Rain	0.20
19	29.61	29.62	29.61	34	35	33	34.0	N. E.	Rain	0.12
20	29.56	29.57	29.62	33	37	33	34.3	N. E.	Rain	0.04
21	29.62	29.59	29.55	33	52	45	43.3	N. W.	Cloudy	
22	29.70	29.74	29.82	40	50	38	42.7	N.	Variable	
23	29.98	29.91	29.85	30	50	32	37.3	S. W.	Variable	
24	29.76	29.80	29.89	35	50	34	39.7	N. W.	Clear	
25	29.90	29.78	29.60	33	57	56	48.7	W'ly	Variable	
26	29.53	29.51	29.49	51	77	65	64.3	S. W.	Variable	
27	29.41	29.50	29.65	58	77	57	64.0	W'ly	Clear	
28	29.75	29.84	29.95	40	41	38	39.7	N. E.	Cloudy	
29	29.95	29.96	29.97	36	44	40	40.0	N. E.	Rain	0.62
30	29.95	29.90	29.81	40	46	40	42.0	N. E.	Cloudy	
Means	29.70	29.70	29.70	35.1	48.0	39.3	...	...	...	3.33
REDUCED TO SEA LEVEL.										
Max.	30.22	30.24	30.26	58	77	65	64.3			
Min.	29.59	29.44	29.43	20	34	26	27.7			
Mean	29.88	29.88	29.88							
Range	0.63	0.80	0.83	38	43	39	36.6			
Mean of month	29.885			...	...	...	40.8			
Extreme range	0.83			...	...	...	57.0			

REMARKS.

7th. Halo about the moon from 7 to 9 P. M.; inner edge well defined; radius 22°.

10th. Halo about the moon at 9 P. M.; air thick and hazy.

May, 1832.

DAYS.	Barometer Sun-rise.	At 1 P. M.	At 10 P. M.	Thermometer Sun-rise.	At 1 P. M.	At 10 P. M.	Daily mean.	Winds.	Weather.	Rain and Snow.
1	29.69	29.56	29.58	41	55	50	48.7	N. W.	Clear	
2	29.72	29.75	29.84	39	57	44	46.7	W'ly	Clear	
3	29.82	29.83	29.81	44	62	47	51.0	S. W.	Variable	
4	29.73	29.62	29.43	46	70	48	54.7	S. W.	Rain	0.45
5	29.33	29.44	29.69	45	50	45	46.7	N. E.	Rain & mist	
6	29.92	29.99	30.12	38	54	42	44.7	N. E.	Variable	
7	30.20	30.21	30.18	36	55	43	44.7	S'ly	Variable	
8	30.09	30.02	29.97	44	65	54	54.3	S. W.	Clear	
9	29.90	29.91	29.93	55	69	56	60.0	S. W.	Little rain	
10	30.06	30.13	30.22	50	64	44	52.7	N. E'ly	Clear	
11	30.23	...	30.22	40	...	44	...	S'ly	Clear	
12	30.04	30.03	29.97	40	76	59	58.3	W'ly	Clear	
13	29.93	29.89	29.89	55	82	60	65.7	W'ly	Clear	
14	29.85	29.79	29.79	58	78	60	65.3	W'ly	Variable	
15	29.73	29.65	29.59	60	66	60	62.0	S. W.	Showery	0.22
16	29.60	29.59	29.70	60	75	60	65.0	W'ly	Clear	
17	29.75	29.65	29.69	52	71	59	60.7	W.	Clear	
18	29.70	29.70	29.68	57	66	50	57.7	W'ly	Variable	
19	29.69	29.66	29.55	51	63	49	54.3	E'ly	Cloudy	
20	29.44	29.45	29.36	54	52	48	51.3	N. E.	Rain	2.25
21	29.18	29.26	29.42	54	63	51	56.0	N. W.	Clear	
22	29.49	29.55	29.74	47	47	46	46.7	W'ly	Cloudy	
23	29.83	29.82	29.82	43	56	44	47.7	N. E.	Variable	
24	29.73	29.69	29.64	42	44	38	41.3	N. E.	Rain	} 0.55
25	29.55	29.56	29.55	36	42	41	39.7	N. E.	R'n & snow	
26	29.47	29.39	29.39	44	61	50	51.7	W'ly	Variable	
27	29.30	29.31	29.47	44	44	44	44.0	N. E.	Rain	0.22
28	29.54	29.59	29.65	45	60	51	52.0	N. W.	Variable	
29	29.70	29.72	29.67	47	68	53	56.0	W'ly	Clear	
30	29.51	29.31	29.33	51	50	46	49.0	S. E.	Rain	0.45
31	29.37	29.50	29.61	50	50	44	48.0	N. E.	Rain	
Means	29.71	29.69	29.73	47.4	60.5	49.4	...	...	...	4.14
REDUCED TO SEA LEVEL.										
Max.	30.41	30.39	30.40	60	82	60	65.7			
Min.	[illegible]	[illegible]	[illegible]	[illegible]	[illegible]	[illegible]	[illegible]			
Mean	29.89	29.86	29.91							
Range	1.05	0.96	0.89	24	40	19	24.4			
Mean of month	29.887			...	...	...	52.4			
Extreme range	1.05			...	...	...	46.0			

REMARKS.

[illegible] M. of the 5th, which prevented observations [illegible] transit of mercury.

Snow on the morning of the 25th, so as to whiten the ground.

June, 1832.

DAYS.	BAROMETER, REDUCED TO 32° F. At 6 A. M.	At 1 P. M.	At 10 P. M.	THERMOMETER. At 6 A. M.	At 1 P. M.	At 10 P. M.	Daily mean.	WINDS	WEATHER.	RAIN AND SNOW IN INCHES OF WATER.
1	29.60	29.60	29.57	47	57	52	52.0	N. E.	Misty	
2	29.49	29.43	29.46	47	64	54	55.0	N. W.	Clear	
3	29.44	...	29.46	46	...	50	...	N. E.	Variable	
4	29.47	29.52	29.59	48	53	46	49.0	N. E.	Cloudy	
5	29.58	29.58	29.61	45	57	49	50.3	N. E.	Cloudy	
6	29.58	29.60	29.60	47	60	53	53.3	N. E'ly	Cloudy	
7	29.60	...	29.66	51	...	52	...	N. E'ly	Cloudy	
8	29.64	29.70	29.80	50	60	55	55.0	E'ly	Cloudy	
9	29.82	29.82	29.82	51	60	52	54.3	S. E.	Variable	
10 •	29.78	29.79	29.82	50	64	52	55.3	S. W.	Va'ble, sh.	0.08
11	29.79	29.76	29.73	52	67	56	58.3	S. E.	Variable	
12	29.72	29.67	29.78	55	85	68	69.3	W'ly	Clear	
13	29.85	...	29.89	59	...	56	...	N. E.	Variable	
14	29.80	29.66	29.59	54	72	65	63.7	W'ly	Clear	
15	29.56	29.48	29.49	63	86	75	74.4	W'ly	Variable	
16	29.48	29.40	29.40	62	88	77	75.7	W'ly	Clear, sh.	0.05
17	29.39	29.36	29.52	72	87	70	76.3	W'ly	Clear	
18	29.54	29.49	29.38	64	74	66	68.0	W.	Clear, sh.	0.20
19	29.50	29.59	29.76	60	64	56	60.0	W'ly	Variable	
20	29.86	29.87	29.90	46	68	58	57.3	W'ly	Clear	
21	29.95	29.98	29.96	54	76	60	63.3	S. W.	Clear	
22	29.95	29.85	29.84	56	76	59	63.4	S. W.	Clear	
23	29.74	29.68	29.71	57	81	69	69.0	N. W.	Clear	
24	29.82	...	29.82	63	...	62	...	W'ly	Clear	
25	29.79	29.73	29.75	63	84	67	71.3	W'ly	Clear	
26	29.74	29.69	29.67	63	83	66	70.7	W'ly	Clear	
27	29.58	29.48	29.46	65	72	68	68.3	S. W.	Cloudy	
28	29.46	29.53	29.69	66	77	62	68.3	W'ly	Clear	
29	29.82	...	29.91	53	...	64	...	W'ly	Clear	
30	29.96	29.93	29.88	57	80	62	66.9	S. W.	Clear	
Means	29.68	29.65	29.68	55.5	71.8	60.0	...	...	...	0.33
REDUCED TO SEA LEVEL.										
Max.	30.14	30.17	30.14	66	88	77	76.3			
Min.	29.57	29.54	29.56	45	53	46	49.0			
Mean	29.86	29.82	29.86							
Range	0.57	0.63	0.58	21	35	31	27.3			
Mean of month	29.847			...	...	...	62.4			
Extreme range	0.63			...	...	...	43.0			

REMARK.

Shower, with thunder and lightning on the afternoon of the 16th; also on afternoon of 18th.

July, 1832.

DAYS.	Barometer Sun-rise.	At 1 P. M.	At 10 P. M.	Thermometer Sun-rise.	At 1 P. M.	At 10 P. M.	Daily mean.	Winds.	Weather.	Rain and Snow.
1	29.81	29.77	29.75	61	81	76	72.7	W'ly	Clear	
2	29.73	29.67	29.56	70	89	72	77.0	W'ly	Clear	
3	29.54	29.48	29.50	69	86	73	76.0	W'ly	Clear	
4	29.68	29.68	29.75	63	86	66	71.7	N'ly	Clear	
5	29.80	29.82	29.79	60	74	62	65.3	S'ly	Clear	
6	29.74	29.79	29.78	58	80	66	68.0	S'ly	Clear	
7	29.61	29.58	29.69	63	83	57	65.7	N. E.	Variable	
8	29.66	29.60	29.63	53	70	59	60.7	N. E.	Cloudy	
9	29.58	29.56	29.51	54	59	53	55.3	N. E.	Rain	0.87
10	29.49	29.53	29.60	51	64	56	57.0	N. E.	Cloudy	
11	29.57	29.53	29.51	51	53	52	52.0	N. E.	Rain	0.60
12	29.51	29.51	29.50	51	64	58	57.7	W'ly	Va'ble, sh.	0.03
13	29.44	29.42	29.47	54	68	59	60.3	W'ly	Variable	
14	29.51	29.56	29.67	51	68	58	59.0	W'ly	Variable	
15	29.74	29.75	29.81	53	72	60	61.7	W'ly	Clear	
16	29.82	...	...	52	...	...	...	W'ly	Clear	
17	...	29.82	29.86	...	77	64	(70.5)	W'ly	Va'ble, sh.	0.20
18	29.86	29.81	29.72	62	80	68	70.0	S. W.	Clear	
19	29.68	29.51	29.43	65	80	70	71.7	W'ly	Clear	
20	29.40	29.38	29.41	64	80	69	71.0	W'ly	Clear	
21	29.38	29.30	29.44	64	77	61	67.3	W'ly	Variable	
22	29.60	29.65	29.77	61	71	63	65.0	N'ly	Clear	
23	29.69	29.83	29.86	57	76	64	65.7	N'ly	Clear	
24	29.84	29.79	29.69	59	74	65	66.0	S'ly	Clear	
25	29.59	29.49	29.48	62	78	65	68.3	S'ly	Va'ble, sh.	0.05
26	29.47	29.47	29.52	60	76	64	66.7	W'ly	Clear	
27	29.65	29.72	29.80	59	76	66	67.0	W'ly	Clear	
28	29.83	29.83	29.84	58	82	65	68.3	W'ly	Clear	
29	29.78	...	28.74	64	...	68	...	W'ly	Clear	
30	29.68	...	29.74	67	...	70	...	W'ly	Variable	
31	29.75	29.77	29.82	70	79	72	73.7	W'ly	Va'ble, sh.	0.07
Means	29.65	29.63	29.65	59.2	70.1	64.0	...	...	...	1.82
REDUCED TO SEA LEVEL.										
Max.	30.04	30.01	30.04	70	89	76	77.0			
Min.	29.56	29.48	29.59	51	53	52	52.0			
Mean	[illegible]	[illegible]	[illegible]							
Range	0.48	0.53	0.45	19	36	24	25.0			
Mean of month	29.923			...	...	...	64.4			
Extreme range	0.56			...	...	...	38.0			

REMARK.

Very clear during solar eclipse of the 27th.

August, 1832.

DAYS.	BAROMETER, REDUCED TO 32° F. Sunrise.	At 1 P. M.	At 10 P. M.	THERMOMETER. Sunrise.	At 1 P. M.	At 10 P. M.	Daily mean.	WINDS.	WEATHER.	RAIN AND SNOW IN INCHES OF WATER.
1	29.86	29.85	29.84	70	80	66	72.0	W'ly	Va'ble, sh.	
2	29.85	29.87	29.87	64	84	70	72.7	W'ly	Variable	
3	29.88	29.82	29.77	64	80	70	71.3	W'ly	Clear	
4	29.78	29.72	29.72	66	84	75	72.7	W'ly	Variable	
5	29.71	29.72	29.76	74	82	71	75.7	S. W'ly	Va'ble, rn.	0.44
6	29.82	29.82	29.88	71	82	69	74.0	W'ly	Va'ble, rn.	0.21
7	29.82	29.80	29.73	71	82	73	75.3	S. W.	Variable	
8	29.63	29.62	29.58	72	82	73	75.7	S. W'ly	Va'ble, rn.	0.11
9	29.57	29.58	29.55	71	75	69	71.7	S. W'ly	Rain	1.52
10	29.35	29.50	29.67	66	78	68	70.7	W'ly	Va'ble, sh.	0.03
11	29.81	29.89	29.95	60	76	65	67.0	N. W.	Clear	
12	29.99	29.97	29.96	61	75	69	68.3	S. W.	Clear	
13	29.98	29.96	29.93	69	83	70	74.0	S. W.	Clear	
14	29.91	29.82	29.82	69	84	73	75.3	S. W.	Clear	
15	29.79	29.71	29.61	71	84	75	76.7	S. W.	Clear	
16	29.58	29.69	29.74	73	66	62	67.0	N. E.	Cloudy, rn.	0.10
17	29.65	29.80	29.89	56	59	56	57.0	N. E.	Rain	0.58
18	29.92	29.94	29.92	51	70	60	60.0	E'ly	Clear	
19	29.80	29.65	29.63	60	71	57	62.7	S. W.	Rain	0.81
20	29.75	29.85	29.93	55	73	63	63.7	N. W.	Clear	
21	29.91	29.84	29.80	62	75	64	67.0	S. W'ly	Variable	
22	29.73	29.68	29.60	60	75	70	68.3	S. W'ly	Va'ble, sh.	0.03
23	29.59	29.58	29.61	67	80	71	72.7	W'ly	Clear	
24	29.64	29.61	29.64	63	76	59	66.0	W'ly	Clear, sh.	0.05
25	29.75	29.74	29.80	47	60	49	55.3	N. W.	Clear	
26	29.81	29.75	29.73	46	68	61	58.3	N. W.	Clear	
27	29.72	29.70	29.74	54	78	62	64.7	N. W.	Clear	
28	29.79	29.79	29.79	60	71	63	64.7	N. W.	Clear	
29	29.84	29.83	29.85	63	76	64	67.7	W'ly	Clear	
30	29.87	29.88	29.83	62	77	66	68.3	S. W.	Clear	
31	29.78	29.68	29.66	65	74	59	66.0	S. W.	Cloudy, sh.	0.04
Means	29.76	29.75	29.76	63.2	76.1	65.9	...	...	...	3.92
REDUCED TO SEA LEVEL.										
Max.	30.17	30.15	30.14	74	84	75	76.7			
Min.	29.53	29.68	29.73	46	59	57	55.3			
Mean	29.94	29.93	29.94							
Range	0.64	0.47	0.41	28	25	18	21.4			
Mean of month	29.937			...	...	...	68.4			
Extreme range	0.64			...	...	...	38.0			

September, 1832.

DAYS.	Sunrise.	At 1 P. M.	At 10 P. M.	Sunrise.	At 1 P. M.	At 10 P. M.	Daily mean.	WINDS.	WEATHER.	RAIN.
1	29.68	29.74	29.80	59	65	54	59.3	N'ly	Cloudy	
2	29.85	29.82	29.83	52	69	58	59.7	N. W.	Clear	
3	29.82	29.81	29.79	53	72	60	61.7	W'ly	Clear	
4	29.75	29.69	29.51	60	63	65	62.7	S. W.	Rain	0.80
5	29.44	29.49	29.60	65	69	54	61.3	W'ly	Clear	
6	29.63	29.60	29.66	51	64	55	56.7	N. W.	Clear	
7	29.67	29.60	29.60	52	70	64	62.0	S. W.	Clear	
8	29.74	29.75	29.75	58	71	59	62.7	S. W.	Clear	
9	29.76	29.81	29.93	58	67	54	59.7	W'ly	Clear	
10	30.05	30.04	30.00	45	65	53	54.3	W'ly	Clear	
11	29.94	39.81	29.64	53	70	64	62.3	S. W.	Clear, rain	0.40
12	29.52	29.60	29.77	63	71	52	62.0	N. W.	Clear	
13	29.86	29.90	29.94	44	64	47	51.7	N. W.	Clear	
14	29.99	29.92	29.91	42	63	52	52.3	W'ly	Clear	
15	29.88	29.82	29.80	52	72	60	61.3	S. W.	Clear	
16	29.73	29.74	29.79	58	75	62	65.0	S. W.	Clear	
17	29.85	29.92	30.01	59	74	60	64.3	S'ly	Clear	
18	30.07	30.01	...	54	72	62	62.7	S'ly	Clear	
19	29.92	29.85	29.82	60	80	69	69.7	S. W.	Clear	
20	29.78	29.74	29.73	63	77	63	67.7	S. W'ly	Clear	
21	29.69	29.52	29.45	63	66	66	65.0	S. E.	Rain	0.79
22	29.56	29.50	29.55	66	70	58	64.7	S. W.	Rain	0.06
23	29.73	29.77	29.85	50	66	50	55.3	N. W.	Clear	
24	29.88	29.83	29.71	44	62	56	54.0	S. W'ly	Variable	
25	29.54	29.47	29.68	55	58	53	55.3	S. W.	Rain	0.40
26	29.82	29.82	29.82	44	62	53	53.0	W'ly	Clear	
27	29.84	29.82	29.84	48	68	59	58.3	W'ly	Clear	
28	29.84	29.83	29.83	59	70	58	62.3	S. W.	Clear	
29	29.76	29.64	29.53	57	61	59	59.0	N. E.	Rain	1.05
30	29.50	29.52	29.60	57	63	62	60.7	N. E.	Cloudy	
Means	29.77	29.74	29.75	54.8	68.0	58.0	...	...	...	3.50
REDUCED TO SEA LEVEL.										
Max.	30.25	30.22	30.19	66	80	69	69.7			
Min.	29.62	29.65	29.63	42	61	47	51.7			
Mean	29.95	29.92	29.93							
Range	0.63	0.57	0.56	24	19	22	18.0			
Mean of month	29.933			...	...	...	60.3			
Extreme range	0.63			...	...	...	38.0			

REMARK.

Frost in the vicinity on the 14th.

October, 1832.

DAYS.	BAROMETER, REDUCED TO 32° F. Sunrise.	At 1 P. M.	At 10 P. M.	THERMOMETER. Sunrise.	At 1 P. M.	At 10 P. M.	Daily mean.	WINDS.	WEATHER.	RAIN AND SNOW IN INCHES OF WATER.
1	29.58	29.54	29.43	61	63	62	62.0	S. E.	Rain	0.63
2	29.41	29.45	29.46	56	65	55	58.7	S. W.	Clear	
3	29.46	29.51	29.53	48	60	53	52.3	W'ly	Clear	
4	29.56	29.55	29.59	48	63	58	56.3	W'ly	Clear	
5	29.71	29.71	29.70	47	65	56	56.0	S. W.	Variable	
6	29.71	29.69	29.65	47	62	50	53.0	E'ly	Variable	
7	29.65	29.67	29.75	46	61	54	53.7	N. E.	Clear	
8	29.86	29.88	29.99	52	60	51	54.3	N. E.	Variable	
9	30.07	30.08	29.99	40	60	50	50.0	N. E.	Clear	
10	29.99	29.86	29.70	50	64	64	59.3	S. W.	Cloudy	
11	29.54	29.50	29.64	63	63	53	59.7	S. W.	Rain	0.38
12	29.77	29.81	29.86	48	63	50	53.7	W'ly	Clear	
13	29.87	29.83	29.81	48	67	57	57.3	W'ly	Clear	
14	29.77	29.74	29.95	57	55	43	51.7	W'ly	Variable	
15	30.13	30.14	30.15	34	56	38	42.7	W'ly	Clear	
16	30.13	30.05	30.03	34	56	47	45.7	S. W.	Clear	
17	29.98	29.88	29.86	48	63	57	56.0	S. W.	Clear	
18	29.72	29.77	29.84	53	73	62	62.7	S. W.	Clear	
19	30.16	30.16	29.98	50	55	52	52.3	N. E.	Cloudy	
20	29.82	29.76	29.62	56	70	63	63.0	S. W.	Variable	
21	29.74	29.85	29.98	55	59	46	53.3	N'ly	Clear	
22	30.06	30.02	29.73	43	46	43	44.0	N. E.	Rain	1.00
23	29.46	29.45	29.60	53	57	46	52.0	W'ly	Variable	
24	29.77	29.77	29.78	37	57	45	46.3	N'ly	Variable	
25	29.75	29.74	29.91	41	53	38	44.0	N'ly	Variable	
26	30.17	30.20	30.24	28	40	32	33.3	N'ly	Clear	
27	30.16	30.00	29.91	29	52	46	42.3	S. W.	Variable	
28	29.92	29.95	30.01	38	42	38	39.3	N'ly	Variable	
29	30.05	30.05	30.08	32	51	40	41.0	N. W.	Clear	
30	30.13	30.08	30.09	38	59	42	46.3	N. W.	Clear	
31	30 06	29.98	29.93	41	63	46	50.0	W'ly	Clear	
Means	29.84	29.82	29.83	45.8	58.8	49.6	...	...	...	2.01
REDUCED TO SEA LEVEL.										
Max.	30.35	30.38	30.42	63	73	64	63.0			
Min.	29.58	29.63	29.61	28	40	32	33.3			
Mean	30.02	30.00	30.01							
Range	0.77	0.75	0.81	35	33	32	29.7			
Mean of month	30.010			...	...	...	51.4			
Extreme range	0.84			...	...	...	45.0			

REMARKS.

First white frost on College Hill on the 15th.

Ice one-fourth of an inch thick on the 26th.

November, 1832.

DAYS.	Sunrise.	At 1 P. M.	At 10 P. M.	Sunrise.	At 1 P. M.	At 10 P. M.	Daily mean.	WINDS.	WEATHER.	RAIN.
1	29.87	29.74	29.68	40	66	54	53.3	S. W.	Clear	
2	29.58	29.64	29.82	54	58	46	52.7	N. W.	Clear	
3	29.94	29.95	29.97	37	54	40	43.7	W.	Clear	
4	29.88	29.80	29.77	39	56	55	50.0	S. W.	Cloudy, r'n	0.07
5	29.76	29.78	29.89	51	63	49	54.3	S. W.	Variable	
6	29.90	29.84	29.69	39	43	43	41.7	N. E.	Rain	0.60
7	29.56	29.58	29.74	43	49	39	43.7	N. W.	Variable	
8	29.87	29.86	29.86	33	39	29	33.7	N. W.	Clear	
9	29.79	29.65	29.58	24	40	34	32.7	N. W.	Clear	
10	29.47	29.51	29.53	38	49	38	41.7	S. W.	Clear	
11	29.53	29.50	29.67	42	54	40	45.3	W'ly	Clear	
12	29.72	29.67	29.64	32	49	42	41.0	W'ly	Clear	
13	29.56	29.42	29.34	43	55	48	48.7	S'ly	Clear	
14	29.52	29.60	29.76	36	37	24	32.3	N. W.	Clear	
15	29.86	29.92	30.08	23	32	22	25.7	N. W.	Clear	
16	30.19	30.17	30.18	18	40	32	30.0	S. W.	Clear	
17	30.17	30.10	29.89	33	50	48	43.7	S'ly	Variable	
18	29.65	29.56	29.60	62	63	55	60.0	S. W.	Rain	1.64
19	29.64	29.60	29.48	52	57	51	53.3	S. W.	Cloudy	
20	29.30	29.43	29.83	50	41	35	42.0	W.	Clear	
21	30.08	30.15	30.07	23	34	33	30.0	N. E.	Clear	
22	29.96	29.75	29.38	39	44	38	40.3	N. E.	Rain	1.15
23	29.39	29.48	29.55	36	44	40	40.0	S. W.	Clear	
24	29.55	29.55	29.57	36	42	34	37.3	S. W.	Variable	
25	29.86	29.95	30.02	28	36	31	31.7	W'ly	Clear	
26	29.98	29.84	29.74	37	52	50	46.3	W'ly	Variable	
27	29.61	29.57	29.68	51	56	44	50.3	S. W.	Cloudy	
28	29.74	29.70	29.74	43	48	40	43.7	W.	Clear	
29	29.82	29.78	29.88	38	48	35	40.3	W'ly	Clear	
30	29.91	29.69	29.53	32	38	35	35.0	N. E.	Rain	
Means	29.75	29.73	29.74	37.2	46.4	38.8	...	...	...	3.46
REDUCED TO SEA LEVEL.										
Max.	30.37	30.35	30.36	62	66	55	60.0			
Min.	29.48	29.60	29.34	18	32	22	25.7			
Mean	29.93	29.91	29.92							
Range	0.89	0.75	1.02	44	34	33	34.3			
Mean of month	29.920			...	...	...	40.8			
Extreme range	1. 03			...	...	...	48.0			

REMARK.

Bright aurora on the night of the 27th.

December, 1832.

Days.	Barometer, reduced to 32° F. Sun-rise	At 1 P. M.	At 10 P. M.	Thermometer. Sun-rise.	At 1 P. M.	At 10 P. M.	Daily mean.	Winds	Weather.	Rain and Snow in Inches of Water.
1	29.35	29.37	29.74	28	26	21	25.0	N. E.	Snow	0.05
2	29.92	29.97	29.94	13	25	23	20.3	W'ly	Clear	
3	29.76	29.60	29.31	26	35	39	33.3	N. E.	Rain	1.80
4	29.34	29.50	29.72	35	40	23	32.7	W'ly	Variable	
5	30.05	30.16	30.30	20	31	20	23.7	N. W.	Clear	
6	30.26	30.16	30.16	22	37	37	32.0	W.	Clear	
7	30.30	30.26	30.17	29	35	33	32.3	N. E.	Variable	
8	29.90	29.81	29.56	43	51	48	47.3	S'ly	Rain }	2.14
9	29.25	29.15	29.48	50	42	38	43.3	N'ly	Rain }	
10	29.74	29.83	29.96	36	44	35	38.3	W'ly	Clear	
11	29.96	29.87	29.75	30	46	40	38.7	S. W.	Variable	
12	29.50	29.47	29.64	40	41	29	36.7	N. E.	Rain	0.33
13	29.80	29.95	30.00	22	25	26	24.3	N.	Cloudy	
14	29.92	29.93	29.83	28	35	39	34.0	W'ly	Mist	
15	29.73	29.62	29.60	38	39	35	37.3	N. E.	Rain	0.15
16	29.75	29.81	29.84	27	30	30	29.0	N.	Cloudy	
17	29.65	29.30	28.75	35	41	35	37.0	N. E.	Rain	0.73
18	28.72	28.77	28.94	35	38	36	36.3	W'ly	Variable	
19	29.03	29.08	29.23	31	35	29	31.7	W'ly	Variable	
20	29.34	29.40	29.54	25	32	24	27.0	W'ly	Clear	
21	29.54	29.50	29.58	19	30	17	22.0	W'ly	Variable	
22	29.70	29.70	29.73	14	20	15	16.3	N. W.	Clear	
23	29.94	30.00	30.01	11	24	21	18.7	N. W.	Variable	
24	30.02	30.00	29.97	19	30	34	27.7	N. W.	Clear	
25	29.87	29.87	30.00	34	39	29	34.0	W.	Clear	
26	30.12	30.11	30.00	24	35	32	30.3	N. E.	Cloudy	
27	29.70	29.47	29.50	34	32	33	33.0	N'ly	Rain	0.43
28	29.61	29.70	29.90	33	34	25	30.7	W'ly	Clear	
29	29.91	29.96	30.28	24	26	18	22.7	W.	Clear	
30	30.43	30.44	30.42	13	28	27	22.7	W'ly	Clear	
31	30.30	30.20	30.15	36	45	45	42.0	W'ly	Variable	
Means	29.75	29.74	29.77	28.2	34.5	30.2	...	...	...	5.63
REDUCED TO SEA LEVEL.										
Max.	30.61	30.62	30.60	50	51	48	47.3			
Min.	28.90	28.95	28.93	11	20	15	16.3			
Mean	29.93	29.92	29.95							
Range	1.71	1.67	1.67	39	31	33	31.0			
Mean of month	29.890			...	...	...	31.0			
Extreme range	1.72			...	...	...	48.0			

REMARK.

The general barometric mean only for this month is corrected for temperature, there being no record of the attached thermometer for the separate observations.

January, 1833.

Days.	Barometer Sun-rise.	At 1 P. M.	At 10 P. M.	Thermometer Sun-rise.	At 1 P. M.	At 10 P. M.	Daily mean.	Winds	Weather	Rain and Snow
1	29.93	29.80	29.94	49	52	46	49.0	S. W.	Rain	0.06
2	30.18	30.23	30.27	34	40	32	35.3	W.	Clear	
3	30.24	30.17	30.30	32	40	41	37.7	S. W.	Rain	0.05
4	30.05	29.94	29.90	41	59	54	51.3	S. W.	Clear	
5	29.87	29.81	29.75	51	63	53	55.7	W'ly	Clear	
6	29.70	29.52	29.52	55	61	49	55.0	W'ly	Cl'dy, spr.	
7	29.60	29.65	29.76	39	38	25	34.0	N. W.	Variable	
8	29.75	29.66	29.47	21	34	29	28.0	N. E.	Cloudy	
9	29.33	29.35	29.40	29	40	29	32.7	N. W.	Clear	
10	29.34	29.24	29.15	31	41	31	34.3	Var.	Cloudy	
11	29.25	29.41	29.73	18	15	10	14.3	N. W.	Clear	
12	29.76	29.81	29.96	12	23	14	16.3	W'ly	Clear	
13	29.94	29.85	29.76	13	29	27	23.0	S. W.	Clear	
14	29.54	29.47	29.84	20	37	19	25.3	W'ly	Clear	
15	30.04	30.05	29.81	14	23	25	20.7	W'ly	Clear	
16	29.05	29.07	29.51	47	47	28	40.7	W'ly	Snow & r'n	1.00
17	30.94	29.11	30.03	12	15	15	14.0	W'ly	Clear	
18	29.83	29.89	29.94	24	31	28	27.7	W'ly	Clear	
19	30.26	30.35	30.32	0	13	10	7.7	N. W.	Clear	
20	30.12	30.03	29.90	26	39	35	33.3	S'ly	Clear	
21	29.78	29.70	29.65	30	43	34	35.7	S'ly	Fog & mist	
22	29.66	29.71	29.80	31	36	33	33.3	N. E.	Mist	
23	29.82	29.83	29.87	35	38	33	35.3	E'ly	Mist	
24	29.80	29.73	29.52	33	37	35	35.0	E'ly	Mist	
25	29.00	29.93	29.15	34	35	32	33.7	N. W.	Clear	
26	29.41	29.58	29.82	27	27	22	25.3	W'ly	Clear	
27	29.94	29.94	29.83	22	33	30	28.3	W'ly	Clear	
28	29.68	29.74	30.02	32	35	18	28.3	W'ly	Clear	
29	30.10	30.07	29.94	19	34	32	28.3	S. W.	Clear	
30	29.66	29.56	29.52	40	50	42	44.0	S'ly	Clear	
31	29.38	29.37	29.58	27	29	13	23.0	N. E.	Snow	
Means	29.74	29.72	29.75	29.0	36.7	29.8	31.8	...	...	1.71
[illegible]										
Max.	30.44	30.53	30.50	55	63	54	[illegible]			
Min.	29.18	29.11	29.33	0	13	10	7.7			
Mean	29.92	29.90	29.93							
Range	1.26	1.42	1.17	55	50	44	48.0			
Mean of month	29.910			...	...	...	31.8			
Extreme range	1.42			...	...	...	63.0			

[illegible]

The general barometric mean only for this month is corrected for temperature, there being no record of the attached thermometer for the separate observations.

February, 1833.

Days.	Barometer, reduced to 32° F. Sun-rise.	At 1 P. M.	At 10 P. M.	Thermometer. Sun-rise.	At 1 P. M.	At 10 P. M.	Daily mean.	Winds.	Weather.	Rain and Snow in Inches of Water.
1	29.63	...	...	10	20	11	13.7	N. W.		
2	29.80	...	...	5	18	15	12.7	N. W.		
3	29.73	...	...	11	23	15	16.3	N. W.		
4	29.77	...	...	10	22	19	17.0	N. W.		
5	29.77	...	...	15	27	19	20.3	N. W.		
6	29.63	...	...	24	34	...	...	S. E.		
7	29.41	...	...	2	13	9	8.0	N. W.		
8	29.87	...	...	5	19	16	13.3	N. W.		
9	29.62	...	...	26	33	29	29.3	N. W.		
10	29.87	...	...	28	40	33	33.7	S. W.		
11	30.00	...	...	25	26	24	25.0	N. E.	Cloudy	
12	29.68	29.57	29.70	29	34	28	30.3	N. E.	Snow & r'n	} 1.05
13	29.74	29.61	29.29	24	31	29	28.0	N. E.	R'n & hail	
14	29.37	29.67	29.95	22	30	20	24.0	N. W.	Clear	
15	30.09	30.03	29.93	16	32	24	24.0	N. E.	Cloudy	
16	30.02	30.02	30.01	20	31	24	25.0	N. W.	Clear	
17	29.89	29.82	29.71	23	41	31	31.7	S. W.	Clear	
18	29.46	29.30	29.43	35	45	36	38.7	S. W.	Variable	
19	29.43	29.41	29.45	34	43	37	38.0	S. W.	Variable	
20	29.45	29.46	29.63	34	46	27	35.7	W'ly	Variable	
21	29.81	29.79	29.86	17	23	20	20.0	N. W.	Clear	
22	29.86	29.73	29.67	22	41	34	31.7	W'ly	Clear	
23	29.66	29.77	29.95	30	45	24	33.0	N. W.	Clear	
24	29.78	29.48	29.21	28	34	16	26.0	N. E.	R'n & snow	0.50
25	29.49	29.66	29.99	5	13	9	9.0	N. W.	Clear	
26	30.15	30.11	29.92	8	28	29	21.7	S. W.	Clear	
27	29.70	29.57	29.87	36	39	20	31.7	W'ly	Variable	
28	30.04	30.11	30.10	13	20	16	16.3	W'ly	Variable	
Means	29.74	29.71	29.75	19.9	30.4	28.0	...	...	...	1.55
REDUCED TO SEA LEVEL.										
Max.	30.33	30.29	30.28	36	46	36	38.7			
Min.	29.55	29.59	29.47	2	13	9	8.0			
Mean	29.92	29.89	29.93							
Range	0.78	0.70	0.81	34	33	27	30.7			
Mean of month	29.913			...	...	...	26.1			
Extreme range	0.86			...	...	...	44.0			

March, 1833.

Days.	Barometer Sun-rise.	At 1 P. M.	At 10 P. M.	Thermometer Sun-rise.	At 1 P. M.	At 10 P. M.	Daily mean	Winds	Weather	Rain and Snow
1	29.95	29.79	29.60	14	17	11	14.0	N. E.	Snow	0.36
2	29.45	29.40	29.75	9	24	—2	10.3	N. W.	Clear	
3	29.91	29.77	29.54	—4	15	18	9.7	W'ly	Variable	
4	29.64	29.72	29.97	11	29	7	12.7	N. W.	Clear	
5	30.13	30.13	29.94	—1	11	12	7.3	W'ly	Clear	
6	29.60	29.58	29.79	12	22	20	18.0	N. E.	Snow	0.14
7	29.90	29.89	29.73	10	34	23	22.3	W.	Variable	
8	29.68	29.61	29.51	27	46	33	34.3	S. W.	Variable	
9	29.47	29.49	29.56	31	41	30	34.0	W.	Clear	
10	29.69	29.78	29.96	30	44	28	34.0	W'ly	Variable	
11	30.02	30.06	30.07	24	33	29	28.7	N. E.	Snow	0.15
12	30.06	29.93	29.76	29	44	40	37.7	N. E.	Mist & rain	0.32
13	29.63	29.67	29.98	38	34	20	30.7	N. W.	Variable	
14	30.13	30.19	30.14	17	30	26	24.3	N'ly	Clear	
15	29.97	29.91	30.02	32	44	32	36.0	S. W'ly	Variable	
16	30.12	30.16	30.26	29	39	26	31.3	W'ly	Clear	
17	30.29	30.28	30.20	20	37	28	28.3	S. W'ly	Clear	
18	30.03	29.92	29.87	39	47	40	42.0	S. W.	Variable	
19	29.85	29.85	29.95	38	48	42	42.7	S. W.	Clear	
20	29.96	29.90	29.75	38	49	43	43.3	S. E'ly	Rain	0.80
21	29.61	29.53	29.36	41	61	51	51.0	S'ly	Variable	
22	29.33	29.34	29.43	44	57	40	47.0	N'ly	Clear	
23	29.63	29.47	29.69	36	54	40	43.3	W'ly	Clear	
24	29.69	29.63	29.55	34	55	40	43.0	S'ly	Clear	
25	29.40	29.34	29.38	35	43	39	39.0	N. E.	Rain	0.20
26	29.49	29.49	29.67	39	42	33	38.0	N. W.	Clear	
27	29.75	29.75	29.77	24	40	29	31.0	N. W.	Clear	
28	29.78	29.71	29.65	23	35	28	28.7	N. W.	Clear	
29	29.60	29.48	29.55	23	43	32	32.7	N. W.	Clear	
30	29.62	29.58	29.76	30	48	38	38.7	N. W.	Clear	
31	29.82	29.74	29.75	38	60	50	49.3	W'ly	Clear	
Means	29.78	29.74	29.77	26.1	39.3	29.9	31.7	...	...	1.97
REDUCED TO SEA LEVEL.										
[illegible]	[illegible]	[illegible]	[illegible]	[illegible]	[illegible]	[illegible]	[illegible]			
Min.	29.51	29.52	29.54	—4	11	—2	7.3			
Mean	29.96	29.92	29.95							
Range	0.96	0.94	0.90	48	50	53	44.7			
Mean of month	29.943			...	...	...	31.7			
Extreme range	0.96			...	...	...	65.0			

April, 1833.

Days.	Barometer, reduced to 32° F. Sun-rise.	At 1 P. M.	At 10 P. M.	Thermometer. Sun-rise.	At 1 P. M.	At 10 P. M.	Daily mean.	Winds.	Weather.	Rain and Snow in Inches of Water.
1	29.79	29.75	29.79	41	68	54	54.3	W'ly	Clear	
2	29.82	29.89	29.88	41	66	42	49.7	W'ly	Clear	
3	29.87	29.83	29.75	37	63	47	49.0	S. W.	Clear	
4	29.59	29.48	29.45	49	58	53	53.3	S'ly	Rain	0.46
5	29.48	29.38	29.59	48	65	43	52.0	S'ly	Variable	
6	29.73	29.78	29.88	38	58	43	46.3	N'ly	Clear	
7	29.96	29.95	29.89	38	62	42	47.3	S'ly	Clear	
8	29.63	29.45	29.42	47	57	48	50.7	S. E'ly	Rain	2.56
9	29.45	29.48	29.68	46	59	47	50.7	N. W.	Clear	
10	29.76	29.78	29.80	48	58	45	50.3	N'ly	Clear	
11	29.83	29.72	29.55	40	55	45	46.7	S. W'ly	Clear	
12	29.35	29.22	29.26	48	61	47	52.0	S'ly	Rain	0.15
13	29.27	29.34	29.48	42	45	36	41.0	N. W.	Clear	
14	29.57	29.57	29.76	33	50	43	42.0	N. W'ly	Clear	
15	29.99	30.10	...	26	42	30	32.7	N. E.	Variable	
16	30.16	30.11	30.04	27	46	36	36.3	N. E.	Clear	
17	...	29.84	29.84	35	45	41	40.3	N. E.	Cloudy	
18	29.87	29.89	...	37	64	49	50.0	N. W.	Clear	
19	30.13	...	30.08	36	62	42	46.3	S'ly	Clear	
20	...	29.86	29.85	40	70	55	55.0	S'ly	Clear	
21	...	29.65	29.52	40	72	54	55.3	S'ly	Clear	
22	...	29.64	29.75	50	62	47	53.0	N. W.	Clear	
23	29.42	29.44	29.55	44	60	39	47.7	S'ly	Cloudy	
24	29.68	29.80	29.87	36	40	31	35.7	N. E.	Cloudy	
25	29.90	29.89	29.89	29	60	43	44.0	N. W'ly	Clear	
26	29.90	29.93	30.03	38	55	38	43.7	N. E'ly	Clear	
27	30.11	30.10	30.08	31	54	38	41.0	N. E'ly	Clear	
28	30.03	29.93	29.87	38	67	53	52.7	N'ly	Clear	
29	29.82	29.75	29.74	53	79	66	66.0	W'ly	Clear	
30	29.75	29.75	30.00	58	82	50	63.3	W'ly	Clear	
Means	29.76	29.73	29.76	40.5	59.5	44.9	48.3	...	...	3.17
REDUCED TO SEA LEVEL.										
Max.	30.34	30.29	30.26	58	82	66	66.0			
Min.	29.45	29.40	29.44	26	40	30	32.7			
Mean										
Range	0.89	0.89	0.82	32	42	36	33.3			
Mean of month			29.930	...	...	...	48.3			
Extreme range			0.94	...	...	...	56.0			

May, 1833.

Days.	Barometer, reduced to 32° F. Sun-rise.	At 1 P. M.	At 10 P. M.	Thermometer. Sun-rise.	At 1 P. M.	At 10 P. M.	Daily mean	Winds.	Weather.	Rain and Snow in Inches of Water.
1	30.02	29.96	29.91	47	65	47	53.0	N. E.	Variable	
2	29.78	29.69	29.88	53	76	51	60.0	W'ly	Clear	
3	30.02	29.94	30.00	38	62	42	47.3	N. E'ly	Clear	
4	30.07	30.07	30.01	38	59	49	49.0	S. W'ly	Variable	
5	29.97	29.94	29.96	46	52	48	48.7	N. E.	Rain	0.05
6	29.97	29.94	29.87	42	64	52	52.7	W'ly	Clear	
7	29.88	29.76	29.76	52	81	63	65.3	W'ly	Variable	
8	29.72	29.61	29.65	63	77	64	68.0	S. W'ly	Variable	
9	29.71	29.78	29.94	62	66	50	59.3	N'ly	Variable	
10	30.02	30.06	30.04	41	60	47	49.3	E'ly	Variable	
11	29.94	29.84	29.88	46	73	60	66.3	E'ly	Fair	
12	29.89	29.85	29.80	61	72	64	65.7	S. W.	Cloudy	
13	29.83	29.77	29.83	62	73	64	66.3	S. W'ly	Variable	
14	29.89	29 89	29.84	63	58	63	61.3	N. E.	Rain	0.06
15	29.75	29.79	29.93	63	70	63	65.3	S. W.	Rain	0.40
16	30.01	29.97	29.95	53	54	49	52.0	N. E.	Rain	0.60
17	29.86	29.80	29.73	50	64	63	59.0	N'ly	Variable	
18	29.71	29.61	29.58	62	82	65	69.7	W'ly	Clear	
19	29.54	29.50	29.62	64	87	71	74.0	W'ly	Variable	
20	29.71	29.79	29.77	50	55	49	51.3	N. E.	Cloudy	
21	29.59	29.51	29.50	49	66	62	59.0	S'ly	Rain	0.53
22	29.55	29.60	29.74	62	75	62	66.3	W'ly	Clear	
23	29.82	29.89	29.94	58	69	63	63.3	W'ly	Variable	
24	30.08	30.12	30.12	52	66	51	56.0	N. E.	Clear	
25	30.10	30.02	29.90	45	68	54	55.7	S'ly	Clear	
26	29.70	29.61	29.65	58	66	56	63.3	S'ly	Rain	0.35
27	29.72	29.75	29.80	53	64	55	57.3	N. E'ly	Cloudy	
28	29.81	29.85	29.87	51	77	56	61.3	N. E'ly	Variable	
29	29.83	29.72	29.53	54	67	57	59.3	N. E'ly	Variable	
30	29.42	29.48	29.70	60	66	55	60.3	W'ly	Clear	
31	29.71	29.72	29.78	50	72	58	60.0	W'ly	Clear	
Means	29.83	29.80	29.82	53.2	67.9	56.2	59.1	...	...	0.99
REDUCED TO SEA LEVEL.										
Max.	30.28	30.30	30.30	64	87	71	74.0			
Min.	29.60	29.66	29.68	38	52	42	47.3			
Mean	30.01	29.97	30.00							
Range	0.68	0.64	0.62	26	35	29	26.7			
Mean of month			29.993	...	...	...	59.1			
Extreme range			0.70	...	...	...	49.0			

June, 1833.

Days.	Barometer, reduced to 32° F. Sun-rise.	At 1 P. M.	At 10 P. M.	Thermometer. At 6 A. M.	At 1 P. M.	At 10 P. M.	Daily mean.	Winds.	Weather.	Rain and Snow in Inches of Water.
1	29.84	29.81	29.87	54	75	61	63.3	W'ly	Clear	
2	29.81	29.60	29.50	61	76	63	66.7	S'ly	Cloudy	0.05
3	29.41	29.47	29.74	68	75	51	64.7	W'ly	Clear	
4	29.88	29.88	29.92	46	68	55	56.3	W'ly	Clear	
5	29.97	29.93	29.89	57	75	58	63.3	W'ly	Clear	
6	29.82	29.75	29.70	58	75	60	64.3	W'ly	Clear	
7	29.62	29.54	29.52	61	79	61	67.0	S. W'ly	Variable	
8	29.56	29.54	29.49	55	66	54	58.3	N'ly	Variable	
9	29.28	29.28	29.42	54	59	50	54.3	W'ly	Clear	
10	29.41	29.31	29.37	46	69	50	55.0	W'ly	Variable	0.05
11	29.35	29.37	29.53	50	61	54	55.0	W'ly	Variable	
12	29.60	29.63	29.76	50	70	56	58.7	W'ly	Clear	
13	29.80	29.75	29.61	53	75	64	64.0	S. W'ly	Shower	0.20
14	29.48	29.43	29.48	66	83	68	72.3	W'ly	Clear	
15	29.54	29.51	29.46	62	75	64	67.0	W'ly	Clear	
16	29.38	29.40	29.43	65	77	64	68.7	W'ly	Clear	
17	29.47	29.54	29.68	60	69	60	63.0	W'ly	Clear	
18	29.81	29.87	29.91	56	71	58	61.7	W'ly	Clear	
19	29.91	29.88	29.90	57	81	59	65.7	W'ly	Clear	
20	29.90	29.93	29.89	60	68	65	64.3	S. W'ly	Rain	0.15
21	29.85	29.86	29.80	66	75	66	69.0	S. W'ly	Rain	2.40
22	29.65	29.68	29.70	62	74	59	65.0	W'ly	Clear	
23	29.71	29.69	29.71	60	81	59	66.7	N. E'ly	Clear	
24	29.69	29.65	29.57	58	69	62	63.0	N. E'ly	Rain }	0.80
25	29.41	29.30	29.39	59	62	54	58.3	S. E'ly	Rain }	
26	29.48	29.54	29.60	50	66	53	56.3	W'ly	Variable	
27	29.68	29.70	29.81	54	63	54	57.0	W'ly	Rain & hail	0.46
28	29.82	29.81	29.78	52	71	60	61.0	W'ly	Clear	
29	29.83	29.83	29.84	55	75	63	64.3	W'ly	Clear	
30	29.85	29.84	29.77	61	81	64	68.7	W'ly	Clear	
Means	29.67	29.63	29.67	57.2	72.1	59.0	62.8	...	...	4.81
REDUCED TO SEA LEVEL.										
Max.	30.15	30.11	30.10	66	83	68	72.3			
Min.	29.46	29.46	29.55	46	61	50	54.3			
Mean	29.85	29.81	29.85							
Range	0.69	0.65	0.55	20	22	18	18.0			
Mean of month			29.837	...	...	...	62.8			
Extreme range			0.69	...	...	...	37.0			

July, 1833.

Days.	Barometer, reduced to 32° F. Sun-rise.	At 1 P. M.	At 10 P. M.	Thermometer. At 6 A. M.	At 1 P. M.	At 10 P. M.	Daily mean.	Winds.	Weather.	Rain and Snow in Inches of Water.
1	29.72	29.70	29.71	67	88	71	75.3	W'ly	Clear	
2	29.67	29.60	29.55	68	81	72	73.7	W'ly	Clear	
3	29.58	29.67	29.67	71	82	67	73.3	N. W'ly	Rain	0.66
4	29.71	29.76	29.86	63	77	66	68.7	W'ly	Clear	
5	29.97	29.96	29.99	61	74	64	66.3	W'ly	Clear	
6	30.01	29.98	29.92	60	76	67	67.7	W'ly	Clear	
7	29.83	29.75	29.71	67	80	70	72.3	W'ly	Variable	
8	29.68	29.61	29.56	63	84	77	74.7	S. W'ly	Variable	
9	...	29.54	29.68	73	78	62	71.0	W'ly	Variable	
10	29.79	29.82	29.82	68	77	65	70.0	W'ly	Clear	
11	29.78	29.68	29.60	63	76	66	68.3	W'ly	Clear	
12	29.55	29.56	29.69	64	79	68	70.3	W'ly	Clear	
13	29.85	29.84	29.83	62	82	68	70.7	W'ly	Clear	
14	29.79	29.70	29.62	70	85	74	76.3	S. W'ly	Variable	
15	29.57	29.59	29.66	72	79	69	73.3	W'ly	Clear	
16	29.68	29.68	29.63	62	75	65	67.3	W'ly	Clear	
17	29.65	29.69	29.79	65	74	64	67.3	W'ly	Clear	
18	29.82	29.85	...	57	74	57	62.7	W'ly	Clear	0.05
19	29.99	29.99	30.00	56	76	66	66.0	W'ly	Clear	
20	29.98	30.00	30.02	65	71	64	66.7	S'ly	Clear	
21	30.00	29.98	29.92	65	76	69	70.0	S. W'ly	Clear	
22	...	29.80	29.91	69	90	78	79.0	W'ly	Clear	
23	30.01	29.98	29.97	66	81	67	71.3	N. E'ly	Clear	
24	29.87	29.71	29.73	67	91	78	78.7	W'ly	Clear	
25	29.92	29.95	...	66	76	64	68.7	W'ly	Clear	
26	30.08	30.04	29.98	56	79	63	66.0	N. W.	Clear	
27	29.88	29.72	29.57	61	83	74	72.7	W'ly	Clear	
28	29.60	29.73	29.92	70	73	60	67.7	W'ly	Clear	
29	29.94	29.88	29.84	56	70	66	64.0	W'ly	Clear	
30	29.58	29.48	29.61	69	76	64	69.7	S. W.	Rain	0.40
31	29.74	29.78	29.79	58	72	60	63.3	W'ly	Clear	
Means	29.80	29.77	29.78	64.5	78.6	67.3	70.1	...	...	1.11
REDUCED TO SEA LEVEL.										
Max.	30.26	30.22	30.20	73	91	78	79.0			
Min.	29.73	29.66	29.73	56	70	60	62.7			
Mean	29.97	29.91	29.95							
Range	0.53	0.56	0.47	17	21	18	16.3			
Mean of month			29.943	...	...	...	70.1			
Extreme range			0.60	...	...	...	35.0			

August, 1883.

Date	Barometer, reduced to 32° F: at 7 A.M.	at 2 P.M.	at 9 P.M.	Thermometer: at 7 A.M.	at 2 P.M.	at 9 P.M.	Daily mean	Wind	Weather	Rain and melted snow, inches of water
[illegible]	[illegible]	[illegible]	[illegible]	[illegible]	[illegible]	[illegible]	[illegible]	[illegible]	[illegible]	[illegible]

Means · Reduced to sea level: Max. · Min. · Mean · Range · Mean of month · Extreme range [illegible]

October, 1883.

Date	Barometer: Sunrise	at 2 P.M.	at 9 P.M.	Thermometer: Sunrise	at 2 P.M.	at 9 P.M.	Daily mean	Wind	Weather	Rain and melted snow, inches of water
[illegible]	[illegible]	[illegible]	[illegible]	[illegible]	[illegible]	[illegible]	[illegible]	[illegible]	[illegible]	[illegible]

Means · Reduced to sea level: Max. · Min. · Mean · Range · Mean of month · Extreme range [illegible]

REMARKS. [illegible]

September, 1883.

Date	Barometer: Sunrise	at 2 P.M.	at 9 P.M.	Thermometer: Sunrise	at 2 P.M.	at 9 P.M.	Daily mean	Wind	Weather	Rain
[illegible]	[illegible]	[illegible]	[illegible]	[illegible]	[illegible]	[illegible]	[illegible]	[illegible]	[illegible]	[illegible]

Means · Reduced to sea level: Max. · Min. · Mean · Range · Mean of month · Extreme range [illegible]

REMARKS. [illegible]

November, 1883.

Date	Barometer: Sunrise	at 2 P.M.	at 9 P.M.	Thermometer: Sunrise	at 2 P.M.	at 9 P.M.	Daily mean	Wind	Weather	Rain
[illegible]	[illegible]	[illegible]	[illegible]	[illegible]	[illegible]	[illegible]	[illegible]	[illegible]	[illegible]	[illegible]

Means · Reduced to sea level: Max. · Min. · Mean · Range · Mean of month · Extreme range [illegible]

REMARKS. [illegible]

December, 1833.

DAYS.	BAROMETER, REDUCED TO 32° F. Sunrise.	At 1 P. M.	At 10 P. M.	THERMOMETER. Sunrise.	At 1 P. M.	At 10 P. M.	Daily mean.	WINDS.	WEATHER.	RAIN AND SNOW IN INCHES OF WATER.
1	29.79	29.75	29.79	33	38	38	36.3	W'ly	Cloudy	
2	29.95	30.02	30.13	34	37	36	35.7	E'ly	Cloudy	
3	30.16	30.16	30.18	34	38	38	36.7	N. E.	Rain	0.06
4	30.16	30.14	30.15	33	36	33	34.0	N. E'ly	Cloudy	
5	30.15	30.12	30.15	32	42	38	37.3	W'ly	Variable	
6	30.15	30.14	30.22	35	38	26	33.0	N. W'ly	Clear	
7	30.30	30.31	30.38	23	35	31	29.7	W'ly	Clear	
8	30.31	30.17	29.76	31	37	43	37.0	E'ly	Rain	0.84
9	29.57	29.64	29.70	35	42	34	37.0	W'ly	Clear	
10	29.71	29.71	29.85	30	36	32	32.7	W'ly	Variable	
11	29.91	29.85	29.92	24	32	23	26.3	W'ly	Clear	
12	29.92	29.96	30.00	17	29	23	23.0	W'ly	Variable	
13	30.07	30.06	30.11	12	27	15	18.0	W'ly	Clear	
14	30.12	30.06	29.93	12	28	29	23.0	N. E.	Cloudy	
15	29.72	29.72	29.93	23	29	27	26.3	N. E.	Cloudy	
16	30.05	30.10	30.09	23	31	34	29.3	N. E'ly	Variable	
17	29.83	29.53	29.36	36	38	36	36.7	N. E.	Rain	1.85
18	29.46	29.47	29.66	39	40	31	36.7	N. E.	Misty	0.17
19	29.82	29.92	29.99	23	30	18	23.7	N. E'ly	Cloudy	
20	30.03	30.03	30.03	15	32	21	22.7	W'ly	Clear	
21	30.01	29.99	29.99	18	31	25	24.7	W'ly	Clear	
22	29.86	29.76	29.89	32	37	31	33.3	N. E'ly	Rain	0.70
23	30.00	30.03	30.03	26	34	33	31.0	N. E'ly	Clear	
24	29.73	29.48	29.57	33	38	31	34.0	N. E.	Rain	0.60
25	29.56	29.44	29.37	30	37	30	32.3	S. W'ly	Variable	
26	29.54	29.65	29.72	31	37	29	32.3	W'ly	Variable	
27	29.69	29.69	29.73	27	31	24	27.3	W'ly	Clear	
28	29.77	29.76	29.79	21	28	27	25.3	W'ly	Clear	
29	29.82	29.86	30.03	25	37	30	30.7	W'ly	Clear	
30	30.13	30.06	30.02	20	31	32	27.7	W'ly	Variable	
31	29.83	29.69	29.65	38	43	34	38.3	S. E'ly	Rain	0.45
Means	29.91	29.88	29.91	27.3	34.8	30.1	...	...	...	4.67
REDUCED TO SEA LEVEL.										
Max.	30.49	30.49	30.56	39	43	43	38.3			
Min.	29.64	29.65	29.64	12	27	15	18.0			
Mean	30.09	30.06	30.09							
Range	0.85	0.84	0.92	27	16	28	20.3			
Mean of month	30.080			...	...	...	30.7			
Extreme range	0.92			...	...	...	31.0			

January, 1834.

DAYS.	Barometer Sunrise	At 1 P. M.	At 10 P. M.	Thermometer Sunrise.	At 1 P. M.	At 10 P. M.	Daily mean.	Winds.	Weather.	Rain and snow.
1	29.78	29.85	29.98	31	37	25	29.3	N. W.	Clear	
2	29.90	29.62	29.38	22	35	46	34.3	S. E'ly	Rain	0.20
3	29.78	29.93	30.14	28	27	18	24.3	N. W.	Clear	
4	30.25	30.26	30.33	12	18	14	14.7	N. W.	Clear	
5	30.19	30.08	30.11	11	16	12	13.0	N. E'ly	Snow	0.05
6	30.14	30.01	29.76	6	18	11	11.7	N'ly	Variable	0.07
7	29.75	29.82	29.85	8	19	20	15.7	N. W'ly	Clear	
8	29.83	29.84	30.00	23	34	27	28.0	W'ly	Clear	
9	30.18	30.17	30.10	15	33	30	26.0	W'ly	Clear	
10	30.10	30.07	30.11	30	40	30	33.3	W'ly	Variable	
11	30.11	30.03	29.94	27	25	21	24.3	N. E.	Rain }	0.80
12	29.68	29.49	29.32	24	31	31	28.7	N. E.	Snow }	
13	29.59	29.79	30.07	30	27	21	26.0	W'ly	Clear	
14	30.18	30.10	30.14	16	30	21	22.3	W'ly	Clear	
15	30.33	30.38	30.48	16	21	13	16.7	W'ly	Clear	
16	30.51	30.45	30.36	10	30	26	22.0	W'ly	Clear	
17	30.13	29.90	29.78	32	44	46	40.7	S. W'ly	Rain	0.20
18	29.75	29.72	29.90	44	51	38	44.3	W'ly	Clear	
19	29.96	29.90	29.86	32	45	36	37.7	W'ly	Variable	
20	29.65	29.54	29.77	36	43	24	34.3	W'ly	Cloudy	
21	29.85	29.79	29.90	14	17	14	15.0	N. W.	Clear	
22	30.00	29.99	30.01	7	15	8	10.0	W'ly	Clear	
23	30.02	29.99	30.04	2	9	6½	5.8	N. W.	Clear	
24	30.06	30.05	30.15	3	11	5½	6.5	N. W.	Clear	
25	30.25	30.25	30.10	8	18	19	15.0	N'ly	Cloudy	
26	29.60	29.24	29.43	22	32	25	26.3	N. E'ly	Snow	0.25
27	29.58	29.58	29.78	18	22	14	18.0	N. W.	Clear	
28	29.92	29.89	29.93	10	28	22	20.0	N. W.	Clear	
29	30.35	30.39	30.52	18	21	18	19.0	N. E.	Clear	
30	30.40	30.20	30.03	17	38	32	29.0	E'ly	Cloudy	
31	29.93	29.88	29.97	31	34	26	30.3	W'ly	Clear	
Means	29.99	29.94	29.98	19.5	28.0	22.6	...	...	...	1.57
REDUCED TO SEA LEVEL.										
Max.	30.69	30.63	30.66	44	51	46				
Min.	29.76	29.42	29.56	2	9	5½				
Mean	30.17	30.12	30.16							
Range	0.93	1.21	1.10	42	42	40½				
Mean of month	30.150			...	...	...	23.3			
Extreme range	1.21			...	...	...	49.0			

REMARK.

18th. Frost quite out of the ground in many places.

February, 1834.

DAYS.	BAROMETER, REDUCED TO 32° F. Sunrise.	At 1 P. M.	At 10 P. M.	THERMOMETER. Sunrise.	At 1 P. M.	At 10 P. M.	Daily mean.	WINDS.	WEATHER.	RAIN AND SNOW IN INCHES OF WATER.
1	30.02	29.97	29.87	23	35	33	30.3	N. E.	Cloudy	
2	29.80	29.84	29.98	28	41	32	33.7	W'ly	Clear	
3	30.11	30.06	29.85	30	40	33	34.3	S. W'ly	Clear	
4	29.60	29.53	29.55	31	47	39	39.0	W'ly	Clear	
5	29.61	29.56	29.55	34	45	38	39.0	W'ly	Variable	
6	29.65	29.81	29.95	32	35	22	29.7	N. W'ly	Clear	
7	29.96	30.00	30.19	13	15	8	12.0	N'ly	Snow	0.18
8	30.24	30.08	30.00	2	23	20	15.0	N. W.	Clear	
9	29.89	29.86	29.77	30	41	34	35.0	S. W'ly	Cloudy	
10	29.97	29.94	29.94	30	35	30	31.7	N. E.	Cloudy	
11	29.86	29.71	29.70	27	38	37	34.0	W'ly	Clear	
12	30.04	30.08	30.08	12	15	13	13.3	N. W.	Clear	
13	30.02	29.88	29.80	12	30	28	23.3	W'ly	Clear	
14	29.70	29.68	29.68	31	45	33	36.3	W'ly	Variable	
15	29.52	29.40	29.39	38	47	46	43.7	S. W.	Cloudy	
16	29.59	29.64	29.94	39	46	35	40.0	W'ly	Variable	
17	30.12	30.15	30.22	34	38	30	34.0	W'ly	Variable	
18	30.29	30.31	30.37	24	43	31	32.7	W'ly	Clear	
19	30.35	30.15	29.94	31	44	44	39.7	S. W'ly	Rain, var.	0.50
20	29.84	29.86	29.96	42	54	38	44.7	W'ly	Clear	
21	29.94	29.84	29.93	31	49	35	38.3	N. E'ly	Clear	
22	9.87	29.84	29.88	33	46	42	40.3	S. E'ly	Clear	
23	9.80	29.73	29.63	41	42	39	40.7	N. E'ly	Cloudy	
24	9.67	29.73	29.83	41	43	37	40.3	N. E'ly	Cloudy	
25	29.66	29.64	29.62	30	33	32	31.7	N. E'ly	Snow	0.45
26	29.67	29.76	29.93	22	29	21	24.0	N. W.	Clear	
27	29.96	29.86	29.77	23	40	30	31.0	W'ly	Clear	
28	29.66	29.56	29.62	27	45	36	36.0	W'ly	Clear	
Means	29.87	29.84	29.86	28.2	38.7	32.0	...	...	...	1.13
REDUCED TO SEA LEVEL.										
Max.	30.53	30.49	30.55	42	54	46	44.7			
Min.	29.70	29.58	29.57	2	15	8	12.0			
Mean	30.05	30.02	30.04							
Range	0.83	0.91	0.98	40	39	38	32.7			
Mean of month	30.037			...	...	...	33.0			
Extreme range	0.98			...	...	...	52.0			

March, 1834.

DAYS.	Barometer Sunrise.	At 1 P. M.	At 10 P. M.	Thermometer Sunrise.	At 1 P. M.	At 10 P. M.	Daily mean.	Winds.	Weather.	Rain and snow.
1	29.68	29.59	29.57	32	43	34	36.3	N'ly	Clear	
2	29.46	29.35	29.47	33	39	28	33.3	S. E'ly	Snow	0.30
3	29.94	29.97	30.01	19	23	20	20.7	W'ly	Clear	
4	29.94	29.86	29.87	26	45	37	36.0	W'ly	Clear	
5	29.91	29.85	29.86	32	54	42	42.7	W'ly	Clear	
6	29.79	29.79	29.84	40	56	46	47.3	S. W'ly	Variable	
7	30.14	30.19	30.23	36	48	36	40.0	N. E'ly	Clear	
8	29.94	29.56	29.65	37	53	46	45.3	S. W.	Rain	0.38
9	30.01	30.08	30.26	32	38	27	32.3	N. W.	Clear	
10	30.49	30.30	30.30	18	35	26	26.3	N. W.	Clear	
11	30.14	29.93	29.77	29	46	42	39.0	W'ly	Variable	
12	29.73	29.59	29.59	36	57	42	45.0	W'ly	Variable	
13	29.90	29.92	29.94	31	41	30	34.0	W'ly	Clear	
14	30.09	29.99	29.91	22	38	32	30.7	S. W'ly	Clear	
15	29.81	29.77	29.86	28	35	32	31.7	N. E.	Snow	0.10
16	29.96	30.00	30.06	26	42	32	33.3	N. E.	Clear	
17	30.09	30.05	30.08	32	43	35	36.7	S. W'ly	Variable	
18	30.17	30.14	30.06	30	50	34	38.0	W'ly	Clear	
19	29.94	29.80	29.82	41	66	56	54.3	W'ly	Clear	
20	29.80	29.80	29.61	48	49	56	51.0	S. W.	Rain	0.32
21	29.46	29.54	29.65	51	46	25	40.7	N. W.	Clear	
22	29.68	29.66	29.77	20	24	22	22.0	N. W.	Clear	
23	29.78	29.70	29.68	18	39	35	30.7	W'ly	Clear	
24	29.66	29.71	29.82	32	44	36	37.3	S. W'ly	Variable	
25	29.88	29.71	29.43	32	37	35	34.7	N. E.	Rain	0.33
26	29.76	29.85	30.05	31	37	24	30.7	N. W.	Clear	
27	30.13	30.13	30.11	18	39	30	29.0	S. W'ly	Clear	
28	30.13	30.05	29.94	30	50	42	40.7	S. W'ly	Clear	
29	29.74	29.53	29.63	40	63	32	45.0	S. W'ly	Clear	
30	29.89	29.88	30.03	19	28	22	23.0	N. W.	Clear	
31	30.13	30.13	30.13	20	42	30	30.7	W'ly	Clear	
Means	29.91	29.85	29.87	30.3	43.5	34.4	...	...	...	1.43
REDUCED TO SEA LEVEL.										
Max.	30.67	30.54	30.48	51	66	56	54.3			
Min.	29.64	29.53	29.61	18	23	20	20.7			
Mean	30.09	30.03	30.05							
Range	1.03	1.01	0.87	33	43	36	33.6			
Mean of month	30.057			...	...	...	36.1			
Extreme range	1.14			...	...	...	48.0			

April, 1834.

DAYS.	BAROMETER, REDUCED TO 32° F. Sun-rise.	At 1 P. M.	At 10 P. M.	THERMOMETER. Sun-rise.	At 1 P. M.	At 10 P. M.	Daily mean.	WINDS.	WEATHER.	RAIN AND SNOW IN INCHES OF WATER.
1	30.11	29.96	29.84	35	43	50	42.7	S. W.	Rain	0.75
2	29.68	29.73	29.89	52	56	44	50.7	S. W.	Rain	0.15
3	30.05	30.13	30.22	38	49	38	41.7	W'ly	Clear	
4	30.30	30.33	30.40	31	46	33	36.7	N. E.	Variable	
5	30.45	30.40	30.39	30	44	32	35.3	N. E.	Variable	
6	30.35	30.33	30.31	29	52	37	39.3	N. E.	Clear	
7	30.31	30.26	30.18	36	62	44	47.3	E'ly	Clear	
8	30.08	29.98	29.89	43	58	50	50.3	E'ly	Cloudy	
9	29.85	29.94	30.03	49	48	40	45.7	N. E.	Rain	0.50
10	30.07	30.10	30.13	37	48	36	40.3	N. E.	Variable	
11	30.10	30.11	30.10	33	61	44	46.0	N. E.	Clear	
12	30.07	30.00	29.93	42	70	57	56.3	S'ly	Clear	
13	29.89	29.84	29.76	55	75	65	65.0	W'ly	Clear	
14	29.81	29.73	29.70	48	60	54	54.0	S. W'ly	Clear	
15	29.59	29.54	29.51	54	75	65	64.7	W'ly	Clear	
16	29.50	29.49	29.49	55	75	55	61.7	W'ly	Clear	
17	29.44	29.49	29.69	51	75	48	58.0	S. W'ly	Clear	
18	29.91	29.94	29.96	37	57	38	44.0	N. E.	Clear	
19	29.98	29.86	29.77	36	56	46	46.0	S. W.	Rain	0.50
20	29.64	29.65	29.76	48	56	45	49.7	S. W'ly	Variable	
21	29.83	29.77	29.69	42	63	50	51.7	S. W'ly	Cloudy	
22	29.84	29.93	29.93	43	42	40	41.7	N. E.	Cloudy	
23	29.73	29.52	29.41	40	43	41	41.3	N. E.	Rain	0.35
24	29.38	29.53	29.64	44	50	38	44.0	N. W.	Clear	
25	29.66	29.60	29.54	34	51	39	41.0	S. W'ly	Variable	
26	29.54	29.50	29.47	29	51	38	39.3	S. W'ly	Clear	
27	29.36	29.20	29.11	37	35	33	35.0	S. W'ly	Snow & r'n	0.68
28	29.30	29.27	29.34	30	52	41	41.0	W'ly	Clear	
29	29.35	29.33	29.33	38	50	44	40.7	W'ly	Variable	
30	29.32	29.29	29.43	41	53	43	45.7	S. W'ly	Showery	0.20
Means	29.82	29.79	29.79	40.6	55.2	44.3	...	...	...	3.13
REDUCED TO SEA LEVEL.										
Max.	30.63	30.58	30.58	55	75	65	65.0			
Min.	29.48	29.38	29.29	29	35	32	35.0			
Mean	30.00	29.97	29.97							
Range	1.15	1.29	1.29	26	40	33	30.0			
Mean of month	29.980			...	...	...	46.7			
Extreme range	1.44			...	...	...	46.0			

REMARKS.

Severe frost on the morning of the 26th.

On the morning of the 28th, the ground was partially covered with sleet and snow.

May, 1834.

DAYS.	BAROMETER, REDUCED TO 32° F. At 6 A. M.	At 1 P. M.	At 10 P. M.	THERMOMETER. At 6 A. M.	At 1 P. M.	At 10 P. M.	Daily mean.	WINDS.	WEATHER.	RAIN AND SNOW IN INCHES OF WATER.
1	29.42	29.52	29.62	40	62	49	50.3	W'ly	Clear	
2	29.62	29.63	29.71	42	63	47	50.7	W'ly	Clear	
3	29.76	29.81	29.86	41	64	51	52.0	W'ly	Clear	
4	29.89	29.88	29.95	48	65	48	53.7	W'ly	Clear	
5	29.97	29.88	29.79	42	64	46	44.0	S. E.	Va'ble, r'n	2.56
6	29.56	29.57	29.77	48	49	45	47.3	N. E'ly	Cloudy	
7	29.78	29.54	29.47	42	48	46	45.3	N. E.	Rain	0.75
8	29.58	29.56	29.52	44	62	55	53.0	S. W'ly	Variable	
9	29.64	29.70	29.72	48	62	52	54.0	W'ly	Clear	
10	29.52	29.52	29.58	49	45	44	46.0	N. E.	Rain	1.50
11	29.70	29.54	29.42	42	62	53	52.3	S. W'ly	Variable	
12	29.32	29.33	29.43	47	49	44	46.7	W'ly	Variable	0.08
13	29.49	29.55	29.59	38	57	37	44.0	W'ly	Variable	
14	29.69	29.76	29.75	32	55	41	42.7	W'ly	Clear	
15	29.73	29.83	29.99	30	42	40	37.3	N. W.	Clear	
16	30.02	30.01	30.04	31	57	45	44.3	W'ly	Clear	
17	30.05	30.05	30.07	38	...	50	...	W'ly	Clear	
18	30.12	30.12	30.08	47	68	56	57.0	W'ly	Clear	
19	29.99	29.90	29.83	53	78	62	64.3	W'ly	Clear	
20	29.85	29.91	29.93	60	69	55	61.3	N'ly	Clear	
21	29.90	29.80	29.80	52	78	66	65.3	S. W'ly	Clear	
22	29.88	29.89	29.96	58	66	53	59.0	S. E'ly	Clear	
23	29.92	29.90	29.86	53	64	49	55.3	N. E'ly	Cloudy	
24	29.76	29.66	29.65	48	71	66	61.7	S'ly	Variable	
25	29.63	29.69	29.73	64	67	53	61.3	N. E.	Cloudy	
26	29.70	29.70	29.65	52	73	57	60.7	S'ly	Variable	
27	29.63	29.61	29.69	54	75	57	55.3	S. W'ly	Variable	0.72
28	29.72	29.72	29.73	51	64	47	54.0	N. E.	Cloudy	
29	29.68	29.67	29.68	47	47	46	46.7	N. E.	Rain	
30	[illegible]	[illegible]	[illegible]	[illegible]	[illegible]	47	[illegible]	N. E.	Cloudy	
31	29.84	29.82	29.79	47	[illegible]	[illegible]	[illegible]	[illegible]	[illegible]	
Means	29.74	29.73	29.76	46.3	61.6	50.5	...	...	...	5.61
REDUCED TO SEA LEVEL.										
Max.	30.30	30.30	30.26	60	78	66	65.3			
Min.	29.50	29.51	29.60	30	42	37	37.3			
Mean	29.92	29.90	29.94							
Range	0.80	0.79	0.66	30	36	29	28.0			
Mean of month	29.920			...	...	...	52.8			
Extreme range	0.80			...	...	...	48.0			

REMARK.

On the mornings of the 14th, 15th, and 16th, severe frost in many places in the vicinity, and in some ice one-eighth of an inch thick.

June, 1834.

DAYS.	BAROMETER, REDUCED TO 32° F. At 5 A. M.	At 1 P. M.	At 10 P. M.	THERMOMETER. At 5 A. M.	At 1 P. M.	At 10 P. M.	Daily mean.	WINDS.	WEATHER.	RAIN AND SNOW IN INCHES OF WATER.
1	29.77	29.72	29.50	56	66	61	61.0	S. W'ly	Rain	0.58
2	29.30	29.13	29.35	61	74	53	62.7	W'ly	Variable	
3	29.37	29.39	29.55	47	64	53	54.7	W'ly	Clear	
4	29.61	29.56	29.51	48	71	55	58.0	S. W'ly	Clear	
5	29.35	29.28	29.47	54	55	52	53.7	N. E.	Rain	1.93
6	29.53	29.61	29.65	52	62	54	56.0	N'ly	Variable	
7	29.62	29.60	29.60	52	68	60	60.0	N. E'ly	Clear	
8	29.60	29.61	29.63	60	80	67	69.0	W'ly	Clear	
9	29.62	29.62	29.62	65	83	75	74.3	W'ly	Clear	
10	29.65	29.77	29.60	67	81	67	71.7	S. W'ly	Clear	
11	29.42	29.40	29.48	65	80	66	70.3	S. W'ly	Variable	0.08
12	29.54	29.61	29.71	53	71	60	61.0	W'ly	Clear	
13	29.69	29.69	29.60	57	69	59	61.7	W'ly	Variable	
14	29.62	29.67	29.87	54	69	53	58.7	W'ly	Clear	
15	29.87	29.84	29.84	50	71	59	60.0	S. W'ly	Clear	
16	29.83	29.77	29.80	57	64	57	59.3	S. E'ly	Rain	0.46
17	29.79	29.76	29.72	52	68	60	60.0	S. E'ly	Variable	
18	29.68	29.40	29.40	57	64	56	59.0	E'ly	Rain	1.30
19	29.35	29.35	29.42	59	71	63	64.3	S. W'ly	Variable	
20	29.48	29.49	29.54	60	74	62	64.7	W'ly	Variable	0.03
21	29.55	29.57	29.61	56	75	65	65.3	W'ly	Clear	
22	29.66	29.62	29.63	58	80	68	68.7	S. W'ly	Clear	
23	29.69	29.71	29.71	67	85	68	73.3	S. W'ly	Clear	
24	29.64	29.58	29.62	67	81	72	73.3	S. W'ly	Variable	
25	29.80	29.88	29.89	63	79	67	69.7	W'ly	Clear	
26	29.84	29.68	29.74	65	81	64	70.0	W'ly	Va'ble, sh'r	0.45
27	29.80	29.81	29.89	56	73	58	62.3	W'ly	Clear	
28	29.93	29.89	29.86	55	69	58	60.7	E'ly	Variable	
29	29.72	29.61	29.58	58	61	58	59.0	N. E.	Rain	0.20
30	29.65	29.69	29.84	57	74	63	64.7	E'ly	Variable	0.07
Means	29.63	29.61	29.64	57.6	72.1	62.1	...	...	...	5.10
REDUCED TO SEA LEVEL.										
Max.	30.11	30.07	30.07	67	85	75	74.3			
Min.	29.48	29.31	29.53	47	55	52	53.7			
Mean	29.81	29.78	29.82							
Range	0.63	0.76	0.54	20	30	23	20.6			
Mean of month	29.803			...	...	...	63.6			
Extreme range	0.80			...	...	...	38.0			

July, 1834.

DAYS.	BAROMETER, REDUCED TO 32° F. At 5 A. M.	At 1 P. M.	At 10 P. M.	THERMOMETER. At 5 A. M.	At 1 P. M.	At 10 P. M.	Daily mean.	WINDS.	WEATHER.	RAIN AND SNOW IN INCHES OF WATER.
1	29.92	29.93	29.86	61	70	61	64.0	E'ly	Misty	
2	29.79	29.71	29.64	64	82	71	72.3	S. W'ly	Rain	0.58
3	29.45	29.59	29.69	71	75	69	71.7	W'ly	Variable	
4	29.70	29.73	29.73	66	80	69	71.7	S. W'ly	Clear	
5	29.71	29.70	29.68	65	80	69	71.3	S'ly	Variable	
6	29.68	29.68	29.67	66	83	73	74.0	S. W'ly	Variable	
7	29.67	29.63	29.67	71	79	74	74.7	S. W'ly	Clear	
8	29.64	29.61	29.67	72	91	82	81.7	W'ly	Clear	
9	29.67	29.65	29.65	76	90	76	80.7	S. W'ly	Clear	
10	29.67	29.63	29.67	75	85	75	78.3	S. W'ly	Clear	
11	29.78	29.81	29.88	67	78	67	70.7	S. W'ly	Variable	
12	29.92	29.94	29.99	63	80	67	70.0	S. W'ly	Clear	
13	30.04	30.08	30.05	64	75	68	69.0	S'ly	Variable	7.00
14	29.91	29.91	29.91	68	82	75	75.0	W'ly	Clear	
15	29.90	29.80	29.81	74	87	76	79.0	W'ly	Clear	
16	29.79	29.74	29.76	74	87	75	78.7	S. W'ly	Clear	
17	29.72	29.63	29.60	74	88	67	76.3	W'ly	Clear	
18	29.88	29.96	30.04	63	72	65	66.6	E'ly	Variable	
19	30.11	30.14	30.15	58	75	61	64.7	N. E.	Clear	
20	30.16	30.13	30.05	57	80	62	65.3	N. E.	Clear	
21	29.96	29.85	29.74	58	78	70	68.7	S. W.	Variable	
22	29.64	29.64	29.72	68	84	74	75.3	W'ly	Clear	
23	29.75	29.77	29.77	68	82	71	73.7	N. W.	Clear	
24	29.74	29.77	29.73	66	80	70	72.0	N. E.	Clear	
25	29.68	29.64	29.64	70	88	84	80.7	S. W.	Clear	
26	29.65	29.64	29.64	78	93	80	83.7	S. W.	Clear	
27	29.63	29.61	29.68	77	90	78	81.7	W.	Clear	
28	29.75	29.76	29.77	76	79	72	75.7	W'ly	Clear	
29	29.71	29.63	29.69	70	78	68	72.0	S. W'ly	Variable	
30	29.79	29.83	29.80	55	72	61	62.7	N. W.	Clear	
31	[illegible]	[illegible]	[illegible]	[illegible]	[illegible]	[illegible]	65.0	S. W'ly	Clear	
Means	29.78	29.77	29.77	67.4	81.2	70.8	...	...	...	7.58
REDUCED TO SEA LEVEL.										
Max.	30.34	30.32	30.33	78	93	80	83.7			
Min.	29.73	29.77	29.78	55	70	61	62.7			
Mean	29.95	29.94	29.94							
Range	0.61	0.55	0.55	23	23	19	21.0			
Mean of month	29.943			...	...	...	73.1			
Extreme range	0.61			...	...	...	38.0			

REMARKS.

The rain on the night of the 12th was most unprecedented. My rain-gauge, holding 6 inches, was running over on the morning of the 13th. From the amount of water collected in open vessels, the whole quantity was judged to be 7 inches.

August, 1834.

DAYS.	BAROMETER, REDUCED TO 32° F. At 5 A. M.	At 1 P. M.	At 10 P. M.	THERMOMETER. At 5 A. M.	At 1 P. M.	At 10 P. M.	Daily mean.	WINDS.	WEATHER.	RAIN AND SNOW IN INCHES OF WATER.
1	29.68	29.73	29.79	63	77	68	69.3	W'ly	Clear	
2	29.80	29.68	29.71	64	83	72	73.0	W'ly	Clear	
3	29.69	29.69	29.73	65	82	69	72.0	E'ly	Clear	
4	29.70	29.68	29.77	65	84	69	72.7	S. W'ly	Clear	
5	29.71	29.64	29.64	65	84	76	75.0	W'ly	Clear	
6	29.69	29.70	29.67	72	86	75	77.6	N'ly	Clear	
7	29.67	29.62	29.56	72	87	78	79.0	S. W'ly	Clear	
8	29.58	29.51	29.54	65	82	69	72.0	W'ly	Clear	
9	29.54	29.56	29.65	65	80	65	70.0	N. E'ly	Clear, r'n	0.35
10	29.70	29.70	29.75	61	78	67	68.7	E'ly	Cloudy	
11	29.71	29.67	29.67	66	81	71	72.6	S. W'ly	Variable	
12	29.64	29.52	29.50	71	85	74	76.7	S. W'ly	Va'ble, r'n	0.50
13	29.53	29.63	29.73	74	72	65	70.3	N. E'ly	Clear	
14	29.75	29.66	29.38	63	75	72	70.0	E'ly	Cloudy	
15	29.38	29.35	29.43	67	74	66	69.0	N. W.	Clear	
16	29.59	29.69	29.82	62	73	63	66.0	N. W.	Variable	
17	29.90	29.84	29.76	56	78	66	66.6	S. W'ly	Va'ble, r'n	0.30
18	29.52	29.57	29.63	69	82	65	72.0	N. W.	Clear	
19	29.64	29.70	29.73	60	63	64	62.3	N. E.	Cloudy	
20	29.68	29.66	29.66	60	69	60	63.0	N. E.	Cloudy	
21	29.66	29.64	29.77	60	70	68	66.0	N. E.	Variable	
22	29.70	29.68	29.69	66	81	69	72.0	N. W'ly	Clear	
23	29.69	29.67	29.68	64	85	69	72.7	N. W.	Clear	
24	29.69	29.68	29.72	67	86	72	75.0	S. W.	Clear	
25	29.78	29.79	29.80	61	72	59	64.0	N. E'ly	Clear	
26	29.80	29.78	29.78	58	75	62	65.0	W'ly	Clear	
27	29.80	29.82	29.85	54	68	58	60.0	N. E.	Clear	
28	29.99	29.93	29.97	57	69	60	62.0	N. E.	Clear	
29	30.03	30.03	30.06	55	73	61	63.0	S. E.	Clear	
30	30.06	30.04	29.99	68	71	62	67.0	N. E.	Clear	
31	29.94	29.92	29.92	58	70	60	62.6	E'ly	Clear	
Means	29.72	29.70	29.72	63.6	77.3	66.9	...	...	...	1.15
REDUCED TO SEA LEVEL.										
Max.	30.24	30.22	30.24	72	87	78	79.0			
Min.	29.56	29.53	29.56	54	63	58	60.0			
Mean	29.89	29.87	29.89							
Range	0.68	0.69	0.68	18	24	20	19.0			
Mean of month			29.883	...	...	...	69.3			
Extreme range			0.71	...	...	...	33.0			

September, 1834.

DAYS.	BAROMETER. Sunrise.	At 1 P. M.	At 10 P. M.	THERMOMETER. Sunrise.	At 1 P. M.	At 10 P. M.	Daily mean.	WINDS.	WEATHER.	RAIN AND SNOW IN INCHES OF WATER.
1	29.89	29.89	29.85	60	67	60	62.3	E'ly	Rain	0.75
2	29.85	29.90	30.01	62	71	60	64.3	E'ly	Variable	
3	30.00	29.95	29.96	60	80	69	69.7	W'ly	Clear	
4	29.84	29.80	29.78	70	86	74	76.7	W'ly	Clear	
5	29.71	29.63	29.57	74	74	72	73.5	S. E'ly	Rain	1.90
6	29.49	29.59	29.74	72	81	66	73.0	W'ly	Clear	
7	29.81	29.83	29.89	63	68	58	63.0	N. E'ly	Cloudy, r'n	0.60
8	29.92	29.86	29.73	60	73	68	67.0	S'ly	Va'ble, r'n	0.35
9	29.52	29.50	29.56	72	77	68	72.3	S. W'ly	Variable	
10	29.45	29.44	29.57	62	71	55	62.7	W'ly	Clear	
11	29.63	29.58	29.84	48	63	48	53.0	W'ly	Clear	
12	29.96	30.03	30.16	43	59	46	49.3	W'ly	Clear	
13	30.31	30.31	30.31	44	64	49	52.3	W'ly	Clear	
14	30.33	30.30	30.22	46	67	53	55.3	S. E'ly	Clear	
15	30.01	30.00	30.06	51	69	56	58.7	W'ly	Clear	
16	30.04	30.04	30.04	53	72	60	61.7	W'ly	Clear	
17	30.02	29.96	29.89	52	76	69	65.7	S. W'ly	Variable	
18	29.79	29.74	29.73	68	77	70	71.7	S'ly	Cloudy	
19	29.73	29.74	29.70	66	76	69	70.3	S'ly	Variable	
20	29.70	29.68	29.69	64	77	68	69.7	S'ly	Clear	
21	29.67	29.67	29.62	61	78	66	68.3	S'ly	Clear	
22	29.71	29.74	29.79	60	73	60	64.3	N. W.	Clear	
23	29.75	29.69	29.69	57	68	66	63.7	N. E'ly	Cloudy, sh.	0.15
24	29.79	29.81	29.86	60	68	58	62.0	N. W.	Clear	
25	29.88	29.83	29.89	58	69	61	62.6	W'ly	Clear	
26	30.03	29.99	30.00	53	68	58	59.7	S'ly	Clear	
27	29.89	29.76	29.69	58	71	62	63.7	S'ly	Variable	
28	29.72	29.80	29.80	61	60	52	57.6	N. E'ly	Cloudy, r'n	0.06
29	29.80	29.85	30.13	43	54	37	44.7	N. W.	Clear	
30	30.26	30.20	30.16	33	54	47	44.7	W'ly	Clear	
Means	29.85	29.84	29.86	57.8	70.4	60.1	...	...	...	3.81
REDUCED TO SEA LEVEL.										
Max.	30.51	30.49	30.49	74	86	74	76.7			
Min.	29.63	29.62	29.69	33	54	37	44.7			
Mean	30.03	30.01	30.04							
Range	0.88	0.87	0.80	41	32	37	32.0			
Mean of month			30.027	...	...	...	62.8			
Extreme range			0.89	...	...	...	53.0			

REMARKS.

Appearances of frost in some places on the morning of the 12th.

White frost in the college yard on the 30th.

October, 1834.

DAYS.	BAROMETER, REDUCED TO 32° F. Sunrise.	At 1 P. M.	At 10 P. M.	THERMOMETER. Sunrise.	At 1 P. M.	At 10 P. M.	Daily mean	WINDS.	WEATHER.	RAIN AND SNOW IN INCHES OF WATER.
1	29.87	29.85	29.63	51	71	68	63.3	S. W.	Rain	0.22
2	29.50	29.44	29.61	72	81	64	72.3	S. W.	Variable	
3	29.75	29.76	29.79	54	70	56	60.0	N. W.	Rain	
4	29.74	29.62	29.50	52	68	65	61.7	S. W.	Clear	0.24
5	29.56	29.70	29.86	54	56	44	51.3	N. W.	Clear	
6	30.04	30.08	30.15	38	56	46	46.7	N. W.	Clear	
7	30.19	30.14	30.11	42	66	55	54.3	S. W.	Variable	
8	30.00	29.96	29.92	54	71	63	62.7	S. W.	Cloudy	
9	29.76	29.56	29.39	62	65	65	64.0	S. W.	Rain	1.33
10	29.55	29.71	30.06	44	50	37	43.7	N. W.	Clear	
11	30.23	30.23	30.23	33	50	42	41.7	N. W.	Clear	
12	30.18	30.06	29.92	38	62	53	51.0	W'ly	Clear	
13	29.78	29.62	29.51	52	70	48	56.7	S. W'ly	Clear	
14	29.52	29.62	29.84	34	43	32	36.3	N. W.	Variable	
15	29.98	30.03	30.18	26	43	34	34.3	N. W.	Clear	
16	30.34	30.31	30.28	28	49	43	40.0	W'ly	Variable	
17	30.18	29.97	29.89	50	64	58	57.3	S. W'ly	Variable	
18	29.81	29.70	29.64	54	71	62	62.3	S. W'ly	Clear	
19	29.52	29.46	29.48	60	70	48	59.3	S. W'ly	Cloudy, r'n	1.30
20	29.55	29.58	29.74	41	47	38	42.0	N. W.	Variable	
21	29.94	29.94	29.97	35	48	37	40.0	N. W.	Clear	
22	29.93	29.77	29.73	34	54	46	44.7	S. W'ly	Variable	
23	29.73	29.69	29.72	43	50	39	44.0	N. W.	Variable	
24	29.93	29.93	30.04	34	47	33	38.0	N. W.	Clear	
25	30.14	30.09	30.14	26	41	31	32.7	N. W.	Clear	
26	30.08	29.88	29.50	32	36	46	38.0	N. E.	Rain	1.55
27	29.71	29.64	29.69	34	52	40	42.0	N. W.	Clear	
28	29.72	29.68	29.83	32	51	41	41.3	N'ly	Clear	
29	29.95	29.98	30.07	30	44	35	36.3	W'ly	Clear	
30	30.14	30.13	30.13	30	44	36	36.7	N. E.	Variable	
31	30.14	30.11	30.12	36	40	37	37.7	N. E.	Cloudy	
Means	29.89	29.85	29.86	42.0	55.8	48.1	...	...	...	4.64
REDUCED TO SEA LEVEL.										
Max.	30.52	30.49	30.46	72	81	68	72.3			
Min.	29.68	29.62	29.64	26	36	31	32.7			
Mean	30.07	30.02	30.04							
Range	0.84	0.87	0.82	46	45	37	39.6			
Mean of month			30.043	...	...	...	48.1			
Extreme range			0.90	...	...	...	55.0			

November, 1834.

DAYS.	BAROMETER. Sunrise.	At 1 P. M.	At 10 P. M.	THERMOMETER. Sunrise.	At 1 P. M.	At 10 P. M.	Daily mean.	WINDS.	WEATHER.	RAIN AND SNOW IN INCHES OF WATER.
1	30.11	30.10	30.11	31	38	28	32.3	N. E.	Variable	
2	30.12	30.05	30.06	27	41	30	32.7	N. W.	Clear	
3	30.07	30.06	30.05	26	43	30	33.0	N. E.	Clear	
4	30.01	29.90	29.79	31	53	47	43.7	W'ly	Clear	
5	29.75	29.73	29.89	51	52	42	48.3	S. W'ly	Cloudy, sh.	0.14
6	29.99	29.97	29.89	36	48	36	40.0	W'ly	Clear	
7	29.73	29.58	29.57	33	51	49	44.3	W'ly	Variable	
8	29.67	29.68	29.93	41	48	34	41.0	W'ly	Clear	
9	30.04	29.99	29.88	28	47	41	38.7	W'ly	Clear	
10	29.78	29.73	29.78	40	52	45	45.7	W'ly	Clear	
11	29.73	29.68	29.76	40	42	35	39.0	N. E.	Rain	0.30
12	29.77	29.68	29.64	35	45	41	40.3	W'ly	Variable	
13	29.77	29.79	29.68	34	46	40	40.0	W'ly	Clear	
14	29.54	29.32	29.33	45	59	53	52.3	S. W.	Variable	
15	29.85	29.97	30.10	23	25	23	23.7	N. E'ly	Variable	
16	30.12	30.16	30.26	23	30	22	25.0	N. E'ly	Variable	
17	30.38	30.33	30.19	20	38	34	30.6	E'ly	Variable	
18	29.72	29.45	29.34	44	48	40	44.0	N. E.	Rain	2.88
19	29.30	29.31	29.34	40	43	39	40.7	N'ly	Cloudy	
20	29.41	29.44	29.45	33	47	36	38.7	N. W.	Clear	
21	29.65	29.64	29.66	32	47	36	38.3	W'ly	Clear	
22	29.70	29.59	29.50	28	46	44	39.3	S. W'ly	Va'ble, sh.	0.07
23	29.36	29.35	29.48	45	48	37	43.3	W'ly	Variable	
24	29.44	29.39	29.37	32	38	32	34.0	W'ly	Variable	
25	29.35	29.35	29.48	27	32	24	27.7	W'ly	Variable	
26	29.59	29.60	29.73	23	36	28	29.0	W'ly	Clear	
27	29.76	29.78	29.80	26	30	24	26.7	W'ly	Clear	
28	29.86	29.85	29.91	26	41	34	33.7	S. W'ly	Clear	
29	29.75	29.64	29.40	34	47	53	44.7	S'ly	Rain	0.11
30	29.61	29.69	29.90	40	46	34	40.0	N. W.	Clear	
Means	29.76	29.73	29.74	33.1	43.5	36.4	...	...	...	3.80
REDUCED TO SEA LEVEL.										
Max.	30.56	30.51	30.44	51	59	53	48.3			
Min.	29.48	29.49	29.52	20	24	22	23.7			
Mean	29.94	29.91	29.92							
Range	1.08	1.02	0.92	31	34	31	24.6			
Mean of month			29.923	...	...	...	37.7			
Extreme range			1.08	...	...	...	39.0			

DAYS.	BAROMETER, REDUCED TO 32° F. Sunrise.	At 1 P. M.	At 10 P. M.	THERMOMETER. Sunrise.	At 1 P. M.	At 10 P. M.	Daily mean.	WINDS. Sunrise.	At 1 P. M.	At 10 P. M.	WEATHER. Sunrise.	At 1 P. M.	At 10 P. M.	RAIN AND SNOW IN INCHES OF WATER.
December, 1834.														
1	30.04	29.90	29.70	32	45	46	41.0	...	S. W'ly	...	...	Clear	...	
2	29.60	29.47	29.44	46	45	40	43.6	...	S. W'ly	...	...	Rain	...	0.10
3	29.45	29.49	29.75	32	39	30	33.7	...	N. W.	...	...	Variable	...	
4	30.05	30.08	30.08	24	32	27	27.7	...	N. W.	...	...	Clear	...	
5	30.02	30.00	30.01	28	38	29	31.7	...	W'ly	...	...	Clear	...	
6	29.46	28.98	29.32	42	55	40	45.7	S. E.	S. W.	W.	Rain	Cleared	Clear	1.50
7	29.80	29.86	29.94	36	45	34	38.3	W.	W.	W.	Clear	Clear	Clear	
8	29.57	29.19	29.46	41	52	41	44.7	S. E'ly	S. W.	W.	Rain	Cloudy	Clear	0.12
9	29.90	29.97	30.08	26	32	23	27.0	N. W.	N. W.	N. W.	Clear	Clear	Clear	
10	30.15	30.11	30.01	18	32	28	26.0	W.	W.	W'ly	Clear	Clear, m.	Clear	
11	29.86	29.76	29.77	27	38	31	32.0	W'ly	S. W.	W'ly	Clear	Clear, m.	Clear, m.	
12	29.79	29.76	29.68	30	33	29	30.7	W'ly	N'ly	N'ly	Clear, m.	Cloudy	Cl'dy, m.	
13	29.40	29.34	29.48	31	33	33	32.3	S. W'ly	S. W'ly	W'ly	Cl'dy, m.	Snow, m.	Cl'dy, m.	
14	29.16	29.38	29.70	34	12½	—4½	14.0	S. W'ly	N. W.	N. W.	Cl'dy, m.	Clear	Clear	
15	29.83	29.81	29.62	—8	9	21	7.3	N. W.	N. W.	S. W'ly	Clear	Var., m.	Cl'dy, m.	
16	29.48	29.50	29.88	28	35	24	29.0	S. W.	W'ly	N. W'ly	Clear, m.	Var., m.	Variable	
17	30.13	30.19	30.20	12	22	17	17.0	N.	N.	N. E.	Variable	Cl'dy, m.	Cloudy	
18	30.19	30.14	30.19	20	30	24	24.7	N. E'ly	N. E'ly	N. E'ly	Cloudy	Variable	Variable	
19	30.22	30.19	30.15	27	34	30	30.3	N. E'ly	N'ly	N. E.	Variable	Variable	Snow	
20	29.95	29.79	29.77	28	34	32	31.3	N. E.	N. W.	N. W.	Cloudy	Variable	Clear	
21	29.98	30.03	30.09	24	25	18	22.3	N. W.	N. W.	N. W.	Clear	Clear	Clear	
22	30.08	30.03	30.03	13	33	30	25.3	N. W.	N'ly	N. E.	Clear	Variable	Cloudy	
23	30.02	30.03	30.02	31	37	25	31.0	W'ly	W'ly	S. W'ly	Variable	Variable	Cloudy	
24	30.03	29.87	29.77	24	29	24	25.7	N. E'ly	N. E.	N. E.	Cloudy	Cloudy	Snow	0.25
25	29.64	29.74	29.98	21	26	8	18.3	N. E.	N. W.	N. W.	Snow	Clear	Clear	
26	29.99	29.85	29.76	8	13	13	11.3	N. E'ly	N. E'ly	N. E'ly	Cloudy	Cloudy	Cloudy	
27	29.75	29.79	29.94	18	25	15	19.3	N. W.	N. W.	N.	Variable	Clear	Clear	
28	30.03	30.09	30.11	10	22	18	16.7	N. W.	N. W.	N'ly	Clear	Clear	Cloudy	
29	30.06	29.95	29.80	18	30	29	25.7	N. E.	N. E.	N. E.	Cloudy	Cloudy	Snow	} 1.00
30	29.42	29.38	29.43	21	30	26	25.7	N. E.	N. E.	N. E.	Snow	Cloudy	Cloudy	
31	29.54	29.54	29.64	20	30	22	24.0	N. W.	N. W.	N. W.	Var., m.	Clear	Clear	
Means	29.83	29.78	29.83	24.6	32.1	25.9	...	...	...	...	...	...	...	2.97
REDUCED TO SEA LEVEL.														
Max.	30.40	30.37	30.38	46	55	46	45.7							
Min.	29.34	29.37	29.50	—8	9	—4½	7.3							
Mean	30.01	29.96	30.01											
Range	1.06	1.00	0.88	54	46	50½	38.4							
Mean of month			30.993	...	...	...	27.5							
Extreme range			0.06	...	...	...	63.0							

REMARKS.

5th. At 10 P. M., haze in the S. W. and S.; wind S'ly; barometer 30.06.

6th. At 6 A. M., wind fresh at S. E.; beginning to rain. 8 A. M. Barom. 29.50. 9 A. M. Barom. 29.40. 10 A. M. Barom. 29.27; heavy rain at intervals. 11 A. M. Wind hauling to S. W., and violent; barom. 29.20. 11½ A. M. Barom. 29.14; blows violently; clouds broken. 12 M. Barom. 29.10; wind farther to westward; sun out. 12½ M. Barom. 29.10; clouds much broken; heavy fog-clouds passing rapidly from S. W. to N. E., pass from about 20° elevation in S. W. to same height N. E., in 2 minutes—some in 2½ and others in 3 minutes; a second stratum of clouds, much higher, moves from a more western point. 1 P. M. Barom. 29.08; wind abated; nearly all clear overhead. 2 P. M. Barom. 29.05; wind still strong from S. W.; heavens covered at short intervals with heavy fog-clouds; rain 1.50 inch. 3½ P. M. Bar. rising, 29.06; clouds passing; wind W. 5 P. M. Barom. 29.10; thick clouds overhead; occasional dashes of rain. 6 P. M. Barom. 29.18; very dark clouds from W.; sky very clear in patches. 10 P. M. Barom. 29.38; clear; wind fresh from W. to N. W.

13th. Wind S. W. Began to snow at 10 A. M. Clouds broken, and stopped snowing at 4 P. M.

14th. At 8 A. M., barom 29.20; ther. 34°; wind S. W'ly; mild, cloudy. 9 A. M. Wind N'ly, brisk; snowing fast; barom. 29.27; ther. 26°. 10 A. M. Snowing; barom. 29.33; ther. 22°.5. 12 M. Clouds broken; sun out; barom. 29.40; ther. 16°; wind N. W'ly. 1 P. M. Wind N. W., brisk; clear; ther. 12°.5; barom. 29.42. 1½ P. M. Barom. 29.45; ther. 10°.5. 4 P. M. Ther. 5°; barom. 29.54. 6 P. M. Ther. —1°; barom. 29.65. 7 P. M. Ther. —2°. 8 P. M. Ther. —3°. 9 P. M. Ther. —4°. 10 P. M. Ther. —4°.75, nearly; barom. 29.72. 11 P. M. Ther. —5°.

15th. At sunrise, ther. —8°; colder than has been known for several years.

24th. Flurry of snow between 9 and 10 A. M. About 3 P. M., began snowing, and continued till night.

29th. Wind N. E.; fine snow occasionally. During night, snow and heavy wind.

30th. At sunrise, snowing fast; wind heavy at N. E. Stopped snowing about 11 A. M. Snow 10 or 11 inches on level, equal to 1 inch of water.

DAYS.	BAROMETER Sunrise.	At 1 P. M.	At 10 P. M.	THERMOMETER Sunrise.	At 1 P. M.	At 10 P. M.	Daily mean.	WINDS Sunrise.	At 1 P. M.	At 10 P. M.	WEATHER Sunrise.	At 1 P. M.	At 10 P. M.	RAIN AND SNOW
January, 1835.														
1	29.78	29.88	29.88	11	16	13	13.3	N. W.	N. W.	N'ly	Clear	Clear	Snow	0.25
2	29.69	29.73	29.88	13	26	20	19.7	N'ly	W'ly	W'ly	Cloudy	Clear	Variable	
3	29.98	30.05	30.17	3	7	—3½	2.2	N. W.	N. W.	N. W.	Variable	Variable	Clear	
4	30.23	30.21	30.21	—9	3½	—3	—2.8	N. W.	N. W.	N. W.	Clear	Clear	Clear	
5	30.21	30.07	30.06	—5½	13	9	5.5	N. W.	N. W.	N. W.	Clear	Clear	Clear	
6	30.07	30.02	30.04	13	5	1	6.3	N. E.	N. E.	N.	Cloudy	Cloudy	Variable	
7	30.05	30.02	30.02	—4½	3	4	0.8	N.	N. W.	N. W.	Clear	Clear	Clear	
8	30.02	30.03	30.06	6	13	14	11.0	N. W.	N. W.	N. W.	Clear	Clear	Clear	
9	30.14	30.12	30.15	8	19	10	12.3	N. W.	N. W.	N. W.	Clear	Clear	Clear	
10	30.17	30.13	30.11	8	27	18	17.3	N. W.	N. W.	W'ly	Clear	Clear	Clear	
11	30.09	30.02	30.02	16	29	24	23.0	N'ly	N'ly	N'ly	Clear	Clear	Clear	
12	29.98	29.91	29.88	20	35	25	26.7	N'ly	W'ly	W'ly	Clear	Clear	Clear	
13	29.80	29.78	29.78	23	40	30	31.0	S. W'ly	S. W'ly	S. W'ly	Clear	Clear	Variable	
14	29.69	29.52	29.45	35	44	39	39.3	S. W'ly	S. W'ly	S. W'ly	Cloudy	Cloudy	Rain	0.25
15	29.73	29.69	29.64	36	46	32	38.0	W'ly	W'ly	S. W'ly	Clear	Clear	Variable	
16	29.28	29.32	29.54	38	45	36	39.7	W'ly	W'ly	W'ly	Rain	Clear	Clear	0.58
17	29.69	29.78	29.86	31	39	34	34.7	W'ly	W'ly	W'ly	Clear	Variable	Cloudy	
18	29.85	29.81	29.84	28	34	24	28.7	W'ly	W'ly	W'ly	Variable	Variable	Clear	
19	29.91	29.86	29.83	16	30	24	23.3	W'ly	N. W'ly	N. W'ly	Clear	Clear	Clear	
20	29.70	29.74	29.81	28	39	28	31.7	W'ly	W'ly	W'ly	S. flurry	Clear	Clear	
21	29.83	29.73	29.45	22	34	34	30.0	N. W'ly	S. W'ly	S. E'ly	Clear	Cloudy	Cloudy	
22	29.18	29.33	29.52	45	39	30	38.0	N. W'ly	N. W.	N. W.	Rain	Clear	Clear	0.30
23	29.54	29.56	29.85	34	45	30	36.3	N. W.	W'ly	N. W.	Clear	Variable	Clear	
24	30.03	30.11	30.22	26	30	26	27.3	N. W.	N. W.	N. W.	Clear	Clear	Clear	
25	30.18	30.07	29.76	18	31	38	29.0	N. W.	S. E'ly	S. E'ly	Clear	Cloudy	Rain	0.62
26	29.50	29.44	29.42	47	53	49	49.7	S. W.	S. W.	S. W.	Cloudy	Cloudy	Rain	0.25
27	29.52	29.60	29.69	40	46	34	40.0	W'ly	N'ly	W'ly	Clear	Clear	Clear	
28	29.74	29.65	29.76	32	38	36	35.3	N. E.	N. E.	N. W.	Rain	Rain	Clear	0.25
29	30.09	30.19	30.09	31	38	30	33.0	N. W.	N. W.	N. W.	Clear	Clear	Clear	
30	30.07	29.85	29.55	30	35	44	36.3	N. E.	N. E.	S. W.	Snow	Rain	Rain	1.00
31	29.09	29.13	29.20	51	48	37	45.3	S. W.	W'ly	N. W.	Rain	Variable	Variable	
Means	29.83	29.82	29.83	22.2	30.6	24.7	...	...	...	...	...	...	...	3.50
REDUCED TO SEA LEVEL.														
Max.	30.41	30.39	30.40	51	53	49	49.7							
Min.	29.17	29.31	29.38	—9	3	—3½	—2.8							
Mean	30.01	30.00	30.01											
Range	1.24	1.08	1.02	60	50	52½	52.5							
Mean of month			30.007	...	...	...	25.9							
Extreme range			1.24	...	...	...	62.0							

The following will present a view of the great diversity in thermometers, placed in different situations, when the weather, as in the present instance, is very cold and very still. Nearly all day of the 3d, all the 4th, and the earlier part of the 5th, there was uncommon stillness in the air—almost a dead calm.

5th. On the morning of the 5th, at or about sunrise, thermometers in this neighborhood varied from 5°.5 below zero to 26° below—the coldest stations all being in valleys, and the warmest on hills.

7th. At sunrise, thermometer 2° above zero. Plunged the bulb about 2 inches beneath the snow, and in about 15 minutes the mercury rose to 13°; plunged it 7 or 8 inches under, and in about 20 minutes the mercury rose to 25°.

19th. At 6½ P. M., observed an unusually bright meteor pass from the star Capella to a point a very little west of Aldebaran; the train of light long and brilliant, of a purplish hue.

29th. The aurora quite bright in the north for several hours in the evening.

31st. Frequent and vivid lightnings and rain before daylight—perhaps from 4 to 5 o'clock.

February, 1835.

DAYS.	BAROMETER, REDUCED TO 32° F.			THERMOMETER.				WINDS.			WEATHER.			RAIN AND SNOW IN INCHES OF WATER.
	Sunrise.	At 1 P. M.	At 10 P. M.	Sunrise.	At 1 P. M.	At 10 P. M.	Daily mean.	Sunrise.	At 1 P. M.	At 10 P. M.	Sunrise.	At 1 P. M.	At 10 P. M.	
1	29.28	29.35	29.45	28	34	24	28.7	N. W.	N. W.	N. W.	Variable	Variable	Clear	
2	29.51	29.66	29.97	24	23	21	22.7	N. W.	N. W.	N. W.	Variable	Clear	Clear	
3	30.07	30.07	30.03	9	20	12	13.7	N. W.	N. W.	N'ly	Clear	Clear	Variable	
4	29.88	29.77	29.79	4	13	6	7.7	N. W.	N. W.	N. W.	Clear	Clear	Clear	
5	29.81	29.77	29.73	7	21	14	14.0	W'ly	N. W'ly	N. W'ly	Clear	Clear	Clear	
6	29.86	29.78	29.68	17	27	26	20.0	S. W'ly	N. E'ly	N. E'ly	Variable	Snow	Snow	0.10
7	29.50	29.50	29.50	27	32	11	23.3	N'ly	N. W.	W'ly	Cloudy	Variable	Variable	
8	29.51	29.49	29.70	2	8	8	6.0	S. W'ly	W'ly	W'ly	Clear	Clear	Clear	
9	30.00	30.01	30.01	4	18	12	11.3	S. W'ly	S. W'ly	W'ly	Clear	Clear	Clear	
10	30.02	30.00	29.99	8	20	12	13.3	N. W'ly	N. W'ly	N'ly	Variable	Clear	Clear	
11	29.82	29.69	29.60	6	29	22	19.0	W'ly	S. W'ly	S. W'ly	Clear	Variable	Cloudy	
12	29.60	29.64	29.74	16	26	17	19.7	W'ly	W'ly	N'ly	Variable	Clear	Clear	
13	29.71	29.59	29.59	17	37	33	29.0	S. W'ly	S. W'ly	S. W'ly	Clear	Cloudy	Cloudy	
14	29.78	29.97	30.28	33	34	16	27.7	W'ly	W'ly	N. W.	Cloudy	Cloudy	Clear	
15	30.39	30.35	30.26	8	18	16	14.0	N. E'ly	N'ly	N'ly	Cloudy	Cloudy	Cloudy	
16	30.17	30.12	30.12	16	27	26	23.0	N. W'ly	N'ly	N. E'ly	Cloudy	Cloudy	Cloudy	
17	29.93	29.81	29.71	28	31	31	30.0	N. E.	N. E.	N. E.	Rain	Rain	Rain	0.85
18	29.54	29.52	29.64	29	34	34	32.3	N. E.	N'ly	N'ly	Cloudy	Cloudy	Cloudy	
19	29.70	29.70	29.86	32	40	32	34.7	S. W'ly	S. W'ly	W'ly	S. flurry	Cloudy	Cloudy	
20	30.06	30.16	30.22	27	35	28	30.0	N. W.	N. W.	N. W.	Clear	Clear	Clear	
21	30.09	29.89	29.83	30	42	36	36.0	S. W'ly	S. W'ly	S. W'ly	Variable	Variable	Clear	
22	29.74	29.64	29.60	36	55	50	47.0	S. W'ly	S. W'ly	W'ly	Clear	Variable	Clear	
23	29.89	30.01	30.10	37	40	32	36.3	N'ly	W'ly	W'ly	Variable	Variable	Cloudy	
24	30.16	30.12	30.13	32	34	30	32.0	N. E.	N. E.	N. E.	Cloudy	Cloudy	Cloudy	
25	30.01	29.86	29.76	32	36	34	34.0	N. E.	S'ly	S. W'ly	Cloudy	Cl'dy, r'n	Cloudy	
26	29.75	29.77	29.87	28	36	24	29.3	S'ly	W'ly	W'ly	Clear	Clear	Cloudy	
27	29.82	29.71	29.58	14	14	12	13.3	N. E.	N. E.	N. E.	Snow	Snow	Snow	0.25
28	29.69	29.71	29.90	0	16	6	7.3	N. W.	N. W.	N. W.	Clear	Clear	Clear	
Means	29.83	29.81	29.84	19.6	28.4	22.3	...	...	...	...	...	...	...	1.20
REDUCED TO SEA LEVEL.														
Max.	30.57	30.53	30.46	37	55	50	47.0							
Min.	29.46	29.53	29.63	0	8	6	6.0							
Mean	30.01	29.99	30.02											
Range	1.11	1.00	0.83	37	47	41	41.0							
Mean of month	30.007			...	...	...	23.5							
Extreme range	1.11			...	...	...	55.0							

REMARKS.

8th. In the Southern and Western States, it appears that this was the coldest day for many years. It was here one of the severest days to be out during the winter thus far.

16th. Hail occasionally through the day.

17th. Ground thickly covered with sleet, walking excessively slippery.

March, 1835.

DAYS.	Bar. Sunrise.	Bar. At 1 P. M.	Bar. At 10 P. M.	Therm. Sunrise.	Therm. At 1 P. M.	Therm. At 10 P. M.	Daily mean.	Wind Sunrise.	Wind At 1 P. M.	Wind At 10 P. M.	Weather Sunrise.	Weather At 1 P. M.	Weather At 10 P. M.	Rain and Snow
1	30.04	30.07	30.12	0	19	6	8.3	N. W.	N. W.	N. W.	Clear	Clear	Clear	
2	30.15	30.13	30.12	—2	21	13	10.7	S. W'ly	S. W'ly	S. W'ly	Clear	Clear	Clear	
3	30.10	30.10	30.19	9	19	4	10.7	S. W'ly	N. W.	N. W.	Clear	Variable	Clear	
4	30.21	30.30	30.39	4	22	15	13.7	N. W.	N. W.	N. W.	Clear	Clear	Clear	
5	30.40	30.39	30.29	9	30	18	19.0	W'ly	W'ly	W'ly	Clear	Clear	Clear	
6	30.21	30.15	30.13	12	35	22	23.0	W'ly	S. W'ly	S. W'ly	Clear	Clear	Clear	
7	30.08	29.93	29.74	20	35	32	29.0	N. E.	N. E.	N. E.	Variable	Rain	Rain	0.50
8	29.61	29.77	29.92	32	31	31	31.3	N. E.	N. E.	N. E.	Misty	Cloudy	Cloudy	
9	29.97	29.97	29.89	28	33	29	30.0	N. E.	N. E.	N. E.	Cloudy	Cloudy	Cloudy	
10	29.74	29.53	29.42	26	32	28	28.7	N. E.	N. E.	N. E.	Cloudy	Rain	Snow	0.75
11	29.64	29.76	29.86	29	39	28	32.0	N'ly	N'ly	W'ly	Variable	Clear	Clear	
12	29.93	29.90	29.80	27	48	32	35.7	N. W'ly	N. W'ly	S. W'ly	Clear	Clear	Clear	
13	29.47	29.46	29.58	34	47	36	39.0	S. W'ly	S. W'ly	S. W'ly	Cloudy	Variable	Clear	
14	29.74	29.76	29.74	32	46	38	38.7	S. W'ly	W'ly	W'ly	Clear	Clear	Clear	
15	29.58	29.59	29.59	36	48	39	41.0	S. W'ly	W'ly	S. W.	Cloudy	Clear	Cloudy	
16	29.44	29.33	29.37	41	53	46	46.7	S. W'ly	S. W.	W'ly	Variable	Clear	Variable	
17	29.28	29.43	29.89	41	46	22	39.7	S. W.	N. W.	N. W.	Rain	Clear	Clear	0.30
18	30.10	30.08	29.99	15	31	26	24.0	N. W.	S. W'ly	S. E'ly	Clear	Clear	Cloudy	
19	29.48	29.04	29.40	32	44	34	36.7	N. E'ly	W'ly	N. W.	Rain	Cloudy	Clear	1.10
20	29.79	29.88	29.85	28	43	37	36.0	N. W.	N. W.	S. W'ly	Clear	Clear	Cloudy	
21	29.59	29.54	29.71	41	61	38	46.7	S. W.	S. W'ly	N. E'ly	Cloudy	Variable	Cloudy	
22	29.57	29.23	29.01	29	32	26	29.0	N. E.	N. E.	N. E.	R'n & h'l	R'n & h'l	R'n & h'l	1.15
23	29.07	29.42	29.79	18	30	22	23.3	N. W.	N. W.	N. W.	Cloudy	Clear	Clear	
24	29 92	30.03	30.02	21	35	30	28.7	W'ly	W.	W.	Clear	Clear	Clear	
25	30.27	30.36	30.40	22	32	26	26.7	N. E'ly	N. E.	N. E.	Variable	Clear	Cloudy	
26	30.30	30.20	29.97	28	42	36	35.3	S. W'ly	S. W'ly	S. W'ly	Variable	Cloudy	Variable	
27	29.78	29.64	29.60	43	48	40	43.7	S. W'ly	S. W.	N. W.	Cloudy	Rain	Clear	0.25
28	29.54	29.51	29.53	36	58	42	45.3	W.	S. W'ly	S'ly	Clear	Variable	Variable	
29	29.59	29.64	29.64	36	38	32	35.3	N. E.	N. E.	N. E.	Misty	Cloudy	Cloudy	
30	29.40	29.29	29.32	30	32	34	32.0	N. E.	N. E'ly	N. E'ly	Snow	Snow	Rain	0.55
31	29.28	29.32	29.47	36	43	42	40.3	N. W'ly	N'ly	N. W'ly	Cloudy	Cloudy	Cloudy	
Means	29.78	29.77	29.80	25.6	37.8	27.2	...	...	...	...	...	...	...	4.60
REDUCED TO SEA LEVEL.														
Max.	30.58	30.57	30.57	43	61	46	46.7							
Min.	29.46	29.41	29.19	—2	19	4	8.3							
Mean	29.96	29.95	29.98											
Range	1.12	1.16	1.38	45	39	42	38.4							
Mean of month	29.963			...	...	...	30.9							
Extreme range	1.39			...	...	...	63.0							

1st. At sunrise, the thermometer at 0° or zero; plunged the bulb 9 inches under a snow-drift, and in 20 minutes it rose to 24°.

2d. Thermometer —2°; several others in the vicinity ranged from —3° to —7°, being all below zero. During the 1st and 2d, the weather was very still.

7th. At sunrise, wind N. E. gentle; a belt of clear sky round the E. and N. E.; nimbus overhead; clouds soon went down in the E and N. E.; wind grew more fresh. At 1 P. M., sprinkling of rain; increases a little till 4 P. M., when it commenced snowing fast, with a strong breeze. At 7 P. M., changed to rain, which continued during the night.

8th. At sunrise, misty. At 8 A. M., barometer began to rise. At 3 P. M., clouds broken in the west; nearly clear. At 5 P. M., clouded over again in the evening.

9th. 1½ inch light snow between 3 and 5 P. M.

10th. Barometer falling in the morning. At 12, began to hail and rain a very little. At 1 P. M., snowing; snowed fast till night, with a driving wind at N. E. At 7 P. M., barometer 29.40; began to rise by 9 P. M., and storm abated. Snow 9 or 10 inches deep, very heavy and damp.

13th. Dash of rain at sunrise.

15th. Clear during the day and pleasant.

16th. Dash of rain at sunrise; also at 9 P. M., with very dark clouds from the W.

17th. Rain at sunrise. Cleared at 10 to 12 A. M. High wind P. M from N. W.

18th. Early part of evening starlight overhead; wind S. E.; heavy cloud stretching from E. round the horizon to S. W. At 9 P. M., thick clouds overhead; wind hauling more to E.; air very raw and chilly. During night, three inches of wet snow from N. E.

19th. At sunrise, rain from E. N. E.; barometer 29.52, and falling fast. Cleared during afternoon; wind brisk at N. W.

21st. Very mild and pleasant during the day; wind S. W'ly. Grew chilly about sunset; wind came to N. E'ly.

22d. Began to rain and hail at 4½ A. M.; strong wind N. E.; barometer 29.62. Continued to rain and hail during the day; heard thunder about noon; lightning and thunder at 5 P. M. Barometer continued falling till 9 P. M., when it stood at 29.03; began to rise immediately; at 9½, stood at 29.05.

27th. Wind changed from S. W. to N. W., about 4 to 5 P. M.

30th. Began snowing 6 to 7 A. M.; wind N. E., very brisk.

April, 1835.

DAYS.	BAROMETER, REDUCED TO 32° F.			THERMOMETER.				WINDS.			WEATHER.			RAIN AND SNOW IN INCHES OF WATER.
	Sunrise.	At 1 P. M.	At 10 P. M.	Sunrise.	At 1 P. M.	At 10 P. M.	Daily mean.	Sunrise.	At 1 P. M.	At 10 P. M.	Sunrise.	At 1 P. M.	At 10 P. M.	
1	29.50	29.52	29.56	42	57	45	48.0	N. W.	N. W.	N. W.	Clear	Clear	Clear	
2	29.57	29.59	29.63	42	55	42	46.3	W'ly	S. W.	S. E'ly	Clear	Variable	Cloudy	
3	29.64	29.69	29.69	40	54	38	44.0	E'ly	E'ly	N. E.	Cloudy	Variable	Rain	1.15
4	29.46	29.51	29.64	38	45	37	36.7	N. E.	N. W'ly	N. E'ly	Cloudy	Cloudy	Cloudy	
5	29.54	29.42	29.39	35	37	37	36.3	N. E.	N. E.	S. W.	Cloudy	Rain	Cloudy	0.25
6	29.39	29.30	29.24	36	52	40	42.7	S. W.	S. W.	S. W.	Variable	Variable	Shower	
7	29.16	29.20	29.37	38	50	40	42.7	W'ly	W'ly	N. W.	Variable	Cloudy	Clear	
8	29.45	29.47	29.50	36	58	42	45.3	N. W.	W'ly	N. W.	Clear	Clear	Clear	
9	29.50	29.50	29.61	42	70	57	56.3	W'ly	W'ly	W'ly	Clear	Variable	Clear	
10	29.75	29.83	29.92	44	66	42	50.7	W'ly	S. W'ly	S'ly	Clear	Clear	Clear	
11	29.98	30.02	30.04	36	60	40	45.3	S. W'ly	S. W'ly	S'ly	Clear	Clear	Clear	
12	30.03	29.98	29.90	32	57	42	43.7	N. W.	N. W.	N. W.	Clear	Clear	Clear	
13	29.77	29.63	29.47	42	51	46	46.3	S. W'ly	S. W.	N. W'ly	Cloudy	Rain	Clear	0.03
14	29.51	20.52	29.61	36	38	28	34.0	N. W.	N. W.	N. W.	Variable	Variable	Clear	
15	29.76	29.74	29.74	26	47	36	36.3	N. W.	N. W.	W'ly	Clear	Clear	Clear	
16	29.65	29.36	29.41	36	32	33	33.7	S. W.	N. E.	N'ly	Cloudy	Snow	Cloudy	0.45
17	29.45	29.60	29.75	29	35	26	30.0	N. W.	N. W.	N. W.	Clear	Clear	Clear	
18	29.89	29.93	30.02	21	36	32	29.7	N. W.	N. W.	N. W.	Clear	Clear	Clear	
19	30.08	29.98	29.67	25	48	44	39.0	N. W.	S. W.	S. W.	Variable	Cloudy	Rain	0.20
20	29.51	29.30	29.27	50	63	50	54.3	S. W.	S. W.	W'ly	Cloudy	Cloudy	Clear	
21	29.51	29.67	29.72	38	52	43	44.7	N. W.	N. W.	S. W.	Clear	Clear	Cloudy	
22	29.63	29.57	29.57	40	52	44	45.3	S. W.	S. E'ly	S. W'ly	Cloudy	Cloudy	Rain	0.28
23	29.56	29.66	29.77	37	52	39	42.7	N. W.	N. W.	N. W.	Clear	Clear	Clear	
24	29.78	29.83	29.93	35	48	37	40.0	N. W.	N. W.	N. W.	Clear	Clear	Clear	
25	29.94	29.88	29.75	33	36	32	33.7	N. W.	S. W.	N. E.	Clear	Snow	Rain	0.80
26	29.76	29.79	29.82	35	38	36	36.3	N. E.	N. E.	N'ly	Cloudy	Rain	Variable	0.05
27	29.86	29.88	29.84	30	55	42	42.3	N'ly	E'ly	E'ly	Clear	Clear	Cloudy	
28	29.37	29.04	29.37	40	43	41	41.3	N. E'ly	S. W'ly	W.	R'n & sn.	Cloudy	Clear	0.85
29	29.62	29.58	29.79	37	63	49	49.7	W'ly	W'ly	W'ly	Clear	Clear	Clear	
30	29.80	29.83	29.76	49	63	51	54.3	W'ly	W'ly	W'ly	Variable	Variable	Variable	
Means	29.65	29.63	29.60	36.7	50.4	40.3	...	...	...	...	...	...	...	4.06
REDUCED TO SEA LEVEL.														
Max.	30.26	30.20	30.22	50	70	57	56.3							
Min.	29.55	29.22	29.45	21	32	26	29.7							
Mean	29.83	29.81	29.84											
Range	0.71	0.98	0.77	29	38	31	26.6							
Mean of month 29.827				...	...	...	41.1							
Extreme range 1.04				...	...	...	49.0							

REMARKS.

3d. Began raining between 8 and 9 P. M.; wind at N. E., growing fresh.

4th. At sunrise, wind N. E.; during the morning, hauled to N and N. W.; towards night, swung back to N. E., and blew heavily during the night. Misty, but no rain.

5th, At sunrise, wind heavy at N. E. Rain occasionally during the day. At 7 or 8 P. M., wind hauled round to S. W. At 9 P. M., clouds broken and stars out. Clear at 10 P. M.

6th. Light shower at 9 P. M.; wind S. W.

13th. Wind S. W.; began to rain at 1 P. M.; wind came to W'ly, and cleared from 4 to 5 P. M. Occasional lightning, from a cloud low in the S. E., between 9 and 10 P. M.

14th and 15th. Very blustering.

16th. At sunrise, wind S. W'ly; began to rain at 6 A. M. Wind soon came to N. E., with copious snow, which continued till 5 P. M.; 2 inches deep.

19th Wind came to S. W. at 8 or 9 A. M.; blew fresh during the day. Began raining moderately between 5 and 6 P. M.; wind very brisk.

20th. Light rain occasionally during the forenoon. Between 8 and 9 P. M., a light shower; wind S. W.; cleared soon after, and wind hauled to N. W.

22d. Light rain from 3 to 8 P. M.; wind S. W'ly and veering to W.

25th. Variable at sunrise; wind N. W'ly. Wind soon hauled to S. W.; clouded up, and began to rain about 10 A. M.; changed to snow at 11. Wind came round to N. E., from 2 to 3 P. M., with rain. Lightning and thunder from 9 to 10 P. M., with moderate rain continued.

26th. Wind N. E.; light rain till about noon; cloudy P. M. At 8 P. M., wind hauling to N., and clouds broken in N. W. Clear overhead between 9 and 10 P. M.

27th. At sunrise, gentle breeze at N'ly; clear. During forenoon, wind came to E'ly. Towards night, began to grow thick and cloudy round the horizon; air raw. 10 P. M., cloudy; light E. wind.

28th. At from 3 to 4 A. M., heavy blow from E., with copious rain. At 10 A. M., rain ceased; clouds beginning to be broken; wind violent, hauling S'ly. At 1 P. M., wind S. W'ly, very heavy. At 4 P. M., wind W'ly, its violence unabated; clouds broken; barometer rising. From 8 to 9 P. M., cleared; wind abating.

29th. At sunrise, clear; wind W'ly. Clouded up, and a dash of rain from 8 to 9 A. M. Clear again before noon.

30th. Variable; sprinkle of rain from 8 to 10 A. M.

May, 1835.

DAYS.	BAROMETER At 6 A. M.	At 1 P. M.	At 10 P. M.	THERMOMETER At 6 A. M.	At 1 P. M.	At 10 P. M.	Daily mean.	WINDS At 6 A. M.	At 1 P. M.	At 10 P. M.	WEATHER At 6 A. M.	At 1 P. M.	At 10 P. M.	RAIN AND SNOW
1	29.76	29.76	29.65	43	58	46	49.0	N. E.	W'ly	S. W.	Rain	Variable	Variable	0.15
2	29.67	29.65	29.75	43	59	48	50.0	W'ly	W'ly	N. W.	Variable	Variable	Clear	
3	29.86	29.84	29.86	40	63	44	49.0	N. W'ly	N. W'ly	S. E'ly	Clear	Clear	Clear	
4	29.90	29.89	29.72	43	58	46	49.0	W'ly	S. W'ly	S'ly	Cloudy	Cloudy	Rain	0.55
5	29.60	29.62	29.76	45	50	46	47.0	E'ly	N. E'ly	N'ly	Rain	Clear	Cloudy	
6	29.73	29.65	29.64	45	54	50	49.7	E'ly	S. W.	S. W'ly	Cloudy	Rain	Clear	0.05
7	29.74	29.73	29.70	42	61	53	52.0	N. W.	N. W.	S. W.	Clear	Clear	Variable	
8	29.58	29.57	29.63	47	45	41	44.3	N. E.	N. E.	W'ly	Cloudy	Cloudy	Variable	
9	29.66	29.63	29.62	36	60	44	46.7	N. W.	S. W.	S. W.	Clear	Variable	Variable	
10	29.58	29.61	29.66	44	56	47	49.0	S. W.	N. E.	W'ly	Cloudy	Clear	Cloudy	
11	29.73	29.72	29.73	42	69	54	55.0	W'ly	W'ly	S. W.	Clear	Clear	Variable	
12	29.72	29.71	29.72	48	63	55	55.3	S. W'ly	W'ly	S. W'ly	Cloudy	Variable	Clear	
13	29.84	29.80	29.77	43	60	45	49.3	N. E.	N. E.	N. E.	Clear	Clear	Clear	
14	29.72	29.62	29.52	42	52	44	46.0	N. E.	E'ly	E'ly	Cloudy	Cloudy	Rain	0.75
15	29.33	29.39	29.41	40	43	40	41.0	N. E.	N'ly	N. W.	Rain	Cloudy	Clear	
16	29.44	29.44	29.51	38	57	47	47.3	S. W.	W.	N. W.	Clear	Variable	Clear	
17	29.53	29.59	29.72	48	66	58	57.3	W'ly	W'ly	W'ly	Variable	Clear	Clear	
18	29.68	29.54	29.80	54	66	59	59.7	W'ly	W'ly	W'ly	Clear	Clear	Clear	
19	29.83	29.75	29.67	51	69	56	58.7	S. W.	S. W.	S. W'ly	Clear	Clear	Clear	
20	29.61	29.58	29.60	54	86	68	69.3	S. W'ly	W'ly	W'ly	Clear	Clear	Cloudy	
21	29.69	29.81	29.87	58	56	49	54.3	N. E'ly	N. E'ly	N. W'ly	Cloudy	Cloudy	Clear	
22	29.91	30.01	30.11	44	55	47	48.7	N. E'ly	N. E'ly	N. E'ly	Clear	Clear	Clear	
23	30.15	30.18	30.17	41	59	48	49.3	N. E'ly	N. E.	N. E.	Clear	Clear	Clear	
24	30.17	29.96	29.95	44	68	56	56.0	S. W'ly	W'ly	W'ly	Clear	Clear	Clear	
25	29.82	29.61	29.55	50	74	69	64.3	W'ly	W'ly	W'ly	Variable	Clear	Clear	
26	29.55	29.53	29.67	65	80	66	70.3	W'ly	W'ly	N. W.	Clear	Clear	Clear	
27	29.78	29.80	29.81	56	73	56	61.7	N. W.	S. W'ly	S. W'ly	Clear	Clear	Clear	
28	29.78	29.74	29.70	56	70	60	62.0	E'ly	E'ly	E'ly	Cloudy	Cloudy	Cloudy	
29	29.50	29.42	29.41	60	71	66	65.7	E'ly	W'ly	W'ly	Cloudy	Cloudy	Clear	
30	29.50	29.59	29.71	65	75	64	68.0	N. W.	N. W.	N. W.	Clear	Variable	Clear	
31	29.81	29.79	29.72	58	75	60	64.3	N. W.	N'ly	S. W.	Clear	Clear	Clear	
Means	29.71	29.69	29.71	47.9	62.9	52.6	...	...	...	...	...	...	...	1.50
REDUCED TO SEA LEVEL.														
Max.	30.35	30.36	30.35	65	86	69	70.3							
Min.	29.51	29.57	29.59	36	43	40	41.0							
Mean	29.89	29.86	29.89											
Range	0.84	0.79	0.76	29	43	29	29.3							
Mean of month 29.880				...	...	...	54.9							
Extreme range 0.85				...	...	...	50.0							

REMARKS.

1st. At sunrise, raining moderately; wind N. E. Rain continued till from 10 to 11 A. M., when wind came round to W'ly.

4th. At sunrise, wind W'ly, very light. During the morning, hauled to S. W'ly; became raw. At 3 P. M., began to rain very gently. From 7 to 8 P. M., wind S'ly, blowing fresh, with rain.

5th. At sunrise, wind E'ly; mist, with some rain. Cloudy during the day; mild.

6th. At sunrise, wind E'ly; mild. At 1 P. M., shower from S. W., equal .05 inch. Cleared, with light breeze from S. W'ly, from 6 to 7 P. M.

8th. At sunrise, wind N. E.; cloudy, mild. Occasional sprinkling of rain during forenoon. At sunset, wind light from W'ly; cloudy. Broken halo round the moon from 9 to 10 P. M.; radius 22°, nearly.

12th. At sunrise, wind S. W'ly; mild, cloudy. Variable during morning. Sprinkling of rain at 1 P. M.; breeze fresh. Dash of rain occasionally from 1 to 4 P. M. At 3 P. M., a violent gust from the N. W., which continued not to exceed two minutes; thick clouds at the time in the W.

14th. At sunrise, mild wind N. E. Cloudy during the morning. Began to rain between 2 and 3 P. M.; wind E'ly, mild. Rain during night.

15th. At sunrise, wind N. E; rain and mist. At 12 M., rain ceased; wind hauling to N. and N. W. Clouds broken and sun out, at 5 P. M.

16th. At sunrise, wind S. W'ly, mild; clear. In the course of the morning, wind hauled more to W; blustering, with heavy clouds from W. Showery from 5 to 6 P. M. Clear evening.

19th. At sunrise, a light breeze from S'ly, while light clouds were passing from N. W. From 8 to 9 A. M., breeze from S'ly became fresh, and continued thus during the day.

20th. Very hot; wind light from W'ly; air thick and sultry. Thunder and lightning, with a light shower, from 6 to 8 P. M.; the main cloud passed to the S.

25th From 8 to 9 P. M., thunder and lightning in the N. E.

28th. Cloudy and foggy during the morning; wind E'ly. Sun came out in the afternoon. Foggy again in the evening.

29th. In morning, cloudy, with mist; wind S'ly. From 11 to 12 A. M., wind came round to W'ly, with a gust, and light shower. Cloudy during the afternoon. Clear in evening.

June, 1835.

DAYS.	BAROMETER, REDUCED TO 32° F. Sun-rise.	At 1 P. M.	At 10 P. M.	THERMOMETER. At 6 A. M.	At 1 P. M.	At 10 P. M.	Daily mean.	WINDS. At 6 A. M.	At 1 P. M.	At 10 P. M.	WEATHER. At 6 A. M.	At 1 P. M.	At 10 P. M.	RAIN AND SNOW IN INCHES OF WATER
1	29.59	29.59	29.72	62	75	64	67.0	S. W.	N. W.	N. W.	Cloudy	Clear	Clear	
2	29.76	29.74	29.73	58	79	69	68.7	N. W.	N. W.	S. W.	Clear	Clear	Clear	
3	29.88	29.92	29.93	65	74	61	66.7	N. E'ly	N. E'ly	S. W'ly	Clear	Clear	Clear	
4	29.92	29.79	29.69	58	77	67	67.3	S. W'ly	S. W'ly	S. W'ly	Variable	Clear	Variable	0.45
5	29.51	29.48	29.48	68	80	66	71.3	S. W.	S. W.	N. W.	Cloudy	Cloudy	Shower	
6	29.64	29.73	29.83	64	74	66	68.0	N. W.	N'ly	N'ly	Clear	Clear	Clear	
7	29.99	30.10	30.20	56	60	50	57.0	N. E.	N. E.	N. E.	Clear	Cloudy	Clear	
8	30.22	30.18	30.12	45	67	50	54.0	S'ly	S'ly	S. W.	Clear	Clear	Clear	
9	30.00	29.88	29.80	50	76	62	62.7	S. W'ly	S. W'ly	S. W'ly	Clear	Clear	Variable	
10	29.76	29.75	29.93	62	80	54	65.3	W'ly	W'ly	N. E.	Variable	Variable	Cl'dy,sh.	0.20
11	29.97	29.90	29.88	54	72	65	63.3	N. E.	S. W'ly	S. W.	Cloudy	Clear	Clear	
12	29.84	29.83	29.80	65	75	68	68.7	S'ly	S. W.	S. W.	Cloudy	Cloudy	Rain	0.50
13	29.75	29.72	29.68	65	78	69	70.7	W'ly	W'ly	W'ly	Cloudy	Clear	Clear	
14	29.63	29.58	29.71	69	77	64	70.0	W'ly	W'ly	N. E.	Clear	Variable	Cloudy	
15	29.86	29.90	29.90	56	64	54	58.0	N. E.	N. E.	N. E.	Cloudy	Clear	Clear	
16	29.87	29.76	29.63	50	71	56	59.0	N. W.	S. W'ly	W'ly	Clear	Clear	Cl'r, sh.	0.10
17	29.54	29.60	29.69	59	72	60	63.7	N. W.	N. W.	N. W.	Clear	Clear	Clear	
18	29.70	29.62	29.64	54	78	62	64.7	N. W.	W'ly	S. W.	Clear	Clear	Clear	
19	29.60	29.49	29.30	61	75	66	67.3	S. W.	S. W'ly	S. W'ly	Clear	Variable	Rain	0.40
20	29.31	29.40	29.63	64	78	65	69.0	N. W.	N. W'ly	N. W.	Clear	Clear	Clear	
21	29.64	29.63	29.76	53	70	54	59.0	N. W.	N. W.	N. W.	Clear	Clear	Clear	
22	29.73	29.65	29.65	46	67	61	58.0	N. W.	N. W.	W'ly	Clear	Clear	Cloudy	
23	29.66	29.70	29.75	55	71	60	62.0	N. W.	N. W.	N. W.	Clear	Clear	Clear	
24	29.75	29.73	29.74	60	76	67	67.7	W'ly	W'ly	S. W'ly	Variable	Clear	Clear	
25	29.76	29.75	29.73	65	78	67	70.0	W'ly	W'ly	S. W'ly	Clear	Variable	Cloudy	
26	29.69	29.67	29.65	62	70	62	64.7	S. W'ly	S. W'ly	N. E.	Rain	Cloudy	Cloudy	0.16
27	29.65	29.65	29.60	60	66	62	62.7	N. E.	N. E.	N. E.	Cloudy	Cloudy	Cloudy	
28	29.52	29.47	29.45	63	79	68	70.0	S. W.	S. W.	S. W.	Misty	Clear	Cloudy	
29	29.40	29.40	29.45	62	77	66	68.3	W'ly	W'ly	W'ly	Clear	Cl'r, sh.	Clear	0.14
30	29.45	29.49	29.62	62	73	54	63.3	W'ly	W'ly	N. W.	Clear	Clear	Clear	
Means	29.72	29.70	29.72	59.1	71.2	59.9	...	...	...	...	...	...	...	1.95
REDUCED TO SEA LEVEL.														
Max.	30.40	30.36	30.38	68	80	69	71.3							
Min.	29.49	29.58	29.48	45	60	50	54.0							
Mean	29.90	29.87	29.90											
Range	0.91	0.78	0.90	23	20	19	17.3							
Mean of month	29.890			...	...	...	64.9							
Extreme range	0.92			...	...	...	30.0							

REMARKS.

1st. At sunrise, wind S. W., rather fresh; cloudy. Showery from 6 to 7 A. M. Wind hauled to N. W. during forenoon, and cleared.

5th. Wind S. W'ly during the day; warm and damp. Thundershower from 6 to 8 P. M., equal .45 inch.

10th. Very hot and sultry during the forenoon; wind W'ly and gentle; the air thick; sun partially obscured. Thundershower from 2 to 5 P. M.; rain .20 inch; wind came to N. E.

11th. At sunrise, wind N. E. Light rain from 9 to 10 A. M. Cleared from 12 M. to 2 P. M.; wind S'ly.

12th. Wind S. W.; cloudy all day; warm and very damp. Commenced raining very gently at 9 P. M. Occasional thunder and lightning during the night. Rain .50 inch.

13th Cloudy in the morning Cleared from 12 M. to 1 P. M. Light shower with thunder, from 5 to 6 P. M.

14th. Wind W'ly during the day. Very warm, and dark clouds from the W. in the afternoon. Wind came to N. E. between 6 and 7 P. M., brisk.

16th. Shower during the night, equal .10 inch.

19th. Clear A. M.; wind light at S. W. Wind freshened towards night; air very damp; fog-clouds from S'ly. Began to rain from 8 to 9 P. M., with thunder; wind very brisk S. W.

29th Shower of rain from W. at 3 P. M., equal .14 inch.

July, 1835.

DAYS.	Sun-rise.	At 1 P. M.	At 10 P. M.	At 6 A. M.	At 1 P. M.	At 10 P. M.	Daily mean.	At 6 A. M.	At 1 P. M.	At 10 P. M.	At 6 A. M.	At 1 P. M.	At 10 P. M.	
1	29.62	29.60	29.62	50	62	54	55.3	N. W.	N. W.	N. W.	Clear	Clear	Clear	
2	29.61	29.47	29.39	50	74	69	64.3	N. W.	N. W.	S. W'ly	Clear	Clear	Clear	
3	29.42	29.42	29.48	64	79	71	71.3	W'ly	W.	S. W'ly	Variable	Clear	Clear	
4	29.55	29.52	29.59	70	88	72	76.7	W'ly	N. W.	W'ly	Clear	Clear	Cloudy	
5	29.61	29.59	29.67	71	84	72	75.7	S. W'ly	S. W'ly	S. W'ly	Clear	Clear	Clear	
6	29.69	29.70	29.75	71	75	65	72.0	S. W'ly	W.	N. W.	Clear	Cloudy	Clear	
7	29.75	29.73	29.71	61	83	68	70.7	S. W'ly	S. W.	S. W.	Clear	Clear	Clear	
8	29.69	29.69	29.75	70	83	68	73.7	W'ly	W'ly	N. E.	Clear	Clear	Variable	
9	29.77	29.77	29.77	64	73	68	68.3	N. E.	N. E.	N. E.	Cloudy	Cloudy	Cloudy	
10	29.78	29.79	29.80	60	67	63	63.3	N. E.	N. E.	N. W.	Rain	Cloudy	Clear	0.28
11	29.87	29.88	29.89	56	75	66	65.7	N. W.	W'ly	S. W'ly	Clear	Clear	Clear	
12	29.91	29.84	29.81	63	75	70	69.3	S. W'ly	S. W'ly	S. W'ly	Clear	Variable	Cloudy	
13	29.70	29.66	29.64	70	84	78	77.3	S. W.	S. W'ly	S. W'ly	Cloudy	Clear	Clear	
14	29.62	29.58	29.62	73	86	76	78.3	S. W.	W'ly	S. W'ly	Clear	Clear	Clear	
15	29.66	29.66	29.66	72	82	70	73.7	S. W.	S. W'ly	W'ly	Cloudy	Variable	Cl'y, r'n	1.63
16	29.48	29.58	29.70	68	77	68	71.0	N. W.	W'ly	N. W.	Variable	Cloudy	Clear	
17	29.75	29.78	29.83	64	78	68	70.0	N. W.	N. W.	N. W.	Clear	Clear	Clear	
18	29.82	29.82	29.81	64	79	70	69.7	N. W.	W'ly	S. W'ly	Clear	Variable	Clear	
19	29.79	29.76	29.75	64	82	70	72.0	W'ly	W'ly	W'ly	Clear	Clear	Clear	
20	29.75	29.78	29.83	67	84	72	74.7	S. W'ly	S. W'ly	S. W'ly	Clear	Variable	Cloudy	
21	29.85	29.87	29.88	70	81	70	73.3	S. W'ly	S. W'ly	S. W'ly	Cloudy	Variable	Clear	
22	29.90	29.89	29.89	64	80	70	71.7	N. W.	N. W.	N. W.	Clear	Clear	Clear	
23	29.89	29.87	29.83	66	81	71	72.7	N. W.	W'ly	W'ly	Clear	Clear	Clear	
24	29.80	29.76	29.76	70	85	74	76.3	N'ly	W'ly	S. W'ly	Clear	Clear	Clear	
25	29.77	29.68	29.64	73	88	74	78.3	S. W'ly	S. W'ly	W'ly	Clear	Clear	Rain	0.18
26	29.73	29.78	29.88	68	74	62	68.0	N. E.	N. E.	N. E'ly	Clear	Clear	Clear	
27	29.96	29.95	29.96	60	75	63	66.0	N. E.	E'ly	E'ly	Clear	Clear	Clear	
28	29.94	29.90	29.88	60	78	67	66.0	S'ly	S'ly	S'ly	Clear	Variable	Cloudy	
29	29.80	29.72	29.70	66	70	68	68.3	S. W'ly	S. W'ly	W'ly	Rain	Rain	Rain	0.60
30	29.62	29.60	29.57	70	80	74	74.7	S. W.	W'ly	W'ly	Cloudy	Clear	Clear	
31	29.58	29.62	29.49	68	78	72	72.7	W'ly	W'ly	W'ly	Variable	Clear	Clear	0.15
Means	29.73	29.72	29.73	65.5	78.7	69.1	...	...	...	...	...	...	...	2.84
REDUCED TO SEA LEVEL.														
Max.	30.14	30.13	30.14	73	88	78	78.3							
Min.	29.60	29.60	29.57	50	62	54	63.3							
Mean	29.90	29.89	29.90											
Range	0.54	0.53	0.57	23	26	24	15.0							
Mean of month	29.897			...	...	...	71.1							
Extreme range	0.57			...	...	...	38.0							

4th. Light shower in the evening.

6th. A heavy thunderstorm passed to the north of us. Fragments of the cloud passed our zenith. Thunder sharp and violent, with only a sprinkling of rain.

9th. Wind N. E. Light rain from 8 to 10 A. M. Clouds broken in afternoon.

10th. Wind N. E Moderate rain in morning. Clouds broken in afternoon. Clear in evening.

14th. Thundershower to N. W. of us. High wind from W'ly in afternoon.

15th. Light shower, with thunder, at sunset. Heavy rain from S. E'ly during the night.

25th. Thundershower from the W., between 9 and 10 P. M.

31st. Light showers, with some thunder, between 8 and 9 P. M.

August, 1835.

Days.	Barometer, reduced to 32° F. Sun-rise.	At 1 P. M.	At 10 P. M.	Thermometer. At 6 A. M.	At 1 P. M.	At 10 P. M.	Daily mean.	Winds. At 6 A. M.	At 1 P. M.	At 10 P. M.	Weather. At 6 A. M.	At 1 P. M.	At 10 P. M.	Rain and Snow in Inches of Water.
1	29.47	29.49	29.58	72	81	66	73.0	W'ly	N. W.	N. W.	Variable	Variable	Clear	
2	29.66	29.65	29.69	63	76	62	67.0	N. W.	N. W.	N. W.	Clear	Clear	Clear	
3	29.67	29.61	29.69	56	74	58	62.7	N. W.	N. W.	N. W.	Clear	Clear	Cl'r, sh.	0.10
4	29.74	29.68	29.74	48	68	56	57.3	N. W.	N. W.	N. W.	Clear	Clear	Clear	
5	29.76	29.77	29.76	52	72	62	62.0	N. W.	N. W.	N. W.	Clear	Clear	Clear	
6	29.76	29.77	29.80	60	71	61	64.0	N. W.	N. E.	S'ly	Variable	Cloudy	Cloudy	
7	29.80	29.80	29.85	57	55	55	55.7	N. E.	N. E.	N. E.	Rain	Rain	Rain	1.50
8	29.88	29.90	29.89	53	72	64	63.0	N. W.	N. W.	S. W.	Clear	Clear	Clear	
9	29.90	29.82	29.79	60	78	69	69.0	S. W'ly	W'ly	W.	Clear	Clear	Clear	
10	29.79	29.79	29.80	65	81	68	71.3	W'ly	S. W'ly	S. W'ly	Clear	Clear	Clear	
11	29.82	29.81	29.82	68	81	74	74.3	S. W.	S. W.	S. W.	Clear	Clear	Variable	
12	29.82	29.83	29.83	72	81	73	75.3	S. W.	S. W.	S. W.	Cloudy	Clear	Cloudy	
13	29.74	29.71	29.69	73	84	74	77.0	S. W.	S. W.	S. W.	Cloudy	Clear	Clear	
14	29.60	29.62	29.77	73	86	68	75.7	S. W.	S. W.	W'ly	Clear	Clear	Variable	
15	29.86	29.88	29.88	63	76	64	67.7	N. E.	N. E.	N. E.	Clear	Clear	Clear	
16	29.69	29.67	29.70	64	78	72	71.3	S'ly	S'ly	S'ly	Cloudy	Cloudy	Cloudy	
17	29.72	29.73	29.75	68	80	70	72.7	S. W.	W'ly	W'ly	Clear	Clear	Clear	
18	29.74	29.65	29.50	67	80	72	73.0	W'ly	S. W.	S'ly	Clear	Clear	Cl'y, sh.	0.15
19	29.48	29.54	29.70	69	78	60	69.0	S. W.	W'ly	N. W.	Clear	Clear	Clear	
20	29.79	29.79	29.69	60	73	66	66.3	N. W.	W'ly	S'ly	Clear	Clear	Clear	
21	29.63	29.48	29.54	66	74	62	67.3	S. W.	S. W.	W'ly	Rain	Clear	Clear	0.15
22	29.65	29.65	29.69	55	70	60	61.7	N. W.	N. W.	N. W.	Clear	Variable	Clear	
23	29.80	29.90	29.91	54	72	61	62.3	N. W.	N. W.	N. W.	Clear	Clear	Clear	
24	29.95	29.93	29.91	54	73	62	63.0	N. W.	S. W'ly	S. W.	Clear	Clear	Clear	
25	29.89	29.82	29.74	59	74	66	66.3	S. W.	S. W.	S. W.	Clear	Clear	Clear	
26	29.69	29.64	29.63	68	73	68	69.0	S. W.	S. W.	S. W.	Cloudy	Rain	Rain	
27	29.63	29.68	29.74	62	77	66	68.3	N. W.	N. W.	N. W.	Clear	Clear	Clear	
28	29.65	29.74	29.78	67	72	72	70.3	S. E.	S. E.	S. W.	Variable	Rain	Rain	0.35
29	29.84	29.82	29.78	70	78	72	73.3	W'ly	W'ly	W'ly	Clear	Clear	Clear	
30	29.65	29.67	29.67	72	76	65	71.0	S. W'ly	W'ly	W'ly	Clear	Clear	Clear	
31	29.66	29.64	29.62	60	74	59	64.3	W'ly	W'ly	W'ly	Clear	Clear	Clear	
Means	29.74	29.73	29.74	62.9	75.4	65.4	...	...	...	...	...	...	...	2.25
REDUCED TO SEA LEVEL.														
Max.	30.13	30.11	30.09	73	86	74	77.0							
Min.	29.65	29.66	29.68	48	55	55	55.7							
Mean	29.91	29.90	29.91											
Range	0.48	0.45	0.41	25	31	19	21.3							
Mean of month 29.907				...	...	...	67.9							
Extreme range 0.48				...	...	...	38.0							

Remarks.

3d. Light showers, with thunder, from 5 to 6 P. M.

4th. At sunrise, thermometer 45°, nearly. Thermometers in the vicinity stood at 42°. Frost in some places in the vicinity.

6th. Showery P. M., with very light wind from E'ly.

11th. Cloudy towards evening, with a sprinkling of rain.

12th. Cloudy in the morning, with light rain. Clear at mid-day, and cloudy at evening with thick fog. Air exceedingly damp.

13th. Foggy in the morning. Air very close and damp.

14th. Light showers from 5 to 6 P. M. Wind hauled more to westward, and became cooler soon after.

16th. Wind S'ly. Cloudy, with mist, in the morning. Showers from 4 to 5 P. M.

18th. Light showers from 4 P. M. until dark, continuing from 5 to 10 minutes.

21st. Light rain, with thunder, from 5 to 6 A. M.; wind S. W. Clear from 9 to 10 A. M. From 4 to 5 P. M., wind hauled more to westward, and grew much cooler; wind fresh.

28th. Wind S. E'ly in the morning. Commenced raining about 10 A. M. Showery till 10 P. M.

September, 1835.

Days.	Barometer. Sun-rise.	At 1 P. M.	At 10 P. M.	Thermometer. Sun-rise.	At 1 P. M.	At 10 P. M.	Daily mean	Winds. Sun-rise.	At 1 P. M.	At 10 P. M.	Weather. Sunrise.	At 1 P. M.	At 10 P. M.	Rain and Snow in Inches of Water.
1	29.81	29.87	29.92	58	65	58	60.3	N. W.	W'ly	N. W.	Clear	Cloudy	Cloudy	
2	29.90	29.92	30.00	58	64	56	59.3	N. E.	N. E.	N. E.	Variable	Variable	Clear	
3	30.01	30.02	30.04	52	74	62	62.7	N. W.	N. W.	N. W.	Clear	Clear	Clear	
4	30.02	30.01	30.03	58	74	64	65.3	N. W.	N. W.	N. W.	Clear	Clear	Clear	
5	29.99	29.88	29.88	62	80	70	70.7	W'ly	W'ly	W'ly	Clear	Clear	Clear	
6	29.78	29.71	29.61	70	84	72	75.3	S. W'ly	S. W'ly	S. W.	Clear	Clear	Clear	
7	29.62	29.66	29.79	70	72	54	65.3	S. W.	S. W'ly	N. W.	Variable	Clear	Clear	
8	29.81	29.76	29.76	45	76	56	59.0	N. W.	W'ly	N. W.	Clear	Clear	Clear	
9	29.74	...	...	58	...	...	...	S. W.	...	...	Clear	...	...	
10	...	29.60	29.69	...	78	61	...	...	S. W.	S. W.	...	Clear	Clear	
11	29.80	29.81	29.82	45	64	56	55.0	N. W.	W'ly	W'ly	Clear	Clear	Clear	
12	29.82	29.81	29.90	51	66	57	58.0	E'ly	E'ly	E'ly	Cloudy	Variable	Variable	
13	29.70	29.69	29.70	57	66	55	59.3	N. E'ly	N. E'ly	S. W'ly	Rain	Cloudy	Clear	0.10
14	29.73	29.74	29.94	51	67	50	56.0	W'ly	W'ly	N. W.	Clear	Variable	Clear	
15	30.08	30.07	30.15	41	62	47	50.0	N. W.	N. W.	N. W.	Clear	Clear	Clear	
16	30.18	30.22	30.25	43	64	48	51.7	N. W.	N'ly	N. E'ly	Clear	Clear	Clear	
17	30.22	30.18	30.17	44	63	49	52.0	N. W.	S. W.	S. W.	Clear	Clear	Clear	
18	30.12	30.05	29.97	42	68	53	54.3	W'ly	S. W.	S. W.	Clear	Clear	Clear	
19	29.84	29.74	29.60	46	68	52	55.3	S. E'ly	S. E'ly	N. E.	Clear	Clear	Cloudy	
20	29.37	29.24	29.40	53	67	58	59.3	N. E.	S. W.	W'ly	Rain	Cloudy	Clear	0.25
21	29.40	29.41	29.52	56	70	61	62.3	S. W.	S. W.	S. W.	Variable	Clear	Clear	
22	29.56	29.74	29.84	51	68	53	57.3	W'ly	W'ly	W'ly	Clear	Clear	Clear	
23	29.93	29.92	29.93	44	66	48	52.7	W'ly	W'ly	W'ly	Clear	Variable	Clear	
24	29.93	29.92	29.92	43	62	50	51.7	W'ly	W'ly	W'ly	Clear	Variable	Variable	
25	29.96	29.98	29.92	44	61	50	51.7	W'ly	W'ly	N'ly	Clear	Variable	Variable	
26	29.98	30.04	30.01	42	63	53	52.7	N. E'ly	N. E'ly	N. E'ly	Clear	Clear	Clear	
27	29.78	29.74	29.66	43	62	50	51.7	N'ly	S'ly	S'ly	Variable	Clear	Clear	
28	29.48	29.46	29.51	42	60	56	52.7	N. E'ly	S'ly	S. W'ly	Variable	Variable	Cloudy	
29	29.61	29.62	29.54	49	62	47	52.7	S. W'ly	W'ly	N. W.	Cloudy	Variable	Rain	0.48
30	29.46	29.40	29.43	40	52	40	54.0	N. W.	N. W.	N. W.	Clear	Clear	Clear	
Means	29.81	29.80	29.82	50.3	67.2	54.7	...	...	...	...	...	...	...	0.83
REDUCED TO SEA LEVEL.														
Max.	30.40	30.40	30.43	70	84	72	75.3							
Min.	29.55	29.42	29.58	40	52	40	44.0							
Mean	30.00	29.97	30.00											
Range	0.95	0.98	0.85	30	32	32	31.3							
Mean of month 29.987				...	...	...	57.4							
Extreme range 1.01				...	...	...	44.0							

Remarks.

13th. Wind N. E'ly at sunrise; cloudy, with occasional rain. Clouds broken through the day. Clear in the evening.

14. Wind W'ly A. M.; weather variable. At 2 or 3 P. M., wind hauled to N. W., and became much cooler. Barometer rose rapidly.

15th. Frost in the vicinity in low places.

19th. Wind light E'ly. Clear till towards night, then cloudy, with wind more to N. E.

20th. Wind N. E., rather fresh. Clouds broken at sunrise. Began to rain very moderately from 7 to 8 A. M. Clouds broken at 1 P. M., with wind S. W. Clear towards night.

26th. First white frost in the College yard.

October, 1835.

DAYS.	BAROMETER, REDUCED TO 32° F. Sun-rise.	At 1 P. M.	At 10 P. M.	THERMOMETER. Sun-rise.	At 1 P. M.	At 10 P. M.	Daily mean.	WINDS. Sun-rise.	At 1 P. M.	At 10 P. M.	WEATHER. Sunrise.	At 1 P. M.	At 10 P. M.	RAIN AND SNOW IN INCHES OF WATER.
1	29.43	29.40	29.33	39	57	55	50.3	N. W.	S. W'ly	S. W.	Clear	Clear	Cloudy	
2	29.37	29.41	29.39	50	66	56	57.3	S. W.	S. W.	S. W.	Clear	Variable	Variable	
3	29.43	29.41	29.53	46	64	47	52.3	S. W.	S. W.	N. W.	Clear	Cloudy	Clear	
4	29.66	29.65	29.65	42	62	58	54.0	N. W.	S. W.	S. W.	Clear	Variable	Cloudy	
5	29.79	29.81	29.76	55	62	62	59.7	S. W.	S. W.	S. W.	Cloudy	Cloudy	Cloudy	
6	29.56	29.50	29.50	65	66	60	63.7	S. E'ly	S'ly	S. W.	Rain	Rain	Cloudy	2.35
7	29.52	29.65	29.77	52	62	48	54.0	W'ly	W'ly	W'ly	Variable	Clear	Clear	
8	29.92	29.92	29.96	42	60	41	47.7	W.	W.	W.	Clear	Clear	Clear	
9	29.92	29.87	29.94	38	56	43	45.7	W.	W.	W.	Clear	Clear	Clear	
10	29.95	29.87	29.84	39	60	49	48.9	W.	S. W.	S. W.	Clear	Clear	Clear	
11	29.72	29.81	30.03	49	62	42	51.0	S. W.	W'ly	N. E.	Clear	Variable	Clear	
12	30.13	30.09	30.07	35	54	44	44.3	W.	W'ly	N. W.	Clear	Clear	Clear	
13	29.99	29.88	29.88	42	64	50	52.0	S. W.	S. W.	S. W.	Clear	Clear	Clear	
14	29.88	29.92	29.93	48	65	51	54.7	S. W.	S. W.	S. W.	Clear	Clear	Foggy	
15	30.01	30.00	30.02	47	61	54	54.0	S. W.	S. W.	S. W.	Foggy	Clear	Foggy	
16	30.05	30.03	30.08	46	65	54	55.0	S. W.	S. W.	S. W.	Clear	Clear	Clear	
17	30.11	30.05	30.05	50	70	57	59.0	S. W.	S. W.	S. W.	Clear	Clear	Clear	
18	30.00	29.96	29.94	57	64	64	61.7	S. W.	S. W.	S. W.	Foggy	Foggy	Foggy	
19	29.96	29.97	30.06	62	74	61	65.7	S. W.	S. W.	S. W.	Foggy	Cloudy	Clear	
20	30.11	30.09	30.10	56	70	62	62.8	S. W.	S. W.	S. W.	Foggy	Clear	Foggy	
21	30.06	30.02	29.99	60	66	57	61.0	N. E.	N. E.	N. E.	Mist	Mist	Mist	
22	30.01	30.01	30.03	57	68	56	60.3	N. E.	W'ly	W'ly	Foggy	Clear	Foggy	
23	30.05	30.00	29.94	53	64	57	58.0	S. W'ly	S. W'ly	S. W'ly	Foggy	Clear	Foggy	
24	29.87	29.84	29.96	57	59	44	53.3	S. W.	N'ly	N. W.	Rain	Cloudy	Clear	0.57
25	30.17	30.13	30.11	34	46	38	39.3	N. W.	N. W.	N. W.	Clear	Clear	Clear	
26	30.08	30.03	30.08	36	56	48	46.7	N. W.	W'ly	W'ly	Clear	Clear	Cloudy	
27	30.18	30.15	30.14	42	58	45	48.3	W'ly	N. E.	W'ly	Clear	Clear	Clear	
28	30.10	29.99	29.96	45	66	55	55.3	W'ly	S. W'ly	W'ly	Cloudy	Clear	Clear	
29	29.95	29.93	29.92	55	71	56	60.7	S. W'ly	S. W.	S. W.	Clear	Clear	Clear	
30	29.92	29.80	29.70	61	69	63	64.3	S. W'ly	S. W.	S. W.	Cloudy	Cloudy	Rain	0.34
31	29.82	29.83	29.97	47	56	44	49.0	N. W.	N. W.	N. W.	Clear	Clear	Clear	
Means	29.89	29.87	29.89	48.6	62.7	52.3	...	...	...	...	...	...	...	3.26
REDUCED TO SEA LEVEL.														
Max.	30.36	30.33	30.32	65	74	64	65.7							
Min.	29.55	29.58	29.51	34	46	38	39.3							
Mean	30.07	30.04	30.07											
Range	0.81	0.75	0.81	31	28	26	26.4							
Mean of month	30.060			...	...	...	54.5							
Extreme range	0.85			...	...	...	40.0							

REMARKS.

5th. Cloudy during the day. Wind at S. W., with occasional dashes of rain.

6th. Heavy blow, and copious rain from the S.

November, 1835.

DAYS.	BAROMETER Sun-rise.	At 1 P. M.	At 10 P. M.	THERMOMETER Sun-rise.	At 1 P. M.	At 10 P. M.	Daily mean.	WINDS Sun-rise.	At 1 P. M.	At 10 P. M.	WEATHER Sunrise.	At 1 P. M.	At 10 P. M.	RAIN AND SNOW
1	30.19	30.23	30.26	30	40	32	34.0	N'ly	N'ly	N'ly	Clear	Clear	Clear	
2	30.20	30.01	30.00	30	54	45	43.0	S. W'ly	S. W'ly	S. W'ly	Clear	Clear	Cloudy	
3	29.90	29.86	29.85	45	60	47	50.7	N. E.	W'ly	W'ly	Cloudy	Variable	Clear	
4	29.88	29.88	29.90	50	67	54	57.0	W'ly	W'ly	W'ly	Clear	Clear	Clear	
5	29.81	29.72	29.73	54	66	58	59.3	W'ly	W'ly	W'ly	Variable	Cloudy	Clear	
6	29.88	29.91	29.94	44	52	43	46.3	W'ly	W'ly	N. E.	Clear	Variable	Cloudy	
7	29.89	29.83	29.85	41	47	45	44.3	N. E.	N. E.	N. E.	Rain	Cloudy	Cloudy	0.20
8	29.88	29.86	29.86	44	50	45	46.3	N'ly	N'ly	N. W.	Variable	Clear	Clear	
9	29.73	29.63	29.60	47	58	50	51.7	S. W'ly	W'ly	W'ly	Cloudy	Variable	Clear	
10	29.82	29.82	29.84	39	49	37	45.0	N. W.	N. W.	N. W.	Clear	Clear	Clear	
11	...	28.93	28.81	...	45	45	...	...	S'ly	W'ly	...	Rain	Clear	0.60
12	28.83	28.84	29.04	37	43	34	38.0	W'ly	W'ly	W'ly	Clear	Variable	Clear	
13	29.31	29.55	29.76	29	34	25	29.3	N. W.	N. W.	N. W.	Clear	Clear	Clear	
14	29.93	29.95	29.92	22	41	38	33.7	N. W.	N. W.	S. W.	Clear	Clear	Variable	
15	29.94	29.89	29.90	45	54	49	49.3	S. W.	S. W.	S. W.	Cloudy	Cloudy	Cloudy	
16	29.64	29.54	29.52	59	62	59	60.0	S. W.	S. W.	W'ly	Cloudy	Cloudy	Cloudy	
17	29.72	29.68	29.72	46	49	34	43.0	W'ly	W'ly	N. W.	Variable	Cloudy	Clear	
18	29.78	29.79	29.81	32	54	44	43.3	W'ly	W'ly	S. W'ly	Clear	Clear	Clear	
19	29.81	29.80	29.78	39	54	49	47.3	S. W'ly	S. W'ly	S. W'ly	Foggy	Clear	Foggy	
20	29.72	29.63	29.46	47	54	63	54.7	S. W'ly	S. W'ly	S. W'ly	Clear	Cloudy	Variable	
21	29.62	29.72	29.88	46	49	40	45.0	W'ly	W'ly	W'ly	Clear	Clear	Cloudy	
22	30.06	30.13	30.21	38	40	28	35.3	W'ly	W'ly	W'ly	Cloudy	Cloudy	Cloudy	
23	29.84	29.70	29.60	25	34	25	28.0	N. E.	N. E.	N. E.	Snow	R'n & sn.	Mist	0.70
24	29.76	29.86	29.91	19	30	27	25.3	N. W.	N. W.	N'ly	Clear	Variable	Cloudy	
25	29.96	29.96	29.97	17	30	24	23.7	N. W.	N. W.	N. W.	Clear	Clear	Clear	
26	29.94	29.86	29.96	20	37	28	28.3	N. W.	W'ly	N. E.	Clear	Variable	Variable	
27	30.07	30.06	29.89	14	23	20	19.0	N'ly	N'ly	N. E.	Variable	Variable	Cloudy	
28	29.78	29.57	29.56	21	31	22	24.7	N. E'ly	N. E.	N. W.	Cloudy	Snow	Clear	0.10
29	29.47	29.50	29.68	21	25	12	19.3	N. W.	N. W.	N. W.	Variable	Clear	Clear	
30	29.82	29.77	29.77	10	21	17	16.0	N. W.	N. W.	N. W.	Cloudy	Snow	Clear	0.12
Means	29.80	29.75	29.77	34.9	45.1	38.3	...	...	...	...	...	...	...	1.72
REDUCED TO SEA LEVEL.														
Max.	30.38	30.41	30.44	59	67	59	60.0							
Min.	29.48	29.11	28.99	10	21	12	16.0							
Mean	29.98	29.93	29.95											
Range	0.90	1.30	1.45	49	46	47	44.0							
Mean of month	29.953			...	...	...	37.7							
Extreme range	1.45			...	...	...	57.0							

REMARKS.

11th. At sunrise, wind light S. E'ly; began to rain at intervals. From 7 to 8 A. M., wind hauled to S'ly, very fresh, with copious rain. From 4 to 5 P. M., wind hauled to W., very high and blustering. Barometer 28.80; began to rise from 5½ to 6 P. M.

The nights of the 12th and 13th were very clear. There was no appearance of the return of the shower of meteors of the 13th of Nov. 1833.

The night of the 14th was cloudy.

15th. Cloudy during the day; wind light, S. W'ly and W'ly. Sprinkling of rain P. M.

16th. At sunrise, wind fresh at S. W. Low fog-clouds passing rapidly.

17th. Weather variable during the day; wind W'ly. Between 10 and 12 P. M., a very uncommon aurora appeared; the whole northern part of the heavens was illuminated; the color of the light varied from a deep red to white; a little after 11 P. M., there was a very extraordinary display of red in the zenith. The magnetic needle was very sensibly agitated.

18th. Clear day; wind W'ly. The aurora again appeared, but far less brilliant than last evening; there was no appearance of red light.

23d. At sunrise, snowing fast; snow two or three inches deep; continued snowing till 10 or 11 A. M., with hail. Mist and hail, with snow intermingled, till evening.

28th. An inch or two of light snow.

30th. Commenced snowing from 11 to 12 A. M.; wind N'ly. Continued snowing moderately till sunset. Snow 1½ to 2 inches deep.

December, 1835.

DAYS.	BAROMETER, REDUCED TO 32° F. Sunrise.	At 1 P. M.	At 10 P. M.	THERMOMETER. Sunrise.	At 1 P. M.	At 10 P. M.	Daily mean.	WINDS. Sunrise.	At 1 P. M.	At 10 P. M.	WEATHER. Sunrise.	At 1 P. M.	At 10 P. M.	RAIN AND SNOW IN INCHES OF WATER.
1	29.82	29.82	29.83	11	26	24	19.0	N. W.	N. W.	N. W.	Clear	Clear	Cloudy	
2	29.88	30.03	30.18	19	13	4	12.0	N. W.	N. W.	N. W.	Clear	Clear	Clear	
3	30.23	30.20	30.11	4	25	15	14.7	N. W.	N. W.	W'ly	Clear	Clear	Clear	
4	29.88	29.62	29.49	21	40	34	32.0	S. W.	S. W.	S. W.	Variable	Cloudy	Cloudy	
5	29.43	29.33	29.43	30	31	17	26.0	S. W.	W'ly	N. W.	Cloudy	Cloudy	Clear	
6	29.52	29.54	29.48	11	21	18	16.7	N. W.	N. W.	W'ly	Clear	Variable	Cloudy	
7	29.57	29.66	29.70	15	21	18	18.0	N. W.	W'ly	N. W.	Clear	Clear	Clear	
8	29.68	29.68	29.78	15	28	20	21.0	W'ly	W'ly	W'ly	Clear	Clear	Clear	
9	29.68	29.50	29.38	15	31	18	21.3	W'ly	N. E.	W'ly	Clear	Cloudy	Cloudy	
10	29.78	29.81	30.04	18	24	13	18.3	N. W.	N. W.	N. W.	Clear	Clear	Cloudy	
11	30.15	30.16	30.17	8	22	20	16.7	N. W.	N. W.	N. W.	Clear	Clear	Clear	
12	30.01	29.88	29.57	25	32	32	29.7	N. E.	N. E.	N. E.	Snow	Sn. & h'l	R'n & h'l	1.25
13	29.67	29.57	29.58	28	30	22	26.8	W'ly	W'ly	N. W.	Variable	Variable	Clear	
14	29.47	29.52	29.37	22	32	22	25.3	W'ly	W'ly	W'ly	Clear	Clear	Clear	
15	29.62	29.59	29.59	8	19	18	15.0	N. W.	N. W.	W'ly	Clear	Variable	Variable	
16	29.63	29.69	29.85	—4	—7	—12	—7.7	N. W.	N. W.	N. W.	Clear	Clear	Clear	
17	30.02	29.99	30.09	—8	5	0	—1.0	N. W.	N. W.	N. W.	Clear	Clear	Clear	
18	30.13	30.13	30.14	—1	14	15	9.3	N. W.	N. W.	W'ly	Variable	Variable	Cloudy	
19	30.15	30.15	30.23	15	24	21	20.0	N'ly	N'ly	N. E'ly	Snow	Cloudy	Cloudy	
20	30.14	30.00	29.84	24	30	29	27.7	N. E.	N. E.	N. E.	Cloudy	Cloudy	Cloudy	
21	29.75	29.73	29.73	36	43	34	37.7	W'ly	W'ly	W'ly	Cloudy	Cloudy	Cloudy	
22	29.71	29.72	29.75	30	35	24	29.7	S. W'ly	W'ly	N. W.	Variable	Variable	Clear	
23	29.99	30.07	30.05	13	24	15	17.3	N. W.	N. W.	N. W.	Clear	Clear	Clear	
24	30.21	30.14	30.09	9	28	26	21.0	W'ly	W'ly	S. W'ly	Clear	Clear	Clear	
25	29.87	29.82	29.75	35	37	37	36.3	S. W'ly	S. W.	S. W.	Rain	Cloudy	Rain	0.40
26	29.60	29.44	29.10	42	42	42	42.0	S. W.	S. W.	N'ly	Rain	Cloudy	Rain	1.60
27	29.25	29.34	29.55	36	33	22	30.3	W'ly	W'ly	W'ly	Clear	Clear	Clear	
28	29.78	29.58	29.80	18	26	22	33.0	W'ly	W'ly	W'ly	Variable	Cloudy	Clear	
29	29.77	29.70	29.63	19	36	34	29.7	W'ly	S. E'ly	E'ly	Clear	Cloudy	Cloudy	
30	29.50	29.40	29.42	34	34	29	32.3	N. E.	N. E.	N. E.	Misty	Misty	Cloudy	
31	29.51	29.56	29.71	27	27	20	24.7	N. W.	N. W.	N. W.	Clear	Clear	Clear	
Means	29.79	29.75	29.76	18.6	26.6	21.1	...	...	...	...	...	...	...	3.25
REDUCED TO SEA LEVEL.														
Max.	30.41	30.38	30.41	42	43	42	42.0							
Min.	29.43	29.52	29.55	—8	—7	—12	—7.7							
Mean	29.97	29.93	29.94											
Range	0.98	0.86	0.86	50	50	54	49.7							
Mean of month	29.947			...	...	...	22.1							
Extreme range	0.98			...	...	...	55.0							

REMARKS.

9th. Cloudy during the early part of the evening, with frequent lightning.

12th. Wind light, N. E. Began to snow from 5 to 6 A. M. During the day, snow and hail in turn.

13th. The ground and trees very thickly covered with ice; many trees broken by its weight. Wind very light from W'ly all day.

14th. In the morning clear, with wind light W'ly. From 12 M. to 1 P. M., hauled round to N'ly, with a flurry of snow. In evening, wind high and blustering, from W'ly.

15th. Wind moderate from W. during the day; high and blustering in the evening.

16th. At sunrise, thermometer at 4° below zero, with the wind brisk and piercing from N. W. Wind strong all day, and cold increasing till sunset, when the thermometer stood at nearly 13° below zero, which is 4° lower than any entry made during the four years past. At 10 P. M., the thermometer stood at 12° below zero; the wind a little abated, but still brisk. The severity of the cold has been excessive during the day.

25th. At sunrise, wind S. W. Very light rain during the morning. Cloudy all day; some rain during the night.

26th. Wind S. W., very light all day. Moderate rain and mist during the morning. Rain increased during the afternoon; heavy at night, with the wind at N. W'ly. Cleared before morning.

27th. Blustering.

30th. Wind N. E; misty all day. Clouds broken and being dispersed from 11 to 12 P. M.

January, 1836.

DAYS.	BAROMETER Sunrise.	At 1 P. M.	At 10 P. M.	THERMOMETER Sunrise.	At 1 P. M.	At 10 P. M.	Daily mean.	WINDS Sunrise.	At 1 P. M.	At 10 P. M.	WEATHER Sunrise.	At 1 P. M.	At 10 P. M.	RAIN AND SNOW
1	29.77	29.75	29.77	16	35	24	25.0	N. W.	W'ly	W'ly	Clear	Variable	Clear	
2	29.81	29.80	29.93	27	41	30	32.7	S. W.	S. W.	W.	Variable	Clear	Clear	
3	30.08	30.16	30.23	24	29	20	24.3	W'ly	N. W'ly	N'ly	Clear	Clear	Clear	
4	30.24	30.12	29.94	27	31	33	30.3	N. E.	E'ly	E'ly	Cloudy	Cloudy	Rain	0.50
5	29.87	29.87	30.00	32	33	32	32.3	N. E.	N. E.	N. E.	Cloudy	Rain	Cloudy	0.25
6	30.17	30.18	30.23	19	21	17	19.0	N. E'ly	N. E'ly	N. E'ly	Cloudy	Cloudy	Cloudy	
7	30.18	30.10	30.01	23	32	32	29.0	N. E.	N. E.	N. E.	Cloudy	Cloudy	Cloudy	
8	29.87	29.76	29.61	32	35	34	33.7	N. E.	E'ly	E'ly	Cloudy	Cloudy	Rain	} 0.60
9	29.40	29.26	29.11	34	26	30	30.0	N. E.	N. E.	N. E'ly	Mist	Hail	Snow	
10	29.07	29.08	29.14	32	34	34	33.3	N. E.	N. E.	N. E.	Rain	Rain	Rain	
11	29.32	29.33	29.39	34	38	35	35.7	N. E.	N. E.	N. W.	Cloudy	Cloudy	Clear	
12	29.45	29.49	29.61	35	42	36	37.7	N. W.	N. W.	N. W.	Variable	Clear	Clear	
13	29.69	29.68	29.71	32	43	30	35.0	N. W.	N. W.	N. W.	Clear	Clear	Clear	
14	29.75	29.75	29.75	30	40	30	33.3	W'ly	W'ly	W'ly	Clear	Clear	Variable	
15	29.77	29.63	29.83	27	31	12	23.3	W'ly	W'ly	N. W.	Clear	Clear	Clear	
16	29.95	29.98	30.00	6	17	9	10.7	N. W.	N. W.	N. W.	Clear	Clear	Clear	
17	29.99	29.90	29.69	8	18	20	15.3	N. E.	N. E.	N. E.	Variable	Cloudy	Snow	} 0.75
18	29.38	29.28	29.49	30	26	25	27.0	N. E.	N. E.	N. W.	Mist	Snow	Clear	
19	29.73	29.71	29.87	18	31	26	25.0	W'ly	W'ly	W'ly	Clear	Clear	Clear	
20	29.93	29.91	30.08	14	25	12	17.0	W'ly	W'ly	W'ly	Clear	Clear	Clear	
21	30.13	30.06	29.88	5	29	33	22.3	W'ly	S. W'ly	S. W'ly	Clear	Clear	Cl'dy, r'n	0.43
22	29.49	29.46	29.69	40	42	26	36.0	S. W.	W'ly	N. W.	Cloudy	Cloudy	Variable	
23	29.87	29.90	30.17	20	22	12	18.0	N. W.	N. W.	N. W.	Variable	Clear	Clear	
24	30.38	30.33	30.08	8	24	18	16.7	N. W.	N. W.	N. E.	Clear	Clear	Snow	} 2.50
25	29.30	29.18	29.60	32	24	20	25.3	N. E.	N. E.	N. W.	Rain	Snow	Clear	
26	29.68	29.74	29.78	15	28	18	20.3	W'ly	W'ly	W'ly	Variable	Variable	Clear	
27	29.82	29.80	29.88	16	23	13	17.3	W'ly	W'ly	W'ly	Clear	Clear	Clear	
28	29.87	29.80	29.82	5	14	5	8.0	N. W.	N. W.	N. W.	Clear	Clear	Clear	
29	29.85	29.85	29.84	2	17	20	13.0	W'ly	W'ly	S. W'ly	Clear	Clear	Variable	
30	29.04	29.78	29.74	24	36	29	29.7	S. W'ly	S. W.	S. W.	Variable	Variable	Variable	
31	[illegible]	[illegible]	[illegible]	[illegible]	[illegible]	[illegible]	[illegible]	S. W.	S. W'ly	N'ly	Snow	Rain	Snow	0.60
Means	29.78	29.74	29.79	22.5	29.7	24.0	...	...	...	...	...	...	...	5.03
REDUCED TO SEA LEVEL.														
Max.	30.56	30.51	30.41	40	43	36	37.7							
Min.	29.25	29.26	29.29	2	14	5	8.0							
Mean	29.90	29.92	29.87											
Range	1.31	1.25	1.12	38	29	31	29.7							
Mean of month	29.917			...	...	...	25.4							
Extreme range	1.31			...	...	...	41.0							

REMARKS.

1st. Variable during the day. Evening beautifully clear.

3d. Clear and pleasant during the day. In the evening, wind came round to N'ly.

4th. Began to snow very moderately about 2 P. M.; soon turned to hail, then to rain, about sunset. Wind all day, light N. E'ly.

5th. Wind light N. E'ly. Rain at intervals during the day. During the night, wind hauled more to N'ly, and became cooler, with a light fall of snow.

6th. Wind moderate, N. E'ly. Cloudy, with some mist.

7th. Wind moderate, N. E'ly. Cloudy.

8th. Wind fresh E'ly all day; increased at night.

9th. Wind heavy from N. E.; misty. Grew cooler, and began to hail from 11 to 12 A. M. Hail and snow, but mostly hail, till 10 P. M., when wind hauled more to E'ly, very heavy; snow and hail continued.

10th. Light rain nearly all day. Wind N. E.

11. Cloudy, with wind hauling to N'ly. From 3 to 5 P. M., clouds broken and wind N. W'ly. Clear late in the evening.

12th. Wind N. W. Variable A. M. Clear P. M. Weather very mild.

13th. Clear, mild, and pleasant.

17th. Light wind N. E. Began to snow moderately at 2 P. M.; snowed till night 4 inches.

18th. Light wind N. E. Misty in morning. Snow from 11 A. M. to 2 P. M. Clouds broken at 4 P. M. Clear and mild in the evening.

19th. Very fine.

20th. Pleasant.

21st. Mild and pleasant during the day. Hazy in S. W. at sunset. Cloudy in evening. Began to rain from 10 to 11 P. M.; rain during night.

22d. Cloudy morning; wind S. W. Clouds broken from 2 to 3 P. M., with wind W'ly.

23d. Weather mostly clear during the day.

24th. At sunrise, wind N. W.; clear. From 1 to [illegible] wind came to S. W'ly. Air grew hazy and [illegible] snowing fast, with wind N. E'ly, from 9 to 10 P. M.

25th. At sunrise, raining, with wind N. E. Snow 5 or 6 inches deep. Rain continued till 10 A. M. to 12 M. From 1 to 2 P. M., wind hauled more to N'ly, and barometer began to rise. From 4 to 5 P. M., wind N. W. Clear in the evening. Quantity of rain and snow, as nearly as could be ascertained, equal to 2.50 inches of water.

31st. At sunrise, wind very light S. W'ly. Began snowing from 7 to 8 A. M.; changed to rain from 11 A. M. to 12 M. From 3 to 4 P. M., wind came to N. W.; grew cooler, with more snow.

DAYS.	BAROMETER, REDUCED TO 32° F.			THERMOMETER.				WINDS.			WEATHER.			RAIN AND SNOW IN INCHES OF WATER.
	Sun-rise.	At 1 P. M.	At 10 P. M.	Sun-rise.	At 1 P. M.	At 10 P. M.	Daily mean.	Sun-rise.	At 1 P. M.	At 10 P. M.	Sunrise.	At 1 P. M.	At 10 P. M.	

February, 1836.

DAYS.	Bar. Sun-rise.	Bar. At 1 P. M.	Bar. At 10 P. M.	Ther. Sun-rise.	Ther. At 1 P. M.	Ther. At 10 P. M.	Daily mean.	Winds Sun-rise.	Winds At 1 P. M.	Winds At 10 P. M.	Weather Sunrise.	Weather At 1 P. M.	Weather At 10 P. M.	Rain and Snow
1	29.24	29.31	29.53	20	25	3	16.0	N'ly	N. W.	N. W.	Cloudy	Variable	Clear	
2	29.61	29.62	29.65	—6	3	—4	—2.3	N. W.	N. W.	N. W.	Clear	Clear	Clear	
3	29.76	29.74	29.81	—3	10	0	2.3	W'ly	W.	W.	Clear	Clear	Clear	
4	29.81	29.81	29.84	0	7	—2	1.7	N. W.	N'ly	N'ly	Cloudy	Cloudy	Variable	
5	29.85	29.82	29.84	—5	6	—3	—0.7	N. W.	N. W.	N. W.	Clear	Clear	Clear	
6	29.92	29.93	30.11	—6	14	8	5.3	N. W.	N. W.	W'ly	Clear	Clear	Clear	
7	30.21	30.20	30.15	5	26	22	17.7	E'ly	E'ly	E'ly	Variable	Variable	Snow	} 1.75
8	29.80	29.29	29.12	30	42	28	33.3	E'ly	S. E'ly	W'ly	Snow	Rain	Clear	
9	29.51	29.56	29.57	25	33	29	29.0	W'ly	S. W'ly	S. W.	Clear	Clear	Variable	
10	29.77	29.80	29.97	23	33	23	26.3	W'ly	W'ly	W'ly	Variable	Clear	Clear	
11	30.17	30.20	30.27	14	28	20	20.7	W'ly	W'ly	W'ly	Clear	Clear	Clear	
12	30.27	30.21	30.07	20	30	28	26.0	N'ly	N'ly	E'ly	Cloudy	Cloudy	Cloudy	
13	29.89	29.71	29.59	30	33	30	31.0	N. E'ly	N. E'ly	N. E.	R'n & h'l	Mist	Mist	0.35
14	29.47	29.44	29.52	22	20	8	16.7	N. W.	N. W.	N. W.	Cloudy	Cloudy	Clear	
15	29.56	29.47	29.42	2	18	14	11.3	W'ly	W'ly	W'ly	Clear	Variable	Cloudy	
16	29.64	29.71	29.86	8	16	8	10.7	N. W.	N. W.	N. W.	Clear	Clear	Clear	
17	29.90	29.85	29.90	4	16	9	9.7	N. W'ly	N. E.	N. E.	Clear	Snow	Snow	0.10
18	30.11	30.10	30.14	1	13	3	5.7	N. W.	N. W.	N. W.	Clear	Clear	Clear	
19	30.17	30.20	30.12	—4	19	16	10.3	N. W.	N. W.	N. E.	Variable	Variable	Cloudy	
20	30.04	29.91	29.80	16	32	28	25.3	N. E.	N. E.	N. E.	Snow	Mist	Rain	} 0.10
21	29.72	29.67	29.66	30	37	39	35.3	N. E'ly	N. E'ly	N. E.	Rain	Rain	Cloudy	
22	29.71	29.70	29.78	31	44	35	36.7	N. W.	N. W.	N. W.	Clear	Clear	Clear	
23	29.89	29.90	29.87	29	45	34	36.0	N. W.	S. W.	S. W.	Clear	Variable	Clear	
24	29.75	29.65	29.26	33	40	42	38.3	N. E.	E'ly	S. E'ly	Cloudy	Cloudy	Rain	0.90
25	29.09	29.35	29.69	37	29	18	28.0	W'ly	W'ly	W'ly	Clear	Variable	Variable	
26	29.80	29.69	29.52	17	16	12	15.0	N. W'ly	N. E'ly	N. E.	Cloudy	Snow	Snow	0.25
27	29.82	29.90	30.08	9	20	14	14.3	N. W.	N. W.	W'ly	Clear	Clear	Clear	
28	30.24	30.25	30.33	10	22	12	14.7	W'ly	W'ly	W'ly	Clear	Clear	Variable	
29	30.36	30.20	29.85	5	34	32	23.7	E'ly	E'ly	E'ly	Variable	Cloudy	Rain	
Means	29.83	29.80	29.80	13.7	24.5	17.4	...	...	...	...	...	...	...	3.45
REDUCED TO SEA LEVEL.														
Max.	30.54	30.43	30.51	37	45	42	38.3			Days.			Days.	
Min.	29.27	29.47	29.30	—6	3	—4	—2.3	S'ly & S. W'ly		2	Clear		12	
Mean	30.01	29.98	29.98					W'ly & N. W'ly		17	Variable		5	
Range	1.27	0.96	1.21	43	42	46	40.6	N. E'ly & E'ly		10	Cloudy		3	
Mean of month	29.990			...	...	...	18.5				Rainy		9	
Extreme range	1.27			...	...	...	51.0							

REMARKS.

2d. Wind brisk N. W'ly.
3d. Wind light W'ly. Cold, but pleasant.
4th. Wind N'ly Air very cold and raw. Flurry of snow from 1 to 2 P. M.
5th and 6th. Cold, but pleasant.
7th. Wind light E'ly all day. Variable A. M. Cloudy P. M.; air raw. Began to snow from 9 to 10 P. M.
8th. At sunrise, wind E'ly; snowing fast. From 9 to 10 A. M., wind hauled more to S. E'ly, with rain. Ceased raining from 3 to 4 P. M. Wind came to W'ly, and cleared in the evening. Quantity of snow and rain, in water, equal to about 1.75 inch.
12th. A little light snow in the morning. Cloudy all day.
13th. Light rain, hail, and mist during the day.
14th. Wind rather blustering and raw all day.
15th. Wind brisk W'ly. Variable A. M. Cloudy, with a flurry of snow, P. M.
17th. At sunrise, clear; wind light N. W'ly. Wind came to N. E'ly, and clouded over from 9 to 10 A. M., and a snow-mist began, and continued increasing till night.
18th. Cold, but not severe.
19th. Two inches of snow during the night.
20th. Very little snow in the morning. Misty, with some rain, during the day.
21st. Very moderate rain at intervals during the day.
22d. Very fine.
23d. Mild and pleasant.
24th. Cloudy and foggy morning. Began to rain from 4 to 5 P. M., and continued during the night.
25th. Wind W'ly, very high; raw and blustering.
26th. Wind N. W'ly at sunrise. Came to N. E'ly, and began to snow from 11 to 12 A. M., and continued till night. Cleared before morning.
27th. Cold, but pleasant.
28th. Clear and pleasant, though cold.
29th. At sunrise, wind light E'ly; variable. Began to snow from 2 to 3 P. M.; turned to rain in the evening.

March, 1836.

DAYS.	Bar. Sun-rise.	Bar. At 1 P. M.	Bar. At 10 P. M.	Ther. Sun-rise.	Ther. At 1 P. M.	Ther. At 10 P. M.	Daily mean.	Winds Sun-rise.	Winds At 1 P. M.	Winds At 10 P. M.	Weather Sunrise.	Weather At 1 P. M.	Weather At 10 P. M.	Rain and Snow
1	29.49	29.38	29.15	34	35	34	34.3	S. W'ly	S. W'ly	S. W'ly	Rain	Cloudy	Rain	1.50
2	29.51	29.56	29.99	24	25	11	20.0	N. W.	W'ly	W'ly	Clear	Clear	Clear	
3	30.01	29.98	29.95	10	27	26	21.0	S. W'ly	S. W'ly	S. W.	Cloudy	Clear	Clear	
4	29.97	29.86	29.66	19	41	32	30.7	S. W'ly	S. W'ly	S. W.	Clear	Clear	Clear	
5	29.36	29.35	29.71	34	43	17	31.3	S. W.	W'ly	N. W.	Cloudy	Clear	Clear	
6	29.81	29.72	29.65	13	32	28	24.3	N. W.	S. W.	S. W.	Variable	Variable	Clear	
7	29.60	29.61	29.61	28	36	26	30.0	S. W.	W'ly	N. W.	Variable	Clear	Clear	
8	29.55	29.55	29.66	24	36	26	28.7	N. E.	N. E.	W'ly	Cloudy	Cloudy	Clear	
9	29.87	29.87	29.87	16	36	31	27.7	N. E'ly	N. E'ly	W'ly	Clear	Clear	Clear	
10	29.78	29.68	29.41	31	40	46	39.0	N. E.	N. E.	S. W.	Clear	Clear	Rain	2.00
11	29.25	29.45	29.57	42	38	30	36.7	S. W'ly	W.	N'ly	Cloudy	Clear	Clear	
12	29.90	29.91	30.11	16	22	15	17.6	W.	W.	N. W.	Clear	Clear	Clear	
13	30.29	30.28	30.10	10	26	26	20.7	N. W.	S. W'ly	S. W'ly	Clear	Variable	Cloudy	
14	29.73	29.72	29.89	40	47	28	38.3	S. W.	S. W'ly	N. W.	Rain	Cloudy	Clear	0.50
15	30.05	30.06	30.16	21	30	23	24.7	N. W.	N. W.	N. W.	Clear	Clear	Clear	
16	30.24	30.16	30.10	17	36	26	26.3	N. W.	N. W.	N. W'ly	Clear	Clear	Clear	
17	29.87	29.66	29.46	30	38	42	36.7	S. W.	S'ly	S. W.	Rain	Mist	Mist	0.10
18	29.56	29.61	29.87	38	38	25	33.7	W'ly	N. W.	N. W.	Clear	Variable	Clear	
19	30.06	30.02	29.94	17	33	26	25.3	N. W.	W'ly	S. W.	Clear	Clear	Cloudy	
20	29.87	29.80	29.81	25	32	24	27.0	W'ly	N. W'ly	N. W.	Variable	Clear	Clear	
21	29.86	29.82	29.80	24	38	28	30.0	W'ly	S. W.	S. W'ly	Clear	Clear	Variable	
22	29.63	29.51	29.43	24	36	28	29.3	E'ly	E'ly	N. E.	Variable	Cloudy	Snow	0.75
23	29.59	29.71	29.91	26	34	23	27.7	W'ly	W'ly	N. W.	Variable	Clear	Cloudy	
24	29.92	29.92	29.92	17	44	33	31.3	W'ly	S. W.	S. W.	Variable	Clear	Variable	
25	29.94	30.05	30.10	26	34	26	28.7	N. W.	N. W.	N. W.	Clear	Clear	Clear	
26	30.22	30.24	30.18	18	34	26	26.0	N. W.	N. W.	N. W.	Clear	Clear	Clear	
27	30.06	29.95	29.86	27	46	36	36.3	S. W.	S. W.	S. W.	Clear	Clear	Variable	
28	29.81	29.84	29.91	35	47	35	39.0	N. E.	N. E.	N. E.	Variable	Variable	Variable	
29	30.02	30.08	30.16	32	39	33	34.6	N. E.	N. E.	N. E.	Snow	Cloudy	Cloudy	0.15
30	30.10	30.16	30.17	28	43	33	34.7	E'ly	E'ly	E'ly	Variable	Cloudy	Cloudy	
31	30.17	30.14	30.08	28	49	36	37.7	N. E'ly	E'ly	N'ly	Clear	Clear	Clear	
Means	29.84	29.83	29.84	24.9	36.6	28.3	...	...	...	...	...	...	...	5.00
REDUCED TO SEA LEVEL.														
Max.	30.47	30.46	30.36	42	49	46	39.0			Days.			Days.	
Min.	29.43	29.53	29.33	10	22	11	17.6	S'ly & S. W'ly		10	Clear		19	
Mean	30.02	30.01	30.02					W'ly & N. W'ly		13	Variable		5	
Range	1.04	0.93	1.03	32	27	35	21.4	N. E'ly & E'ly		8	Cloudy		2	
Mean of month	30.017			...	...	...	30.0				Rainy		5	
Extreme range	1.14			...	...	...	39.0							

REMARKS.

1st. Rainy at intervals during the day. Heavy rain at night.
2d. Cold, searching wind W'ly.
3d. At sunrise, wind S. W'ly; cloudy. Flurry of snow from 7 to 8 A. M. Clear day.
4th. Mild and fine.
5th. Foggy at sunrise. Cleared from 9 to 10 A. M. Wind came round to N. W. Blustering and cold towards night.
10th. At sunrise, wind very light N. E.; cloudy, with some mist. In afternoon, wind came round to S'ly. Began to rain from 4 to 5 P. M., with wind S. W. Heavy rain and high wind in evening. Rain estimated at 2 inches.
11th. Cloudy at sunrise; wind S. W'ly. From 8 to 9 A. M., wind came to W'ly. Continued blustering during the day; weather clear. River opened by the boats, after being frozen up since the 27th of January.
12th. Cold and blustering.
13th. Weather raw and cold, with the wind brisk at S. W. Snow during the night, with rain in the morning.
14th. Light wind at sunrise; wind S. W'ly. Cloudy during the day.
15th. Air raw and blustering.
16th. Pleasant day.
17th. Light rain at intervals during the day; wind light S. W. Blustering in the evening.
18th. Very blustering.
19th. Pleasant morning. Raw and chilly, with wind S. W., in afternoon.
20th. Wind raw and chilly.
21st. Wind light W'ly; chilly.
22d. At sunrise, wind light E'ly, with clouds in the E. At 12 M., cloudy and raw. Began to snow from 4 to 5 P. M., with wind light at N. E.
23d. Pleasant day.
24th. Very pleasant. Flurry of snow during the night.
25th. Pleasant.
26th. Cool, but pleasant.
27th. Wind fresh from S. W.; air raw.
28th. Wind light N. E'ly. Weather mild.
29th. Light snow at sunrise. Cloudy during the day.
30th. Cloudy, with E'ly wind.
31st. Very pleasant day.

April, 1836.

DAYS.	BAROMETER, REDUCED TO 32° F. Sun-rise.	At 1 P. M.	At 10 P. M.	THERMOMETER. Sun-rise.	At 1 P. M.	At 10 P. M.	Daily mean.	WINDS. Sun-rise.	At 1 P. M.	At 10 P. M.	WEATHER. Sunrise.	At 1 P. M.	At 10 P. M.	RAIN AND SNOW IN INCHES OF WATER.
1	29.95	29.89	29.87	33	54	36	41.0	W'ly	W'ly	W'ly	Clear	Clear	Clear	
2	29.78	29.77	29.73	35	52	40	42.3	W'ly	W'ly	S. W'ly	Variable	Cloudy	Cloudy	
3	29.66	29.64	29.64	33	56	39	42.7	S. W'ly	S. W'ly	S'ly	Variable	Clear	Cloudy	
4	29.63	29.61	29.56	32	48	40	40.0	N'ly	E'ly	N. E'ly	Foggy	Cloudy	Cloudy	
5	29.64	29.71	29.81	32	42	30	34.7	N. E.	N. E'ly	N. E'ly	Variable	Clear	Clear	
6	29.83	29.83	29.93	24	43	28	31.7	N. E.	W'ly	N. W.	Variable	Clear	Cloudy	
7	29.96	29.96	29.97	20	42	32	31.3	N. W.	N. W.	N. W.	Clear	Clear	Clear	
8	29.99	29.99	29.67	30	44	48	40.7	W'ly	S. W.	S. W.	Clear	Cloudy	Cloudy	
9	29.71	29.67	29.64	48	61	53	54.0	S. W.	S. W.	S. W.	Cloudy	Cloudy	Cloudy	
10	29.51	29.42	29.70	53	53	34	46.7	S. W.	S. W.	N. W.	Cloudy	Cloudy	Clear	
11	29.86	29.90	29.99	26	44	31	33.7	N. W.	N. W.	N. W.	Clear	Clear	Cloudy	
12	30.14	30.18	30.20	21	43	32	32.0	N. W.	N. W.	S. W.	Clear	Clear	Clear	
13	30.21	30.14	29.72	31	41	38	36.7	S. W.	S. E.	S. E.	Cloudy	Cl'dy, r'n	Cl'dy, r'n	1.70
14	29.37	29.44	29.53	36	45	43	41.3	N. W.	N. W.	N. W.	Clear	Clear	Clear	
15	29.55	29.66	29.84	39	42	33	38.0	N. W.	N. E.	N. W.	Cloudy	Cloudy	Clear	
16	29.97	30.04	30.07	33	51	36	40.0	N. E.	N. E.	S. W.	Cloudy	Clear	Clear	
17	30.12	30.14	30.14	34	52	36	40.7	S. W.	S. W.	S. W.	Variable	Clear	Clear	
18	30.05	29.93	29.82	36	64	51	50.3	S. W.	S'ly	S'ly	Variable	Variable	Rain	0.40
19	29.84	29.95	30.02	54	56	47	52.3	S. W.	N. W'ly	N. E.	Variable	Cloudy	Cloudy	
20	30.13	30.19	30.18	42	60	38	46.6	N. E.	N. E'ly	N. E'ly	Variable	Clear	Variable	
21	29.87	29.76	29.58	39	59	46	48.0	N. E.	N. E.	N. E.	Mist	Variable	Cloudy	0.10
22	29.43	29.69	29.98	42	40	32	38.0	W'ly	W'ly	N. W.	Cloudy	Clear	Clear	
23	29.98	29.98	29.93	28	50	44	40.7	S. W.	S. W.	W.	Variable	Variable	Clear	
24	29.93	30.08	30.19	38	45	36	39.6	N. W.	N. W.	N. W.	Clear	Clear	Clear	
25	30.36	30.30	30.17	25	48	36	36.3	N. W.	S. W.	S. W.	Clear	Clear	Variable	
26	29.90	29.70	29.58	44	68	62	58.0	S. W.	S. W.	S. W.	Rain	Clear	Clear	
27	29.59	29.56	30.01	60	61	46	55.7	N. W.	N. W.	N. W.	Clear	Clear	Clear	
28	30.11	30.12	30.12	40	61	58	53.0	N. W.	S. W.	S. W.	Clear	Clear	Variable	
29	30.10	29.92	29.82	59	51	59	56.3	S. W.	S. W.	S. W.	Rain	Rain	Misty	0.10
30	30.08	30.12	30.13	42	61	46	44.7	N. E.	N. E.	N'ly	Cloudy	Variable	Clear	
Means	29.87	29.87	29.88	36.9	51.3	41.0	...	...	...	...	...	...	...	2.30
REDUCED TO SEA LEVEL.										Days.			Days.	
Max.	30.54	30.48	30.38	60	68	62	58.0	S'ly & S. W'ly		11	Clear		15	
Min.	29.55	29.62	29.74	20	40	28	31.3	W'ly & N. W'ly		11	Variable		5	
Mean	30.05	30.05	30.06					N. E'ly & E'ly		8	Cloudy		7	
Range	0.99	0.86	0.64	40	28	34	26.7				Rainy		3	
Mean of month	30.053			...	...	...	43.1							
Extreme range	0.99			...	...	...	48.0							

REMARKS.

1st. Very pleasant.
2d. Pleasant.
3d. Very pleasant.
19th. Sprinkling of rain from N. E. in afternoon.
21st. Variable during the day; wind N. E. Light rain at night.
22d. Wind W'ly, very blustering. Auroral meteor in the evening; brushes of faint white light shooting quite up to the zenith.
23d. Wind S. W'ly and W'ly; raw and blustering.
24th. Weather raw and blustering.
26th. Showery in morning; very mild. Clear in afternoon. Fresh wind in the evening.
27th. Very fine.
28th. Pleasant day.
29th. Showery; weather mild.

May, 1836.

DAYS.	BAROMETER. At 6 A. M.	At 1 P. M.	At 10 P. M.	THERMOMETER. At 6 A. M.	At 1 P. M.	At 10 P. M.	Daily mean	WINDS. At 6 A. M.	At 1 P. M.	At 10 P. M.	WEATHER. At 6 A. M.	At 1 P. M.	At 10 P. M.	RAIN AND SNOW IN INCHES OF WATER.
1	30.13	30.02	29.92	44	62	53	53.0	W'ly	S. W.	S. W.	Clear	Clear	Clear	
2	29.82	29.68	29.62	50	76	68	64.7	S. W.	S. W.	S. W.	Clear	Clear	Cloudy	
3	29.50	29.48	29.52	66	81	47	64.7	S. W'ly	S. W'ly	N. E.	Variable	Clear	Rain	0.56
4	29.49	29.55	29.74	48	70	54	57.3	N. E.	N. W.	N. W.	Variable	Clear	Clear	
5	29.82	29.82	29.86	42	64	50	52.0	N. W.	N. W.	N. W.	Clear	Clear	Clear	
6	29.92	29.91	29.87	44	64	50	52.7	N. W.	S'ly	S'ly	Clear	Clear	Clear	
7	29.82	29.72	29.57	50	61	52	54.3	S. W.	S. W.	S. W.	Variable	Rain	Rain	1.10
8	29.56	29.81	29.81	48	60	47	51.7	N'ly	N'ly	N. W'ly	Variable	Clear	Clear	
9	29.86	29.93	29.97	41	64	46	50.3	N'ly	N. E'ly	S'ly	Clear	Clear	Clear	
10	29.97	29.96	29.96	44	72	50	55.3	W'ly	S. W'ly	S. W.	Clear	Clear	Clear	
11	29.91	29.80	29.76	50	79	56	61.7	S. W'ly	S. W'ly	S. W.	Clear	Clear	Clear	
12	29.60	29.57	29.43	54	75	58	62.3	S. W.	S. W.	S. W.	Clear	Clear	Cloudy	
13	29.32	29.50	29.85	60	62	42	54.7	S. W.	N. W.	N. E.	Cloudy	Clear	Cloudy	
14	30.07	30.07	30.09	34	56	44	44.7	N. E'ly	N. E'ly	S. W'ly	Clear	Clear	Clear	
15	30.09	30.10	30.02	44	62	47	51.0	S. W.	S. W.	S. W.	Clear	Clear	Clear	
16	29.92	29.80	29.76	50	76	60	62.0	S. W.	S. W.	S. W.	Clear	Clear	Cloudy	
17	29.72	29.72	29.72	58	80	62	66.7	S. W'ly	S. W.	S. W.	Clear	Clear	Clear	
18	29.80	29.78	29.78	59	79	66	68.0	W'ly	N. W.	S. W.	Clear	Variable	Clear	
19	29.90	29.89	29.99	56	74	60	63.3	N. W.	N. W.	N. E.	Clear	Clear	Clear	
20	30.10	30.00	29.90	50	68	56	58.0	N. E.	S'ly	S'ly	Clear	Variable	Rain	
21	29.75	29.63	29.63	61	81	72	71.3	W'ly	W'ly	W'ly	Clear	Clear	Clear	
22	29.69	29.72	29.71	54	64	48	55.3	N. E.	N. E.	N. E.	Cloudy	Clear	Cloudy	
23	29.63	29.62	29.68	48	63	48	53.0	N. E.	N. E.	N. E.	Cloudy	Cloudy	Cloudy	
24	29.73	29.75	29.73	47	53	44	48.0	N. E.	N. E.	N. E.	Cloudy	Cloudy	Rain	0.65
25	29.60	29.62	29.76	46	55	46	49.0	N. E.	N. E.	N. E.	Cloudy	Cloudy	Cloudy	
26	29.82	30.02	30.05	46	49	43	46.0	N. E.	N. E.	N. E.	Cloudy	Cloudy	Cloudy	
27	30.03	30.03	29.98	40	46	44	43.3	N. E.	N. E'ly	N. E.	Cloudy	Cloudy	Cloudy	
28	29.88	29.82	29.76	44	56	48	49.3	N. E.	N. E.	N. E.	Cloudy	Cloudy	Cloudy	
29	29.74	29.79	29.88	50	53	47	50.0	N. E.	N. E.	N. E.	Cloudy	Cloudy	Cloudy	
30	29.90	29.90	30.05	43	46	42	43.7	N. E.	N. E.	N. E.	Rain	Cloudy	Cloudy	0.20
31	30.03	30.01	29.95	42	56	30	45.7	N. E.	N. E.	N. E.	Variable	Clear	Clear	
Means	29.81	29.81	29.82	48.8	64.7	51.2	...	...	...	...	...	...	...	2.51
REDUCED TO SEA LEVEL.										Days.			Days.	
Max.	30.31	30.28	30.27	66	81	72	71.3	S'ly & S. W'ly		12	Clear		17	
Min.	29.50	29.66	29.61	34	46	39	43.3	W'ly & N. W'ly		6	Variable		2	
Mean	29.99	29.90	30.00					N. E'ly & E'ly		13	Cloudy		8	
Range	0.81	0.62	0.66	32	35	33	28.0				Rainy		4	
Mean of month	29.990			...	...	...	54.9							
Extreme range	0.81			...	...	...	47.0							

REMARKS.

1st. Very fine.
2d. Very pleasant. Cloudy towards night, with light shower at sunset. Thunder and light shower in the evening.
3d. Variable morning; wind S. W'ly. Very hot from 10 A. M. to 4 P. M., when wind came to N. E., and began to grow cooler.
4th, 5th, and 6th. Very fine.
7th. Began to rain at 1 P. M. Wind S. W., mild.
8th. Pleasant during the day. At sunset, wind light S. W'ly. In evening, diffused light round the north; at about 9½ o'clock, beams of faint white light shot up from the east, or a little to the south of east, half way to the zenith. At 9¾ o'clock, a beautiful bow or belt of white light extended from said point in the east, across the heavens, south of the zenith, and terminated a little to the north of west. It descended on each side to within 6° or 8° of the horizon, and terminated conically. The belt was broadest in the central portions; it moved slowly to the south. At 10 o'clock, the middle of it passed through the northern part of the Sickle, the Dolphin, Arcturus, &c. At 10½ o'clock, it had entirely disappeared. It very much resembled the bow seen in August, 1827.
11th. Very fine.
12th. Beautiful day. Towards sunset, cloudy and damp, with wind S'ly.
13th. Warm and rather sultry morning; wind S. W'ly. Wind hauled W'ly towards noon. From noon to 1 P. M., came round to N'ly, and soon to N. E., with a gust. Very suddenly changed from warm to cold. Barometer rose rapidly.
15th. Beautiful day. The eclipse of the sun commenced and terminated a little later than the computed time; the duration very nearly the same—that is, only 5½ seconds longer.
16th. Clear during the day. Wind very brisk at S. W., and cloudy in evening.
18th. Mostly clear during the day. Heavy gust from S. W., at from 5½ to 6 P. M., with thunder.
20th. Clear morning. Variable afternoon. Began to rain at 10 P. M. Rained but little.
24th. Began to rain from 9 to 10 P. M.
25th. From 9 to 10 P. M., observed two currents of clouds passing the moon; the lower from N. E. rapidly, the higher from W'ly.
26th. Air very raw and cold.
27. Still cold, with occasional mist and sprinkling of rain
28th. Wind N. E.; occasional mist.
29th. Wind N. E.; occasional sprinkling P. M.
30th. Wind N. E.; rain in the morning. Clouds broken in the evening.

June, 1836.

DAYS.	Barometer, reduced to 32° F. At 6 A. M.	At 1 P. M.	At 10 P. M.	Thermometer. At 6 A. M.	At 1 P. M.	At 10 P. M.	Daily mean.	Winds. At 6 A. M.	At 1 P. M.	At 10 P. M.	Weather. At 6 A. M.	At 1 P. M.	At 10 P. M.	Rain and Snow in Inches of Water
1	29.89	29.85	29.86	37	64	48	49.7	N. E.	N. E'ly	N. E'ly	Clear	Clear	Clear	
2	29.86	29.87	29.91	46	70	52	56.0	N. E'ly	S. E'ly	S. E'ly	Clear	Clear	Clear	
3	29.91	29.91	29.90	49	68	53	56.7	N. E'ly	E'ly	E'ly	Variable	Cloudy	Cloudy	
4	29.85	29.83	29.84	51	58	54	54.3	N. E'ly	N. E'ly	N. E.	Cloudy	Rain	Cloudy	0.20
5	29.88	29.93	29.97	54	68	54	58.7	N. E.	N. E'ly	N. E.	Misty	Clear	Cloudy	
6	29.96	29.98	29.97	54	64	56	58.0	N. E.	N. E.	N. E.	Misty	Rain	Cloudy	0.35
7	29.96	29.93	29.90	55	65	63	61.0	N. E.	N. E.	N. E'ly	Misty	Rain	Misty	0.10
8	29.84	29.82	29.82	63	79	69	70.3	N. E'ly	N. E'ly	S. W.	Misty	Variable	Clear	
9	29.82	29.81	29.87	65	82	73	73.3	S. W.	W'ly	W'ly	Clear	Clear	Clear	
10	29.92	29.94	29.96	60	70	60	63.3	N. E.	N. E.	N. E.	Clear	Clear	Clear	
11	29.88	29.78	29.68	60	76	69	68.3	S. W.	S. W.	S. W.	Foggy	Variable	Cloudy	
12	29.72	29.74	29.80	68	76	65	69.7	N. W.	N. W.	N. W.	Clear	Clear	Clear	
13	29.92	29.93	29.96	56	71	57	61.3	N. W.	S. E'ly	W'ly	Clear	Variable	Clear	
14	29.96	29.90	29.80	51	67	52	56.7	N'ly	E'ly	N. E.	Variable	Variable	Clear	
15	29.74	29.72	29.90	50	74	54	59.3	N. W.	N. W.	N. W.	Clear	Clear	Clear	
16	29.96	29.90	29.82	49	71	62	60.7	N. W.	S. W.	S. W.	Clear	Clear	Clear	
17	29.74	29.71	29.73	65	83	58	68.7	W'ly	S. W'ly	N. E.	Clear	Clear	Rain	0.90
18	29.73	29.69	29.61	57	66	62	61.7	N. E.	S. W'ly	S. W'ly	Cloudy	Cloudy	Cloudy	
19	28.59	29.58	29.58	70	84	68	74.0	W'ly	W'ly	N. E'ly	Variable	Variable	Rain	} 0.30
20	29.70	29.72	29.73	55	55	52	54.0	N'ly	N. E.	N. E.	Rain	Misty	Cloudy	
21	29.70	29.66	29.72	40	54	49	50.7	N. E.	N. E.	N. E.	Rain	Misty	Cloudy	0.85
22	29.74	29.76	29.82	48	55	50	51.0	N. E.	N. E.	N. E.	Cloudy	Variable	Cloudy	
23	29.83	29.85	29.92	50	56	50	52.0	N. E.	N. E.	N. E.	Cloudy	Cloudy	Cloudy	
24	29.93	29.92	29.93	49	53	50	50.7	N. E.	N. E.	N. E.	Misty	Misty	Misty	
25	29.92	29.92	29.93	52	56	50	52.7	N. E.	N. E.	N. E.	Misty	Rain	Rain	0.45
26	29.93	29.91	29.88	51	58	52	53.7	N. E.	N. E.	N. E.	Misty	Cloudy	Rain	0.10
27	29.82	29.80	29.77	50	66	54	56.7	N. E.	N. E.	N. E.	Cloudy	Clear	Clear	
28	29.72	29.70	29.71	50	75	64	63.0	N. E.	S. E'ly	S'ly	Clear	Clear	Clear	
29	29.73	29.76	29.79	64	74	60	66.0	N. E.	E'ly	S'ly	Variable	Clear	Clear	
30	29.80	29.78	29.73	57	76	64	65.7	S. E'ly	S. E'ly	S. E'ly	Variable	Clear	Clear	
Means	29.83	29.82	29.83	54.5	67.8	57.5	...	...	...	...	...	...	...	3.25
REDUCED TO SEA LEVEL.										Days.			Days.	
Max.	30.14	30.16	30.15	70	84	73	74.0	S'ly & S. W'ly		2	Clear		12	
Min.	29.77	29.76	29.76	37	53	48	49.7	W'ly & N. W'ly		7	Variable		6	
Mean	30.01	29.99	30.01					N. E'ly & E'ly		21	Cloudy		4	
Range	0.37	0.40	0.39	33	31	25	24.3				Rainy		8	
Mean of month	30.003			...	...	...	59.9							
Extreme range	0.40			...	...	...	47.0							

REMARKS.

8th. Foggy in the morning; wind N. E'ly, very light. Nearly calm during the day. Towards night, the wind, after *being N. E. with small and very transient deviations for 18 days*, came round to S. W. Clear in the evening.

9th. Wind light S'ly, W'ly, and N. W'ly; very warm.

11th. Wind S. W.; cloudy. Sprinkling at intervals in afternoon. Wind very fresh in the evenings.

12th. Beautiful day. Wind light at N. W.

13th. Wind N. W'ly in morning. At 20 minutes before 12, a very well defined halo was observed around the sun, with a radius of little more than 22°. The inner edge of the halo was dilute red; the middle and exterior white. Breadth more than a degree. This continued for about two hours, being occasionally obscured by light fleecy clouds from the west. The arc of a second halo, at the distance of about 46°, was occasionally visible in the south, which was fainter and less perfectly defined than the first.

17th. Thundershower from N. W. in afternoon. Rain began to fall at about 20 minutes before 5, and continued with great violence for 15 minutes. Showery in the evening.

18th. Wind S. W'ly; cloudy.

19th. Wind W'ly; variable. Sun out at intervals; very hot. Rain at night.

20th. Wind N. E. Rain in the morning; cool. Cloudy in afternoon.

21st. Wind N. E., brisk all day. Rain in the morning. Misty, with occasional light showers or sprinkling during the day.

22d. Wind N. E. Cloudy for the most part. Quite cool.

23d. Wind N. E. Cloudy and misty. Continues cool. For the last three days, fire has been comfortable.

24th. Wind light N. E. Misty all day.

25th. Wind light N. E'ly. Misty in the morning. Rain in the afternoon and evening.

26th. Wind light N. E. Misty during the day. Rain in the evening.

30th. Wind S. E'ly; warm. Sun smoke red towards evening.

July, 1836.

DAYS.	Barometer At 6 A. M.	At 1 P. M.	At 10 P. M.	Thermometer At 6 A. M.	At 1 P. M.	At 10 P. M.	Daily mean.	Winds At 6 A. M.	At 1 P. M.	At 10 P. M.	Weather At 6 A. M.	At 1 P. M.	At 10 P. M.	Rain and Snow in Inches of Water
1	29.73	29.71	29.71	64	80	73	72.3	S'ly	W'ly	W'ly	Clear	Clear	Clear	
2	29.73	29.77	29.78	57	82	71	70.0	W'ly	W'ly	W'ly	Clear	Clear	Variable	
3	29.83	29.83	29.83	67	78	66	70.3	S. W.	S. W.	S. E'ly	Variable	Clear	Clear	
4	29.83	29.78	29.73	67	78	70	71.7	S. W.	S. W.	S. W.	Foggy	Cloudy	Rain	0.10
5	29.73	29.73	29.71	71	85	72	76.0	S. W.	S'ly	W'ly	Variable	Clear	Clear	
6	29.70	29.70	29.68	70	83	74	75.7	S. W.	W'ly	W'ly	Variable	Clear	Clear	
7	29.71	29.72	29.73	72	86	78	78.7	W'ly	W'ly	W'ly	Clear	Clear	Clear	
8	29.74	29.72	29.70	74	89	76	79.7	W'ly	W'ly	S. W'ly	Clear	Clear	Clear	
9	29.70	29.68	29.67	70	79	70	73.0	S. W.	S. E'ly	S'ly	Cloudy	Clear	Foggy	
10	29.68	29.67	29.74	68	75	66	69.7	S. W'ly	S. W.	N. E.	Cloudy	Rain	Rain	0.35
11	29.78	29.80	29.81	65	63	62	63.3	N. E.	N. E.	N. E.	Cloudy	Rain	Cloudy	0.20
12	29.81	29.79	29.78	60	73	63	65.3	N. E.	N. E.	N. E.	Cloudy	Variable	Cloudy	
13	29.79	29.75	29.75	61	73	66	66.7	N. E.	N. E.	N. E.	Cloudy	Cloudy	Cloudy	
14	29.73	29.72	29.71	63	82	72	72.3	N. E.	S'ly	S'ly	Misty	Variable	Variable	
15	29.78	29.80	29.89	68	66	62	65.3	N. E.	N. E.	N. E.	Cloudy	Cloudy	Cloudy	
16	29.89	29.90	29.92	60	65	55	60.0	N. E.	N. E.	N. E.	Cloudy	Clear	Clear	
17	29.91	29.92	29.96	52	64	58	58.0	N. E.	N. E.	N. E.	Clear	Clear	Clear	
18	30.00	29.97	29.97	58	77	64	66.3	N. E'ly	N'ly	S. E'ly	Clear	Clear	Clear	
19	29.96	29.85	29.75	62	80	70	70.7	N. W'ly	N. W.	S. W'ly	Clear	Clear	Clear	
20	29.73	29.68	29.67	70	81	75	75.3	W'ly	W'ly	W'ly	Clear	Clear	Clear	
21	29.62	29.58	29.39	70	83	68	73.7	S. W.	S. W.	S. W.	Clear	Clear	Rain	0.25
22	29.34	29.43	29.57	68	77	64	69.7	S. W.	N. W.	N. E'ly	Variable	Clear	Clear	
23	29.68	29.71	29.75	54	74	62	63.3	N. E.	S. E'ly	S. W'ly	Clear	Clear	Clear	
24	29.75	29.73	29.72	62	74	68	68.0	S. W.	S. W.	S. W.	Variable	Cloudy	Rain	0.10
25	29.73	29.77	29.79	68	78	70	72.0	N. E.	S. W.	S. W.	Cloudy	Variable	Cloudy	
26	29.73	29.71	29.76	67	66	64	65.7	S. W.	N'ly	N. E.	Rain	Cloudy	Cloudy	0.38
27	29.81	29.82	29.83	58	75	65	66.0	N'ly	N. W.	S. W.	Clear	Clear	Clear	
28	29.84	29.83	29.83	64	74	64	67.3	S. W.	S. W.	S. W.	Variable	Clear	Clear	
29	29.79	29.71	29.64	64	71	65	66.7	S. W.	S. W.	S. W.	Variable	Cloudy	Cloudy	
30	29.54	29.50	29.58	66	75	70	70.3	S. W.	S. W.	N. W.	Rain	Clear	Clear	0.15
31	29.68	29.75	29.78	65	78	68	70.3	N. E.	N. E.	S. E'ly	Clear	Clear	Clear	
Means	29.75	29.74	29.74	64.6	76.3	67.5	...	...	...	...	...	...	...	1.53
REDUCED TO SEA LEVEL.										Days.			Days.	
Max.	30.18	30.15	30.15	74	89	78	79.7	S'ly & S. W'ly		13	Clear		17	
Min.	29.52	29.61	29.57	52	63	55	58.0	W'ly & N. W'ly		9	Variable		2	
Mean	29.92	29.91	29.91					N. E'ly & E'ly		9	Cloudy		5	
Range	0.66	0.54	0.58	22	26	23	21.7				Rainy		7	
Mean of month	29.913			...	...	...	69.5							
Extreme range	0.66			...	...	...	37.0							

REMARKS.

1st Wind very light W'ly. Atmosphere filled with smoky exhalations, and the sun of a deep smoke red. During a part of the day, while the wind at the surface was W'ly, an upper current came from the N. E., as was evident by light clouds crossing the sun's disk.

2d. Warm and sultry. Sun continues red. Air smoky.

3d. Weather warm. Wind light S. E'ly in the afternoon. Corruscations of the aurora borealis appeared shooting nearly up to the zenith a little before 10 P. M.

4th and 5th. Weather warm. Wind light S. W'ly and W'ly.

6th. Very warm. Fine breeze from W'ly in the afternoon.

7th. Very hot. Fine breeze from W'ly in the afternoon and evening.

10th. Wind S. W'ly in the morning. Began to rain gently about noon. In the afternoon, wind hauled more to W'ly. From 5 to 6 P. M., wind came round to N. E., with fine rain and mist.

16th. Wind N. E. Cloudy morning; broke away from 11 to 12 A. M. Wind high and blustering in the afternoon. Cold for the season.

18th. Wind light N. E'ly and N'ly, in the morning; S. E'ly towards night at the surface of the earth, while an upper current carried the clouds from the N. W.

21st. Began to rain gently about 10 P. M., and continued during the night

24th. Began to rain very moderately at 6 P. M., and continued through the night.

30th. Rain in the morning; wind light S. W. Cleared about noon. From 6 to 7 P. M., wind came round to N. W. Aurora borealis in the evening—not very bright.

August, 1836.

Days.	Barometer, reduced to 32° F. Sun-rise.	At 1 P. M.	At 10 P. M.	Thermometer. Sun-rise.	At 1 P. M.	At 10 P. M.	Daily mean.	Winds. Sun-rise.	At 1 P. M.	At 10 P. M.	Weather. Sunrise.	At 1 P. M.	At 10 P. M.	Rain and Snow in Inches of Water.
1	29.80	29.74	29.83	67	82	72	73.7	S. W.	S. W.	N. W.	Clear	Clear	Clear	
2	29.88	29.89	29.92	65	73	64	67.3	N. E.	N. E.	S. E'ly	Clear	Clear	Clear	
3	29.90	29.88	29.79	64	76	66	68.7	S'ly	S'ly	S. W.	Clear	Clear	Clear	
4	29.68	29.74	29.85	70	80	64	71.3	W'ly	W'ly	N. W.	Variable	Clear	Clear	
5	29.99	30.00	30.04	61	74	63	66.0	W'ly	W'ly	W'ly	Variable	Clear	Clear	
6	30.05	30.04	29.99	60	68	57	61.7	S. W.	S. W.	S. W.	Cloudy	Cloudy	Rain	0.10
7	29.98	29.89	29.89	55	72	65	64.0	N. W.	S'ly	S'ly	Clear	Clear	Clear	
8	29.85	29.79	29.70	65	81	72	72.7	W'ly	W'ly	W'ly	Clear	Clear	Clear	
9	29.78	29.83	29.89	55	65	53	57.7	N. E.	N. E.	N. E.	Rain	Clear	Clear	0.05
10	29.90	29.88	29.90	50	71	58	59.7	N. E.	S. E'ly	S'ly	Clear	Variable	Variable	
11	29.87	...	29.75	55	...	60	...	S. W.	...	S. W.	Variable	...	Cloudy	
12	29.76	29.73	29.83	62	63	61	62.0	N. E.	N. E.	N. E.	Cloudy	Cloudy	Cloudy	
13	29.80	29.74	29.69	55	72	65	64.0	N. W.	N. W.	S. W'ly	Cloudy	Cloudy	Variable	
14	29.60	29.61	29.62	65	76	67	69.3	S. W.	S. W.	N. W.	Rain	Variable	Clear	0.15
15	29.73	29.74	29.78	60	72	64	65.3	N. W.	N. W.	N. W.	Clear	Clear	Clear	
16	29.79	29.80	29.82	58	75	63	65.3	N. W.	N. W.	N. E.	Clear	Clear	Clear	
17	29.85	29.89	29.89	57	75	60	64.0	N'ly	N. E.	N. E.	Clear	Clear	Clear	
18	29.90	29.79	29.76	53	74	63	63.3	N. E.	S'ly	S'ly	Clear	Clear	Cloudy	
19	29.65	29.56	29.59	64	68	68	66.7	S. W.	S. W.	S. W.	Cloudy	Rain	Cloudy	0.07
20	29.62	29.68	29.79	65	71	57	64.3	N. W.	W'ly	W'ly	Variable	Clear	Clear	
21	29.87	29.79	29.79	52	71	59	60.7	N. W.	S. W'ly	S. W'ly	Clear	Clear	Clear	
22	29.75	29.75	29.83	60	74	56	63.3	S. W.	W'ly	N. W.	Cloudy	Clear	Clear	
23	29.90	29.90	29.90	50	66	53	56.3	N. W.	N. W.	N. W.	Clear	Variable	Clear	
24	29.96	29.98	30.00	50	74	56	60.0	N. W.	W'ly	W'ly	Clear	Clear	Clear	
25	30.00	29.99	29.95	55	75	63	64.3	S. W.	S. W'ly	S. W'ly	Clear	Clear	Variable	
26	29.86	29.80	29.75	60	78	67	68.3	S. W.	S. W.	S. W.	Clear	Variable	Variable	
27	29.73	29.73	29.74	66	79	68	71.0	W'ly	S. W.	S. W.	Clear	Clear	Clear	
28	29.78	29.79	29.81	67	76	67	70.0	S. W.	S. W.	S. W.	Foggy	Clear	Clear	
29	29.82	29.78	...	67	75	68	70.0	S. W.	S. W.	S. W.	Cloudy	Cloudy	Rain	0.35
30	...	...	29.59	69	76	55	66.7	S. W.	S. W.	N. W.	Cloudy	Variable	Clear	
31	29.70	29.75	29.75	51	71	59	60.3	N. W.	N. W.	W'ly	Clear	Clear	Clear	
Means	29.82	29.81	29.81	59.8	73.4	62.7	...	...	...	...	...	...	...	0.72
REDUCED TO SEA LEVEL.														
Max.	30.23	30.22	30.22	70	82	72	73.7							
Min.	29.78	29.74	29.77	50	63	53	56.3							
Mean	29.99	29.98	29.98											
Range	0.45	0.48	0.45	20	19	19	17.4							
Mean of month	29.983			...	...	...	65.2							
Extreme range	0.49			...	...	...	32.0							

Winds	Days.
S'ly & S. W'ly	15
W'ly & N. W'ly	11
N. E'ly & E'ly	5

Weather	Days.
Clear	20
Variable	4
Cloudy	2
Rainy	5

Remarks.

1st. Dash of rain from W'ly at 9 P. M.

2d. Aurora borealis observed from 9 to 10 P. M.; not brilliant: diffused light, with faint and occasional corruscations.

3d. Wind fresh S. W. in the evening.

8th. Very warm, with the wind W'ly.

9th. From 2 to 4 A. M., the wind came round to the N E., with a pretty heavy blow, and rapid fall of temperature from 72° to 55°.

18th. Wind light N. E. in the morning: in the afternoon, fresh S'ly. Cloudy towards night.

21st. Diffused aurora from 8 to 12 P. M.

September, 1836.

Days.	Barometer Sun-rise.	At 1 P. M.	At 10 P. M.	Thermometer Sun-rise.	At 1 P. M.	At 10 P. M.	Daily mean.	Winds Sun-rise.	At 1 P. M.	At 10 P. M.	Weather Sunrise.	At 1 P. M.	At 10 P. M.	Rain and Snow in Inches of Water.
1	29.70	29.62	29.67	62	74	58	64.7	S. W.	S. W.	S. W'ly	Cloudy	Variable	Rain	0.10
2	29.83	29.84	29.93	50	66	53	56.3	N. W.	N. W.	N. W.	Clear	Clear	Clear	
3	29.95	29.92	29.90	52	68	60	60.0	N. W.	W'ly	S. W.	Variable	Clear	Clear	
4	29.83	29.78	29.72	62	78	67	69.0	S. W.	S. W.	S. W.	Clear	Variable	Clear	
5	29.64	29.70	29.79	68	66	56	63.3	S. W.	N. E.	N. E.	Variable	Rain	Cloudy	
6	29.95	30.01	30.10	42	57	43	47.3	N. E.	N. E.	N. E.	Clear	Clear	Clear	
7	30.12	30.11	30.09	38	66	50	51.3	N. E.	N. E.	N. E.	Clear	Clear	Clear	
8	30.02	29.97	29.91	50	62	54	55.3	N. E.	N. E.	E'ly	Cloudy	Cloudy	Cloudy	
9	29.84	29.81	29.86	56	79	70	68.3	W'ly	W'ly	N. E.	Cloudy	Clear	Cl'y, r'n	0.35
10	30.02	30.06	30.10	54	54	50	52.7	N. E.	N. E.	N. E.	Cloudy	Cloudy	Mist, r'n	0.13
11	30.02	30.00	29.95	52	71	66	63.0	N. E.	S. W'ly	S. W.	Mist	Cloudy	Cloudy	
12	29.95	29.94	29.99	64	74	66	68.0	S. W.	S. W.	S. W.	Cloudy	Cloudy	Cloudy	
13	30.01	30.05	30.06	64	75	64	67.7	S. W.	S. W.	S. W.	Cloudy	Cloudy	Cloudy	
14	30.02	29.97	29.88	61	79	70	70.0	S. W.	W'ly	N. W.	Cloudy	Clear	Clear	
15	30.04	30.02	30.04	68	75	66	69.7	N. W.	N. E.	N. E.	Cloudy	Clear	Clear	
16	30.05	30.04	30.03	60	69	58	62.3	N. E.	N. E.	N. E.	Clear	Clear	Variable	
17	30.00	29.94	29.79	60	64	63	62.3	S. W.	S. W.	W'ly	Cloudy	Cloudy	Clear	
18	29.78	29.79	29.81	62	74	65	67.0	W'ly	W'ly	S. W.	Clear	Clear	Foggy	
19	29.81	29.77	29.76	64	81	76	73.7	W'ly	W'ly	W'ly	Clear	Clear	Clear	
20	29.72	29.75	29.79	72	84	72	76.0	W'ly	W'ly	W'ly	Clear	Clear	Clear	
21	29.97	29.94	29.99	58	71	60	63.0	N. E.	N. E.	N. E'ly	Variable	Variable	Cloudy	
22	29.95	29.89	29.84	54	72	64	63.3	E'ly	S'ly	S. W.	Variable	Clear	Cloudy	
23	29.75	29.76	29.79	64	68	60	64.0	S. W'ly	N. E.	N. E.	Cloudy	Rain	Cloudy	0.10
24	29.82	29.77	29.63	60	72	64	65.3	N. E.	N. E'ly	S. W.	Cloudy	Cloudy	Cloudy	
25	29.57	29.67	29.76	60	63	48	57.0	N. W.	N. W.	N. W.	Clear	Clear	Clear	
26	29.75	29.74	29.71	46	61	52	53.0	N. W.	N. W.	N. W.	Clear	Clear	Clear	
27	29.52	29.28	29.31	53	61	51	55.0	S. W.	S. W.	N. W.	Cloudy	Variable	Variable	
28	29.37	29.52	29.62	46	48	42	45.3	N. W.	N. E.	N. E.	Cloudy	Variable	Clear	
29	[illegible]	[illegible]	[illegible]	42	41	41	41.3	N. E.	N. E.	N. W.	Rain	Rain	Clear	0.35
30	[illegible]	[illegible]	[illegible]	[illegible]	[illegible]	[illegible]	[illegible]	[illegible]	[illegible]	[illegible]	[illegible]	[illegible]	[illegible]	
Means	29.85	29.84	29.85	55.9	67.6	59.0	...	...	...	...	...	...	...	1.03
REDUCED TO SEA LEVEL.														
Max.	30.30	30.29	30.28	72	84	76	76.0							
Min.	29.55	29.41	29.49	34	41	41	41.3							
Mean	30.03	30.01	30.03											
Range	0.75	0.88	0.79	38	43	35	34.7							
Mean of month	30.023			...	...	...	60.6							
Extreme range	0.89			...	...	...	50.0							

Winds	Days.
S'ly & S. W'ly	8
W'ly & N. W'ly	10
N. E'ly & E'ly	12

Weather	Days.
Clear	14
Variable	5
Cloudy	6
Rainy	5

Remarks.

5th. At sunrise, wind S W.; warm and damp From 9 to 10 A. M., wind came to N. E. Rain from noon to 2 P. M.

6th. Considerable frost at sunrise.

7th. Severe frost in the vicinity.

9th. Wind W'ly during the day. Cloudy towards night. Wind came to N. E. from 7 to 9 P. M. At 11 P. M., began to rain.

17th. Wind S. W.: air damp. Sprinkling of rain from 1 to 2 P. M. Wind came to W'ly, and cleared in the evening.

29th. Wind N. E. Began to rain about 6 A. M. and continued moderately till 9 to 10 P. M., and cleared.

30th. First white frost in the College yard, and very abundant.

October, 1836.

DAYS.	BAROMETER, REDUCED TO 32° F. Sunrise.	At 1 P. M.	At 10 P. M.	THERMOMETER. Sunrise.	At 1 P. M.	At 10 P. M.	Daily mean.	WINDS. Sunrise.	At 1 P. M.	At 10 P. M.	WEATHER. Sunrise.	At 1 P. M.	At 10 P. M.	RAIN AND SNOW IN INCHES OF WATER.	REMARKS.
1	29.97	30.00	...	44	59	52	51.7	S'ly	S'ly	S'ly	Cloudy	Cloudy	Cloudy		
2	...	...	...	52	74	64	63.3	S. W.	S. W.	S. W.	Cloudy	Cloudy	Cloudy		2d. High wind from S. W.
3	...	29.63	29.67	50	58	46	51.3	N. E'ly	N. E.	N. E.	Clear	Clear	Clear		
4	29.64	29.53	29.62	44	48	42	44.7	N. E.	N. E.	N. E.	Cloudy	Cloudy	Cloudy		4th. Wind very fresh at N. E.; raw and chilly.
5	29.42	29.24	29.22	44	53	46	47.7	N. E.	S. W.	S. W.	Rain	Rain	Clear	1.00	5th. At sunrise, wind very fresh at N. E., with heavy rain. From noon to 1 P. M., wind came to S. W. Variable in the afternoon with occasional showers. Clear in the evening.
6	29.32	29.42	29.62	44	52	44	46.7	W'ly	W'ly	W'ly	Clear	Clear	Clear		
7	29.74	29.72	29.82	40	57	46	47.6	S. W'ly	W'ly	W'ly	Clear	Clear	Cloudy		Light frosts on the mornings of 7th, 8th, and 9th.
8	29.92	29.93	30.01	40	50	42	46.0	W'ly	W'ly	N. W.	Clear	Clear	Clear		
9	30.01	30.02	30.02	38	55	45	46.0	N. W.	N. W.	N. W.	Clear	Clear	Clear		
10	30.04	30.03	30.10	34	50	35	39.7	N. W.	N. W.	N. W.	Clear	Clear	Clear		
11	30.17	30.14	30.03	32	47	40	39.6	N. E.	N. E.	N. E.	Variable	Cloudy	Cloudy		
12	29.54	29.22	29.39	44	55	40	46.3	N. E.	N. E.	W'ly	Rain	Rain	Cloudy	1.10	12th. Rain began about 1 A. M., with high wind at N. E'ly. Wind and rain continued until from 5 to 6 P. M. Wind came round to W'ly, very high and blustering. Cleared during the night.
13	29.73	29.74	29.79	37	57	46	46.7	N. W.	N. W.	N. W.	Clear	Clear	Clear		
14	29.76	29.70	29.65	47	64	55	55.3	S. W.	S. W.	S. W.	Clear	Clear	Var., sh.	0.10	14th. Shower from 11 to 12 P. M.
15	29.55	29.66	29.72	53	66	44	54.8	S. W.	S. W.	W'ly	Clear	Clear	Clear		
16	29.74	29.60	29.63	39	60	47	48.7	N. E.	S. E'ly	S. W.	Variable	Cloudy	Clear		16th. Wind N. E. at sunrise; S'ly at noon and afternoon. Light showers from 2 to 4 P. M.
17	29.74	29.78	29.75	36	55	44	45.0	S. W.	S. W.	W'ly	Clear	Clear	Clear		
18	29.97	29.97	30.07	34	49	34	39.0	N. W.	N. W.	N. W.	Clear	Clear	Clear		
19	30.03	29.82	29.63	33	57	60	50.0	S. E'ly	S'ly	S. W.	Cloudy	Cloudy	Cloudy		19th. Wind high S. W. in the evening.
20	29.39	29.18	29.50	63	65	39	55.7	S. W.	S. W.	N. W.	Cloudy	Rain	Clear	0.15	20th. Wind S. W. in the morning, very high and blustering, with occasional dashes of rain. Wind changed suddenly to N. W.; from 1 to 2 P. M., and lulled. Clear and beautiful in the evening.
21	29.54	29.54	29.82	38	46	31	38.3	N. W.	N. W.	N. W.	Variable	Variable	Clear		
22	29.85	29.92	30.02	28	46	36	36.7	N. W.	N. W.	W'ly	Clear	Clear	Clear		22d. Ice this morning ⅜ of an inch thick.
23	30.00	29.95	29.91	36	62	52	50.0	S. W.	S. W.	S. W.	Clear	Clear	Cloudy		
24	29.81	29.71	29.76	47	66	57	56.7	S. W.	S. W.	W'ly	Variable	Clear	Clear		
25	29.90	29.93	29.93	28	38	28	31.3	N. W.	N. W.	N. W.	Clear	Clear	Clear		
26	29.73	29.68	29.64	24	38	29	30.3	N'ly	N'ly	N. W.	Clear	Clear	Clear		26th. Weather blustering, and very cold for the season.
27	29.58	29.49	29.54	22	42	28	30.7	W'ly	W'ly	W'ly	Variable	Clear	Clear		
28	29.65	29.63	29.56	24	44	42	36.7	W'ly	W'ly	S. W.	Clear	Clear	Cloudy		
29	29.55	29.54	29.79	42	50	32	41.3	S. W.	S. W.	N. W.	Clear	Variable	Clear		
30	30.01	30.00	29.99	30	40	28	32.7	N. W.	N. W.	N. W.	Variable	Clear	Clear		
31	30.13	30.09	30.10	24	41	29	31.3	N. W.	N. W.	N. W.	Clear	Clear	Clear		
Means	29.77	29.73	29.77	38.4	53.2	42.0	...	...	...	...	...	...	...	2.35	
REDUCED TO SEA LEVEL.										Days.			Days.		
Max.	30.35	30.32	30.28	63	74	64	63.3	S'ly & S. W'ly		11	Clear		18		
Min.	29.50	29.36	29.40	22	38	28	30.3	W'ly & N. W'ly		15	Variable		5		
Mean	29.95	29.90	29.95					N. E'ly & E'ly		5	Cloudy		5		
Range	0.85	0.96	0.88	41	36	36	33.0				Rainy		3		
Mean of month	29.933			...	...	...	44.6								
Extreme range	0.99			...	...	...	52.0								

November, 1836.

DAYS.	BAROMETER. Sunrise.	At 1 P. M.	At 10 P. M.	THERMOMETER. Sunrise.	At 1 P. M.	At 10 P. M.	Daily mean.	WINDS. Sunrise.	At 1 P. M.	At 10 P. M.	WEATHER. Sunrise.	At 1 P. M.	At 10 P. M.	RAIN AND SNOW.	REMARKS.
1	30.07	29.99	29.95	23	45	33	33.7	N. W'ly	S'ly	S'ly	Clear	Clear	Clear		
2	29.83	29.72	29.52	29	46	41	38.7	S. E'ly	N. E.	N. E.	Clear	Cloudy	Rain	} 1.65	2d. Wind N. E. Began to rain at about 4 P. M. Wind very fresh in the evening.
3	29.41	29.43	29.63	32	36	34	34.0	N. E.	N. E'ly	N. W.	R'n & sn.	Cloudy	Clear	}	3d. At sunrise, rain and snow. Snow continued till noon; wind more N'ly. Light rain and mist in the afternoon. Clear in evening; wind N. W. Quantity of rain and snow equal to 1.65 inch of water.
4	29.69	29.72	29.75	34	42	33	36.3	N. W.	N. W.	N. W.	Cloudy	Cloudy	Cloudy		
5	29.74	29.75	29.75	33	41	35	36.3	N. W.	N. W.	N. W.	Cloudy	Variable	Cloudy		
6	29.74	29.73	29.73	29	42	32	34.3	N. W.	N. W.	N. W.	Variable	Variable	Clear		
7	29.80	29.82	29.85	28	50	36	38.0	N. W.	N. W.	N. W.	Clear	Clear	Clear		
8	29.90	29.92	29.98	36	46	35	39.0	W'ly	S. W'ly	S. W.	Cloudy	Clear	Clear		8th. At sunrise, cloudy; wind S. W'ly. Began to rain moderately from 8 to 9 A. M; rained but little. Clear in the afternoon.
9	30.07	30.23	30.32	30	45	34	36.3	N'ly	N. E.	N. E.	Clear	Clear	Clear		
10	30.32	30.23	30.29	35	48	35	39.3	S. E'ly	E'ly	E'ly	Cloudy	Clear	Clear		
11	30.07	29.97	29.91	42	53	51	48.7	S'ly	S. W.	S. W.	Rain	Cloudy	Cloudy		
12	29.72	29.57	29.59	56	57	51	54.7	S. E'ly	S'ly	S. W.	Cloudy	Rain	Clear	1.05	12th. At sunrise, wind S. E'ly. Began to rain from 7 to 8 A. M., and rained till noon. Cloudy in the afternoon. Clear in the evening.
13	29.70	29.75	29.84	40	51	38	43.0	W'ly	N. W.	N. W.	Clear	Clear	Clear		
14	29.90	29.85	29.61	36	46	40	40.7	N. E.	N. E.	N. E.	Cloudy	Cloudy	Rain	1.40	14th. Rain began about 2 P. M.; wind N. E.
15	29.53	29.48	29.54	34	35	36	35.0	N. E.	N. E.	N. W.	Mist	Rain	...	0.15	15th. Light rain from 7 to 10 A. M.
16	29.59	29.67	29.68	35	46	40	40.3	W'ly	S. W.	S. W'ly	Variable	Clear	Rain	0.05	16th. Light shower in the evening; wind W'ly.
17	29.72	29.77	29.90	35	46	37	39.3	W'ly	W'ly	N. W.	Variable	Cloudy	Variable		17th. Light rain and snow from 10 to 11 A. M.; wind N. W.
18	30.03	30.05	30.18	28	39	32	33.0	N. W'ly	N. W.	N. W.	Clear	Clear	Clear		
19	30.30	30.29	30.28	22	38	29	29.7	N. W.	N. W.	N. W.	Clear	Clear	Clear		
20	30.24	30.17	30.10	30	46	36	37.3	S. W'ly	S. W.	S. W.	Variable	Cloudy	Variable		
21	29.80	29.50	29.56	36	53	47	45.3	S. E.	S. E.	S. W.	Rain	Rain	Clear	0.95	21st. Rain commenced at about 6 A. M.; wind S. E'ly. Continued to rain copiously, with heavy wind, till 1 to 2 P. M. Cleared in the evening from 9 to 10.
22	29.63	29.61	29.53	39	50	38	42.3	S. W.	W'ly	N. W.	Clear	Variable	Clear		
23	29.40	29.33	29.25	32	46	34	37.3	W'ly	W'ly	W'ly	Clear	Clear	Cloudy		
24	29.31	29.23	29.36	30	36	27	31.0	N. W.	W'ly	N. W.	Clear	Cloudy	Clear		
25	29.35	29.35	29.47	21	28	16	21.7	N. W.	N. W.	N. W.	Clear	Variable	Clear		25th. Wind N. W'ly. Cold and blustering, with a flurry of snow in the afternoon.
26	29.46	29.50	29.57	14	27	19	20.0	N. W.	N. W.	N. W.	Clear	Clear	Clear		
27	29.72	29.74	29.84	14	27	20	20.3	N. W.	N. W.	N. W.	Clear	Clear	Clear		
28	29.82	29.77	29.78	16	31	22	23.0	N. W.	N. W.	N. W.	Clear	Clear	Clear		
29	29.66	29.52	29.50	20	27	28	25.0	N'ly	N'ly	N'ly	Variable	Cloudy	Cloudy		29th. Flurry of snow from 1 to 2 P. M. Wind raw at N'ly.
30	29.49	29.44	29.34	22	35	33	30.0	N. W.	S. W'ly	S. W.	Clear	Variable	Cloudy		
Means	29.77	29.74	29.75	30.4	41.9	34.1	...	...	...	...	...	...	...	5.25	
REDUCED TO SEA LEVEL.										Days.			Days.		
Max.	30.50	30.47	30.50	56	57	51	54.7	S'ly & S. W'ly		7	Clear		12		
Min.	29.49	29.41	29.43	14	27	16	20.0	W'ly & N. W'ly		16	Variable		7		
Mean	29.95	29.92	29.93					N. E'ly & E'ly		7	Cloudy		5		
Range	1.01	1.06	1.07	42	30	35	34.7				Rainy		6		
Mean of month	29.933			...	...	...	35.4								
Extreme range	1.09			...	...	...	43.0								

December, 1836.

DAYS.	BAROMETER, REDUCED TO 32° F. Sunrise.	At 1 P. M.	At 10 P. M.	THERMOMETER. Sunrise.	At 1 P. M.	At 10 P. M.	Daily mean.	WINDS. Sunrise.	At 1 P. M.	At 10 P. M.	WEATHER. Sunrise.	At 1 P. M.	At 10 P. M.	RAIN AND SNOW IN INCHES OF WATER.
1	29.36	29.41	29.66	32	35	21	29.3	N. W'ly	N. W'ly	N. W.	Cloudy	Cloudy	Clear	
2	29.79	29.78	29.77	9	26	19	18.0	N. W.	N. W.	N. W.	Clear	Clear	Clear	
3	29.80	29.76	29.78	21	33	31	28.3	N. W.	N. W.	W'ly	Clear	Variable	Variable	
4	29.90	29.89	29.88	30	41	33	34.7	W'ly	W'ly	W'ly	Variable	Clear	Clear	
5	29.75	29.61	29.67	40	48	36	41.3	S. W'ly	S. W.	S. W.	Cloudy	Variable	Clear	
6	29.76	29.80	29.95	31	37	23	30.3	S. W'ly	N. W.	N. W.	Clear	Variable	Clear	
7	30.03	29.98	29.95	13	26	19	19.3	N'ly	N. W.	N. W.	Variable	Variable	Clear	
8	29.92	...	29.98	16	...	30	...	N. W.	N. W.	N. W.	Clear	Clear	Clear	
9	30.01	29.96	29.94	26	49	35	36.7	S. W.	S. W.	S. W.	Clear	Clear	Clear	
10	29.84	29.68	29.65	36	48	42	42.0	S. W.	S. W.	S'ly	Variable	Cloudy	Rain	0.05
11	29.78	29.79	29.75	37	46	33	38.7	N. W.	N. W.	N. W.	Clear	Clear	Clear	
12	29.73	29.79	29.91	33	45	36	38.0	W'ly	S. W'ly	N. W.	Variable	Clear	Clear	
13	29.91	29.79	29.40	31	42	44	39.0	W'ly	S'ly	S. E'ly	Variable	Variable	Rain	1.05
14	28.03	29.02	29.34	44	43	32	39.7	W'ly	W'ly	W'ly	Cloudy	Variable	Variable	
15	29.60	29.69	29.90	24	27	19	23.3	N. W.	N. W.	N. W.	Clear	Clear	Clear	
16	30.03	30.02	30.03	13	29	25	22.3	N. W.	N. W.	N. E.	Clear	Clear	Cloudy	
17	29.65	29.19	29.35	34	50	36	40.0	E'ly	S'ly	W'ly	Rain	Rain	Variable	1.20
18	29.71	29.83	30.07	28	33	26	29.0	N. W.	N. W.	N. W.	Clear	Clear	Clear	
19	30.36	30.43	30.46	20	33	24	25.7	N. W.	N. W.	S. W.	Clear	Clear	Clear	
20	30.42	30.33	30.14	22	39	40	33.7	W'ly	S. W.	S'ly	Clear	Variable	Rain	} 1.33
21	29.64	29.43	29.83	47	50	22	39.7	S'ly	S'ly	N. W.	Rain	Rain	Clear	
22	30.25	30.27	30.39	10	18	11	13.0	N. W.	N. W.	N. W.	Clear	Clear	Clear	
23	30.37	30.26	30.08	9	22	34	21.7	N. W.	N. E.	S. W'ly	Clear	Clear	Sn. & r'n	0.04
24	30.12	30.20	30.27	26	38	28	30.7	W'ly	W'ly	S. W'ly	Clear	Clear	Clear	
25	30.28	30.19	30.10	32	38	39	36.3	N. E.	N. E.	N. E'ly	Cloudy	Misty	Misty	
26	29.89	29.77	29.83	49	51	32	44.0	S. E'ly	S. E'ly	N. W'ly	Rain	Rain	R'n & sn.	1.18
27	29.95	30.02	30.16	14	18	7	13.0	N. W.	N. W.	N. W.	Clear	Clear	Clear	
28	30.17	30.13	30.01	2	14	9	8.3	N. W.	N. W.	N. W.	Clear	Variable	Clear	
29	29.78	29.66	29.69	12	28	26	22.0	N. W.	W'ly	N'ly	Variable	Variable	Cloudy	
30	29.98	30.02	30.18	5	7	0	4.0	N. W.	N. W.	N. W.	Clear	Clear	Clear	
31	30.19	30.10	29.98	0	11	13	8.0	N. W.	N. W.	W'ly	Clear	Clear	Cloudy	
Means	29.90	29.86	29.90	24.0	34.2	26.6	...	...	...	...	...	...	...	4.85
REDUCED TO SEA LEVEL.														
Max.	30.60	30.61	30.64	49	57	44	44.0							
Min.	29.21	29.20	29.52	0	7	0	4.0							
Mean	30.08	30.04	30.08											
Range	1.39	1.41	1.12	49	44	44	40.0							
Mean of month	30.067			...	...	...	28.3							
Extreme range	1.44			...	...	...	57.0							

Winds	Days.
S'ly & S. W'ly	6
W'ly & N. W'ly	20
N. E'ly & E'ly	5

Weather	Days.
Clear	17
Variable	5
Cloudy	5
Rainy	4

REMARKS.

10th. Very light rain at intervals in afternoon. Wind light S'ly.

17th. Snow before 6 A. M.; then rain; wind E'ly. Wind hauled to S. E'ly, with rain and blow, during morning. In afternoon, wind came to S. W'ly, and storm abated.

20th. Began to rain very moderately at 10 P. M. Wind heavy at S. W'ly during the night, with but little rain.

21st. Commenced raining with violence from 6 to 7 A. M. Continued to rain at intervals, with heavy wind from S'ly, till 2 P. M., when wind hauled to S. W. From 3 to 4 P. M., wind came to N. W. At 6 P. M., clear, with wind brisk at N. W.

23d. Cloudy afternoon; wind N. E. From 5 to 6 P. M., wind came to S'ly, with flurry of snow, which passed into rain, and continued for a short time.

January, 1837.

DAYS.	BAROMETER. Sunrise.	At 1 P. M.	At 10 P. M.	THERMOMETER. Sunrise.	At 1 P. M.	At 10 P. M.	Daily mean.	WINDS. Sunrise.	At 1 P. M.	At 10 P. M.	WEATHER. Sunrise.	At 1 P. M.	At 10 P. M.	RAIN AND SNOW.
1	29.63	29.46	29.27	29	37	34	33.3	S. W.	S. W.	S. W.	Snow	Rain	Cloudy	0.40
2	29.13	29.01	28.89	17	25	9	17.0	N'ly	N. W.	N. W'ly	Cloudy	Cloudy	Cloudy	
3	28.93	29.03	29.28	2	8	4	4.7	N. W.	W'ly	W'ly	Clear	Clear	Clear	
4	29.30	29.25	29.36	0	17	12	9.3	W'ly	S. W'ly	S. W'ly	Clear	Clear	Clear	
5	29.23	29.19	29.26	12	17	9	12.7	S. W'ly	N. W.	N. W'ly	Clear	Variable	Clear	
6	29.22	29.07	29.10	9	25	25	19.7	N. W.	N. W.	N'ly	Cloudy	Cloudy	Clear	
7	29.25	29.22	29.27	22	28	24	24.7	N. W.	N. W.	N. W.	Variable	Variable	Variable	
8	29.28	29.34	29.40	21	28	24	24.3	N. W.	N. W.	N. W.	Clear	Clear	Clear	
9	29.47	29.42	29.56	19	31	19	23.0	N. W'ly	N. W'ly	N. W.	Clear	Clear	Clear	
10	29.53	29.50	29.49	21	28	28	25.7	N'ly	N. W'ly	S. W'ly	Variable	Cloudy	Cloudy	
11	29.59	29.55	29.67	21	31	26	26.0	N. W'ly	N. W.	N. W.	Clear	Clear	Clear	
12	29.68	29.72	29.77	22	34	23	26.3	N. W.	N. W.	N. W.	Clear	Clear	Clear	
13	29.87	29.85	29.80	17	24	11	17.3	N. W.	N. W.	N. W.	Clear	Clear	Clear	
14	29.78	29.76	29.78	5	12	7	8.0	N. W.	N. W.	N. W.	Clear	Clear	Clear	
15	29.57	29.52	29.56	4	14	15	11.3	N. W.	N. W.	W'ly	Clear	Clear	Clear	
16	29.58	29.54	29.55	15	25	21	20.3	W'ly	W'ly	W'ly	Clear	Clear	Clear	
17	29.53	29.52	29.58	18	28	16	20.7	W'ly	W'ly	N. W.	Clear	Clear	Clear	
18	29.59	29.59	29.61	10	27	18	18.3	N. W.	N. W.	N. W.	Clear	Clear	Clear	
19	29.62	29.62	29.64	17	32	21	23.3	W'ly	W'ly	N. W.	Clear	Clear	Clear	
20	29.68	29.66	29.66	19	34	25	26.0	N. W'ly	N. W.	N. W.	Clear	Clear	Variable	
21	29.36	29.21	28.57	26	31	32	29.7	N. E.	N. E.	N. E.	Cloudy	Snow	Sn. & r'n	1.00
22	28.46	28.56	28.91	23	24	21	22.7	N. E.	N. E'ly	N. W.	Cloudy	Snow	Clear	
23	29.38	29.46	29.59	16	22	15	17.7	N. W.	N. W.	N. W.	Clear	Clear	Clear	
24	29.63	29.60	29.68	14	28	24	22.0	W'ly	W'ly	W'ly	Clear	Clear	Cloudy	
25	29.77	29.77	29.89	14	20	10	14.7	W'ly	N. W.	N. W.	Variable	Clear	Clear	
26	29.93	29.88	29.87	2	17	7	8.7	N. W.	N. W.	N. W.	Clear	Variable	Clear	
27	29.93	29.89	29.85	4	30	28	20.7	N. W.	S. W.	S. W.	Clear	Clear	Cloudy	
28	29.57	29.44	29.67	29	37	27	31.0	S. E.	W'ly	N. W.	Snow	Variable	Clear	
29	29.87	29.84	29.83	22	33	28	27.7	W'ly	S. W.	S. W.	Clear	Clear	Clear	
30	20.73	29.64	29.65	33	44	36	37.7	S. W.	S. W.	S. W.	Variable	Variable	Cloudy	
31	29.55	29.51	29.65	34	36	36	35.3	N. E.	N. E.	N. E.	Rain	Rain	Cloudy	
Means	29.50	29.47	29.51	16.7	26.7	20.5	...	...	...	...	...	...	...	1.40
REDUCED TO SEA LEVEL.														
Max.	30.11	30.07	30.09	34	44	36	37.7							
Min.	28.64	28.74	28.75	0	8	4	4.7							
Mean	29.08	29.05	20.60											
Range	1.47	1.23	1.34	34	36	32	33.0							
Mean of month	29.673			...	...	...	21.3							
Extreme range	1.47			...	...	...	44.0							

Winds	Days.
S'ly & S. W'ly	5
W'ly & N. W'ly	23
N. E'ly & E'ly	3

Weather	Days.
Clear	21
Variable	2
Cloudy	3
Rainy	5

REMARKS.

6th. Very blustering, with a flurry of snow in the morning.

7th. Very blustering and raw.

8th. Pleasant. Wind rather brisk N. W.

17th. Day pleasant. Evening remarkably pleasant.

18th, 19th, and 20th. Very pleasant.

21st. Began to snow from 9 to 10 A M.—wind N. E.—and continued during the day, intermixed with hail and some rain. Wind fresh, and sometimes violent, during the night.

22d. Wind N E'ly. The air full of fine needles of ice and snow. At 8 A. M., barometer 28.50; began to rise from 9 to 10 A. M. Wind hauled more to N'ly. Cleared during the night.

23d. Pleasant.

24th. Pleasant. Wind light to W'ly. Cloudy in evening. Flurry of snow in the night.

25th. Extraordinary aurora borealis with red light.

28th. A light fall of snow from S. E. in the morning. Cleared in the afternoon; wind N. W.

February, 1837.

DAYS.	BAROMETER, REDUCED TO 32° F. Sunrise.	At 1 P. M.	At 10 P. M.	THERMOMETER. Sunrise.	At 1 P. M.	At 10 P. M.	Daily mean.	WINDS. Sunrise.	At 1 P. M.	At 10 P. M.	WEATHER. Sunrise.	At 1 P. M.	At 10 P. M.	RAIN AND SNOW IN INCHES OF WATER.
1	29.60	29.47	29.44	33	37	36	35.3	S. W.	S. W.	W'ly	Misty	Misty	Clear	
2	29.53	29.48	29.55	26	29	20	25.0	W'ly	W'ly	W'ly	Clear	Clear	Clear	
3	29.61	29.64	29.74	10	19	16	15.0	W'ly	W'ly	W'ly	Clear	Clear	Clear	
4	29.84	29.82	29.92	18	31	23	24.0	W'ly	W'ly	W'ly	Variable	Clear	Cloudy	
5	30.10	30.11	30.09	16	21	21	19.3	N. E.	N. E.	N. E.	Snow	Snow	Cloudy	
6	30.03	30.02	30.01	21	33	23	25.7	N. E.	N. E.	N. E.	Cloudy	Cloudy	Clear	
7	29.83	29.65	29.38	23	35	36	31.3	S. W.	S. W.	S. W.	Cloudy	Cloudy	Cloudy	
8	29.45	29.52	29.61	26	27	24	25.7	N'ly	N. E.	N. E.	Cloudy	Cloudy	S. flurry	
9	29.77	29.76	29.71	18	22	13	17.7	N. E.	N. E.	N. E.	Variable	Cloudy	Clear	
10	29.62	29.54	29.61	12	35	27	24.7	N'ly	N. W.	N. W.	Clear	Clear	Clear	
11	29.71	29.77	29.85	21	35	25	27.0	N. W.	W'ly	N. W.	Clear	Clear	Clear	
12	29.76	29.55	29.42	23	37	29	29.7	W'ly	W'ly	W'ly	Clear	Clear	Clear	
13	29.46	29.66	30.08	18	8	—1	8.3	N. W.	N. W.	N. W.	Clear	Clear	Clear	
14	30.20	30.08	29.94	—2	19	26	14.7	N. W.	N. W.	S. W'ly	Clear	Clear	Cloudy	
15	29.67	29.57	29.50	30	38	36	34.7	S. W.	S. W.	S. W.	Rain	Cloudy	Cloudy	0.10
16	29.61	29.65	29.63	36	40	30	35.3	S. W.	N. E.	N. E.	Variable	Cloudy	Snow	
17	29.16	29.16	29.59	26	11	—3	11.3	N. E.	N. E.	W'ly	Snow	Snow	Variable	0.30
18	29.99	30.03	30.04	—4	12	7	5.0	N. W.	N. W.	N. W.	Clear	Clear	Clear	
19	29.98	29.97	29.97	11	33	23	22.3	N. W.	N. W'ly	W'ly	Clear	Clear	Clear	
20	29.90	29.80	29.64	21	41	29	30.3	S. W.	S'ly	S. W.	Clear	Variable	Clear	
21	29.50	29.44	29.75	30	33	30	31.0	N. E'ly	N. E.	N'ly	Snow	Snow	Cloudy	0.25
22	29.97	29.94	30.00	23	36	30	29.7	N. W.	N. W.	N. W.	Clear	Clear	Clear	
23	29.80	29.47	28.86	30	31	32	31.0	S. W.	S. E.	E'ly	Cloudy	Snow	Rain	0.75
24	29.04	29.26	29.46	29	37	26	30.7	N. W.	W'ly	N. W.	Variable	Clear	Clear	
25	29.59	29.60	29.66	23	36	32	30.3	N. W.	N. W.	W'ly	Clear	Clear	Clear	
26	29.84	29.91	29.96	24	33	23	26.7	N. W.	N. W.	N. .	Clear	Clear	Clear	
27	29.65	29.48	28.98	30	39	35	34.7	S'ly	S. W.	S. W	Variable	Cloudy	Rain	1.25
28	28.91	29.25	29.68	26	18	10	18.0	N. W.	N. W.	N. W.	Cloudy	Clear	Clear	
Means	29.66	29.60	29.68	21.3	29.7	23.5	...	...	...	...	...	...	...	2.65
REDUCED TO SEA LEVEL.														
Max.	30.38	30.29	30.27	36	41	36	35.3							
Min.	29.09	29.43	29.16	—4	8	—3	5.0							
Mean	29.86	29.78	29.86											
Range	1.29	0.86	1.11	40	33	39	30.3							
Mean of month	29.833			...	...	...	24.7							
Extreme range	1.29			...	...	...	45.0							

Winds	Days.
S'ly & S. W'ly	5
W'ly & N. W'ly	15
N. E'ly & E'ly	8

Weather	Days.
Clear	15
Variable	3
Cloudy	3
Rainy	7

REMARKS.

1st. Misty during the day. Cleared from 9 to 10 A. M.

5th. Wind raw at N. E. The air filled with fine snow during the day; not enough to cover the ground.

7th. Wind light from S. W. Air damp and raw.

13th. Wind high and blustering at N. W. Cold very severe.

15th. Light rain for an hour or two in the morning. Wind S. W'ly.

16th. Morning exceedingly mild; wind S W. Wind came round E'ly and N. E., from noon to 2 P. M., and grew raw. Began to snow from 5 to 6 P. M.

17th. At sunrise, light snow from N. E., with heavy wind; thermometer at 26°; growing colder. Light snow continued the greater part of the day, and the cold increased till sunset; thermometer at 4°. Wind came round to W'ly. Barometer rose rapidly.

18th. Mars was in occultation by the south limb of the moon, commencing at about three minutes after 5 P. M., and continuing from fifteen to twenty minutes—the exact time was not observed.

27th. Began to rain moderately from 1 to 2 P. M.; wind light S. W. Rain continued during the afternoon and greater part of the night; then wind came round to N'ly, with snow and heavy blow.

March, 1837.

DAYS.	BAROMETER. Sunrise.	At 1 P. M.	At 10 P. M.	THERMOMETER. Sunrise.	At 1 P. M.	At 10 P. M.	Daily mean.	WINDS. Sunrise.	At 1 P. M.	At 10 P. M.	WEATHER. Sunrise.	At 1 P. M.	At 10 P. M.	RAIN AND SNOW IN INCHES OF WATER.
1	29.88	29.90	30.08	9	20	8	12.3	N. W.	W'ly	N. W.	Clear	Clear	Clear	
2	30.19	30.16	30.13	4	18	14	12.0	N. W.	N. W.	N. W.	Clear	Clear	Clear	
3	30.03	29.99	30.08	11	20	8	13.0	N'ly	N. W.	N. W.	Variable	Clear	Clear	
4	30.19	30.19	30.19	5	21	14	13.3	N. W.	N. W.	N. W.	Clear	Clear	Clear	
5	30.14	30.06	30.11	17	36	21	24.7	S. W.	S. W.	N. W.	Cloudy	Snow	Clear	0.10
6	30.13	30.18	30.13	15	35	24	24.7	N. W.	N. W.	N. W.	Clear	Clear	Clear	
7	30.11	30.10	30.09	22	44	32	36.0	S. W.	S. W.	S. W.	Clear	Variable	Clear	
8	30.11	30.07	30.02	32	36	34	34.0	S. E.	S. E.	S. E.	Variable	Cloudy	Cloudy	
9	29.95	29.95	29.96	35	38	34	35.7	E'ly	N. E.	N. E.	Cloudy	Rain	Rain	1.50
10	30.01	30.02	30.05	34	35	32	33.0	N. E.	N. E.	N. W.	Rain	Rain	Clear	
11	30.18	30.19	30.17	28	35	28	30.3	N. W.	N. W.	N. W.	Clear	Clear	Clear	
12	30.20	30.15	30.04	24	40	32	32.0	N. W.	S. W.	S. W.	Clear	Clear	Cloudy	
13	29.85	29.73	29.49	32	43	47	40.7	S. E'ly	S'ly	S. W.	Cloudy	Rain	Rain	0.88
14	29.43	29.63	29.93	43	39	28	36.7	W'ly	N. W.	N. W.	Variable	Clear	Clear	
15	30.06	30.03	30.03	22	32	26	26.7	N. E'ly	N. E.	N. W.	Variable	Clear	Clear	
16	30.16	30.15	30.15	18	31	26	25.0	N. W.	N. W.	N. W.	Clear	Clear	Clear	
17	30.17	30.09	29.99	22	44	32	32.7	W'ly	S. W.	S. W.	Clear	Clear	Clear	
18	29.70	29.53	29.31	33	49	41	41.0	S. W.	S. W.	S. W.	Variable	Cloudy	Cloudy	
19	29.38	29.44	29.70	30	34	22	28.7	N. W.	N. W.	N. W.	Variable	Clear	Clear	
20	29.86	29.91	29.96	19	33	29	27.0	N. W.	N. W.	N. W.	Variable	Cloudy	Cloudy	
21	30.00	30.01	30.03	27	38	32	32.3	N. E.	N. E.	N. E.	Variable	Cloudy	Cloudy	
22	29.89	29.80	29.75	31	35	33	33.0	N. E.	N. E.	N. E.	Mist	Rain	Rain	0.64
23	29.67	29.76	29.89	33	34	33	33.3	N. E.	N. E.	N. E.	Rain	Mist	Cloudy	
24	29.95	29.94	29.95	31	43	31	35.0	N. E.	N. E.	N. E.	Variable	Clear	Clear	
25	29.95	29.86	29.82	28	51	42	40.3	N. W.	S. W'ly	S. W.	Clear	Clear	Clear	
26	29.87	29.89	29.89	36	43	33	37.3	N'ly	N. W.	N. W.	Clear	Clear	Clear	
27	29.85	29.76	29.63	28	42	26	35.3	N. W.	N. W.	N. W.	Variable	Cloudy	Cloudy	
28	29.63	29.52	29.40	35	44	40	39.7	W'ly	S. E'ly	S. E'ly	Rain	Variable	Mist	0.05
29	29.48	29.58	29.70	39	42	30	37.0	N. W.	N. W.	N. W.	Cloudy	Clear	Clear	
30	29.86	29.83	29.88	21	34	28	37.7	N. W.	N. W.	N. W.	Clear	Clear	Clear	
31	29.91	29.89	29.75	24	42	34	33.3	N. E'ly	N. E'ly	S. E'ly	Clear	Variable	Cloudy	
Means	29.93	29.91	29.91	25.4	36.4	29.1	...	...	...	...	...	...	...	3.17
REDUCED TO SEA LEVEL.														
Max.	30.38	30.37	30.35	43	49	47	41.0							
Min.	29.56	29.62	29.58	4	18	8	12.0							
Mean	30.11	30.09	30.09											
Range	0.82	0.75	0.77	39	31	39	29.0							
Mean of month	30.097			...	...	...	30.3							
Extreme range	0.82			...	...	...	47.0							

Winds	Days.
S'ly & S. W'ly	7
W'ly & N. W'ly	14
N. E'ly & E'ly	10

Weather	Days.
Clear	18
Variable	1
Cloudy	5
Rainy	7

5th. Light snow at intervals during the morning. Cleared from 4 to 5 P. M.

6th. Pleasant.

7th. Mild and pleasant.

8th. Cloudy for the most part during the day. Wind light from S. E., with sprinkling of rain in the afternoon and evening.

9th. Rain, with wind light at E'ly, nearly all day.

10th. Rain, with wind light N. E'ly, all day.

11th. Very pleasant.

12th. Pleasant. Raw towards night. Wind S. W.

18th. Cloudy during the day. Wind S.W., with sprinkling of rain in the afternoon. During the night, wind came to N. W., blustering and cool.

19th. Very blustering.

31st. Began to rain moderately from 10 to 11 P. M. Wind S. E'ly.

April, 1837.

Days.	Barometer, reduced to 32° F. At 6 A. M.	At 1 P. M.	At 10 P. M.	Thermometer. At 6 A. M.	At 1 P. M.	At 10 P. M.	Daily mean.	Winds. At 6 A. M.	At 1 P. M.	At 10 P. M.	Weather. At 6 A. M.	At 1 P. M.	At 10 P. M.	Rain and Snow in Inches of Water.
1	29.35	29.24	29.44	41	41	33	38.3	S. E'ly	W'ly	N. W.	Rain	Variable	Clear	1.62
2	29.55	29.58	29.60	29	41	32	34.0	N. W.	N. W.	N. W.	Clear	Clear	Clear	
3	29.52	29.37	29.47	32	52	34	42.7	S. W.	S. W.	N. W.	Variable	Cloudy	Clear	
4	29.54	29.61	29.63	31	44	33	36.0	N. W.	N. W.	N. W.	Clear	Clear	Clear	
5	29.62	29.53	29.50	27	47	36	36.7	N. W.	N. W.	N. W.	Clear	Clear	Clear	
6	29.63	29.65	29.70	34	56	40	43.3	N. W.	N. W.	W'ly	Clear	Clear	Clear	
7	29.74	29.70	29.65	32	56	41	43.0	N. W.	S'ly	S. W.	Clear	Clear	Cloudy	
8	29.14	28.98	29.98	48	55	42	48.3	S. W.	S. W.	W'ly	Rain	Foggy	Clear	1.85
9	29.09	29.11	29.27	39	46	38	41.0	W'ly	W'ly	W'ly	Variable	Cloudy	Clear	
10	29.35	29.34	29.53	34	46	36	33.7	W'ly	N. W.	N. W.	Variable	Variable	Clear	
11	29.62	29.72	29.87	35	54	41	43.3	N. W.	N. W.	N. W.	Clear	Clear	Clear	
12	29.91	29.82	29.81	37	58	44	46.3	N. W.	N. W.	N. W.	Clear	Clear	Clear	
13	29.72	29.58	29.49	41	63	46	50.0	N. W.	N. W.	S. W.	Foggy	Clear	Clear	
14	29.29	29.23	29.27	44	50	40	47.3	W'ly	N. W.	W'ly	Cloudy	Clear	Clear	
15	29.42	29.52	29.61	38	42	44	41.3	S. W.	N. W.	S. W.	Clear	Clear	Clear	
16	29.55	29.30	29.05	42	52	44	46.0	N. E.	E'ly	N. W.	Cloudy	Rain	Cloudy	
17	29.21	29.27	29.41	40	51	42	44.3	W.	N. W.	N. W.	Clear	Clear	Clear	
18	29.49	29.51	29.54	36	46	40	40.7	N. W.	Var.	S. W.	Cloudy	Cloudy	Clear	0.53
19	29.57	29.54	29.63	36	44	42	40.7	W.	W.	W.	Clear	Clear	Clear	
20	29.63	29.56	29.57	34	54	46	44.7	W.	W.	S. W.	Clear	Variable	Cloudy	
21	29.60	29.57	29.62	36	49	43	42.7	N. W.	N. W.	N. W.	Clear	Variable	Cloudy	
22	29.62	29.71	29.77	35	46	42	42.3	N. W.	N. W.	N. W.	Variable	Variable	Variable	
23	29.80	29.78	29.79	34	49	40	41.0	N. W.	S.	S. W.	Variable	Cloudy	Cloudy	
24	29.64	29.60	29.54	38	40	38	38.7	N. E.	N. E.	N. E.	Cloudy	Cloudy	Cloudy	
25	29.50	29.47	29.48	39	48	43	43.3	N.	N'ly	N'ly	Foggy	Cloudy	Variable	
26	29.49	29.47	29.61	40	54	46	46.7	N. W.	N. W.	N. W.	Cloudy	Cloudy	Cloudy	
27	29.66	29.71	29.86	39	62	43	48.0	W'ly	W.	E'ly	Clear	Clear	Clear	
28	29.97	30.02	30.07	42	68	50	53.3	S'ly	S. W.	S. W.	Clear	Clear	Clear	
29	30.07	30.00	29.90	46	71	51	56.0	S. W.	S. W.	S. W.	Clear	Clear	Clear	
30	29.82	29.74	29.59	50	70	50	56.7	S. W.	S. W.	N. E.	Clear	Haze	Rain	0.65
Means	29.57	29.54	29.61	37.6	52.0	41.4	...	...	...	...	...	...	...	4.65
REDUCED TO SEA LEVEL.														
Max.	30.25	30.20	30.25	50	71	51	56.7							
Min.	29.27	29.29	29.23	27	40	32	34.0							
Mean	29.75	29.72	29.79											
Range	0.98	0.91	1.02	23	31	19	22.7							
Mean of month	29.753			...	...	...	43.7							
Extreme range	1.02			...	...	...	44.0							

Winds. Days.
S'ly & S. W'ly 8
W'ly & N. W'ly 19
N. E'ly & E'ly 3

Weather. Days.
Clear 15
Variable 7
Cloudy 4
Rainy 4

REMARKS.

1st. At sunrise, wind light S'ly, with rain. From 8 to 10 A. M., heavy rain and high wind. Wind came round to W'ly, from noon to 1 P. M., and the rain ceased. Barometer began to rise about 3 P. M.

3d. Wind S. W. in the morning. Came round to N. W. towards night, with a gust of wind; colder.

8th. Thunder, with heavy rain and wind heavy at S. W. Rain continued till 10 A. M., then foggy. At 2 P. M., thunder, with very heavy shower of rain and hail, which continued about 20 minutes. From 4 to 5 P. M., the barometer stood at 28.96. Began to rise from 6 to 7 P. M.; wind came to W'ly, and clear. Quantity of rain equal to 1.85 inch.

9th. Wind W'ly, blustering and raw.

14th. At 6 A. M., wind W'ly. Sprinkling of rain.

19th. Shower.

23d. Slight sprinkling of rain in afternoon.

24th. Rain mixed with a little snow.

May, 1837.

Days.	Barometer. At 6 A. M.	At 1 P. M.	At 10 P. M.	Thermometer. At 6 A. M.	At 1 P. M.	At 10 P. M.	Daily mean.	Winds. At 6 A. M.	At 1 P. M.	At 10 P. M.	Weather. At 6 A. M.	At 1 P. M.	At 10 P. M.	Rain and Snow in Inches of Water.
1	29.51	29.67	29.93	42	43	28	37.7	N. E.	N. W.	N. W.	Cloudy	Clear	Clear	
2	30.03	29.94	29.88	28	48	40	38.7	N. W.	S. W.	S. W.	Clear	Clear	Cloudy	
3	29.54	29.40	29.60	48	75	56	59.7	S. W.	W.	S. W.	M't & r'n	Cl., var.	Variable	
4	29.76	29.80	29.80	42	60	48	50.0	N. W.	N. W.	W'ly	Clear	Clear	Clear	0.23
5	29.71	29.51	29.45	46	55	60	53.7	E'ly	S'ly	S. W.	Cloudy	Cloudy	Rain	0.42
6	29.33	29.40	29.50	58	76	52	62.0	S. W.	S. W.	N. W.	Variable	Clear	Variable	0.14
7	29.69	29.77	29.87	45	54	44	47.7	N. W.	W'ly	N. W.	Clear	Clear	Clear	
8	30.02	30.02	30.02	38	56	42	45.3	N. E.	N. E.	S. W.	Clear	Clear	Clear	
9	30.03	29.92	29.78	38	57	50	48.3	S. W.	S. W.	S. W.	Clear	Cloudy	Cl'dy, r'n	0.70
10	29.63	29.63	29.73	46	52	49	49.0	N. E.	N. E.	W'ly	Rain	Cloudy	Cloudy	0.42
11	29.77	29.82	29.88	48	69	48	55.0	W'ly	W'ly	S. W.	Variable	Clear	Clear	
12	29.93	29.94	30.00	45	69	49	54.3	S. W.	S. W.	S. W.	Clear	Clear	Clear	
13	30.02	30.02	29.92	48	57	54	53.0	S. W.	S'ly	S'ly	Cloudy	Cloudy	Cloudy	
14	29.82	29.77	29.75	54	72	58	61.3	S. W.	S. W.	S. W.	Cloudy	Clear	Variable	
15	29.83	29.83	29.84	54	54	47	51.7	S. W.	N. E.	N. E.	Foggy	Mist	Mist	
16	29.75	29.72	29.70	44	84	56	61.3	N. E.	E'ly	S. E'ly	Rain	Rain	Rain	2.13
17	29.62	29.64	29.71	54	69	56	59.7	S'ly	S'ly	S. W.	Rain	Clear	Clear	0.33
18	29.76	29.79	29.80	53	65	55	57.7	S. W.	S. W.	S. W.	Clear	Variable	Rain	
19	29.70	29.62	29.56	56	63	57	58.7	S. E'ly	S'ly	S'ly	Rain	Cloudy	Rain	0.50
20	29.56	29.53	29.64	53	68	48	56.3	S. W.	S. W.	W'ly	Cloudy	Clear	Clear	
21	29.73	29.83	29.84	46	73	56	58.3	S. W.	S. W.	S. W.	Clear	Clear	Clear	
22	29.81	29.74	29.64	54	59	54	55.7	S. W.	S. E'ly	S. E.	Variable	Rain	Cloudy	0.86
23	29.70	29.73	29.90	48	66	54	56.0	N. W.	N. W.	N. W.	Clear	Clear	Clear	
24	30.00	29.89	29.95	48	69	50	55.7	N. W.	S. W.	S. W.	Clear	Clear	Rain	
25	29.77	29.71	29.60	49	52	45	48.7	S. E'ly	N. E.	N. E.	Mist	Rain	Rain	1.55
26	29.42	29.51	29.61	45	52	47	48.0	N. E.	N. E.	N'ly	Mist	Mist	Clear	
27	29.63	29.62	29.75	47	70	56	57.7	N. W.	W'ly	W'ly	Clear	Clear	Clear	
28	29.87	29.90	29.90	48	61	52	53.7	N. W.	N. W.	N. W.	Clear	Clear	Clear	
29	29.90	29.89	29.86	46	66	56	56.0	N. W.	N. W.	N. W.	Clear	Clear	Clear	
30	29.50	29.86	29.84	51	70	59	60.0	W'ly	O. W.	O. W.	Clear	Clear	Cloudy	
31	29.84	29.88	29.83	59	80	64	67.7	S. W.	S. W.	W'ly	Cloudy	Clear	Clear	
Means	29.75	29.75	29.77	47.7	63.4	51.3	...	...	...	...	...	...	...	7.28
REDUCED TO SEA LEVEL.														
Max.	30.21	30.20	30.20	59	80	64	67.7							
Min.	29.51	29.58	29.63	28	43	28	37.7							
Mean	29.93	29.92	29.95											
Range	0.70	0.72	0.67	31	37	36	30.0							
Mean of month	29.933			...	...	...	54.1							
Extreme range	0.70			...	...	...	52.0							

Winds. Days.
S'ly & S. W'ly 15
W'ly & N. W'ly 8
N. E'ly & E'ly 7

Weather. Days.
Clear 16
Variable 3
Cloudy 3
Rainy 9

REMARKS.

1st. At sunrise, wind N. E.; cloudy. From 8 to 9 A. M., wind came to N. W., with gust and sprinkling of rain; very cool.

2d. The ground frozen hard. Ice formed more than a quarter of an inch thick.

5th. Thundershower from 4 to 5 A. M. Cloudy during the day. Thunder and rain from 8 to 10 P. M.

6th. Variable. Shower from 4 to 6 P. M.; wind W'ly.

9th. Heavy rain during the night.

11th. Wind N. E. Rain in the morning. Clear in the afternoon. Cloudy and sprinkling of rain in the evening.

13th. Wind S'ly. Cloudy, with occasional sprinkling of rain.

14th. Cloudy at sunrise. Clear from 7 to 8 A. M.

16th. Very heavy rain. Wind E'ly and S. E.

18th. Rain in the evening.

19th. Warm rain from S'ly.

22d. Commenced raining from 8 to 9 A. M.; wind S. W'ly. Wind came round to E'ly and S. E'ly in the afternoon, with pretty heavy rain.

June, 1837.

DAYS.	BAROMETER, REDUCED TO 32° F. At 6 A. M.	At 1 P. M.	At 10 P. M.	THERMOMETER. At 6 A. M.	At 1 P. M.	At 10 P. M.	Daily mean.	WINDS. At 6 A. M.	At 1 P. M.	At 10 P. M.	WEATHER. At 6 A. M.	At 1 P. M.	At 10 P. M.	RAIN AND SNOW IN INCHES OF WATER
1	29.85	29.83	29.83	64	82	66	70.7	S. W.	S. W.	S. W.	Clear	Clear	Clear	
2	29.84	29.79	29.78	65	80	64	69.7	S. W.	S. E'ly	S. W.	Clear	Clear	Clear	
3	29.68	...	...	62	76	...	...	S. W.	S. W.	S. W.	Foggy	Clear	Clear	
4	...	...	...	65	80	74	73.0	N. W.	N. W.	W'ly	Clear	Clear	Clear	
5	...	29.28	29.41	64	72	64	66.7	N. W.	N. W.	N. W.	Clear	Variable	Clear	
6	29.47	29.48	29.48	59	80	61	66.7	N'ly	N. W.	S. W.	Clear	Clear	Clear	
7	29.39	29.42	29.42	56	79	61	65.7	S. W.	S. E.	S. W.	Clear	Clear	Variable	
8	29.48	29.51	29.61	58	67	60	61.7	N. E.	N. E.	N. E.	Cloudy	Cloudy	Cloudy	
9	29.70	29.76	29.85	60	68	53	60.3	N. E.	N. E.	N. E.	Misty	Cloudy	Variable	
10	29.89	29.89	29.90	50	53	46	49.7	N. E.	N. E.	N. E.	Cloudy	Cloudy	Variable	
11	29.84	29.78	29.78	45	64	52	53.7	N. E.	N. E.	S. W'ly	Variable	Clear	Clear	
12	29.78	29.72	29.74	52	72	57	60.3	S. W.	S. W.	S. W.	Misty	Variable	Cloudy	
13	29.72	29.70	29.69	56	65	58	59.7	S. W.	S. W.	S. W.	Rain	Cloudy	Clear	
14	29.70	29.67	29.65	56	74	61	63.7	S. W.	S. W.	S. W.	Clear	Clear	Clear	
15	29.61	29.61	29.60	60	66	59	61.7	S. W.	N. E.	N. E.	Cloudy	Rain	Variable	
16	29.66	29.65	29.66	55	72	54	60.3	N. E.	S. W.	S'ly	Clear	Clear	Cl'dy, r'n	} 0.66
17	29.60	29.58	29.61	54	63	50	55.7	N. E.	N. E.	N. E.	Rain	Cloudy	Cloudy	
18	29.65	29.66	29.70	48	64	57	56.3	N. E.	N. E.	N. E.	Cloudy	Clear	Clear	
19	29.70	29.69	29.69	56	78	59	64.3	W'ly	W'ly	W'ly	Clear	Clear	Clear	
20	29.58	29.39	29.30	58	62	60	60.0	S'ly	S. E'ly	W'ly	Rain	Rain	Clear	0.96
21	29.40	29.43	29.39	58	72	60	63.3	W'ly	S. W.	S. W.	Clear	Variable	Rain	
22	29.40	29.50	29.70	55	75	72	67.3	N. W.	N. W.	N. W.	Rain	Clear	Clear	1.10
23	29.83	29.85	29.88	64	81	63	69.3	N. W.	S. W.	S. W.	Clear	Clear	Clear	
24	29.85	29.74	29.68	63	70	64	65.7	S. W.	S. W.	S. W.	Cloudy	Cloudy	Cloudy	
25	29.65	29.61	29.68	64	79	69	70.7	S. W.	W'ly	S. W.	Cloudy	Variable	Variable	
26	29.79	29.78	29.83	61	75	64	66.7	S. W.	W'ly	W'ly	Clear	Clear	Foggy	
27	29.82	29.74	29.63	62	74	67	67.7	S. W.	S. W.	S. W.	Foggy	Variable	Rain	0.10
28	29.73	29.78	29.86	63	67	64	64.7	N. W.	N. W.	N. W.	Clear	Clear	Clear	
29	29.84	29.84	29.66	63	79	65	69.0	N. W.	W'ly	S. W.	Clear	Clear	Cloudy	
30	29.63	29.55	29.58	64	82	75	73.7	W'ly	S. W.	S. W.	Cloudy	Clear	Clear	
Means	29.67	29.65	29.66	58.7	72.4	61.4	...	...	...	...	...	...	...	2.82
REDUCED TO SEA LEVEL.														
Max.	30.07	30.07	30.08	65	82	75	73.7							
Min.	29.57	29.46	29.48	45	62	50	49.7							
Mean	29.85	29.82	29.84											
Range	0.50	0.61	0.60	20	20	25	24.0							
Mean of month	29.837			...	...	...	64.2							
Extreme range	0.62			...	...	...	37.0							

Winds	Days.
S'ly & S. W'ly	15
W'ly & N. W'ly	8
N. E'ly & E'ly	7

Weather	Days.
Clear	16
Variable	5
Cloudy	3
Rainy	6

REMARKS.

16th. Heavy rain during the night.

20th. Heavy rain S. E'ly during the forenoon.

21st. Very clear in the morning; wind W'ly. Overcast with clouds about 11 A. M. Cloudy in afternoon. Began to rain about 8 P M.; air very still. Rained during the night.

22d. At sunrise, wind N. W.; raining moderately. Ceased raining about 9 A. M; cleared by noon. Clear in afternoon.

24th. Cloudy, with the wind brisk at S. W. Occasional sprinkling of rain. Air very damp.

27th. Occasional showers in afternoon.

July, 1837.

DAYS.	Barometer At 6 A. M.	At 1 P. M.	At 10 P. M.	Thermometer At 6 A. M.	At 1 P. M.	At 10 P. M.	Daily mean.	Winds At 6 A. M.	At 1 P. M.	At 10 P. M.	Weather At 6 A. M.	At 1 P. M.	At 10 P. M.	Rain
1	29.56	29.52	29.52	75	88	77	80.0	W'ly	S. W.	S. W.	Clear	Clear	Clear	
2	29.62	29.68	29.78	70	78	65	71.0	N. W.	N. W.	N. W.	Clear	Clear	Clear	
3	29.72	29.65	29.53	62	72	64	66.0	N. W.	N'ly	S. W.	Clear	Cloudy	Rain	0.05
4	29.53	29.54	29.57	60	76	64	66.7	N. W.	N. W.	N. W.	Clear	Clear	Clear	
5	29.55	29.49	29.45	61	70	63	64.7	N. W.	S. W.	S. W.	Clear	Rain	Clear	
6	29.50	29.51	29.55	60	77	65	67.3	S. W.	S. W.	S. W.	Cloudy	Clear	Clear	
7	29.59	29.63	29.65	64	76	65	67.3	S. W.	S. W.	S. W.	Variable	Clear	Variable	
8	29.61	29.59	29.66	65	76	67	69.3	S. W.	S. W.	S. W.	Cloudy	Clear	Clear	
9	29.73	29.79	29.81	60	72	61	64.3	N. W.	N. W.	N. W.	Clear	Clear	Clear	
10	29.79	29.74	29.74	59	75	61	65.0	N. W.	N. W.	N. W.	Clear	Clear	Clear	
11	29.71	29.66	29.68	58	81	63	67.3	N. W.	N. W.	S. W.	Clear	Clear	Rain	0.55
12	29.79	29.80	29.89	60	71	57	62.7	N. E.	N. E.	N. E.	Variable	Clear	Variable	
13	29.89	29.90	29.81	57	73	59	63.0	N. E.	S. W.	S'ly	Variable	Clear	Variable	
14	29.74	29.60	29.59	59	81	68	69.7	S. W.	S. W.	S. W.	Clear	Clear	Variable	
15	29.63	29.47	29.58	67	82	68	72.3	S. W.	S. W.	W'ly	Clear	Clear	Shower	0.23
16	29.65	29.71	29.82	64	77	64	68.3	N. W.	N. W.	N. W.	Clear	Clear	Clear	
17	29.95	29.99	29.98	60	76	68	68.0	N. W.	N. W.	W'ly	Clear	Clear	Clear	
18	30.00	29.93	29.94	62	83	68	71.0	W'ly	W'ly	S. W.	Clear	Clear	Clear	
19	29.85	29.77	29.70	67	84	70	73.7	S. W.	S. W'ly	S. W'ly	Clear	Clear	Shower	
20	29.67	29.68	29.71	70	82	69	73.7	W'ly	W'ly	N. W.	Clear	Clear	Clear	
21	29.77	29.77	29.77	62	77	64	67.7	N. W.	N. W.	N. W.	Clear	Clear	Clear	
22	29.82	29.80	29.79	58	76	62	65.3	N. W.	N. W.	N. W.	Clear	Clear	Clear	
23	29.75	29.74	29.68	60	76	66	67.3	S. W.	S. W.	S. W.	Clear	Cloudy	Cloudy	
24	29.58	29.51	29.45	66	75	64	68.3	S. W.	S. W.	W'ly	Cloudy	R'n, s'hr	Clear	0.45
25	29.45	29.45	29.48	62	74	64	66.7	N. W.	N. W.	N. W.	Clear	Clear	Clear	
26	29.48	29.48	29.46	58	74	65	65.7	N. W'ly	N'ly	S. W'ly	Variable	Clear	Clear	
27	29.45	29.48	29.57	62	78	70	70.0	N. W'ly	N. W.	N. W.	Clear	Clear	Clear	
28	29.65	29.65	29.67	63	79	67	69.7	N. W.	N. W.	N'ly	Clear	Clear	Rain	0.10
29	29.63	29.68	29.81	64	64	58	62.0	N. E.	N. E.	N. E.	Variable	Cloudy	Clear	
30	29.83	29.81	29.81	58	73	62	64.3	N. E.	S. E'ly	S. W.	Clear	Clear	Cloudy	
31	29.74	29.70	29.69	63	73	70	68.7	S. W.	S. W.	S. W.	Cloudy	Cloudy	Cloudy	
Means	29.68	29.67	29.68	62.4	76.1	65.1	...	...	...	...	...	...	...	1.38
REDUCED TO SEA LEVEL.														
Max.	30.18	30.11	30.12	75	88	77	73.7							
Min.	29.63	29.63	29.63	57	64	57	62.0							
Mean	29.85	29.84	29.85											
Range	0.55	0.48	0.49	18	24	20	11.7							
Mean of month	29.847			...	...	...	67.9							
Extreme range	0.55			...	...	...	31.0							

Winds	Days.
S'ly & S. W'ly	12
W'ly & N. W'ly	16
N. E'ly & E'ly	3

Weather	Days.
Clear	17
Variable	6
Cloudy	3
Rainy	5

1st. Aurora in the evening; was seen first from 8 to 9 o'clock; the northern portion of the heavens was pretty strongly illuminated. At 10½ P. M., the light extended nearly round to the S., and began to shoot up toward the zenith from all quarters. The coruscations were not in the form of slender needles, as they most frequently are, but broad sheets or waves, which followed each other with great rapidity from 30° or 40° altitude up to the zenith; or, more exactly, to a point S. E of the zenith, or very nearly in the magnetic pole The light began to assume at times a reddish hue, which grew more and more intense, sometimes, for two or three minutes, presenting a pretty deep red, which seems chiefly spread over a broad belt spanning the heavens from N. W. to S. E. It continued till 11½ P. M., when it was much faded. Was not further observed.

19th. Light shower in evening.

23d. Clear at sunrise. Clouded before noon, with occasional sprinkling. Variable in afternoon. Cloudy in evening.

24th. Thundershower from 2 to 3½ P. M., and another from 8 to 9 P. M. Clear before 10 P. M.

28th. Showery in the evening.

29th. Aurora in the evening. Diffused light round the north; not brilliant.

August, 1837.

DAYS.	BAROMETER, REDUCED TO 32° F. At 6 A. M.	At 1 P. M.	At 10 P. M.	THERMOMETER. At 6 A. M.	At 1 P. M.	At 10 P. M.	Daily mean.	WINDS. At 6 A. M.	At 1 P. M.	At 10 P. M.	WEATHER. At 6 A. M.	At 1 P. M.	At 10 P. M.	RAIN AND SNOW IN INCHES OF WATER.	REMARKS.
1	29.73	29.73	29.73	66	83	69	72.7	W'ly	W'ly	S. W.	Clear	Clear	Clear		
2	29.73	29.71	29.66	70	86	75	77.0	S. W.	S. W.	S. W.	Clear	Clear	Cloudy		
3	29.57	29.47	29.49	73	82	65	73.3	S. W.	S. W.	Calm	Variable	Cl'y, sh'r	Clear	0.85	3d. Variable during the day. A copious shower, with some thunder, from 4 to 6 P. M.
4	29.58	29.63	29.68	62	73	64	66.3	N. W.	N. W.	N. W.	Clear	Clear	Clear		
5	29.84	29.88	30.01	54	70	58	60.7	N. W.	N. W.	N. W.	Clear	Clear	Clear		
6	30.16	30.15	30.13	54	74	59	62.3	N. W.	N. W.	W'ly	Clear	Clear	Clear		
7	30.11	30.04	29.96	59	72	68	66.3	W'ly	W'ly	S. W.	Clear	Rain	Cloudy		7th. Light shower and mist during the day, with the wind W'ly and S. W'ly.
8	29.89	29.87	29.84	68	82	72	74.0	S. W.	S. W.	S. W.	Clear	Variable	Cloudy		
9	29.72	29.57	29.42	70	77	73	73.3	S. W.	S. W.	S. W.	Misty	Shower	Clear	0.27	9th. Showery during the day.
10	29.59	29.79	29.99	72	70	63	61.3	W'ly	N. E.	N. E.	Clear	Cloudy	Cloudy		
11	29.51	29.72	29.77	59	76	60	65.0	N. E.	N. E.	N'ly	Cloudy	Cloudy	Cloudy		11th. Sprinkling of rain in the evening.
12	29.80	29.80	29.79	56	65	61	60.7	N'ly	N. E.	N. E.	Cloudy	Cloudy	Cloudy		12th. Sprinkling in the morning and mist, and some rain in afternoon.
13	29.80	29.85	29.88	58	66	60	61.3	N.	N.	N.	Cloudy	Cloudy	Cloudy		
14	29.89	29.89	29.85	60	70	62	64.0	N. E.	S. E.	E.	Cloudy	Cloudy	Cloudy		
15	29.85	29.85	29.84	58	67	64	63.0	N. E.	N. E.	N. E.	Cloudy	Cloudy	Cloudy		15th. Misty from 12 M. to 4 P. M.
16	29.83	29.81	29.80	62	66	64	65.3	S. W.	S. W.	S. W.	Cloudy	Cloudy	Cloudy		
17	29.78	29.78	29.74	62	69	66	65.7	S. W.	S. W.	S. W.	Variable	Clear	Clear		
18	29.70	29.73	29.73	64	67	70	67.0	S. E.	S. E.	S. E.	Rain	Rain	Cloudy	0.43	
19	29.78	29.70	29.68	74	80	76	76.7	S. W.	N. W.	N. W.	Clear	Clear	Clear		
20	29.70	29.78	29.64	63	74	60	65.7	N. W.	N. E.	N. E.	Clear	Clear	Cloudy		
21	29.54	29.49	29.46	58	73	58	63.0	N. E.	N. E.	N. E.	Cloudy	Clear	Clear		
22	29.42	29.39	29.49	62	75	56	64.3	S'ly	W'ly	N. W.	Foggy	Variable	Clear		
23	29.54	29.59	29.65	51	68	56	58.3	N. W.	N. W.	N. W.	Clear	Clear	Clear		
24	29.70	29.69	29.69	49	71	60	60.0	N. W.	W'ly	S. W.	Clear	Clear	Clear		24th. Thermometer 47° at sunrise.
25	29.70	29.72	29.82	56	63	58	59.0	W'ly	W'ly	N. E.	Clear	Rain	Clear	0.05	25th. Light shower, with thunder, from 12 M. to 1 P. M. Light showers, also, at intervals in the afternoon.
26	29.90	29.85	29.79	54	70	64	62.7	S'ly	S. W.	S. W.	Cloudy	Clear	Cl'dy, r'n	0.40	26th. Rain during the night, with lightning.
27	29.62	29.53	29.64	66	78	67	70.3	S. W.	S. W.	N. W.	Misty	Variable	Clear		
28	29.56	29.59	29.65	60	70	59	63.0	N. W.	N. W.	N. W.	Clear	Clear	Clear		
29	29.65	29.62	29.59	53	75	64	64.0	N. W.	N. W.	N. W.	Clear	Clear	Variable		
30	29.38	29.27	29.43	68	84	60	70.7	S. W.	W'ly	N. E.	Clear	Clear	Cloudy		30th. Clear at sunrise. Showers from 9 to 10 A. M. Severe tempest, with heavy thunder and copious rain, from 4 to 6 P. M.; wind W'ly. In the evening, wind N. E.; cloudy.
31	29.55	29.60	29.62	57	67	54	59.3	N. W.	N. W.	N. W.	Clear	Variable	Clear		
Means	29.71	29.71	29.72	61.3	73.0	63.4	...	...	...	...	...	...	...	2.00	
REDUCED TO SEA LEVEL.															
Max.	30.34	30.33	30.31	74	86	76	77.0			Days.			Days.		
Min.	29.56	29.45	29.64	49	63	54	58.3	S'ly & S. W'ly		8	Clear		15		
Mean	29.88	29.88	29.89					W'ly & N. W'ly		13	Variable		4		
Range	0.78	0.88	0.67	25	23	22	18.7	N. E'ly & E'ly		10	Cloudy		7		
Mean of month	29.883			...	...	...	65.9				Rainy		5		
Extreme range	0.89			...	...	...	35.0								

September, 1837.

DAYS.	BAROMETER. Sunrise.	At 1 P. M.	At 10 P. M.	THERMOMETER. Sunrise.	At 1 P. M.	At 10 P. M.	Daily mean.	WINDS. Sunrise.	At 1 P. M.	At 10 P. M.	WEATHER. Sunrise.	At 1 P. M.	At 10 P. M.	RAIN AND SNOW IN INCHES OF WATER.	REMARKS.
1	29.71	29.73	29.80	50	66	55	57.0	N. W.	N. W.	N. E.	Clear	Clear	Clear		
2	29.80	29.79	29.70	50	64	53	55.7	N. E.	N. E.	N. E.	Clear	Variable	Clear		
3	29.74	29.81	29.94	48	70	54	57.3	N. W.	N. W.	N. W.	Clear	Clear	Clear		
4	30.05	30.11	30.15	45	68	50	54.3	N. W.	N. W.	N. W.	Clear	Clear	Clear		
5	30.19	30.18	30.27	49	73	56	59.3	N. W.	S. W'ly	S. W.	Clear	Clear	Clear		
6	30.19	30.16	30.14	50	76	56	60.7	S. W.	S. W.	S. W.	Clear	Clear	Clear		
7	30.07	30.01	29.94	55	72	60	62.3	S. W.	S. W.	S. W.	Clear	Clear	Clear		
8	29.89	29.86	29.85	60	76	63	66.3	S. W.	S. W.	S. W.	Foggy	Variable	Clear		
9	29.85	29.83	29.84	56	78	60	64.7	S. W.	S. W.	S. W.	Clear	Clear	Clear		
10	29.84	29.78	29.73	60	76	68	68.0	S. W.	S. W.	S. W.	Variable	Variable	Clear		
11	29.64	29.56	29.48	68	82	68	72.7	S. W.	S. W.	S. W.	Misty	Clear	Cloudy		
12	29.47	29.47	29.57	57	67	55	59.7	N. W.	N. W.	N. W.	Clear	Clear	Clear		
13	29.66	29.71	29.82	46	62	51	59.7	N. W.	N. W.	N. W.	Clear	Clear	Clear		
14	29.87	29.89	29.92	42	68	53	53.0	N. W.	S. W'ly	W'ly	Clear	Clear	Clear		14th. At sunrise, thermometer 42°; light frost in the vicinity.
15	29.98	29.99	30.00	44	64	50	54.3	N. W.	N. E.	N. E.	Clear	Clear	Clear		
16	30.00	29.95	29.94	48	67	55	52.7	N. E'ly	N. E'ly	N. E.	Clear	Cloudy	Variable		
17	29.85	29.79	29.75	54	76	65	65.0	N. E'ly	E'ly	S'ly	Variable	Variable	Variable		
18	29.69	29.58	29.51	63	78	69	70.0	S'ly	S'ly	W'ly	Foggy	Misty	Clear		18th. Wind S'ly. Foggy, with mist, during the day; the air very sultry. Cleared in the evening, with wind W'ly.
19	29.65	29.69	29.76	60	64	52	58.7	W'ly	W'ly	N. W.	Variable	Clear	Clear		
20	29.94	29.98	30.04	43	64	49	52.0	N. W.	N. W.	N. W.	Clear	Clear	Clear		
21	30.13	30.17	30.17	41	67	47	51.7	N. W.	E.	E.	Clear	Clear	Clear		21st. Aurora in the evening.
22	30.12	29.87	29.80	49	68	54	57.0	N. E.	S'ly	S'ly	Clear	Clear	Clear		
23	29.75	29.80	30.00	52	65	49	55.3	N. W.	N. W.	N. W.	Clear	Clear	Clear		23d. Wind N. W., very blustering Aurora in the evening.
24	30.11	30.16	30.15	40	63	48	50.3	N. W.	N. W.	S. W.	Clear	Clear	Clear		24th. Pleasant. Aurora in the evening.
25	30.11	30.04	29.97	39	71	53	54.3	S. W.	S. W.	S. W.	Clear	Clear	Clear		25th. Light frost in the vicinity.
26	29.85	29.80	29.82	52	70	63	61.7	S. W.	S. W.	W'ly	Clear	Cloudy	Clear		
27	29.90	29.99	30.03	51	63	51	55.0	N. E.	E'ly	N. E.	Clear	Variable	Cloudy		
28	30.00	29.90	29.80	51	62	63	58.7	N. E.	W'ly	S. W.	Cloudy	Cloudy	Cloudy		
29	29.82	29.90	29.95	62	58	50	56.7	W'ly	N. E.	N. E.	Clear	Cloudy	Cloudy		
30	29.92	29.81	29.65	53	54	53	53.3	N. E.	N. E.	E'ly	Cloudy	Rain	Rain		
Means	29.89	29.89	29.88	51.0	67.7	55.7	...	...	...	...	...	...	...	0.48	
REDUCED TO SEA LEVEL.															
Max.	30.37	30.36	30.45	68	82	69	72.7			Days.			Days.		
Min.	29.65	29.65	29.75	39	54	47	50.3	S'ly & S. W'ly		12	Clear		19		
Mean	30.07	30.06	30.06					W'ly & N. W'ly		10	Variable		7		
Range	0.72	0.71	0.70	29	28	22	22.4	N. E'ly & E'ly		8	Cloudy		3		
Mean of month	30.063			...	...	...	58.5				Rainy		1		
Extreme range	0.80			...	...	...	42.0								

October, 1837.

DAYS.	BAROMETER, REDUCED TO 32° F. Sun-rise.	At 1 P. M.	At 10 P. M.	THERMOMETER. Sun-rise.	At 1 P. M.	At 10 P. M.	Daily mean.	WINDS. Sun-rise.	At 1 P. M.	At 10 P. M.	WEATHER. Sunrise.	At 1 P. M.	At 10 P. M.	RAIN AND SNOW IN INCHES OF WATER.	REMARKS.
1	29.55	29.59	29.70	55	70	58	61.0	N. W.	N. W.	N. W.	Cloudy	Clear	Clear		
2	29.75	29.71	29.67	49	71	61	60.3	S. W'ly	S. W.	S. W.	Clear	Clear	Clear		
3	29.82	29.81	29.86	45	62	44	50.3	N. W.	N. W.	N. E.	Clear	Clear	Cloudy		
4	29.93	29.94	30.06	34	46	35	38.3	N. W.	N. W.	N. W.	Clear	Clear	Clear		4th. First white frost in the College yard.
5	30.07	29.96	29.76	29	52	50	43.7	N. W.	S. W'ly	S. W'ly	Clear	Cloudy	Rain		5th. Severe frost. Ice in open vessels more than one-eighth of an inch thick.
6	29.68	29.63	29.68	53	60	44	52.3	S. W.	S. W.	N. W.	Cloudy	Cloudy	Clear		
7	29.82	29.78	29.81	36	57	46	46.3	N. W.	N. W.	W'ly	Clear	Clear	Clear		
8	29.92	29.97	30.14	42	50	37	43.0	N. W.	N. W.	N. W.	Clear	Clear	Clear		
9	30.30	...	...	29	...	...	...	N. W.	...	...	Clear	...	...		
10	...	...	...	...	...	...	...	...	...	...	...	...	...		
11	...	29.86	29.92	...	74	60	...	...	W'ly	W'ly	...	Clear	Cloudy		
12	29.86	29.74	29.68	50	72	61	61.0	W'ly	S. W.	S. W.	Clear	Clear	Rain	} 0.86	
13	29.72	29.81	30.06	42	40	30	37.3	N. E.	N'ly	N. W.	Rain	Cloudy	Clear		13th. Rain and snow in the forenoon; wind N. E. Cleared in the afternoon.
14	30.15	30.20	30.17	23	44	35	34.0	N. W'ly	N. W.	W'ly	Clear	Clear	Clear		
15	30.09	...	29.99	33	...	52	...	S. W.	...	S. W.	Clear	...	Clear		
16	29.98	30.00	30.11	52	63	50	55.0	S. W.	N. W.	N. W.	Cloudy	Clear	Clear		
17	30.21	30.16	30.07	43	59	45	49.0	N. W.	S. W.	W'ly	Clear	Clear	Clear		
18	29.82	29.63	29.55	45	68	62	58.3	S. W.	S. W.	S. W.	Clear	Clear	Clear		
19	29.77	29.85	29.96	59	54	38	50.3	S. W.	N. E.	N. W.	Cloudy	Cloudy	Clear		
20	29.82	29.58	29.55	46	53	53	50.7	S'ly	S. E'ly	S'ly	Cloudy	Rain	Variable		
21	29.70	29.75	29.87	44	55	38	45.7	W'ly	N. W.	N. W.	Clear	Clear	Clear		
22	29.94	29.89	29.85	30	51	44	41.7	N. W.	S. E'ly	S. W.	Clear	Clear	Clear		22d. Aurora; bright from 6½ to 8 P. M, shooting up towards the zenith in long, slender needles.
23	29.81	29.80	29.80	48	67	55	56.7	S. W.	S. W.	S. W.	Clear	Clear	Foggy		
24	29.80	29.79	29.83	55	65	61	60.3	S. W.	S. W.	W'ly	Foggy	Variable	Foggy		
25	29.81	29.82	29.94	60	65	50	58.3	N. E.	N. E.	N. E.	Cloudy	Cloudy	Variable		
26	29.90	29.90	29.86	49	51	48	49.3	N. E.	N. E.	N. E.	Cloudy	Misty	Rain	0.43	
27	29.75	29.60	29.64	48	52	45	48.3	N. E.	N. E.	N. W.	Misty	Misty	Variable		27th. Wind N. E. Mist and light rain during the day. Stars appearing at 10 P. M.; wind N. W'ly.
28	29.82	29.91	29.88	36	46	36	39.3	N. W.	N. W.	N. W.	Variable	Clear	Clear		
29	29.91	29.91	29.83	31	34	34	33.0	N. E.	N. E.	N. E.	Cloudy	Cloudy	Cloudy		
30	29.69	29.67	29.83	30	47	40	39.0	N'ly	N'ly	N. W.	Variable	Variable	Clear		
31	29.94	29.93	29.88	36	41	37	38.0	N. E.	N. E.	N. E.	Variable	Variable	Variable		
Means	29.84	29.83	29.87	42.4	56.0	46.5	...	...	...	...	...	...	...	1.29	
REDUCED TO SEA LEVEL.															
Max.	30.48	30.40	30.35	59	74	62	65.0			Days.			Days.		
Min.	29.73	29.76	29.73	23	34	30	29.0	S'ly & S. W'ly		8	Clear		19		
Mean	30.05	30.00	30.05					W'ly & N. W'ly		12	Variable		4		
Range	0.75	0.64	0.62	36	40	32	26.0	N. E'ly & E'ly		10	Cloudy		5		
Mean of month	30.033			...	...	...	48.3				Rainy		2		
Extreme range	0.75			...	...	...	51.0								

November, 1837.

DAYS.	Sun-rise.	At 1 P. M.	At 10 P. M.	Sun-rise.	At 1 P. M.	At 10 P. M.	Daily mean.	Sun-rise.	At 1 P. M.	At 10 P. M.	Sunrise.	At 1 P. M.	At 10 P. M.		
1	29.69	29.62	29.62	30	51	38	39.7	N. W.	N. W.	N. W.	Variable	Clear	Clear		
2	29.63	29.62	29.63	33	51	36	40.0	N. W.	N. W.	N. W.	Variable	Clear	Clear		
3	29.86	29.82	29.84	31	50	42	41.0	N. W.	N. W.	N. W.	Clear	Clear	Clear		
4	29.80	29.71	29.70	36	61	44	47.0	W'ly	S. W.	S. W.	Clear	Clear	Clear		
5	29.42	29.28	29.22	50	61	60	57.0	S. W.	S. W'ly	S. W.	Rain	Cloudy	Variable	0.10	
6	29.32	29.43	29.54	50	50	40	46.7	W'ly	N. W.	N. W.	Clear	Clear	Variable		
7	29.36	29.51	29.73	40	49	37	42.0	W'ly	N. W.	N. W.	Clear	Clear	Clear		
8	29.99	30.02	30.14	28	35	26	29.7	N. W.	N. W.	N. W.	Clear	Clear	Clear		
9	30.24	30.17	29.96	22	35	36	31.0	N. W.	N. W.	S. W.	Clear	Cloudy	Cloudy		
10	29.71	29.72	29.97	48	58	36	47.3	S. W.	W'ly	N. W.	Cloudy	Clear	Clear		
11	30.05	29.96	29.77	27	46	46	39.7	N'ly	S'ly	S. E'ly	Clear	Clear	Cloudy		
12	29.34	29.27	29.55	54	54	44	50.7	S. E.	W'ly	N. W.	Rain	Cloudy	Clear	0.45	
13	29.68	29.76	29.76	31	40	33	34.7	N. W.	...	N. E.	Clear	Clear	Variable		
14	29.60	29.48	29.52	31	24	27	27.3	N. E.	N. E.	N. E'ly	Snow	Snow	Cloudy	0.50	14th. Began to snow about sunrise. Wind brisk N. E. Continued to snow, with driving wind and cold, till from 8 to 9 P. M. Severe storm for the season.
15	29.75	29.79	29.99	20	34	24	26.0	N. W.	N. W.	N. W.	Clear	Clear	Clear		
16	30.15	30.11	30.10	18	42	28	29.3	N. W.	N. W.	N. W.	Clear	Clear	Clear		
17	30.21	30.21	30.17	29	42	36	35.7	N. W.	N. W.	S. W.	Clear	Clear	Variable		
18	30.14	30.08	30.01	36	52	44	44.0	S. W.	S. W.	S. W.	Variable	Variable	Clear		
19	29.83	29.86	30.01	54	57	50	53.7	S. W.	W'ly	W'ly	Cloudy	Clear	Cloudy		
20	29.92	29.82	29.80	42	67	59	56.0	S. W.	S. W.	S. W.	Variable	Clear	Clear		
21	29.76	29.71	29.66	50	69	57	58.7	S. W.	S. W.	S. W.	Clear	Clear	Clear		
22	29.48	29.26	28.95	50	57	55	54.0	S. W.	S. E'ly	S. E'ly	Foggy	Foggy	Misty		22d. Wind light S. E'ly, with heavy fog. Occasional mist and rain during the day.
23	28.77	28.88	29.19	38	40	30	33.3	W'ly	W'ly	W'ly	Clear	Variable	Clear		23d. Wind W'ly; very blustering.
24	29.29	...	29.34	28	...	30	29.0	W'ly	...	N. E.	Clear	...	Snow	} 0.90	
25	29.21	29.15	29.46	25	26	18	23.0	N. E.	N. E.	W'ly	Snow	Cloudy	Clear		25th. Driving snow-storm from N. E. during the night, and continued, without much abatement, till from 8 to 9 A. M. Eight or nine inches of moist snow, equal to 0.9 inch of water. Cloudy, with light snow in the air, during the greater part of the day. Clear in the evening.
26	29.73	29.80	29.91	11	24	13	16.0	N. W.	N. W.	N. W.	Clear	Clear	Clear		
27	30.12	30.16	30.26	13	28	18	19.7	N. W.	W'ly	N. W.	Clear	Clear	Clear		
28	30.29	30.26	30.25	13	38	33	28.0	W'ly	S. W.	S. W.	Clear	Clear	Clear		
29	30.21	30.12	29.89	38	47	44	43.0	S. W.	S. W.	S. W.	Cloudy	Clear	Clear		
30	29.90	29.92	29.98	43	54	42	46.3	S. W.	S. W.	S. W.	Clear	Clear	Variable		
Means	29.74	29.74	29.73	33.9	46.2	37.5	...	...	...	...	...	...	...	1.95	
REDUCED TO SEA LEVEL.															
Max.	30.47	30.44	30.44	54	69	60	58.7			Days.			Days.		
Min.	29.39	29.33	29.37	11	24	13	16.0	S'ly & S. W'ly		8	Clear		21		
Mean	29.92	29.92	29.91					W'ly & N. W'ly		17	Variable		3		
Range	1.08	1.11	1.07	43	45	47	42.7	N. E'ly & E'ly		5	Cloudy		1		
Mean of month	29.917			...	...	...	39.2				Rainy		5		
Extreme range	1.14			...	...	...	58.1								

December, 1837.

Days.	Barometer, reduced to 32° F. Sunrise.	At 1 P. M.	At 10 P. M.	Thermometer. Sunrise.	At 1 P. M.	At 10 P. M.	Daily mean.	Winds. Sunrise.	At 1 P. M.	At 10 P. M.	Weather. Sunrise.	At 1 P. M.	At 10 P. M.	Rain and Snow in Inches of Water.
1	29.95	29.84	29.83	36	49	43	42.7	S. W'ly	S. W'ly	W'ly	Variable	Cloudy	Clear	
2	29.79	29.76	29.68	42	47	46	45.0	N. E'ly	N. E'ly	N. E'ly	Cloudy	Cloudy	Misty	
3	29.48	29.52	29.59	44	48	44	45.3	S'ly	S. W'ly	N. W.	Cloudy	Cloudy	Variable	
4	29.69	29.69	29.72	32	47	34	37.7	W'ly	W'ly	N. W.	Cloudy	Variable	Clear	
5	29.98	29.98	30.03	28	36	28	30.7	N. W.	N. W.	N. W.	Clear	Clear	Hazy	
6	30.07	30.00	29.89	25	37	32	31.3	N. W.	N. W.	S. W.	Clear	Clear	Clear	
7	29.85	29.83	29.78	29	40	30	33.0	N. W.	N. W.	N. W.	Clear	Clear	Cloudy	
8	29.50	29.41	29.64	31	40	18	29.7	S. W.	W'ly	N. W.	Clear	Clear	Clear	
9	29.86	29.86	29.82	14	26	24	21.3	N. W.	N. W.	N. E.	Cloudy	Variable	Variable	
10	29.60	29.43	29.32	22	31	28	27.0	N. E.	N. E'ly	N. E.	Cloudy	Snow	Snow	0.75
11	29.40	29.39	29.50	22	32	26	26.7	N'ly	N'ly	N. W.	Cloudy	Cloudy	Clear	
12	29.50	29.52	29.59	22	33	24	26.3	W.	W'ly	N. W.	Clear	Clear	Clear	
13	29.67	29.66	29.75	22	31	23	25.3	N. W.	N. W.	N. W.	Clear	Clear	Clear	
14	29.68	29.66	29.70	10	22	10	14.0	N. W.	N. W.	N. W.	Clear	Clear	Clear	
15	29.78	29.82	29.98	4½	19	12	11.8	N. W.	N. W.	N. W.	Clear	Clear	Clear	
16	30.06	30.03	30.04	7	25	16	16.0	N. W.	N. W'ly	N. W.	Clear	Variable	Variable	
17	30.07	29.99	29.88	14	21	26	30.3	N. W.	N. E'ly	N. E'ly	Variable	Cloudy	Cloudy	
18	29.45	28.70	29.15	35	50	37	40.7	S. E.	S. W.	N. W'ly	Rain	Rain	Cloudy	1.80
19	29.41	29.38	29.41	31	37	30	32.7	N. W.	N. W.	N. W.	Clear	Variable	Variable	
20	29.43	29.48	29.63	22	21	12	18.3	N. W.	N. W.	N. W.	Clear	Clear	Clear	
21	29.69	29.71	29.74	8	21	13	14.0	N. W.	N. W.	N. W.	Clear	Clear	Clear	
22	29.84	29.87	30.06	5	19½	10	11.3	N. W.	N. W.	N. W.	Clear	Clear	Clear	
23	30.11	30.17	30.15	8	27	24	19.7	N. W.	S. W'ly	S. W.	Clear	Clear	Cloudy	
24	30.02	29.86	29.82	27	33	29	29.7	S'ly	S. E'ly	N. E.	Snow	Cloudy	Cloudy	
25	29.83	29.81	29.78	23	36	33	30.7	W'ly	W'ly	S. W.	Clear	Clear	Clear	
26	29.65	29.53	29.84	33	45	28	35.3	S. W.	S. W.	N. W.	Cloudy	Variable	Clear	
27	30.15	30.20	30.21	19	26	22	22.3	N. W.	N. W.	N. E.	Clear	Clear	Cloudy	
28	30.01	29.87	29.87	25	39	30	31.3	N. E.	S'ly	N. W.	Cloudy	Cloudy	Clear	
29	29.86	29.87	29.79	25	40	35	33.3	W'ly	W'ly	S. W'ly	Clear	Clear	Clear	
30	29.78	29.82	29.93	31	47	33	37.0	S. W'ly	W'ly	N. W.	Clear	Clear	Clear	
31	29.96	29.99	30.08	30	39	34	34.3	N. W.	W'ly	N. E.	Variable	Variable	Cloudy	
Means	29.78	29.73	29.78	23.4	34.3	26.9	...	...	...	...	...	...	...	2.55
REDUCED TO SEA LEVEL.														
Max.	30.33	30.38	30.39	44	50	46	45.3							
Min.	29.58	29.57	29.33	4½	19½	10	11.3							
Mean	29.96	29.91	29.96											
Range	0.75	0.81	1.06	39½	30½	36	34.0							
Mean of month	29.943			...	...	...	28.2							
Extreme range	1.06			...	...	...	45.0							

Winds	Days.
S'ly & S. W'ly	4
W'ly & N. W'ly	21
N. E'ly & E'ly	6

Weather	Days
Clear	16
Variable	7
Cloudy	6
Rainy	2

REMARKS.

1st. The aurora considerably bright during the evening; for a short time, brilliant corruscations of red light.

5th. Very clear at sunrise. Soon after dark, the moon appeared with a halo around it, distant about 22½°. The air soon began to be perceptibly hazy. The disk of the moon was dimmed, and the stars disappeared one after another, till, at 10 o'clock, the moon was much obscured by increasing vapor, and the bow became extinct.

On the following morning, the weather was mild and beautiful.

8th. Cloudy and blustering in the afternoon with wind W'ly. Came to N. W., and cleared in the evening; much cooler.

9th. Wind came to N. E., from 1 to 2 P. M., very light. Clouded up towards night. Flurry of snow in the night.

10th. Began to snow from 7 to 8 P. M.; wind very light N. E.; snow damp. Continued to snow till from 10 to 12 P. M. Snow from six to seven inches, equal to 0.75 of an inch of water.

17th. Began snowing from 1 to 2 P. M.; wind light at N. E.

18th. At 5 A. M., raining moderately; wind light at S. E. At sunrise, rain increasing; wind as before; barometer 29.48. At 10 A. M., wind hauling to S. with increased force, and heavy rain. At 12 M., wind S'ly, pretty strong, and rain still heavy. At from 12 M. to 1 P. M., rain abating, clouds broken, and the sun out for a few minutes. At 1 P. M., wind S. W., moderate; rain nearly over; barometer 28.74. At 2 P. M., wind light S. W.; clouds broken; barometer 28.60. At 3 P. M., wind S. W.; raining moderately; barometer 28.60. At 3½ P. M., wind W'ly; barometer beginning to rise. At 4 P. M., barometer 28.67, rising fast; wind hauling round to N. W.

January, 1838.

Days.	Barometer Sunrise.	At 1 P. M.	At 10 P. M.	Thermometer Sunrise.	At 1 P. M.	At 10 P. M.	Daily mean.	Winds Sunrise.	At 1 P. M.	At 10 P. M.	Weather Sunrise.	At 1 P. M.	At 10 P. M.	Rain and Snow
1	30.15	30.17	30.16	33	40	34	35.7	N. E.	N. E.	N. E.	Misty	Cloudy	Cloudy	
2	30.09	30.03	29.93	34	41	37	37.3	N. E'ly	S. W.	S. W.	Cloudy	Variable	Variable	
3	29.84	29.79	29.87	35	50	39	41.3	S. W.	S. W.	W'ly	Clear	Clear	Clear	
4	29.96	30.02	30.07	40	48	40	42.7	S. E.	N. E.	N. E.	Cloudy	Variable	Variable	
5	29.93	29.74	29.69	42	58	52	50.7	S. W'ly	S. W.	S. W.	Foggy	Variable	Variable	
6	29.89	29.94	30.04	38	47	34	39.7	W'ly	W'ly	W'ly	Clear	Clear	Clear	
7	29.93	29.92	29.79	29	45	44	39.3	S. W'ly	S. W.	S. W.	Foggy	Clear	Foggy	
8	29.64	29.65	29.95	46	45	32	41.0	S. W.	N. W.	N. W.	Variable	Cloudy	Variable	
9	30.09	30.05	29.93	22	35	33	30.0	N. E.	N. E.	N. E'ly	Clear	Cloudy	Misty	
10	29.88	29.84	29.91	34	35	22	30.3	S. W.	N. W.	N. W.	Variable	Clear	Variable	
11	29.99	29.99	30.01	14	20	15	16.3	N. W.	N. W.	N. W.	Clear	Clear	Clear	
12	30.06	30.05	30.12	17	31	23	23.7	N. W.	W'ly	W'ly	Clear	Clear	Clear	
13	30.07	30.00	30.04	22	39	32	31.0	W'ly	S. W'ly	S. W'ly	Clear	Clear	Clear	
14	29.97	29.83	29.68	30	46	40	38.7	S. W'ly	S. W'ly	S. W.	Clear	Clear	Variable	
15	29.36	29.41	29.72	44	41	32	39.0	S. W.	W.N.W	W.N.W	Rain	Clear	Clear	0.33
16	29.86	29.78	29.80	31	43	41	38.3	W'ly	S. W.	S. W.	Clear	Clear	Clear	
17	29.74	29.65	29.59	42	56	54	50.7	S. W.	S. W.	W'ly	Variable	Cloudy	Variable	
18	29.76	29.76	29.72	41	46	37	41.3	S. W'ly	N. E.	N. E.	Foggy	Foggy	Misty	
19	29.35	29.12	29.48	34	38	25	32.3	N. E.	N. E.	N. W.	Rain	Rain	Clear	1.00
20	29.89	30.00	30.09	18	26	18	20.7	N. W.	N. W.	N. W.	Clear	Clear	Clear	
21	30.05	29.94	29.98	17	28	26	23.7	W'ly	W'ly	N. E'ly	Variable	Cloudy	Clear	
22	30.12	30.07	30.10	16	25	16	19.0	N. E.	N. E.	N. W.	Variable	Variable	Clear	
23	30.14	30.09	30.07	12	30	28	23.3	N. W.	N. E'ly	S. E'ly	Clear	Clear	Variable	
24	30.15	30.10	30.11	25	40	29	31.3	S. W.	S. W.	S. W.	Clear	Clear	Clear	
25	30.21	30.20	30.11	28	38	34	33.3	S. W.	S. W.	E'ly	Cloudy	Clear	Cloudy	
26	29.85	29.74	29.93	38	53	40	43.7	S. W'ly	S. W.	W'ly	C'y, f'g, r	Variable	Clear	0.33
27	29.94	29.92	29.38	34	37	35	35.3	N. E.	N. E.	N. E.	Cloudy	Cloudy	Rain	1.04
28	29.16	29.20	29.44	33	42	34	36.3	W'ly	S. W.	N. W.	Variable	Variable	Variable	
29	29.55	29.38	29.66	24	26	15	21.7	W'ly	W'ly	N. W.	Variable	Variable	Clear	
30	29.71	29.68	29.75	10	14	6	10.0	N. W.	N. W.	N. W.	Clear	Clear	Clear	
31	[illegible]	[illegible]	[illegible]	[illegible]	[illegible]	[illegible]	[illegible]	[illegible]	[illegible]	[illegible]	[illegible]	[illegible]	[illegible]	
Means	29.90	29.84	29.87	28.6	38.0	30.9	...	...	...	...	...	...	...	2.70
REDUCED TO SEA LEVEL.														
Max.	30.39	30.38	30.34	42	58	54	50.8							
Min.	29.34	29.30	29.56	3	14	6	10.0							
Mean	30.08	30.02	30.05											
Range	0.95	1.08	0.78	39	44	48	40.8							
Mean of month	30.050			...	...	...	32.5							
Extreme range	1.09			...	...	...	55.0							

Winds	Days.
S'ly & S. W'ly	11
W'ly & N. W'ly	11
N. E'ly & E'ly	9

Weather	Days.
Clear	12
Variable	11
Cloudy	4
Rainy	4

5th. Wind brisk from S. W. in afternoon. From 6 to 8 P. M., very blustering, with heavy clouds from S. W. and sprinkling of rain. At 10 P. M., moon out; wind more moderate

8th. Very mild in the morning; wind S. W. From 11 A. M. to 12 M., wind came round to W., and thence, in an hour or so, to N. W., with dashes of rain, heavy clouds, and blusterings. In the evening, partially clear; wind at the surface light from N. W., while the clouds come from S. W.

9th. Wind came to N. E. early in the morning A little snow and mist at intervals during the day; wind light.

15th. At sunrise, wind S. W.; warm; raining moderately. From 9 to 10 A. M., wind came to about W. N. W., and continued blustering through the day.

17th. Wind S. W., very fresh; came round to W'ly in afternoon, and subsided; partially clear. Two or three very light showers during the day —just enough to wet the ground.

18th. At sunrise, very thick fog; wind light S. W'ly. At 1 P. M., wind light N. E.; fog thick. Misty in the evening. Considerable rain during the night. Frost entirely out of the ground in many places.

19th. At sunrise, raining moderately; wind N. E. From 11 to 12 A. M., wind hauled N'ly, and continued to swing till 2 P. M., when it reached the S. W., much increased in strength, with heavy dashes of rain. At 4 P. M., the clouds became broken; wind hauled to W'ly, and soon to N. W., very high and gusty. At sunset, there were two strata of clouds, which seemed to be very close together, both low and heavy, though broken, and both in pretty rapid motion—the lower from N. W., the upper from S. W. Clear at 6 P. M.; barometer rising rapidly. Wind high and very blustering during the night. Rain 1.00 inch.

27th. Wind light N. E. in morning; cloudy. Began to hail gently from 3 to 4 P. M.; wind still [illegible] to freshen. Rain and wind heavy during the evening. Rain ceased, and wind came to W'ly, before morning.

28th. At sunrise, weather mild and pleasant. Frost out of the ground in most places.

29th. Very blustering all day. Flurry of snow from 11 A. M. to 2 P. M. Weather changed to severe cold

30th. Wind blustering, and severe cold

February, 1838.

DAYS.	BAROMETER, REDUCED TO 32° F. Sun-rise.	At 1 P. M.	At 10 P. M.	THERMOMETER. Sun-rise.	At 1 P. M.	At 10 P. M.	Daily mean.	WINDS. Sun-rise.	At 1 P. M.	At 10 P. M.	WEATHER. Sunrise.	At 1 P. M.	At 10 P. M.	RAIN AND SNOW IN INCHES OF WATER.
1	30.01	29.96	29.87	5	24	19	16.0	N. W.	N. W.	N. W.	Clear	Clear	Cloudy	
2	29.75	29.67	29.66	12	23	10	15.0	N. W.	N. W.	W'ly	Variable	Cloudy	Clear	
3	29.56	29.47	29.45	8	14	10	10.7	N. E.	N'ly	N'ly	Cloudy	Cloudy	Cloudy	
4	29.42	29.43	29.48	5	18	13	12.0	N. W.	N. W.	N. W.	Variable	Variable	Clear	
5	29.52	29.47	29.55	8	23	14	15.0	S. W.	W'ly	W'ly	Clear	Clear	Clear	
6	29.72	29.72	29.83	9	26	19	18.0	N. W.	N. W.	N. W.	Clear	Clear	Clear	
7	29.93	29.90	29.74	12	31	33	25.3	W'ly	S. W.	S. W.	Clear	Clear	Cloudy	
8	29.41	29.40	29.43	44	39	33	35.3	S. W'ly	N. W'ly	N. E.	Cloudy	Cloudy	Cloudy	.25
9	29.34	29.28	29.30	31	34	28	31.0	N. E.	N. E'ly	W'ly	Snow	Sn. & r'n	Variable	.10
10	29.45	29.45	29.50	23	29	24	25.3	N. W.	N. W.	N. W.	Clear	Clear	Cl'y, var.	0
11	29.49	29.43	29.40	19	35	23	25.7	N. W.	W'ly	N. E.	Clear	Variable	Snow	0.50
12	29.75	29.84	29.87	10	24	22	18.7	N. W.	N. W.	S. W.	Clear	Clear	Variable	
13	29.90	29.84	29.64	26	38	32	32.0	S. W.	S. W.	E'ly	Variable	Clear	Rain	0.60
14	29.58	29.67	29.89	28	29	15	24.0	N. W.	N. W.	N. W.	Variable	Clear	Clear	
15	29.91	29.81	29.68	8	16	14	12.7	N. E.	N. E.	N'ly	Cloudy	Snow	Cloudy	0.25
16	29.38	29.31	29.68	12	20	16	16.0	N. E.	N. E.	N'ly	Misty	Misty	Snow	0.62
17	29.32	29.71	29.74	4	10	4	6.0	N. W.	N. W.	N. W.	Clear	Clear	Clear	
18	29.66	29.53	29.47	4	24	16	14.7	N. W'ly	W'ly	W'ly	Clear	Clear	Clear	
19	29.44	29.36	29.43	13	22	13	16.0	W'ly	W'ly	W'ly	Clear	Clear	Clear	
20	29.45	29.42	29.47	10	18	8	12.0	W'ly	W'ly	N. W.	Clear	Clear	Clear	
21	29.52	29.55	29.68	5	19	12	12.0	N. W.	N. W.	N. W.	Clear	Clear	Clear	
22	29.79	29.78	29.79	10	26	16	17.3	N. W.	N. W.	N. W.	Clear	Clear	Clear	
23	29.77	29.67	29.65	9	29	17	18.3	N. W.	W'ly	W'ly	Clear	Clear	Clear	
24	29.60	29.57	29.67	15	28	14	19.0	W'ly	W'ly	N. W.	Clear	Clear	Clear	
25	29.73	29.70	29.68	2	16	11	9.7	W'ly	N. W.	N. W.	Clear	Clear	Clear	
26	29.73	29.73	29.86	4	19	5	9.3	N. W.	N. W.	N. W.	Variable	Variable	Clear	
27	29.89	29.87	29.87	1	23	15	13.0	N. W.	N. W.	N'ly	Clear	Clear	Cloudy	
28	29.88	29.83	29.83	7	25	22	18.0	N. W.	N'ly	W'ly	Clear	Clear	Clear	
Means	29.64	29.62	29.65	12.3	24.4	17.0	...	...	...	...	...	...	...	2.32
REDUCED TO SEA LEVEL.														
Max.	30.19	30.14	30.07	28	39	33	35.3			Days.			Days.	
Min.	29.50	29.46	29.48	1	10	4	6.0	S'ly & S. W'ly		3	Clear		19	
Mean	29.82	29.80	29.83					W'ly & N. W'ly		19	Variable		2	
Range	0.69	0.68	0.59	27	29	29	29.3	N. E'ly & E'ly		6	Cloudy		2	
Mean of month	29.817			...	...	...	17.9				Rainy		5	
Extreme range	0.73			...	...	...	38.0							

REMARKS.

1st. Wind N. W. in morning, S.W'ly in afternoon; came to N. W. again in evening; light all day.

2d. Cloudy in morning. Clear in afternoon. Wind moderate N. W.

3d. Very raw and cold. Flurry of snow towards night. Wind moderate.

4th. Variable in morning, with a flurry of snow. Very clear in afternoon and evening. Brilliant aurora of red light seen at 5 A. M., shooting up from the N. E. towards the zenith, and also from the W. Light round the N.; some corruscations, but not brilliant.

Night of 7th. Shower, equal 0.25 inch of water.

9th. Began to snow very moderately from 6 to 7 A. M.; wind light N. E. Snow, mixed with a little rain, continued very moderately during a greater part of the day. 0.10 inch of water.

11th. Very pleasant morning; nearly clear; wind light W'ly. Clouded up, and flurry of snow, from 11 to 12 A. M. At 1 P. M., sun out; wind S. W.; very mild. From 4 to 5 P. M., began to snow; wind soon came to N. E. At 6 P. M. and after, wind growing fresh, and snow blowing. Wind came to N. W., and cleared before morning. About 6 inches light, dry snow fallen, equal 0.5 inch of water.

13th. Rain during the night from E'ly. Clear before morning.

15th. Began to snow about sunrise; wind light N. E. Snow continued till from 12 M. to 1 P. M.—about 2 inches. Wind came more to N'ly. Cloudy afternoon. From 2 to 3 snows in the night.

16th. Fine mist in the morning, which froze as it fell; wind light N. E. Began to hail and snow about 1 P. M., and continued during the afternoon and evening. Wind came to N. W. before morning, and cleared.

17th. Very severe cold; the wind cutting from N. W.

18th. Very blustering.

19th. Very blustering.

20th. Blustering. River closed against the boat by ice.

21st. Blustering. Brilliant aurora in evening.

22d. Weather milder and more pleasant.

23d. Pleasant.

24th. Pleasant in morning. Cloudy and flurry of snow in afternoon.

March, 1838.

DAYS.	BAROMETER Sun-rise.	At 1 P. M.	At 10 P. M.	THERMOMETER Sun-rise.	At 1 P. M.	At 10 P. M.	Daily mean.	WINDS Sun-rise.	At 1 P. M.	At 10 P. M.	WEATHER Sunrise.	At 1 P. M.	At 10 P. M.	RAIN AND SNOW
1	29.83	29.84	29.86	20	29	23	24.0	N. W'ly	N. E.	N. E.	Clear	Variable	Clear	
2	29.88	29.89	29.93	15	26	22	21.0	N. E'ly	N. E'ly	N'ly	Clear	Clear	Clear	
3	30.06	30.10	30.15	27	35	23	28.3	N. E.	N. E.	N. E.	Cloudy	Clear	Clear	
4	30.20	30.18	30.15	17	36	26	26.3	N. W.	N. E.	W'ly	Clear	Clear	Clear	
5	29.95	29.74	29.32	18	38	40	32.0	S. E.	S. E.	S. E'ly	Cloudy	Cloudy	Rain	1.00
6	29.46	29.62	29.76	35	46	36	39.0	W'ly	W'ly	W'ly	Clear	Clear	Variable	
7	29.77	29.76	29.78	34	33	32	33.0	N. E.	N. E.	N. E.	Cloudy	Snow	Rain	
8	29.75	29.72	29.60	32	36	31	33.0	N. E.	N. E.	N. E.	Cloudy	Cloudy	Snow	1.00
9	29.68	29.79	29.90	26	38	34	32.7	N. E.	N. W.	N. W.	Snow	Clear	Clear	
10	29.95	29.95	29.94	34	44	35	37.7	N. W.	N'ly	N. W.	Cloudy	Cloudy	Clear	
11	29.85	29.76	29.73	35	48	33	38.7	S'ly	S. W'ly	S. W.	Cloudy	Variable	Clear	
12	29.74	29.78	29.91	31	46	34	37.0	W'ly	N'ly	N. E.	Clear	Clear	Clear	
13	29.98	29.98	29.94	28	48	34	36.7	N. E.	S. W'ly	S. W'ly	Clear	Clear	Clear	
14	29.93	29.87	29.87	30	49	34	37.7	N. W'ly	E'ly	N. E.	Clear	Clear	Clear	
15	29.73	29.62	29.60	35	49	38	40.7	E'ly	N. E'ly	N. E.	Clear	Clear	Clear	
16	29.63	29.67	29.76	38	52	41	43.7	N. W.	N. E.	S'ly	Clear	Clear	Clear	
17	29.83	29.87	29.84	35	38	34	35.7	N. E.	N. E.	N. E.	Variable	Cloudy	Cloudy	
18	29.67	29.63	29.55	31	32	28	30.3	N. E.	N. E.	N. E.	Snow	Snow	Snow	0.50
19	29.43	29.38	29.35	28	38	34	33.3	N. E.	E'ly	S'ly	Cloudy	Cloudy	Clear	
20	29.39	29.45	29.54	36	56	36	42.7	S. W.	S. W.	S. W.	Clear	Variable	Clear	
21	29.58	29 81	30.04	35	45	31	37.0	W'ly	N. E'ly	E'ly	Cloudy	Variable	Clear	
22	30.09	30.16	30.09	34	46	33	37.7	N. E'ly	S. E'ly	E'ly	Variable	Variable	Misty	
23	30.10	30.12	30.04	35	42	36	37.7	N'ly	S. E'ly	S'ly	Misty	Cloudy	Misty	
24	29.77	29.65	29.81	37	61	43	47.0	S. W.	S. W'ly	N. W.	Variable	Variable	Clear	
25	30.03	30.04	29.99	30	41	34	35.0	N. W.	N. W.	N. W.	Clear	Clear	Clear	
26	29.94	29.92	29.93	35	51	38	41.3	N. E'ly	N. W'ly	N. W.	Clear	Clear	Clear	
27	29.98	29.92	29.92	29	43	27	33.0	N. E.	S. E'ly	S. E'ly	Clear	Cloudy	Snow	0.20
28	29.94	29.93	29.75	25	42	29	32.0	E'ly	S. E'ly	S. W'ly	Cloudy	Cloudy	Cloudy	
29	29.32	29.13	29.46	30	40	30	33.3	S. E'ly	S. W.	N. E'ly	Snow	Cloudy	Cloudy	
30	29.32	29.27	29.39	30	44	34	36.0	N. W.	N. W.	N. W.	Cloudy	Variable	Variable	
31	29.46	29.42	29.47	27	43	32	34.0	N. W.	N. W.	N. W.	Clear	Clear	Clear	
Means	29.78	29.77	29.78	30.1	42.4	32.7	...	...	...	...	...	...	...	2.70
REDUCED TO SEA LEVEL.														
Max.	30.38	30.36	30.33	38	61	43	47.0			Days.			Days.	
Min.	29.40	29.31	29.50	15	26	22	21.0	S'ly & S. W'ly		4	Clear		14	
Mean	29.96	29.95	29.96					W'ly & N. W'ly		7	Variable		5	
Range	0.98	1.05	0.83	23	35	21	26.0	N. E'ly & E'ly		20	Cloudy		6	
Mean of month	29.957			...	...	...	35.1				Rainy		6	
Extreme range	1.07			...	...	...	46.0							

REMARKS.

4th. Very pleasant.

5th. Wind S E'ly. Began to rain from 3 to 4 P. M. Wind and rain heavy in the evening. Cleared, with wind W'ly, before morning. Rain 1.00 inch.

6th. Halo about the moon in the evening; wind light W'ly; came to N. E. before morning.

7th. Began to snow early in the forenoon, with wind N. E Snow and rain in the afternoon and evening.

8th. Wind N. E. Cloudy, with some mist during the day. At 5½ P. M., began to snow, and continued through the night. 6 or 7 inches of damp snow.

9th. Cleared from 8 to 9 A. M. Wind came to N. W.

10th. Cloudy in morning. Clear in afternoon, mild and pleasant.

11th and 12th. Mild and pleasant.

13th. Very mild and pleasant.

15th and 16th. Mild and pleasant.

17th. Wind N. E., brisk and raw, increasing towards night, and cloudy. Wind continued heavy during the night.

18th. Snow began to fall about 6 A. M.; wind heavy N. E. Snow continued till after 10 P. M., but ceased before morning.

24th. Wind light S. W. in morning; mild and pleasant. Wind came to W., and then to N. W., in afternoon; gusty and blustering.

27th. Began to snow moderately from 3 to 4 P. M.; wind light S. E'ly. Snow till night, nearly 2 inches.

April, 1838.

DAYS.	BAROMETER, REDUCED TO 32° F. At 6 A. M.	At 1 P. M.	At 10 P. M.	THERMOMETER. At 6 A. M.	At 1 P. M.	At 10 P. M.	Daily mean.	WINDS. At 6 A. M.	At 1 P. M.	At 10 P. M.	WEATHER. At 6 A. M.	At 1 P. M.	At 10 P. M.	RAIN AND SNOW IN INCHES OF WATER
1	29.48	29.38	29.38	28	44	35	35.7	N. W.	W'ly	N. W.	Clear	Clear	Clear	
2	29.33	29.25	29.31	26	43	32	33.7	N. W.	N. W.	N. W.	Clear	Clear	Clear	
3	29.28	29.29	29.34	31	44	33	36.0	N. W.	N. W.	N. W.	Clear	Clear	Cloudy	
4	29.45	29.53	29.63	33	50	38	40.3	W'ly	N. W.	N. W.	Variable	Clear	Clear	
5	29.73	29.76	29.78	30	55	40	41.7	W'ly	N. W.	S. W.	Clear	Clear	Clear	
6	29.77	29.63	29.68	34	67	54	51.7	S. W.	S. W.	W'ly	Clear	Clear	Variable	
7	29.82	29.84	29.90	40	51	35	42.0	N. E'ly	N. E.	N. E.	Variable	Clear	Clear	
8	29.92	29.89	29.71	30	54	42	42.0	N. E.	S. E'ly	S. E'ly	Clear	Clear	Rain	0.70
9	29.39	29.34	29.42	42	57	44	47.7	S. W'ly	W'ly	N. W.	Cloudy	Clear	Clear	
10	29.43	29.41	29.58	44	45	38	42.3	W'ly	N. W.	N. W.	Cloudy	Variable	Clear	
11	29.61	29.61	29.60	32	45	36	37.7	S. W.	E'ly	W'ly	Variable	Rain	Variable	0.20
12	29.73	29.77	29.85	32	48	38	39.3	N'ly	N'ly	N. W.	Clear	Clear	Clear	
13	29.88	29.88	29.90	35	57	44	45.3	N'ly	S. W'ly	S. W'ly	Clear	Variable	Cloudy	
14	29.88	29.71	29.85	32	32	29	31.0	N. E.	N'ly	N. W.	Snow	Snow	Clear	0.20
15	29.86	29.75	29.65	23	43	34	33.3	N. W.	W'ly	S. W'ly	Clear	Clear	Variable	
16	29.75	29.90	30.03	24	32	25	27.0	N. W.	N. W.	N. W.	Clear	Clear	Clear	
17	30.10	30.03	29.90	23	44	33	33.3	N. W.	S'ly	S. W'ly	Clear	Variable	Rain	0.25
18	29.64	29.53	29.41	37	52	55	48.0	S. W.	S. W.	S. W.	Cloudy	Cloudy	Cl'dy, r'n	1.00
19	29.36	29.34	29.48	50	55	44	49.7	S. W.	W'ly	W'ly	Cloudy	Cloudy	Cloudy	
20	29.72	29.76	29.87	30	42	30	34.0	N. W.	N. W.	N. W.	Clear	Clear	Clear	
21	29.94	29.92	29.83	24	42	34	33.3	N. W.	N. W.	S. W.	Clear	Clear	Clear	
22	29.64	29.41	29.46	36	64	56	52.0	S. W'ly	S. W'ly	S. E'ly	Clear	Clear	Clear	
23	29.67	29.71	29.81	32	47	38	39.0	N'ly	N. W.	N. W.	Clear	Clear	Cloudy	
24	29.88	29.89	29.89	26	40	28	31.3	N. E.	N. E.	S. W'ly	Cloudy	Cloudy	Clear	
25	29.94	29.91	29.93	27	51	36	38.0	N. W.	S. E'ly	S. W.	Clear	Clear	Clear	
26	29.83	29.71	29.57	38	44	42	41.3	S. W.	S. E'ly	S. E'ly	Cloudy	Rain	Cloudy	0.35
27	29.45	29.48	29.57	46	62	48	52.0	S. W.	S. W.	N. W.	Cloudy	Cloudy	Clear	
28	29.64	29.60	29.55	48	57	50	51.7	N. W.	S. E.	S. E'ly	Variable	Cloudy	Cloudy	
29	29.50	29.47	29.47	45	59	47	50.3	N. E'ly	E'ly	S'ly	Cloudy	Clear	Variable	
30	29.66	29.70	29.81	42	50	40	44.0	W'ly	W'ly	N. W.	Clear	Variable	Clear	
Means	29.67	29.65	29.67	34.3	49.2	39.3	...	...	...	...	...	...	...	2.70
REDUCED TO SEA LEVEL.														
Max.	30.28	30.21	30.21	50	67	56	52.0			Days.			Days.	
Min.	29.46	29.43	29.49	23	32	25	27.0	S'ly & S. W'ly		7	Clear		16	
Mean	29.85	29.83	29.85					W'ly & N. W'ly		15	Variable		5	
Range	0.82	0.78	0.72	27	35	31	25.0	N. E'ly & E'ly		8	Cloudy		3	
Mean of month	29.843			...	...	...	40.8				Rainy		6	
Extreme range	0.85			...	...	...	44.0							

REMARKS.

1st. Pleasant, but rather cool.
2d Cool and blustering. 3d. Blustering; raw.
4th Pleasant day. 5th. Very pleasant.
6th. Very pleasant and warm. Wind in the evening fresh W'ly.
7th. Wind N. E. Mild and pleasant.
8th. Wind rather brisk and raw S. E'ly. Clear morning. Cloudy afternoon. Began to sprinkle about 6 P. M. Very moderate rain in evening.
9th. Cloudy morning; wind W'ly. Clear and pleasant afternoon.
10th. Cloudy morning. Clear afternoon. Wind blustering and cool.
11th. Began to rain moderately from 9 to 10 A. M.; Wind light S. W'ly. Rain continued moderately during the day. Wind light E'ly in afternoon. Clouds broken in evening: wind light W'ly.
12th. Pleasant; rather cool.
13th Pleasant morning. Cloudy afternoon. Sprinkling of rain from 7 to 8 P. M.; clouds heavy.
14th. Began to snow moderately from 4 to 6 A. M.; wind light N. E. Snow continued nearly all day, sometimes covering the ground and then melting. Cleared in the evening.
15th. Wind raw and blustering during the day. Ther. in the vicinity stood at 18° at sunrise.
16th. Wind N. W.; very cold and blustering.
17th Clear morning. Cloudy afternoon. Began to hail about 5 P. M. Rain in the evening.
18th. Cloudy all day, with wind S. W., with some dashes of rain. Wind heavy in the evening. Heavy rain during the night.
19th. Wind light W'ly. Cloudy, with occasional sprinkling of rain.
20th. Cool but pleasant.
21st. Pleasant, though cold. The ground frozen hard in the morning.
22d. Mild, pleasant day; warm for the season.
23d. Pleasant, but cool.
24th. Cloudy morning; wind light N. E. Wind S. W'ly towards night; raw and cold.
25th. Wind light S'ly and S. W'ly the greater part of the day. Weather cool.
26th. Wind light S. E'ly, with light rain and mist all day.
27th and 28th. Cloudy for the most part. Winds light.
29th. Wind light S. E'ly during the greater part of the day. Air raw, but not cold.
30th. Pleasant; wind fresh W'ly. Aurora borealis in the evening, shooting up towards the zenith with considerable brightness, notwithstanding the light of the moon.

May, 1838.

DAYS.	BAROMETER At 6 A. M.	At 1 P. M.	At 10 P. M.	THERMOMETER At 6 A. M.	At 1 P. M.	At 10 P. M.	Daily mean.	WINDS At 6 A. M.	At 1 P. M.	At 10 P. M.	WEATHER At 6 A. M.	At 1 P. M.	At 10 P. M.	RAIN AND SNOW
1	29.94	29.90	29.87	36	60	46	47.3	N. W.	N. W.	W'ly	Clear	Clear	Clear	
2	29.89	29.80	29.70	40	58	46	48.0	N. W.	S. W.	S. W.	Clear	Variable	Cloudy	
3	29.42	29.50	29.62	42	42	38	40.7	E'ly	N. E.	N. W.	Rain	Cloudy	Clear	0.40
4	29.63	29.69	29.76	38	47	40	41.7	N. E'ly	N. E.	N. E.	Clear	Variable	Cloudy	
5	29.63	29.56	29.36	37	44	48	43.0	N. E.	N. E.	S. E.	Rain	Rain	Rain	1.10
6	29.42	29.55	29.61	48	57	46	50.3	S. W.	S. W.	S. W.	Variable	Clear	Variable	
7	29.55	29.58	29.61	44	62	47	51.0	S. W'ly	S. W'ly	S. W.	Clear	Clear	Clear	
8	29.58	29.54	29.51	47	64	50	43.7	W'ly	S. E'ly	S'ly	Clear	Clear	Cloudy	
9	29.51	29.52	29.53	44	56	46	48.7	W'ly	S. W'ly	W'ly	Cloudy	Variable	Var., r'n	0.30
10	29.55	29.55	29.61	43	57	40	46.7	W'ly	S. W'ly	W'ly	Variable	Shower	Foggy	0.13
11	29.62	29.62	29.63	37	57	44	46.0	N. W.	N. W.	N. W.	Clear	Variable	Clear	
12	29.61	29.56	29.50	43	63	52	52.7	W'ly	S. W.	S. W.	Clear	Clear	Clear	
13	29.52	29.54	29.71	46	65	48	53.0	N. W.	N. W.	N. E.	Clear	Clear	Clear	
14	29.85	29.86	29.94	44	64	46	51.3	N. E.	S. E'ly	S. W.	Clear	Clear	Clear	
15	29.94	29.93	29.91	44	71	55	56.7	S. W.	S. W.	S. W.	Clear	Clear	Clear	
16	29.85	29.75	29.62	52	70	60	60.7	S. W.	S. W.	S. W.	Clear	Variable	R'n, sh'r	
17	29.57	29.57	29.57	58	72	60	63.3	S. W.	S. W.	S. E'ly	Cl'y, sh'r	Clear	Cloudy	
18	29.40	29.47	29.60	45	43	44	44.0	N. E.	N. E.	N. E.	Rain	Cloudy	Clear	0.50
19	29.56	29.60	29.66	42	61	46	49.7	E'ly	S. E.	S. W.	Clear	Clear	Clear	
20	29.69	29.62	29.65	44	70	56	56.7	S. W'ly	S. W.	S. W.	Clear	Clear	Clear	
21	29.70	29.70	29.72	50	73	59	60.7	S. W.	S. W.	S. W.	Clear	Clear	Clear	
22	29.73	29.72	29.74	58	67	63	62.7	S. W.	S. W.	S. W.	Cl'y, sh'r	Cloudy	Cloudy	0.15
23	29.78	29.79	29.71	57	73	60	63.3	S. W.	S. E.	S. E.	Cloudy	Clear	Rain	0.30
24	29.59	29.55	29.53	60	73	60	64.3	S. W.	S. W.	S. W.	Cloudy	Cloudy	Cloudy	
25	29.52	29.42	29.41	57	59	54	56.7	N. W.	N. E.	S. W.	Cloudy	Cloudy	Clear	
26	29.50	29.54	29.58	45	64	47	52.0	W'ly	S. W.	S. W.	Clear	Variable	Clear	
27	29.57	29.56	29.56	48	70	52	56.7	N. W.	S'ly	S'ly	Clear	Variable	Clear	
28	29.51	29.51	29.56	52	70	53	58.3	W'ly	S. E'ly	S. W.	Clear	Clear	Clear	
29	29.62	29.66	29.69	50	67	56	57.7	W'ly	S. E'ly	S. W.	Clear	Variable	Clear	
30	29.71	29.70	29.69	53	66	55	58.0	N. E.	N. E.	N. E.	Clear	Clear	Clear	
31	29.74	29.70	29.73	55	74	63	64.0	N. W.	N. W'ly	N. E.	Clear	Clear	Clear	
Means	20.63	29.63	29.64	47.0	62.5	50.9	...	...	...	...	...	...	...	3.88
REDUCED TO SEA LEVEL.														
Max.	30.12	30.11	30.12	60	74	63	64.0			Days.			Days.	
Min.	29.58	29.60	29.54	36	42	38	40.7	S'ly & S. W'ly		16	Clear		17	
Mean	29.81	29.80	29.82					W'ly & N. W'ly		6	Variable		4	
Range	0.54	0.51	1.58	24	32	25	23.3	N. E'ly & E'ly		9	Cloudy		3	
Mean of month	29.810			...	...	...	53.6				Rainy		7	
Extreme range	0.58			...	...	...	38.0							

REMARKS.

1st. Pleasant.
2d. Clear morning. Cloudy afternoon.
3d. Rain in morning; wind N. E'ly, brisk. Clouds broken in afternoon. Clear in the evening.
4th. Wind fresh N. E. Cloudy for the most part. Air rather raw and cold.
5th. Incessant rain during the day. Wind moderate N. E'ly. Late in the afternoon, wind hauled more E'ly, and increased. At sunset, high wind S. E., and very heavy rain in the evening.
6th. Mild and pleasant.
7th. Very pleasant.
8th. Pleasant. Air rather raw towards night. Light wind S'ly.
9th. Wind light W'ly and S. W'ly, with fine showers through the day.
10th. Wind light W'ly and S. W'ly. Showers, with some hail.
11th. Pleasant. Alternate clouds and sunshine.
12th. Pleasant. Wind light S. W. nearly all day.
13th. Very pleasant. Aurora in the evening, not very bright.
14th. Very pleasant.
15th. Very pleasant. Wind light S. W.
16th. Clear morning; very pleasant; wind light S. W. Cloudy towards night; wind fresh. Began to sprinkle about 10 P. M.; wind heavy S. W.
17th. Showery in morning; wind light S. W. Clear afternoon. Cloudy evening; wind S. E'ly. Rain during the night.
18th. Moderate rain during the morning; wind fresh N. E. Cloudy afternoon.
19th. Pleasant. Wind S. E'ly the greater part of the day.
20th. Pleasant, with wind fresh at S. W.
21st. Warm and pleasant.
22d. Thundershower at about 4 A. M., equal 0.15 inch of water; wind fresh S. W. Cloudy, and air very damp all day.
23d. Thick fog in the morning. Sun out at noon. Cloudy towards night. Began to rain from 5 to 6 P. M.; wind moderate S. E. Wind fresh, with rain, in the evening.
24th. Wind light S. W., and cloudy all day. Light shower from 5 to 6 P. M.
25th. Wind N. W'ly at sunrise; soon came to N. E., and then (in afternoon), to S. W'ly. Cloudy, with occasional light showers. Clear at 10 P. M.; wind S. W'ly, hauling to W.
26th. Rather cool, but not unpleasant.
27th Pleasant.
28th, 29th, 30th, and 31st. Very pleasant.

June, 1838.

DAYS.	BAROMETER, REDUCED TO 32° F. At 6 A. M.	At 1 P. M.	At 10 P. M.	THERMOMETER. At 6 A. M.	At 1 P. M.	At 10 P. M.	Daily mean.	WINDS. At 6 A. M.	At 1 P. M.	At 10 P. M.	WEATHER. At 6 A. M.	At 1 P. M.	At 10 P. M.	RAIN AND SNOW IN INCHES OF WATER.
1	29.75	29.78	29.79	59	76	57	64.0	E'ly	S. E'ly	S. W.	Clear	Clear	Clear	
2	29.69	29.74	29.72	59	73	61	64.3	S'ly	S. W'ly	W'ly	Cloudy	Clear	Clear	
3	29.73	29.74	29.74	60	75	64	66.3	N. W.	S. W.	S. W.	Clear	Variable	Clear	
4	29.70	29.66	29.61	60	75	61	65.3	S. W.	S. W.	S. W.	Clear	Clear	Foggy	
5	29.25	29.20	29.27	60	66	58	61.3	S. E'ly	N. W'ly	N. W.	Rain	Rain	Clear	1.45
6	29.35	29.42	29.44	58	76	60	64.3	W'ly	S. W.	S. W.	Clear	Clear	Cloudy	
7	29.30	29.27	29.43	60	65	60	61.7	S. W.	S. W.	N. W.	Cloudy	Cloudy	Clear	
8	29.55	29.58	29.78	60	75	64	66.3	N. W.	N. W.	W'ly	Clear	Clear	Clear	
9	29.89	29.90	29.88	59	76	62	65.7	N. W.	S. W.	S. W.	Clear	Clear	Clear	
10	29.84	29.81	29.76	64	91	75	76.7	W'ly	W'ly	S. W.	Clear	Clear	Clear	
11	29.77	29.72	29.70	67	86	74	75.7	S. W.	S. W.	S. W.	Clear	Clear	Clear	
12	29.68	29.67	29.66	72	87	74	77.7	S. W'ly	S. W'ly	S. W.	Clear	Clear	Var., sh.	0.15
13	29.68	29.66	29.72	73	87	73	77.7	S. W'ly	S. W'ly	N. E.	Clear	Clear	Cloudy	
14	29.74	29.73	29.74	71	83	72	75.3	S. W'ly	S. E'ly	S. W.	Clear	Clear	Clear	0.25
15	29.79	29.77	29.80	72	87	71	76.7	S. W'ly	S. W'ly	S. W'ly	Clear	Clear	Clear	
16	29.79	29.77	29.75	71	83	69	74.3	S. W'ly	S. W'ly	S. W.	Clear	Clear	Clear	
17	29.70	29.65	29.59	68	81	68	72.3	S. W'ly	S. W'ly	S. W.	Clear	Clear	Shower	0.20
18	29.59	29.58	29.66	66	59	55	60.0	N. E.	N. E.	N. E.	Cloudy	Cloudy	Cloudy	
19	29.77	29.88	29.93	55	68	54	59.0	N. E.	N. E.	N. E'ly	Clear	Clear	Clear	
20	29.90	29.93	29.89	50	74	57	60.3	N. E.	S. E'ly	S. W'ly	Clear	Clear	Clear	
21	29.87	29.79	29.74	58	83	62	67.7	S. W.	S. W.	S. W'ly	Variable	Clear	Clear	
22	29.69	29.65	29.67	66	83	66	71.7	S. W.	N'ly	N. W.	Variable	Shower	Clear	0.65
23	29.74	29.75	29.74	64	76	65	68.3	N. E.	N. E.	S. W.	Clear	Clear	Cloudy	
24	29.68	29.63	29.72	65	79	69	71.0	S. W.	S. W.	S. W.	Variable	Variable	Cloudy	
25	29.58	29.58	29.54	68	77	65	70.0	N. E.	E'ly	N. W.	Misty	Cloudy	Shower	0.60
26	29.58	28.58	29.70	64	76	64	68.0	N. W.	N. W.	N. W.	Clear	Clear	Clear	
27	29.83	29.83	29.84	59	77	65	67.0	N. W.	N. W.	N. W.	Clear	Clear	Clear	
28	29.79	29.63	29.55	66	70	67	67.7	S'ly	S. E'ly	N. W.	Cloudy	Rain	Clear	
29	29.55	...	...	70	...	...	70.0	W'ly	...	...	Clear	...	...	
30	...	...	29.85	...	...	64	64.0	...	...	N. E.	...	...	Cloudy	
Means	29.68	29.67	29.67	63.6	77.2	64.4	...	...	...	...	...	...	...	3.30
REDUCED TO SEA LEVEL.														
Max.	30.08	30.11	30.07	73	91	75	77.7			Days.			Days.	
Min.	29.43	29.38	29.45	50	59	57	59.0	S'ly & S. W'ly		16	Clear		21	
Mean	29.86	29.84	29.85					W'ly & N. W'ly		7	Variable		5	
Range	0.65	0.73	0.62	23	32	18	18.7	N. E'ly & E'ly		7	Cloudy		3	
Mean of month	29.850			...	...	...	68.4				Rainy		1	
Extreme range	0.73			...	...	...	41.0							

REMARKS.

1st. Pleasant.
2d. Cloudy at sunrise; wind S'ly, with sprinkling of rain. From 10 to 11 A. M., cleared, with wind S. W'ly. Pleasant in afternoon.
3d. Very pleasant.
4th. Pleasant. Cloudy towards night. Mist and fog in evening; wind light S. W.
5th. Rain during the morning; ceased about noon. Cloudy in afternoon. Clear in evening.
6th. Pleasant.
7th. Cloudy through the day; wind S. W'ly. Cleared in the evening, with wind N. W.
8th. Very pleasant.
9th. Pleasant.
10th. Fine breeze from W'ly. Sun excessively burning. The warmest day since July 26, 1831. Thermometer 91°.
11th. Pleasant; very warm.
12th. Very warm. Wind fresh S. W'ly. Light thundershower about 6 P. M.
13th. Very warm. At 8 P. M., sprinkling of rain with thunder, and change of wind from S. W. to N. E.
14th. Very warm. Wind fresh S'ly and S. E'ly. Copious shower, with some thunder, from 5 to 6 P. M.
15th. Very warm, with wind fresh—sometimes approaching to high wind—from S. W'ly.
16th. Pleasant.
17th. Warm. Wind fresh S. W. Sun considerably obscured by clouds. Thundershower from 7 to 8 P. M. Clear at 10 P. M.
18th. Very cool, with wind brisk from N. E., and cloudy.
19th, 20th, and 21st. Pleasant.
22d. Pleasant in morning. Thunder from 2 to 3 P. M.
23d. Pleasant.
24th. Cloudy for the most part. Sprinkling of rain from 5 to 6 P. M.
25th. Mist, with wind N. E., in morning. Clouds broken in afternoon. Thundershower from 7 to 8 P. M.
26th. Pleasant. Aurora began from 9 to 10 P. M.; continued for more than an hour.
27th. Pleasant.
28th. Wind S'ly. Moderate rain at intervals during the day.
29th and 30th. Pleasant.

July, 1838.

DAYS.	BAROMETER At 6 A. M.	At 1 P. M.	At 10 P. M.	THERMOMETER At 6 A. M.	At 1 P. M.	At 10 P. M.	Daily mean.	WINDS At 6 A. M.	At 1 P. M.	At 10 P. M.	WEATHER At 6 A. M.	At 1 P. M.	At 10 P. M.	RAIN
1	29.83	29.82	29.78	66	75	69	70.0	S. E'ly	S. E'ly	S. E'ly	Misty	Cloudy	Cloudy	
2	29.78	29.73	29.71	69	85	72	75.3	S'ly	S. W.	S. W.	Clear	Variable	Clear	
3	29.69	29.66	29.65	72	85	75	77.3	N. W'ly	N. W.	N. W.	Clear	Clear	Clear	
4	29.67	29.68	29.68	73	86	76	78.3	N. W.	S. W.	S. W.	Clear	Clear	Clear	
5	29.67	29.65	29.62	73	92	79	81.3	S. W.	S. W.	S. W.	Clear	Variable	Clear	0.05
6	29.66	29.68	29.66	70	82	71	74.3	N. W.	N. W.	N. W.	Clear	Clear	Clear	
7	29.68	29.68	29.70	70	83	70	74.3	N. W.	N. W.	N. W.	Clear	Clear	Clear	
8	29.77	29.77	29.72	65	80	69	71.3	N. E.	E'ly	S. E'ly	Clear	Clear	Clear	
9	29.65	29.59	29.57	73	93	81	82.3	S. W.	N. W.	W'ly	Clear	Clear	Clear	
10	29.58	29.59	29.59	76	88	74	79.3	N. W.	S. E'ly	S'ly	Variable	Clear	Variable	
11	29.56	29.50	29.51	77	93	83	84.3	S. W'ly	W'ly	W'ly	Clear	Clear	Clear	
12	29.55	29.63	29.74	76	85	73	78.0	N. W.	N. W.	N. W.	Cloudy	Variable	Cloudy	
13	29.78	29.79	29.93	65	83	66	71.3	N. E.	N. E.	N. E.	Rain	Cloudy	Clear	
14	29.98	29.96	29.92	65	82	72	73.0	N. E.	N. W.	S. W'ly	Clear	Clear	Clear	
15	29.88	29.75	29.70	70	83	74	75.7	S. W.	S. W.	S. W.	Clear	Variable	Clear	
16	29.64	29.61	29.66	72	85	71	76.0	W'ly	W'ly	N. W.	Clear	Variable	Clear	
17	29.71	29.71	29.80	70	81	70	73.7	N'ly	N. E.	N. W.	Clear	Clear	Clear	
18	29.85	29.80	29.75	65	83	69	72.3	S. W'ly	S. W.	S. W.	Foggy	Variable	Rain	0.18
19	29.67	29.68	29.70	71	84	73	76.0	N. W.	N. W.	N. W.	Clear	Clear	Clear	
20	29.69	29.69	29.63	68	81	72	73.7	N. W.	S. W.	S. W.	Variable	Clear	Shower	0.05
21	29.49	29.50	29.67	70	84	65	73.0	N. W.	N. W.	N. W.	Clear	Clear	Clear	
22	29.79	29.80	29.84	62	76	65	67.7	N. W.	N. W.	N'ly	Clear	Variable	Clear	
23	29.86	29.88	29.88	58	76	65	66.3	N'ly	N. E.	N'ly	Variable	Variable	Clear	
24	29.88	29.82	29.78	62	78	67	69.0	N'ly	S. W.	S. W.	Variable	Clear	Cloudy	
25	29.74	29.66	29.64	66	75	72	71.0	S. W.	S. W.	S. W.	Rain	Cloudy	Cloudy	0.18
26	29.64	29.66	29.66	70	82	67	73.0	S. W.	S. W.	S. W.	Clear	Cloudy	Rain	0.20
27	29.67	29.69	29.77	65	80	69	71.3	S. W.	E'ly	S'ly	Clear	Clear	Clear	
28	29.77	29.60	29.59	70	87	75	77.3	W'ly	S. W.	W'ly	Clear	Clear	Clear	
29	29.59	29.53	29.50	76	94	80	83.3	W'ly	W'ly	W'ly	Clear	Clear	Clear	
30	29.56	29.57	29.60	77	92	77	82.0	W'ly	W'ly	W'ly	Clear	Clear	Clear	
31	29.62	29.63	29.60	70	81	69	73.3	W'ly	W'ly	W.	Clear	Clear	Clear	
Means	29.70	29.69	29.70	69.4	83.7	71.9	...	...	...	...	...	...	...	0.63
REDUCED TO SEA LEVEL.														
Max.	30.16	30.14	30.11	77	96	83	84.3			Days.			Days.	
Min.	29.67	29.68	29.68	58	75	65	66.3	S'ly & S. W'ly		10	Clear		21	•
Mean	29.87	29.86	29.87					W'ly & N. W'ly		16	Variable		7	
Range	0.49	0.46	0.43	19	21	18	18.0	N. E'ly & E'ly		5	Cloudy		2	
Mean of month	29.867			...	...	...	75.0				Rainy		1	
Extreme range	0.49			...	...	...	36.0							

REMARKS.

1st. Cloudy, with S. E'ly wind. Sprinkling of rain in afternoon.
2d. Pleasant. 3d. Very warm; sun burning.
4th. Clear, and very burning sun all day.
5th. Burning sun in morning. Fresh breeze at 1 P. M., S. W. Ther. 92°, with sun obscured. Light thundershower from 10 to 11 P. M.
6th. Very pleasant.
7th. Very pleasant. Fresh breeze N. W.
8th. Very pleasant.
9th. Fresh breeze N. W'ly and W'ly; very hot.
10th. Very warm. Wind light in morning. In afternoon, fresh breeze from S. E'ly.
11th. Very hot, with fresh breeze from W'ly all day. Cumulus clouds in afternoon, but no rain.
12th. Pleasant. Sun much obscured by clouds in morning.
13th. Very light shower in morning. Clear in afternoon and evening. Wind light N. E.
14th. Very pleasant.
15th. Clear in morning. Sun mostly obscured in afternoon. Wind moderate S. W.
16th. Clear in morning; sun very hot. Sun mostly obscured in afternoon, with sprinkling of rain from 3 to 5 o'clock. Clear in evening.
17th. Very pleasant.
18th. Clear in morning; wind moderate S. W. Cloudy in afternoon, with light showers.
19th. Very pleasant.
20th. Cloudy in morning. Sun out hot in middle of the day. Cloudy towards night, with wind rather brisk S. W. Light showers in evening, with thunder.
21st. Very pleasant. Warm, but a fresh breeze from N. W.
22d. Cool, but very pleasant.
23d. Pleasant. Sun much obscured by clouds.
24th. Variable in morning. Clear awhile about noon. Cloudy, with fresh S. W. wind, towards night and in evening.
25th. Fine showers in the morning. Cloudy all day. Wind light S. W.
26th. Clear in morning. Cloudy for most part in afternoon. Began to rain from 8 to 9 P. M., with very light S. W'ly wind.
27th and 28th. Pleasant.
29th. Excessively hot. Wind W'ly, rather fresh at mid-day. Ther. 96° in the shade at 2½ P. M. Very light shower from 5 to 6 P. M.
30th. Pleasant. Fresh breeze from W'ly during the afternoon and evening.
31st. Very pleasant.

August, 1838.

DAYS.	Barometer, reduced to 32° F. At 6 A. M.	At 1 P. M.	At 10 P. M.	Thermometer. At 6 A. M.	At 1 P. M.	At 10 P. M.	Daily mean.	Winds. At 6 A. M.	At 1 P. M.	At 10 P. M.	Weather. At 6 A. M.	At 1 P. M.	At 10 P. M.	Rain and Snow in Inches of Water.
1	29.58	29.54	29.59	72	86	74	77.3	S. W.	W'ly	W'ly	Variable	Clear	Clear	
2	29.73	29.73	29.81	65	78	68	70.3	N. E'ly	N'ly	N. W.	Variable	Variable	Clear	
3	29.88	29.91	29.94	63	78	67	69.3	N. E'ly	N. E.	S. W.	Variable	Clear	Clear	
4	29.98	29.92	29.86	65	84	75	74.7	N. W'ly	W'ly	N. W.	Clear	Clear	Clear	
5	29.82	29.64	29.68	72	92	77	80.3	W'ly	W'ly	S. W.	Clear	Clear	Cloudy	
6	29.58	29.55	29.61	74	94	69	79.0	S. W.	W'ly	N. E'ly	Cloudy	Cl'r, sh.	Cloudy	0.90
7	29.64	29.63	29.67	69	83	74	75.3	S. E'ly	S. W.	S. W.	Cloudy	Clear	Clear	
8	29.84	29.88	29.90	70	82	70	74.0	N. E'ly	N. E'ly	S. W.	Clear	Clear	Clear	
9	29.90	29.87	29.82	67	78	71	72.0	S. W.	S. W.	S. W.	Cloudy	Clear	Cloudy	
10	29.78	29.78	29.79	70	73	66	69.7	S. W.	N. E.	N. E.	Cloudy	Cloudy	Cloudy	
11	29.80	29.71	29.63	65	74	70	69.7	N. E.	S. W.	S. W.	Cloudy	Cloudy	Rain	0.10
12	29.52	29.56	29.66	70	83	70	74.3	S. W.	W'ly	N. W.	Clear	Clear	Clear	
13	29.75	29.76	29.81	65	82	68	71.8	N. W.	N. W.	N. W.	Clear	Clear	Clear	
14	29.92	29.98	29.98	58	72	61	63.7	N. E'ly	N. E'ly	N. E'ly	Clear	Clear	Clear	
15	29.99	29.93	29.88	58	80	66	68.0	N. W.	S. W.	S. W.	Clear	Clear	Cloudy	
16	29.81	29.75	29.51	63	71	70	68.0	S. W.	S. W.	S. E.	Cloudy	Cloudy	Rain	
17	29.36	29.37	29.54	70	80	66	72.0	N. W.	N. W.	N. W.	Clear	Clear	Clear	
18	39.58	29.67	...	61	79	72	70.7	N. W.	N. W.	N. W.	Clear	Clear	Clear	
19	...	...	...	62	75	64	67.0	W'ly	W'ly	N. W'ly	Clear	Clear	Clear	
20	...	...	...	59	74	63	65.3	W'ly	W'ly	W'ly	Variable	Clear	Clear	
21	...	...	29.95	66	80	71	72.3	S. W.	S. W.	S. W.	Clear	Clear	Clear	
22	29.94	29.93	29.97	69	83	71	74.3	S. W'ly	S. E.	S'ly	Clear	Clear	Clear	
23	29.97	29.92	29.89	67	85	72	74.7	S. W'ly	S. W.	S'ly	Variable	Clear	Clear	
24	29.69	29.75	29.71	72	88	78	79.3	S. W.	S. W.	W'ly	Cloudy	Clear	Variable	
25	29.68	29.61	29.56	72	91	68	67.0	W'ly	S. W.	W'ly	Clear	Clear	Rain	2.05
26	29.47	29.49	29.67	67	74	56	65.7	N. W.	N. W.	N. W.	Clear	Clear	Clear	
27	29.70	29.70	29.60	49	67	59	68.3	N. W.	N. W.	N. W.	Clear	Variable	Cloudy	
28	29.49	29.51	29.68	57	75	64	65.3	N. W.	N. W.	N. W.	Variable	Clear	Clear	
29	29.81	29.85	29.88	54	74	64	64.0	N. W.	N. W.	S. W.	Clear	Clear	Clear	
30	29.85	29.84	...	64	78	...	71.0	S. W.	S. W.	...	Variable	Clear	Rain	
31	...	...	29.74	...	...	60	60.0	...	...	N. W.	...	...	Clear	0.50
Means	29.74	29.73	29.75	65.2	79.8	68.1	...	...	...	...	...	...	...	3.55
REDUCED TO SEA LEVEL.														
Max.	30.17	30.16	30.16	74	94	78	79.3							
Min.	29.54	29.55	29.69	49	67	56	58.3							
Mean	29.91	29.90	29.92											
Range	0.63	0.61	0.47	25	27	22	21.0							
Mean of month	29.910			...	...	...	71.0							
Extreme range	0.63			...	...	...	45.0							

Winds	Days.
S'ly & S. W'ly	11
W'ly & N. W'ly	15
N. E'ly & E'ly	5

Weather	Days.
Clear	22
Variable	6
Cloudy	3
Rainy	4

REMARKS.

1st. Very pleasant.
2d. Sun a good deal obscured by clouds. Weather pleasant.
3d. Wind N'ly and N. E'ly. Sun much obscured during morning. Clear at intervals in afternoon. Light shower from 5 to 6 P. M.
4th. Pleasant.
5th. Very burning sun in morning. Sun much obscured after 4 P. M., with fresh breeze from S. W. Cloudy, and wind fresh, in evening.
6th. Clear for the most part, and very hot, in morning. Heavy dash of rain, with a gust of wind from W'ly, at 3 P. M. Heavy thundershower from 4 to 5 P. M., from E'ly, equal 0.90 inch of water.
7th. Pleasant.
8th. Pleasant. Wind N. E'ly and S. W'ly, P. M.
9th. Cloudy morning. Clear from 9 A. M. to 1 or 2 P. M.; then cloudy, with wind fresh at S. W. Sprinkling of rain in evening
10th. Cloudy all day. Wind S. W. early; from 9 to 10 A. M., came to N. E.
11th. Cloudy all day. Wind N. E. in morning, S. W. in afternoon. Began to rain moderately at 9 P. M
12th and 13th. Very pleasant.
14th. Cool and pleasant.
15th. Pleasant.
16th. Cloudy all day, with occasional dashes of rain. Wind S. W. A. M.; S. E'ly P. M., increasing
17th. Very pleasant.
18th, 19th, 20th, and 21st. Pleasant.
22d Pleasant. Aurora in the evening, not very bright.
23d. Pleasant.
24th. Cloudy in morning. Sun frequently obscured during the day. Very hot.
25th. Clear and very hot till 4 to 5 P. M., when there was a gust of wind and heavy clouds from the N. W. and N., which was soon followed by very heavy rain with thunder and lightning, continued, with short intervals, till 11 P. M.; amount, 2.05 inches.
26th. Pleasant.
27th. Cool. Clear in morning. Cloudy, and sprinkling of rain in afternoon.
28th and 29th. Pleasant.
30th. Pleasant in morning. Violent thunder-gust and heavy rain from 3½ to 5 P. M. A whirlwind passed the S. W. side of the city at 3½ P. M., of such violence as to unroof and demolish buildings.
31st. Very pleasant, but cool.

September, 1838.

DAYS.	Barometer. At 6 A. M.	At 1 P. M.	At 10 P. M.	Thermometer. At 6 A. M.	At 1 P. M.	At 10 P. M.	Daily mean.	Winds. At 6 A. M.	At 1 P. M.	At 10 P. M.	Weather. At 6 A. M.	At 1 P. M.	At 10 P. M.	Rain and Snow in Inches of Water.
1	29.45	29.43	29.49	58	75	67	66.7	W'ly	S. W.	S. W.	Rain	Clear	Clear	0.30
2	29.64	29.72	29.89	58	65	52	58.3	N. W.	N. W.	N. W.	Clear	Clear	Clear	
3	30.00	29.96	30.00	44	63	50	52.3	N. W.	N. W.	N. W.	Clear	Clear	Clear	
4	30.01	30.00	30.00	44	66	56	55.3	N. W.	N. W.	N. W.	Clear	Clear	Clear	
5	29.96	29.93	29.93	52	76	70	66.0	N. W.	N. W.	N. W.	Clear	Clear	Clear	
6	30.03	30.02	30.02	63	76	62	67.0	W'ly	N. W'ly	N. W.	Clear	Clear	Clear	
7	29.96	29.92	29.89	60	80	69	69.7	W'ly	W'ly	W'ly	Clear	Clear	Clear	
8	30.03	30.03	30.05	59	70	54	61.0	N. E.	N. E.	N. E.	Clear	Clear	Clear	
9	30.04	29.99	29.96	54	71	58	61.0	N. E.	N. E.	S. W.	Variable	Clear	Clear	
10	29.93	29.83	29.81	56	76	66	66.0	S. W.	S. W.	S. W.	Clear	Clear	Clear	
11	29.75	29.72	29.75	66	78	66	70.0	S. W.	S. W.	N. E.	Clear	Variable	Variable	
12	29.74	29.73	29.61	54	57	56	55.7	N. E.	N. E.	N. E.	Rain	Misty	Rain	} 3.20
13	29.17	29.46	29.84	59	67	58	61.3	N'ly	N. W.	N. W.	Rain	Clear	Clear	
14	29.87	29.96	29.93	56	73	60	63.0	W'ly	W'ly	N. W.	Clear	Clear	Clear	
15	29.93	29.91	29.98	55	73	60	62.7	N'ly	N. E.	N. E.	Clear	Clear	Variable	
16	29.98	29.99	29.95	55	63	50	56.0	N. E.	N. E.	N. E.	Clear	Clear	Cloudy	
17	29.80	29.74	29.66	53	58	58	56.3	N. E.	N. E.	N. E.	Cloudy	Cloudy	Cloudy	
18	29.56	29.49	29.47	58	71	63	64.0	N. E.	N. E.	N. W.	Cl'dy, fog	Cloudy	Variable	
19	29.44	29.49	29.65	60	69	55	61.3	N. W.	N. W.	N. W.	Clear	Clear	Clear	
20	29.81	29.81	29.85	48	68	56	57.3	N. W.	N. W.	N. W.	Clear	Clear	Clear	
21	29.90	29.89	29.87	57	67	67	63.7	S. W.	S. W.	S. W.	Cloudy	Cloudy	Rain	0.55
22	29.79	29.77	29.73	67	73	68	69.3	S. W'ly	S. W'ly	S. W'ly	Cloudy	Cloudy	Cloudy	
23	29.60	29.53	29.63	68	68	50	62.0	S. W'ly	W'ly	N. W.	Misty	Rain	Clear	0.38
24	29.80	29.83	29.92	44	67	52	54.3	W'ly	W'ly	W'ly	Clear	Clear	Clear	
25	30.00	30.10	30.18	47	69	58	58.0	S. W'ly	S. W'ly	S. W.	Clear	Clear	Variable	
26	30.24	30.25	30.15	52	60	56	56.0	N. E.	N. E.	N. E.	Cloudy	Rain	Rain	1.43
27	29.99	29.97	29.96	59	62	58	59.7	N. E.	N. E'ly	N. E'ly	Misty	Cloudy	Cloudy	
28	29.94	29.90	29.83	57	67	62	62.0	N. E.	N. E.	S. W.	Cloudy	Cloudy	Cloudy	
29	[illegible]	[illegible]	[illegible]	[illegible]	[illegible]	[illegible]	[illegible]	S'ly	S'ly	N. W'ly	Rain	Rain	Cloudy	0.90
30	29.70	29.89	29.75	56	71	[illegible]	[illegible]	[illegible]	[illegible]	[illegible]	[illegible]	[illegible]	[illegible]	
Means	29.82	29.82	29.84	58.0	68.9	59.0	...	...	...	...	...	...	...	6.76
REDUCED TO SEA LEVEL.														
Max.	30.42	30.43	30.36	68	80	70	70.0							
Min.	29.35	29.61	29.65	44	57	50	52.3							
Mean	30.00	29.99	30.02											
Range	1.07	0.82	0.71	24	23	20	17.7							
Mean of month	30.003			...	...	...	61.4							
Extreme range	1.08			...	...	...	36.0							

Winds	Days.
S'ly & S. W'ly	7
W'ly & N. W'ly	12
N. E'ly & E'ly	11

Weather	Days.
Clear	17
Variable	1
Cloudy	5
Rainy	7

REMARKS.

1st. Showers in the morning. Cleared from 9 to 10 A. M.
2d. Cool, but pleasant.
3d, 4th, 5th, 6th, 7th, 8th, 9th, & 10th. Pleasant.
11th. Weather variable, but mild.
12th. Wind fresh N. E. Moderate rain all day. Heavy rain in the night, with light wind.
13th. Very heavy rain in the morning; wind N. E. Rain ceased from 8 to 9 A. M. Cleared from 10 to 12 A. M. Clear in afternoon. Diffused aurora in the evening; pretty bright.
14th. Pleasant. Aurora visible through the night, sometimes shooting up towards the zenith with considerable brightness.
15th. Pleasant.
16th. Cool, but pleasant.
17th. Cloudy. Wind moderate N. E., with occasional sprinkling of rain.
18th. Cloudy. Wind moderate N. E. Cleared from 5 to 7 P. M.
19th. Very pleasant.
20th. Very pleasant. Faint aurora in the evening.
21st. Cloudy in morning, with wind light S. W., and occasional sprinkling of rain. Began raining gently from 1 to 2 P. M., and continued so for the greater part of the afternoon and evening. Showery during the night.
22d. Cloudy, with some mist, in the morning. Cloudy, with wind fresh S. W'ly, in the afternoon.
23d. Showery in morning; wind moderate W'ly. Steady rain in afternoon. Cleared from 8 to 9 P. M.
24th and 25th. Pleasant.
26th. Wind light N. E all day. Misty and wet in morning. Moderate rain in afternoon. Heavy rain at night.
27th. Wind light N. E'ly all day. Weather mild and cloudy.
[illegible] N. E. in morning; S'ly [illegible] the night.
29th. Moderate rain during the greater part of the day, with wind light S'ly. From 5 to 6 P. M., wind came to N. W'ly.
30th. Very pleasant.

October, 1838.

DAYS.	BAROMETER, REDUCED TO 32° F. Sunrise.	At 1 P. M.	At 10 P. M.	THERMOMETER. Sunrise.	At 1 P. M.	At 10 P. M.	Daily mean.	WINDS. Sunrise.	At 1 P. M.	At 10 P. M.	WEATHER. Sunrise.	At 1 P. M.	At 10 P. M.	RAIN AND SNOW IN INCHES OF WATER.
1	29.82	29.83	29.82	54	73	62	63.0	N. W'ly	W'ly	S'ly	Clear	Clear	Clear	
2	29.84	29.78	29.72	54	72	60	62.0	S. W.	S. W.	S. W.	Clear	Clear	Clear	
3	29.59	29.54	29.69	60	69	48	59.0	S. W.	W'ly	N. W.	Variable	Variable	Clear	
4	29.84	29.81	29.80	42	59	50	50.3	N. W.	N. W.	S. W.	Clear	Clear	Clear	
5	29.70	29.65	29.66	54	68	58	60.0	S. W.	W'ly	W'ly	Clear	Clear	Clear	
6	29.61	29.48	29.47	56	69	61	62.0	S. W.	S. W.	S. W.	Clear	Clear	Clear	
7	29.51	29.69	29.83	53	55	42	50.0	N. W'ly	N. W.	N. E.	Rain	Clear	Clear	0.40
8	29.81	29.71	29.70	36	51	37	41.3	N. W.	N. W.	N. W.	Clear	Clear	Clear	
9	29.65	29.64	29.65	33	56	46	45.0	N. W.	N. W.	S. W'ly	Clear	Clear	Clear	
10	29.64	29.57	29.43	42	52	46	46.7	N. E'ly	N. E'ly	N. E.	Clear	Cloudy	Rain	0.10
11	29.28	29.30	29.56	50	56	46	50.7	S. W'ly	S. W'ly	S. W'ly	Cloudy	Cloudy	Clear	
12	29.66	29.60	29.50	45	59	46	50.0	S. W'ly	S. W'ly	W'ly	Variable	Cloudy	Rain	0.40
13	...	...	29.72	...	...	37	37.0	N. W.	N. W.	N. W.	Clear	Clear	Clear	
14	29.69	29.60	29.60	38	61	57	52.0	S. W.	S. W.	S. W.	Variable	Variable	Cloudy	
15	29.44	29.39	29.50	57	64	54	61.7	S. W.	S. W.	S'ly	Foggy	Rain	Clear	0.15
16	29.74	29.80	29.92	42	55	42	46.3	N. W.	W'ly	N. W.	Clear	Clear	Clear	
17	30.01	30.02	30.15	39	53	40	44.0	N. W'ly	N. W.	N. W.	Clear	Clear	Clear	
18	30.16	30.10	30.06	33	53	43	43.0	N. W.	N. W.	W'ly	Clear	Clear	Clear	
19	30.04	29.91	29.61	40	46	51	45.7	N. E'ly	N. E'ly	S. E'ly	Cloudy	Rain	Rain	1.73
20	29.49	29.51	29.58	44	55	46	48.3	N. W.	N. W.	N. W.	Clear	Clear	Clear	
21	29.61	29.61	29.63	40	52	46	46.0	N. W.	N. W.	N. W.	Clear	Variable	Cloudy	
22	29.71	29.73	29.86	46	49	38	44.3	N. W'ly	N. W.	N. W.	Clear	Cloudy	Clear	
23	29.92	29.98	29.96	34	53	44	43.7	N. W.	N. W.	W'ly	Clear	Clear	Clear	
24	29.82	29.53	29.36	42	46	41	43.0	S. W'ly	N. E.	N. E.	Rain	Rain	Rain	0.95
25	29.42	29.43	29.47	41	48	43	44.0	N. W.	W'ly	W'ly	Variable	Variable	Clear	
26	29.66	29.71	29.80	38	52	39	43.0	N. W.	N. W.	N. W.	Clear	Clear	Clear	
27	29.76	29.53	29.73	35	51	39	41.7	S. E'ly	W'ly	W'ly	Variable	Rain	Clear	0.16
28	29.70	29.61	29.42	34	46	33	37.7	S. W.	S. W.	N. E.	Variable	Variable	Rain	0.72
29	29.44	29.49	29.72	33	43	31	35.7	N. W.	N. W.	N. W.	Clear	Clear	Clear	
30	29.78	29.77	29.77	30	44	36	36.7	N. W.	N. W.	N. W.	Clear	Clear	Clear	
31	29.73	29.71	29.97	30	47	28	35.0	N. W.	N. W.	N. W.	Cloudy	Cloudy	Variable	
Means	29.70	29.67	29.70	42.5	55.2	44.9	...	...	...	...	...	...	...	4.61
REDUCED TO SEA LEVEL.														
Max.	30.34	30.28	30.33	60	73	62	63.0			Days.			Days.	
Min.	29.46	29.48	29.60	30	43	28	35.0	S'ly & S. W'ly		7	Clear		17	
Mean	29.88	29.84	29.88					W'ly & N. W'ly		21	Variable		4	
Range	1.88	1.80	1.73	30	30	34	28.0	N. E'ly & E'ly		3	Cloudy		2	
Mean of month	29.867			...	...	...	47.5				Rainy		8	
Extreme range	1.88			...	...	...	45.0							

REMARKS.

1st and 2d Very pleasant.

3d. Variable till 3½ or 4 P. M., when the wind changed from W'ly to N. W., with a shower, and soon cleared.

4th. Very pleasant. 5th. Pleasant.

6th. Pleasant in the morning. Wind very fresh S. W. in the afternoon.

7th. Rain till 9 A. M.; wind N. W'ly. Cleared from 11 to 12 A. M. Clear and cool in afternoon.

8th. Pleasant.

9th. First white frost in the College yard, rather light. Pleasant day.

10th. Variable in morning; wind light N. E. Cloudy in afternoon; wind increasing. Began to rain moderately from 5 to 6 P. M.

11th. Variable in morning. Cloudy and dashes of rain in afternoon. Clear in evening.

12th. Variable in morning. Cloudy in afternoon. Began to rain moderately at 4 P. M.; heavy rain from 5 to 6 P. M. Partially clear in evening.

13th. Pleasant. 14th. Wind rather fresh S. W.

15th. Wind light S. W.; moderate rain at intervals. Cleared from 9 to 10 P. M.

16th. Pleasant. Aurora in the evening—not brilliant.

17th. Pleasant.

18th. Pleasant; light frost in morning.

19th. Wind N. E. in morning; cloudy with sprinkling. Wind more E'ly towards noon, with moderate rain. Wind came to S. E'ly towards night; rain increasing; heavy in the evening.

20th. Pleasant.

21st. Wind light N. W. Cloudy a large part of the day.

22d. Wind light N. W. Sun much obscured by clouds.

23d. Pleasant.

24th. Moderate rain all day. Commenced from 6 to 7 A. M., with wind S. W'ly, which came to N. E., and continued light all day. Cleared from 10 to 11 P. M.; wind N. W.

25th. Variable. Heavy clouds from the west, with thunder and sprinkling of rain at sunset.

26th. Pleasant.

27th. Variable in morning; wind S. E'ly and S'ly, with light showers from 11 A. M. to 1 P. M. From 1½ to 2 P. M., heavy gusts of wind, with copious rain, hail of the size of buckshots, and some thunder. Clear in the evening.

28th. Variable in morning. Rain—wind light N. E.—afternoon and evening.

29th and 30th. Pleasant.

31st. Cloudy at sunrise, the ground white with snow just fallen. Variable and raw during day.

November, 1838.

DAYS.	BAROMETER. Sunrise.	At 1 P. M.	At 10 P. M.	THERMOMETER. Sunrise.	At 1 P. M.	At 10 P. M.	Daily mean.	WINDS. Sunrise.	At 1 P. M.	At 10 P. M.	WEATHER. Sunrise.	At 1 P. M.	At 10 P. M.	RAIN AND SNOW IN INCHES OF WATER.
1	30.10	30.03	29.81	19	33	30	27.3	N. W.	N. W.	S'ly	Clear	Clear	Snow	
2	29.71	29.74	29.83	34	49	38	40.3	W'ly	W'ly	W'ly	Clear	Clear	Clear	
3	29.86	29.88	29.88	36	52	43	43.7	W'ly	S. W'ly	S. W'ly	Clear	Clear	Clear	
4	29.77	29.68	29.67	51	57	53	53.7	S. W'ly	S. W'ly	S. W.	Cloudy	Rain	Rain	} 1.95
5	29.52	29.37	29.20	53	56	52	53.7	S. W.	S. E.	N. E.	Rain	Rain	Rain	
6	29.34	29.51	29.92	47	46	30	41.0	W'ly	W'ly	W'ly	Clear	Clear	Clear	
7	30.01	30.06	29.99	28	44	40	37.3	W'ly	S'ly	S. E'ly	Clear	Cloudy	Cloudy	
8	29.73	29.57	29.46	56	61	61	59.3	S. E.	S. W.	S'ly	Rain	Rain	Cloudy	1.10
9	29.51	29.60	29.84	42	45	28	38.3	N. W.	N. W.	N. W.	Variable	Variable	Clear	
10	30.21	30.29	30.47	22	33	24	26.3	N. W.	N. W.	N. W.	Clear	Clear	Clear	
11	30.59	30.57	30.50	21	34	30	28.3	N. W.	N. W.	N. E.	Clear	Clear	Clear	
12	30.34	30.25	30.16	25	41	34	33.3	N. W.	S. W'ly	S. W.	Clear	Clear	Clear	
13	30.01	29.93	29.87	37	53	54	48.0	S. W.	S. W.	S. W.	Variable	Cloudy	Rain	0.10
14	29.93	29.90	29.99	52	63	48	54.7	W'ly	W'ly	W'ly	Clear	Clear	Clear	
15	30.02	29.91	29.84	42	45	45	44.0	N. E.	N. E.	N. E.	Cloudy	Rain	Rain	0.35
16	29.66	29.53	29.85	45	61	36	47.3	S. W.	S. W.	N. W.	Cloudy	Cloudy	Cloudy	
17	29.93	29.95	30.03	30	39	28	32.3	N. W.	N. W.	N. W.	Clear	Clear	Clear	
18	30.06	29.93	29.61	25	39	32	32.0	N. E.	N. E.	N. E.	Clear	Cloudy	R'n & sn.	0.15
19	29.67	29.76	29.85	30	35	25	30.0	N. W.	N. W.	N. W.	Clear	Clear	Clear	
20	29.82	29.78	29.75	24	35	31	30.0	N. W.	N. W.	S. W.	Clear	Clear	Variable	
21	29.85	29.88	29.74	28	35	35	32.7	N. W.	N. W.	W'ly	Clear	Clear	Clear	
22	29.68	29.61	29.73	35	43	34	37.3	W'ly	S. W.	S. W.	Variable	Variable	Clear	
23	29.74	29.68	29.76	33	41	33	35.7	S. W.	S. W.	S. W.	Cloudy	Clear	Variable	
24	29.79	29.79	29.96	22	27	8	19.0	N'ly	N. W'ly	N. W.	Cloudy	Clear	Clear	
25	29.96	29.89	29.89	4	17	12	11.0	N. W.	N. W.	N. W.	Clear	Clear	Clear	
26	29.89	29.88	29.94	6	20	14	13.3	N. W.	N. W.	N. W.	Clear	Clear	Clear	
27	29.87	29.77	29.74	16	32	30	26.0	S. W'ly	S. W'ly	W'ly	Variable	Cloudy	Cloudy	
28	29.70	29.65	29.80	32	38	22	30.7	S. W'ly	N. W'ly	N. W.	Cloudy	Clear	Clear	
29	29.92	29.75	29.72	12	24	26	20.7	N. W.	N. W.	N. W.	Clear	Clear	Clear	
30	29.72	29.75	29.77	22	39	30	30.3	N. W.	N. W.	W'ly	Clear	Clear	Clear	
Means	29.86	29.83	29.88	31.0	41.2	33.5	...	...	...	...	...	...	...	3.65
REDUCED TO SEA LEVEL.														
Max.	30.77	30.75	30.68	56	63	61	59.3			Days.			Days.	
Min.	29.52	29.55	29.38	4	17	8	11.0	S'ly & S. W'ly		9	Clear		18	
Mean	30.04	30.01	30.06					W'ly & N. W'ly		17	Variable		3	
Range	1.25	1.20	1.30	52	46	53	48.3	N. E'ly & E'ly		4	Cloudy		3	
Mean of month	30.037			...	...	...	35.3				Rainy		6	
Extreme range	1.39			...	...	...	59.0							

REMARKS.

1st. Clear and cold during the day. Cloudy in the evening, with wind S. W'ly. Halo round the moon from 6 to 7 P. M. Snow and hail about 10 P. M. for a short time.

2d and 3d. Pleasant.

4th. Cloudy in morning. Rain in afternoon; wind light S. W'ly.

5th. Moderate rain, with hardly any intermission, all day. At sunrise, wind light S. W.; then came to S. E., to E., and N. E.

6th. Blustering.

7th. Clear at sunrise. Variable in morning. Cloudy in afternoon and evening.

8th. Rain the greater part of the day. Wind heavy at nearly S.

9th. Weather variable.

10th. Very clear. Wind cold and rather brisk from N. W.

11th. Very clear at sunrise; ther. 21°; barom. 30.64. Cirrus clouds A. M. Bar. 30.67 at 10 A. M. Wind light N. E., P. M.; hazy and cirrus clouds in various directions. Barom. extraordinarily high.

12th. Very pleasant. Aurora in evening, not very bright. Wind light S. W'ly. Clouds lying round the N. and N. E.

13th. Wind light S. W. all day; air damp; clouds watery. Began to rain moderately from 8 to 9 P. M.

14th. Clear and pleasant. Aurora, not bright.

15th. Cloudy A. M.; wind light N. E. Moderate rain in afternoon and evening.

16th. Cloudy, with occasional light rain, during the day. Clear evening, with change of wind from S. W. to N. W.

17th. Clear and pleasant.

18th. Clear at sunrise; wind light N. E. Clouded up before noon. Began to snow from 4 to 5 P. M.; turned to rain from 9 to 10 P. M.; wind more E'ly.

19th. Snow an inch deep. Clear and pleasant, though cool.

20th. Clear A. M. Variable P. M. 21st. Clear.

22d. Wind S. W'ly. Air raw; cloudy for the most part. Evening clear and pleasant.

23d. Pleasant.

24th. Cloudy; wind N'ly. Cleared A. M.; wind came more to N. W.; light all day. Cold increased fast towards night and in the evening.

25th. Wind moderate N. W. Clear; very cold.

26th. Wind moderate N. W. Cold severe.

27th. Cloudy for the most part; air raw. Flurry of snow from 8 to 9 P. M.

28th. Cloudy A. M. Clear P. M. Pleasant.

29th. Cold A. M. More mild and pleasant P. M.

30th. Pleasant.

December, 1838.

Days.	Barometer, reduced to 32° F. Sunrise.	At 1 P. M.	At 10 P. M.	Thermometer. Sunrise.	At 1 P. M.	At 10 P. M.	Daily mean.	Winds. Sunrise.	At 1 P. M.	At 10 P. M.	Weather. Sunrise.	At 1 P. M.	At 10 P. M.	Rain and Snow in Inches of Water.
1	29.59	29.49	29.43	21	39	40	33.3	W'ly	S. W.	S. W.	Variable	Variable	Cloudy	
2	29.50	29.34	29.40	32	47	36	38.3	W'ly	W'ly	W'ly	Clear	Clear	Variable	
3	29.74	29.82	30.02	26	33	22	27.0	N. W.	N. W.	N. W.	Clear	Clear	Clear	
4	30.06	30.08	30.01	15	34	30	26.3	N. W.	N. E.	N. E.	Clear	Cloudy	Clear	
5	29.78	29.63	29.33	33	41	44	39.3	N. E.	S'ly	S. W'ly	Foggy	Misty	Cloudy	
6	29.49	29.53	29.57	34	34	22	30.0	N. W.	N. W.	N. W.	Clear	Clear	Clear	
7	29.59	29.53	29.62	18	37	34	29.7	N. W.	S. W'ly	S. W.	Clear	Clear	Clear	
8	29.38	29.29	29.50	34	37	28	33.0	S. W.	W'ly	N. W.	Variable	Rain	Clear	0.30
9	29.81	29.86	29.96	18	22	19	19.7	N. W.	N. W.	N. W.	Clear	Clear	Cloudy	
10	30.01	29.96	29.93	14	24	20	19.3	N. W.	W'ly	W'ly	Clear	Clear	Cloudy	
11	29.88	29.80	29.61	18	32	36	28.7	N. W.	W'ly	S. W.	Clear	Cloudy	Clear	
12	29.48	29.49	29.97	32	36	15	27.7	S. W'ly	W'ly	N. W.	Clear	Clear	Clear	
13	30.18	30.18	30.12	8	22	20	16.7	N. W.	S. W'ly	W'ly	Clear	Clear	Clear	
14	29.97	29.84	29.71	32	43	36	37.0	S. W'ly	S. W'ly	W'ly	Variable	Clear	Clear	
15	29.62	29.62	29.74	31	45	34	36.7	S. W'ly	S. W'ly	S. W.	Clear	Clear	Clear	
16	29.94	30.00	30.03	24	22	13	19.7	N. W.	N. W.	N. W.	Clear	Clear	Clear	
17	30.00	29.94	29.78	8	27	26	20.3	N. W.	S. W'ly	S. W.	Clear	Variable	Cloudy	
18	29.48	29.43	29.45	36	45	34	38.3	S. W.	S. W.	W'ly	Cloudy	Clear	Clear	
19	29.49	29.54	29.61	30	38	25	31.0	S. W.	N. W'ly	N'ly	Variable	Variable	Cloudy	
20	29.62	29.65	29.59	22	24	16	20.7	N'ly	N. W.	N. W.	Variable	Variable	Clear	
21	29.42	29.37	29.40	26	32	26	28.0	S. W'ly	W'ly	W'ly	Variable	Variable	Clear	
22	29.37	29.25	29.31	26	39	32	32.3	N. E'ly	S. E.	W'ly	Snow	Cloudy	Clear	0.15
23	29.17	29.08	29.22	26	35	18	26.3	S. E'ly	W'ly	W'ly	Variable	Variable	Clear	
24	29.56	29.74	30.01	8	11	11	10.0	N. W.	N. W.	N. W.	Clear	Clear	Clear	
25	30.02	29.94	29.85	13	29	29	20.3	S. W'ly	S. W'ly	W'ly	Clear	Clear	Clear	
26	29.76	29.75	29.86	27	33	14	24.7	W'ly	W'ly	N. W.	Cloudy	Variable	Clear	
27	29.93	29.91	29.97	10	26	18	18.0	N. W.	W'ly	W'ly	Clear	Clear	Variable	
28	30.17	30.12	29.99	10	22	17	16.3	N. W.	N. W.	S. W'ly	Clear	Clear	Clear	
29	29.39	29.05	29.45	31	38	20	29.7	S. E.	W'ly	N. W.	Snow	Cloudy	Clear	0.63
30	29.81	29.93	30.08	8	17	9	11.3	N. W.	W'ly	W'ly	Clear	Clear	Clear	
31	30.29	30.36	30.54	10	23	13	15.3	N. W.	W'ly	W'ly	Clear	Clear	Clear	
Means	29.72	29.70	29.74	22.0	31.8	24.4	...	...	...	...	...	...	...	1.08
REDUCED TO SEA LEVEL.														
Max.	30.47	30.54	30.72	36	47	44	39.3			Days.			Days	
Min.	29.35	29.26	29.50	8	11	9	10.0	S'ly & S. W'ly		9	Clear		20	
Mean	29.90	29.88	29.93					W'ly & N. W'ly		20	Variable		7	
Range	1.12	1.28	1.22	28	36	35	29.3	N. E'ly & E'ly		2	Cloudy		1	
Mean of month	29.903			...	...	...	26.1				Rainy		3	
Extreme range	1.46			...	...	...	39.0							

Remarks.

1st. Weather mild.
2d. Clear A. M. Variable P. M. Weather mild.
3d. Pleasant.
4th. Clear A. M. Cloudy towards night. Weather mild.
5th. Heavy fog. with some mist. 6th. Fine.
7th. Fine. An unusual number of shooting stars in the evening; thirty were observed in the space of half an hour.
8th. Variable at sunrise; wind fresh S. W. Began to rain from 11 to 12 A. M.; wind increasing and hauling to W. Rain ceased from 2 to 3 P. M. Clear evening; wind N. W., fresh.
9th. Clear, with the wind brisk and cutting from N. W. Cloudy evening.
10th. Clear for the most part; cold. Cloudy evening.
11th. Pleasant. Temperature rising all day.
12th. Mild A. M.; wind S. W'ly. Wind came to N. W., with heavy gust from 3 to 5 P. M. Thermometer fell rapidly, and barometer rose rapidly.
13th. Clear. Wind light S. W'ly.
14th. Mild and pleasant.
15th. Very mild and pleasant.
16th. Pleasant, though cold.
17th. Pleasant A. M. Cloudy towards night. Light fall of snow, commencing at 10 P. M.
18th. Cloudy at sunrise; cleared before noon. Clear P. M. Ground covered with snow, which disappeared A. M.
19th. Wind light. Weather mild.
20th. Wind light. Sun much obscured by clouds.
21st. Wind light W'ly. Weather mild. Sun considerably obscured by clouds.
22d. Began to snow moderately from 5 to 6 A. M. Wind light N. E. Wind hauled to S. E'ly, and snow ceased, before 10 A. M. Wind W'ly, and cloudy, P. M.
23d. Variable at sunrise; wind very light S. E'ly. Snowed fast from 9 to 10 A. M. Cloudy P. M.; wind W'ly; blustering. Very blustering evening; cold.
24th. Clear and cold; piercing wind.
25th. Very pleasant.
26th. Pleasant. Wind light W'ly. Sun considerably obscured by clouds. 27th. Pleasant.
28th. Pleasant. A bright fog bow around the moon all the evening.
29th. At sunrise, snow 2 to 3 inches deep, quite damp. Snow and rain till about 10 A. M.; wind S. E'ly. Wind came to W'ly before noon. Cleared P. M. Blustering evening; wind N. W.
30th. Clear and cold. Wind light W'ly. Still and clear evening.
31st. Clear, with wind quite light W'ly all day.

January, 1839.

Days.	Barometer Sunrise.	At 1 P. M.	At 10 P. M.	Thermometer Sunrise.	At 1 P. M.	At 10 P. M.	Daily mean.	Winds Sunrise.	At 1 P. M.	At 10 P. M.	Weather Sunrise.	At 1 P. M.	At 10 P. M.	Rain and Snow
1	30.62	30.63	30.62	5	23	19	15.7	N. W.	N. W.	N. W.	Clear	Clear	Clear	
2	30.53	30.46	30.40	17	22	26	21.7	N'ly	N. E.	S. E.	Variable	Variable	Variable	
3	30.29	30.17	30.15	26	36	30	30.7	N. E'ly	N. E'ly	N. E'ly	Variable	Variable	Cloudy	
4	30.05	30.04	30.06	31	32	30	31.0	N. E.	N. E.	N. E.	Snow	Misty	Cloudy	0.20
5	30.10	30.12	30.17	28	32	23	27.7	N. E.	N. E.	N. E.	Misty	Cloudy	Clear	
6	30.20	30.22	30.26	23	32	26	27.0	N'ly	N'ly	N. E.	Variable	Clear	Clear	
7	29.98	29.76	29.49	28	37	36	33.7	S'ly	S. W.	S. W.	Cloudy	Misty	Cloudy	
8	29.35	29.55	29.91	36	39	26	33.7	W'ly	N. W.	N. W.	Variable	Clear	Clear	
9	30.13	30.10	30.05	16	28	26	23.3	N. W.	N. W.	W.	Clear	Clear	Cloudy	
10	29.85	29.75	29.74	36	42	36	38.0	S. W.	S. W.	W'ly	Cloudy	Clear	Clear	
11	29.80	29.82	29.85	40	52	39	43.7	S. W.	S. W.	S. W.	Clear	Clear	Cloudy	
12	29.73	29.57	29.72	40	53	36	43.0	S. W.	S. W.	N. W.	Foggy	Clear	Clear	
13	30.01	30.00	29.96	27	33	31	30.3	N. W.	N. W.	N. W.	Clear	Clear	Clear	
14	29.81	29.84	29.91	34	36	22	30.7	W'ly	N'ly	N'ly	Cloudy	Cloudy	Cloudy	
15	29.94	29.90	29.90	12	22	14	16.0	N. E'ly	N. E.	N. W.	Variable	Variable	Clear	
16	29.89	29.88	29.88	11	26	22	19.7	N. E'ly	N. E'ly	N. E'ly	Clear	Clear	Clear	
17	29.96	29.99	30.00	23	39	29	30.3	N. E'ly	S. E'ly	S'ly	Clear	Clear	Clear	
18	29.97	29.93	29.84	27	41	34	24.0	S. W'ly	S. W'ly	S. W.	Cloudy	Cloudy	Rain	
19	29.75	29.65	29.67	30	38	14	27.3	W'ly	W'ly	N. W.	Variable	Clear	Clear	
20	29.87	...	29.72	4½	...	24	...	N. W.	...	S. W.	Clear	Clear	Clear	
21	29.59	29.54	29.63	24	32	18	24.7	W'ly	N. W.	N. W.	Variable	Variable	Clear	
22	29.64	29.51	29.34	4	21	24	16.3	N. W.	N. W.	W'ly	Clear	Variable	Snow	
23	29.16	29.23	29.67	22	19	—6	11.7	W'ly	N. W.	N. W.	Cloudy	Clear	Clear	
24	29.99	29.97	30.05	—8	10	12	4.7	N. W.	N. W.	W'ly	Clear	Clear	Variable	
25	30.08	30.04	29.96	15	37	33	28.3	S. W'ly	S. W.	S. E'ly	Clear	Variable	Variable	
26	29.66	29.34	28.70	43	49	40	44.0	S. E'ly	S. E.	S. E.	Cloudy	Cloudy	Rain	0.56
27	29.04	29.09	29.21	29	33	22	28.0	W'ly	W'ly	N. E.	Clear	Clear	Cloudy	
28	29.17	29.04	29.15	8	24	19	17.0	N. W.	N. W.	N. W.	Variable	Clear	Variable	
29	29.33	28.35	29.47	16	28	18	20.7	N. W.	N. W.	N. W.	Clear	Clear	Clear	
30	29.50	29.55	30.02	18	31	19	22.7	W'ly	S. W.	W'ly	Clear	Cloudy	Clear	
31	29.82	29.84	29.95	16	27	22	21.7	W'ly	W'ly	W'ly	Clear	Clear	Clear	
Means	29.83	29.80	29.81	22.0	32.5	24.7	...	...	...	...	...	...	...	0.76
REDUCED TO SEA LEVEL.														
Max.	30.80	30.81	30.80	43	53	40	44.0			Days.			Days.	
Min.	29.22	29.22	28.88	—8	10	—6	4.7	S'ly & S. W'ly		7	Clear		17	
Mean	30.01	29.90	29.99					W'ly & N. W'ly		16	Variable		8	
Range	1.58	1.59	1.92	51	43	46	39.3	N. E'ly & E'ly		8	Cloudy		4	
Mean of month	29.993			...	...	...	26.3				Rainy		2	
Extreme range	1.93			...	...	...	61.0							

Remarks.

1st. Wind light N. W'ly. Clear. 2d. Wind light.
3d. Mild and pleasant. Wind light N. E.
4th. Snow in morning, turning to mist from 9 to 10 A. M. Cloudy P. M. Mild; wind light N. E.
5th. Weather mild. Wind light N. E. all day.
6th. Variable A. M.; wind N'ly. Clear P. M.; wind N. E.; light all day.
7th. Fog and mist A. M. Mist and some rain P. M. Wind light S. W'ly during day; grew heavy and blustering in evening, with some rain.
8th. At sunrise, wind S. W'ly, with occasional dashes of rain. From 9 to 10 A. M., wind came to W'ly and N. W., and cleared. Clear P. M.
9th. Clear and pleasant. Hazy early in the evening. Flurry of snow at night.
10th. Pleasant. Brilliant aurora in evening.
11th. Unusually mild and pleasant. Cl'dy ev'ng.
12th. Do. do. Wind S. W'ly. From 6 to 7 P. M., wind came to N. W., gusty and cooler.
13th. Pleasant.
14th. Cloudy; raw. Aurora in even'g, not bright.
15th. Wind rather brisk N'ly and N. E'ly. Sun much obscured. Air pretty cold.
16th. Wind light N. E'ly. Very clear.
17th. Very pleasant.
18th. Cloudy for the most part; mild. Very moderate rain commenced from 8 to 9 P. M.
19th. Cl'dy at sunrise. Cleared from 8 to 9 A. M.; mild; wind W'ly. Wind came to N. W.; grew cold. Very blustering and cold evening. Aurora bright.
20th. Cold, but clear.
21st. Variable during day. Flurry of snow from N. from 5 to 6 P. M. Clear at 10 P. M.; growing cold.
22d. Began to snow moderately from 5 to 6 P. M.
23d. Light snow 1½ in. deep, at sunrise; mild; wind W'ly; air full of snow. About noon, wind came to N. W.; heavy gust, filling the air with snow from the ground; grew colder. At sunset, ther. +4°; at 10 P. M., —6°, with piercing N. W. wind.
24th. Wind light N. W'ly, inclining W'ly towards night. 25th. Mild.
26th. Cloudy at sunrise; wind fresh S. E'ly; bar. 29.70; indications of rain. Wind increased A. M., with mist and rain. Heavy dashes of rain at 2 P. M. Wind increased to a gale in evening, with rain. Bar. at 9 P. M., 28.77. Stationary not more than 30 minutes; began to rise by 10 P. M. Wind hauling to S. W. and abated; clouds thin.
27th. Clear and pleasant during day; wind W'ly. Cloudy evening; wind fresh N. E.
28th. Raw and cold. Flurry of snow from 6 to 7 P. M. 29th. Pleasant.
30th. Clear at sunrise; wind W'ly. Hail from 11 to 12 A. M.; wind S. W. Var. P. M. Clear evening.
31st. Pleasant.

February, 1839.

DAYS.	BAROMETER, REDUCED TO 32° F. Sunrise.	At 1 P. M.	At 10 P. M.	THERMOMETER. Sunrise.	At 1 P. M.	At 10 P. M.	Daily mean.	WINDS. Sunrise.	At 1 P. M.	At 10 P. M.	WEATHER. Sunrise.	At 1 P. M.	At 10 P. M.	RAIN AND SNOW IN INCHES OF WATER.
1	29.96	29.85	29.80	16	26	19	20.3	N. E.	N. E.	N. E.	Cloudy	Variable	Snow	
2	29.76	29.70	29.70	16	27	14	19.0	N. E'ly	N. E'ly	W'ly	Cloudy	Cloudy	Clear	
3	29.61	29.58	29.53	13	28	29	23.3	W'ly	W'ly	S. W.	Clear	Clear	Clear	
4	29.62	29.68	29.82	26	26	18	23.3	N. W.	N. E.	N. W.	Cloudy	Snow	Clear	0.20
5	29.94	29.85	29.90	7	18	9	11.3	N. W.	N. W.	N. W.	Clear	Clear	Clear	
6	29.98	29.93	30.03	6	15	9	10.0	W'ly	W'ly	W'ly	Clear	Clear	Clear	
7	30.19	30.18	29.93	2	22	29	17.7	S. W'ly	S. W.	S. W.	Clear	Variable	Cloudy	
8	29.83	29.64	29.62	29	52	40	40.3	S. W'ly	S. W.	W'ly	Variable	Variable	Cloudy	
9	29.55	29.71	30.08	32	26	12	23.3	N. E.	N. E.	N'ly	Snow	Cloudy	Clear	
10	30.17	30.10	30.02	7	22	22	17.0	N. W'ly	N. W.	N. E'ly	Variable	Variable	Cloudy	
11	29.92	29.78	29.90	22	26	21	23.0	N. E.	N. E.	N. E.	Cloudy	Cloudy	Snow	
12	30.14	30.13	30.16	17	27	21	21.7	N. W'ly	N. W'ly	N. W.	Variable	Clear	Clear	
13	30.16	30.09	30.07	21	34	28	27.7	S. W'ly	S'ly	S. W.	Clear	Clear	Clear	
14	30.00	29.96	29.94	30	33	33	32.0	N. E'ly	N. E.	N. E.	Misty	Misty	Cloudy	
15	29.95	29.93	29.94	30	37	32	33.0	N. E'ly	S. W'ly	S'ly	Cloudy	Cloudy	Cloudy	
16	29.95	29.94	29.88	32	35	32	33.0	S. W.	N. W.	N. E'ly	Misty	Cloudy	Misty	
17	29.83	29.81	29.84	32	36	32	33.3	N. E.	N. E.	N. E.	Cloudy	Cloudy	Snow	0.15
18	29.82	29.80	29.91	27	31	27	28.3	N. E.	N. E.	N. W.	Cloudy	Cloudy	Clear	
19	30.06	30.01	30.00	20	34	28	27.3	N. W.	N. W.	W'ly	Clear	Clear .	Clear	
20	29.94	29.93	29.95	30	43	32	35.0	S. W.	W'ly	S. W.	Variable	Clear	Clear	
21	30.04	30.04	30.06	30	44	34	36.0	N. E.	E'ly	E'ly	Variable	Variable	Snow	} 0.30
22	30.06	30.08	30.07	32	34	34	33.3	E'ly	E'ly	E'ly	Misty	Misty	Cloudy	
23	29.98	29.98	30.05	33	37	32	34.0	N. E.	N. E.	N. E.	Cloudy	Cloudy	Cloudy	
24	30.13	30.11	30.10	31	38	36	35.0	N. E.	N. E.	E'ly	Variable	Variable	Cloudy	
25	29.90	29.66	29.60	34	39	35	36.0	S. E.	S. E.	N. W.	Rain	Rain	Clear	0.30
26	29.71	29.66	29.45	32	45	33	36.7	N. W.	E'ly	N. E.	Clear	Clear	Rain	0.55
27	29.21	29.32	29.34	33	45	38	38.7	N. W.	N. W.	S. E'ly	Cloudy	Cloudy	Cloudy	
28	29.43	29.41	29.10	30	45	34	36.3	S'ly	S'ly	N. E.	Clear	Variable	Snow	
Means	29.89	29.85	29.85	23.9	33.0	26.8	...	...	...	...	...	...	...	1.50
REDUCED TO SEA LEVEL.										Days.			Days	
Max.	30.37	30.36	30.34	34	52	40	40.3							
Min.	29.39	29.50	29.28	2	15	9	10.0	S'ly & S. W'ly		7	Clear		7	
Mean	30.07	30.03	30.03					W'ly & N. W'ly		9	Variable		7	
Range	0.98	0.86	1.06	32	37	31	30.3	N. E'ly & E'ly		12	Cloudy		7	
Mean of month	29.390			...	...	...	27.9				Rainy		7	
Extreme range	1.09			...	...	...	50.0							

REMARKS.

1st. Wind light N. E. all day. Cloudy for the most part. Began to snow moderately from 3 to 4 P. M.—about 1 inch, light.
2d. Mild A. M.; wind light N. E'ly. Cloudy P. M. wind W'ly. Clear evening.
3d. Clear; rather blustering.
4th. Cloudy morning. Flurry of snow from noon to 2 P. M. Clear evening
5th. Cold, with wind light N. W. all day.
6th. Blustering, and cold severe.
7th. Clear and pleasant A. M. Hazy P. M. Cl'dy evening. Wind fresh S. W.; thor. rising; barom. falling.
8th. Mild; wind light S. W'ly. Cloudy evening, with appearances of rain.
9th. Rain and snow at sunrise. Light snow A. M. Cloudy P. M. Clear evening. Snow nearly all melted as it fell.
10th. Wind light N'ly.
11th. Cloudy and moderate, though rather raw. Began to snow moderately from 8 to 9 P. M.
12th. Ground just covered with snow. Mild.
13th. Mild and pleasant.
14th. Light mist all day. Mild.
15th. Cloudy, with some mist. Wind light and weather mild.
16th. Cloudy, with some mist. Moderate.
17th. Cloudy and damp. Wind light N. E. Weather moderate.
18th. Cloudy, with wind light N. E all day. Wind came to N. W., and cleared in evening.
19th. Pleasant.
20th. Very pleasant.
21st. Variable till evening, then cloudy. Began to mist and snow from 8 to 9 P. M.
22d. Wet snow an inch deep, at sunrise. Mist during the morning.
23d. Weather mild.
24th. Very mild.
25th. Moderate rain A. M.; wind light S. E'ly. Cloudy P. M. Clear evening, with wind light N. W. Very mild.
26th. Mild. Air rather raw towards night. Began to rain—wind light N. E.—from 7 to 8 P. M.
27th. Mild.
28th Mild. Variable through the day. Cloudy evening. Began to snow and rain at about P. M. Wind N. E., growing rather fresh.

March, 1839.

DAYS.	BAROMETER Sunrise.	At 1 P. M.	At 10 P. M.	THERMOMETER Sunrise.	At 1 P. M.	At 10 P. M.	Daily mean.	WINDS Sunrise.	At 1 P. M.	At 10 P. M.	WEATHER Sunrise.	At 1 P. M.	At 10 P. M.	RAIN AND SNOW
1	29.20	29.40	29.65	32	38	30	33.3	N. W.	N. W.	N. W.	Clear	Clear	Clear	
2	29.54	...	...	29	52	41	40.7	S. W'ly	...	...	Clear	Variable	Cloudy	
3	...	...	...	23	22	7	17.3	N. E.	N. E.	N. W.	Snow	Cloudy	Clear	0.25
4	30.07	30.07	30.06	5	24	18	15.7	W'ly	W'ly	W'ly	Clear	Clear	Clear	
5	29.97	29.88	29.99	15	32	24	23 7	W'ly	S. W.	N. W.	Clear	Clear	Clear	
6	30.08	30.06	29.96	23	42	34	33.0	W'ly	S. W.	S. W.	Clear	Clear	Clear	
7	29.80	29.68	29.65	32	51	33	38.7	S. W.	S. W.	S. W.	Clear	Clear	Clear	
8	29.53	29.33	29.03	32	47	36	38.3	S. W.	S. W.	E'ly	Clear	Variable	Rain	1.25
9	29.05	29.13	29.31	32	43	34	36.3	W'ly	W'ly	W'ly	Variable	Clear	Clear	
10	29.44	29.47	29.61	31	31	26	29.3	N. W.	N. W.	N. W.	Variable	Clear	Clear	
11	29.57	29.66	29.81	18	33	30	27.0	N. W.	N. W.	N'ly	Clear	Clear	Cloudy	
12	29.99	30.00	30.15	24	45	34	34.3	N. W.	N. W.	N. W.	Clear	Clear	Clear	
13	30.15	30.15	30.03	28	45	34	35.7	N. W.	S. E'ly	S'ly	Clear	Clear	Clear	
14	29.83	29.74	29.86	34	42	32	36.0	S. W.	S. W.	N. W.	Cloudy	Rain	Clear	
15	29.90	29.94	30.00	24	40	30	31.3	N. W.	N. W.	W'ly	Clear	Clear	Clear	
16	30.00	29.94	29.89	30	45	36	37.0	S. W.	S. W.	S. W.	Clear	Variable	Clear	
17	29.90	29.90	29.89	34	47	39	40.0	W'ly	W'ly	S. W'ly	Clear	Clear	Clear	
18	29.80	29.71	29.67	37	54	37	42.7	S. W.	S. W.	N. E.	Misty	Variable	Cloudy	
19	29.68	29.68	29.93	34	37	33	34.7	N. E.	N. E.	N. E.	Misty	Cloudy	Clear	
20	30.01	30.04	30.01	27	31	28	28.7	N. E.	N. E.	N. E.	Cloudy	Cloudy	Hail	
21	29.89	29.79	29.69	27	33	34	31.3	N. E.	E'ly	E'ly	Cloudy	Misty	Misty	
22	29.55	29.49	29.55	33	46	39	39.3	N. E.	N'ly	N. W.	Misty	Cloudy	Variable	
23	29.49	29.40	29.43	34	49	39	40.7	N. W.	N. W.	N. E.	Variable	Variable	Variable	
24	29.59	29.62	29.62	30	45	36	37.0	N. W.	N. W.	N. W.	Clear	Clear	Clear	
25	29.63	29.58	29.73	32	40	28	33.3	N. E'ly	N. W.	N. W.	Cloudy	Variable	Clear	
26	29.77	29.70	29.69	24	48	36	36.0	N. W.	N. W.	W'ly	Clear	Clear	Clear	
27	29.58	29.43	29.57	43	64	52	53.0	S. W.	S. W.	N. W.	Clear	Clear	Clear	
28	29.71	29.79	29.81	45	64	38	49.0	W'ly	S. E.	E'ly	Clear	Clear	Clear	
29	29.67	29.63	29.52	37	48	37	40.7	N. E.	N. E.	N. E'ly	Cloudy	Cloudy	Cloudy	
30	29.74	29.82	30.13	37	41	28	35.3	N. W.	N. W.	N. W.	Cloudy	Cloudy	Clear	
31	30.31	30.33	30.27	24	43	32	33.0	N. W.	N'ly	S'ly	Clear	Clear	Clear	
Means	29.75	29.74	29.77	29.3	42.6	32.7	...	...	...	...	...	...	...	1.50
REDUCED TO SEA LEVEL.										Days.			Days.	
Max.	30.49	30.51	30.45	45	64	52	53.0							
Min.	29.38	29.31	29.21	5	22	7	15.7	S'ly & S. W'ly		12	Clear		17	
Mean	29.93	29.92	29.95					W'ly & N. W'ly		12	Variable		7	
Range	1.11	1.20	1.24	40	42	45	37.3	N. E'ly & E'ly		8	Cloudy		5	
Mean of month	29.933			...	...	...	34.9				Rainy		2	
Extreme range	1.30			...	...	...	59.0							

REMARKS.

1st. Rather blustering.
2d. Warm, with S'ly wind, in morning. Wind came to N. E., and began to snow, late at night.
3d. Snow in morning; wind N. E. Wind came to N. W., and grew colder fast. Clear. From 2 to 3 inches of snow.
4th. Clear and cold.
5th. Clear and cool. Faint aurora in evening.
6th. Pleasant. Wind brisk S. W. in evening.
7th. Very pleasant.
8th. Clear morning; wind S'ly; hazy. Clouded over, and began to rain moderately, from 2 to 3 P. M. Rain increased, and continued through the evening.
9th. Pleasant. Ground covered with snow in the morning; melted soon.
10th. Blustering and cold.
11th. Rather blustering and cold.
12th and 13th. Pleasant.
14th. Moderate rain in morning.
15th, 16th, and 17th. Pleasant.
18th. Cloudy, with snow, in morning Variable in afternoon. Wind came to N. E. towards night, with some mist.
19th. Cloudy all day, with some mist in morning. Flurry of hail from 4 to 5 P. M., and cleared; wind N E.
20th Cloudy; wind raw N. E. Began to hail at 9 P. M.
21st. Wind light E'ly Mist most of the day.
22d. Mild.
23d. Weather mild.
24th. Very pleasant.
25th. Cloudy at sunrise; wind N. E'ly. Snowed moderately from 8 to 12 A. M. Variable in afternoon. Clear in evening.
26th. Very pleasant.
27th. Very mild and pleasant.
28th. Very mild and pleasant. Wind S'ly at 10 A. M.; S. E'ly at 1 P. M.; E'ly in evening. Air rather hazy.
29th. Wind light N. E'ly, inclining to N'ly towards night.
30th. Air raw. Cloudy during the day. Clear in evening.
31st. Cool, but very pleasant.

April, 1839.

DAYS.	Barometer, reduced to 32° F. At 6 A. M.	At 1 P. M.	At 10 P. M.	Thermometer. At 6 A. M.	At 1 P. M.	At 10 P. M.	Daily mean.	Winds. At 6 A. M.	At 1 P. M.	At 10 P. M.	Weather. At 6 A. M.	At 1 P. M.	At 10 P. M.	Rain and Snow in Inches of Water
1	30.04	29.99	29.85	27	52	38	39.0	S'ly	S'ly	S'ly	Clear	Clear	Variable	
2	29.93	29.98	30.04	37	49	33	39.7	N. E.	N. E.	N. E.	Variable	Clear	Clear	
3	30.06	30.04	30.02	37	49	39	41.7	N. E.	N. E.	N. E.	Cloudy	Cloudy	Clear	
4	29.96	29.94	29.92	33	62	45	46.7	N. E.	S'ly	S'ly	Clear	Clear	Clear	
5	29.96	30.00	30.06	37	62	38	45.7	S. W.	N. E.	N. E.	Clear	Clear	Foggy	
6	30.07	29.90	29.78	38	62	48	49.3	S. W'ly	S. W.	S. W.	Foggy	Clear	Clear	
7	29.62	29.49	29.49	46	73	61	60.0	S. W.	W'ly	N. W.	Variable	Hazy	Clear	
8	29.74	29.72	29.79	36	51	40	42.3	N. W.	N. W.	N. W.	Clear	Clear	Clear	
9	29.84	29.87	29.92	32	53	37	40.7	N. W.	N. E.	S'ly	Clear	Clear	Clear	
10	29.93	29.88	29.84	33	57	45	45.0	S. W'ly	S. W.	S. W.	Clear	Clear	Clear	
11	29.80	29.73	29.72	43	63	53	53.0	S. W.	S. W.	S. W.	Variable	Clear	Cloudy	
12	29.62	29.60	29.49	52	44	40	45.3	S. W.	N. E.	N. E.	Rain	Rain	Rain	} 2.50
13	29.46	29.51	29.59	38	37	35	36.7	N. E.	N. E.	N. E.	Cloudy	Rain	Cloudy	
14	29.60	29.60	29.65	32	34	34	33.3	N. E.	N. E.	N. E.	H'l & r'n	R'n & sn.	Rain	0.35
15	29.57	29.45	29.38	34	41	36	37.0	N. E.	N'ly	N'ly	Cloudy	Cloudy	Rain	0.10
16	29.25	29.21	29.25	36	57	46	46.3	N. W.	N. W.	N. W.	Variable	Clear	Variable	} 0.30
17	29.24	29.11	29.15	40	37	38	38.3	N. E.	N. E.	N'ly	Cloudy	Rain	R'n & sn.	
18	29.23	29.32	29.57	38	51	54	47.7	N. W.	N. W.	N. W.	Cloudy	Clear	Clear	
19	29.56	29.54	29.50	49	63	52	54.7	N. W.	W'ly	W'ly	Clear	Clear	Clear	
20	29.47	29.48	29.72	54	58	38	50.0	N'ly	N. W.	N'ly	Cloudy	Variable	Clear	
21	29.86	29.89	29.94	34	52	37	41.0	N'ly	N'ly	S'ly	Clear	Clear	Clear	
22	30.02	30.06	30.08	36	66	46	49.3	W'ly	S. E.	S. W.	Clear	Clear	Clear	
23	30.13	30.15	30.13	40	60	48	49.3	S. W.	S. E'ly	S. W.	Clear	Clear	Hazy	
24	30.13	30.07	29.92	46	64	52	54.0	S. W.	S. W.	S. W.	Variable	Clear	Clear	
25	29.82	29.70	29.69	50	66	50	55.3	S'ly	S'ly	N. W.	Cloudy	Variable	Clear	
26	29.66	29.69	29.72	48	60	52	53.3	N. W.	N'ly	N. W.	Variable	Clear	Clear	
27	29.72	29.61	29.59	44	69	50	54.3	S. W.	W'ly	W'ly	Clear	Clear	Variable	
28	29.60	29.59	29.78	56	64	42	54.0	W'ly	N. E.	N. E.	Clear	Hazy	Cloudy	
29	29.88	29.99	29.93	46	45	44	45.0	N. E.	E'ly	N. E.	Cloudy	Cloudy	Cloudy	} 0.38
30	29.81	29.72	29.71	43	66	52	53.7	N. E.	E'ly	S. E.	Cloudy	Variable	Cloudy	
Means	29.75	29.72	29.74	40.5	55.6	44.1	...	...	...	...	...	...	...	3.63
REDUCED TO SEA LEVEL.										Days			Days.	
Max.	30.31	30.33	30.31	56	73	61	60.0	S'ly & S. W'ly		8	Clear		15	
Min.	29.41	29.29	29.33	27	34	33	33.3	W'ly & N. W'ly		8	Variable		5	
Mean	29.93	29.90	29.92					N. E'ly & E'ly		14	Cloudy		4	
Range	0.90	1.04	0.98	29	39	28	26.7				Rainy		6	
Mean of month	29.917			...	...	...	46.7							
Extreme range	1.04			...	...	...	46.0							

REMARKS.

1st. Pleasant. Wind light S'ly.

2d. Pleasant. Wind moderate N. E'ly. At 28 or 30 min. past 8 P. M., an unusually bright meteor was seen to pass from the vicinity of Sirius, 20° or 30° in the direction nearly of the centre of Lepus. It was visible 3 or 4 seconds, and disappeared behind a neighboring house. Its brightness exceeded that of Jupiter or Venus; color greenish white. It was seen through a window from a room with two lamps in. No noise was heard; no luminous train was observed.

3d. Cloudy. Wind steady and moderate at N. E. Clear evening.

4th. Very pleasant.

5th. Warm and pleasant.

6th. Foggy A. M. Clear and mild P. M.

7th. Very warm. At 1 P. M., thick haze; sun obscured; ther. 73°. Wind came to N. W'ly, with a gust from 4 to 5 P. M. Evening clear and rather windy

8th. Very pleasant. Rather blustering P. M.

9th. Ground frozen in the morning. Pleasant but cool through the day.

10th. Very blustering. Air filled with dust.

11th. Variable in morning. Clear at mid-day. Cloudy towards evening, with wind quite fresh and increasing.

12th. At sunrise, wind light S. W'ly with moderate rain. From 9 to 10 A. M., wind came to N. E.; grew cooler; rain and wind increased. Rain continued all day and evening. Wind heavy at 10 P. M.

13th. Rain at intervals through the day.

14th. Hail, snow, and rain in morning, which continued during the forenoon. Light rain, rather drizzling in afternoon; very raw and cold.

15th. Cloudy in morning; wind N'ly. Rain moderate after 5 P. M.

16th. Cloudy at sunrise; cleared soon. Pleasant.

17th. Rain and snow

23d. Clear through the day. Evening foggy.

25th. Sprinkling of rain at sunrise. About 5 P. M., wind shifted from S. E. to N. and N. E., with a shower of rain. Wind then came to N. W., and cleared.

29th. Began to rain very moderately at 9 A. M., and continued till 1 P. M.

30th. Foggy in the morning. Showery in the afternoon and evening.

May, 1839.

DAYS.	Barometer At 6 A. M.	At 1 P. M.	At 10 P. M.	Thermometer At 6 A. M.	At 1 P. M.	At 10 P. M.	Daily mean.	Winds At 6 A. M.	At 1 P. M.	At 10 P. M.	Weather At 6 A. M.	At 1 P. M.	At 10 P. M.	Rain and Snow in Inches of Water
1	29.70	29.70	29.60	50	58	50	52.7	E'ly	N. E.	E'ly	Cloudy	Rain	Rain	} 0.40
2	29.57	29.58	29.53	50	66	54	56.7	S. E.	S. E.	S'ly	Cloudy	Clear	Sh'r, fog	
3	29.30	29.50	29.63	56	50	44	50.0	S. W.	N. W.	N. W.	Cloudy	Clear	Clear	
4	29.74	29.78	29.92	36	51	41	42.7	N. W.	N. W.	N. W.	Clear	Clear	Clear	
5	29.92	29.81	29.70	40	57	48	48.3	S. W'ly	S. W.	S. W.	Clear	Clear	Cloudy	
6	29.87	30.07	30.02	43	61	50	51.3	W'ly	W'ly	S. W.	Clear	Clear	Clear	
7	30.15	30.05	30.20	40	58	42	46.7	N. E.	N. E.	S'ly	Clear	Variable	Clear	
8	30.28	30.21	29.95	34	57	52	47.7	S. W.	S. W.	S. W.	Clear	Variable	Cloudy	
9	29.94	29.96	30.06	51	69	55	58.3	S. W.	N. E.	W'ly	Clear	Variable	Clear	
10	30.20	30.19	30.16	42	64	44	50.0	N. E.	N. E.	S. W.	Clear	Variable	Clear	
11	30.10	30.07	30.08	42	64	44	50.0	N. E.	N. E.	S. W.	Clear	Clear	Clear	
12	30.10	30.05	30.01	45	65	51	53.7	N. W.	S'ly	S'ly	Clear	Clear	Clear	
13	30.02	30.00	29.94	47	69	55	57.0	S. W'ly	S. W'ly	S. W.	Clear	Variable	Variable	
14	29.72	29.65	29.74	58	58	58	58.0	S'ly	S'ly	N. W.	Rain	Rain	Clear	2.18
15	29.93	29.91	29.90	57	70	56	61.0	N. W.	S. W.	S. W.	Clear	Clear	Clear	
16	29.90	29.89	29.87	57	71	61	63.0	W'ly	S. W.	S. W.	Clear	Clear	Clear	
17	29.94	29.96	29.96	59	67	58	61.3	W'ly	S. W'ly	S. W.	Cloudy	Variable	Clear	
18	30.03	30.01	30.00	53	70	57	60.0	W'ly	W'ly	S. W.	Rain	Clear	Clear	0.36
19	30.04	29.97	29.90	57	73	64	64.7	W'ly	W'ly	W'ly	Clear	Clear	Clear	
20	29.83	29.78	29.94	62	78	56	65.3	W'ly	W'ly	N. E.	Clear	Clear	Clear	
21	30.00	29.96	29.87	49	68	55	57.3	S. E'ly	S. W'ly	S. W.	Clear	Clear	Cloudy	
22	29.87	29.96	30.12	51	51	47	49.7	N. E.	N. E.	N. E.	Rain	Cloudy	Variable	
23	30.21	30.29	30.27	46	64	49	53.0	N. E.	N. E.	N. E.	Variable	Clear	Variable	
24	30.21	30.12	30.07	46	54	51	50.3	N. E.	N. E.	N. E.	Rain	Misty	Cloudy	0.20
25	29.98	29.89	29.83	51	66	56	58.3	N. E.	W'ly	W'ly	Cloudy	Variable	Foggy	
26	29.89	29.87	29.85	62	76	60	66.0	W'ly	S. E.	S'ly	Clear	Clear	Clear	
27	29.83	29.79	29.74	59	68	60	62.3	S'ly	S'ly	S'ly	Variable	Variable	Rain	0.40
28	29.61	29.60	29.60	60	73	60	64.3	S'ly	S. W'ly	S. W'ly	Misty	Variable	Cloudy	
29	29.61	29.63	29.66	60	70	58	62.7	S. E'ly	S. E'ly	S. W.	Shower	Variable	Variable	0.25
30	29.66	29.69	29.80	56	69	57	60.7	N. W.	N. W.	N. W.	Clear	Clear	Clear	
31	29.81	29.81	29.77	51	64	48	54.3	N. W.	S. W.	N. W.	Clear	Variable	Clear	
Means	29.90	29.89	29.89	50.6	64.5	52.9	...	...	...	...	...	...	...	3.79
REDUCED TO SEA LEVEL.										Days.			Days.	
Max.	30.46	30.47	30.45	62	78	64	66.0	S'ly & S. W'ly		16	Clear		17	
Min.	29.48	29.68	29.71	34	50	41	42.7	W'ly & N. W'ly		4	Variable		4	
Mean	30.07	30.07	30.07					N. E'ly & E'ly		11	Cloudy		3	
Range	0.98	0.89	0.74	28	28	23	23.3				Rainy		7	
Mean of month	30.070			...	...	...	56.0							
Extreme range	0.99			...	...	...	44.0							

REMARKS.

1st. Showery throughout the day.

2d. Foggy, and some showers, in the forenoon.

3d. Clear. Wind brisk W'ly and N. W'ly.

4th. Clear. Wind fresh and cool.

5th. Clear Wind very blustering and cool. Cloudy in evening, with dashes of rain.

6th. Rather blustering and cool.

7th. Very chilly in afternoon, with S'ly wind.

8th. Clear in the morning, with a heavy white frost. Air damp, with appearances of rain, in afternoon.

9th. Warm; variable during the middle of day.

10th. Pleasant. Aurora in the evening, not very bright.

11th, 12th, and 13th. Pleasant.

14th. Very heavy rain in morning; wind about S. Cloudy, with occasional light showers, in afternoon. Clear from 7 to 8 P. M.

15th. Very pleasant. Aurora in the evening, not brilliant.

16th. Very pleasant in morning. Variable in afternoon. Very light shower from 5 to 6 P. M.

17th. Cloudy in the morning, with a little rain. Clear towards night.

18th. Cloudy in the morning, rain having fallen during the night. Clear in afternoon.

19th. Very pleasant.

20th. Very pleasant. From 6 to 7 P. M., thunder, with sprinkling of rain, and change of wind from W'ly to N. E. Clear in evening.

21st. Very pleasant. Air chilly towards night.

22d. Sprinkling of rain in the morning. Cloudy during the day.

23d. Cool.

24th. Rain and mist. Wind light N. E. Air cool.

25th. Rain in morning. Variable in afternoon.

26th. Pleasant.

27th. Variable in morning; sunshine and clouds. Showers, commencing at 5 P. M.

28th. Clouds and mist for the most part.

29th. Heavy shower from 5 to 6 A. M. Variable during the day.

30th and 31st. Very pleasant.

June, 1839.

DAYS.	BAROMETER, REDUCED TO 32° F. At 6 A. M.	At 1 P. M.	At 10 P. M.	THERMOMETER. At 6 A. M.	At 1 P. M.	At 10 P. M.	Daily mean.	WINDS. At 6 A. M.	At 1 P. M.	At 10 P. M.	WEATHER. At 6 A. M.	At 1 P. M.	At 10 P. M.	RAIN AND SNOW IN INCHES OF WATER
1	29.74	29.73	29.81	46	53	44	47.7	N. E.	N. E.	N. E.	Clear	Cloudy	Clear	
2	29.82	29.84	29.84	47	59	49	51.7	N. E.	N. E.	S. W.	Clear	Cloudy	Clear	
3	29.85	29.87	29.93	52	65	54	57.0	W'ly	S. W.	W'ly	Cloudy	Cloudy	Variable	
4	29.98	30.00	30.02	52	68	53	57.7	E'ly	E'ly	E'ly	Clear	Clear	Variable	
5	29.93	29.62	29.74	48	52	49	49.7	N. E.	N. E.	N. E.	Rain	Rain	Misty	0.55
6	29.78	29.80	29.92	50	63	58	57.0	N. W.	N. W.	N. W.	Cloudy	Variable	Clear	
7	30.00	30.08	30.16	53	75	62	63.3	N. W.	N. W.	N. E.	Clear	Clear	Clear	
8	30.21	30.18	30.08	62	74	64	66.7	S. W'ly	S. E'ly	S. W.	Clear	Variable	Variable	
9	29.89	29.79	29.69	63	81	70	71.3	S. W.	S. W.	S. W'ly	Cloudy	Variable	Var., sh.	0.20
10	29.66	29.69	29.78	62	75	68	68.3	N. W.	N. W.	N. W.	Clear	Clear	Clear	
11	29.74	29.73	29.83	64	78	62	68.0	S. W.	S. W.	N. E.	Variable	Clear	Clear	
12	29.93	29.98	29.99	52	68	56	58.7	N. W.	N. W.	N. W.	Clear	Clear	Clear	
13	29.90	29.79	29.84	52	66	50	56.0	N. W'ly	S. W'ly	N. E.	Variable	Variable	Cloudy	
14	29.90	29.89	29.95	46	70	56	57.3	N. W.	N. W.	N. W.	Clear	Clear	Clear	
15	29.94	29.89	28.85	52	72	56	60.0	N. W.	S'ly	S'ly	Clear	Clear	Clear	
16	29.70	29.67	29.76	56	67	53	58.7	S. W.	N. W.	N. W.	Rain	Clear	Clear	0.28
17	29.80	29.82	29.93	56	74	64	64.7	N. W.	W'ly	S. W.	Clear	Clear	Variable	
18	29.93	29.84	29.65	62	73	66	67.0	S. W.	S. W.	S. W.	Variable	Cloudy	Rain	0.38
19	29.65	29.72	29.89	62	66	54	60.7	N. W.	N. W.	N. W.	Clear	Clear	Clear	
20	29.87	29.86	29.89	57	76	62	61.7	W'ly	S. W'ly	W'ly	Clear	Clear	Clear	
21	29.84	29.77	29.78	66	82	66	71.3	W'ly	S. W'ly	S. W'ly	Clear	Clear	Foggy	
22	29.71	29.70	29.79	56	60	59	58.3	N. E.	N. E.	N. W'ly	Misty	Misty	Clear	
23	29.83	29.84	29.93	59	77	63	66.3	W'ly	W'ly	W'ly	Clear	Clear	Clear	
24	29.99	30.02	30.07	54	72	61	62.3	N. W.	N. W.	W'ly	Clear	Variable	Cloudy	
25	30.04	30.03	30.09	60	76	64	66.7	W'ly	W'ly	W'ly	Cloudy	Clear	Clear	
26	30.09	30.08	30.05	62	76	65	67.7	S. W'ly	S. W'ly	S. W.	Clear	Variable	Clear	
27	30.08	30.01	29.98	63	78	66	69.0	S. W'ly	S. W.	S. W.	Clear	Clear	Variable	
28	29.88	29.78	29.79	60	60	58	59.3	N. E.	N. E.	N. W'ly	Rain	Rain	Variable	0.90
29	29.83	29.84	29.92	58	75	68	67.0	N. W'ly	S. W'ly	N. W.	Variable	Clear	Clear	
30	30.02	30.05	30.11	68	77	66	70.3	W'ly	W'ly	S'ly	Clear	Clear	Clear	
Means	29.88	29.86	29.90	56.7	70.3	59.5	...	...	...	...	...	...	...	2.31
REDUCED TO SEA LEVEL.														
Max.	30.39	30.36	30.34	68	82	70	71.3			Days.			Days.	
Min.	29.85	29.80	29.83	46	52	44	51.7	S'ly & S. W'ly		16	Clear		15	
Mean	30.06	30.04	30.08					W'ly & N. W'ly		7	Variable		7	
Range	0.54	0.56	0.51	22	30	26	19.6	N. E'ly & E'ly		6	Cloudy		3	
Mean of month	30.060			...	...	...	62.16				Rainy		5	
Extreme range	0.59			...	...	...	36.00							

REMARKS.

1st. Wind N. E'ly. Cool, with sprinkling of rain in afternoon.
2d. Very cool and cloudy, with wind N. E'ly.
3d. Cool; cloudy for the most part.
4th. Pleasant, rather cool.
5th. Rain and mist all day.
6th. Cloudy for the most part. Cool and rather blustering.
7th. Clear and warm.
8th. A good deal cloudy. Wind fresh S. W. in the afternoon and evening.
9th. Cloudy for the most part, and very warm. Shower, with lightning in the evening.
10th, 11th, and 12th. Very pleasant.
13th. Cloudy in the afternoon. Some rain in the evening.
14th. Very pleasant, though cool.
15th. Pleasant.
16th. Shower in the morning. Very cool during the day and evening.
17th. Wind fresh from N. W. and W'ly.
18th. Wind brisk S. W'ly all day. Cloudy. Moderate rain began from 4 to 5 P. M.; continued in the evening, with pretty heavy wind.
19th. Cool and rather blustering, but very clear.
20th. Very pleasant.
21st. Very warm, but pleasant.
22d. Wind N. E. in the morning, with occasional rain. Cloudy in afternoon. Clear in evening.
23d. Very pleasant.
24th. Clear in morning. Cloudy in afternoon and evening, with sprinkling of rain.
25th. Cloudy in the morning. Clear through the day and evening.
26th and 27th. Very pleasant.
28th. Wind E'ly, inclining to N. E., with copious rain. Wind came to N'ly and N. W. in the evening, and stars appeared.
29th. Pleasant.
30th. Very pleasant.

July, 1839.

DAYS.	BAROMETER At 6 A. M.	At 1 P. M.	At 10 P. M.	THERMOMETER At 6 A. M.	At 1 P. M.	At 10 P. M.	Daily mean.	WINDS At 6 A. M.	At 1 P. M.	At 10 P. M.	WEATHER At 6 A. M.	At 1 P. M.	At 10 P. M.	RAIN AND SNOW
1	30.20	30.18	30.19	64	82	65	70.3	W'ly	W'ly	W'ly	Clear	Clear	Clear	
2	30.19	30.14	30.00	66	80	71	72.3	S. W.	S. W.	S. W.	Clear	Clear	Cloudy	
3	29.77	29.79	29.85	68	72	68	69.3	S'ly	S. W.	S. W.	Rain	Cloudy	Clear	1.05
4	29.90	29.88	29.94	68	81	67	72.3	S. W.	S. W.	S. W.	Clear	Clear	Clear	
5	29.99	30.00	30.02	60	73	68	67.0	N'ly	W'ly	S. W'ly	Variable	Variable	Cloudy	
6	30.00	29.97	29.98	62	67	63	64.0	N. E.	N. E.	S'ly	Cloudy	Cloudy	Clear	
7	29.96	29.96	29.98	63	76	64	67.7	S. W.	S. W.	N. W.	Variable	Clear	Cl'r, sh.	0.15
8	29.99	29.98	29.95	63	77	67	69.0	S. W.	S. W.	S. W.	Clear	Clear	Clear	
9	29.92	29.89	29.88	65	72	65	67.3	S. W.	S. W.	W'ly	Foggy	Shower	Clear	0.80
10	29.88	29.83	29.81	63	84	72	73.0	S. W.	S. W.	S. W.	Clear	Clear	Variable	
11	29.77	29.77	29.72	71	77	71	73.0	S. W.	S. W.	S. W.	Cl'r, sh.	Cloudy	Cl'dy, r'n	0.62
12	29.68	29.69	29.74	67	77	67	70.3	S. W.	S. W.	S. W.	Clear	Clear	Clear	
13	29.83	29.83	29.89	64	77	69	70.0	S. W.	S. W'ly	N. W.	Clear	Clear	Clear	
14	29.90	29.88	29.84	64	74	66	64.0	N. W.	W'ly	S. W.	Clear	Shower	Variable	
15	29.74	29.75	29.79	64	75	64	67.7	W'ly	W'ly	S. W.	Variable	Variable	Shower	0.25
16	29.93	29.92	30.04	63	79	66	69.3	N. W.	W'ly	S. W.	Clear	Clear	Clear	
17	30.15	30.16	30.17	66	79	70	71.7	S. W.	S. W.	S. W.	Clear	Clear	Clear	
18	30.20	30.19	30.18	68	81	71	66.7	S. W.	S. W.	S. W.	Clear	Clear	Clear	
19	30.20	30.17	30.16	71	84	74	76.3	S. W.	S. W.	S. W'ly	Clear	Clear	Clear	
20	30.17	30.12	30.08	72	88	75	78.3	S. W.	S. W.	S. W.	Clear	Clear	Variable	
21	30.04	30.01	29.97	72	78	74	74.7	S. W.	S. W.	S. W.	Rain	Cloudy	Variable	0.10
22	29.93	29.92	29.92	74	83	72	76.3	S. W.	S. W.	S. W.	Cloudy	Variable	Rain	0.12
23	29.90	29.89	29.96	73	83	71	75.7	W'ly	W'ly	N. W.	Clear	Clear	Clear	
24	30.02	30.01	30.01	67	79	70	72.0	N. E'ly	E'ly	W'ly	Clear	Clear	Variable	
25	29.94	29.86	29.84	68	78	70	72.0	S'ly	S. E'ly	S'ly	Cloudy	Cloudy	Cloudy	
26	29.81	29.78	29.81	70	80	75	75.0	W'ly	N. W'ly	N. W.	Cloudy	Clear	Clear	
27	29.91	29.91	29.93	68	81	70	73.0	N. W.	N. W.	N. W.	Clear	Clear	Variable	
28	29.98	29.97	29.97	64	79	70	71.0	N. E.	S. E.	S'ly	Clear	Clear	Clear	
29	29.95	29.93	29.96	70	80	71	73.7	S. W.	S. W.	S. W.	Cloudy	Clear	Variable	
30	29.98	29.96	29.97	71	81	73	75.0	S. W.	S. W.	S. W.	Clear	Clear	Clear	
31	29.94	29.87	29.80	72	77	69	72.7	S. W.	S. W.	W'ly	Cloudy	Cl'dy, r'n	Clear	2.17
Means	29.96	29.94	29.95	67.1	78.5	69.3	...	...	...	...	...	...	...	5.26
REDUCED TO SEA LEVEL.														
Max.	30.38	30.37	30.37	74	88	75	78.3			Days.			Days.	
Min.	29.86	29.87	29.90	60	72	63	64.0	S'ly & S. W'ly		22	Clear		18	
Mean	30.14	30.12	30.13					W'ly & N. W'ly		6	Variable		3	
Range	0.52	0.50	0.47	14	16	12	14.3	N. E'ly & E'ly		3	Cloudy		2	
Mean of month	30.130			...	...	...	71.66				Rainy		8	
Extreme range	0.52			...	...	...	28.00							

REMARKS.

1st. Very pleasant, though burning sun.
2d. Pleasant.
3d. Copious rain in morning from S'ly. Cloudy in afternoon. Clear in evening.
4th. Very pleasant. 5th. Pleasant.
6th. Cloudy till towards night. Clear in the evening, with wind S'ly.
7th. Fog-clouds in morning; then clear. Copious shower from 3 to 4 P. M. Clear in evening.
8th. Very pleasant.
9th. Foggy early; then clear for the most part of morning. Copious shower from noon to 1 P. M. Showers in afternoon, with severe thunder. Clear evening.
10th. Wind light S. W'ly. Very warm.
11th. Clear in morning. From 11 to 12 A. M., copious shower, with a heavy gust and violent thunder. Variable in afternoon. Mist in evening. Rain during night.
12th. Pleasant.
13th. Sprinkling of rain, with distant thunder, from 11 to 12 A. M., with change of wind from S. W. to W'ly and N. W.
14th. Clear in morning. Light shower in afternoon, with some thunder.
15th. Variable in morning. Cl'dy in afternoon. Moderate rain in evening. Wind S. W.
16th, 17th, 18th, and 19th. Very pleasant.
20th. Very warm, with fresh breeze at S. W. all day and evening.
21st. Moderate rain A. M. Cloudy during day.
22d. Va'ble during day. Moderate rain evening.
23d. Very pleasant. Cumulus cloud abundant
24th. Very pleasant.
25th. Cloudy for the most part. Lower strata of clouds from S'ly, upper from W'ly, all P. M.
26th and 27th. Pleasant.
28th. At 6 P. M., clear; wind very light N. E.; dew-point 64°. At 1 P. M., dew-point 64°; at 3 P. M., 68°; at 5 P. M., 70½°, temp. 75°; at 9 P. M., dew-point 69°, temp. 70°. From 10 A. M. to 5 P. M., wind S. E'ly; from 1 to 4 P. M., quite fresh. Air in the mean time hazy; and at times distinct cirrus clouds from the N. W.
29th. At 6 A. M., wind light S. W. Clouds thick; broken cumuli from W.; temp. 70°; dew-point 67°. Wind light S. W. all day. Upper clouds from W.
30th. Fine. Light cirrus clouds, pretty high, from W'ly and N. W'ly, P. M.; wind brisk at S. W.
31st. At 6 A. M., wind S. W.; dew-point 70°; temp. 73°; cloudy At 1 P. M., clouds became thicker; dew-point rose to 73°, and temp. to 77°. Began to rain at 1½ P. M. Heavy rain at 4½ P. M. Wind brisk W'ly in the evening.

August, 1839.

DAYS.	BAROMETER, REDUCED TO 32° F. At 6 A. M.	At 1 P. M.	At 10 P. M.	THERMOMETER. At 6 A. M.	At 1 P. M.	At 10 P. M.	Daily mean.	WINDS. At 6 A. M.	At 1 P. M.	At 10 P. M.	WEATHER. At 6 A. M.	At 1 P. M.	At 10 P. M.	RAIN AND SNOW IN INCHES OF WATER.
1	29.90	29.88	29.94	66	76	64	68.7	N. W'ly	N. W'ly	N. W.	Clear	Clear	Clear	
2	29.98	30.00	29.93	60	73	67	66.7	N. W.	S. W'ly	S. W'ly	Variable	Cloudy	Cloudy	
3	29.92	29.91	29.97	64	77	70	70.3	W'ly	N. W.	N. W.	Clear	Clear	Clear	
4	30.08	30.08	30.08	61	74	66	63.7	N. E.	N. E.	S. W.	Clear	Clear	Clear	
5	30.07	30.04	30.04	65	78	69	70.7	S. W.	S. W'ly	N. W.	Variable	Clear	Clear	
6	30.08	30.08	30.07	66	80	72	72.7	W'ly	S. W'ly	S. W.	Clear	Clear	Cloudy	
7	30.05	29.95	29.95	76	83	68	75.7	S. W.	S. W.	N. W.	Cloudy	Clear	Clear	
8	29.95	29.88	29.76	64	76	68	69.3	N'ly	S'ly	S'ly	Clear	Cloudy	Cloudy	
9	29.63	29.54	29.70	69	80	66	71.7	S. W.	S. W.	N. W.	Cloudy	Clear	Clear	0.10
10	29.81	29.83	29.90	58	76	66	66.7	W'ly	N. W.	N. W.	Clear	Clear	Clear	
11	30.01	30.03	30.05	63	76	70	69.7	N. W.	S. W.	S. W.	Clear	Clear	Clear	
12	30.07	30.08	30.03	66	70	70	68.7	S'ly	S. W.	S. W.	Cloudy	Cloudy	Shower	
13	30.06	30.08	30.15	63	74	65	67.3	N. W.	N. W.	E'ly	Rain	Clear	Clear	
14	30.19	30.18	30.16	60	71	60	63.7	N. E.	N. E.	N. E.	Cloudy	Cloudy	Clear	
15	30.14	30.16	30.15	59	68	58	61.7	N. E.	N. E.	N. E.	Clear	Cloudy	Cloudy	
16	30.11	30.06	30.01	58	61	57	58.7	N. E.	E. N. E.	N. E'ly	Cloudy	Rain	Rain	} 0.90
17	30.01	30.04	30.05	58	64	62	61.3	N. E.	N. E.	N. E'ly	Cloudy	Variable	Cloudy	}
18	30.06	30.04	30.04	60	73	65	66.0	N. E.	N. E.	N. E.	Cloudy	Variable	Variable	1.00
19	30.05	30.04	30.04	65	75	64	68.0	N. E.	S. E'ly	S. W'ly	Foggy	Clear	Clear	
20	30.05	29.95	29.92	62	76	67	68.3	S'ly	S. E.	S'ly	Clear	Clear	Clear	
21	29.92	29.89	29.90	67	80	72	73.0	W'ly	S'ly	S. W.	Clear	Clear	Clear	
22	29.89	29.86	29.86	70	85	70	75.0	S. W.	S. W.	S. W.	Clear	Clear	Clear	
23	29.86	29.86	29.90	70	84	71	75.0	S. W.	S. W.	S. W.	Clear	Variable	Clear	
24	29.94	29.91	29.89	72	81	70	74.3	S. W.	S. E'ly	S. W.	Cloudy	Clear	Clear	
25	29.84	29.82	29.83	70	83	74	75.7	S. W.	S. W.	S. W.	Cloudy	Clear	Clear	
26	29.87	29.89	29.85	68	80	69	72.3	N. W.	S. W.	S. W.	Clear	Clear	Clear	
27	29.77	29.72	29.69	72	85	76	77.7	S. W.	S. W.	S. W.	Variable	Clear	Clear	
28	29.77	29.83	29.97	68	74	60	66.7	N. W'ly	N. W'ly	W'ly	Cloudy	Clear	Clear	
29	30.03	30.03	29.96	50	58	53	53.7	N.	N. E.	N. E.	Cloudy	Cloudy	Cloudy	
30	29.98	29.86	29.77	53	53	50	52.0	E'ly	N. E.	N. E.	Rain	Rain	Rain	} 3.00
31	29.64	29.90	30.04	51	64	54	56.3	N. W.	N. W.	N. W.	Rain	Cloudy	Clear	}
Means	29.96	29.95	29.95	63.7	74.4	65.5	...	...	...	...	...	...	...	5.00
REDUCED TO SEA LEVEL.														
Max.	30.37	30.36	30.34	76	85	76	77.7							
Min.	29.81	29.72	29.87	50	53	50	52.0							
Mean	30.14	30.13	30.13											
Range	0.56	0.64	0.47	26	32	26	25.7							
Mean of month	30.133			...	...	...	67.9							
Extreme range	0.65			...	...	...	35.0							

Winds	Days.
S'ly & S. W'ly	14
W'ly & N. W'ly	6
N. E'ly & E'ly	11

Weather	Days.
Clear	14
Variable	7
Cloudy	6
Rainy	4

REMARKS.

1st. Very pleasant. From 11 A. M. to 4 P. M., cirro-cumulus clouds sparsely scattered, then fading into cirrus.

2d. Wind light. Variable A. M. Cloudy for most part P. M.

3d. Very pleasant. Clouds, cumulus.

4th. Wind light N. E., A. M.; nearly cloudless. Wind light S. W'ly, P. M.; clear. Day very fine.

5th. Very pleasant; sun hot.

6th. Clear A. M. Cloudy P. M., with appearance of rain. Wind fresh S. W.

7th. Rain in morning (light showers).

8th. Very moderate rain from 3 to 6 P. M.

9th. Foggy and thunder in morning; some rain. Cleared off about 10 A. M., or half clear. Wind changed about 3 P. M., and began to grow cooler.

12th. Drizzling showers began about 10 A. M. Showery P. M. Heavy rain during the night.

13th. Rain ceased from 5 to 6 A. M. Variable in morning. Clear in afternoon.

14th. Cloudy for the most part. Clear and cool in evening.

15th. Clear at 6 A. M. Clouds gathered pretty thick from 7 to 8 A. M. Cloudy P. M., and thick cloudy evening. Wind moderate N. E.

16th. At 6 A. M., wind fresh N. E.; clouds rather broken. Began to sprinkle from noon to 1 P. M. Rather moderate rain afternoon and evening.

17th. Wind light N. E. and N. E'ly all day. Occasional sunshine.

18th. Wind light. Some mist and fog in morning. Variable through the day.

19th. Calm morning and foggy. Cleared from 8 to 9 A. M. Wind light S. E'ly. Clear P. M.

20th and 21st. Clear and warm.

22d. Very burning sun all day. Refreshing breeze in afternoon and evening.

23d. Very burning sun all day.

24th. Clear and hot.

25th. Burning sun nearly all day. Breeze moderate S. W.

26th. Pleasant.

27th. Very hot. Heavy cumulus clouds towards night; some thunder, but no rain. The abundance of high stratus clouds in the morning indicated rain to the west.

28th. Light shower at 4 A. M. Pleasant and clear for the great part of the day.

29th. Cold and cloudy, with wind N. E., all day.

30th. Cold mist in morning. Began to rain from 10 to 12 A. M.; wind very fresh. Rain and wind very heavy P. M. and night; almost a gale.

31st. Mist in morning; wind N'ly. Cloudy all day. Clear evening; wind N. W. Faint aurora at the north in early part of evening.

September, 1839.

DAYS.	BAROMETER. At 6 A. M.	At 1 P. M.	At 10 P. M.	THERMOMETER. At 6 A. M.	At 1 P. M.	At 10 P. M.	Daily mean.	WINDS. At 6 A. M.	At 1 P. M.	At 10 P. M.	WEATHER. At 6 A. M.	At 1 P. M.	At 10 P. M.	RAIN AND SNOW IN INCHES OF WATER.
1	30.15	30.20	30.20	50	69	58	59.0	N. W.	N. W.	E'ly	Clear	Clear	Clear	
2	30.21	30.19	30.18	53	74	64	63.7	N. W.	N. W.	N. W.	Clear	Clear	Clear	
3	30.20	30.17	30.17	58	75	64	65.7	N. W.	N. W.	N. W.	Clear	Clear	Clear	
4	30.17	30.14	30.10	62	76	65	67.7	N. W.	N. W.	N. W.	Clear	Clear	Clear	
5	30.00	29.87	29.80	65	75	66	68.7	S. E.	S. E.	S'ly	Cloudy	Cloudy	Clear	
6	29.84	29.80	29.72	63	79	69	67.0	S. W.	S. W.	W'ly	Clear	Clear	Clear	
7	29.78	29.73	29.80	67	78	62	69.0	W.	S. E.	N. E.	Clear	Clear	Foggy	
8	29.83	29.82	29.77	58	63	68	63.0	N. E.	N. E.	S. E.	Cl'dy,fog	Cloudy	Rain	1.38
9	29.73	29.72	29.64	68	78	71	72.3	S'ly	S. W.	S. W.	Cl'dy,fog	Variable	Clear	
10	29.72	29.73	29.73	68	77	63	69.3	S. W.	W'ly	N. W.	Clear	Variable	Clear	
11	29.79	29.78	29.86	55	70	55	60.0	N. W.	S. W.	N. W.	Clear	Clear	Clear	
12	29.89	29.89	29.80	51	69	56	58.7	W.	W'ly	N. W.	Clear	Clear	Clear	
13	29.94	...	29.98	52	...	52	...	W.	...	N. W.	Clear	Variable	Clear	
14	30.20	30.20	30.27	45	66	52	54.3	N. W.	W'ly	S. W.	Clear	Clear	Clear	
15	30.27	30.25	30.17	45	70	64	59.7	N. W.	S. W.	S. W.	Clear	Clear	Variable	
16	30.10	30.05	30.02	62	76	68	68.7	S. W.	S. W.	S. W.	Clear	Clear	Rain	
17	29.95	29.92	29.93	66	75	66	69.0	N. E.	S. W.	S. W.	Foggy	Clear	Variable	
18	29.78	29.77	29.72	64	78	68	70.0	E'ly	S. W.	S. W.	Rain	Clear	Variable	0.45
19	29.70	29.69	29.89	62	74	62	66.0	W'ly	W'ly	W.	Clear	Clear	Clear	
20	29.91	29.93	29.93	62	74	63	66.3	W.	W'ly	W.	Clear	Clear	Clear	
21	29.98	29.97	29.99	63	78	66	69.0	W'ly	W'ly	W'ly	Clear	Clear	Clear	
22	29.95	29.83	29.76	63	78	66	69.0	S. W'ly	S. W.	S. W.	Foggy	Clear	Variable	
23	29.59	29.60	...	64	73	...	...	W'ly	W'ly	...	Clear	Clear	...	
24	29.70	29.71	29.71	50	66	58	58.0	N. W.	N. W.	S. W.	Clear	Clear	Clear	
25	29.74	29.75	29.65	54	67	64	61.7	S. W.	S. W.	S. W.	Clear	Cloudy	Cloudy	
26	29.56	29.55	29.85	54	59	47	53.3	N. W.	W'ly	N. W.	Cloudy	Variable	Clear	
27	29.93	29.82	29.86	40	64	63	55.7	N. W.	N. W.	S. W.	Clear	Clear	Cl'dy, r'n	
28	29.94	29.95	30.00	41	54	44	46.3	N. W.	N. W.	N. W.	Clear	Clear	Clear	
29	30.01	30.00	30.04	40	50	48	40.0	N. W.	N. W.	S. W'ly	Variable	Clear	Clear	
30	30.07	30.07	30.13	42	56	48	48.7	N. W.	N. W.	N. W.	Variable	Cloudy	Clear	
Means	29.92	29.90	29.92	56.2	70.7	60.7	...	...	...	...	...	...	...	1.83
REDUCED TO SEA LEVEL.														
Max.	30.45	30.43	30.45	68	79	69	72.3							
Min.	29.74	29.73	29.82	40	54	44	46.3							
Mean	30.10	30.08	30.10											
Range	0.71	0.70	0.63	28	25	25	26.0							
Mean of month	30.093			...	...	...	62.5							
Extreme range	0.72			...	...	...	39.0							

Winds	Days.
S'ly & S. W'ly	12
W'ly & N. W'ly	14
N. E'ly & E'ly	4

Weather	Days.
Clear	15
Variable	10
Cloudy	3
Rainy	2

REMARKS.

1st. Very pleasant; almost cloudless; cool.

2d. Very pleasant.

3d. Very pleasant. Brilliant aurora; first noticed a little after 9 P. M., radiating from almost all points of the horizon, but most brilliantly from N. E'ly and N. W'ly. Color varying from pretty deep red to white. A splendid corona was formed in the neck of the Swan.

4th. Very fine. Faint aurora at N., in evening.

5th. Very damp; occasional rain. Clear even'g

6th. Very pleasant.

7th. Clear and very warm, with wind S'ly and W'ly till about 4 P. M., when it came to N. E., and grew cool very fast, and became foggy at sunset.

8th. Wind N. E. Showery during the day, with thunder. Evening, wind S E. Rain during night.

9th. Foggy and very sultry A. M. Hot sun towards night; wind light S. W'ly.

10th. Clear and warm A. M. Var. P. M. Wind came more to N. W.; grew cooler. Clear evening.

11th and 12th Pleasant.

13th. Pleasant A. M. Var. P. M., with sprinkling of rain. Clear evening.

14th. Very pleasant. Aurora low in N., in evening—not brilliant; continued all night. At 3 A. M. (15th), luminous needles were shooting to the height of about 20°, and the merry-dancers playing upon them with great beauty.

15th. Wind very light N. W. at sunrise; came to S. W. fresh, in morning; same in afternoon.

16th. Wind S. W. Air very damp. A light shower from 10 to 11 P. M.

17th. Pleasant.

18th. Rain early in morning. Variable P. M.

19th, 20th, and 21st. Very pleasant.

22d. Foggy morning; wind very light S. W. Fog cleared from 8 to 9 A. M. Wind very fresh P. M. and evening.

23d. Pleasant. 24th. Very pleasant.

25th. Clear and pleasant A. M. Cloudy P. M. Sprinkling of rain in evening; wind fresh S. W.

26th. Cloudy and sprinkling of rain in morning; wind N. W. and raw. Cleared towards noon. Very blustering in afternoon. Barometer rose fast. Very cool evening.

27th. Frost in some places in the vicinity. Clear A. M. Variable P. M. Sprinkling in the evening. Wind S. W., very blustering. Rain during the night, and wind came to N. W.

28th and 29th. Pleasant.

30th. Cloudy, with some sprinkling of rain in afternoon.

DAYS.	BAROMETER, REDUCED TO 32° F. Sunrise.	At 1 P. M.	At 10 P. M.	THERMOMETER. Sunrise.	At 1 P. M.	At 10 P. M.	Daily mean.	WINDS. Sunrise.	At 1 P. M.	At 10 P. M.	WEATHER. Sunrise.	At 1 P. M.	At 10 P. M.	RAIN AND SNOW IN INCHES OF WATER.
October, 1839.														
1	30.21	30.21	30.21	39	58	46	47.7	N. W.	N. W.		Clear	Clear	Variable	
2	30.11	30.00	29.90	40	64	56	53.3	N. W.	W.	S. W.	Clear	Clear	Variable	
3	29.80	29.70	29.58	53	70	63	62.0	W.	S. W.	W.	Clear	Clear	Cloudy	
4	29.74	29.73	30.10	56	64	42	54.0	S. W'ly	N. W.	W.	Clear	Clear	Clear	
5	30.32	30.40	30.50	34	56	36	42.0	N'ly	N'ly	S. E.	Clear	Clear	Clear	
6	30.56	30.55	30.53	32½	55	44	43.8	N'ly	E'ly	N. E.	Clear	Clear	Clear	
7	30.42	30.36	30.27	37	62	51	50·0	W'ly	S. W.	S. W.	Clear	Variable	Variable	
8	30.17	30.10	30.11	44	68	54	55.3	S. W.	S. W.	S. W.	Clear	Clear	Clear	
9	30.04	29.98	29.95	53	65	55	57.7	N. E.	N. E.	N. E.	Variable	Clear	Clear	
10	29.88	...	29.93	52	...	63	...	N. E.	...	N. W.	Variable	...	Clear	
11	30.13	30.13	30.15	47	63	50	53.3	N. W.	N. W.	S. W'ly	Clear	Clear	Variable	
12	30.12	30.11	30.00	48	57	52	52.3	E'ly	S. E.	S. y	Variable	Cloudy	Rain	0.25
13	29.85	29.85	29.84	58	70	62	63.3	S. W.	S. W.	S.	Cloudy	Cloudy	Cloudy	
14	29.87	29.90	29.91	56	54	51	53.7	E'ly	N. E'ly	N. E.	Rain	Rain	Rain	} 2.60
15	29.97	30.02	30.10	48	48	49	48.3	N. E.	N. E.	N. E.	Rain	Rain	Variable	
16	30.22	30.23	30.27	46	62	48	52.0	N. W.	S. W.	S. W.	Clear	Clear	Clear	
17	30.28	30.20	30.16	44	64	52	53.3	N. W.	S. E'ly	S'ly	Clear	Clear	Clear	
18	30.16	30.09	30.05	48	70	56	58.0	S. W.	S. W.	S. W.	Clear	Clear	Clear	
19	29.94	29.81	29.83	60	66	56	60.7	S. W.	S. W.	E.	Rain	Rain	Rain	0.90
20	30.12	30.30	30.45	38	40	33	37.0	N'ly	N'ly	N. E.	Cloudy	Cloudy	Clear	
21	30.57	30.57	30.57	27	42	31	33.3	N. E'ly	N. E.	N. E.	Clear	Clear	Clear	
22	30.49	30.43	30.40	26	48	40	38.0	N. E.	S. E'ly	S. W.	Clear	Clear	Clear	
23	30.34	30.20	30.12	40	59	52	50.3	S. W.	S. W.	S. W.	Clear	Clear	Clear	
24	29.90	29.83	29.89	52	72	59	61.0	S. W.	S. W.	W'ly	Clear	Clear	Clear	
25	30.07	30.12	30.20	44	59	44	49.0	N. W.	N. W.	W'ly	Clear	Clear	Clear	
26	30.22	30.21	30.18	38	57	46	47.0	N. W.	S. W.	E.	Clear	Clear	Clear	
27	30.08	29.99	30.00	51	66	52	56.3	S. W.	S. W.	W.	Clear	Clear	Clear	
28	29.90	29.78	29.81	52	66	58	58.7	S. W.	S. W.	W.	Cloudy	Cloudy	Clear	
29	29.89	29.86	29.83	44	68	48	53.3	N. W.	N. W.	W.	Clear	Clear	Clear	
30	29.80	29.72	29.68	42	56	48	48.7	W'ly	S. W.	S. W.	Clear	Clear	Cloudy	
31	29.67	29.64	29.74	43	51	46	46.7	N. W.	N. E.	S. E.	Cloudy	Variable	Cloudy	
Means	30.09	30.07	30.07	44.9	60.0	49.8	...	...	...	...	...	...	...	3.75
REDUCED TO SEA LEVEL.														
Max.	30.75	30.75	30.75	60	72	63	63.0							
Min.	29.85	29.82	29.76	26	40	31	33.3							
Mean	30.27	30.25	30.25											
Range	0.90	0.93	0.99	34	32	32	29.7							
Mean of month	30.257			...	...	...	51.5							
Extreme range	0.99			...	...	...	46.0							

Winds	Days.
S'ly & S. W'ly	13
W'ly & N. W'ly	6
N. E'ly & E'ly	12

Weather	Days.
Clear	20
Variable	4
Cloudy	3
Rainy	4

REMARKS.

1st, 2d, and 3d. Pleasant.

4th. Pleasant. Cool towards night.

5th. Pleasant. First white frost in the College yard.

6th and 7th. Copious white frost. Pleasant day.

8th and 9th. Very pleasant.

10th and 11th. Mild and pleasant.

12th. Cloudy P. M., with rain in evening.

13th. Cloudy and sultry.

14th. Rainy day. In morning, wind E'ly and warm; hauled more to N. E., and grew colder.

15th. Rain all day. Clouds broken and partially clear in the evening.

16th. Beautiful day. Very clear and mild.

17th and 18th. Very pleasant.

19th. Moderate rain all day. Wind light S. W. and very warm. From 9 to 10 P. M., wind came to N. E, and became blustering and cooler.

20th. Cloudy till near night. Wind N'ly and N. E'ly, very raw and cold.

21st. Pleasant, but cool.

22d, 23d, 24th, 25th, 26th, and 27th. Very pleasant.

28th. Cloudy in morning; sun very red in afternoon. Clear in evening

29th and 30th. Very pleasant.

31st. Cloudy for the most part. Mild.

November, 1839.

DAYS.	Barometer Sunrise.	At 1 P. M.	At 10 P. M.	Thermometer Sunrise.	At 1 P. M.	At 10 P. M.	Daily mean	Winds Sunrise.	At 1 P. M.	At 10 P. M.	Weather Sunrise.	At 1 P. M.	At 10 P. M.	Rain and Snow
1	29.75	29.74	29.81	43	46	41	43.3	N. W.	N. W.	N. W.	Variable	Variable	Cloudy	
2	29.87	29.89	29.92	36	43	38	39.0	N. W.	N. E.	N. E.	Clear	Variable	Cloudy	
3	29.99	29.97	30.00	36	42	37	38.3	N'ly	N. E'ly	N. E.	Cloudy	Cloudy	Cloudy	
4	30.00	29.97	29.99	29	44	32	35.0	N. E.	N. E.	N. E.	Clear	Clear	Clear	
5	29.96	29.92	29.69	26	50	41	39.0	N. E.	S. E.	E'ly	Clear	Clear	Rain	} 1.00
6	29.43	29.34	29.36	48	57	42	49.0	S. E'ly	S. W.	N. W.	Rain	Clear	Clear	
7	29.40	29.39	29.43	36	50	40	42.0	N. W.	W'ly	W'ly	Clear	Clear	Cloudy	
8	29.49	29.48	29.75	34	47	37	39.3	N. W'ly	N. W'ly	N. W.	Clear	Variable	Clear	
9	29.82	29.81	29.88	32	41	34	35.7	N. W.	N. W'ly	N. W.	Variable	Clear	Variable	
10	29.89	29.92	29.98	30	37	30	32.3	N. W.	N. W.	N. W.	Variable	Variable	Clear	
11	30.04	30.04	30.08	27	43	31	33.7	N. W.	N. W.	N. W.	Clear	Clear	Clear	
12	30.09	30.06	30.06	28	47	34	36.3	N. E.	N. E.	N. E.	Clear	Clear	Clear	
13	30.03	29.99	30.02	34	48	38	40.0	N. E.	S. E'ly	E'ly	Cloudy	Variable	Clear	
14	29.97	29.92	29.82	38	50	57	48.3	N. E.	N. E.	S. E'ly	Cloudy	Rain	Rain	0.35
15	29.77	...	29.77	57	...	57	...	S. W.	S. W.	S. W.	Cloudy	Cloudy	Cloudy	
16	30.03	30.05	30.15	41	50	38	43.0	N. W.	N. W.	W'ly	Cloudy	Clear	Clear	
17	30.17	30.09	29.92	35	47	44	42.0	N. W.	N. W.	S. W.	Clear	Clear	Cloudy	
18	29.74	29.67	29.63	40	46	38	41.3	N. W.	N. W'ly	W'ly	Clear	Clear	Clear	
19	29.42	29.41	29.50	34	45	34	37.7	N. W.	N. W.	N. W.	Clear	Clear	Clear	
20	29.57	29.56	29.75	29	36	26	23.7	N. W.	N. W.	N. W.	Clear	Clear	Clear	
21	29.90	29.93	30.21	22	27	20	23.0	N. W.	N. W.	N. W.	Clear	Clear	Clear	
22	30.38	30.45	30.55	19	30	18	22.3	N. W.	N. W.	N. W.	Clear	Clear	Clear	
23	30.57	30.55	30.56	17	34	27	26.0	N. W.	N. W.	S. W'ly	Clear	Clear	Clear	
24	30.50	30.43	30.13	31	41	46	39.3	S. E.	S. E.	S'ly	Cloudy	Rain	Rain	} 0.95
25	29.83	29.67	29.82	52	54	34	46.7	S. E.	S. W.	W'ly	Rain	Rain	Clear	
26	30.08	30.12	30.24	16	23	19	19.3	N. W.	N. W.	N. W.	Clear	Clear	Clear	
27	30.24	30.20	30.20	23	33	32	29.3	S. W.	S. W.	S. W.	Variable	Variable	Clear	
28	30.19	30.20	30.20	30	41	32	34.3	S. W.	S. W.	W'ly	Variable	Cloudy	Clear	
29	30.19	30.16	30.17	26	44	34	34.7	N. W.	N. W'ly	N'ly	Clear	Variable	Clear	
30	30.15	30.13	30.13	30	44	36	36.7	N. W'ly	N. W'ly	N. W.	Clear	Clear	Clear	
Means	29.95	29.93	29.96	32.6	42.8	35.9	...	...	...	...	...	...	...	2.30
REDUCED TO SEA LEVEL.														
Max.	30.75	30.73	30.74	57	57	57	57.0							
Min.	29.58	29.59	29.54	16	23	18	19.3							
Mean	30.13	30.11	30.14											
Range	1.17	1.14	1.20	41	34	39	37.7							
Mean of month	30.127			...	...	...	37.1							
Extreme range	1.21			...	...	...	41.0							

Winds	Days.
S'ly & S. W'ly	7
W'ly & N. W'ly	15
N. E'ly & E'ly	8

Weather	Days.
Clear	13
Variable	9
Cloudy	3
Rainy	5

REMARKS.

1st. Sprinkling of rain in the morning. Variable during the day. Sprinkling of rain at night. Air raw.

2d. Weather raw and cold.

3d. Cloudy and raw.

4th. Clear and cool.

5th. Clear in morning. Variable in afternoon, with wind S. E'ly Wind increased in the evening, with rain.

6th. At sunrise, wind E'ly, with some rain; soon came round, for a short time, to N'ly and N. W'ly; then fell back to E'ly; then S'ly and S. W., and cleared before noon.

7th and 8th. Pleasant.

9th. Raw and cold.

10th. Cool. Variable day. Clear evening.

11th. Pleasant.

12th and 13th. Very pleasant.

14th. Cloudy in morning. Moderate rain in afternoon and evening.

15th. Warm and cloudy, with occasional sprinkling of rain.

16th. Very fine day; air very clear. The planet Venus easily seen at mid-day with the naked eye.

17th. Very pleasant in morning. Cloudy in afternoon, and sprinkling of rain in evening.

18th and 19th. Very pleasant.

20th. Clear and blustering. Wintery.

21st. Clear and cold. Very wintery.

22d. Clear and cold.

23d. Clear and pleasant, and more moderate. Wind changed from N. W. to S. W. in afternoon.

24th. Cloudy in morning, with wind S. E'ly, light. Rain from 11 to 12 A. M. Intervals of moderate rain in afternoon and evening, with wind increasing.

25th. Rain in morning, with wind S. E., early; then S. W. From 2 to 3 P. M., wind came to W'ly, and rain ceased. Clouds broke away at sunset, and evening very clear, with wind fresh W'ly.

26th. Clear and cold. Wind fresh.

27th. Variable in morning and afternoon. Clear in evening.

28th. Variable; mostly cloudy, but mild. Clear in evening.

29th. Mild and pleasant.

30th. Very mild and pleasant.

December, 1839.

DAYS.	BAROMETER, REDUCED TO 32° F. Sunrise	At 1 P. M.	At 10 P. M.	THERMOMETER. Sunrise.	At 1 P. M.	At 10 P. M.	Daily mean.	WINDS. Sunrise.	At 1 P. M.	At 10 P. M.	WEATHER. Sunrise.	At 1 P. M.	At 10 P. M.	RAIN AND SNOW IN INCHES OF WATER.
1	30.09	30.03	30.03	37	44	41	40.7	N. E.	N. E.	N. E.	Cloudy	Cloudy	Cloudy	
2	30.04	30.04	30.07	40	42	40	40.7	N. E.	N. E.	N. E.	Cloudy	Cloudy	Cloudy	
3	30.03	29.94	29.90	40	40	40	40.0	N. E.	N. E.	N. E.	Cloudy	Misty	Cloudy	
4	29.91	29.74	29.80	40	45	43	42.7	N. E.	N. E.	N. E.	Cloudy	Variable	Variable	
5	29.74	29.69	29.90	36	48	42	42.0	N. E.	N. E.	N. E.	Clear	Clear	Clear	
6	29.98	29.96	30.02	37	49	37	41.0	N. E.	N. E.	N. E.	Clear	Clear	Cloudy	
7	29.95	29.92	29.95	38	46	42	42.0	N. E.	N. E.	E.	Cloudy	Cloudy	Cloudy	
8	29.88	29.76	29.71	42	46	44	44.0	N. E.	N. E.	N. E.	Misty	Rain	Rain	0.80
9	29.53	29.23	29.06	41	43	40	41.3	N. E.	N. E.	N. W.	Cloudy	Misty	Cloudy	
10	29.55	29.57	29.65	34	42	33	36.3	S. W.	S. W.	S. W.	Clear	Clear	Clear	
11	29.73	29.75	29.78	31	41	34	35.3	W'ly	W'ly	W'ly	Clear	Clear	Clear	
12	...	29.22	29.40	46	49	36	43.7	S. E'ly	S. W.	W'ly	Rain	Variable	Clear	1.50
13	29.57	29.73	29.87	33	38	31	34.0	W'ly	W'ly	W'ly	Clear	Clear	Clear	
14	30.08	30.08	29.91	28	36	30	31.3	N. W'ly	N. W.	N. E.	Clear	Clear	Cloudy	
15	29.49	29.11	29.05	32	32	32	32.0	N. E.	N. E.	N. E.	Snow	Snow	Cloudy	} 1.50
16	29.15	29.19	29.47	28	31	28	29.0	N'ly	N'ly	N'ly	Snow	Snow	Variable	
17	29.70	29.74	29.89	24	29	17	23.3	N. W.	N. W.	N. W.	Clear	Clear	Clear	
18	29.82	29.81	29.82	14	28	13	18.3	N. W.	N. W.	N. W.	Clear	Clear	Clear	
19	29.82	29.86	29.94	7	20	7	11.3	N. W.	N. W.	N. W.	Clear	Clear	Clear	
20	29.96	29.92	29.92	4	17	14	11.7	N. W.	N. W.	N. W.	Clear	Clear	Clear	
21	29.93	29.91	30.00	12	26	17	18.3	N. W.	N. W.	N. W.	Clear	Clear	Clear	
22	29.97	29.86	29.63	17	30	32	26.3	N. E.	E'ly	E'ly	Clear	Variable	Cloudy	
23	29.53	29.51	29.67	30	26	26	27.3	N. E.	N. E.	N. E.	Snow	Snow	Cloudy	0.20
24	29.77	29.80	29.84	27	35	27	29.7	N. E.	N'ly	N. E.	Cloudy	Cloudy	Cloudy	
25	29.85	29.90	29.99	26	32	20	26.0	N'ly	N. W.	N. W.	Cloudy	Clear	Clear	
26	30.06	30.10	30.14	15	29	22	22.0	N. W.	N. W.	N. W.	Clear	Clear	Clear	
27	30.16	30.10	29.63	20	34	35	29.7	N. W.	E'ly	S. E'ly	Clear	Variable	Rain	1.12
28	28.90	28.61	28.64	35	39	33	35.7	S'ly	S'ly	W'ly	Variable	Cloudy	Clear	
29	28.85	28.87	29.00	27	29	21	25.7	W'ly	W'ly	W'ly	Variable	Clear	Clear	
30	29.30	29.36	29.66	13	17	15	15.0	W'ly	N. W.	N. W.	Clear	Clear	Clear	
31	29.88	29.91	29.97	10	20	9	13.0	N. W.	N. W.	N. W.	Clear	Clear	Clear	
Means	29.74	29.68	29.72	27.9	34.9	29.1	...	...	...	...	...	...	...	5.12
REDUCED TO SEA LEVEL.														
Max.	30.34	30.28	30.25	40	49	44	44.0			Days.			Days.	
Min.	29.03	28.79	28.82	4	17	7	11.3	S'ly & S. W'ly		6	Clear		15	
Mean	29.92	29.86	29.90					W'ly & N. W'ly		10	Variable		5	
Range	1.31	1.49	0.43	36	32	37	32.7	N. E'ly & E'ly		15	Cloudy		6	
Mean of month			29.713	...	...	...	30.6				Rain and snow . .		6	
Extreme range			1.55	...	...	...	45.0							

REMARKS.

1st. Cloudy. Wind N. E.; very fresh in evening.
2d. Wind fresh all day. Thick clouds.
3d. Wind fresh all day, with some mist.
4th. Wind fresh all day. Stars out in evening.
5th. Wind fresh all day. Mostly clear.
6th. Very mild and pleasant.
7th. Cloudy. Wind E., P. M., with sprinkling of rain in evening.
8th. Mist in morning. Moderate rain began from 11 to 12 A. M.; continued through P. M. and night. Wind light N. E. Frost all out of the ground for a week past.
9th. Misty A. M. Cloudy P. M. From 6 to 8 P. M., wind came to S'ly and S. W'ly, with lightning and rain. At 9 P. M., wind W'ly; rain over,
10th and 11th. Mild and pleasant.
12th. Heavy rain till 10 to 11 A. M.; wind S. E'ly. Cloudy P. M. Clear evening; wind brisk W'ly.
13th. Wind very high and blustering A. M.
14th. Mild, wind N. W'ly. Evening very hazy. Moon at first surrounded by a bow, and then shining but dimly through dense vapor.
15th. At daylight, moist snow falling fast—wind brisk N. E—continuing till 2 P. M. Bar. at 4 P. M., 29.05; stationary till near 7 P. M., when it began to rise slowly. No frost in the ground.
16th. Additional snow in morning. Air full of snow during day, without much accumulation.
17th and 18th. Very pleasant.
19th. Wind moderate N. W. Cold, but pleasant. Very clear.
20th. Wind moderate N. W. Cold, but evening more mild. Very clear.
21st. Very calm in morning. Pleasant all day.
22d. Wind light N. E. in morning; before noon, came nearly to E., and freshened; quite fresh in evening.
23d. Wind fresh N. E. Air full of snow, which fell about 2 or 3 inches deep.
24th. Very mild.
25th. Cloudy at sunrise; wind N'ly. Cleared from 10 to 11 A. M. Very mild and pleasant.
26th. Pleasant.
27th. Wind E'ly, P. M. Cloudy towards night; wind more to S. E., and very heavy, with heavy rain in the night, beginning about 10 P. M.
28th. Clouds broken in morning. Vanes pointing E'ly, but the clouds coming from S'ly. Bar. very low in the morning; continued to sink till 5 to 6 P. M., when it stood at 28.63. Clear evening; wind fresh W'ly.
29th. Blustering.
30th. Blustering, and severe to be out.
31st. Clear and cold, yet with some clouds.

January, 1840.

DAYS.	BAROMETER Sunrise.	At 1 P. M.	At 10 P. M.	THERMOMETER Sunrise.	At 1 P. M.	At 10 P. M.	Daily mean.	WINDS Sunrise.	At 1 P. M.	At 10 P. M.	WEATHER Sunrise.	At 1 P. M.	At 10 P. M.	RAIN AND SNOW
1	29.88	29.84	29.80	2	9	2	4.3	N. W.	N. W.	N. W.	Clear	Clear	Clear	
2	29.75	29.68	29.75	—3	10	7	4.7	N. W.	N. W.	N. W.	Clear	Clear	Clear	
3	29.79	29.77	29.77	4	18	8	10.0	N. W.	W'ly	W'ly	Clear	Clear	Clear	
4	29.75	29.72	29.73	12	22	15	16.3	W'ly	S. W'ly	N. W.	Clear	Clear	Clear	
5	29.70	29.66	29.67	14	26	22	20.7	W'ly	W'ly	W. by S.	Clear	Clear	Clear	
6	29.69	29.71	29.82	20	32	17	23.0	W. by S.	W. by S.	N. W.	Clear	Variable	Clear	
7	29.84	29.84	29.86	16	29	17	20.7	N. W.	N. W'ly	N. W.	Clear	Clear	Clear	
8	29.80	29.66	29.72	14	29	18	20.3	N. W.	N'ly	N. W.	Variable	Clear	Clear	
9	29.80	29.79	29.69	14	32	24	23.3	N. W.	N. W.	S. W'ly	Clear	Clear	Clear	
10	29.66	29.62	29.64	22	34	31	29.0	N. W'ly	N. W.	N. W.	Clear	Clear	Variable	
11	29.74	29.77	29.86	30	28	20	26.0	N. E.	N. E.	N. E.	Snow	Snow	Cloudy	0.10
12	29.89	29.90	29.99	12	16	14	14.0	N. E.	N'ly	N'ly	Cloudy	Cloudy	Cloudy	
13	29.85	29.71	29.72	18	26	22	22.0	W'ly	S. W.	W'ly	Cloudy	Snow	Clear	0.15
14	29.62	29.52	29.43	20	33	30	27.7	W'ly	W'ly	S. W.	Clear	Variable	Snow	
15	29.36	29.31	29.41	22	27	8	19.0	S. W.	N. W.	N. W.	Cloudy	Cloudy	Cloudy	
16	29.67	29.70	29.82	—4	6	—3	—0.3	N. W.	N. W.	W'ly	Clear	Clear	Clear	
17	29.90	29.87	29.88	—4	9	2	2.3	W'ly	W'ly	W'ly	Clear	Clear	Clear	
18	29.89	29.83	29.87	—2	11	4	4.3	W'ly	N. W.	N. W.	Clear	Clear	Clear	
19	29.90	29.88	29.73	7	24	21	17.3	W'ly	S. W'ly	S. W'ly	Clear	Clear	Cloudy	
20	29.78	29.74	29.73	21	32	26	29.7	W'ly	W'ly	W'ly	Cloudy	Clear	Variable	
21	29.59	29.60	29.84	30	40	25	31.7	S. W'ly	W'ly	N. W'ly	Variable	Cloudy	Clear	
22	29.93	29.84	29.71	14	19	28	20.3	N. E'ly	N. E'ly	N. E.	Cloudy	Snow	Snow	} 1.75
23	28.96	28.91	29.36	34	29	22	28.3	N. E.	N. W.	N. W.	Rain	Cloudy	Clear	
24	29.67	29.75	29.91	9	16	10	11.7	S. W'ly	W'ly	W'ly	Clear	Clear	Clear	
25	30.06	30.04	30.10	6	18	11	11.7	W'ly	W'ly	W'ly	Clear	Clear	Clear	
26	30.20	30.25	30.27	6	15	9	10.0	W'ly	W'ly	N. W.	Clear	Clear	Clear	
27	30.20	30.13	30.17	14	22	14	16.7	N. W.	W'ly	W'ly	Cloudy	Cloudy	Clear	
28	30.19	30.11	29.96	14	24	22	20.0	N. W.	N. W.	E'ly	Cloudy	Snow	Cloudy	} 0.80
29	29.89	29.84	29.66	28	38	33	33.0	E'ly	S. E.	S. E'ly	Sprink'g	Misty	M't & r'n	
30	29.40	29.31	29.10	33	37	40	36.7	N. E'ly	N. E.	W'ly	Misty	Misty	Cloudy	
31	29.62	29.75	29.96	26	31	24	27.0	W'ly	W'ly	W'ly	Clear	Clear	Variable	
Means	29.77	29.74	29.77	14.5	23.9	17.5	...	...	...	...	...	...	...	2.80
REDUCED TO SEA LEVEL.														
Max.	30.38	30.43	30.45	34	38	40	36.7			Days.			Days.	
Min.	29.54	29.49	29.28	—4	6	—3	—0.3	S'ly & S. W'ly		13	Clear		13	
Mean	29.96	29.92	29.95					W'ly & N. W'ly		12	Variable		8	
Range	0.84	0.94	1.17	38	32	43	37.0	N. E'ly & E'ly		6	Cloudy		4	
Mean of month			29.940	...	...	...	18.6				Rainy		6	
Extreme range			1.17	...	...	...	44.0							

1st. Wind brisk N. W. Very cold.
2d. Wind moderate. Very cold.
3d. Wind moderate; N. W., A. M.; W'ly, P. M. Aurora in evening considerably bright; was noticed from 5 to 6 A. M. next day.
4th. Wind moderate W'ly and S. W'ly during day. At night, came more to N. W., and increased. Aurora quite bright, with occasional corruscations.
5th. More moderate. Aurora as before.
6th, 7th, 8th, 9th, and 10th. Very pleasant.
11th. Snowed gently, with wind light N. E.
12th. Raw and cold.
13th. Cloudy at sunrise; wind W'ly. Came to S. W'ly, and snowed moderately from 10 A. M. to 3 P. M. Clear evening; wind light W'ly; pleasant.
14th. Mostly clear A. M.; wind light W'ly. Cloudy P. M.; wind more to S. W. Began to snow moderately about 7 P. M.
15th. An inch of light snow on ground. Clouds broken. Wind came to N. W. before noon. Colder towards night. Moon dimly seen through clouds.
16th. Very cold, but still, and not unpleasant.
17th. Very clear, with light W'ly winds.
18th. Wind light and variable A. M., with some clouds. Clear P. M.; wind N. W'ly. Thermometers in the street fell to —9°, —10°, and —11°. It has been very still for two or three days.
19th. Very pleasant. Wind a little fresh towards night, about W. S. W., and cloudy evening.
20th. Mostly clear. Wind W. S. W. to W. N. W.
21st. Mild. Wind W'ly; frequent clouds. Towards night, wind came more to N. W.; cleared.
22d. Cloudy A. M.; wind light N. E'ly. Moderate snow all day and even'g, beginning about 10 A. M.
23d. At sunrise, wind light N. E'ly; raining. Rain ceased about 11 A. M.; wind came to N'ly, and soon to N. W. Cloudy P. M. Clear evening.
24th. Clear, and rather severe wind, varying from W. S. W. to W. N. W.
25th. Cold.
26th. Cold, but not severe, wind being light.
27th. Cloudy A. M. and P. M. Clear evening.
28th. Cloudy A. M. Began to snow moderately from 10 to 11 A. M.; wind light N. W'ly. In afternoon, wind came to N. E., then to E'ly; snow continued; wind very light.
29th. Sprinkling of rain in morning, on 1½ or 2 inches of fresh snow. Mist through the day, with occasional sprinkling of rain. Rain during night.
30th. Wind N. E'ly, light. Mist all day, with occasional sprinkling. Thunder and lightning from 8 to 9 P. M. Cleared, with wind W'ly about 11 P. M. Aurora in the north.
31st. Pleasant.

February, 1840.

DAYS.	BAROMETER, REDUCED TO 32° F. Sun-rise	At 1 P. M.	At 10 P. M.	THERMOMETER. Sun-rise.	At 1 P. M.	At 10 P. M.	Daily mean.	WINDS. Sun-rise.	At 1 P. M.	At 10 P. M.	WEATHER. Sunrise.	At 1 P. M.	At 10 P. M.	RAIN AND SNOW IN INCHES OF WATER.
1	30.02	29.95	30.03	24	21	18	21.0	W'ly	N. E.	N. W.	Snow	Snow	Clear	
2	30.08	30.04	29.87	10	25	14	16.3	N. W.	N. W.	S. W.	Clear	Clear	Clear	
3	29.67	29.70	29.77	10	22	11	14.3	N. W.	N. W.	N. W.	Clear	Clear	Clear	
4	29.89	29.93	30.12	0	5	0	1.7	N. W.	N. W.	N. W.	Clear	Clear	Clear	
5	30.20	30.17	30.11	—5	20	24	13.7	W'ly	S. W'ly	S. W.	Clear	Variable	Variable	
6	30.08	30.04	30.00	24	37	38	33.0	S. W.	S. W.	S. W.	Clear	Clear	Clear	
7	29.81	29.89	30.04	42	48	34	41.3	S. W.	W'ly	W'ly	Rain	Clear	Clear	
8	29.95	29.83	29.79	29	36	35	33.3	S'ly	N'ly	N. E'ly	Rain	Misty	Misty	1.55 (7th–10th)
9	29.80	29.73	29.65	35	44	35	38.0	N. E'ly	W'ly	N. E'ly	Foggy	Variable	Rain	
10	29.41	29.29	29.23	35	42	39	38.7	N. E'ly	N. E'ly	S. W'ly	Foggy	Foggy	Foggy	
11	29.43	29.46	29.56	34	32	26	30.7	N'ly	N'ly	N. W.	Cloudy	Clear	Clear	
12	29.75	29.76	29.87	19	33	32	28.0	N. W.	N. W.	W'ly	Clear	Clear	Clear	
13	29.82	29.90	30.20	32	43	31	35.3	W'ly	N. W.	N. W.	Variable	Variable	Clear	
14	30.30	30.18	29.65	29	36	42	35.7	N. E.	E'ly	S. E.	Cloudy	Cloudy	Rain	0.50 (14th–15th)
15	29.46	29.79	30.09	36	34	24	31.3	N. W.	N. W.	N. W.	Cloudy	Clear	Clear	
16	30.30	30.27	30.25	17	29	25	23.7	N. W.	N. W.	S'ly	Clear	Clear	Clear	
17	30.08	30.06	30.13	29	48	36	37.7	S. W'ly	W'ly	W'ly	Clear	Clear	Clear	
18	30.21	30.19	30.12	30	44	38	37.3	N. E'ly	N. E.	E'ly	Cloudy	Cloudy	Cloudy	
19	30.07	30.02	30.02	36	51	39	42.0	E'ly	S'ly	S. E'ly	Foggy	Variable	Foggy	
20	29.95	29.84	29.67	36	61	52	49.7	S. W.	S. W.	S. W.	Variable	Clear	Cloudy	
21	29.91	30.08	30.22	46	51	35	44.0	S. W.	N. W.	N. W.	Clear	Clear	Clear	
22	30.17	30.08	29.92	29	48	42	39.7	N'ly	S'ly	S. W.	Variable	Clear	Cloudy	
23	29.78	29.73	29.58	52	57	50	53.0	S'ly	S'ly	S. W'ly	Cloudy	Cloudy	Variable	
24	29.67	29.73	29.78	42	40	31	37.7	N. W.	N. W.	N. W.	Cloudy	Cloudy	Variable	
25	29.78	29.77	29.80	26	34	28	29.3	N. W.	W'ly	S. W.	Variable	Snow	Clear	
26	29.79	29.63	29.57	26	45	40	37.0	S'ly	S. W'ly	S. W'ly	Variable	Variable	Variable	
27	29.81	29.85	29.97	36	34	32	34.0	N. E.	N. E.	N. E.	Cloudy	Cloudy	Cloudy	
28	29.94	29.85	29.75	32	40	40	37.3	N. E.	S. W.	S. W.	Cloudy	Cloudy	Cloudy	
29	29.88	29.88	29.86	36	44	37	39.0	N. W'ly	N. W.	N. W.	Clear	Clear	Clear	
Means	29.90	29.88	29.88	28.5	38.1	32.0	...	...	...	...	...	...	...	2.05
REDUCED TO SEA LEVEL.														
Max.	30.48	30.45	30.43	52	61	52	49.7							
Min.	29.59	29.47	29.41	—5	5	0	1.7							
Mean	30.08	30.06	30.06											
Range	0.89	0.98	1.02	57	56	52	48.0							
Mean of month	30.067			...	...	...	32.9							
Extreme range	1.07			...	...	...	66.0							

Prevailing winds from some point between—

	Days.
N. & E.	7
E. & S.	1
S. & W.	9
W. & N.	12

	Days.
Clear	11
Variable	7
Cloudy	6
Rain or snow fell on	5

REMARKS.

1st. In the morning, wind light, a little S of W, with gentle snow. Before noon, wind came to about N. N. E, and snow continued during the day. Cleared from 8 to 9 P. M. About 3 inches of light dry snow.
2d. Very pleasant.
3d. Clear, but cold, with wind brisk at N. W.
4th. Very piercing wind at N W. Cold severe
5th. Cold in the morning, but not severe, the wind being light W'ly.
6th. Very mild and pleasant. Wind increasing at 10 P. M. at S. W.
7th. Moderate rain from sunrise till 10 A. M.; wind S. W. Wind came more to W., and cleared about noon. Aurora considerably bright in the evening.
8th. Wind variable. Light rain in the morning Mist in the afternoon.
9th. Foggy in morning. Variable in afternoon; sun out at intervals. Pretty heavy rain in evening.
10th. Mist and fog all day. Wind very light N. E'ly in morning, and S. W'ly in afternoon. Shower in evening.
11th. Cloudy until evening, with wind blustering at N'ly, a little W. Cleared in the evening; wind very fresh N. W.
12th. Very pleasant.
13th. Very mild. Variable day. Clear evening.
14th. At sunrise, wind moderate N. E.; cloudy. Before noon, wind came to E., and then to S E., with sprinkling of rain in afternoon. Rain, with heavy wind at S. E, in the evening.
15th. At sunrise, wind brisk at N. W., barometer rising, and some rain. Very blustering during day. River opened by cutting through the ice.
16th. Pleasant. 17th. Very pleasant.
18th. Mild. Wind light N'ly and N. E'ly in morning; then E'ly in afternoon and evening.
19th. Very mild. Sun out in middle of day.
20th. Very mild. Wind brisk S. W. in evening
21st and 22d. Very pleasant.
23d. Mild and pleasant morning. Rather raw afternoon, with cool fog from S'ly towards night.
24th. Mild, without much sun.
25th. Very moderate snow from 9 A. M. till 1 P. M.; wind W'ly. Cleared towards night; wind more S. W'ly.
26th. Mild; cloudy for the most part.
27th. Some snow and rain in morning. Cloudy in afternoon and evening.
28th. Mild and cloudy.
29th. Pleasant. Frost generally out of ground.

March, 1840.

DAYS.	BAROMETER At 6 A. M.	At 1 P. M.	At 10 P. M.	THERMOMETER At 6 A. M.	At 1 P. M.	At 10 P. M.	Daily mean.	WINDS At 6 A. M.	At 1 P. M.	At 10 P. M.	WEATHER At 6 A. M.	At 1 P. M.	At 10 P. M.	RAIN AND SNOW
1	29.89	29.86	29.74	35	44	37	38.7	N. E.	N. E.	N. E.	Cloudy	Cloudy	Rain	
2	29.64	29.63	29.72	36	49	44	43.0	W'ly	S. E.	S'ly	Cloudy	Clear	Clear	
3	29.73	29.64	29.57	34	48	44	42.0	S. W.	S. W.	S'ly	Clear	Cloudy	Rain	
4	29.42	29.30	29.16	44	68	44	52.0	S'ly	S. W.	S. W.	Cloudy	Variable	Clear	
5	29.11	29.13	29.27	44	44	32	40.0	N. W.	N. W.	N. W.	Variable	Clear	Clear	
6	29.40	29.21	29.26	29	48	42	39.7	N. W.	N. W.	N. W.	Clear	Clear	Clear	
7	29.39	29.11	29.50	33	37	14	28.0	N. W.	W'ly	N. W.	Clear	Variable	Clear	
8	29.66	29.64	29.50	8	31	27	22.0	N. W.	N. W.	S. W.	Clear	Clear	Clear	
9	29.25	29.12	29.19	31	43	36	36.7	S. W.	S. W.	S. W.	Variable	Variable	Clear	
10	29.24	29.09	29.32	34	55	27	38.7	S. W.	S'ly	N. W.	Cloudy	Variable	Clear	
11	29.46	29.49	29.71	18	26	21	21.7	N. W.	N. W.	N. W.	Clear	Clear	Clear	
12	29.81	29.77	29.74	18	37	25	26.7	N. W.	W'ly	N. W.	Variable	Variable	Clear	
13	29.66	29.64	29.79	23	32	30	28.3	N. W.	N. W'ly	N. W.	Variable	Clear	Clear	
14	29.89	29.88	29.94	25	38	27	30.0	N. W.	N. W.	N. W.	Clear	Clear	Clear	
15	29.82	29.64	29.50	25	36	33	31.3	S. W'ly	S. W.	S. W.	Clear	Snow	Cloudy	
16	29.60	29.61	29.68	31	44	33	36.0	N. W.	N. W.	S. W.	Clear	Clear	Clear	
17	29.58	29.44	29.59	32	32	32	32.0	S. E'ly	N. E.	N. E.	Cloudy	Snow	Cloudy	0.15
18	29.79	29.82	29.86	28	45	38	37.0	N. W.	S'ly	S. E'ly	Clear	Clear	Cloudy	
19	29.88	29.84	29.78	30	51	40	40.3	S. W.	S. E'ly	S. E'ly	Clear	Clear	Cloudy	
20	29.80	29.79	29.79	34	43	41	39.3	N. E'ly	N. E'ly	S. E'ly	Rain	Cloudy	Cloudy	1.00
21	29.80	29.76	29.84	41	48	32	40.3	N. W'ly	N. W.	N. W.	Cloudy	Clear	Clear	
22	29.99	30.00	30.00	24	32	27	27.7	N. W.	N. W.	N. W.	Clear	Clear	Clear	
23	30.04	29.98	29.94	24	43	32	33.0	N. E.	S. E.	N. E.	Cloudy	Cloudy	Cloudy	
24	29.74	29.44	29.13	31	30	28	29.7	E'ly	E'ly	N. E.	Cloudy	Snow	Sn. & h'l	0.75
25	29.25	29.29	29.54	25	35	28	29.3	N. N. E.	N. N. E.	N'ly	Cloudy	Cloudy	Clear	
26	29.36	29.40	29.61	22	34	28	28.0	N.	N. W.	N. W.	Cloudy	Clear	Clear	
27	29.80	29.79	29.85	30	49	40	39.7	W'ly	S. W.	S. W.	Clear	Clear	Clear	
28	29.88	29.89	29.88	40	49	45	44.7	S. W.	S. W.	S. W.	Cloudy	Cloudy	Rain	
29	29.76	29.65	29.67	46	53	48	49.0	S. W.	S. W.	S. W.	Cloudy	Cloudy	Cloudy	
30	29.58	29.38	29.21	42	53	53	49.3	S. W.	S. S. W.	S. S. W.	Foggy	Rain	Rain	1.60
31	29.23	29.42	29.64	40	45	38	41.0	W'ly	W'ly	W'ly	Clear	Clear	Clear	
Means	29.63	29.63	29.61	30.9	42.7	34.4	...	...	...	...	...	...	...	3.50
REDUCED TO SEA LEVEL.														
Max.	30.22	30.16	30.12	46	68	53	52.0							
Min.	29.29	29.29	29.31	8	26	14	21.7							
Mean	29.81	29.81	29.79											
Range	0.93	0.87	0.81	38	42	39	30.3							
Mean of month	29.803			...	...	...	36.0							
Extreme range	0.93			...	...	...	60.0							

Prevailing winds from some point between—

	Days.
N. & E.	5
E. & S.	4
S. & W.	10
W. & N.	12

	Days.
Clear	11
Variable, Cloudy	10
Rain or snow fell on	10

REMARKS.

1st. Cloudy, with wind moderate N. E. Moderate rain began from 8 to 9 P. M.; soon ceased.
2d. Very pleasant.
3d. Wind light S. W'ly Quite cloudy. Moderate rain began from 9 to 10 P. M.; wind light S'ly.
4th. Very warm. Sky a good deal covered. Thunder from 11 to 12 P. M., and frequent lightning during the night, with some rain.
5th. Very blustering. Evening clear, with diffused aurora, low, and somewhat bright.
6th. Blustering; wind N. W.
7th. Very blustering; frequent clouds, with occasional rain. Flurry of snow from 2 to 3 P. M. Wind hauled from W'ly to N. W.; grew colder.
8th Severe cold and piercing wind in morning.
9th. Mild.
10th. Variable; mild. From 3 to 5 P. M., wind changed from S. W. to N. W., and grew colder.
11th. Cold rather severe. Wind brisk N. W.
12th. Wind moderate W'ly.
13th. Rather raw.
14th. Cool, but pleasant.
14th Clear at sunrise, with wind light S. W'ly. Clouded up before noon, and began to snow very moderately, which continued till evening.
16th. Very pleasant.
17th. At sunrise, wind light S. E'ly; before 10 A. M., came to N. E., and began to snow moderately, which continued till night without gaining much on the ground.
18th. Pleasant. Ground covered with snow in the morning, which disappeared before noon.
19th. Pleasant.
20th. Mild. Cloudy for the most part.
21st. Pleasant.
22d. Very clear, but blustering wind and cold.
23d. Raw and unpleasant.
24th. Began to snow and hail moderately from 7 to 8 A. M.; wind light, about E. N. E. Snow and hail during the day; wind nearly the same. In the evening, wind more to N. E., pretty heavy.
25th. Snow about 3 inches deep; very damp. Cloudy; wind light N. N. E'ly. Clear evening.
28th and 27th. Pleasant.
28th. Cloudy in morning. Sprinkling in afternoon. Rain in evening.
29th. Wind fresh S. W. Heavy clouds, with some rain.
30th. Foggy in morning. Began to rain from 10 to 11 A. M.; wind rather fresh, about S. S. W. rain continued in afternoon and evening, wind increasing to very fresh in the evening.
31st. Clear at sunrise; wind W'ly, fresh. From 8 to 9 A. M., clouded and rained moderately. Rather blustering.

April, 1840.

DAYS.	BAROMETER, REDUCED TO 32° F. At 6 A. M.	At 1 P. M.	At 10 P. M.	THERMOMETER. At 6 A. M.	At 1 P. M.	At 10 P. M.	Daily mean.	WINDS. At 6 A. M.	At 1 P. M.	At 10 P. M.	WEATHER. At 6 A. M.	At 1 P. M.	At 10 P. M.	RAIN AND SNOW IN INCHES OF WATER
1	29.75	29.73	29.62	34	36	34	34.7	S. W'ly	E'ly	N. E'ly	Clear	Snow	Rain	0.30
2	29.74	...	29.91	34	...	34	34.0	N. W.	N. W.	N. W.	Clear	Clear	Clear	
3	29.94	29.70	29.58	30	53	47	43.3	W'ly	S. W.	S. W.	Clear	Clear	Clear	
4	29.34	29.27	29.47	47	53	44	47.3	S. W.	S. W.	N. W.	Cloudy	Cloudy	Clear	
5	29.61	29.63	29.71	35	51	41	42.3	N. W.	N. W.	N. W.	Clear	Clear	Clear	
6	29.85	29.80	29.86	32	47	35	38.0	N. W.	N. W.	N. W.	Clear	Clear	Clear	
7	29.92	29.96	29.98	30	43	33	35.3	N. W.	N. W.	N. W.	Clear	Clear	Clear	
8	30.09	30.05	30.13	28	46	30	34.7	N. W.	N. W.	N. W.	Clear	Clear	Clear	
9	30.23	30.22	30.17	30	47	33	36.7	W'ly	S'ly	S. W.	Clear	Clear	Clear	
10	30.09	...	30.01	38	...	50	...	S. W.	...	S. W.	Cloudy	...	Clear	
11	30.03	30.00	29.96	47	67	55	56.3	S. W.	S. W.	S. W.	Clear	Variable	Shower	
12	29.86	29.73	29.51	54	58	58	56.7	S. W.	S. W.	S. W.	Cloudy	Rain	Rain	1.80
13	29.70	29.84	30.04	42	54	44	46.7	N. W'ly	N. W.	N. W.	Clear	Clear	Clear	
14	30.11	30.02	29.84	40	53	44	45.7	N. W.	N. W.	S. W'ly	Clear	Clear	Cloudy	
15	29.86	29.79	29.80	44	64	45	51.0	S. W.	S. W.	S'ly	Variable	Variable	Clear	
16	29.83	29.83	29.84	40	61	44	48.3	N. W.	S. W.	S'ly	Clear	Clear	Clear	
17	29.86	29.82	29.80	44	60	49	51.0	S'ly	S'ly	S. W.	Foggy	Clear	Clear	
18	29.74	29.63	29.58	54	69	57	60.0	S. W.	S. W.	S. W.	Variable	Clear	Variable	
19	29.76	29.85	29.95	51	55	42	49.3	N. E'ly	N'ly	N'ly	Cloudy	Variable	Clear	
20	29.97	29.90	30.06	38	63	44	48.3	S'ly	S. W.	N. W.	Cloudy	Clear	Clear	
21	30.07	30.11	30.13	35	54	38	42.3	N. E.	N. E.	N. E.	Clear	Clear	Clear	
22	30.12	29.97	...	38	57	...	...	S. W'ly	S. W.	...	Clear	Variable	Rain	
23	...	...	...	...	...	...	...	...	...	...	...	...	...	
24	...	...	29.80	...	75	58	...	...	...	S. W.	...	...	Clear	
25	29.90	29.84	29.80	52	67	56	58.3	N. E.	S'ly	S'ly	Clear	Clear	Foggy	
26	29.71	29.59	29.52	57	74	60	63.7	S. W.	S. W.	W'ly	Foggy	Variable	Rain	
27	29.50	...	30.19	50	...	40	...	N. W.	...	N. W.	Clear	...	Clear	
28	30.33	30.30	30.29	36	57	44	45.7	N. W.	S. W.	S'ly	Clear	Clear	Variable	
29	30.09	29.91	29.70	44	56	46	48.3	E'ly	E'ly	E'ly	Rain	Misty	Rain	1.35
30	29.42	29.43	29.59	46	68	56	56.7	N. W'ly	N. W'ly	W'ly	Cloudy	Clear	Clear	
Means	29.87	29.84	29.85	41.1	57.2	45.0	...	...	...	...	...	...	...	3.45
REDUCED TO SEA LEVEL.														
Max.	30.51	30.48	30.47	57	75	58	66.5							
Min.	29.52	29.45	29.65	28	36	30	34.0							
Mean	30.05	30.02	30.03											
Range	0.99	1.03	0.82	29	39	28	32.5							
Mean of month	30.033			...	...	...	47.8							
Extreme range	1.06			...	...	...	47.0							

Prevailing winds from some point between—

	Days.
N. & E.	3
E. & S.	2
S. & W.	15
W. & N.	9

	Days.
Clear	12
Variable / Cloudy	12
Rain or snow fell on	6

(1 day omitted.)

REMARKS.

1st. Clear at sunrise; wind S. W'ly. Clouded, and began to snow from 10 to 11 A. M., wind hauling to S E, then to E'ly and N. E. Snow continued through the day, with rain in the evening.

2d. Cool, but pleasant.

3d. Pleasant. Wind very fresh S. W.

4th. In morning, wind fresh S. W.; came to N. W., with a gust and heavy clouds, from 1 to 2 P. M. Clear evening. Diffused aurora, considerably bright.

5th. Very blustering wind, N. W.

6th, 7th, 8th, 9th. Cool, but pleasant.

10th. Morning cloudy for the most part. Clear in afternoon; blustering.

11th. Warm and springlike. Clear in morning. Cloudy in afternoon. Shower in evening.

12th. Mist in the morning. Began to rain from 10 to 11 A. M. Heavy rain during the remainder of the day and evening, with high wind at S. W.

13th. Fine weather.

14th. Pleasant.

15th. Mild and pleasant.

16th and 17th. Very pleasant.

18th. Very warm, and yet very blustering.

19th. Pleasant.

20th. Pleasant. Wind came to N. W., and grew cooler towards night.

21st. Pleasant, but cool.

22d. Clear morning. Cloudy and rain in afternoon and evening.

23d. Cloudy in morning. Pleasant and warm in afternoon.

24th. Pleasant and very warm.

25th. Pleasant.

26th. Foggy in morning. Sun out from 8 to 10 A. M. Thunder and sprinkling of rain before noon. Clear in afternoon. Cloudy, with some rain, in evening.

27th. Pleasant; cooler.

28th. Very pleasant.

29th. Moderate rain nearly all day; increased in evening. In the morning, wind light S E'ly, or from E. to S. E. In the afternoon and night, wind more E'ly.

May, 1840.

DAYS.	BAROMETER. At 6 A. M.	At 1 P. M.	At 10 P. M.	THERMOMETER. At 6 A. M.	At 1 P. M.	At 10 P. M.	Daily mean.	WINDS. At 6 A. M.	At 1 P. M.	At 10 P. M.	WEATHER. At 6 A. M.	At 1 P. M.	At 10 P. M.	RAIN
1	29.47	29.29	29.39	54	69	48	57.0	S'ly	S. W'ly	W'ly	Variable	Shower	Clear	
2	29.57	29.55	29.56	42	65	49	52.0	N. W.	W'ly	W'ly	Clear	Clear	Cloudy	
3	29.55	29.51	29.45	52	73	56	60.3	S. W.	S. W.	S. W.	Clear	Clear	Cloudy	} 0.68
4	29.10	28.96	29.03	51	57	44	50.7	E'ly	N. E.	N. E.	Rain	Cloudy	Cloudy	
5	29.21	29.32	29.41	40	45	36	40.3	N. W'ly	N. W'ly	N. W.	Misty	Rain	Rain	0.47
6	29.53	29.52	29.54	40	58	40	46.0	N. W.	N. W.	N. W.	Cloudy	Variable	Variable	
7	29.56	29.56	29.67	43	57	46	48.7	N. W.	N. W.	N. W.	Clear	Clear	Clear	
8	29.81	29.82	29.84	40	53	...	...	N.	N. E.	...	Clear	Variable	...	
9	29.77	29.65	29.52	...	...	38	...	...	...	N. E.	...	...	Rain	0.95
10	29.50	29.53	29.60	38	45	45	42.7	N. E.	N. E.	N'ly	Cloudy	Cloudy	Cloudy	
11	29.62	29.67	29.75	44	56	44	48.0	N. E'ly	N. E.	S. W'ly	Clear	Clear	Clear	
12	29.74	29.73	29.77	41	63	48	50.8	S. W.	S. W.	S'ly	Clear	Clear	Clear	
13	29.82	29.82	29.86	45	67	50	54.0	E'ly	S. E'ly	S'ly	Clear	Clear	Clear	
14	29.88	29.84	29.82	45	69	52	55.3	S. W.	S. E'ly	S. E'ly	Clear	Clear	Clear	
15	29.71	29.56	29.63	52	75	57	61.3	S. W.	S. W.	W'ly	Clear	Clear	Shower	0.25
16	29.81	29.83	29.91	52	72	58	60.7	N. W.	W'ly	S. W'ly	Clear	Clear	Clear	
17	29.90	29.88	29.80	55	77	64	65.3	S. W.	S. W.	S. W.	Clear	Clear	Clear	
18	29.74	29.66	29.67	62	88	72	74.0	S. W.	S. W.	S. W.	Clear	Clear	Clear	
19	29.80	29.88	29.90	54	65	52	57.0	N. E.	N. E.	N. E.	Variable	Clear	Cloudy	
20	29.89	29.80	29.73	51	68	56	58.3	N. E.	N. E.	N. E.	Cloudy	Cloudy	Cloudy	
21	29.55	29.46	29.45	51	51	44	48.7	N. E.	N. E.	N. E.	Rain	Rain	Rain	1.00
22	29.47	29.59	29.67	47	55	53	51.7	N'ly	N. E'ly	N. W.	Cloudy	Cloudy	Variable	
23	29.80	29.83	29.93	56	74	54	61.3	N. W'ly	N. E'ly	N. E.	Variable	Clear	Clear	
24	30.10	30.14	30.17	50	66	53	56.3	N. E.	S. E'ly	S'ly	Cloudy	Clear	Clear	
25	30.23	30.21	30.20	50	67	51	56.0	S. W'ly	S. E'ly	S'ly	Clear	Clear	Clear	
26	30.11	30.03	30.04	50	68	55	57.7	S. W'ly	S. W'ly	S. W.	Clear	Clear	Clear	
27	29.84	29.73	29.67	55	75	66	65.3	S. W.	S. W.	S. W.	Clear	Clear	Clear	
28	29.63	29.57	29.54	63	83	68	71.3	W'ly	S. W.	S. W.	Clear	Clear	Clear	
29	29.54	29.58	29.67	64	74	59	65.7	S. W'ly	N. E.	E'ly	Clear	Clear	Clear	
30	[illegible]	[illegible]	[illegible]	[illegible]	76	[illegible]	62.7	N. E.	E'ly	S. W.	Clear	Clear	Clear	
31	[illegible]	[illegible]	[illegible]	[illegible]	[illegible]	[illegible]	[illegible]	[illegible]	[illegible]	[illegible]	[illegible]	[illegible]	[illegible]	
Means	29.69	29.67	29.69	53.2	66.2	52.4	...	...	...	...	...	...	...	3.85
REDUCED TO SEA LEVEL.														
Max.	30.41	30.39	30.38	64	88	72	71.3							
Min.	29.28	29.14	29.21	38	45	36	40.0							
Mean	29.87	29.88	29.87											
Range	1.13	1.25	1.14	26	43	36	31.3							
Mean of month	29.877			...	...	...	57.3							
Extreme range	1.27			...	...	...	52.0							

Prevailing winds from some point between—

	Days.
N. & E.	11
E. & S.	5
S. & W.	11
W. & N.	4

	Days.
Clear	20
Variable / Cloudy	8
Rain fell on	8

REMARKS.

1st. Variable. Light shower from 2 to 3 P. M., with thunder.

2d. Pleasant.

3d. Very fine. Heavy rain during the night.

4th. Some rain.

5th. Mist in morning. Moderate rain in afternoon and evening; wind N. W.

6th. Variable.

7th. Pleasant, but cool.

8th. Clear in morning. Cloudy in afternoon, with wind brisk at N. E.

9th. Heavy N. E. storm all day, and cold for the season.

10th. Raw N. E'ly weather.

11th. Pleasant, but cool.

12th and 13th. Very fine.

14th. Very fine and warm.

15th. Fine in morning. Showers in afternoon.

16th and 17th. Very fine.

18th. Weather clear, and excessively warm for the season. Wind rather fresh S. W. Thermometer at 88° in the shade.

19th and 20th. Variable.

21st. Moderate rain nearly all day. Rain increased in the evening, and grew colder, with wind freshening.

22d. Some rain in morning. Cloudy in afternoon. Partly clear in evening.

23d. Warm and pleasant.

24th. Pleasant. Air rather damp.

25th. Fine.

26th and 27th. Very fine.

28th. Very fine and very warm.

29th. Fine. Wind N. E'ly the greater part of the day. Brilliant aurora in the evening, with frequent corruscations.

30th and 31st. Weather continues fine.

June, 1840.

DAYS.	BAROMETER, REDUCED TO 32° F. At 6 A. M.	At 1 P. M.	At 10 P. M.	THERMOMETER. At 6 A. M.	At 1 P. M.	At 10 P. M.	Daily mean.	WINDS. At 6 A. M.	At 1 P. M.	At 10 P. M.	WEATHER. At 6 A. M.	At 1 P. M.	At 10 P. M.	RAIN AND SNOW IN INCHES OF WATER
1	29.69	29.70	29.76	54	67	49	56.7	N'ly	S. W.	N. E.	Cloudy	Cloudy	Rain	
2	29.92	29.92	29.94	45	67	54	55.3	N. E.	S. E.	N. E.	Cloudy	Cloudy	Cloudy	
3	29.83	29.75	29.66	54	62	61	59.0	S. E.	S. E.	S'ly	Cloudy	Cloudy	Cloudy	
4	29.50	29.48	29.42	62	69	62	64.3	S'ly	S. W.	S. W.	Rain	Cloudy	Cloudy	1.68
5	29.41	29.49	29.62	60	78	68	68.7	N. W'ly	W'ly	W'ly	Variable	Clear	Clear	
6	29.69	29.68	29.68	63	78	66	69.0	N. W.	W'ly	S. W.	Clear	Clear	Clear	
7	29.68	29.64	29.71	66	75	55	65.3	S. W.	S. W.	N'ly	Clear	Cloudy	Shower	0.33
8	29.79	29.85	29.91	51	64	60	58.3	N'ly	N'ly	S. W.	Cloudy	Cloudy	Variable	
9	29.96	29.98	29.98	62	73	64	66.3	N. W'ly	N. W'ly	N. W'ly	Clear	Clear	Clear	
10	29.99	29.96	29.93	60	80	68	69.3	N. W.	N. W.	S. W.	Clear	Clear	Clear	
11	29.84	29.77	29.71	64	78	69	70.3	S. W.	S. W.	S. W.	Clear	Clear	Clear	
12	29.62	29.56	29.54	67	85	74	75.3	S. W.	N. W.	N. W.	Clear	Clear	Variable	
13	29.48	29.43	29.61	70	81	60	70.3	S. W.	N. W.	N. W.	Variable	Clear	Clear	
14	29.68	29.68	29.70	60	74	63	65.7	N. W.	N. W.	N. W.	Clear	Clear	Clear	
15	29.69	29.65	29.64	60	71	57	62.7	N. W.	N. W.	N. W.	Variable	Variable	Clear	
16	29.73	29.78	29.82	53	71	61	61.7	N. W.	N. W.	N. W.	Clear	Clear	Clear	
17	29.89	29.87	29.87	59	78	66	67.7	N. W.	N. W.	W'ly	Clear	Clear	Clear	
18	29.89	29.80	29.65	61	68	65	64.7	S. W.	S. E.	S. E'ly	Clear	Cloudy	Cloudy	
19	29.48	29.40	29.39	60	72	56	62.7	W'ly	W'ly	N. W.	Cloudy	Clear	Clear	
20	29.30	...	29.49	54	...	59	...	W'ly	...	N'ly	Cloudy	...	Cloudy	
21	29.60	29.59	29.59	57	74	63	64.7	N. W.	N. W.	S'ly	Clear	Clear	Clear	
22	29.61	29.58	29.70	64	76	69	69.7	S. W.	S. W.	W'ly	Clear	Variable	Clear	
23	29.84	29.87	29.87	63	83	64	70.0	N'ly	S. W'ly	S. W'ly	Clear	Variable	Clear	
24	29.80	29.77	29.60	64	82	72	72.7	S. W.	W'ly	W'ly	Clear	Clear	Clear	
25	29.58	29.57	29.58	72	76	63	70.3	N.	E'ly	E'ly	Clear	Clear	Clear	
26	29.79	29.82	29.82	58	77	62	65.7	E'ly	S. E'ly	E'ly	Clear	Clear	Clear	
27	29.79	29.77	29.72	62	73	67	67.3	N. E.	N. E.	N. E'ly	Cloudy	Rain	Rain	} 0.90
28	...	29.64	29.65	...	75	71	...	...	N. E.	N. E.	...	Rain	Variable	}
29	29.67	29.66	29.66	71	83	72	75.3	S'ly	S. W'ly	S. W'ly	Clear	Clear	Cloudy	
30	29.62	29.61	29.61	72	84	71	75.7	S'ly	S. W'ly	S. W.	Misty	Clear	Variable	
Means	29.70	29.70	29.70	61.0	75.0	63.9	...	...	...	...	...	...	...	2.89
REDUCED TO SEA LEVEL.								Prevailing winds from some point between—						
Max.	30.17	30.14	30.16	72	85	74	75.7			Days.			Days.	
Min.	29.48	29.58	29.57	45	82	49	55.3	N. & E.		4	Clear		12	
Mean	29.88	29.87	29.88					E. & S.		4	Variable		} 7	
Range	0.69	0.56	0.59	27	23	25	20.4	S. & W.		9	Cloudy		}	
Mean of month 29.877				...	...	...	66.3	W. & N.		13	Rain fell on . .		11	
Extreme range 0.69				...	...	...	40.0							

REMARKS.

1st. Began raining moderately from 4 to 5 P. M.
2d. Cloudy, with occasional sprinkling of rain.
3d. Foggy and damp. Heavy rain during the night.
4th. Heavy rain early. Foggy during the day.
5th and 6th. Very fine.
7th. Clear early. Clouded before 9 A. M., and showery during the day; wind S. W'ly. Wind came to N. W., and grew cool towards night.
8th. Cloudy. Mist in morning.
9th, 10th, and 11th. Very fine.
12th. Very warm, but a fine breeze from N. W. in afternoon.
13th. At 3 A. M., thunder, with sprinkling of rain. Light showers from 9 to 11 A. M. Clear towards night, and cooler. Very clear in evening.
14th. Very fine.
15th. Variable in the morning. Clear towards night. Very clear and pleasant in the evening.
16th and 17th. Very fine.
18th. Clear in the morning. Cloudy in the afternoon, with wind S. S. E. nearly, and occasional very light showers.
19th. Mostly fine.
20th. Light showers in morning. Variable in afternoon. Clear in evening.
21st. Fine.
22d. Fine in morning. Very light shower from 5 to 6 P. M. Clear in evening.
23d. Very fine.
24th. Very fine. Sun very burning.
25th and 26th. Fine.
27th. Moderate rain from N. E. commenced about noon, and continued at intervals through afternoon and evening.
28th. Light showers in morning. Cloudy in afternoon. Very sultry.
29th. Very fine.
30th. Very misty in the morning. Clear and drier by noon.

July, 1840.

DAYS.	BAROMETER. At 6 A. M.	At 1 P. M.	At 10 P. M.	THERMOMETER. At 6 A. M.	At 1 P. M.	At 10 P. M.	Daily mean.	WINDS. At 6 A. M.	At 1 P. M.	At 10 P. M.	WEATHER. At 6 A. M.	At 1 P. M.	At 10 P. M.	RAIN
1	29.60	29.60	29.67	68	80	70	72.7	N. W.	W.	N. W.	Clear	Clear	Clear	
2	29.79	29.81	29.88	60	76	66	67.3	N. W.	N. W.	N. W.	Clear	Clear	Variable	
3	29.88	29.93	29.93	60	67	60	62.3	N. E.	N. E.	N. E.	Cloudy	Sprink'g	Cloudy	
4	...	...	...	...	...	...	...	...	...	...	...	...	...	
5	...	...	...	...	...	...	...	...	...	...	...	...	...	
6	...	...	...	...	...	...	...	...	...	...	...	...	...	
7	30.00	29.92	29.91	63	71	64	66.0	N. E.	N. E.	N. E.	Cloudy	Cloudy	Cloudy	
8	29.90	29.88	29.82	64	78	67	69.7	N. E.	W'ly	S. W.	Cloudy	Variable	Variable	0.25
9	29.68	29.57	29.58	70	84	68	74.0	S. W.	S. W.	N. W.	Rain	Variable	Variable	
10	29.59	29.52	29.71	68	82	67	72.3	W.	W.	W.	Clear	Clear	Clear	
11	29.79	29.80	29.77	62	80	69	70.3	N. E.	W'ly	W'ly	Clear	Clear	Clear	
12	29.77	29.77	29.75	70	89	70	76.3	W'ly	S. E'ly	S'ly	Clear	Clear	Clear	
13	29.74	29.67	29.64	68	80	72	73.3	S. W.	S. W.	S. W.	Cloudy	Variable	Cl'y, sh'r	0.20
14	29.45	29.42	29.50	72	80	74	75.3	S. W.	S. W.	S. W.	Cloudy	Cloudy	Clear	
15	29.63	29.67	29.70	70	86	76	77.3	N. W.	S. W.	S. W.	Clear	Clear	Clear	
16	29.77	29.77	29.77	74	87	74	78.3	S. W.	S. W.	S. W.	Clear	Clear	Clear	
17	29.78	29.76	29.76	72	90½	74	78.7	S. W.	S. W.	S. W.	Clear	Clear	Clear	
18	29.76	29.76	29.73	74	76	74	74.7	S. W.	S. W.	S. W.	Cloudy	Shower	Clear	0.81
19	29.63	29.51	29.60	74	80	68	74.0	S. W.	S. W.	W'ly	Variable	Shower	Var., sh.	0.57
20	29.71	29.75	29.76	58	73	62	64.3	N. W.	N. W.	N. W.	Clear	Clear	Clear	
21	29.76	29.75	29.78	58	76	69	67.7	N. W.	N. W.	S. W.	Clear	Clear	Clear	
22	29.89	29.88	29.88	64	78	69	70.3	W'ly	S. W.	S. W.	Clear	Clear	Clear	
23	29.88	29.80	29.73	66	80	71	72.3	S. W.	S. W.	S. W.	Clear	Clear	Cloudy	
24	29.53	29.38	29.55	70	74	69	71.0	S. E'ly	N'ly	N. W.	Rain	Variable	Cloudy	1.55
25	29.72	29.81	29.87	69	79	68	68.7	N'ly	W'ly	S. W'ly	Variable	Variable	Clear	
26	29.89	29.90	29.92	68	84	71	74.3	S. W'ly	S. W'ly	S. W.	Clear	Clear	Clear	
27	29.95	29.97	29.95	70	80	69	73.0	S. W.	S. W.	S. W.	Variable	Clear	Clear	
28	29.91	29.80	29.67	69	79	70	72.7	S. W.	S. E'ly	S. W.	Clear	Clear	Cl'r, sh'r	
29	29.61	29.67	29.70	70	83	72	75.0	N. W.	N. W'ly	N. W.	Variable	Clear	Clear	
30	29.80	29.84	29.85	68	83	69	73.3	N. W.	S. W'ly	S. W.	Clear	Clear	Clear	
31	29.88	29.87	29.88	68	80	72	73.3	S. W.	S. W.	S. W.	Clear	Clear	Clear	
Means	29.76	29.77	29.76	67.4	79.8	69.4	...	...	...	...	...	...	...	3.38
REDUCED TO SEA LEVEL.								Prevailing winds from some point between—						
Max.	30.18	30.15	30.13	74	90½	76	78.7			Days.			Days.	
Min.	29.63	29.60	29.68	58	67	60	62.3	N. & E.		4	Clear		13	
Mean	29.93	29.94	29.93					E. & S.		2	Variable		} 6	
Range	0.55	0.55	0.45	16	23½	16	16.4	S. & W.		16	Cloudy		}	
Mean of month 29.933				...	...	...	72.2	W. & N.		6	Rain fell on . .		9	
Extreme range 0.58				...	...	...	32.0				(3 days omitted.)			

REMARKS.

1st and 2d. Very fine.
3d. Cloudy, with frequent sprinklings.
7th. Cloudy and rather cool, with light rain occasionally during morning.
8th. Pleasant, though for the most part cloudy.
9th. Moderate rain in morning; wind light S. W. Wind came to N.W., with heavy clouds, and grew cooler about sunset.
10th and 11th. Very fine.
12th. Wind light E'ly in morning; more S. E'ly and fresh in afternoon. Sun excessively hot all day.
13th. Cloudy in the morning and evening, with sprinkling of rain. Shower in the night.
14th. Cloudy in the morning; then hot sun. Thunder-clouds from noon to 3 P. M. A light shower between 1 and 2 P. M., which was quite heavy in the immediate vicinity. Very clear in the evening.
15th. Clear, and very hot sun.
16th. Very fine and very warm.
17th. Very hot, notwithstanding a fine breeze all day from S. W.
18th. Cloudy, but very warm, in the morning. Fine shower, with light thunder, from 1 to 3 P. M.
19th. Shower from 3 to 5 A. M., with light thunder. Thundershower about noon, equal to 0.25 inch of water. Shower again about 6 P. M., equal to 0.32 inch of water. Very hot sun part of the day. Wind fresh from S. W.
20th, 21st, and 22d. Very fine.
23d. Clear in morning. Cloudy in afternoon towards night. Air very damp; wind fresh S. W., with appearances of rain.
24th. Rain, with wind S. E'ly. Rain heavy from 8 to 10 A. M. Wind came to N'ly, and partly clear by 1 P. M. Rain equal to 1.55 inch of water. Hot sun at intervals during afternoon.
25th. Variable for the most part. Sun very hot at times.
26th and 27th. Very fine.
28th. Very fine. Shower during the night.
29th. Fine. Aurora in the evening, not bright.
30th. Very fine.
31st. Fine.

August, 1840.

DAYS.	BAROMETER, REDUCED TO 32° F. At 6 A. M.	At 1 P. M.	At 10 P. M.	THERMOMETER. At 6 A. M.	At 1 P. M.	At 10 P. M.	Daily mean.	WINDS. At 6 A. M.	At 1 P. M.	At 10 P. M.	WEATHER. At 6 A. M.	At 1 P. M.	At 10 P. M.	RAIN AND SNOW IN INCHES OF WATER.
1	29.81	29.73	29.77	68	70	69	69.0	N. E.	N. E.	N. W'ly	Rain	Rain	Variable	1.05
2	29.82	29.81	29.72	68	77	72	72.3	N. W.	S'ly	S'ly	Variable	Shower	Cloudy	
3	29.73	29.68	29.69	71	78	73	74.0	S. W.	S. W.	S. W.	Cloudy	Cloudy	Cloudy	} 0.25
4	29.67	29.62	29.60	68	83	75	75.3	S. W.	S. W.	S. W.	Cloudy	Clear	Cloudy	
5	29.56	29.53	29.53	73	80	73	75.3	W'ly	N. W.	S. W.	Variable	Clear	Clear	
6	29.61	29.53	29.45	64	78	66	69.3	S. W.	S'ly	S. W.	Clear	Clear	Var., sh.	0.40
7	29.50	29.53	29.57	64	76	64	68.7	S. W.	S. W.	W'ly	Cloudy	Clear	Clear	
8	29.59	29.58	29.64	61	75	68	68.0	S. W.	S. W.	N. W.	Clear	Clear	Clear	
9	29.75	29.78	29.83	62	79	65	68.7	N. W.	N. W.	N. W.	Clear	Variable	Clear	
10	29.89	29.92	29.90	57	74	65	65.3	N. W.	N. W.	N. W.	Clear	Variable	Clear	
11	29.89	29.81	29.77	62	76	71	69.7	N. W.	S. W.	S. W.	Clear	Variable	Variable	
12	29.73	29.69	29.66	68	83	74	75.0	S. W.	S. W.	S. W.	Cloudy	Clear	Cl'y, sh'r	0.10
13	29.62	29.61	29.58	69	75	73	72.3	S. W.	S. W.	S. W.	Cloudy	Rain	Rain	} 1.05
14	29.45	29.47	29.60	72	80	70	74.0	S. W.	S. W.	S. W.	Rain	Clear	Clear	
15	29.62	29.77	29.87	65	79	67	70.3	N. W.	W.	N. W.	Clear	Clear	Clear	
16	29.99	30.01	30.04	60	71	62	64.3	N. W.	N. E.	N. E.	Clear	Cloudy	Clear	
17	30.09	30.12	30.10	58	78	66	67.3	N. E'ly	S'ly	S. W'ly	Clear	Clear	Clear	
18	30.10	30.07	30.05	62	79	64	68.3	S. W.	S. W.	S. W.	Variable	Clear	Clear	
19	29.99	29.89	29.82	62	79	71	70.7	S. W.	S. W.	S. W.	Variable	Clear	Clear	
20	29.79	...	...	70	82	74	75.3	S. W.	...	...	Clear	...	...	
21	...	...	...	70	83	73	75.3	...	S. W'ly	...	...	...	...	
22	...	29.77	29.72	70	82	75	75.7	...	S. W.	S. W.	...	Clear	Variable	
23	29.71	...	29.56	73	...	75	74.0	S. W.	...	S. W.	Clear	...	Var., sh.	0.35
24	29.57	29.58	29.64	72	82	69	...	W'ly	W'ly	W'ly	Clear	Clear	Clear	
25	29.68	29.68	29.77	75	78	64	72.3	N. W'ly	N. W'ly	N. W.	Clear	Clear	Clear	
26	29.82	29.84	29.84	58	77	65	66.7	N. W.	N. W.	N. W.	Clear	Clear	Clear	
27	29.86	29.84	29.86	61	76	67	69.0	N. W'ly	W'ly	S. W.	Clear	Clear	Clear	
28	29.89	29.88	29.86	59	79	66	68.0	S. W.	S. W.	S. W.	Clear	Clear	Clear	
29	29.91	29.91	29.91	61	77	65	67.7	N'ly	S'ly	S. W'ly	Cloudy	Clear	Clear	
30	29.90	29.85	29.80	64	80	70	71.3	S. W.	S. W.	S. W.	Clear	Clear	Clear	
31	29.71	29.67	29.64	70	78	72	73.3	S. W.	S. W.	S. W.	Variable	Cloudy	Clear	
Means	29.77	29.76	29.75	65.7	78.1	69.1	...	...	...	...	...	...	...	3.20

REDUCED TO SEA LEVEL.							
Max.	30.28	30.30	30.28	75	83	75	75.3
Min.	29.63	29.65	29.63	57	70	62	64.3
Mean	29.94	29.93	29.92				
Range	0.65	0.65	0.65	18	23	13	11.0
Mean of month	29.930			...	...	...	71.0
Extreme range	0.65			...	...	...	26.0

Prevailing winds from some point between—

	Days.
N. & E.	2
E. & S.	1
S. & W.	20
W. & N.	8

	Days.
Clear	10
Variable } Cloudy }	13
Rain fell on	8

REMARKS.

1st. Steady rain from N. E. during the morning. Variable in the afternoon and evening.
2d. Variable in the morning. Light showers from 1 to 3 P. M.
3d. Light showers in the morning. Heavy shower at 5 P. M.
4th. High wind.
6th. Lightning, and a thundershower in the night.
7th to 11th. Very fine.
12th. Fine. Very burning sun about mid-day.
13th. Showery through the day; wind fresh S. W. Heavy rain during the night.
14th. Rain early. Cloudy in morning. Clear towards night.
15th. Very fine.
16th. Variable in the morning. Clear and fine in the afternoon.
17th, 18th, and 19th. Very fine.
20th and 21st. Very sultry and hot.
22d. Fine. Some fog in the morning.
23d. Fine in the morning. Heavy clouds and frequent lightning in the evening, with sprinkling of rain. Heavy shower during the night.
24th to 30th. Very fine.
31st. Variable. Occasional sprinkling of rain.

September, 1840.

DAYS.	BAROMETER At 6 A. M.	At 1 P. M.	At 10 P. M.	THERMOMETER At 6 A. M.	At 1 P. M.	At 10 P. M.	Daily mean.	WINDS At 6 A. M.	At 1 P. M.	At 10 P. M.	WEATHER At 6 A. M.	At 1 P. M.	At 10 P. M.	RAIN
1	29.72	...	...	60	...	...	...	N. W.	...	...	Clear	...	...	
2	...	...	...	60	...	...	...	N. W.	...	...	...	...	Shower	0.30
3	29.71	...	29.75	61	...	58	...	N. W.	...	N. W.	Variable	...	Clear	
4	29.85	29.87	29.87	50	72	58	60.0	N. W.	N. W.	N. E.	Clear	Variable	Cloudy	
5	29.96	29.72	29.68	56	56	55	55.3	N. E.	N. E.	N. E.	Rain	Rain	Cloudy	0.70
6	29.71	29.72	29.83	56	68	58	60.7	N'ly	N. W.	N. W.	Cloudy	Variable	Clear	
7	29.89	29.90	29.91	56	75	63	64.7	N. W.	N. W.	S. W.	Clear	Clear	Clear	
8	29.90	29.81	29.78	57	76	65	62.7	S. W.	S. W.	S. W.	Clear	Variable	Variable	
9	29.73	29.70	29.68	66	74	69	69.7	S. W.	S. W.	S. W.	Rain	Cloudy	Cloudy	
10	29.58	29.54	29.50	67	77	64	69.3	S. W.	S. W.	S. W.	Cloudy	Variable	Rain	0.25
11	29.57	29.60	29.62	58	66	55	59.7	N. W.	S. E.	N. W.	Variable	Rain	Variable	0.25
12	29.74	29.79	29.94	49	64	52	55.0	N. W.	N. W.	N. W.	Clear	Clear	Clear	
13	30.00	30.00	29.99	44	63	51	52.7	N. W.	N. W.	N. W.	Clear	Clear	Clear	
14	29.87	29.82	29.81	44	66	55	55.0	N. W.	N. W.	N. W.	Clear	Clear	Clear	
15	29.75	29.74	29.78	54	72	59	65.0	N. W'ly	N. W.	N. W.	Clear	Clear	Clear	
16	29.84	29.84	29.89	53	73	60	62.0	N. W.	S. E'ly	S. E'ly	Clear	Clear	Clear	
17	29.90	29.83	29.79	60	74	62	65.3	S'ly	S. E'ly	S. E'ly	Foggy	Clear	Clear	
18	29.73	29.72	29.68	62	74	67	67.7	S. W'ly	S'ly	S'ly	Clear	Clear	Cloudy	
19	29.51	29.48	29.49	64	68	56	62.7	S. E.	W'ly	N. W.	Rain	Clear	Clear	0.95
20	29.39	29.29	29.30	50	70	62	60.7	W'ly	W'ly	S. W'ly	Clear	Clear	Cloudy	
21	29.40	29.50	29.73	52	59	45	52.0	N. W.	N. W.	N. W.	Clear	Clear	Clear	
22	29.90	29.95	29.95	38	58	45	47.0	N. W.	N. W.	N. W.	Clear	Clear	Clear	
23	29.91	29.90	29.92	42	73	54	56.3	W'ly	W'ly	W'ly	Clear	Clear	Clear	
24	30.07	30.12	30.12	48	57	46	50.3	N'ly	N. E.	N. E.	Clear	Cloudy	Clear	
25	30.10	30.07	30.06	40	64	50	51.3	N. E.	N. E.	S. E.	Clear	Clear	Clear	
26	30.04	...	29.92	46	...	52	...	S'ly	S. W'ly	S. W'ly	Clear	Clear	Clear	
27	29.80	29.70	...	52	72	71	66.3	S. W.	S. W.	S. W.	Foggy	Variable	Rain	0.50
28	29.75	29.79	29.87	56	66	47	56.3	N. W.	N. W.	N. W.	Clear	Clear	Clear	
29	[illegible]	[illegible]	[illegible]	[illegible]	[illegible]	54	55.0	N. W.	N. W.	N. W.	Clear	Clear	Clear	
30	[illegible]	[illegible]	[illegible]	[illegible]	71	62	[illegible]	N. W.	S. W.	S. W.	Clear	Clear	Variable	
Means	29.83	29.81	29.84	53.1	68.2	56.9	...	...	...	...	...	...	...	2.95

REDUCED TO SEA LEVEL.							
Max.	31.04	31.02	31.02	67	77	69	69.7
Min.	29.57	29.47	29.48	40	56	45	47.0
Mean	30.01	29.98	30.02				
Range	1.47	1.55	1.54	27	21	24	22.7
Mean of month	30.003			...	...	...	59.4
Extreme range	1.57			...	...	...	37.0

Prevailing winds from some point between—

	Days.
N. & E.	4
E. & S.	2
S. & W.	10
W. & N.	14

	Days.
Clear	17
Variable } Cloudy }	5
Rain fell on	8

REMARKS.

1st. Fine. Sun very hot, and ground very dry.
2d. Fine. Sun very hot, and ground very dry. Fine shower in the evening.
3d. Very fine. Pleasantly cool.
4th. Fine.
5th. Steady rain during morning. Occasional rain in afternoon. Wind light N. E., and quite cool.
6th. Variable, but pleasant. Evening very mild and clear.
7th Very fine.
8th. Pleasant.
9th. Very light rain in the morning. Cloudy through the day.
10th. Cloudy in the morning. Light shower and gust at 3 P. M. Shower in the evening.
11th. Variable in the morning. Showery in the afternoon.
12th. Fine, but cool.
13th. Very fine, though cool.
14th and 15th. Very fine.
16th. Fine.
17th. Fine. Fog in the morning.
18th. Fine. Heavy rain during the night, with thunder.
19th. Rain in morning. Cleared before noon.
20th. Very blustering. Cloudy, with appearances of rain in the evening.
21st. Clear and cool. Wind fresh N. W. Faint aurora all night.
22d. Very fine.
23d and 24th. Fine.
25th and 26th. Very fine.
27th. Foggy in the morning; variable. Rain moderate in the evening.
28th. Cool but pleasant.
29th and 30th. Mild and pleasant.

October, 1840.

DAYS	BAROMETER, REDUCED TO 32° F. Sunrise.	At 1 P. M.	At 10 P. M.	THERMOMETER. Sunrise.	At 1 P. M.	At 10 P. M.	Daily mean.	WINDS. Sunrise.	At 1 P. M.	At 10 P. M.	WEATHER. Sunrise.	At 1 P. M.	At 10 P. M.	RAIN AND SNOW IN INCHES OF WATER.
1	29.89	29.92	29.98	56	57	56	56.3	N. E.	N. E.	N. E.	Misty	Misty	Misty	
2	29.89	29.98	29.96	52	67	62	60.3	N. E.	N. E.	N. E.	Misty	Misty	Misty	
3	29.81	29.70	29.74	63	72	58	64.3	S'ly	S. W.	W'ly	Misty	M't & r'n	Cloudy	0.25
4	29.82	29.91	29.89	43	62	50	51.7	W'ly	W'ly	S. W.	Clear	Clear	Clear	
5	29.90	29.81	29.82	48	68	54	56.7	S. W.	S. W.	S. W.	Clear	Clear	Clear	
6	29.90	29.75	29.75	52	73	59	64.3	S. W.	S. W.	S. W.	Clear	Clear	Clear	
7	29.90	29.91	30.00	56	64	49	56.3	S. W.	N. E.	N. E.	Clear	Clear	Clear	
8	30.04	29.98	29.99	43	68	53	54.7	N. E.	S. W.	S. W.	Clear	Clear	Clear	
9	29.91	29.99	30.04	53	60	46	53.0	S. W.	N. E.	N. E.	Clear	Cloudy	Cloudy	
10	30.04	30.02	29.97	36	56	44	45.3	N'ly	N'ly	S. W'ly	Clear	Clear	Clear	
11	29.80	29.60	29.36	50	58	62	56.7	S. W.	S. W.	S. W.	Cloudy	Rain	Cloudy	0.20
12	29.19	29.30	29.41	63	65	49	59.0	S. W.	W'ly	N. W.	Clear	Clear	Variable	
13	29.53	29.69	29.70	37	53	44	64.7	N. W.	N. W.	W'ly	Clear	Clear	Clear	
14	29.63	29.60	29.62	46	67	56	56.3	S. W'ly	S. W.	W'ly	Clear	Clear	Clear	
15	29.75	...	29.90	44	...	38	...	N.	...	N. W.	Clear	...	Clear	
16	29.96	30.01	30.07	34	47	36	39.0	N. W.	N. W.	N. W.	Clear	Clear	Clear	
17	30.16	30.15	30.16	31½	53	41	41.7	N. E.	N. E'ly	S. W'ly	Clear	Variable	Variable	
18	30.17	30.16	30.15	41	57	50	49.3	W'ly	S. W.	S. W.	Variable	Cloudy	Variable	
19	30.04	29.97	29.93	50	59	60	56.3	S. W.	S. E.	S'ly	Cloudy	Misty	Cloudy	
20	29.83	29.79	29.81	63	67	63	64.3	S. W.	S. W.	S. W.	Rain	Misty	Cloudy	} 2.37
21	29.79	29.68	29.42	58	60	52	56.7	N. E.	N. E.	N. E.	Rain	Rain	Rain	
22	29.36	29.55	29.80	48	52	39	46.3	N. W.	N. W.	N. W.	Cloudy	Clear	Clear	
23	29.80	29.68	29.59	37	60	54	50.3	S. W.	S. W.	S. W.	Clear	Clear	Clear	
24	29.80	29.86	29.90	42	53	44	46.3	W'ly	N. W.	N. W.	Clear	Clear	Clear	
25	29.86	29.69	29.59	38	44	40	40.7	N. E.	N. E.	N. E.	Variable	Cloudy	Var., sn.	0.15
26	29.41	29.46	29.61	32	39	35	35.3	W'ly	W'ly	W'ly	Cloudy	Clear	Clear	
27	29.98	30.03	30.10	30	43	32	35.0	W'ly	W'ly	W'ly	Clear	Clear	Clear	
28	30.11	30.02	29.96	31	49	51	43.7	S. E.	S. E.	S'ly	Cloudy	Rain	Variable	} 22.0
29	29.97	29.79	29.57	50	60	60	56.7	S. E.	S. E.	S. E'ly	Rain	Rain	Cloudy	
30	29.39	29.34	29.44	60	65	53	59.3	S'ly	S. W'ly	W'ly	Rain	Misty	Variable	
31	29.60	29.53	29.55	46	52	43	47.0	N. W.	N. W.	N'ly	Variable	Cloudy	Variable	
Means	29.81	29.79	29.80	46.2	58.3	49.4	...	...	...	...	...	...	...	5.17
REDUCED TO SEA LEVEL.														
Max.	30.35	30.34	30.34	63	73	63	64.7							
Min.	29.37	29.48	29.54	30	43	32	35.0							
Mean	29.99	29.96	29.98											
Range	0.98	0.86	0.80	33	30	31	29.7							
Mean of month	29.967			...	...	...	51.3							
Extreme range	0.98			...	...	...	43.0							

Prevailing winds from some point between—

	Days.
N. & E.	7
E. & S.	3
S. & W.	14
W. & N.	7

	Days.
Clear	13
Variable, Cloudy	} 10
Rain or snow fell on	8

REMARKS.

1st and 2d. Wind light N. E. Mist all day.
3d. Mist through the day. Wind S. W'ly, rather fresh. Showers about sunset.
4th to 8th. Very fine.
9th. Cloudy for the most part.
10th. Fine.
11th. Cloudy in the morning. Light rain in the afternoon, with some mist.
12th to 15th. Fine.
16th. First white frost in the College yard—very slight. The day fine.
17th. Pretty severe frost. Weather fine.
18th. Mild. Cloudy for the most part.
19th. Cloudy, with frequent mist.
20th. Light rain in the morning. Cloudy, with occasional mist, through the day.
21st. Moderate rain nearly all day; wind light N. E. Rain continued through the night.
22d. Cloudy in the morning. Cleared in the afternoon. Fine in the evening.
23d and 24th. Very fine.
25th. Cold. Raw N. E. wind, with sprinkling of rain and some hail. During the night, wind came to N. W. and W'ly, with snow nearly an inch deep.
26th. At sunrise, wind blustering from W'ly. Ground covered with snow. Thermometer 32°. Snow remained on the roofs of the houses all day.
27th. Cool, but pleasant.
28th. Wind S. E. Sprinkling of rain in afternoon.
29th. Cloudy, with some rain. Wind fresh S. E.; became more fresh at night, with heavy rain.
30th. Rain and mist in the morning; wind S. by W. nearly. Clouds broken in the afternoon, and clear some part of the evening.
31st. Variable, with the wind light N. W. and N'ly.

November, 1840.

DAYS	BAROMETER Sunrise.	At 1 P. M.	At 10 P. M.	THERMOMETER Sunrise.	At 1 P. M.	At 10 P. M.	Daily mean.	WINDS Sunrise.	At 1 P. M.	At 10 P. M.	WEATHER Sunrise.	At 1 P. M.	At 10 P. M.	RAIN AND SNOW
1	29.80	29.84	29.99	35	49	40	41.3	N. W.	N. W.	N. W.	Clear	Clear	Clear	
2	30.15	30.18	30.19	32	50	38	40.0	N. W.	N. E.	E'ly	Clear	Clear	Clear	
3	30.07	29.98	29.94	34	51	43	42.7	N. E.	N. E.	N. E.	Clear	Variable	Variable	
4	29.90	29.87	29.89	43	48	43	44.7	N. E.	N. E.	N. E.	Cloudy	Cloudy	Variable	
5	29.80	29.76	29.74	43	50	44	49.0	N. E.	N. E.	N. E.	Cloudy	Variable	Variable	
6	29.65	29.60	29.74	44	51	47	47.3	N. E.	N. E'ly	N. E.	Cloudy	Cloudy	Variable	
7	29.85	29.87	29.90	44	44	45	44.3	N. E.	N. E.	N. E.	Cloudy	Cloudy	Variable	
8	29.85	29.74	29.61	45	50	50	48.3	N. E.	E'ly	E'ly	Cloudy	Cloudy	Rain	1.45
9	29.39	29.34	29.39	50	56	50	52.0	N. E.	E'ly	N. E.	Rain	Misty	Rain	} 1.15
10	29.54	29.60	29.65	38	45	44	42.3	N. E.	N.	N. by E.	Rain	Variable	Cloudy	
11	29.74	29.79	29.81	41	44	42	42.3	N. by E.	N. E'ly	N. by E.	Misty	Cloudy	Cloudy	
12	29.77	29.74	29.59	43	46	44	44.3	N. E'ly	N. E'ly	N'ly	Cloudy	M't & r'n	Cloudy	0.40
13	29.55	29.49	29.59	42	50	41	44.3	N. W.	N. W.	N. W.	Clear	Clear	Clear	
14	29.70	29.70	29.71	32	46	37	38.3	N. W.	N. W.	N. W.	Clear	Clear	Clear	
15	29.49	29.39	29.59	38	49	36	41.0	E'ly	S. W'ly	N. W.	Rain	Cloudy	Clear	0.50
16	29.65	29.64	29.66	28	41	34	34.3	N. W.	W'ly	W'ly	Clear	Cloudy	Cloudy	
17	29.71	29.66	29.66	27	40	37	35.7	W'ly	W'ly	W'ly	Clear	Clear	Variable	
18	...	...	29.38	...	...	30	...	W'ly	N'ly	N. E.	Variable	Cloudy	Snow	
19	29.29	28.36	29.49	26	35	26	29.7	N. W.	N. W.	N. W.	Snow	Variable	Clear	} 0.75
20	29.62	29.64	29.78	28	34	25	29.0	N. W.	N. W.	N. W.	Clear	Clear	Clear	
21	29.91	29.90	29.94	20	37	32	29.7	N. W.	N. W.	N. W.	Clear	Clear	Clear	
22	29.96	29.85	29.75	26	33	35	31.3	N. E.	N. E.	N. E.	Variable	Cloudy	Rain	1.00
23	29.38	29.36	29.50	35	30	32	32.3	N.	N.	N. W.	Misty	Misty	Clear	
24	29.80	29.82	29.90	32	43	36	37.0	N. W.	N. W'ly	N. W.	Clear	Variable	Variable	
25	29.80	29.69	29.50	36	46	33	39.0	W'ly	S'ly	N. E.	Cloudy	Cloudy	R'n & sn.	0.10
26	29.46	29.53	29.60	32	38	34	34.7	N. W.	N. W.	N. E.	Cloudy	Variable	Cloudy	
27	29.67	29.73	29.84	28	32	26	29.3	N. W.	N. W.	N. W.	Clear	Clear	Clear	
28	29.89	29.86	29.81	25	39	32	32.0	W'ly	W'ly	W'ly	Cloudy	Variable	Clear	
29	29.81	29.74	29.59	30	47	43	40.0	S. W'ly	S'ly	S'ly	Variable	Clear	Variable	
30	29.56	29.40	29.51	42	58	36	45.3	S. W.	S. W.	W'ly	Clear	Clear	Clear	
Means	29.71	29.69	29.70	35.1	44.6	37.8	...	...	...	...	...	...	...	5.35
REDUCED TO SEA LEVEL.														
Max.	30.33	30.36	30.37	50	58	50	52.0							
Min.	29.47	29.52	29.56	20	30	25	29.0							
Mean	29.89	29.87	29.88											
Range	0.86	0.84	0.81	30	28	25	23.0							
Mean of month	29.880			...	...	...	39.2							
Extreme range	0.90			...	...	...	38.0							

Prevailing winds from some point between—

	Days.
N. & E.	13
E. & S.	2
S. & W.	3
W. & N.	12

	Days.
Clear	9
Variable, Cloudy	} 12
Rain or snow fell on	9

REMARKS.

1st. Fine.
2d. Very fine.
3d. Fine; clear for the most part. Evening hazy. Bow about the moon. Air raw.
4th and 5th. Cloudy for the most part.
6th. Cloudy for the most part. Wind fresh; increased at night.
7th. Cloudy. Air damp and raw.
8th. Cloudy, with occasional rain in evening.
9th. Rain in the morning and evening.
10th. Rain in the morning. Clouds broken at noon. Variable in the afternoon and evening.
11th. Mist at intervals. Wind raw at about N. by E. all day.
12th. Rain in the afternoon; wind about N. N. E. Cloudy in the evening; wind N. N. W.
13th. Fine. Aurora in the evening, considerably bright till the rising of the moon at about 8½ o'clock.
14th. Very fine. Hazy in the evening. Rain during the night.
15th. Rain in the morning; wind E'ly. Wind came to S. and S. W. before 1 P. M.; then to W., and before night to N. W. Clear in the evening. Aurora not bright.
16th and 17th. Fine.
18th. Wind W'ly in the morning; hazy. Wind came to N'ly before noon, with clouds increasing, and to N. E. before night. Began to snow about 5½ P. M.
19th. Seven or eight inches of snow in the morning.
20th and 21st. Fine.
22d. Variable in the morning. Began to rain at 2 P. M., and continued moderately through the afternoon and night.
23d. Mist all day; wind N'ly. Clear in the evening.
24th. Weather mild.
25th. Wind very variable—W'ly, S'ly, S. E'ly, N'ly, and N. E'ly. Commenced raining moderately from 5 to 6 P. M.
26th. Weather variable.
27th and 28th. Weather variable and raw.
29th. Mild and pleasant.
30th. Mild and pleasant. Wind S. W., which became fresh in the afternoon and evening.

December, 1840.

DAYS.	BAROMETER, REDUCED TO 32° F. Sunrise.	At 1 P. M.	At 10 P. M.	THERMOMETER. Sunrise.	At 1 P. M.	At 10 P. M.	Daily mean.	WINDS. Sunrise.	At 1 P. M.	At 10 P. M.	WEATHER. Sunrise.	At 1 P. M.	At 10 P. M.	RAIN AND SNOW IN INCHES OF WATER.
1	29.91	30.01	30.11	22	29	20	23.7	N. W.	N. W.	N. W.	Clear	Variable	Clear	
2	30.14	30.10	30.06	15	37	31	27.7	N. W.	S. W.	W'ly	Clear	Clear	Clear	
3	30.02	30.02	30.17	31	44	31	35.3	S. W.	S. W.	W'ly	Clear	Clear	Clear	
4	30.27	30.30	30.28	16	26	20	21.3	N. W.	N. E.	N. E.	Clear	Variable	Cloudy	
5	30.22	30.21	30.21	17	18	18	17.7	N. E.	N'ly	N. E.	Snow	Cloudy	Cloudy	} 0.75
6	30.17	30.00	29.80	18	30	30	26.0	N. E'ly	N. E'ly	N. E'ly	Cloudy	Snow	Sn. & h'l	
7	29.96	29.95	30.06	21	32	24	25.7	N'ly	N'ly	N. W.	Variable	Variable	Clear	
8	30.06	29.95	29.84	17	36	32	28.3	N. W.	S'ly	S. W'ly	Clear	Clear	Variable	
9	29.81	29.80	29.75	27	43	32	34.0	W'ly	W'ly	W'ly	Clear	Clear	Clear	
10	29.63	29.57	29.68	37	44	36	39.0	S. E'ly	S. W.	S. W.	Cloudy	Clear	Clear	
11	29.80	29.90	30.02	29	37	26	30.7	N. W.	N. W.	N. W.	Clear	Clear	Clear	
12	30.05	30.01	29.80	18	38	38	31.3	N. W.	S. E.	S. E.	Clear	Cloudy	Cloudy	
13	29.40	29.29	29.39	49	52	42	47.7	S. E.	S. W.	W'ly	Rain	Cloudy	Clear	0.75
14	29.47	29.40	29.50	36	45	36	39.0	W'ly	W'ly	W'ly	Clear	Clear	Clear	
15	29.52	29.54	29.54	36	45	44	41.7	S. W.	S. W.	S. W'ly	Clear	Clear	Variable	
16	29.49	29.53	29.39	38	47	31	38.7	S. W.	N. W.	N. E.	Clear	Clear	R'n & sn.	0.25
17	29.40	29.46	29.60	27	28	21	25.3	N. W.	N. W.	N. W.	Clear	Clear	Clear	
18	29.71	29.71	29.73	13	24	12	16.3	N. W.	N. W.	N. W.	Clear	Clear	Clear	
19	29.72	29.70	29.75	12	27	24	21.0	W'ly	W'ly	W'ly	Clear	Clear	Clear	
20	29.85	29.84	29.87	19	32	26	25.7	W'ly	N. W.	N. W.	Clear	Clear	Clear	
21	29.75	29.81	29.92	20	29	15	21.3	N. W.	N. W.	N. W.	Clear	Clear	Clear	
22	29.77	29.45	29.40	18	36	29	27.7	S'ly	S. W'ly	W'ly	Snow	Cloudy	Variable	0.15
23	29.69	29.80	29.64	14	21	24	19.7	N. W.	N. W.	W'ly	Clear	Clear	Variable	
24	29.46	29.59	29.71	29	26	11	22.0	S. W.	N. W.	N. W.	Clear	Clear	Clear	
25	29.80	29.80	29.81	4	15	7	12.0	N. W.	N. W.	N. W.	Clear	Clear	Clear	
26	29.72	29.53	29.33	9	26	32	19.0	N. E.	N. E.	E'ly	Cloudy	Snow	Snow	1.10
27	29.34	29.40	29.47	22	22	22	22.0	N. E.	N. E.	N. E.	Cloudy	Cloudy	Cloudy	
28	29.62	...	29.80	14	...	22	18.0	N. W.	...	N. W.	Clear	...	Clear	
29	29.92	29.94	29.97	20	35	32	29.0	S. W.	S. W.	S'ly	Clear	Clear	Cloudy	
30	30.00	29.97	29.96	31	40	33	34.7	S. W.	S. E.	N. E'ly	Variable	Cloudy	Cloudy	
31	29.90	29.83	29.84	31	40	34	35.0	N. E.	N. E.	W'ly	Snow	Cloudy	Cloudy	0.10
Means	29.79	29.78	29.79	22.9	33.4	26.9	...	...	...	...	...	...	...	3.10

REDUCED TO SEA LEVEL.	Sunrise.	At 1 P. M.	At 10 P. M.	Sunrise.	At 1 P. M.	At 10 P. M.	Daily mean.
Max.	30.45	30.48	30.46	49	52	44	47.7
Min.	29.52	29.47	29.51	4	15	7	12.0
Mean	29.97	29.96	29.97				
Range	0.93	1.01	0.95	45	37	37	35.7
Mean of month	29.967			...	...	...	27.7
Extreme range	1.01			...	...	...	48.0

Prevailing winds from some point between—

	Days.
N. & E.	6
E. & S.	2
S. & W.	8
W. & N.	15

	Days
Clear	19
Variable } Cloudy }	5
Rain or snow fell on	7

REMARKS.

1st and 2d. Fine.
3d. Very fine.
4th. Raw and cold. Wind brisk N. and N. E.
5th. Light snow in the morning. Cold and blustering through the day.
6th. Cloudy in the morning; wind about E.N E., very fresh. Began to snow from 12 to 1 o'clock, and continued through the afternoon and evening.
7th. Pleasant. Snow five or six inches deep in the morning, rather wet.
8th to 11th. Fine.
12th. Cloudy. Wind S. E. in the afternoon, with appearances of rain.
13th. Heavy wind from S. E., and rain in the morning. Cloudy in the afternoon. Clear in the evening; wind W'ly.
14th. Fine.
15th. Very fine.
16th. Clear and pleasant in morning. Cloudy towards night. Began to rain and snow about 6 P. M.; wind N. E.
17th. About three inches of snow in the morning. Day fine.
18th. Cold, and rather blustering.
19th. Cold, but pleasant.
20th. Cool, but pleasant.
21st. Clear and cold.
22d. Snow in the morning. Cloudy in the afternoon. Variable in the evening. Snow from two to three inches deep.
23d. Cold, but fine. Variable in the evening.
24th. Wind S. W. at sunrise. Flurry of snow from 9 to 10 A. M., and wind came to N. W., and grew colder.
25th. Clear and cold. Wind light.
26th. Cloudy in the morning. Began to snow from 8 to 9 A. M., and continued moderately all day and evening.
27th. Ground covered with heavy snow six or seven inches deep.
28th. Pleasant.
29th. Mild and pleasant.
30th. Very mild.
31st. Very mild. Snow in the morning.

January, 1841.

DAYS.	BAROMETER Sunrise.	At 1 P. M.	At 10 P. M.	THERMOMETER Sunrise.	At 1 P. M.	At 10 P. M.	Daily mean.	WINDS Sunrise.	At 1 P. M.	At 10 P. M.	WEATHER Sunrise.	At 1 P. M.	At 10 P. M.	RAIN AND SNOW
1	29.91	29.72	29.00	18	23	37	26.0	N. E'ly	N. E.	E'ly	Variable	Snow	Rain	0.90
2	29.20	29.27	29.40	21	27	19	22.3	S. W.	S. W'ly	W'ly	Clear	Clear	Clear	
3	29.42	29.46	29.64	15	19	7	13.7	N. W.	N. W.	N. W.	Clear	Clear	Clear	
4	29.87	29.95	30.08	2	16	5	7.7	N. W.	N. W.	N. W.	Clear	Clear	Clear	
5	30.34	30.35	30.40	0	21	20	13.7	N. W.	W'ly	N. E.	Clear	Variable	Cloudy	
6	30.32	30.19	30.13	34	40	42	38.7	S. E.	S. E.	S. E.	Rain	Rain	Cloudy	} 2.00
7	30.00	29.88	29.78	45	50	48	47.7	S'ly	S. E'ly	S'ly	Rain	Cloudy	Rain	
8	29.72	29.77	29.81	47	53	40	46.7	S'ly	S'ly	N'ly	Cloudy	Variable	Cloudy	
9	29.83	29.85	29.90	35	39	35	36.3	N'ly	N. E.	N. E.	Cloudy	Cloudy	Cloudy	
10	29.93	29.89	29.88	32	34	33	33.0	N. E.	N. E.	N. E.	Cloudy	Cloudy	Cloudy	
11	29.83	29.67	29.49	33	40	36	36.3	N. E.	N. E.	N. E'ly	Misty	Rain	Cloudy	0.20
12	29.69	29.78	29.96	35	41	31	35.7	W'ly	W'ly	N. W.	Clear	Clear	Clear	
13	30.03	29.95	29.88	31	33	28	30.7	S. W.	N. E.	N. E.	Cloudy	Snow	Snow	0.70
14	30.01	30.07	30.14	20	26	22	22.7	N'ly	N'ly	N'ly	Variable	Variable	Cloudy	
15	30.11	30.00	29.99	21	32	32	28.3	N'ly	W'ly	N. E'ly	Variable	Variable	R'n & sn.	
16	30.12	30.10	30.13	32	40	35	35.7	N. W.	N. W.	N. E.	Clear	Clear	Cloudy	
17	29.83	29.59	29.49	43	47	49	46.3	S. E.	S. E.	W'ly	Rain	Rain	Variable	1.15
18	29.79	29.99	30.26	28	25	14	22.3	N. W.	N. W.	N. W.	Clear	Clear	Clear	
19	30.49	30.49	30.54	12	22	19	17.7	N. W.	N. W.	N. E'ly	Clear	Clear	Hazy	
20	30.54	30.44	30.31	18	26	26	23.3	N. E'ly	N. E.	N. E.	Cloudy	Clear	Cloudy	
21	29.79	29.49	29.42	32	35	32	33.0	N. E.	N. E.	N. E.	Rain	Rain	Cloudy	0.70
22	29.52	29.54	29.59	30	35	26	30.3	N. W.	N. W.	N. W.	Variable	Clear	Clear	
23	29.60	29.59	29.66	24	31	30	28.3	N. W.	N. W.	N. W.	Cloudy	Cloudy	Cloudy	
24	29.73	29.72	29.59	28	36	38	34.0	N. W.	S'ly	S. E'ly	Cloudy	Cloudy	Rain	
25	29.57	29.55	29.64	31	45	35	37.0	W'ly	S. W.	W'ly	Clear	Variable	Clear	
26	29.89	29.92	29.89	30	40	34	34.7	N. W.	W'ly	S. W'ly	Clear	Clear	Cloudy	
27	29.69	29.62	29.63	32	43	36	37.0	W'ly	W'ly	W'ly	Cloudy	Cloudy	Clear	
28	29.80	29.85	30.03	34	42	32	36.0	W'ly	W'ly	N. W.	Clear	Clear	Clear	
29	30.07	29.99	29.75	28	31	32	30.3	N. E.	N. E.	N. E.	Variable	Snow	Snow	0.80
30	29.72	29.61	29.79	27	36	24	29.0	W'ly	W'ly	N. W.	Clear	Clear	Clear	
31	29.82	29.71	29.63	22	39	33	31.3	S. W'ly	S. W'ly	S. W'ly	Clear	Clear	Clear	
Means	29.87	29.84	29.83	27.2	34.4	30.0	...	...	...	...	...	...	...	6.45

REDUCED TO SEA LEVEL.	Sunrise.	At 1 P. M.	At 10 P. M.	Sunrise.	At 1 P. M.	At 10 P. M.	Daily mean.
Max.	30.72	30.67	30.72	47	53	48	47.7
Min.	29.38	29.45	29.18	0	16	5	7.7
Mean	30.05	30.02	30.01				
Range	1.34	1.22	1.54	47	37	43	40.0
Mean of month	30.023			...	...	...	30.5
Extreme range	1.54			...	...	...	53.0

Prevailing winds from some point between—

	Days.
N. & E.	11
E. & S.	4
S. & W.	6
W. & N.	10

	Days.
Clear	10
Variable } Cloudy }	11
Rain or snow fell on	10

REMARKS.

1st. Variable at sunrise. Clouded, and began to snow from 1 to 2 P. M., pretty fast; turned to rain in the evening, with wind light E'ly.
2d. Clear and pleasant.
3d. Clear and cold.
4th. Very clear and cold, and calm.
5th. Very still and cold. Ther. at zero in the morning. Thermometers in low situations, —7°, —8°, and —10°.
6th. Light wind nearly all day. Wind light S. E'ly, and foggy.
7th. Very warm and showery. In the evening, wind brisk, with rain.
8th. Very warm and damp. Frost out of the ground in many places. Wind changed from S'ly to N'ly in the evening.
9th. Cloudy and mild.
10th. Cloudy all day, with some mist.
11th. Mist and occasional rain during the day and evening.
12th. Wind W'ly, very blustering.
13th. At sunrise, wind light S. W., and cloudy. Began to snow from 8 to 9 A. M., and wind came to N. E. Snow continued all day and evening.
14th. In morning, 6 or 7 inches of compact snow. Cloudy for the most part, and raw.
15th. Variable. Light rain and snow in evening.
16th. Very pleasant.
17th. Began to rain about sunrise, with wind S. E. Rain continued all day; heavy in afternoon, with wind brisk S. W'ly. Barometer began to rise from 8 to 9 P. M. Some stars appeared.
18th. Grew cold. Wind fresh N. W.
19th. Wind very light. Barometer extraordinarily high. Hazy in the evening.
20th. Wind very light N. E. Raw in afternoon; wind increasing. Snow towards morning.
21st. Rain and snow; turned to rain; continued through morning. Cloudy afternoon and evening.
22d. Fine. 23d. Cloudy and mild.
24th. Cloudy. Wind S'ly and S. E'ly in the afternoon, and raw. Began to rain moderately from 7 to 8 P. M.
25th. Variable. Cloudy early in the evening, with some rain. Clear at 10 P. M.
26th. Clear through day. Cloudy in evening.
27th. Mild through the day and cloudy. Very clear in the evening.
28th. Very fine day.
29th. At sunrise, wind light from N. E. Mostly cloudy. Began to snow from 11 to 12 A. M. Snow continued through afternoon.
30th. Pleasant. Ground covered with about four or five inches of wet snow.
31st. Very fine.

February, 1841.

DAYS.	BAROMETER, REDUCED TO 32° F. Sun-rise.	At 1 P. M.	At 10 P. M.	THERMOMETER. Sun-rise.	At 1 P. M.	At 10 P. M.	Daily mean.	WINDS. Sun-rise.	At 1 P. M.	At 10 P. M.	WEATHER. Sunrise.	At 1 P. M.	At 10 P. M.	RAIN AND SNOW IN INCHES OF WATER.
1	29.66	29.51	29.16	30	35	24	29.7	W'ly	N. E.	N. E.	Variable	Cloudy	Snow	1.25
2	29.40	29.59	29.62	17	27	20	21.3	N. W'ly	W'ly	W'ly	Clear	Clear	Cloudy	
3	29.40	29.43	29.79	33	32	18	27.7	S. W.	N. W'ly	N. W.	Cloudy	Clear	Clear	
4	30.00	29.99	30.00	12	28	20	20.0	N. W.	N. W.	N. W.	Clear	Clear	Clear	
5	29.97	29.87	29.76	15	35	23	24.3	W'ly	W'ly	W'ly	Variable	Clear	Clear	
6	29.74	29.69	29.75	22	40	30	30.7	W'ly	W'ly	W'ly	Variable	Variable	Clear	
7	29.90	29.89	29.89	27	40	27	31.3	W'ly	W'ly	W'ly	Variable	Clear	Clear	
8	29.99	29.99	29.99	21	30	24	28.3	N. W.	N. W.	N. W.	Clear	Clear	Clear	
9	29.90	29.79	29.60	18	40	29	29.0	N. W.	W'ly	N. E.	Clear	Cloudy	Snow	0.25
10	29.47	29.45	29.60	27	35	18	23.3	N. W'ly	W'ly	N. W.	Clear	Clear	Clear	
11	29.68	29.62	29.62	9	24	12	15.0	N. W.	N. W.	N. W.	Clear	Clear	Clear	
12	29.66	29.59	29.58	2	15	6	7.7	N. W.	N. W.	N. W.	Clear	Clear	Clear	
13	29.50	29.46	29.60	2	17	14	7.7	N. W.	N. W.	N. W.	Clear	Clear	Clear	
14	29.63	29.64	29.57	10	24	12	15.3	N. W.	W'ly	N'ly	Clear	Clear	Clear	
15	29.51	29.50	29.63	9	19	11	13.0	N. W.	N. W.	N. W.	Variable	Variable	Clear	
16	29.63	29.61	29.63	14	29	22	21.7	S. W'ly	S. W'ly	S. W.	Clear	Clear	Clear	
17	29.55	29.54	29.70	25	31	22	29.3	N. E.	N. E.	N. E.	Snow	Cloudy	Cloudy	
18	29.87	29.83	29.73	14	25	22	20.3	N. W'ly	N. W.	N. W.	Clear	Clear	Clear	
19	29.42	29.25	29.31	28	38	30	32.0	S. W.	S. W'ly	N. W.	Variable	Cloudy	Variable	
20	29.43	29.37	29.36	17	32	27	25.7	W'ly	W'ly	W'ly	Clear	Clear	Clear	
21	29.29	29.26	29.39	30	45	36	37.0	W'ly	S. W.	W'ly	Clear	Clear	Variable	
22	29.43	29.43	29.33	29	33	30	30.7	N'ly	N'ly	W'ly	Cloudy	Variable	Cloudy	
23	29.10	29.09	29.67	36	43	16	31.7	S. W.	S. W.	N. W.	Clear	Clear	Clear	
24	29.92	29.91	29.92	12	27	15	18.0	N. W.	N. W.	N. W.	Clear	Variable	Clear	
25	30.01	29.98	29.94	12	30	28	23.3	W'ly	S. E.	W'ly	Clear	Clear	Clear	
26	29.90	29.84	29.81	30	44	34	36.0	S. W.	S. W.	S'ly	Cloudy	Clear	Clear	
27	29.60	29.37	29.51	34	42	35	37.0	E'ly	N. E'ly	N. W.	Rain	Misty	Clear	
28	29.65	29.69	29.71	30	44	35	36.3	W'ly	W'ly	W'ly	Clear	Clear	Clear	
Means	29.65	29.61	29.65	20.2	32.2	22.9	...	...	...	...	...	...	...	1.50
REDUCED TO SEA LEVEL.														
Max.	30.19	30.17	30.12	36	45	36	37.0							
Min.	29.28	29.27	29.34	2	15	6	7.7							
Mean	29.83	29.79	29.83											
Range	0.91	0.90	0.78	34	30	30	29.3							
Mean of month	29.827			...	...	...	25.1							
Extreme range	0.92			...	...	...	43.0							

Prevailing winds from some point between—

	Days.
N. & E.	4
E. & S.	1
S. & W.	8
W. & N.	15

	Days.
Clear	16
Variable } Cloudy }	8
Rain or snow fell on	4

REMARKS.

1st. Mild and calm in the morning. Began to snow from 3 to 4 P. M. Snow thick, and the wind very fresh in the evening. Nine or ten inches of snow fell during the night.

2d. Fine.

3d. Dash of rain from 11 to 12 A. M., with gust, and change of wind from S. W'ly to N. W'ly.

4th. Very fine. Halo round the moon in the evening.

5th. Fine. Total eclipse of the moon in the evening.

6th. Very mild. Wind light W'ly.

7th. Very mild and pleasant.

8th. Very fine. Aurora considerably bright from 7 to 8½ P. M., when the approach of the moon extinguished it.

9th. Mild. Began to snow from 8 to 9 P. M.

10th. About three inches of snow on the ground. Fine during the day. Grew cold at night.

11th. Very clear.

12th. Very clear and cold. Wind light; more fresh at night.

13th. Clear and cold. Wind fresh in the morning, light in the afternoon.

14th. Clear and cold

15th. Variable and cold.

16th. Fine and milder.

17th. Flurry of snow in the morning. Cloudy during the afternoon, with mist and snow in the air.

18th. Fine.

19th. Cloudy for the most part. Weather mild.

20th. Fine.

21st. Very fine.

22d. Mild. Aurora in the evening considerably bright.

23d. Mild in the morning; wind light S. W. From 3 to 4 P. M., wind came to N. W., with a marked change of temperature.

24th. Clear for the most part.

25th and 26th. Very fine.

27th. Rainy in the morning; wind light N. E'ly. Cleared in the afternoon; mild.

28th. Very fine.

March, 1841.

DAYS.	BAROMETER. Sun-rise.	At 1 P. M.	At 10 P. M.	THERMOMETER. Sun-rise.	At 1 P. M.	At 10 P. M.	Daily mean.	WINDS. Sun-rise.	At 1 P. M.	At 10 P. M.	WEATHER. Sunrise.	At 1 P. M.	At 10 P. M.	RAIN AND SNOW.
1	29.65	29.59	29.62	34	47	37	39.3	W'ly	W'ly	W'ly	Clear	Cloudy	Clear	
2	29.75	29.78	29.78	35	45	30	36.7	N'ly	N. E'ly	N. E.	Clear	Clear	Hazy	
3	29.69	29.59	29.58	30	43	33	35.3	N. E.	N. E.	N. E.	Cloudy	Cloudy	Cloudy	
4	29.72	29.79	29.94	27	32	20	26.3	N. W.	N. W.	N. W.	Clear	Clear	Clear	
5	30.12	30.12	30.14	11	25	20	18.7	N. W.	N. W.	N. W.	Clear	Clear	Clear	
6	30.15	30.00	29.60	19	35	30	28.0	N. E.	S. E'ly	N. E'ly	Variable	Cloudy	Snow	0.75
7	29.11	29.16	29.29	37	42	36	38.3	S. W'ly	W'ly	W'ly	Cloudy	Variable	Variable	
8	29.27	29.31	29.55	30	39	28	32.3	W'ly	W'ly	N. W.	Cloudy	Cloudy	Variable	
9	29.62	29.85	29.99	26	42	31	33.0	W'ly	W'ly	W'ly	Clear	Clear	Clear	
10	29.99	29.96	29.86	30	38	32	33.3	W'ly	S. W'ly	S. W'ly	Variable	Cloudy	Snow	0.15
11	29.80	29.79	30.00	29	39	26	31.3	N. W.	S. W.	N. W.	Clear	Clear	Clear	
12	30.12	30.07	29.87	19	36	26	27.0	N. W.	N. E.	N. E.	Clear	Cloudy	Cloudy	
13	29.12	28.90	29.20	28	38	28	31.3	E'ly	S. W'ly	W'ly	Snow	Clear	Clear	1.00
14	29.36	29.47	29.60	21	34	32	29.0	N. W.	N. W.	N. W.	Clear	Clear	Clear	
15	29.85	29.90	30.00	20	26	21	22.3	N. W.	N. W.	N. W.	Clear	Clear	Clear	
16	30.01	29.98	30.07	17	26	20	21.0	N. E.	N. E.	N'ly	Cloudy	Snow	Variable	0.33
17	30.21	30.16	30.11	16	27	20	21.0	N.	N. E.	N. E.	Variable	Clear	Clear	
18	29.95	29.84	29.71	21	33	35	29.7	N. E.	N. E.	N. E.	Cloudy	Cloudy	Cloudy	
19	29.74	29.74	29.79	33	57	44	44.7	N.	N. W.	N. W.	Clear	Clear	Clear	
20	29.79	29.68	29.69	34	63	49	48.7	S. W.	S. W'ly	W'ly	Clear	Clear	Clear	
21	29.74	29.78	29.99	40	46	34	40.0	W'ly	W.	N. W.	Clear	Clear	Clear	
22	30.11	30.12	30.06	26	46	35	35.7	N. W.	S'ly	S'ly	Clear	Clear	Hazy	
23	29.79	29.63	29.50	38	54	49	47.0	S. W.	S. W.	S. W.	Cloudy	Cloudy	Rain	0.33
24	29.69	29.69	29.70	34	54	41	43.0	N. W.	N. W.	N. W.	Clear	Clear	Clear	
25	29.87	29.88	29.90	36	54	49	46.3	N. W.	S. W.	S. W.	Clear	Clear	Clear	
26	29.84	29.79	29.76	38	60	52	50.0	S. W.	S. W.	S. W.	Clear	Clear	Clear	
27	29.75	29.73	29.70	51	63	48	54.0	S. W.	S. E.	S'ly	Clear	Clear	Variable	
28	29.63	29.66	29.79	47	60	44	50.3	S. W.	N. E.	N. E.	Cloudy	Cloudy	Cloudy	
29	29.85	29.69	29.43	37	36	33	35.3	N. E.	N. E.	N. E.	Rain	Rain	Cloudy	0.30
30	29.52	29.72	29.99	31	32	23	28.7	N. E.	N. E.	N. E.	Cloudy	Cloudy	Clear	
31	30.11	30.05	30.00	19	38	31	29.3	N. W.	N. W.	S'ly	Clear	Clear	Clear	
Means	29.78	29.72	29.77	29.5	42.3	33.4	...	...	...	...	...	...	...	2.86
REDUCED TO SEA LEVEL.														
Max.	30.39	30.34	30.32	51	63	52	54.0							
Min.	29.29	29.34	29.38	11	25	20	18.7							
Mean	29.96	29.90	29.95											
Range	1.10	1.00	0.94	40	38	32	35.3							
Mean of month	29.937			...	...	...	35.1							
Extreme range	1.10			...	...	...	52.0							

Prevailing winds from some point between—

	Days.
N. & E.	9
E. & S.	2
S. & W.	10
W. & N.	10

	Days.
Clear	17
Variable } Cloudy }	5
Rain or snow fell on	9

REMARKS.

1st. Very fine.

2d. Very fine. Halo about moon in evening.

3d Cloudy for the most part; mild. In evening, wind N. E., while the clouds came from W'ly.

4th. Very fine.

5th. Very clear, but cold.

6th. Cloudy in the morning; wind light N. E; came to E'ly and S. E. before noon, and clouds continued. Began to snow from 4 to 5 P. M., with wind about E. N. E., very fresh. Heavy wind, rain, and snow during the night.

7th. Cloudy. Wet under foot. Weather mild.

8th. In the morning, ground covered with four or five inches of damp snow, which fell during the night. Weather blustering.

9th. Pleasant.

10th. Cloudy. Flurry of snow in the afternoon, and snow in the evening.

11th. Three or four inches of light snow fell during the previous night. Pleasant during day.

12th. Raw and unpleasant. Snow during the night, with a heavy blow from N. E'ly.

13th. In the morning, ground covered with wet snow, four or five inches deep on an average, considerably drifted. Storm moderated. From 10 to 12 A. M., wind came round to S. W'ly. Cleared in the afternoon; still blustering.

14th. Pleasant, but cool.

15th. Wind brisk N. W., and cold quite severe.

16th. At sunrise, cloudy; wind N. E., rather light. Began to snow from 9 to 10 A. M.; wind increased, with driving snow all day. Cleared in the evening.

17th. Raw and cold.

18th. Cloudy, with slight sprinkling of rain.

19th. Very fine.

20th. Uncommonly mild.

21st. Very fine. In the afternoon, wind changed W'ly to N. W., and grew cooler.

22d. Fine.

23d. Wind S. W'ly, and damp during the day. Began to rain from 4 to 5 P. M. Rain, with thunder, in the evening.

24th. Very fine. Aurora in the evening—low and not very bright.

25th, 26th, and 27th. Very fine.

28th. Cloudy and mild.

29th. Light rain at intervals all day.

30th. Raw and cold.

31st. Clear and cold.

April, 1841.

DAYS.	BAROMETER, REDUCED TO 32° F. Sunrise.	At 1 P. M.	At 10 P. M.	THERMOMETER. Sunrise.	At 1 P. M.	At 10 P. M.	Daily mean.	WINDS. Sunrise.	At 1 P. M.	At 10 P. M.	WEATHER. Sunrise.	At 1 P. M.	At 10 P. M.	RAIN AND SNOW IN INCHES OF WATER.
1	29.80	29.64	29.73	34	48	41	41.0	S. W.	S. W.	S. W.	Cloudy	Variable	Clear	
2	29.75	29.73	29.27	34	60	51	48.3	S. W.	S. W.	S. W.	Foggy	Clear	Rain	0.75
3	29.58	29.73	29.92	34	44	37	38.3	N. W.	N. W.	N. W.	Clear	Clear	Clear	
4	30.01	29.89	29.65	34	50	45	43.0	S'ly	S. E.	S. E.	Clear	Cloudy	Rain	} 1.00
5	29.26	29.49	29.65	48	56	47	50.3	N. W.	N. W.	S. W.	Cloudy	Clear	Clear	
6	29.74	29.80	29.92	40	52	36	42.7	N. W.	N. W.	N. W.	Clear	Clear	Clear	
7	29.96	29.85	29.71	36	51	38	41.7	W'ly	S. W.	S. W'ly	Cloudy	Cloudy	Rain	0.33
8	29.60	29.59	29.68	37	51	41	43.0	W'ly	W'ly	S. E'ly	Cloudy	Variable	Clear	
9	29.69	...	...	41	...	...	...	W'ly	...	...	Cloudy	Rain	Cloudy	0.15
10	...	...	29.74	...	...	31	...	...	...	N. E.	...	...	Cloudy	
11	29.88	29.97	30.06	25	36	26	29.0	N. E.	N. E.	N. E.	Cloudy	Clear	Clear	
12	30.11	29.87	29.84	24	37	32	31.9	N. E.	E'ly	N. E'ly	Variable	Cloudy	Snow	} 1.75
13	29.61	29.57	29.62	28	32	30	30.0	N. E'ly	N.	N. W.	Snow	Snow	Clear	
14	29.64	29.68	29.79	27	45	36	36.0	N. W.	N. W.	N. W.	Variable	Clear	Clear	
15	29.92	30.07	30.21	30	42	34	35.3	N. W.	N. W.	N. W.	Clear	Clear	Clear	
16	30.26	30.24	30.16	31	47	37	38.3	N. W.	W'ly	S. W.	Clear	Clear	Clear	
17	30.01	29.85	29.71	40	46	45	43.7	S. W.	S. W.	S. W.	Variable	Rain	Cloudy	} 0.55
18	29.34	29.26	29.55	45	57	35	45.7	S. W.	N. W.	N. W.	Rain	Clear	Clear	
19	29.75	29.83	29.81	31	47	38	38.7	N. W.	W'ly	S. W.	Clear	Clear	Clear	
20	29.95	30.01	30.02	43	52	46	47.0	S. W.	S'ly	S. W.	Variable	Cloudy	Cloudy	
21	29.94	29.68	29.69	48	48	44	46.7	S. E.	N. E.	N. E.	R'n, cl'y	Rain	Cloudy	
22	29.82	29.92	29.96	40	40	40	40.0	N. E.	N. E.	N. E.	Cloudy	Rain	Cloudy	
23	29.96	30.00	29.98	40	46	42	42.7	N. E.	N. E.	N. E.	Rain	Cloudy	Cloudy	
24	29.94	29.89	29.89	44	57	50	50.3	N. E.	N. E.	N. E.	Cloudy	Cloudy	Cloudy	
25	29.92	29.98	29.96	43	46	40	43.0	N. E.	N. E.	N. E.	Cloudy	Cloudy	Cloudy	} 3.25
26	28.95	29.76	29.61	41	53	50	48.0	N. E.	N. E.	S'ly	Cloudy	Cloudy	Fog, cl'y	
27	29.51	29.45	29.58	48	50	42	46.7	S'ly	S. W.	N. W.	Fog, cl'y	Rain	Clear	
28	29.66	29.67	29.65	35	58	50	47.7	N. W.	N. W.	N. W.	Clear	Clear	Clear	
29	29.66	29.52	29.28	44	68	46	52.7	N. W.	S. W.	S. E.	Clear	Variable	Rain	
30	28.74	28.77	28.86	44	48	43	44.3	N. E.	N. W.	N. W.	Rain	Cloudy	Variable	
Means	29.72	29.74	29.74	37.5	48.7	40.4	...	...	...	...	...	...	...	7.78
REDUCED TO SEA LEVEL.								Prevailing winds from some point between—		Days.			Days.	
Max.	30.44	30.42	30.39	48	68	51	52.7	N. & E.		10	Clear		8	
Min.	28.92	28.95	29.04	24	32	26	29.0	E. & S.		1	Variable } Cloudy }		7	
Mean	29.90	29.92	29.92					S. & W.		10	Rain or snow fell on		16	
Range	1.52	1.47	1.35	24	36	25	23.7	W. & N.		10				
Mean of month	29.913			...	...	...	42.2							
Extreme range	1.52			...	...	...	44.0							

REMARKS.

1st. Cloudy, with some rain, in the morning. Clear in the afternoon and evening.

2d. Foggy in the morning. Clear in afternoon. Thunder and lightning, with a heavy gust and rain, from 9 to 11 P. M.

3d. Fine, but cool.

4th. Clear in morning. Cloudy in afternoon. Rain in evening, with strong wind from S. E.

5th and 6th. Fine.

7th. Cloudy in morning. Began to rain very moderately from 3 to 4 P. M.

8th. Cloudy in morning. Clear in afternoon.

9th. Light showers during the day.

10th. Cold and raw, with wind at N. E.

11th. Very raw and cold.

12th. Cold and raw. Wind brisk N. E'ly, varying to E'ly. Began to snow from 8 to 9 P. M., and continued all night, with a heavy N. E'ly wind.

13th. Snow very deep and still snowing. Wind came to N. W. at 4 or 5 P. M.; snow ceased. Snow, though rather moist, is somewhat drifted, and, by measurement in different places, is believed to be, on the average, 16 or 18 inches deep. It is by far the heaviest fall of snow during the winter. Including what was absorbed by the ground, the snow must have been equal to 1.75 inch of water.

14th. Variable. Clear at noon. Flurry of rain and snow at sunset. Clear at 9 P. M.

15th and 16th. Fine.

17th. Partly cloudy in the morning. Began to rain moderately from 8 to 9 A. M. Cloudy in the afternoon and evening, but no rain.

18th. Rain in the morning; wind S. W. Wind came to N. W., and cleared from 11 to 12 A. M. Clear in the afternoon, and very gusty.

19th. Aurora borealis in the evening.

21st. Began to rain during the past night, and continued till 2 P. M.

22d. Began to rain at 10½ A. M., and continued moderately till 4½ P. M.

23d. Light rain last night and this morning. Foggy.

24th. Light rain last night.

25th. Rained again this morning before sunrise.

26th. Wind changed from N. E. to S. W. about 4½ P. M., and then to about S. Evening calm and foggy.

27th. Foggy in the morning. Began to rain at 10½ A. M., and continued moderately till 3 P. M., and then came up clear.

28th. Very fine.

29th. Began to rain at 8½ P. M.

30th. Rained all last night; sometimes heavily.

May, 1841.

DAYS.	BAROMETER. At 6 A. M.	At 1 P. M.	At 10 P. M.	THERMOMETER. At 6 A. M.	At 1 P. M.	At 10 P. M.	Daily mean	WINDS. At 6 A. M.	At 1 P. M.	At 10 P. M.	WEATHER. At 6 A. M.	At 1 P. M.	At 10 P. M.	RAIN.
1	28.99	29.15	29.39	42	52	46	46.7	N. W.	N. W.	N. W.	Cloudy	Cloudy	Cloudy	
2	29.47	29.48	29.29	41	56	34	43.7	W'ly	S. W.	N. W.	Clear	Variable	Clear	
3	29.20	29.45	29.59	36	45	37	49.3	N. W.	N. W.	N. W.	Cl'dy, r'n	Clear	Clear	0.50
4	29.56	29.53	29.60	34	54	42	43.3	N. W.	N. W.	N. W.	Clear	Clear	Clear	
5	29.62	29.64	29.67	39	59	45	47.7	N. W.	S'ly	S. W.	Clear	Clear	Cloudy	
6	29.60	29.60	29.69	43	50	42	45.0	S. E.	S. W.	N. W.	Misty	Misty	Clear	
7	29.84	29.82	29.84	42	64	52	52.7	N. W.	W'ly	S. W'ly	Clear	Clear	Cloudy	
8	29.79	29.77	29.81	46	52	46	48.0	N. E.	N. E.	N. E.	Rain	Cloudy	Clear	0.10
9	29.92	29.91	29.89	45	66	50	53.7	N. W.	W'ly	S. W.	Clear	Clear	Clear	
10	29.73	29.51	29.29	48	52	50	50.0	S'ly	S. E.	S'ly	Rain	Rain	Cloudy	1.25
11	29.13	29.10	29.22	46	62	50	52.7	N'ly	W'ly	W'ly	Cloudy	Cloudy	Clear	
12	29.29	29.29	29.49	46	67	50	54.3	W'ly	W'ly	N. W.	Clear	Variable	Variable	
13	29.50	29.54	29.58	43	61	44	49.3	N. W.	N. W.	S. W.	Clear	Variable	Clear	
14	29.60	29.59	29.68	40	66	48	51.3	S'ly	S'ly	S'ly	Clear	Clear	Cloudy	
15	29.80	29.79	29.86	41	59	45	48.3	N. W.	S'ly	S'ly	Clear	Clear	Clear	
16	29.87	29.85	29.81	42	63	48	51.0	W'ly	W'ly	S. W'ly	Clear	Variable	Clear	
17	29.50	29.39	29.51	46	60	48	51.3	S. W'ly	S. W.	N. W.	Clear	Cloudy	Clear	
18	29.51	29.46	29.63	44	55	47	48.7	N. W.	N. W.	N. W.	Clear	Cloudy	Cloudy	
19	29.67	29.68	29.79	44	56	46	48.7	N. E.	N'ly	S'ly	Clear	Cloudy	Variable	
20	29.76	29.75	29.75	44	69	59	57.3	W'ly	W'ly	W'ly	Clear	Clear	Clear	
21	29.78	29.78	29.82	59	80	65	68.0	W'ly	W'ly	S. W.	Clear	Variable	Clear	
22	29.92	29.93	29.93	59	75	59	64.3	S. W.	S. W.	S. W.	Variable	Variable	Cloudy	
23	29.92	29.88	29.84	60	70	64	64.7	S. W.	S. W.	S. W.	Cl'y, sh'r	Cloudy	Clear	0.33
24	29.88	29.84	29.88	62	75	63	66.7	S. W.	S. W'ly	S. W.	Clear	Clear	Clear	
25	29.86	29.85	29.84	61	73	64	66.0	S. W.	S. W.	S. W.	Clear	Clear	Clear	
26	29.78	29.74	29.78	62	68	61	63.7	S. W.	S. W.	S. W.	Cloudy	Cloudy	Foggy	
27	29.86	29.88	29.90	60	70	62	64.0	S. W.	S. W.	S. W.	Foggy	Misty	Cloudy	
28	29.88	29.85	29.81	60	73	65	66.0	S. W.	S. W.	W'ly	Rain	Cloudy	Clear	
29	29.83	29.83	29.84	62	79	53	64.7	S. W.	S'ly	N. E.	...	Clear	Cloudy	
30	[illegible]	[illegible]	[illegible]	[illegible]	[illegible]	[illegible]	[illegible]	N. E.	N. E.	N. E.	Cloudy	Clear	Clear	
31	29.89	29.80	29.80	44	66	46	52.0	N. E.	N. E.	N. E.	Clear	Clear	Clear	
Means	29.67	29.66	29.70	48.2	63.2	51.0	...	...	...	...	...	...	...	2.18
REDUCED TO SEA LEVEL.								Prevailing winds from some point between—		Days.			Days.	
Max.	30.10	30.11	30.11	62	80	65	68.0	N. & E.		4	Clear		10	
Min.	29.17	29.28	29.40	34	45	34	43.3	E. & S.		1	Variable } Cloudy }		8	
Mean	29.85	29.83	29.88					S. & W.		17	Rain fell on		13	
Range	0.93	0.83	0.71	28	35	31	24.7	W. & N.		9				
Mean of month	29.853			...	...	...	54.1							
Extreme range	0.94			...	...	...	46.0							

REMARKS.

1st. Cold and raw. Wind N. W. Occasional sprinkling of rain.

2d. Showery from 2 to 5 P. M. At 8 P. M., wind N. W., and clear.

3d. Light rain last night. Air full of snow for several hours in the morning. Cleared in the afternoon, and very blustering all day.

4th. Clear, but cool.

5th. Pleasant.

6th. Misty in the morning; wind S. W. Wind came to N. W towards night, and cleared.

7th. Pleasant. Clouded over towards night.

8th Moderate rain in the morning. Clear in the evening; wind N. E.

9th. Very fine.

10th. Rain steady and pretty copious nearly all day.

11th. Cloudy in morning. Clear in evening.

12th. Pleasant. Cloudy towards night.

13th. Fine.

14th. Clear in the morning. Cloudy in the afternoon. Shower from 6 to 7 P. M.

15th. Fine.

16th. Changeable. Light shower from 10 to 11 A. M.

17th. Variable. Sprinkling of rain in the morning. Gust from 3 to 4 P. M. Wind changed from S. W. to N. W.

18th. Cloudy for the most part. Rather blustering. Sprinkling of rain in the evening.

19th. Cloudy for the most part.

20th. Very fine. The first day which has been warm for the season.

21st. Very warm.

22d. Warm. Cloudy in the afternoon. Sprinkling of rain in the evening.

23d. Cloudy in the morning. Thundershower from 8 to 9 A. M. Sun out in the afternoon. Clear and warm in the evening.

24th and 25th. Very fine.

[illegible] day. Stars out in the evening. Halo round the moon.

27th. Cloudy, with sprinkling of rain in the afternoon.

28th. Shower from 6 to 7 A. M. Cloudy through the day. Clear in the evening.

29th. Very warm in the morning. Hot sun.

30th. Cloudy in the morning. Clear in the afternoon and evening, and cool.

31st. Wind light N. E. Weather cool. Day and evening nearly cloudless. Frost in the vicinity this morning.

June, 1841.

DAYS.	Barometer, reduced to 32° F. At 6 A. M.	At 1 P. M.	At 10 P. M.	Thermometer. At 6 A. M.	At 1 P. M.	At 10 P. M.	Daily mean.	Winds. At 6 A. M.	At 1 P. M.	At 10 P. M.	Weather. At 6 A. M.	At 1 P. M.	At 10 P. M.	Rain and Snow in Inches of Water
1	29.74	29.69	29.64	42	66	54	54.0	N.	S. E'ly	S. E'ly	Cloudy	Clear	Clear	
2	29.60	29.52	29.59	55	75	62	64.0	W'	N. W.	W'ly	Clear	Clear	Clear	
3	29.64	29.62	29.68	55	71	61	62.3	N. E.	N. W.	N. W.	Clear	Clear	Clear	
4	29.65	29.64	29.58	55	75	66	65.3	N. W.	S. W.	S. W.	Clear	Clear	Clear	
5	29.49	29.47	29.72	67	86	59	70.7	W'ly	N. W.	N. E.	Clear	Clear	Clear	
6	29.84	29.83	29.84	55	65	58	58.7	N. E.	N. E.	N. E.	Clear	Clear	Clear	
7	29.74	29.68	29.60	55	81	67	67.7	S'ly	S. W.	S. W.	Clear	Clear	Clear	
8	29.61	29.60	29.59	71	90	81	80.7	'ly	N. W'ly	N. W.	Clear	Clear	Clear	
9	29.67	29.68	29.70	60	74	60	64.7		N. E.	N. E.	Cloudy	Clear	Cloudy	
10	29.70	29.67	29.64	61	76	69	68.7	E.	S. W.	S. W.	Cloudy	Clear	Variable	
11	29.49	29.41	29.36	67	87	76	76.7	W.	S. W.	S. W.	Clear	Clear	Clear	
12	29.38	29.51	29.61	67	74	64	68.3	'ly	N'ly	S'ly	Clear	Clear	Clear	
13	29.63	29.62	29.59	62	74	62	65.7		S. W.	S. W.	Cloudy	Cloudy	Cloudy	
14	29.59	29.58	29.57	62	75	63	66.7	W.W.	S. W.	S. W.	Variable	Clear	Cl'y, sh'r	0.25
15	29.50	29.49	29.54	62	75	66	67.7	S.W.	S. W.	N. W.	Cloudy	Cloudy	Clear	
16	29.66	29.66	29.78	61	76	64	67.0	N.	N'ly	N. W.	Clear	Clear	Clear	
17	29.87	29.88	29.88	59	78	67	68.0	N'	N. E.	S. W.	Clear	Clear	Clear	
18	29.92	29.90	29.90	63	70	58	63.7	S'ly	S'ly	S. E.	Variable	Cloudy	Cloudy	
19	29.87	29.82	29.73	57	65	58	60.0	S. E.	E'ly	N. E'ly	Cl'dy, r'n	Cloudy	Rain	0.53
20	29.73	...	29.85	55	...	57	...	N. E'ly	...	N. E.	Clear	...	Cloudy	
21	29.92	29.92	29.91	52	71	61	61.3	N. E'ly	N. E'ly	S. W.	Clear	Clear	Clear	
22	29.90	29.87	29.80	59	70	65	64.7	S.	S. W.	S. W.	Clear	Cloudy	Cloudy	
23	29.72	29.68	29.64	66	76	71	71.0	S.	S. W.	S. W.	Clear	Clear	Clear	
24	29.64	29.69	29.78	70	73	64	69.0	N.	N. E.	N. E.	Cloudy	Cloudy	Cloudy	
25	29.82	29.80	29.80	60	71	66	65.7	N.	N. E.	N. E.	Misty	Cloudy	Cloudy	
26	29.75	29.67	29.68	62	77	72	70.3	S. W	S. W.	S. W.	Rain	Cloudy	Clear	0.20
27	29.69	29.70	29.71	73	80	73	75.3	S. W.	S. W.	S. W.	Cloudy	Cloudy	Cloudy	
28	29.64	29.67	29.67	71	81	72	74.7	S. W'ly	S. W'ly	W'ly	Cloudy	Variable	Clear	
29	29.68	29.65	29.62	72	85	80	79.0	W'ly	W'ly	W'ly	Clear	Clear	Clear	
30	29.66	29.56	29.57	78	90	79	82.3	W'ly	W'ly	S. W.	Clear	Clear	Clear	
Means	29.69	29.67	29.68	61.8	76.1	65.8	...	...	...	...	...	...	...	0.98
REDUCED TO SEA LEVEL.														
Max.	30.10	30.10	30.09	78	90	81	82.3							
Min.	29.56	29.59	29.54	42	65	54	54.0							
Mean	29.87	29.84	29.86											
Range	0.54	0.51	0.55	36	25	27	28.3							
Mean of month	29.857			...	...	...	67.9							
Extreme range	0.56			...	...	...	48.0							

Prevailing winds from some point between—

	Days.
N. & E.	9
E. & S.	1
S. & W.	14
W. & N.	6

	Days.
Clear	15
Variable } Cloudy }	7
Rain fell on	8

REMARKS.

1st. Cloudy in the morning. Cool all day.
2d. Very fine in the morning. Heavy dash of rain for five minutes at 5 P. M.
3d. Very fine all day and evening.
4th. Very fine.
5th. Very warm. From 3 to 4 P. M., the wind changed from N. W. to N. E., and grew cooler.
6th. Fine.
7th. Fine. Very burning sun.
8th. Excessively hot.
9th. Cloudy the greater part of the day. From 2 to 3 P. M., a sprinkling of rain.
10th. Fine for the most part.
11th. Fine. Sun very hot.
12th. Fine.
13th. Cloudy. Sprinkling of rain from 10 to 11 A. M.
14th. Mostly cloudy. Lightning and thunder in the evening. Shower during the night.
15th. Cloudy, with occasional sprinkling of rain.
16th and 17th. Fine.
18th. Cloudy in the morning. Began to rain gently from 3 to 4 P. M., and continued till sunset.
19th. Moderate rain at intervals during the day and evening.
20th. Clear in the morning; wind N. E. Cloudy in the afternoon; cool.
21st. Fine.
22d. Fine in the morning. Cloudy in the afternoon.
23d. Fine.
24th. Wind light N. E. Weather cloudy.
25th. Cloudy.
26th. Moderate rain at intervals in the morning. Clear towards night and in the evening.
27th. Very sultry.
28th. Cloudy in the morning. Clear in the afternoon and evening.
29th. Very burning sun all day. Fresh breeze from W'ly.
30th. Very burning sun. From 4 to 5 P. M., a thunder-cloud passed a few miles to north of us. The wind followed to the N. and N. E., very cool and refreshing, and continued to E. and S., and became fixed at S. W. in the evening; very fresh, but warm.

July, 1841.

DAYS.	Barometer. At 6 A. M.	At 1 P. M.	At 10 P. M.	Thermometer. At 6 A. M.	At 1 P. M.	At 10 P. M.	Daily mean.	Winds. At 6 A. M.	At 1 P. M.	At 10 P. M.	Weather. At 6 A. M.	At 1 P. M.	At 10 P. M.	Rain and Snow in Inches of Water
1	29.57	29.56	29.57	77	72	71	73.3	S. W.	N'ly	N. W'ly	Clear	Rain	Clear	0.33
2	29.63	29.63	29.72	66	78	62	68.7	N. W.	N. W.	N. W.	Clear	Clear	Clear	
3	29.74	...	...	56	...	...	...	N. W.	...	...	Clear	...	...	
4	...	...	...	...	...	...	...	...	...	...	...	...	...	
5	...	...	...	...	...	...	...	...	...	...	...	...	Shower	1.75
6	...	29.62	29.59	...	82	71	...	...	S. W.	S. W.	...	Clear	Cloudy	
7	29.61	29.62	29.61	66	79	71	70.3	S. W.	S. W.	S. W.	Sh'r, cl'r	Clear	Cloudy	0.20
8	29.62	29.64	29.71	64	74	65	67.7	N. W.	N. W.	N. W.	Clear	Clear	Clear	
9	29.81	29.79	29.71	60	76	67	67.7	N. W.	W'ly	S. W.	Clear	Clear	Clear	
10	29.59	...	...	65	...	65	...	S. W.	...	N. W.	Cloudy	...	Clear	
11	29.69	...	29.61	60	...	63	...	N. W.	...	N. W.	Clear	...	Clear	
12	29.62	29.59	29.59	56	78	65	66.3	N. W.	N. W.	N. W.	Clear	Clear	Clear	
13	29.62	29.66	29.67	61	78	71	70.0	N. W.	S'ly	S. W'ly	Clear	Clear	Clear	
14	29.70	29.69	29.68	67	83	71	73.7	S. E'ly	S'ly	W'ly	Clear	Clear	Shower	2.00
15	29.63	29.60	29.59	71	84	74	76.3	W'ly	S. W.	W'ly	Cloudy	Clear	Clear	
16	...	...	...	...	...	...	...	...	...	...	...	...	...	
17	29.72	29.80	29.81	66	72	64	67.3	N. E.	N. E.	N. E.	Clear	Clear	Clear	
18	29.83	...	29.82	64	...	64	...	N. W.	...	S. W'ly	Clear	Clear	Clear	
19	29.83	29.81	29.87	62	80	70	70.7	S. W'ly	S. W'ly	S. W.	Clear	Clear	Clear	
20	29.98	30.03	30.06	68	80	71	73.0	N. E.	N. E.	S'ly	Clear	Clear	Clear	
21	30.09	30.01	29.97	67	82	72	73.7	S. W.	S. W.	S. W.	Clear	Clear	Clear	
22	29.94	29.85	29.76	67	83	75	75.0	S. W.	S. W.	S. W.	Clear	Cl'r, sh'r	Clear	0.10
23	29.77	29.75	29.80	74	87	65	78.7	S. W.	W'ly	N. E.	Hazy	Variable	Cloudy	
24	29.86	29.83	29.83	64	80	72	72.0	N. E.	E'ly	S'ly	Cloudy	Variable	Cloudy	
25	29.78	29.66	29.60	73	84	76	77.7	S. W'ly	S. W.	S. W.	Rain	Clear	Clear	0.10
26	29.60	29.67	29.77	73	80	65	72.7	N. W.	W.	N. W.	Variable	Clear	Clear	
27	29.80	29.74	29.70	60	77	66	67.7	N. W.	W.	N. W.	Clear	Clear	Clear	
28	29.60	29.62	29.77	64	74	62	66.7	S. W.	'ly	N. W.	Rain	Clear	Clear	0.10
29	29.82	29.78	29.71	54	72	62	62.7	N. W.	W.	N. W.	Clear	Clear	Clear	
30	29.72	29.70	29.72	62	77	67	68.7	W'ly	N.'ly	S. W.	Clear	Clear	Clear	
31	29.68	29.67	29.64	62	65	59	62.0	N. E.	N. E.	N. E.	Rain	Rain	Rain	0.55
Means	29.73	29.73	29.72	64.8	78.2	67.8	...	...	...	...	...	...	...	5.13
REDUCED TO SEA LEVEL.														
Max.	30.27	30.21	30.24	77	87	76	78.7							
Min.	29.75	29.74	29.75	54	65	59	56.0							
Mean	29.90	29.90	29.89											
Range	0.52	0.45	0.49	23	22	17	22.7							
Mean of month	29.897			...	...	...	70.0							
Extreme range	0.53			...	...	...	33.0							

Prevailing winds from some point between—

	Days.
N. & E.	4
E. & S.	1
S. & W.	12
W. & N.	11

	Days.
Clear	16
Variable } Cloudy }	2
Rain fell on	10

(3 days omitted.)

REMARKS.

1st. Very hot in the morning Fine shower from noon to 1½ P. M. Clear in the evening.
2d. Fine. Evening cool.
5th. Thunder, with very heavy rain, from 10 to 11 P. M.
6th. Wind very fresh S. W. in the evening.
7th. Shower from 1 to 2 A. M. Clear for the most part during the day. Cloudy in the evening.
8th and 9th. Very fine.
10th. Light showers in the morning. Clear in the afternoon and evening.
11th, 12th, and 13th. Very fine.
14th. Fine during the day. Very powerful rain from 9 to 11 P. M., with thunder and lightning.
15th. Fine.
16th. Sprinkling of rain, with thunder in the afternoon.
17th to 22d. Very fine.
23d. Very hot in the morning; wind W'ly. Thunder, with a light shower, at 2 P. M.; wind came to N. E., and became cooler.
24th. Pleasant.
25th. Light shower in the morning. Sun out at noon. Cloudy, with appearances of rain, in the afternoon and evening.
26th and 27th. Very fine.
28th. Light shower in the morning; then pleasant.
29th and 30th. Very fine.
31st. Wind N. E. Moderate rain all day.

August, 1841.

DAYS.	BAROMETER, REDUCED TO 32° F.			THERMOMETER.				WINDS.			WEATHER.			RAIN AND SNOW IN INCHES OF WATER.
	At 6 A. M.	At 1 P. M.	At 10 P. M.	At 6 A. M.	At 1 P. M.	At 10 P. M.	Daily mean.	At 6 A. M.	At 1 P. M.	At 10 P. M.	At 6 A. M.	At 1 P. M.	At 10 P. M.	
1	29.69	29.70	29.84	60	65	56	60.3	N. E.	N. E.	N. E.	Cloudy	Cloudy	Clear	
2	29.90	29.94	29.97	57	76	67	66.7	N. W.	S. W'ly	S. W.	Clear	Clear	Clear	
3	29.99	29.97	29.95	64	80	66	70.0	S. W.	S. W.	S. W.	Clear	Clear	Clear	
4	29.91	29.83	29.77	65	87	74	75.3	S. W.	S. W.	S. W.	Clear	Clear	Variable	
5	29.71	29.70	29.67	71	84	72	75.7	N. W'ly	S. W'ly	S'ly	Variable	Clear	Rain	
6	29.68	29.67	29.70	67	76	66	69.7	N. E'ly	N. E'ly	N. E.	Variable	Clear	Cloudy	
7	29.74	29.77	...	61	82	...	...	N. E.	N. E.	...	Cloudy	Clear	...	
8	...	...	...	...	...	...	...	...	...	...	...	...	...	
9	...	29.80	29.77	...	73	73	...	...	S. W.	S. W.	...	Rain	Clear	0.25
10	29.83	29.84	29.85	71	81	74	75.3	S. W.	S. W.	S. W.	Clear	Clear	Cloudy	
11	29.77	29.78	29.80	70	68	65	67.7	E'ly	N'ly	N. E'ly	Rain	Cloudy	Cloudy	1.40
12	29.78	29.81	29.78	65	78	72	71.7	N. E.	W'ly	S. W.	Cloudy	Clear	Cloudy	
13	29.78	29.76	29.75	68	78	69	71.7	S. W'ly	S. W.	S. W.	Cloudy	Variable	Clear	
14	29.80	29.85	29.87	65	67	64	65.3	N. E.	N. E.	N. E.	Variable	Variable	Variable	
15	30.05	30.11	30.10	62	75	64	67.0	N. E.	S. E.	S. W.	Variable	Clear	Clear	
16	30.11	30.07	30.02	54	73	69	65.3	N. W.	S'ly	W'ly	Clear	Clear	Clear	
17	29.94	29.89	29.87	62	78	73	71.0	W'ly	S. E.	S. W.	Clear	Clear	Clear	
18	29.85	29.82	29.80	66	81	70	72.3	S. W.	S. W.	S. W.	Clear	Clear	Clear	
19	29.79	29.75	29.77	69	82	74	75.0	S. W.	S. E.	S'ly	Variable	Variable	Cloudy	1.10
20	29.78	29.78	29.79	70	83	74	75.7	W'ly	S. E.	S. W.	Clear	Variable	Cloudy	
21	29.79	29.78	29.72	71	84	74	76.3	S. W.	S. W.	S. W.	Clear	Clear	Clear	
22	29.69	29.67	29.74	73	70	67	70.0	S. W.	N'ly	N. W.	Rain	Cloudy	Clear	0.20
23	29.80	29.88	29.91	60	72	61	64.3	N. W.	N. E.	N. E'ly	Clear	Clear	Clear	
24	30.04	30.04	30.04	55	74	64	64.3	N. W.	W'ly	S. W'ly	Clear	Clear	Clear	
25	30.06	30.00	30.08	56	75	61	64.0	W'ly	S. W.	W'ly	Clear	Clear	Clear	
26	29.94	29.88	29.85	58	76	62	65.3	W'ly	S. W.	W.	Clear	Clear	Cloudy	} 2.17 (26th–30th)
27	29.85	29.84	...	56	69	...	...	N. E.	N. E.	...	Cloudy	Rain	Rain	
28	...	29.88	29.94	57	70	67	65.7	N. E.	N. E.	N. E.	Rain	Clear	Cloudy	
29	29.94	29.98	29.96	68	73	68	69.7	N. E'ly	N. E.	N. E.	Cloudy	Cloudy	Rain	
30	29.92	29.80	29.76	68	70	68	68.7	E'ly	E'ly	E'ly	Rain	Rain	Misty	
31	29.73	29.71	29.72	66	74	64	68.0	W'ly	N. E'ly	N. E'ly	Cloudy	Cloudy	Cloudy	
Means	29.85	29.84	29.88	63.9	75.8	67.8	...	...	...	...	...	...	...	5.12
REDUCED TO SEA LEVEL.														
Max.	30.29	30.29	30.28	73	87	74	76.3							
Min.	29.84	29.85	29.85	54	65	56	60.3							
Mean	30.02	30.01	30.05											
Range	0.45	0.44	0.43	19	22	18	16.0							
Mean of month	30.023			...	...	...	69.2							
Extreme range	0.45			...	...	...	33.0							

Prevailing winds from some point between—

	Days.
N. & E.	11
E. & S.	4
S. & W.	12
W. & N.	3

	Days.
Clear	10
Variable } Cloudy }	10
Rain fell on	10

(1 day omitted.)

REMARKS.

1st. Rain in the forenoon. Cloudy in the afternoon. Clear in the evening.
2d. Very fine.
3d. Fine. Very hot sun.
4th. Many clouds and haze during the day, with moderate rain at 10 P. M., and continued only for a short time.
5th. Hazy, and occasional appearances of rain towards night. Hot sun at mid-day.
6th, 7th, and 8th. Fair.
9th. Wind fresh S. W.; cloudy. Began to rain from 9 to 10 A. M., and was showery through the day.
10th. Very warm and sultry. Began to rain about 10 P. M., and rained all night.
11th. Rain continued till between 8 and 9 A. M.; then cloudy.
12th. Clear for the most part, and pleasant.
13th to 16th. Pleasant.
17th. Air smoky and hazy.
18th. Foggy in the morning.
20th. Heavy shower, with thunder, from 2 to 3 P. M.
21st. Very hot.
22d. Shower in the morning; wind S. W. Wind changed to N'ly, from 10 to 11 A. M. Cloudy in the afternoon. Clear in the evening.
23d. Cool and pleasant.
24th and 25th. Very fine.
26th. Fine day.
27th. Moderate rain towards evening; wind S. E.
28th. Mist and some rain in the morning; wind N. E. Rain again towards night.
29th. Cloudy, with occasional rain. Wind light N. E.

September, 1841.

DAYS.	BAROMETER Sunrise.	At 1 P. M.	At 10 P. M.	THERMOMETER Sunrise.	At 1 P. M.	At 10 P. M.	Daily mean.	WINDS Sunrise.	At 1 P. M.	At 10 P. M.	WEATHER Sunrise.	At 1 P. M.	At 10 P. M.	RAIN AND SNOW
1	29.61	...	29.63	62	...	64	...	W'ly	W'ly	W'ly	Cloudy	Clear	Clear	
2	29.67	29.66	29.63	63	79	73	71.7	W'ly	S. W'ly	S. W.	Clear	Clear	Clear	
3	29.67	29.68	29.67	73	79	72	74.7	S. W.	S. W.	S. W.	Clear	Clear	Clear	
4	29.55	29.42	29.43	71	81	68	73.3	S. W.	W'ly	W'ly	Cloudy	Variable	Var., sh.	0.30
5	29.50	29.57	29.68	65	74	64	67.7	N. E.	N. E.	N. E.	Cloudy	Cloudy	Misty	
6	29.74	29.78	29.82	60	64	61	61.7	N. E.	N. E.	N. E.	Cloudy	Cloudy	Misty	
7	29.86	29.85	29.85	62	71	59	63.3	N. E.	N. E.	N. E.	Cloudy	Clear	Clear	
8	29.84	29.81	29.81	57	69	58	61.3	N. E.	N. E.	N. E.	Clear	Clear	Clear	
9	29.84	29.84	29.91	57	68	58	61.0	N. E.	N. E.	N. E.	Variable	Cloudy	Clear	
10	29.90	29.86	...	57	68	...	...	N. E.	N. E.	...	Misty	Cloudy	...	
11	...	...	29.75	...	...	64	...	...	...	S. W.	...	...	Variable	
12	29.75	29.75	29.78	64	77	69	70.0	S. W.	S. W.	N. E'ly	Clear	Variable	Cloudy	
13	29.78	29.80	29.79	65	65	61	63.7	N. E.	N. E.	N. E.	Misty	Misty	Misty	
14	29.84	29.86	29.89	56	70	59	61.7	N'ly	N. E'ly	N. W.	Clear	Clear	Clear	
15	30.00	30.02	30.06	54	70	57	60.3	N. W.	N. W.	N. E'ly	Clear	Clear	Clear	
16	30.07	30.04	30.04	52	67	55	58.0	N. E'ly	N'ly	N. E'ly	Clear	Clear	Variable	
17	29.96	29.91	29.83	52	67	60	59.7	N. E.	N. E.	E'ly	Variable	Variable	Misty	
18	29.80	29.76	29.79	55	70	62	62.1	N'ly	N. E.	N. E'ly	Cloudy	Clear	Clear	
19	29.85	29.82	29.90	56	66	56	59.3	N'ly	N. E.	N. E.	Clear	Cloudy	Clear	
20	29.90	29.90	29.89	52	68	60	60.0	E'ly	S'ly	S. W.	Clear	Clear	Clear	
21	29.90	29.89	29.87	56	69	59	61.3	N. E'ly	N. E'ly	N. E.	Cloudy	Variable	Cloudy	
22	29.75	29.72	29.66	55	66	58	59.3	N. E.	N. E.	N. E.	Variable	Cloudy	Cloudy	
23	29.64	29.64	29.69	58	71	66	65.0	N. E.	N. E.	N. E'ly	Cloudy	Cloudy	Cloudy	
24	29.70	29.67	29.64	64	72	69	68.3	S. E'ly	S. E'ly	S. E'ly	Cloudy	Misty	Rain	} 0.70 (24th–25th)
25	29.49	29.29	29.34	68	73	61	67.3	S. E'ly	S'ly	W'ly	Rain	Rain	Clear	
26	29.49	29.50	29.58	57	70	62	63.0	S. W'ly	S. W.	W'ly	Clear	Clear	Clear	
27	29.76	29.79	29.80	52	68	56	58.7	N. W.	W'ly	W'ly	Clear	Clear	Clear	
28	29.82	29.75	29.68	52	72	66	63.3	W'ly	S. W.	S. W.	Clear	Clear	Variable	
[illegible]	[illegible]	[illegible]	[illegible]	[illegible]	[illegible]	[illegible]	[illegible]	[illegible]	[illegible]	[illegible]	[illegible]	Rain	Rain	[illegible]
30	29.59	29.50	29.61	50	58	48	52.0	N'ly	N'ly	N. W.	Cloudy	Cloudy	Clear	
Means	29.75	29.74	29.74	[illegible]	[illegible]	61.4	...	...	...	...	...	...	...	2.05
REDUCED TO SEA LEVEL.														
Max.	30.25	30.22	30.24	73	81	73	74.7							
Min.	29.67	29.47	29.52	50	58	48	52.0							
Mean	29.93	29.91	29.92											
Range	0.58	0.75	0.72	23	23	25	22.7							
Mean of month	29.920			...	...	...	63.3							
Extreme range	0.78			...	...	...	33.0							

Prevailing winds from some point between—

	Days.
N. & E.	11
E. & S.	4
S. & W.	13
W. & N.	2

	Days.
Clear	10
Variable } Cloudy }	14
Rain fell on	6

1st. Variable. Light shower in the afternoon.
2d. Very fine.
3d. Very warm.
4th. Variable. Shower from 10 to 11 A. M. Thundershower from 8 to 9 P. M.
5th. Cloudy for the most part.
6th. Cloudy all day, with some mist.
7th. Cool. Very clear in the evening.
8th and 9th. Very fine, but cool.
10th. Cloudy.
11th. Cloudy, with mist, in the morning. Clear in the afternoon.
12th. Clear in the morning. Cloudy in the afternoon.
13th. Misty through the day. Some rain.
14th, 15th, and 16th. Pleasant.
17th. Mild, with indications of rain.
18th and 19th. Pleasant.
20th. Very pleasant.
21st. Variable.
22d. Cloudy, and rather raw.
23d. Cloudy.
24th. Cloudy. Rain in the evening.
25th. Rainy.
26th and 27th. Very pleasant.
28th. Very fine.
29th. Cloudy in the morning. Began to rain moderately from noon to 1 P. M. Rain in the evening, with wind changed from S. W. to N. E.
30th. Clouds and mist in the morning. Cloudy [illegible] N. W.

October, 1841.

DAYS.	BAROMETER, REDUCED TO 32° F. Sunrise.	At 1 P. M.	At 10 P. M.	THERMOMETER. Sunrise.	At 1 P. M.	At 10 P. M.	Daily mean.	WINDS. Sunrise.	At 1 P. M.	At 10 P. M.	WEATHER. Sunrise.	At 1 P. M.	At 10 P. M.	RAIN AND SNOW IN INCHES OF WATER.
1	...	...	29.99	...	...	45	...	...	...	N. W.	...	...	Clear	
2	30.05	30.06	30.05	38	52	46	45.3	N. W.	N. E.	N. E.	Clear	Variable	Cloudy	
3	29.86	29.69	29.55	45	48	38	43.7	N. E.	N. E.	N. E.	Rain	Rain	Rain	} 2.50
4	29.41	29.55	29.73	34	42	42	39.3	N'ly	N'ly	N. W'ly	R'n & sn.	Misty	Cloudy	
5	29.80	29.81	29.84	42	47	43	44.0	N'ly	N'ly	N'ly	Cloudy	Misty	Rain	
6	29.82	29.81	29.79	43	50	46	46.3	N. W'ly	N'ly	N. W'ly	Cloudy	Cloudy	Clear	
7	29.76	29.69	29.71	46	60	47	51.0	N. W.	N. W.	E'ly	Clear	Clear	Variable	
8	29.71	29.63	29.59	47	59	53	53.0	E'ly	E'ly	E'ly	Cloudy	Cloudy	Cloudy	
9	29.59	29.59	29.67	57	59	47	54.3	N. W.	N. W.	N. W.	Rain	Clear	Clear	
10	29.80	29.78	29.89	42	59	45	48.3	N. W.	W'ly	N. W.	Clear	Clear	Clear	
11	29.90	29.79	29.59	38	62	55	51.7	W'ly	S. W.	S. W.	Cloudy	Variable	Cloudy	
12	29.59	29.53	29.55	60	65	53	59.3	S. W.	S. W.	N. W.	Cloudy	Cloudy	Clear	
13	29.65	29.66	29.76	45	55	43	47.7	N. W.	N. W.	N. W.	Cloudy	Clear	Clear	
14	29.80	...	29.78	36	...	39	...	N. W.	N. W.	N. W.	Clear	Clear	Clear	
15	29.77	29.64	29.57	37	49	50	45.3	N. W'ly	S. W.	W'ly	Clear	Cloudy	Clear	
16	29.64	29.70	...	43	68	44	51.7	N. W.	N. W.	W'ly	Clear	Cloudy	Cloudy	
17	29.88	...	29.87	38	...	39	...	N. W.	...	N. W.	Clear	...	Clear	
18	29.86	...	...	34	...	39	...	N. W.	...	N. W.	Clear	...	Clear	
19	29.75	29.63	29.60	32	51	44	42.3	N. W.	N. W.	W'ly	Clear	Clear	Clear	
20	29.48	29.24	29.18	42	45	46	44.3	S. W.	N. E'ly	N. E'ly	Cloudy	Rain	Cloudy	0.70
21	29.11	29.10	29.21	37	47	41	41.7	N. W.	N. W.	N. W.	Clear	Clear	Clear	
22	29.24	29.27	29.43	37	52	44	44.3	W'ly	W'ly	W'ly	Clear	Variable	Variable	
23	29.58	29.57	29.60	48	52	42	54.0	N. W.	W'ly	N. W.	Cloudy	Cloudy	Clear	
24	29.54	29.39	29.61	45	52	39	45.3	S. W'ly	S. W'ly	W'ly	Cloudy	Clear	Clear	
25	29.70	29.70	29.89	32	39	28	33.0	N. W.	N. W.	N. W.	Clear	Variable	Clear	
26	29.85	29.67	29.69	26	49	45	40.0	N. W.	S. W.	S. W.	Clear	Clear	Clear	
27	29.86	29.87	30.08	38	52	35	41.7	S. W.	S. W.	N. W.	Clear	Clear	Clear	
28	30.24	30.26	30.27	28	42	31	33.7	N. W.	N'ly	N. W.	Clear	Clear	Clear	
29	30.23	30.14	30.09	30	52	50	44.0	W'ly	S. W.	S. W.	Cloudy	Cloudy	Variable	
30	30.06	30.02	30.06	50	68	49	55.7	S. W.	S. W.	S. W.	Clear	Clear	Clear	
31	...	...	30.10	...	62	51	...	...	S. E.	S. W.	...	Clear	Clear	
Means	29.70	29.72	29.75	40.3	53.3	43.8	...	...	...	...	...	...	...	3.20
REDUCED TO SEA LEVEL.														
Max.	30.42	30.44	30.45	60	68	55	59.3							
Min.	29.29	29.28	29.36	26	39	28	33.0							
Mean	29.88	29.89	29.93											
Range	1.13	1.16	1.09	34	29	27	26.3							
Mean of month			29.900	...	...	...	45.8							
Extreme range			1.17	...	...	...	31.0							

Prevailing winds from some point between—

	Days.
N. & E.	7
E. & S.	1
S. & W.	9
W. & N.	14

	Days.
Clear	13
Variable } Cloudy }	11
Rain or snow fell on	7

REMARKS.

1st. Very fine, but cool.
2d. Variable and cool.
3d. Very severe N. E. storm; heavy wind.
4th. Rain and snow. Wind a little W. of N., and very high. Snow in the air, and also on fences, and the roofs of houses.
5th. Cloudy, with mist. Rain moderate in the evening.
6th. Cloudy till evening; then clear.
7th. Pleasant.
8th. Cloudy.
9th. Light rain in the morning. Clear in the afternoon. Aurora in evening—not very bright.
10th. Pleasant.
11th. Mild and pleasant. Slight frost.
12th. Warm, damp, and cloudy in the morning; wind S. W. Wind came to N. W., and cleared in the evening.
13th. Very fine. Evening uncommonly clear.
14th. White frost this morning in College yard. Day very fine.
15th. Light frost in College yard. From 10 to 12 A. M., wind came to S. W. From noon to 3 P. M., very gusty, with some rain; wind heavy. Clear in the evening; wind W'ly.
16th and 17th. Pleasant.
18th. Frost. Day fine.
19th. Ice one-eighth of an inch thick. Day fine.
20th. Moderate rain in the morning. Misty and cloudy P. M.
21st. The day fine.
22d. Mild.
23d. Cloudy for the most part.
24th. Shower about daylight. Pleasant through the day.
25th. Cool, but pleasant.
26th. Wind S. W., very blustering.
27th and 28th. Very pleasant.
29th. Mild Sun much obscured by clouds.
30th. Very fine.

November, 1841.

DAYS.	Barometer Sunrise.	At 1 P. M.	At 10 P. M.	Thermometer Sunrise.	At 1 P. M.	At 10 P. M.	Daily mean.	Winds Sunrise.	At 1 P. M.	At 10 P. M.	Weather Sunrise.	At 1 P. M.	At 10 P. M.	Rain and snow
1	30.06	29.97	29.89	53	68	55	58.7	S. W.	S. W.	S. W.	Clear	Clear	Clear	
2	29.70	29.63	29.64	57	63	49	56.3	S. W.	S. W.	S. W.	Clear	Rain	Clear	
3	29.64	29.64	29.51	42	59	44	48.3	S. W.	S. W.	S. W.	Clear	Clear	Clear	
4	29.49	29.45	29.39	36	49	46	43.7	S. E.	S. E.	E'ly	Foggy	Cloudy	Cl'y, sh'r	0.35
5	29.26	29.39	29.49	44	45	38	42.3	N. W.	N. W.	N. W.	Cloudy	Cloudy	Clear	
6	29.54	29.60	29.79	40	47	38	41.7	N. W.	N. W.	N. W.	Clear	Cloudy	Clear	
7	...	...	29.94	...	...	34	...	...	...	N. W.	...	...	Clear	
8	29.91	29.74	29.76	31	35	35	33.7	N'ly	E'ly	N. W.	Cloudy	Rain	Clear	0.20
9	30.07	30.11	30.23	35	41	32	36.0	N'ly	N'ly	N. E'ly	Cloudy	Variable	Clear	
10	30.30	30.27	30.25	30	35	27	30.7	N. E'ly	N'ly	N'ly	Clear	Clear	Clear	
11	30.23	29.97	29.80	22	45	34	33.7	N. W.	N. W.	N. W.	Clear	Clear	Clear	
12	29.58	29.35	29.26	34	36	36	35.3	N. W.	N. E.	N'ly	Variable	Rain	Clear	0.60
13	29.21	29.19	29.36	35	46	39	40.0	N. W.	S. W.	N'ly	Clear	Variable	Cloudy	
14	29.41	29.34	29.30	36	47	44	42.3	N. W.	N. W.	N. W.	Clear	Clear	Variable	
15	29.17	29.13	29.16	36	45	38	39.7	N. W.	N. W.	N. W.	Clear	Variable	Variable	
16	29.26	29.26	29.36	30	35	32	32.3	N. W.	N. W.	N. W.	Clear	Clear	Clear	
17	29.47	...	29.53	34	...	32	...	N. W.	W'ly	N. W.	Clear	Variable	Clear	
18	29.61	29.58	29.70	27	36	26	29.7	N. W.	N. W.	N. W.	Clear	Clear	Clear	
19	29.80	29.80	29.73	24	39	36	33.0	N. W.	N. E.	E'ly	Clear	Cloudy	Rain	} 1.35
20	29.62	...	...	36	...	35	...	N. E.	...	N. W.	Rain	...	Variable	
21	29.90	...	...	32	...	34	...	N. W.	N. W.	N. W.	Clear	Clear	Clear	
22	29.85	29.78	29.48	34	47	56	45.7	S. E'ly	S. E'ly	S'ly	Misty	Rain	Rain	0.80
23	29.53	29.55	29.63	52	52	43	49.0	N. W.	W'ly	W'ly	Clear	Clear	Clear	
24	29.75	29.74	29.86	34	45	34	37.7	N. W.	N. W.	N. W.	Clear	Clear	Clear	
25	29.71	29.86	29.66	32	42	34	36.0	N. W.	N. E.	N. E.	Clear	Cloudy	Rain	0.15
26	29.45	29.39	29.49	40	39	34	37.7	N. E.	N'ly	N'ly	Misty	Misty	Cloudy	
27	...	29.71	29.95	26	27	22	25.0	N. W.	N. W.	N. W.	Clear	Cloudy	Clear	
28	30.12	30.15	30.12	19	30	24	24.3	N. W.	N'ly	N'ly	Clear	Cloudy	Cloudy	
29	29.84	29.63	29.71	22	22	22	22.0	N'ly	N. E'ly	N. W.	Snow	Snow	Variable	1.00
30	29.93	29.96	30.03	18	30	18	22.0	N. W.	N. W.	N. W.	Clear	Clear	Clear	
Means	29.69	29.66	29.68	34.2	42.5	35.7	...	...	...	...	...	...	...	4.45
REDUCED TO SEA LEVEL.														
Max.	30.48	30.45	30.43	57	68	56	58.7							
Min.	29.35	29.31	29.34	18	22	18	22.0							
Mean	29.87	29.84	29.86											
Range	1.13	1.14	1.09	39	46	38	36.7							
Mean of month			29.857	...	...	...	37.5							
Extreme range			1.07	...	...	...	50.0							

Prevailing winds from some point between—

	Days.
N. & E.	10
E. & S.	1
S. & W.	4
W. & N.	15

	Days.
Clear	11
Variable } Cloudy }	9
Rain or snow fell on	10

REMARKS.

1st. Very fine. Evening perfectly mild and clear.
2d. At sunrise, nearly clear. Before 9 A. M., became cloudy, with heavy fog, with mist and some rain. Cleared towards night. Evening beautifully clear and mild.
3d. Very fine. Shower in the night.
4th. Cloudy. Cold fog in the morning.
5th. Cloudy during the day, with sprinkling of rain. Occasionally clear in the evening.
6th. Rather raw and blustering.
7th. Rather raw. Very fine in the evening.
8th. Cloudy in the morning; wind N'ly. Began to snow about 8 A. M. Continued to snow till from 10 to 11 A. M., and turned to rain, which continued moderately, with wind E'ly, till near night. Wind came to N. W., and clear evening.
9th. Cold and raw.
10th. Very cool for the season.
11th. Very pleasant, but cool.
12th. Moderate rain from 10 A. M. to 4 P. M.; wind N. E'ly. Partly clear in the evening.
13th. Variable.
14th. Clear and pleasant.
15th. Variable.
16th. Very blustering and severe.
17th. Variable. Cloudy, clear, spitting of snow. then of rain. Evening beautifully clear.
18th. Cool. Brilliant aurora all the evening; seemed to attain a maximum of brightness at 11½ o'clock; chiefly merry dancers, sometimes gathering into quite a brilliant corona near the zenith.
19th. Cloudy in the afternoon; wind N. E. and E'ly. Rain began from 7 to 8 P. M.
20th. Rainy all day.
21st. Clear and very fine.
22d. Mist in the morning, gradually increasing to rain at noon. Rain in the afternoon. Steady and heavy rain in the evening.
23d. Fine.
24th. Very fine.
25th. Variable in the morning. Cloudy in the afternoon, with light rain in the evening.
26th. Misty through the day.
27th. Very cold for the season.
28th. Very raw, and snowy air.
29th. Cold, driving snow-storm all day; began at 3 or 4 A. M., and continued till 7 or 8 P. M. Clouds broken, and the moon out, at 10 P. M. Snow deep, and considerably drifted.
30th. Snow 7 or 8 inches deep on the level. Day pleasant.

December, 1841.

DAYS.	BAROMETER, REDUCED TO 32° F. Sunrise.	At 1 P. M.	At 10 P. M.	THERMOMETER. Sunrise.	At 1 P. M.	At 10 P. M.	Daily mean.	WINDS. Sunrise.	At 1 P. M.	At 10 P. M.	WEATHER. Sunrise.	At 1 P. M.	At 10 P. M.	RAIN AND SNOW IN INCHES OF WATER.
1	30.11	30.10	30.05	22	36	30	29.3	N. W.	N. W.	S. W'ly	Clear	Clear	Cloudy	
2	30.04	30.05	30.09	30	43	32	35.0	W.	W'ly	N. W.	Clear	Clear	Clear	
3	30.04	29.88	29.36	31	42	45	39.3	W'ly	S. E'ly	S. E.	Cloudy	Rain	Rain	1.25
4	29.14	28.96	28.97	47	50	41	46.0	S. W'ly	W'ly	W'ly	Clear	Clear	Clear	
5	28.99	...	29.00	36	...	38	...	N. W.	...	S. W.	Variable	...	Cloudy	
6	29.21	29.26	29.47	36	38	31	35.0	W'ly	N. W.	N. W.	Clear	Clear	Clear	
7	29.66	...	29.85	26	...	26	...	N. W.	N. W.	N. W.	Clear	Clear	Clear	
8	29.95	29.90	29.90	24	34	35	31.0	N. W.	S. W'ly	S. W'ly	Clear	Clear	Clear	
9	29.71	29.66	29.69	42	46	43	43.7	S. W.	S. W.	S. W.	Cloudy	Cloudy	Cloudy	
10	29.71	...	29.46	35	...	48	...	N. E.	...	S. E'ly	Clear	...	Rain	0.68
11	29.33	29.21	29.29	49	54	43	48.7	S. W.	S. W.	N. W.	Misty	Clear	Cloudy	
12	29.47	29.53	29.75	40	46	34	40.0	N. W'ly	N. W.	N. W.	Variable	Clear	Clear	
13	29.94	29.89	29.87	26	40	34	33.3	N. W.	N. W.	S. E'ly	Clear	Clear	Clear	
14	29.68	29.54	29.58	36	46	40	40.7	S. E'ly	S. E'ly	N. W.	Cloudy	Rain	Clear	0.70
15	29.69	29.74	29.78	35	48	42	41.7	N. W.	N. W.	W'ly	Clear	Clear	Cloudy	
16	29.70	29.68	29.60	39	44	36	39.7	N. E'ly	N. E'ly	N. E.	Cloudy	Cloudy	Rain	} 1.85
17	29.33	29.10	29.13	36	36	27	33.0	N. E.	N. E.	N'ly	Rain	Misty	Cloudy	}
18	29.04	29.13	29.40	22	22	15	19.7	N. W.	N. W.	N. W.	Snow	Snow	Variable	0.10
19	29.62	29.69	29.76	14	26	25	21.7	N. W.	W'ly	W'ly	Clear	Variable	Clear	
20	29.85	29.81	29.86	27	32	27	28.7	W'ly	S. W'ly	N. W.	Cloudy	Variable	Cloudy	
21	29.90	29.95	30.15	19	31	12	20.7	N. E.	N. W'ly	N. W.	Snow	Cloudy	Clear	0.10
22	30.36	30.44	30.51	5	17	8	10.0	N. W.	N. W.	N. W.	Clear	Clear	Clear	
23	30.49	30.38	30.07	11	26	34	23.7	N. E'ly	E'ly	E'ly	Cloudy	Cloudy	Cloudy	
24	29.57	29.66	...	47	44	27	39.3	S. W.	W'ly	N. W.	Rain	Clear	Variable	1.18
25	29.83	29.82	29.95	30	35	22	29.0	W'ly	N. W.	N. W.	Cloudy	Clear	Cloudy	
26	29.93	29.92	29.96	13	25	20	19.3	N. W.	N. W.	N. W.	Clear	Clear	Clear	
27	30.03	30.00	30.03	17	33	26	25.3	N. W.	N. W.	S. W.	Clear	Variable	Variable	
28	30.00	29.90	30.05	31	38	30	33.0	S. W.	S. W.	W.	Cloudy	Snow	Variable	
29	30.05	30.06	30.16	28	38	29	31.7	N. W.	N. W.	N. W.	Variable	Cloudy	Clear	
30	30.13	29.94	29.76	29	37	32	32.7	S. W.	S. W.	E'ly	Variable	Cloudy	Snow	
31	29.76	29.64	29.69	32	38	30	33.3	N. W.	W'ly	W'ly	Clear	Clear	Variable	
Means	29.75	29.75	29.73	29.5	38.0	31.0	...	...	...	...	...	...	...	5.86
REDUCED TO SEA LEVEL.														
Max.	30.67	30.56	30.69	49	54	48	48.7							
Min.	29.17	29.14	29.15	5	17	8	10.0							
Mean	29.93	29.93	29.91											
Range	1.50	1.42	1.54	44	37	40	38.7							
Mean of month	29.923			...	...	...	32.8							
Extreme range	1.55			...	...	...	49.0							

Prevailing winds from some point between—

	Days.
N. & E.	4
E. & S.	2
S. & W.	8
W. & N.	17

	Days
Clear	10
Variable } Cloudy }	10
Rain or snow fell on	11

REMARKS.

1st. Pleasant.
2d. Very pleasant.
3d. Cloudy in the morning, and very damp; wind very light W'ly, but soon hauled S'ly and S. E. Began to rain moderately from 11 to 12 A. M. Rain and wind increased to a heavy storm in the evening. Cleared during the night, with wind at S. W.
4th. Pleasant.
5th. Variable; rather blustering.
6th, 7th, and 8th. Fine.
9th. Mild.
15th. Cloudy for the most part. Began to rain moderately from 4 to 5 P. M.
11th. Mild and pleasant.
12th and 13th. Pleasant.
14th. Cloudy in the morning; wind S. E. Began to rain from 10 to 11 A. M., and continued—at times heavy—till 4 or 5 P. M., when the wind came to N. W. and cleared. Evening very clear, with faint aurora.
15th. Pleasant.
16th. Began to rain from 2 to 3 P. M.; wind N. E. Rain continued in the evening and during the night; wind increasing to a gale.
17th. Heavy storm, with wind N. E., all day.
18th. Snowed moderately, with the wind brisk at N. W., all day. Clouds broken in the evening. Two inches of dry snow.
19th. Variable; raw and blustering.
20th. Pleasant.
21st. Cold. Light snow in the morning; abou two inches.
22d. Cold, but pleasant. Wind light N. W.
23d. Air raw, and indications of rain. Heavy wind and rain during the night. Wind S. W.
24th. Rain in the morning. Cleared from 10 to 11 P. M.
25th. Pleasant.
26th. Very fine, though cool.
27th. Mild and pleasant. Very bright and well defined halo round the moon from 10 P. M.
28th. Moderate snow in the morning; 1½ to [illegible] inches deep. Clear and mild in the evening.
29th. Pleasant. Halo around the moon in the evening.
30th. Cloudy in the morning. Began to snow moderately from 3 to 4 P. M.
31st. Mild and pleasant.

January, 1842.

DAYS.	BAROMETER Sunrise.	At 1 P. M.	At 10 P. M.	THERMOMETER Sunrise.	At 1 P. M.	At 10 P. M.	Daily mean.	WINDS Sunrise.	At 1 P. M.	At 10 P. M.	WEATHER Sunrise.	At 1 P. M.	At 10 P. M.	RAIN AND SNOW
1	29.96	29.85	29.64	17	32	35	28.0	N. W.	S. W.	S. W.	Clear	Cloudy	Clear	
2	29.44	29.31	29.32	34	43	39	38.7	S. W.	W'ly	S. W'ly	Clear	Variable	Cloudy	
3	29.70	29.75	29.91	10	15	15	13.3	N. W.	W'ly	W'ly	Clear	Clear	Clear	
4	29.72	29.48	29.63	18	37	27	27.3	N. E.	W'ly	W'ly	Snow	Clear	Variable	0.25
5	30.01	30.05	30.30	22	24	10	18.7	N. W.	N. W.	N. W.	Clear	Clear	Clear	
6	30.36	30.27	29.85	3	24	34	20.3	N. W.	S. W.	S. E.	Clear	Variable	Rain	0.65
7	29.43	29.43	29.67	46	46	36	42.7	W'ly	W'ly	W'ly	Cloudy	Cloudy	Cloudy	
8	30.00	29.98	29.83	24	36	34	31.3	N. E'ly	N. E.	N. E.	Clear	Clear	Cloudy	
9	29.64	29.74	29.99	38	46	35	39.7	S. W'ly	W'ly	W'ly	Cloudy	Clear	Cloudy	
10	29.98	29.98	30.00	32	35	31	32.7	S. W.	S. W.	W'ly	Snow	Cloudy	Clear	0.10
11	29.93	29.85	29.68	27	35	33	31.7	W'ly	S. W.	W'ly	Cloudy	Cloudy	Cloudy	
12	29.57	29.51	29.56	28	38	32	32.7	W'ly	W'ly	W'ly	Clear	Cloudy	Cloudy	
13	29.91	29.96	30.08	16	11	6	11.0	N. W.	N. W.	N. W.	Clear	Clear	Clear	
14	29.90	29.61	29.50	14	40	38	30.7	S'ly	S. W.	S. W.	Variable	Cloudy	Clear	
15	29.55	29.51	29.62	31	36	25	30.7	W'ly	N. W.	N. W.	Clear	Clear	Clear	
16	29.66	...	29.75	19	...	24	...	N. W.	...	N. W.	Clear	...	Clear	
17	29.85	29.79	29.76	24	38	36	32.7	N. W.	S. W'ly	W'ly	Clear	Variable	Clear	
18	29.82	29.85	29.88	33	46	34	37.7	S. W.	S'ly	S. W'ly	Clear	Clear	Clear	
19	29.89	29.78	29.77	32	45	37	38.0	S. W.	S. E.	S'ly	Foggy	Clear	Clear	
20	29.69	29.63	29.56	36	49	42	42.3	S. W.	S'ly	S. W'ly	Clear	Clear	Cloudy	
21	29.24	29.08	29.29	47	49	35	43.7	S'ly	S. E'ly	W'ly	Rain	Foggy	Clear	0.30
22	29.55	29.56	29.86	28	33	18	26.3	W'ly	W'ly	N. W.	Clear	Clear	Clear	
23	30.10	30.13	30.26	12	18	10	13.3	W'ly	W'ly	N. W.	Clear	Clear	Clear	
24	30.38	30.31	30.21	4	16	14	11.3	N. W.	N. W.	W'ly	Clear	Clear	Clear	
25	29.98	29.81	29.71	22	37	32	30.3	S. W.	S. W.	S. W.	Clear	Variable	Clear	
26	29.67	29.57	29.44	30	43	33	35.3	S. W.	S. W.	S. W.	Clear	Clear	Clear	
27	29.25	29.40	29.90	33	35	21	29.7	W'ly	W'ly	N. W.	Snow	Clear	Clear	
28	30.17	30.05	...	20	33	36	29.7	W'ly	W'ly	S. W.	Clear	Clear	Clear	
29	29.73	29.64	29.58	44	52	39	45.0	S. W.	S. W.	S. W.	Cloudy	Variable	Foggy	
30	[illegible]	[illegible]	[illegible]	[illegible]	[illegible]	[illegible]	[illegible]	W'ly	W'ly	W'ly	Variable	Clear	Clear	
31	29.72	29.55	29.40	34	46	50	43.3	S. W.	S. W.	S. W.	Variable	Cloudy	Cloudy	
Means	29.70	29.70	29.75	26.5	36.2	29.9	...	...	...	...	...	...	...	1.30
REDUCED TO SEA LEVEL.														
Max.	30.56	30.49	30.48	47	52	50	45.0							
Min.	29.42	29.26	29.47	3	11	6	11.0							
Mean	29.96	29.91	29.93											
Range	1.14	1.23	1.01	44	41	44	34.0							
Mean of month	29.933			...	...	...	30.9							
Extreme range	1.30			...	...	...	49.0							

Prevailing winds from some point between—

	Days.
N. & E.	1
E. & S.	2
S. & W.	18
W. & N.	10

	Days.
Clear	11
Variable } Cloudy }	12
Rain or snow fell on	8

1st. Pleasant and mild.
2d. Mild and pleasant. Wind brisk W'ly.
3d. Cold. Wind brisk and cutting.
4th. Snow in the morning Clear and mild in the afternoon. From two to three inches of snow
5th. Fine, though cool.
6th. Clear in the morning; hazy towards noon Cloudy in the afternoon, with wind S'ly and inclining to S. E. Began to snow and rain from [illegible] to 8 P. M.; soon turned to pure rain.
7th. Rain in the morning. Cloudy in the afternoon and evening.
8th. Mild. Clear in the morning. Cloudy late in the afternoon and in the evening. Dash of snow from 8 to 9 P. M.
9th. Pleasant.
10th. From one to two inches of light snow in the morning.
11th. Very mild. Cloudy, with occasional appearances of snow in the air.
12th. Very mild.
13th. At sunrise, wind brisk N. W.; ther. 16° and falling fast. At 9 A. M., ther. 10°. At 11 A. M. ther. 9°. At 1 P. M., 11°. At 10 P. M., 6°; clea and very still.
14th. Wind fresh from S. W.
15th. Pleasant. Aurora in the evening; diffused light of considerable brightness, withou corruscations.
16th. Pleasant.
17th. Very pleasant.
18th. Very pleasant. The air mild and soft a May.
19th. Unusually mild and pleasant.
20th. Mild through the day. Cloudy at 11 P. M.
21st. Light rain in the morning. Cloudy in the afternoon. Wind changed from S. W. to about W. from 4 to 5 P. M. Quite gusty in the evening, and clear.
22d. Wind strong and blustering from the west [illegible] evening, and colder.
23d. Pleasant, though cold.
24th. Cold.
25th. Blustering.
26th. Pleasant.
27th. Flurry of snow from 7 to 9 A. M. Clear in the afternoon.
28th. Pleasant.
29th. Mild and pleasant.
30th. Very pleasant.

February, 1842.

DAYS.	BAROMETER, REDUCED TO 32° F. Sunrise.	At 1 P. M.	At 10 P. M.	THERMOMETER. Sunrise.	At 1 P. M.	At 10 P. M.	Daily mean.	WINDS. Sunrise.	At 1 P. M.	At 10 P. M.	WEATHER. Sunrise.	At 1 P. M.	At 10 P. M.	RAIN AND SNOW IN INCHES OF WATER.
1	29.73	29.89	30.06	30	43	30	34.3	W'ly	N. W.	N. W.	Clear	Clear	Clear	
2	30.15	30.05	29.94	26	42	41	36.3	N. W.	S. W.	S. W.	Clear	Clear	Clear	
3	29.70	29.58	29.58	48	54	55	52.3	S. W.	S. W.	S. W.	Rain	Cloudy	Cloudy	0.88
4	29.38	29.48	29.35	58	56	47	53.7	S. W.	N. E.	N. E.	Cloudy	Cloudy	Rain	0.10
5	29.27	29.16	29.71	48	52	34	44.7	W'ly	N. W.	W'ly	Cloudy	Clear	Clear	
6	29.96	29.85	29.71	30	43	44	39.0	W'ly	S. W.	S. W.	Clear	Clear	Clear	
7	29.60	29.49	29.36	44	48	42	44.7	S. W.	S. W.	S. W.	Cloudy	Rain	Rain	0.12
8	29.30	29.27	29.44	34	42	20	32.0	N'ly	N. W.	N. W.	Cloudy	Cloudy	Clear	
9	29.88	29.92	29.87	9	20	24	17.7	N'ly	W'ly	S. W.	Clear	Clear	Variable	
10	29.85	29.90	29.97	27	40	31	32.7	S. W.	S. E'ly	S. E'ly	Clear	Clear	Clear	
11	30.03	30.00	29.84	27	45	38	36.7	S. E.	S. E.	S. E.	Clear	Variable	Clear	
12	29.59	29.61	29.88	47	53	36	45.3	S. W.	N. W.	N. W.	Rain	Variable	Clear	
13	29.84	29.69	29.46	30	39	38	35.7	N. W.	N. E.	E'ly	Variable	Variable	Cloudy	
14	29.33	29.26	29.45	42	48	23	37.7	W'ly	W'ly	N. W.	Variable	Clear	Clear	
15	29.81	29.89	30.03	9	21	17	15.7	N. W.	N. W.	N. W.	Clear	Clear	Clear	
16	29.80	29.91	28.51	28	39	44	37.0	S. E.	S. E.	S. E.	Cloudy	Cloudy	Rain	0.60
17	28.85	29.21	29.75	20	22	18	20.0	W'ly	W'ly	W'ly	Cloudy	Cloudy	Clear	
18	30.04	30.04	29.88	18	33	39	30.0	W'ly	S. W.	S. W.	Clear	Clear	Variable	
19	29.61	29.29	29.81	43	53	25	40.3	S.	S. W.	N. W.	Rain	Cloudy	Clear	1.40
20	30.12	30.12	30.10	20	30	27	25.7	N. W.	N. W.	W'ly	Clear	Clear	Variable	
21	29.94	29.89	29.91	21	35	26	27.3	S. W'ly	S. W'ly	W'ly	Clear	Clear	Clear	
22	29.87	29.80	29.81	21	35	26	27.3	N'ly	S. W.	N. W.	Clear	Clear	Clear	
23	29.92	29.89	29.90	21	38	29	29.3	N'ly	W'ly	S. W'ly	Clear	Clear	Clear	
24	29.90	29.87	30.04	32	47	32	37.0	S. W.	S. W.	N'ly	Clear	Clear	Clear	
25	30.27	30.29	30.31	22	34	27	27.7	N'ly	E'ly	N. E.	Clear	Clear	Clear	
26	30.21	30.10	29.75	30	32	34	32.0	N E by E	E'ly	E'ly	Cloudy	Rain	Rain	0.95
27	29.64	29.63	29.66	30	37	36	34.3	N'ly	N'ly	N. W.	Cloudy	Sn. & r'n	Clear	
28	29.82	29.88	29.98	33	41	34	36.0	N. W.	N'ly	N. W.	Clear	Clear	Clear	
Means	29.76	29.75	29.75	30.3	40.1	32.7	...	...	...	...	...	...	...	4.05
REDUCED TO SEA LEVEL.														
Max.	30.45	30.47	30.49	58	56	55	53.7							
Min.	29.03	29.34	28.69	9	20	17	15.7							
Mean	29.94	29.93	29.93											
Range	1.42	1.13	1.80	49	36	38	38.0							
Mean of month	29.933			...	...	...	34.4							
Extreme range	1.80			...	...	...	49.0							

Prevailing winds from some point between—

	Days.
N. & E.	4
E. & S.	3
S. & W.	10
W. & N.	11

	Days.
Clear	12
Variable, Cloudy	5
Rain or snow fell on	11

REMARKS.

1st and 2d. Very pleasant.
3d. Rainy.
4th. At sunrise, wind fresh S. W.; ther. 58°. At 10 A. M., wind light; ther. 60°. Before 1 P. M., wind came to N. E., and ther. fell to 56°. Cloudy during the day, with occasional light rain. In the evening, rain increased.
5th. Cloudy in the morning, with some rain. Gusty during the day. Clear evening. Frost out of the ground in many places.
6th. Pleasant.
7th. Light rain occasionally during the day and evening.
8th. Cloudy, with occasional flurries of snow. Grew cold in the evening, with wind very brisk at N. W. Frost generally out of the ground, but began to freeze about sunset.
9th. Pleasant, though cool.
10th. Pleasant.
11th. Very pleasant.
12th. Very pleasant. Sprinkling of rain in the morning.
13th. Mild. Air damp.
14th. Mild through the day. Wind came to N. W., very fresh, and grew cold in the evening. Frost out of the ground in most places.
15th. Cold, but fine.
16th. Cloudy at sunrise; wind light S. E'ly. Wind increased, with dashes of rain in afternoon. Rain, with very heavy wind, in evening. At 10½ P. M., bar. 28.61; wind considerably abated; rain light. At 11 P. M., bar. 28.60, and still falling.
17th. At 5 A. M., wind heavy from W'ly, with flurry of snow on the ground. At 7 A. M., wind about W. S. W., and rather abated. Very blustering all day. Wind generally a little to the south of west.
18th. Mild.
19th. Raining moderately at 6 A. M., with wind nearly S. Wind came more to S. W., and heavy rain in the morning. Cleared towards night, with wind at N. W.
20th. Pleasant.
21st to 24th. Very pleasant.
25th. Pleasant.
26th. Rainy. A little hail in morning. Steady rain in afternoon and evening.
27th. Light snow, mixed with some rain, in the morning. Cleared towards night.
28th. Very pleasant.

March, 1842.

DAYS.	BAROMETER Sunrise.	At 1 P. M.	At 10 P. M.	THERMOMETER Sunrise.	At 1 P. M.	At 10 P. M.	Daily mean.	WINDS Sunrise.	At 1 P. M.	At 10 P. M.	WEATHER Sunrise.	At 1 P. M.	At 10 P. M.	RAIN AND SNOW
1	29.99	29.89	29.80	34	48	40	40.7	S'ly	S. W.	S. W.	Clear	Cloudy	Cloudy	
2	29.59	29.39	29.22	43	51	53	49.0	S. W.	S. W.	S. W.	Cloudy	Cloudy	Cloudy	
3	29.61	29.50	29.62	47	64	50	53.7	W'ly	W'ly	W'ly	Variable	Clear	Clear	
4	29.60	29.54	29.51	46	68	50	54.7	S. E'ly	S. W.	S. E'ly	Cloudy	Clear	Variable	
5	29.40	29.61	29.89	46	40	35	40.3	S. W.	N. E.	N. E.	Variable	Cloudy	Cloudy	
6	29.97	29.96	29.91	33	34	36	34.3	N. E.	N. E.	N. E.	Misty	Shower	Shower	0.52
7	29.71	29.70	29.80	35	46	35	38.7	N. W.	N. W'ly	N'ly	Cloudy	Variable	Cloudy	
8	30.02	30.07	30.11	31	41	34	35.3	N'ly	N'ly	W'ly	Clear	Clear	Clear	
9	29.90	29.65	29.41	36	48	46	43.3	S. W.	S. W.	S. W.	Variable	Cloudy	Cloudy	
10	29.37	29.34	29.56	45	66	45	52.0	S. W.	S. W.	N'ly	Cloudy	Variable	Variable	
11	29.51	29.42	29.74	42	40	23	35.0	N. E.	N. E.	N. W.	Cloudy	Cloudy	Clear	
12	30.11	30.16	30.17	15	27	24	22.0	N. W.	N. W.	N. W.	Clear	Clear	Clear	
13	30.02	...	29.92	27	38	32	32 3	S. W.	S. W'ly	S. W.	Cloudy	Cloudy	Clear	
14	29.96	29.92	29.94	27	45	34	35.3	N. W'ly	N. W'ly	W'ly	Variable	Variable	Clear	
15	29.91	29.86	29.85	31	50	36	39.0	N. W.	S'ly	S. W.	Clear	Variable	Clear	
16	29.99	30.00	29.98	31	42	38	37.0	N. W.	N. W.	S. W.	Clear	Clear	Clear	
17	29.71	29.55	29.66	41	55	50	48.7	S. W.	S. W.	S. W'ly	Cloudy	Variable	Clear	
18	29.85	29.89	29.94	40	54	40	44.7	N. W.	N. W.	N. W.	Clear	Clear	Clear	
19	29.84	29.66	29.59	35	58	52	48.3	S. W.	S. W.	S. W.	Clear	Clear	Clear	
20	29.73	29.60	29.65	44	60	49	51.0	S. W.	W'ly	W'ly	Clear	Clear	Variable	
21	29.90	29.90	29.92	27	47	36	36.7	N.	N. E.	S'ly	Clear	Variable	Variable	
22	29.81	29.75	29.84	31	32	28	30.3	N. E.	N. E.	N. E.	Snow	Rain	Snow	0.50
23	29.97	30.00	30.04	21	27	23	23.7	N.	N. N. E.	N.	Clear	Cloudy	Clear	
24	30.11	30.08	30.06	21	40	33	31.3	N. W.	N. W.	S'ly	Clear	Clear	Variable	
25	29.89	29.74	29.57	32	33	34	33.0	E'ly	E'ly	N. E.	Sn. & r'n	R'n & h'l	Rain	0.80
26	29.53	29.53	29.71	32	47	36	38.3	N. W.	N. W.	N. W.	Cloudy	Variable	Clear	
27	29.84	29.79	29.65	36	52	45	44.3	N. W.	N. W'ly	S. W.	Clear	Clear	Clear	
28	29.59	29.67	29.94	40	45	33	39.3	N.N.W.	N. W.	N. W.	Clear	Clear	Clear	
29	30.09	30.03	29.99	30	48	38	38.7	N. W.	S. E.	S. W.	Clear	Clear	Cloudy	
30	29.68	29.45	29.47	40	52	46	46.0	S. W.	S. W.	S. W.	Cloudy	Cloudy	Cloudy	
31	29.52	29.58	29.86	40	38	25	34.3	N. W.	N'ly	N. W.	Clear	Rain	Clear	0.25
Means	29.79	29.74	29.78	34.8	4[illegible].3	38.0	...	...	...	...	...	...	...	2.07
REDUCED TO SEA LEVEL.														
Max.	30.29	30.34	30.35	47	68	53	54.7							
Min.	29.55	29.52	29.40	15	27	23	22.0							
Mean	29.97	29.92	29.96											
Range	0.74	0.82	0.95	32	41	30	32.7							
Mean of month	29.950			...	...	...	39.7							
Extreme range	0.95			...	...	...	53.0							

Prevailing winds from some point between—

	Days.
N. & E.	7
E. & S.	1
S. & W.	12
W. & N.	11

	Days.
Clear	8
Variable, Cloudy	15
Rain or snow fell on	8

1st. Pleasant. Copious white frost in morning.
2d. Foggy morning. Appearances of rain.
3d. Pleasant.
4th. Very warm for the season. Frost out of the ground generally.
5th. In the morning, wind S. W.; from 10 to 10½ A. M., very blustering, with heavy clouds and dashes of rain, and change of wind suddenly from S. W. to N. E.
6th. Mist, with occasional approach to rain during the day. Copious shower about 10 P. M., with thunder and lightning.
7th. Cloudy, with occasional dashes of rain.
8th. Very pleasant.
9th. Cloudy, with appearances of rain.
10th. Very mild.
11th. Wind N. E., raw. From 3 to 4 P. M, a flurry of snow; wind came to N. W., and cleared.
12th. Very clear.
13th. Weather raw.
14th. Mild and pleasant.
15th. Very mild and pleasant. Wind light S'ly and S. W'ly during the day.
16th. Prevailing wind N. W.; rather cool, and raw.
17th. Very pleasant.
18th. Very fine. Hazy in the evening. A well-defined halo round the moon from 7½ to 8 P. M.
19th. Unusually fine. In the evening, wind light from S. W'ly. Light clouds passing the moon from the north of west.
20th. Very pleasant.
21st. Pleasant.
22d. Moderate snow nearly all day.
23d. The ground covered with snow blown into drifts—perhaps two inches deep on the average—which, in the fields, continued during the day.
24th. Very pleasant in the morning. Towards night, wind came to S'ly; very raw. Halo round the moon in the evening
25th. Very stormy. Snow, rain, and hail—altogether and separately.
26th. Blustering, with many clouds. Very clear in the evening.
27th. Very fine.
28th. Rather blustering, and raw.
29th. In the morning, wind N. W.; then N., N. E., and E., and so to S. E at 2 P. M. In the evening, wind S. W., and cloudy.
30th. Light rain from 3 to 5 P. M.
31st Pleasant in the morning. Blustering, with rain and some snow, in the afternoon. Clear in the evening, and blustering and cold.

April, 1842.

DAYS.	BAROMETER, REDUCED TO 32° F. At 6 A. M.	At 1 P. M.	At 10 P. M.	THERMOMETER. At 6 A. M.	At 1 P. M.	At 10 P. M.	Daily mean.	WINDS. At 6 A. M.	At 1 P. M.	At 10 P. M.	WEATHER. At 6 A. M.	At 1 P. M.	At 10 P. M.	RAIN AND SNOW IN INCHES OF WATER.
1	30.07	30.05	30.08	23	33	30	28.7	N. W.	N. W.	N. W.	Clear	Clear	Clear	
2	29.99	29.80	29.72	35	55	53	47.7	S. W.	S. W.	S. W.	Cloudy	Clear	Clear	
3	29.69	29.72	29.84	54	70	52	58.7	S. W.	W.	N. W.	Cloudy	Hazy	Rain	
4	29.99	30.02	30.02	35	38	35	36.0	N. E.	E'ly	E'ly	Rain	Rain	Cloudy	0.70
5	29.91	29.82	29.89	34	38	36	36.0	N. E.	N. E.	N. E.	Rain	Cloudy	Cloudy	
6	29.99	29.95	29.90	36	57	46	46.3	N. E.	S. E'ly	S. E'ly	Clear	Clear	Clear	
7	29.82	29.64	29.60	46	54	42	47.3	S'ly	N. W'ly	N. E.	Cloudy	Cloudy	Rain	0.24
8	29.64	29.69	29.75	41	45	39	41.7	N. E.	N. E.	N. E.	Cloudy	Cloudy	Cloudy	
9	29.77	29.76	29.79	36	40	36	37.3	N. E.	N. E.	N. E.	Cloudy	Cloudy	Cloudy	
10	29.78	29.75	29.69	35	48	42	41.7	N. E.	N. E	N. E.	Cloudy	Variable	Clear	
11	29.59	29.59	29.66	47	64	51	54.0	S. W.	N. W.	N. E'ly	Clear	Clear	Clear	
12	29.76	29.72	29.82	42	55	42	46.3	N'ly	N. W.	N. W.	Variable	Clear	Clear	
13	29.94	29.91	29.84	34	54	42	43.3	N. E.	N. E.	S. E'ly	Clear	Clear	Rain	
14	29.62	29.58	29.71	38	43	42	41.0	N. E.	N. E.	N'ly	Rain	Cloudy	Variable	
15	29.79	29.77	29.79	40	59	49	49.3	S. W'ly	S. W.	S. W.	Clear	Clear	Variable	
16	29.90	29.92	29.98	40	52	42	44.7	N. W.	N. W.	N. W.	Clear	Clear	Clear	
17	30.11	30.09	30.10	40	54	41	45.0	N. E.	N. E.	S. E.	Clear	Clear	Cloudy	
18	30.03	29.99	29.78	36	38	38	37.3	E'ly	N. E.	N. E.	Rain	Rain	Misty	0.63
19	29.65	29.50	29.45	40	42	41	41.0	N. E.	N. E.	N. E.	Misty	Misty	Misty	
20	29.44	29.52	29.75	44	60	46	50.0	N. W'ly	N. W.	N. E'ly	Cloudy	Variable	Variable	
21	29.90	29.89	29.86	45	62	47	51.3	N. E.	S'ly	S'ly	Clear	Clear	Clear	
22	29.72	29.58	29.45	48	80	63	63.7	S'ly	S. W.	S. W.	Clear	Clear	Clear	
23	29.59	29.74	29.89	57	63	46	55.3	N. by E.	N. E.	S. W.	Clear	Clear	Clear	
24	29.94	29.86	29.90	44	59	48	50.3	N. W.	S'ly	S. W.	Clear	Cloudy	Hazy	
25	29.77	29.68	29.68	48	54	46	49.3	S. W.	N. E.	N. E.	Cloudy	Cloudy	Cloudy	
26	29.63	29.48	29.35	44	50	44	46.0	N. E.	N. E.	N. E.	Cloudy	Misty	Rain	0.53
27	29.21	29.20	29.35	45	61	46	50.7	N. W.	N. .	'ly	Cloudy	Clear	Clear	
28	29.40	29.39	29.51	44	55	42	47.0	N. W.	N. W.	W.	Clear	Cloudy	Clear	
29	29.60	29.53	29.61	42	58	47	49.0	W'ly	N. W.	W'ly	Clear	Clear	Clear	
30	29.65	29.60	29.55	44	64	50	52.7	W'ly	S. W'ly	S. W.	Clear	Clear	Clear	
Means	29.76	29.75	29.74	41.2	53.5	44.1	...	...	...	...	...	...	...	2.10
REDUCED TO SEA LEVEL.														
Max.	30.29	30.27	30.28	57	80	63	63.7							
Min.	29.39	29.38	29.53	23	33	30	28.7							
Mean	29.94	29.93	29.92											
Range	0.90	0.89	0.75	34	47	33	35.0							
Mean of month	29.930			...	...	...	46.3							
Extreme range	0.91			...	...	...	57.0							

Prevailing winds from some point between—

	Days.
N. & E.	13
E. & S.	1
S. & W.	6
W. & N.	10

	Days.
Clear	13
Variable / Cloudy	8
Rain fell on	9

REMARKS.

1st. Pleasant.
2d. Very pleasant. Wind brisk in the evening.
3d. Warm and sultry. Sprinkling of rain in the afternoon; wind N. W.
4th. Moderate rain during the greater part of the day. Wind light, about E. N. E.
5th. Moderate rain at intervals during the day.
6th. Weather fine.
7th. Cloudy. Moderate rain from 4 to 7 or 8 P. M.
8th. Air damp and raw.
9th. Cloudy and raw. Wind fresh.
10th. Clouds broken at noon. Clear towards night and evening. Aurora in the north—not very bright.
11th and 12th. Fine.
13th. Clear in the morning; wind N. E. and E'ly. In the afternoon, wind S'ly and S. E'ly. Cloudy towards night; began to rain moderately from 9 to 10 P. M.
14th. Rain in the morning. Cleared towards night.
15th, 16th, and 17th. Fine.
18th. Rainy. Wind N. E., cold.
19th. Heavy mist, mixed with some rain, for the greater part of the day and evening. Wind light, about N. N. E.
20th. Fine.
21st. Very pleasant.
22d. Clear and very warm.
23d. Very fine.
24th. Pleasant.
25th. Wind changed from S. W. to N. E., from 8 to 10 A. M.
26th. Misty through the day. Heavy showers in the evening.
27th. Fine day.
28th. Fine for the most part.
29th and 30th. Fine.

May, 1842.

DAYS.	BAROMETER At 6 A. M.	At 1 P. M.	At 10 P. M.	THERMOMETER At 6 A. M.	At 1 P. M.	At 10 P. M.	Daily mean.	WINDS At 6 A. M.	At 1 P. M.	At 10 P. M.	WEATHER At 6 A. M.	At 1 P. M.	At 10 P. M.	RAIN
1	29.51	29.41	29.32	50	63	53	55.3	S. W.	S. E'ly	S. W'ly	Clear	Variable	Clear	
2	29.33	29.37	29.44	50	56	49	51.7	N. W.	S. W.	N. W.	Clear	Rain	Clear	0.10
3	29.60	29.67	29.65	46	49	42	45.7	N. E.	N. E.	N. E.	Cloudy	Cloudy	Cloudy	
4	29.60	29.69	29.83	41	52	47	46.7	N. E.	N. E.	N. W.	Rain	Cloudy	Clear	
5	29.95	29.93	29.90	46	65	51	54.0	N. W.	S. W.	S. W.	Clear	Clear	Clear	
6	29.82	...	29.67	49	...	61	...	S. W'ly	...	S. W.	Clear	Clear	Clear	
7	29.80	29.83	29.86	43	55	46	48.0	N. W.	N. W.	N. W.	Clear	Clear	Clear	
8	29.84	29.72	29.67	38	60	51	49.7	N. W.	S. W.	S. W.	Clear	Variable	Rain	0.10
9	29.48	29.49	29.57	46	50	41	45.7	S. W.	N. W.	N. W.	Cloudy	Cloudy	Shower	
10	29.53	29.53	29.48	40	49	48	45.7	N. W.	S. W.	S. W.	Clear	Cloudy	Clear	
11	29.49	29.40	29.45	48	74	58	60.0	S. W.	S. W.	W'ly	Clear	Clear	Rain	0.68
12	29.54	29.57	29.71	50	64	50	54.7	N. W.	W'ly	W'ly	Clear	Clear	Clear	
13	29.75	29.63	29.55	46	63	57	55.3	S. E'ly	S. E'ly	S'ly	Clear	Clear	Cloudy	
14	29.73	29.74	29.80	46	62	51	53.0	N. W.	N. W.	N. E.	Clear	Clear	Clear	
15	29.82	29.81	29.72	49	63	50	54.0	N. E.	S. E'ly	S. E'ly	Clear	Variable	Cloudy	
16	29.69	29.66	29.76	44	68	55	55.7	N. W.	S. W.	S. W'ly	Clear	Clear	Clear	
17	29.94	29.96	30.01	53	74	54	60.3	S'ly	S. E'ly	S. W.	Clear	Clear	Clear	
18	30.01	29.99	29.94	50	70	55	58.3	S'ly	S'ly	S'ly	Clear	Clear	Clear	
19	29.87	29.71	29.95	56	76	49	60.3	S. W'ly	S. W.	N. E'ly	Clear	Variable	Rain	0.72
20	30.09	30.11	30.09	38	37	38	37.7	N. E.	N. E.	N. E.	Rain	Rain	Clear	
21	30.09	30.01	29.95	36	65	47	49.3	W'ly	S. W.	S. W.	Clear	Clear	Clear	
22	29.80	29.67	29.61	45	63	56	54.7	S. W.	S'ly	S. W.	Variable	Clear	Cloudy	
23	29.56	29.63	29.77	56	56	50	54.0	S. W.	N. E.	N. E.	Cloudy	Cloudy	Clear	
24	29.85	29.81	29.71	44	63	52	53.0	N. E.	S. E'ly	S'ly	Foggy	Cloudy	Rain	
25	29.67	29.56	29.59	54	69	55	59.3	W'ly	N. W.	N. W.	Cloudy	Clear	Clear	
26	29.64	29.69	29.74	55	73	57	61.7	W'ly	W'ly	W'ly	Clear	Clear	Clear	
27	29.76	29.69	29.63	53	58	56	55.7	N. E.	N. E.	S. E'ly	Cloudy	Rain	Cloudy	0.10
28	29.63	29.63	29.68	54	74	62	63.3	S. W.	W'ly	S. W.	Clear	Clear	Clear	
29	29.73	29.67	29.56	56	65	56	59.0	N. E.	S. E'ly	N. E.	Variable	Rain	Rain	1.00
30	29.39	29.34	29.38	51	54	55	53.3	N. E.	N. E.	N. W.	Cloudy	Rain	Clear	0.70
31	29.49	29.59	29.64	51	...	...	...	N. W.	...	...	Clear	...	Clear	
Means	29.70	29.68	29.70	47.0	61.7	51.7	...	...	...	...	...	...	...	3.40
REDUCED TO SEA LEVEL.														
Max.	30.27	30.29	30.27	56	76	62	63.3							
Min.	29.51	29.52	29.50	36	37	38	37.7							
Mean	29.88	29.85	29.88											
Range	0.76	0.77	0.77	20	39	24	25.6							
Mean of month	29.870			...	...	...	53.8							
Extreme range	0.79			...	...	...	40.0							

Prevailing winds from some point between—

	Days.
N. & E.	7
E. & S.	5
S. & W.	12
W. & N.	7

	Days.
Clear	11
Variable / Cloudy	7
Rain fell on	13

REMARKS.

1st. Pleasant. Shower from 8 to 9 P. M.
2d. Cloudy for the most part, with sprinkling of rain.
3d. Cloudy, with appearances of rain.
4th. Light rain from N. E. for a while in the morning. Light showers from 5 to 6 P. M., with wind from W'ly.
5th. Very fine.
6th. Fine.
7th. Very fine.
8th. Considerable white frost in the College yard this morning. Pleasant in the morning. Cloudy in the afternoon. Light rain began from 7 to 8 P. M.
9th. Cool. Cloudy, with some rain, in the morning. Clear from 7 to 9 P. M. Light shower before 10 P. M.
10th. Cloudy, cool, and raw.
11th. Fine during the day. Heavy thunder-shower from 7 to 10 P. M.
12th. Fine.
13th. Fine for the greater part of the day. Towards night, the air grew raw. Sprinkling of rain in the evening.
14th. Fine.
15th. Clear in the morning. Cloudy in the afternoon, and raw.
16th, 17th, and 18th. Fine.
19th. Fine in the morning. Cloudy in the afternoon. Began to rain from 5 to 6 P. M. Rain in the evening.
20th. Storm of rain, hail, and snow intermixed —from the N. E.—during a large part of the forenoon. Storm ceased in the afternoon. Clear in the evening.
21st. Copious white frost in the College yard this morning, and the ground frozen quite hard in many places in the vicinity. Fine during the day.
22d. Pleasant.
23d. Cloudy. Fog and mist till 5 or 6 P. M. Clear in the evening.
24th. Fog and clouds. Sprinkling of rain in the evening.
25th. Cloudy in the morning. Clear in the afternoon and evening.
26th. Fine.
27th. Cloudy, with sprinkling of rain at times during the day.
28th. Fine.
29th. Light rain in the afternoon and evening. Heavy rain in the night.
30th. Rain in the morning. Cloudy in the afternoon. Cleared in the evening.
31st. Fine.

June, 1842.

DAYS.	Barometer, reduced to 32° F. At 6 A. M.	At 1 P. M.	At 10 P. M.	Thermometer. At 6 A. M.	At 1 P. M.	At 10 P. M.	Daily mean.	Winds. At 6 A. M.	At 1 P. M.	At 10 P. M.	Weather. At 6 A. M.	At 1 P. M.	At 10 P. M.	Rain and Snow in Inches of Water.
1	29.76	29.79	29.89	52	70	70	64.0	N. W.	N. W.	S. E.	Clear	Clear	Clear	
2	29.96	29.96	29.95	52	73	54	59.7	N. W.	E'ly	E'ly	Clear	Clear	Clear	
3	29.95	29.95	29.89	49	69	52	56.7	N. W.	S. E'ly	S. E'ly	Clear	Clear	Clear	
4	29.80	29.72	29.68	46	75	64	61.7	N. E.	S. E'ly	S. W.	Clear	Clear	Variable	
5	29.68	29.60	29.54	66	79	66	70.3	S. W'ly	S. W.	S. W.	Cloudy	Clear	Clear	
6	29.56	29.60	29.78	66	74	54	64.7	N. W.	N. W.	N. W.	Clear	Variable	Clear	
7	30.03	30.04	30.13	44	63	50	52.3	N. W.	N. W.	S. W.	Clear	Clear	Clear	
8	30.22	30.24	30.22	49	64	52	55.0	N. W.	S. W.	S. W.	Cloudy	Clear	Cloudy	
9	29.95	29.76	29.68	54	67	62	61.0	S. E.	S. E'ly	S. W.	Rain	Rain	Clear	} 2.00
10	29.55	29.46	29.45	62	73	62	65.7	S. W.	S'ly	S. W.	Fog, r'n	Variable	Clear	}
11	29.53	29.66	29.83	52	46	43	47.0	N. W.	N. W.	N. W.	Cloudy	Cloudy	Clear	
12	29.98	29.94	29.95	45	69	51	55.0	N. W.	W'ly	S. W.	Clear	Clear	Clear	
13	29.90	29.88	29.84	54	71	63	62.7	S. W.	S. W.	S. W.	Clear	Variable	Rain	0.95
14	...	...	29.90	63	...	64	...	S. W.	S. W.	S. W.	Cloudy	Cloudy	Rain	} 4.50
15	29.86	29.85	29.84	64	75	74	71.0	S. W.	S. W.	S. W.	Rain	Showery	Rain	}
16	29.71	29.64	29.67	66	77	70	71.0	S. W.	S. W.	S. W.	Cloudy	Cloudy	Cloudy	
17	29.67	29.67	29.71	67	76	70	71.0	S. W.	S. W.	S. W.	Clear	Cloudy	Variable	
18	29.75	29.76	29.73	67	73	66	68.7	S. W.	S. W.	S. W.	Foggy	Rain	Cloudy	0.97
19	29.50	29.51	29.52	66	83	71	73.3	S. W.	S. W.	S. W.	Misty	Variable	Clear	
20	29.60	29.63	29.71	67	78	68	71.0	W.	W'ly	N. W'ly	Variable	Clear	Variable	
21	29.81	29.82	29.78	58	77	63	66.0	N. W.	N. W.	S. W'ly	Clear	Clear	Clear	
22	29.71	29.63	29.59	62	80	70	70.7	N. W.	S. W.	S. W.	Clear	Clear	Clear	
23	29.68	29.70	29.62	62	58	56	58.7	N. E.	N. E.	N. E.	Cloudy	Rain	Cloudy	0.33
24	29.62	29.65	...	58	70	...	...	N. W.	N.	...	Variable	Clear	...	
25	...	29.69	29.59	...	76	62	...	...	S. W.	S. W.	Clear	Clear	Rain	0.30
26	...	29.40	29.41	62	78	74	71.3	S. W.	S. W.	S. W.	Cloudy	Variable	Cloudy	
27	29.52	29.61	...	60	67	...	...	N.	N. E.	...	Clear	Clear	Rain	0.60
28	29.64	...	29.61	56	...	64	...	N. E.	...	S. W.	Cloudy	...	Clear	
29	29.63	...	...	64	...	...	...	S. W.	...	...	Clear	...	...	
30	...	29.84	...	...	78	...	...	...	S. E'ly	...	...	Clear	...	
Means	29.75	29.76	29.75	58.3	71.8	62.1	...	...	...	...	...	...	...	9.65
REDUCED TO SEA LEVEL.														
Max.	30.40	30.42	30.40	67	83	74	73.3							
Min.	29.68	29.58	29.59	44	46	43	47.0							
Mean	29.93	29.93	29.93											
Range	0.72	0.84	0.81	23	37	31	26.3							
Mean of month	29.930			...	...	...	64.1							
Extreme range	0.84			...	...	...	40.0							

Prevailing winds from some point between—

	Days.
N. & E.	3
E. & S.	4
S. & W.	16
W. & N.	8

	Days.
Clear	8
Variable } Cloudy }	13
Rain fell on	9

REMARKS.

1st. Fine.
2d, 3d, and 4th. Very fine.
5th. Cloudy in the morning. Clear in the afternoon.
6th and 7th. Fine.
8th. Moderately fine.
9th. Heavy rain in the morning; wind E'ly and S. E'ly. From 1 to 2 P. M., wind came to S. W., and rain ceased. Clear in the evening.
10th. Showery and warm.
11th. Cloudy through the day; wind brisk N. W., and very cool. Clear in evening; breeze light.
12th. At sunrise, thermometer 41°; brisk breeze at N. W., which probably prevented frost. The day fine, but cool.
13th. Clear in the morning. Variable in the afternoon. Began to rain from 9 to 10 P. M. Heavy rain during the night.
14th. Cloudy. Showery in the evening.
15th. Warm and showery through the day and evening. Very heavy rain during night. Rain gauge found running over on the morning of the 16th; gauge holds 3½ inches. From the quantity of water caught in open vessels, it is probable that nearly 4½ inches fell during the night.
16th. Warm, damp, and sultry.
17th. Warm and sultry.
18th. Moderate rain through the day; continued during the night.
19th. Sunshine and clouds in turn. Very warm.
20th. Fine.
21st. Very fine.
22d. Fine.
23d. Moderate rain nearly all day. Cloudy in the evening.
24th. Variable.
25th. Rain.
26th. Variable.
27th. Clear during the day. Heavy rain during the night, with wind at N. E.
28th. Pleasant.

July, 1842.

DAYS.	Barometer. At 6 A. M.	At 1 P. M.	At 10 P. M.	Thermometer. At 6 A. M.	At 1 P. M.	At 10 P. M.	Daily mean.	Winds. At 6 A. M.	At 1 P. M.	At 10 P. M.	Weather. At 6 A. M.	At 1 P. M.	At 10 P. M.	Rain.
1	29.78	29.77	29.80	69	78	71	72.7	S. W.	S. W.	S. W.	Foggy	Clear	Cloudy	
2	29.88	29.86	...	72	82	...	...	S. W.	S. W'ly	...	Variable	Clear	...	
3	...	...	...	...	...	...	...	...	...	...	...	...	...	
4	...	...	...	...	...	...	...	...	...	...	...	...	...	
5	...	...	29.72	...	...	71	...	...	...	S. W.	...	...	Cloudy	
6	29.72	29.71	29.78	70	75	67	70.7	S. W.	S. W.	S. W.	Cloudy	Rain	Cloudy	0.15
7	29.93	29.94	29.93	63	76	66	68.3	N. W.	W'ly	S. E'ly	Clear	Clear	Cloudy	
8	29.90	29.85	29.81	64	78	70	70.7	N. E.	S. E.	S. W'ly	Foggy	Cloudy	Cloudy	
9	29.75	29.74	29.82	72	82	72	75.3	S. W.	S. W.	S. W.	Cloudy	Cloudy	Cloudy	
10	29.91	29.93	29.94	64	73	63	66.7	N. W.	N. E.	E'ly	Cloudy	Clear	Clear	
11	29.95	29.93	29.93	58	78	64	66.7	N. E.	E'ly	S. W.	Clear	Clear	Clear	
12	29.92	29.84	29.78	64	79	66	69.7	S. W.	S'ly	S. W.	Clear	Clear	Clear	
13	29.73	29.67	29.66	66	84	74	74.7	S. W.	S. W.	W'ly	Clear	Clear	Clear	
14	29.66	29.66	29.68	74	86	74	78.0	S. W.	S. W.	S. W.	Clear	Clear	Cloudy	
15	29.70	29.73	29.76	74	82	70	75.3	S. W.	S. W.	N'ly	Variable	Cloudy	Showery	0.55
16	29.74	29.71	29.69	69	77	70	72.0	N. E.	N. E.	N. E.	Cloudy	Cloudy	Variable	
17	29.66	29.64	29.63	68	86	74	76.0	N. W.	N. W.	W'ly	Clear	Clear	Clear	
18	29.63	29.62	29.68	74	86	71	77.0	S. W.	S. W.	S. W.	Clear	Clear	Clear	
19	29.69	29.66	29.60	72	85	74	77.0	S. W.	S. W.	S. W.	Clear	Clear	Cloudy	
20	29.59	29.67	29.87	74	77	66	72.3	S. W.	S. W.	N. W.	Cloudy	Shower	Clear	0.15
21	30.04	30.03	30.03	60	76	63	66.3	N. E.	W'ly	S. W.	Clear	Clear	Clear	
22	30.04	30.02	29.99	62	78	63	60.7	N. W.	N. W.	S. W.	Clear	Clear	Clear	
23	29.98	29.97	29.92	64	80	72	72.0	S. W.	S. W.	S. W.	Clear	Clear	Clear	
24	29.87	29.75	29.81	72	88	71	77.0	S. W.	S. W.	N. W.	Clear	Clear	Variable	
25	29.95	29.95	29.93	59	71	64	64.7	N. W.	N. W.	N. W.	Clear	Clear	Clear	
26	29.91	29.81	29.77	64	85	76	75.0	S. W.	S. W.	S. W.	Cloudy	Clear	Clear	
27	29.70	29.67	28.76	73	90	73	78.7	N. W.	S. W.	N. W.	Clear	Clear	Clear	
28	29.88	29.87	29.90	66	81	71	72.7	N. E.	S. W.	S. W.	Clear	Clear	Clear	
29	29.95	29.90	29.80	70	80	73	74.3	S. W.	S. W.	S. W.	Variable	Clear	Cloudy	
30	29.68	29.53	29.50	73	90	77	80.0	S. W.	S. W.	S. W.	Clear	Clear	Clear	
31	29.46	29.45	29.67	76	87	64	75.7	S. W.	S. W.	N. E.	Clear	Cl'r, sh'r	Cl'dy, r'n	0.63
Means	29.81	29.80	29.80	68.1	81.1	69.6	...	...	...	...	...	...	...	1.48
REDUCED TO SEA LEVEL.														
Max.	30.22	30.21	30.21	76	90	77	80.0							
Min.	29.64	29.63	29.68	58	71	63	64.7							
Mean	29.98	29.97	29.97											
Range	0.58	0.58	0.53	18	19	14	15.3							
Mean of month	29.973			...	...	...	72.9							
Extreme range	0.59			...	...	...	32.0							

Prevailing winds from some point between—

	Days.
N. & E.	3
E. & S.	1
S. & W.	21
W. & N.	4

	Days.
Clear	13
Variable } Cloudy }	9
Rain fell on	7

(2 days omitted.)

REMARKS.

1st. Very warm and damp.
2d to 5th. Mostly cloudy, with wind S. W'ly.
6th. Light rain at intervals.
7th. Fine.
8th. Cloudy, and very damp.
9th. Cloudy, with occasional sprinkling of rain.
10th. Cloudy in the morning. Clear in the afternoon.
11th and 12th. Very fine.
13th. Very fine. Fresh breeze and burning sun.
14th. Fine.
15th. Variable. Copious shower at 2 P. M., and again at 8 P. M.
16th. Cloudy for the most part. Wind light N. E.
17th. Very hot sun. Very little air.
18th. Very fine.
19th. Fine.
20th. Showery in the morning. Clouds broken in the afternoon. Clear in the evening, with wind about W. N. W.
21st, 22d, and 23d. Very fine.
24th. Very hot in the morning. Cloudy in the afternoon, with light shower at 3 o'clock, accompanied with thunder. Light shower again from 7 to 8 P. M.
25th. Fine, though cool.
26th. Fine.
27th. Clear and very hot in the morning. Overcast at 2 P. M. Thunder and sprinkling of rain from 4 to 5 P. M. Clear in the evening. Breeze fresh S. W. most of the day.
28th. Fine.
29th. Fine. Cloudy, with light mist, at sunset.
30th. Fine. Wind very fresh W'ly or W. S. W. all day.
31st. Clear in the morning and very hot, though with a fresh breeze from S. W'ly. Copious shower from 2 to 3 P. M. Showery till night.

August, 1842.

Days.	Barometer, reduced to 32° F. At 6 A. M.	At 1 P. M.	At 10 P. M.	Thermometer. At 6 A. M.	At 1 P. M.	At 10 P. M.	Daily mean.	Winds. At 6 A. M.	At 1 P. M.	At 10 P. M.	Weather. At 6 A. M.	At 1 P. M.	At 10 P. M.	Rain and Snow in Inches of Water.
1	29.75	29.79	29.86	56	70	57	61.0	N. W.	N. W.	N. W.	Variable	Clear	Clear	
2	29.94	29.98	30.01	52	69	62	61.0	N. W.	N. W.	N. W.	Clear	Clear	Clear	
3	30.01	...	30.02	58	76	65	66.3	N. W.	N. W.	N. W.	Clear	Clear	Cloudy	
4	30.03	29.99	29.97	62	68	60	63.3	N. E.	N. E.	N. E.	Cloudy	Cloudy	Cloudy	
5	29.96	29.94	29.99	58	71	70	66.3	N. E.	N. E.	S. W.	Rain	Cloudy	Rain	} 0.83
6	30.01	30.01	29.98	71	81	71	74.3	S. W.	S. W.	S. W.	Rain	Clear	Cloudy	
7	29.93	29.90	29.83	71	74	74	73.0	S. W.	S. W.	S. W.	Cloudy	Rain	Cloudy	1.30
8	29.77	29.74	29.76	71	75	68	71.3	N. W.	N. E.	N. E.	Cloudy	Cloudy	Clear	
9	29.88	29.89	29.89	68	78	69	71.7	N. E.	E.	S'ly	Cloudy	Cloudy	Cloudy	
10	29.94	29.92	29.93	70	79	69	72.7	S. W.	S. W.	S. W.	Variable	Clear	Clear	
11	29.95	29.93	29.93	68	77	70	71.7	S. W.	S. W.	S. W.	Variable	Cloudy	Variable	
12	29.92	29.91	29.92	68	68	67	67.7	E'ly	N. E.	N. E'ly	Cloudy	Rain	Variable	0.52
13	29.95	29.95	29.90	62	66	61	63.0	N. E.	N. E.	N. E.	Cloudy	Cloudy	Cloudy	
14	29.83	...	29.75	64	...	64	...	N. E.	...	N. E.	Cloudy	Shower	Variable	0.20
15	29.78	...	...	64	...	...	...	N. E.	...	...	Cloudy	...	...	
16	...	...	29.78	...	...	68	...	...	...	S. W.	...	...	Variable	
17	29.79	29.77	29.80	68	80	70	72.7	S. W.	S. W.	S. W.	Cloudy	Clear	Variable	
18	29.76	29.75	29.75	70	76	72	72.7	S. W.	S. W.	S. W.	Cl'y, sh'r	Cloudy	Cloudy	0.25
19	29.75	29.73	29.71	72	82	72	75.3	S. W.	S. W.	S. W.	Cloudy	Clear	Clear	
20	29.78	29.79	29.82	66	79	69	71.3	N. W.	N. W.	W'ly	Clear	Clear	Clear	
21	...	...	30.01	...	...	66	...	...	...	N. E'ly	...	...	Clear	
22	...	...	...	...	...	...	...	...	...	...	...	...	...	
23	...	...	...	...	...	...	...	...	...	...	...	...	...	
24	...	...	...	...	...	...	...	...	...	...	...	...	...	
25	...	...	...	...	...	...	...	...	...	...	...	...	...	
26	...	...	...	...	...	...	...	...	...	...	...	...	...	
27	...	...	...	...	...	...	...	...	...	...	...	...	...	
28	...	...	...	...	...	...	...	...	...	...	...	...	...	
29	...	...	29.69	...	...	63	...	...	...	N. W.	...	...	Clear	0.25
30	29.82	29.86	29.91	56	72	62	63.3	N. W.	N. E'ly	S'ly	Clear	Clear	Clear	
31	30.00	30.00	30.01	61	72	63	65.3	S. W'ly	S. E'ly	S'ly	Clear	Clear	Clear	
Means	29.88	29.88	29.85	64.6	74.4	66.6	...	...	...	...	...	...	...	3.35

Reduced to sea level.	At 6 A. M.	At 1 P. M.	At 10 P. M.	Therm. At 6 A. M.	At 1 P. M.	At 10 P. M.	Daily mean.
Max.	30.21	30.19	30.20	72	82	74	75.3
Min.	29.93	29.91	29.87	52	66	57	61.0
Mean	30.05	30.05	30.02				
Range	0.28	0.28	0.33	20	16	17	14.3
Mean of month	30.040			...	...	...	68.5
Extreme range	0.34			...	...	...	30.0

Prevailing winds from some point between— (Days.)
N. & E. . . . 9
E. & S. . . . 1
S. & W. . . . 9
W. & N. . . . 5

(Days.)
Clear 8
Variable . . . . } 8
Cloudy . . . . }
Rain fell on . . 8
(7 days omitted.)

Remarks.

1st. Clear for the most part, and very cool.
2d. Clear.
3d. Fine.
4th. Cloudy. Wind moderate N. E.
5th. Moderate rain at intervals in the morning; wind N. E. From 2 to 3 P. M., wind came to S'ly and S. W.; clouds broken. Sun appeared afterwards; warm and showery. At 3 P. M., thermometer 74°.
6th. Rain early in the morning. Clear at noon. Variable in the afternoon. Foggy in the evening. Copious shower during the night.
7th. Heavy showers during the day and night.
8th. Cloudy, with wind light N. E., most of the day. Clear in the evening.
9th. Wind light and variable. Sun out at times.
10th and 11th. Pleasant.
12th. Heavy thunder and rain from noon to 2 P. M.
13th. Cloudy and cool. Wind moderate.
14th. Copious shower from 4 to 5 P. M.
15th. Light shower at 9 P. M.
16th. Pleasant, though cloudy.
17th. Pleasant.
18th. Heavy shower from 10 to 11 A. M.
19th and 20th. Very fine.
21st. Fine day.
29th. Copious shower between 2 and 3 P. M.
30th and 31st. Very fine.

September, 1842.

Days.	Barometer. Sunrise.	At 1 P. M.	At 10 P. M.	Thermometer. Sunrise.	At 1 P. M.	At 10 P. M.	Daily mean.	Winds. Sunrise.	At 1 P. M.	At 10 P. M.	Weather. Sunrise.	At 1 P. M.	At 10 P. M.	Rain and Snow in Inches of Water.
1	30.01	29.96	29.93	63	76	65	68.0	S. W.	S. W.	S. W.	Variable	Cloudy	Clear	
2	29.90	29.85	29.85	64	78	69	70.3	S. W.	W'ly	S. W.	Clear	Clear	Clear	
3	29.84	29.78	29.74	72	82	73	75.7	S. W.	S. W.	S. W.	Cloudy	Clear	R'n, sh'r	
4	29.90	...	29.92	64	...	62	...	N. W.	...	N. E.	Clear	...	Clear	
5	29.72	29.64	29.69	64	73	66	67.7	S. E.	S. W.	N. W.	Misty	Rain	Clear	
6	29.85	...	29.85	58	...	59	...	N. W.	N. W.	N. W.	Clear	Clear	Clear	
7	29.81	...	...	54	...	62	...	N. W.	...	N. W.	Variable	...	Clear	
8	29.82	29.84	29.85	58	...	...	...	...	...	E'ly	Clear	Clear	Sprink'g	
9	29.77	29.59	29.67	55	53	54	54.0	N. E'ly	N. E'ly	N. W.	Rain	Rain	Clear	1.00
10	29.82	...	29.88	52	...	55	...	N. W.	N. W.	N. W.	Clear	Clear	Clear	
11	29.89	29.69	29.58	55	67	66	62.7	S. W.	S. W.	S. W.	Cloudy	Rain	Hazy	
12	29.50	29.47	29.44	70	83	74	75.7	W'ly	W'ly	W'ly	Clear	Clear	Clear	
13	29.33	29.32	29.60	73	79	60	70.7	S. W'ly	W'ly	N. E.	Clear	Cloudy	Clear	
14	29.73	...	29.85	58	...	56	...	N. E.	N. E.	N. E.	Cloudy	Variable	Clear	
15	29.87	29.85	29.83	56	58	55	56.3	N. E.	N. E.	N. E.	Cloudy	Cloudy	Misty	
16	29.79	29.76	29.75	55	64	60	59.7	N. E.	N. E.	N. E.	Cloudy	Rain	Cloudy	0.40
17	29.79	29.76	29.76	59*	72	56	62.3	N. W.	N. W.	N. W.	Cloudy	Clear	Clear	
18	29.76	29.70	29.66	52	69	55	58.7	N. W.	W'ly	N. W.	Clear	Variable	Clear	
19	29.64	29.64	29.76	51	63	50	54.7	N. W.	N. W.	N. W.	Clear	Variable	Cl'r, sh'r	
20	29.82	29.81	29.81	46	63	48	52.3	N. W.	N. W.	N. W.	Clear	Clear	Clear	
21	29.68	29.56	29.54	44	63	50	52.3	N. W.	S. W.	S. W.	Variable	Cloudy	Clear	
22	29.61	29.65	29.71	42	55	42	46.3	N. W.	N. W.	N. W.	Clear	Clear	Clear	
23	...	...	...	38	...	...	...	N. W.	...	...	Clear	...	...	
24	...	...	29.92	38	...	50	...	...	...	W'ly	...	...	Clear	
25	30.00	30.00	29.99	43	64	50	52.3	N. W.	N. W.	N. W.	Clear	Clear	Clear	
26	30.05	30.03	29.99	45	67	51	54.3	N. W.	N. W.	N. W.	Clear	Clear	Clear	
27	29.97	29.90	29.80	45	72	56	57.7	N. W.	S. W.	S. W.	Clear	Clear	Clear	
28	29.71	29.68	29.70	57	74	60	63.7	S. W.	S. W.	S. W.	Variable	Clear	Clear	
29	[illegible]	[illegible]	[illegible]	[illegible]	[illegible]	[illegible]	[illegible]	N. W.	[illegible]	[illegible]	Clear	Variable	Clear	
30	29.84	29.79	[illegible]	[illegible]	61	55	54.0	N. E.	S'ly	S'ly	Variable	Cloudy	Clear	
Means	29.70	29.74	29.77	54.4	68.2	57.5	...	...	...	...	...	...	...	1.40

Reduced to sea level.	Sunrise.	At 1 P. M.	At 10 P. M.	Therm. Sunrise.	At 1 P. M.	At 10 P. M.	Daily mean.
Max.	30.23	30.21	30.17	73	83	74	75.7
Min.	29.51	29.50	29.62	38	53	42	46.3
Mean	29.97	29.91	29.95				
Range	0.72	0.71	0.55	35	30	32	29.4
Mean of month	29.943			...	...	...	60.0
Extreme range	0.73			...	...	...	45.0

Prevailing winds from some point between— (Days.)
N. & E. . . . 7
E. & S. . . . 0
S. & W. . . . 9
W. & N. . . . 14

(Days.)
Clear 10
Variable . . . . } 12
Cloudy . . . . }
Rain fell on . . 8

Remarks.

1st. Pleasant.
2d. Very pleasant.
3d. Fine. Wind very fresh S. W'ly.
4th. Very pleasant.
5th. Showery in the morning. Clear in the evening.
6th and 7th. Very fine.
8th. Very fine. Cloudy evening. Sprinkling of rain began about 11 P. M.
9th. Rain nearly all day. Cleared in the evening.
10th. Very pleasant.
11th. Cloudy, with sprinkling of rain.
12th. Pleasant and very warm.
13th. Sprinkling of rain in the afternoon. Wind came to N. E.
14th. Pleasant.
15th. Cloudy, with occasional rain.
16th. Wind light N. E., with occasional showers.
17th and 18th. Pleasant.
19th. Variable. Occasional showers during the day. Clear in the evening.
20th. Very fine, but cool.
21st. Variable. Heavy shower for a few minutes from 3 to 4 P. M.
22d. Frost in some places in the vicinity this morning. Wind rather fresh N. W'ly all day, and quite cool.
23d. No frost apparent, the night being windy.
24th. First white frost in the College yard. The day pleasant.
25th and 26th. Very fine.
27th. Fine.
28th. Very fine.
29th and 30th. Variable.

DAYS.	BAROMETER, REDUCED TO 32° F. Sunrise.	At 1 P. M.	At 10 P. M.	THERMOMETER. Sunrise.	At 1 P. M.	At 10 P. M.	Daily mean.	WINDS. Sunrise.	At 1 P. M.	At 10 P. M.	WEATHER. Sunrise.	At 1 P. M.	At 10 P. M.	RAIN AND SNOW IN INCHES OF WATER.
October, 1842.														
1	29.77	29.71	29.62	49	71	56	58.7	N. W.	W'ly	W'ly	Clear	Clear	Clear	
2	29.62	29.56	29.59	59	72	54	61.7	S. W'ly	S. W.	N. W.	Cloudy	Clear	Clear	
3	29.70	29.63	29.69	47	64	54	55.0	W'ly	W'ly	N. W.	Variable	Clear	Clear	
4	29.74	29.73	29.79	43	63	48	51.3	W'ly	W'ly	N. W.	Clear	Clear	Clear	
5	29.87	29.86	29.99	39	55	43	45.7	N. W.	N. W.	N. W.	Clear	Clear	Clear	
6	30.10	30.09	30.09	36	57	44	45.7	N. E.	N. E'ly	N. W.	Clear	Clear	Clear	
7	30.08	29.99	29.96	42	64	50	52.0	S. W'ly	S. W'ly	S. W'ly	Clear	Clear	Clear	
8	29.86	29.78	29.73	50	68	58	58.7	S. W'ly	S. W.	S. W.	Clear	Clear	Clear	
9	29.64	29.46	29.37	58	71	64	64.3	S. W.	S. W.	S. W.	Cloudy	Cloudy	Cloudy	
10	29.62	29.69	29.71	48	68	49	55.0	W'ly	W'ly	W'ly	Clear	Clear	Clear	
11	29.67	29.54	29.49	48	63	52	54.3	S. W.	S. W.	S'ly	Clear	Clear	Clear	
12	29.50	29.50	29.70	51	62	49	54.0	S. W'ly	W'ly	W'ly	Clear	Clear	Clear	
13	29.81	29.84	29.88	41	62	47	50.0	N. W.	N. W.	S. W.	Clear	Clear	Clear	
14	29.88	29.78	29.70	40	62	52	51.3	N. W.	S'ly	S'ly	Clear	Variable	Cloudy	
15	29.39	29.29	29.41	60	64	52	58.7	S. E'ly	S. W.	N. W.	Rain	Cloudy	Clear	0.36
16	29.62	29.66	29.66	43	60	53	52.0	W'ly	N. W'ly	W'ly	Clear	Clear	Clear	
17	29.74	29.83	29.99	50	62	47	53.0	S. W'ly	S. W.	N. W.	Clear	Clear	Clear	
18	29.92	...	29.54	42	...	65	...	N. W.	...	S. W.	Variable	...	Variable	
19	29.64	29.68	29.82	47	54	40	47.0	N. W.	N. W.	N. W.	Cloudy	Clear	Clear	
20	29.84	29.84	29.89	36	48	39	41.0	N'ly	N'ly	N. W.	Clear	Cloudy	Clear	
21	30.01	29.94	29.88	35	48	40	41.0	N. W.	N. W.	N. W.	Clear	Clear	Clear	
22	29.85	29.68	29.62	38	59	55	50.7	N. W.	S. W.	S. W.	Clear	Cloudy	Cloudy	
23	29.54	29.60	29.78	50	60	44	51.3	N. W'ly	N. W'ly	N. W.	Rain	Variable	Clear	
24	29.89	29.88	29.88	40	64	54	52.7	N. W.	N. W.	S'ly	Clear	Clear	Cloudy	
25	29.74	29.58	29.54	57	61	55	57.7	S. E'ly	S'ly	S'ly	Variable	Rain	Cloudy	0.80
26	29.68	29.68	29.79	46	54	40	46.7	N. W.	N. W.	N. W.	Cloudy	Clear	Clear	
27	29.80	29.91	30.10	36	53	41	43.3	N. W.	N. W.	N. W.	Clear	Clear	Clear	
28	30.24	30.21	30.19	35	51	41	42.3	N. W.	N. W.	N. W.	Clear	Clear	Clear	
29	30.15	30.05	30.09	36	58	48	47.3	N. E.	W'ly	N. W'ly	Clear	Clear	Clear	
30	30.16	30.15	30.20	37	51	38	42.0	N. W.	N. W.	N. E.	Clear	Clear	Clear	
31	30.23	30.15	30.13	32	51	40	41.0	N. E.	N. E.	N. E.	Clear	Clear	Clear	
Means	29.81	29.77	29.80	44.2	60.0	48.8	...	...	...	...	...	...	...	1.16
REDUCED TO SEA LEVEL.														
Max.	30.42	30.39	30.38	60	72	64	64.3							
Min.	29.57	29.47	29.55	32	48	38	41.0							
Mean	29.99	29.94	29.98											
Range	0.85	0.92	0.83	28	24	26	23.3							
Mean of month	29.970			...	...	...	51.0							
Extreme range	0.95			...	...	...	40.0							

Prevailing winds from some point between—

	Days.
N. & E.	2
E. & S.	1
S. & W.	12
W. & N.	16

	Days.
Clear	20
Variable / Cloudy	7
Rain fell on	4

REMARKS.

1st. Very fine.
2d. Cloudy in the morning. Very clear in the evening.
3d. Very fine.
4th. Fine.
5th to 8th. Very fine.
9th. Cloudy, with occasional sprinkling of rain.
10th and 11th. Pleasant.
12th and 13th. Very fine.
14th. Fine for the most part.
15th. Rainy in the morning. Variable through the day. Clear in the evening.
16th and 17th. Very fine.
18th. Pleasant during the day. Cloudy and variable in the evening. Wind S. W., very brisk, nearly a gale.
19th. Very fine.
20th and 21st. Fine.
22d. Cloudy for the most part.
23d. Sprinkling of rain early in the morning, from N. W. Variable in the afternoon. Clear in the evening.
24th. Pleasant.
25th. Wind fresh S'ly and S. E'ly in the morning. Began to rain moderately from 1 to 2 P. M. Moderate rain, with high wind, most of the afternoon. Wind lulled in the evening.
26th. Pleasant.
27th to 30th. Very fine.
31st. Fine.

DAYS.	BAROMETER Sunrise.	At 1 P. M.	At 10 P. M.	THERMOMETER Sunrise.	At 1 P. M.	At 10 P. M.	Daily mean.	WINDS Sunrise.	At 1 P. M.	At 10 P. M.	WEATHER Sunrise.	At 1 P. M.	At 10 P. M.	RAIN AND SNOW
November, 1842.														
1	29.95	29.93	29.98	36	60	46	47.3	S. W'ly	W'ly	N'ly	Clear	Clear	Clear	
2	29.95	30.02	30.09	44	51	39	44.7	N'ly	N. W'ly	N'ly	Variable	Clear	Clear	
3	30.20	30.15	30.12	30	47	38	38.3	N'ly	N'ly	N. W.	Clear	Clear	Clear	
4	30.10	30.01	30.01	31	50	40	40.3	N. W.	N. W.	W'ly	Clear	Clear	Clear	
5	30.00	29.94	29.89	38	60	48	48.7	N. W.	W'ly	S. W.	Clear	Clear	Clear	
6	29.85	29.76	29.71	44	60	58	54.0	W'ly	S. E'ly	W'ly	Clear	Clear	Cloudy	
7	29.62	29.61	29.60	49	58	48	51.7	W'ly	W'ly	E'ly	Clear	Clear	Variable	
8	29.51	29.29	29.41	45	47	38	43.3	N. E.	N. E.	N. E.	Rain	Rain	Cloudy	} 1.12
9	29.61	29.59	29.56	39	49	45	44.3	N. E.	N. E.	N. E.	Cloudy	Cloudy	Rain	
10	29.62	29.63	29.72	39	48	38	41.7	N. W.	N. W.	N. W.	Clear	Clear	Clear	
11	29.72	29.73	29.91	39	47	38	41.3	N. W.	N. W.	N. W.	Cloudy	Cloudy	Clear	
12	29.92	29.91	29.85	39	47	42	42.7	N. W.	N. W.	W'ly	Cloudy	Cloudy	Rain	0.27
13	29.79	29.81	29.90	41	44	38	41.0	N. W.	N. W.	N'ly	Cloudy	Cloudy	Variable	
14	29.91	29.79	29.56	37	45	47	43.0	E'ly	S. E'ly	S. E'ly	Cloudy	Rain	Cloudy	0.50
15	29.70	29.71	29.83	40	49	36	41.7	N. W.	N. W.	N. W.	Clear	Clear	Clear	
16	29.80	29.73	29.78	34	40	34	36.0	N'ly	N. E'ly	N. E'ly	Cloudy	Cloudy	Clear	
17	29.80	29.79	29.64	30	44	40	38.0	N'ly	N. E.	N. E.	Clear	Variable	Rain	} 0.38
18	29.06	28.99	29.31	56	53	32	47.0	S. E'ly	W'ly	N. W.	Rain	Clear	Clear	
19	29.50	29.51	29.68	26	36	32	31.3	N'ly	W'ly	W'ly	Clear	Clear	Clear	
20	29.90	29.89	29.91	29	38	32	33.0	W'ly	W'ly	W'ly	Clear	Clear	Variable	
21	29.97	29.95	30.01	27	39	28	31.3	W'ly	W'ly	N. W.	Clear	Clear	Clear	
22	30.07	30.06	30.06	26	40	27	31.0	N. W.	N. W.	N. W.	Clear	Clear	Clear	
23	30.07	30.01	29.91	25	42	33	33.3	N. W.	S. W.	E'ly	Clear	Clear	Clear	
24	29.60	29.39	29.80	38	37	35	36.7	N. E.	N. W.	N. W.	Rain	Rain	Clear	0.80
25	30.07	29.99	29.94	30	41	38	36.3	N. W.	S. E.	N'ly	Clear	Clear	Cloudy	
26	29.99	29.97	29.89	30	42	30	34.0	N. W.	N. W.	N. W.	Clear	Clear	Clear	
27	29.46	29.39	29.60	36	35	24	31.7	S. W.	N. W.	N. W.	Snow	Clear	Clear	
28	29.80	29.81	29.94	20	28	23	23.7	N. W.	N. W.	N. W.	Clear	Clear	Clear	
29	30.03	30.02	30.16	18	26	22	22.0	N. W.	N. W.	N. W.	Clear	Clear	Clear	
30	30.15	29.97	29.17	23	29	32	28.0	N. W.	N. E.	N. E.	Cloudy	Cloudy	R'n & sn.	0.75
Means	29.82	29.78	29.80	34.6	44.4	36.7	...	...	...	...	...	...	...	3.82
REDUCED TO SEA LEVEL.														
Max.	30.38	30.33	30.34	56	60	58	54.0							
Min.	29.24	29.17	29.35	18	26	22	22.0							
Mean	30.00	29.96	29.98											
Range	1.14	1.16	0.99	38	34	36	32.0							
Mean of month	29.980			...	...	...	38.6							
Extreme range	1.21			...	...	...	42.0							

Prevailing winds from some point between—

	Days.
N. & E.	5
E. & S.	3
S. & W.	3
W. & N.	19

	Days.
Clear	14
Variable / Cloudy	9
Rain or snow fell on	7

REMARKS.

1st, 2d, and 3d. Fine.
4th and 5th. Very fine.
6th and 7th. Pleasant.
8th. Moderate rain nearly all day, with wind N. E. Wind came to N. W. in the evening; cloudy.
9th. Cloudy in the morning and afternoon. Rain in the evening, with thunder.
10th. Pleasant.
11th. Cloudy day. Evening very clear.
12th. Cloudy in the morning. Moderate rain in the evening.
13th. Pleasant.
14th. Moderate rain.
15th. Fine.
16th. Cloudy. Cleared from 8 to 9 P. M.
17th. Clear in the morning. Cloudy in the afternoon. Moderate rain in the evening.
18th. Rain in the morning. Clear in the afternoon. Wind blustering all day and evening.
19th. Blustering, but clear.
20th. Clear. Wind fresh.
21st. Fine. Aurora quite bright from 7 to 8 P. M.
22d. Clear and fine.
23d. Fine.
24th. Rain in the morning; wind N. E. Wind came to N. W. from noon to 1 P. M., with rain and some snow—the first for the season—which continued but for a short time. Evening clear.
25th. Pleasant.
26th. Fine.
27th. At sunrise, cloudy; mild wind S. W., with some snow in the air. Before 11 A. M., the wind hauled to W'ly, grew cooler, and became very blustering. Cleared in the evening, with wind at N. W.; cold and very blustering.
28th. Clear and cold.
29th. Clear.
30th. Cloudy at sunrise; wind N. W., light. Before noon, wind came to N. E. At 3 P. M., commenced snowing moderately; wind still light. Storm increased in the evening. At 10 and 11 P. M., rain and snow, with the wind very heavy, and barometer 29.27 (at 10½ P. M.), and slowly falling. At sunrise (Dec. 1st), barometer 29.10, and rising; wind N. W'ly, with the air full of snow.

December, 1842.

DAYS.	BAROMETER, REDUCED TO 32° F. Sunrise.	At 1 P. M.	At 10 P. M.	THERMOMETER. Sunrise.	At 1 P. M.	At 10 P. M.	Daily mean.	WINDS. Sunrise.	At 1 P. M.	At 10 P. M.	WEATHER. Sunrise.	At 1 P. M.	At 10 P. M.	RAIN AND SNOW IN INCHES OF WATER.
1	29.01	29.20	29.50	33	33	28	31.3	N. W.	N. W.	N. W.	Snow	Cloudy	Clear	
2	29.93	29.96	29.97	24	31	25	26.7	N. W.	N. W.	N. W.	Clear	Clear	Clear	
3	29.66	29.64	29.68	37	45	38	40.0	S. W.	S. W.	W'ly	Cloudy	Cloudy	Clear	
4	29.70	29.67	29.60	37	46	46	43.0	N. W.	S. W'ly	S. W'ly	Cloudy	Cloudy	Cloudy	
5	29.60	29.59	29.64	42	44	35	40.3	S. W.	S. W.	S. W.	Very cl'y	Cloudy	Rain	0.33
6	30.10	30.12	30.19	28	29	23	26.7	N. W.	N. W.	N'ly	Clear	Clear	Cloudy	
7	30.02	29.90	29.90	26	37	29	30.7	N'ly	N. W'ly	N. W.	Cloudy	Clear	Clear	
8	29.90	29.84	29.70	29	30	32	30.3	N. W.	N. E.	N. E'ly	Cloudy	Snow	Cloudy	} 0.67
9	29.42	29.47	29.67	35	29	30	31.3	N. E.	N. E.	N. W'ly	Rain	Snow	Clear	
10	29.94	30.07	30.16	30	27	27	28.0	N. E.	N. W.	N. W.	Cloudy	Clear	Clear	
11	30.07	29.94	29.91	28	33	31	30.7	N. W.	N. W.	N'ly	Cloudy	Cloudy	Cloudy	
12	30.00	30.01	30.16	30	32	23	28.3	N. W.	N. W.	N. W.	Variable	Variable	Cloudy	} 0.60
13	30.16	29.91	29.57	24	32	32	29.3	N. E'ly	N. E.	N. E.	Cloudy	Snow	Snow	
14	29.42	...	...	24	...	...	...	N. W.	...	...	Snow	...	...	
15	30.06	30.07	30.10	...	...	25	...	N. W.	N. W.	N. W.	Clear	Clear	Clear	
16	30.00	29.87	29.79	24	33	27	28.0	W'ly	W'ly	W'ly	Clear	Cloudy	Variable	
17	29.73	29.70	29.40	21	25	27	24.3	N. W.	N. W.	S. W.	Clear	Clear	Clear	
18	29.25	29.24	29.52	28	34	17	26.3	S. W.	W'ly	N. W.	Clear	Snow	Clear	
19	29.64	29.51	29.66	14	28	27	23.0	N. W.	S. W.	S. W.	Clear	Cloudy	Clear	
20	29.92	29.94	29.86	24	35	30	29.7	N. W.	W'ly	S. W.	Clear	Clear	Clear	
21	29.80	29.60	29.16	31	38	45	38.0	N. E.	N. E.	E'ly	Cloudy	Rain	Rain	1.33
22	29.16	29.23	29.40	40	43	29	37.3	W'ly	W'ly	N. E.	Cloudy	Variable	Snow	
23	29.70	29.74	29.93	21	23	17	20.3	N. W.	N. W.	N. W.	Clear	Clear	Clear	
24	30.24	30.34	30.43	7	14	10	10.3	N. W.	N. W.	N. W.	Clear	Clear	Clear	
25	30.41	30.27	30.31	18	33	29	26.7	N. W.	N. E.	N. W'ly	Cloudy	Cloudy	Variable	
26	30.30	...	30.17	24	...	34	...	N. W.	...	N. W.	Clear	...	Variable	
27	30.12	30.02	30.02	34	37	33	34.7	N. W.	N. W.	N. W.	Cloudy	Cloudy	Cloudy	
28	30.14	30.22	30.22	25	27	17	23.0	N. W.	N. W.	N. W.	Clear	Clear	Clear	
29	30.15	29.99	29.72	13	22	28	21.0	N. W.	N. E.	N. E.	Variable	Cloudy	Snow	} 1.00
30	29.11	29.06	29.24	38	36	32	35.3	S. E.	S. W.	N. W.	Rain	Cloudy	Clear	
31	29.45	29.52	29.70	27	26	18	23.7	N. W.	N. W.	N. W.	Cloudy	Clear	Clear	
Means	29.81	29.78	29.81	27.2	32.2	28.1	...	...	...	...	...	...	...	3.93
REDUCED TO SEA LEVEL.														
Max.	30.59	30.52	30.61	42	46	46	43.0							
Min.	29.19	29.24	29.34	7	14	10	10.3							
Mean	29.99	29.96	29.99											
Range	1.40	1.28	1.27	35	32	36	32.7							
Mean of month	20.980			...	...	...	29.2							
Extreme range	1.42			...	...	...	39.0							

Prevailing winds from some point between—

	Days.
N. & E.	5
E. & S.	0
S. & W.	8
W. & N.	18

	Days.
Clear	7
Variable } Cloudy }	13
Rain or snow fell on	11

REMARKS.

1st. Wind N. W. at sunrise. About three inches of wet snow, and air still filled with snow.
2d and 3d. Fair.
4th. Cloudy.
5th. Cloudy. Rain in the evening.
6th. Pleasant, but cold.
7th. Cloudy. Began to snow at 9 A. M. Not enough snow to cover the ground. Clear towards night.
8th. Cloudy in the morning. Snowed moderately in the afternoon.
9th. Rain during previous night. Continued, mixed with snow, moderately through the greater part of the day. Clear in the evening.
10th. Pleasant.
11th. Cloudy. Wind very light; nearly calm.
12th. Variable. Circle round the moon.
13th. Began to snow from noon to 1 P. M.
14th. Ground covered with snow and water. My thermometer got broken by the water collecting in the bottom of the tin case and freezing.
15th. Very fine.
16th and 17th. Pleasant.
18th. Blustering. Flurry of snow at 2 P. M. Wind soon came to N. W., and grew cold.
19th. Cold in the morning. Pleasant towards evening. At 10 P. M., wind light S. W'ly. Clouds at the same time coming from the N. W.
20th. Pleasant.
21st. Began to rain moderately at 7 A. M.; more copiously in the evening.
22d. Mild.
23d. One and a half inch of light snow. Clear and cold.
24th. Cold, but not unpleasant. Very little air stirring.
25th. Cloudy, with some snow. Nearly calm.
26th. Very fine.
27th. Cloudy, but mild.
28th. Fine.
29th. Wind light N. E. during the day. Became a fresh breeze, approaching to strong wind, at 10 P. M., when snow commenced falling. Barometer 29.81, and falling pretty fast. After considerable snow had fallen, which was much drifted, the wind came to S. E., and the snow changed to rain, which continued till morning.
30th. Ground covered with wet snow and snow-water. Storm ceased from 8 to 9 A. M. Cloudy in the afternoon. Clear in the evening.
31st. Cloudy in the morning. Very clear and cold in the evening.

January, 1843.

DAYS.	BAROMETER. Sunrise.	At 1 P. M.	At 10 P. M.	THERMOMETER. Sunrise.	At 1 P. M.	At 10 P. M.	Daily mean.	WINDS. Sunrise.	At 1 P. M.	At 10 P. M.	WEATHER. Sunrise.	At 1 P. M.	At 10 P. M.	RAIN AND SNOW.
1	29.91	29.97	30.10	17	28	21	22.0	N. W.	N. W.	N. W.	Clear	Clear	Clear	
2	30.11	29.91	29.68	14	17	17	16.0	N. E.	N. E.	N. E.	Cloudy	Snow	Cloudy	
3	29.51	29.57	30.00	21	27	12	20.0	N'ly	N. W.	N. W.	Snow	Clear	Clear	
4	30.11	30.05	30.09	8	22	16	15.3	N. W.	S. W.	W'ly	Clear	Cloudy	Clear	
5	30.07	30.00	30.02	22	37	38	32.3	S. W'ly	S. W.	N. E.	Cloudy	Cloudy	Rain	
6	30.09	30.09	30.10	30	35	34	33.0	N. E.	N. E.	N. E.	Cloudy	Clear	Misty	
7	30.09	30.08	30.04	34	37	36	35.7	N. E.	N. E.	N. E.	Cloudy	Cloudy	Misty	
8	29.95	29.91	29.89	38	49	49	45.3	N. E'ly	S. W.	S'ly	Misty	Cloudy	Cloudy	
9	30.05	29.99	30.04	48	52	45	48.3	S. W'ly	S'ly	S'ly	Foggy	Misty	Misty	
10	30.08	30.00	29.97	43	51	47	47.0	N. W'ly	Misty	S. W.	Foggy	Cloudy	Variable	
11	29.94	29.92	29.96	48	52	43	47.7	S. W.	N. W.	N. W.	Misty	Cloudy	Misty	
12	29.85	29.78	29.68	40	43	42	41.7	N. E'ly	N. E'ly	N. W'ly	Misty	Misty	Misty	
13	29.52	29.39	29.35	38	41	42	40.3	N. E'ly	N. E'ly	W'ly	Rain	Cloudy	Variable	0.25
14	29.46	29.49	29.50	34	35	31	33.3	W'ly	W'ly	W'ly	Clear	Cloudy	Cloudy	
15	29.76	29.79	29.84	32	37	36	35.0	S. W'ly	W'ly	W'ly	Variable	Variable	Clear	
16	...	30.19	30.31	26	33	27	28.7	N'ly	N. W.	N. W.	Clear	Clear	Clear	
17	30.50	30.50	30.55	20	30	25	25.0	N. W.	N. E.	N. E.	Clear	Clear	Clear	
18	30.41	30.25	30.19	26	42	37	35.0	S. W.	S. W.	S. W.	Clear	Clear	Clear	
19	30.09	30.00	29.98	30	48	45	41.0	S. W.	S. W.	S. W.	Clear	Cloudy	Clear	
20	29.98	29.98	30.06	44	54	40	46.0	S. W.	S. W.	N. W.	Clear	Clear	Clear	
21	30.01	29.82	29.68	36	47	44	42.3	S. W.	S'ly	S. W.	Variable	Cloudy	Clear	
22	29.61	29.52	29.56	44	50	38	42.7	W.	W'ly	N. W.	Clear	Clear	Clear	
23	29.57	29.43	29.15	34	40	37	37.0	N. W.	N. W.	S. W'ly	Clear	Variable	Cloudy	
24	29.00	28.92	29.03	37	45	33	38.3	S. W.	N. W'ly	N. W.	Variable	Cloudy	Variable	
25	29.23	29.23	29.48	27	35	23	28.3	N. W.	N. W.	N. W.	Clear	Clear	Clear	
26	29.81	29.81	29.96	20	32	23	25.0	N. W.	N. W.	N. W.	Clear	Clear	Clear	
27	30.01	29.95	29.92	18	35	33	28.7	N. W.	S. W.	S. W.	Clear	Cloudy	Cloudy	
28	29.70	29.62	29.72	32	31	30	31.0	N. E.	N. E.	N. E.	Rain	Misty	Cloudy	0.35
29	29.97	30.02	30.04	19	28	23	23.3	N. W.	N. W.	N. W.	Clear	Clear	Clear	
30	30.01	29.94	29.89	20	38	32	30.0	N. W.	S. W.	S. W.	Clear	Clear	Clear	
31	29.70	29.45	29.15	34	50	44	42.7	N. E.	S. E.	W'ly	Cloudy	Cloudy	Clear	
Means	29.87	29.86	29.84	30.1	38.7	33.6	...	...	...	...	...	...	...	0.60
REDUCED TO SEA LEVEL.														
Max.	30.68	30.68	30.73	48	54	49	48.3							
Min.	29.18	29.10	29.21	8	17	12	15.3							
Mean	30.05	30.04	30.02											
Range	1.50	1.58	1.52	40	37	37	33.0							
Mean of month	30.037			...	...	...	34.2							
Extreme range	1.63			...	...	...	46.0							

Prevailing winds from some point between—

	Days.
N. & E.	7
E. & S.	1
S. & W.	13
W. & N.	10

	Days.
Clear	10
Variable } Cloudy }	12
Rain or snow fell on	9

1st. Fine, though cool.
2d. Cloudy. Wind light N. E. Flurry of snow from 1 to 2 P. M.
3d. Cold. Wind brisk N. W. Flurry of snow in the morning.
4th. Fine for the most part.
5th. Cloudy, but mild. Began to rain very moderately from 7 to 8 P. M. Amount of rain not more than enough to wet the surface of ground.
6th. Cloudy, with mist in the evening.
7th. Misty. Wind light N. E.
8th. Mild. Cloudy, occasionally broken.
9th. Very foggy. Heavy mist and occasional sprinkling of rain.
10th. Fog, mist, and light rain at sunrise. Clouds broken in the evening.
11th. Heavy mist and fog for the greater part of the day.
12th. Very mild, with mist and occasional sprinkling of rain.
13th. Moderate rain at sunrise; ceased from 9 to 10 A. M. Clouds broken in the evening.
14th. Pleasant. Cloudy in the afternoon.
15th. Variable; sunshine and clouds throughout the day. Very clear in the evening.
16th. Very fine.
17th. Very fine. Evening beautifully clear and calm.
18th, 19th, and 20th. Very fine.
21st. Pleasant and warm. Frost out of ground, and farmers ploughing in the vicinity.
22d. Very fine.
23d. Very mild and pleasant. Starlight early in the evening. Cloudy at 10 P. M.; quite calm.
24th. Variable; mild. Rather blustering in the evening.
25th. Fine. Rather blustering in the evening.
26th. Fine.
27th. Variable; mild. Wind very light.
28th. Rain, hail, mist, and snow during the greater part of the day.
29th. Ground barely covered with sleet and snow, which mostly disappeared during the day.
30th. Very fine.
31st. At sunrise, wind light N. E., with mist. Clouds and mist continued during morning, and wind hauled to E'ly and freshened. In the afternoon, wind brisk S. E., with dashes of rain. From 7 to 8 P. M., wind S. E., blowing a gale.

February, 1843.

DAYS.	BAROMETER, REDUCED TO 32° F. Sunrise.	At 1 P. M.	At 10 P. M.	THERMOMETER. Sunrise.	At 1 P. M.	At 10 P. M.	Daily mean.	WINDS. (DIRECTION AND FORCE.) Sunrise.	At 1 P. M.	At 10 P. M.	WEATHER. (TENTHS CLOUDY.) Sunrise.	At 1 P. M.	At 10 P. M.	RAIN AND SNOW IN INCHES OF WATER.
1	29.30	29.08	29.17	40	34	31	35.0	S'ly 1	N. E. 1	N. W. 2	Rain	Snow	0	1.08
2	29.56	29.66	29.92	17	14	9	13.3	S. W. 2	N. W. 4	N. W. 2	2	0	0	
3	30.11	30.06	30.06	6	26	23	18.3	W. 1	W'ly 0	S'ly 0	0	8	10	
4	30.06	30.04	30.08	20	34	27	27.0	N. W. 1	S. W'ly 1	N. E'ly 1	1	0	8	
S 5	29.87	29.50	28.83	24	31	33	29.3	N. E. 2	N. E. 4	N. E. 5	10	Snow	Rain	2.20
6	28.84	28.89	29.13	27	29	16	24.0	W by S. 1	N. W'ly 3	N. W'ly 4	10	9	2	
7	29.26	29.38	29.67	12	17	12	13.7	N. W. 2	N. W'ly 3	W. 2	2	0	5	
8	29.67	29.67	29.93	14	21	16	17.0	W'ly 1	W'ly 3	W'ly 2	0	8	0	
9	30.06	30.11	30.21	7	22	8	12.3	W'ly 1	W'ly 2	W'ly 0	0	4	0	
10	30.31	30.32	30.27	2	15	20	12.3	N. W. 1	N. W. 1	N. E. 1	0	0	10	
11	29.61	29.41	29.66	37	43	32	37.3	S. E. 3	S. W. 1	W'ly	Rain	Misty	0	1.00
S 12	29.71	29.67	29.95	30	38	21	29.7	S. W. 0	W. 3	N. W. 1	10	1	4	
13	30.05	30.01	30.05	19	24	22	21.7	N. E. 1	N. E. 1	N. E. 1	10	10	10	
14	30.02	29.96	29.72	16	24	27	22.3	N. E. 1	N. E. 2	N. 2	Snow	Snow	Snow	} 0.72
15	29.29	29.21	29.44	16	20	16	17.3	N. 2	N. W. 2	N. W. 3	Hail	Hail	0	
16	29.65	29.77	29.88	10	20	10	13.3	W. 2	N. W. 2	N. W. 1	0	2	0	
17	29.96	29.92	29.86	2	20	15	12.3	N. W. 1	N. W. 2	W. 1	0	0	5	
18	30.01	30.06	30.11	6	24	15	15.0	N. W. 1	W'ly 1	W'ly 0	0	2	Snow	} 0.27
S 19	30.03	29.87	29.65	18	26	24	22.7	N. E. 1	N. 1	N. E. 1	10	10	Rain	
20	29.45	29.46	29.46	31	39	31	33.7	S'ly 1	N. W. 1	N. W. 1	Foggy	2	5	
21	29.35	29.26	29.38	24	26	23	24.3	N. 2	N. 1	N. W. 1	10	10	2	
22	29.50	29.40	29.29	22	38	28	29.3	W'ly 1	S. W. 1	W'ly 1	1	10	2	
23	29.60	29.61	29.66	14	21	16	17.0	N. W. 3	N. W. 3	N. W. 1	0	1	0	
24	29.67	29.57	29.58	14	26	19	19.7	W. 1	W'ly 1	W'ly 1	8	0	0	
25	29.61	29.54	29.54	13	34	24	23.7	N. W. 1	S. W. 1	S. W. 1	0	0	0	
S 26	29.60	29.63	29.69	30	37	32	33.0	W. 1	W. 2	W. 1	0	0	0	
27	29.57	29.50	29.71	24	32	24	26.7	N. E. 2	N'ly 1	N. W. 2	Snow	10	0	
28	29.90	29.89	29.79	17	34	29	26.7	N. W. 1	N. W. 1	S. W'ly 1	0	0	Hazy	
Means	29.70	29.66	29.70	18.3	27.5	21.5	...	1.4	1.7	1.4	4.8	4.6	4.0	5.27
									1.5			4.5		
REDUCED TO SEA LEVEL.														
Max.	30.49	30.50	30.45	40	43	33	37.3	Prevailing winds from some point between— Days.						
Min.	29.02	29.07	29.01	2	14	8	12.3						Days.	
Mean	29.89	29.84	29.88					N. & E. 6			Clear 8			
Range	1.47	1.43	1.44	38	29	25	25.0	E. & S. 0			Variable . . . } 6			
Mean of month			29.870	...	...	...	22.4	S. & W. 8			Cloudy . . . . }			
Extreme range			1.49	...	...	...	41.0	W. & N. 14			Rain or snow fell on 14			

REMARKS.

1st. Early in morning, wind S'ly, with moderate rain. Before noon, wind came to N. E.; rain turned to snow, which continued till towards night, when wind came to N. W'ly, and cleared in evening.

2d. Flurry of snow at 10 A. M. Wind changed from S. W. to N. W., and grew cold.

3d. Hazy during the day. Wind came to S. W. and S'ly, very light, in afternoon. Haze thickened to clouds in evening. Flurry of snow during night.

4th. Pleasant.

5th. Began to snow gently at 10 A. M.; wind light N. E. At 1 P. M., snowed very fast, wind increased to that of a pretty heavy storm; both continued till 5 P. M., when the snow, having become more and more moist, began to be mixed with rain. In evening, rain and snow—chichy rain, though moderate; wind unabated. At 12 P. M., wind much abated. Bar. ranged from 28.97, at 8¾ P. M., to 28 88 at midnight.

6th. Blustering. Occasional flurries of snow.

7th. Cold. Hazy in the evening.

8th. Rather severe. Cloudy during the day.

9th. Pleasant for cold weather.

10th. Clear in morning; pleasant, though cold. Cloudy in afternoon. Wind came to N. E. at 8 P. M.

11th. Rainy at sunrise; wind S. E., which came round to S. W. from 9 to 10 A. M. Clouds broken at 3 P. M. Very clear in the evening.

12th. Pleasant.

13th. Thin clouds all day, with snow in the air

14th. Moderate snow nearly all day, quite dry in morning, but became moist in evening.

15th. Fine hail nearly all day. Clouds became broken at sunset. Very clear in the evening.

16th and 17th. Pleasant.

18th. Pleasant in the morning. Cloudy towards night About an inch of light snow during night.

19th. Raw and unpleasant. Air full of fine mist or congealed vapor. Moderate rain in evening.

20th. Foggy at sunrise; wind S'ly. Wind came to S. W. and W., A. M. Sun came out warm.

21st. Clouds broken at sunset.

22d. Clear and pleasant at sunrise. Clouded up by 10 A. M. Began to snow moderately from 2 to 3 P. M., continued till 8 or 9 P. M.; then clear.

23d. About 1½ or 2 inches of light snow.

24th, 25th, and 26th. Pleasant.

27th. Air full of snow from 7 to 11 A. M., without much more than covering the ground. Cleared in the afternoon; wind N. W., fresh in evening.

28th. Pleasant. Flurry of snow during night.

March, 1843.

DAYS.	Barometer Sunrise.	At 1 P. M.	At 10 P. M.	Thermometer Sunrise.	At 1 P. M.	At 10 P. M.	Daily mean.	Winds Sunrise.	At 1 P. M.	At 10 P. M.	Weather Sunrise.	At 1 P. M.	At 10 P. M.	Rain and snow
1	29.57	29.49	29.54	24	35	22	27.0	W. 1	N. W. 2	N. W. 2	0	7	0	
2	29.61	29.65	29.80	16	23	16	18.3	N. W. 3	N. W. 3	N. W. 3	0	0	0	
3	29.87	29.80	29.81	12	22	15	16.3	N. W. 2	N. W. 3	N. W. 2	0	0	0	
4	29.87	29.77	29.70	13	24	19	18.7	N. W. 1	N. W. 3	N. W. 2	4	0	0	
S 5	29.61	29.50	29.58	14	27	20	20.3	N. W. 2	N. W. 4	N. W. 2	0	0	0	
6	29.71	29.69	29.80	16	24	20	20.0	N. W. 2	N. W. 3	N. W. 4	0	0	0	
7	29.82	29.76	29.84	17	28	22	22.3	N. W. 3	N. W. 4	N. W. 3	0	0	0	
8	29.88	29.81	29.80	17	35	31	27.7	N. W. 2	N. W. 2	N. W. 1	0	0	5	
9	29.85	29.87	29.94	25	41	32	32.7	N. W. 1	N. W. 1	N. W. 1	0	4	5	
10	29.98	29.92	29.75	30	37	32	33.0	N. E. 1	E'ly 1	E'ly 3	8	10	Rain	0.60
11	29.40	29.52	29.74	34	40	33	35.7	N'ly 1	N. W'ly 1	N. W. 2	Misty	1	0	
S 12	29.98	29.93	30.02	25	36	33	31.3	N. W. 2	N. W. 2	N. W'ly 2	0	0	10	
13	29.90	29.63	29.15	33	33	34	33.3	N. E. 2	E'ly 3	N. E. 3	10	R'n, h'l	Rain	0.80
14	29.36	29.55	29.66	26	27	26	26.3	N. W. 4	W'ly 6	N. W. 5	0	0	0	
15	29.56	29.40	29.73	31	41	29	33.7	S. W. 2	S. W. 3	N. W. 3	5	5	5	
16	29.87	29.81	29.61	27	37	30	31.3	W'ly 2	N. E. 2	N. E. 4	7	4	Snow	} 0.75
17	28.80	28.75	29.23	35	36	29	33.3	E'ly 5	W'ly 4	W'ly 4	Rain	Snow	0	
18	29.29	29.32	29.44	23	33	25	27.0	W'ly 4	W. 5	W'ly 3	0	0	0	
S 19	29.43	29.42	29.50	19	34	26	26.3	N. W. 2	N. W. 2	N. W. 2	0	4	0	
20	29.54	29.52	29.60	20	35	27	27.3	N. W. 2	N. W. 3	N. W. 2	0	3	0	
21	29.65	29.69	29.72	28	36	31	31.7	N. W. 1	N. W. 2	N. W. 2	0	2	10	
22	29.69	29.59	29.53	21	40	30	30.3	N. W. 1	S. W. 1	S'ly 1	0	4	6	
23	29.40	29.21	29.19	26	32	14	24.0	E. 2	S. E'ly 3	N. W. 5	8	Snow	0	} 0.10
24	29.11	29.40	29.66	16	36	26	26.0	N. W. 3	N. W. 3	N. W. 2	Snow	0	0	
25	29.76	29.69	29.69	25	36	28	29.7	W'ly 2	S. W. 2	W. 2	8	4	2	
S 26	29.70	29.81	30.05	24	33	26	27.7	N. W. 3	N. W. 3	W'ly 2	0	0	0	
27	30.14	30.09	30.02	22	43	32	32.3	N. W. 2	S'ly 2	E'ly 2	0	9	10	
28	29.63	29.18	28.94	37	45	46	42.7	S. E. 3	S. E. 5	S. W'ly 3	Rain	Rain	Misty	3.33
29	29.20	29.56	29.80	34	40	34	36.0	N. W. 3	N. W. 3	N. W. 2	5	0	0	
30	29.93	30.03	30.12	30	42	33	35.0	N. W. 1	N. W. 2	N. E'ly 2	0	0	10	
31	30.12	30.04	29.93	28	36	30	31.3	N. E. 2	N. E. 2	N. E. 2	10	10	Snow	
Means	29.65	29.62	29.67	24.1	34.4	27.5	...	2.2	2.7	2.5	3.4	3.4	3.2	5.58
									2.6			3.3		
REDUCED TO SEA LEVEL.														
Max.	30.32	30.27	30.30	37	45	46	42.7	Prevailing winds from some point between— Days.						
Min.	28.98	28.93	29.12	12	22	14	16.3						Days.	
Mean	29.83	29.80	29.85					N. & E. 3			Clear 13			
Range	1.34	1.34	1.18	25	23	32	26.4	E. & S. 3			Variable . . . } 11			
Mean of month			29.827	...	...	...	28.7	S. & W. 5			Cloudy . . . . }			
Extreme range			1.39	...	...	...	34.0	W. & N. 20			Rain or snow fell on 7			

1st. Pleasant.

2d. Wind brisk, and cold pretty severe.

3d and 4th. Cold and severe.

5th. Cold and blustering. A beam of light first seen in the west this evening which resembled the tail of a comet.

6th. Cold and blustering. Aurora, not bright.

7th. Blustering. After sunset, a beam or brush of light appeared in the west; presumed to be the tail of a comet; the body was below the horizon; the tail became visible 3° or 4° above horizon, 10° or 15° S. of W., and inclined S., making with horizon an angle of 30° or 35°, and 40° or 45° in length. At narrowest point near horizon, it was about 2° wide, and at broadest point, towards upper extremity, it was, perhaps, 4° or 5° broad. Was seen on evening of 5th. Visible till about 8 o'clock.

8th. Weather fine. Evening cloudy and hazy. The comet not visible.

9th. Very fine. The comet again visible.

10th. Cloudy A. M. Gentle snow P. M. Moderate rain in the evening.

11th. Clouds and mist A. M. Clear P. M. The comet very distinct, notwithstanding the increased light of the moon.

12th. Fine.

13th. Moderate rain and hail all day.

14th. Blustering and severe. Comet visible.

15th. Blustering. Comet faintly visible.

16th. Variable. Wind N. E.; heavy in evening.

17th. Heavy snow and rain last night. Bar. fell to 28.74 by 11 A. M. Wind W'ly; very blustering. Cleared in evening. Comet very brilliant.

18th. Clear and cold. Comet brilliant; nucleus about 2° S. E. of Eta Eridoni, and upper end of tail a few degrees beyond the head of the Hare or Lepus. A bright meteor was seen, which seemed to explode near Musca, or the Fly, leaving a train of light visible with a telescope for 10 minutes.

19th. Fine, though cool. Comet very bright.

20th and 21st. Pleasant. Clouds prevented the comet from being seen well.

22d. Pleasant. Comet still obscured by clouds.

23d. Snow. Cleared in evening. Comet visible.

24th. Pleasant. Evening very clear. Comet declining a little in brightness.

25th. Flurry of snow early in the evening.

26th. Pleasant. Comet visible.

27th. Appearances of storm.

28th. Violent storm. Bar. lowest at 10 P. M.

29th. Clear evening. Comet visible, but faint. aurora in the north—not very bright.

30th. Pleasant.

31st. Began to rain and hail at 7 P. M.; turned to snow before 10 P. M.

April, 1843.

DAYS.	BAROMETER, REDUCED TO 32° F. At 6 A. M.	At 1 P. M.	At 10 P. M.	THERMOMETER. At 6 A. M.	At 1 P. M.	At 10 P. M.	Daily mean.	WINDS. (DIRECTION AND FORCE.) At 6 A. M.	At 1 P. M.	At 10 P. M.	WEATHER. (TENTHS CLOUDY.) At 6 A. M.	At 1 P. M.	At 10 P. M.	RAIN AND SNOW IN INCHES OF WATER.
1	29.64	29.50	29.60	31	34	32	32.3	N. E. 2	N. E. 3	N. W. 2	Rain	Rain	7	0.70
S 2	29.72	29.80	29.88	25	36	31	30.7	N. W. 3	N. W. 3	N. W. 2	0	0	0	
3	29.94	29.95	30.00	28	39	32	33.0	N. W. 2	N. W. 2	N. W. 1	0	0	0	
4	30.04	30.05	30.03	25	42	34	33.7	N. W. 1	N. E. 1	N. E. 1	0	5	10	
5	29.95	...	29.65	32	...	32	...	N. E. 1	N. E. 1	N. E. 3	10	Rain	Rain	0.44
6	29.51	29.54	29.62	35	46	37	39.3	N. W. 2	N. W. 2	N. W. 2	6	0	0	
7	29.62	29.64	29.66	34	45	41	40.0	N. W. 2	N. W. 2	N. W. 2	0	0	2	
8	29.51	29.19	29.23	39	57	45	47.0	S. W. 2	S. W. 2	W'ly 2	10	8	2	
S 9	29.19	29.14	29.20	40	52	40	44.0	S. W. 1	N. W. 1	N. W. 1	8	5	0	
10	29.35	29.41	29.52	37	41	35	37.7	N. W. 2	N. W. 2	N. W. 1	2	10	0	
11	29.63	29.64	29.63	34	48	44	42.0	N. W. 1	N. W. 3	N. W. 2	0	0	8	
12	29.80	29.83	29.91	38	60	47	48.3	N. W. 1	N. W. 1	S. W. 1	0	0	0	
13	29.94	29.95	30.00	36	55	44	45.0	S'ly 2	S'ly 2	S'ly 1	0	0	5	
14	30.00	29.99	29.98	47	59	52	52.7	S'ly 1	S. E. 1	S. E. 1	10	Rain	10	
15	29.83	29.80	29.78	55	59	53	55.7	S. E. 2	S. E. 2	S'ly 1	10	10	10	
S 16	29.78	29.71	29.71	54	67	50	57.0	S'ly 1	S. E'ly 1	S. W. 1	10	6	2	
17	29.68	29.78	29.82	50	45	40	45.0	N. E. 1	N. E. 2	N. E. 3	Misty	Misty	Rain	} 0.95
18	29.88	29.93	29.99	40	38	36	38.0	N. E. 2	N. E. 3	N. E. 3	Misty	Rain	10	
19	29.99	29.98	29.95	36	39	39	38.0	N. E. 4	N. E. 3	...	10	10	10	
20	29.93	29.91	29.92	39	50	40	43.0	N. E. 2	N. E. 2	N. E'ly 1	10	9	0	
21	29.94	29.89	29.88	40	62	46	49.3	N'ly 1	N'ly 1	S'ly 1	0	0	0	
22	29.89	29.90	29.92	49	65	47	53.7	S. E. 1	S. E. 1	S'ly	8	0	0	
S 23	29.85	29.72	29.60	47	49	51	49.0	S. E. 1	S. E. 2	S'ly 2	Rain	Rain	10	2.00
24	29.51	29.44	29.55	49	66	56	57.0	S'ly 1	W'ly 1	N. W. 1	Misty	5	10	
25	29.58	29.55	29.72	51	53	48	50.7	N. E'ly 2	N. E. 2	N. E. 2	Misty	7	Misty	
26	29.78	29.74	29.71	50	61	55	55.3	N. E. 1	N. E. 1	N. E. 1	Misty	Misty	Misty	
27	29.51	29.31	29.35	53	55	49	52.3	S'ly 1	S. W.	N. E. 1	Misty	Rain	10	0.25
28	29.56	29.59	29.59	46	66	54	55.3	N. W. 1	N. W.	N. W.	4	0	0	
29	29.76	29.83	29.92	49	54	45	49.3	N. E. 1	N. E. 2	S. E. 1	8	5	10	
S 30	29.93	29.86	29.73	42	51	50	47.7	S. E. 1	E'ly 3	S. E'ly 3	9	10	Rain	
Means	29.74	29.71	29.73	41.0	51.5	43.5	...	1.6	1.9	1.6	6.5	5.7	5.5	4.34
									1.7			5.9		

REDUCED TO SEA LEVEL.							
Max.	30.22	30.23	30.21	55	67	56	57.0
Min.	29.37	29.32	29.38	25	34	31	30.7
Mean	29.92	29.89	29.91				
Range	0.85	0.91	0.83	30	33	25	20.3
Mean of month	29.907			...	...	...	45.3
Extreme range	0.91			...	...	...	42.0

Prevailing winds from some point between—	Days.
N. & E.	11
E. & S.	5
S. & W.	4
W. & N.	10

	Days.
Clear	10
Variable / Cloudy	} 11
Rain fell on	9

REMARKS.

1st. Rain, hail, and snow. Cleared partially at 8 P. M. Ground covered with snow and sleet.
2d. Pleasant, but rather blustering.
3d. Fine.
4th. Mild, and a little spring-like.
5th. Began to snow moderately from 7 to 8 A. M.; soon turned to rain, which continued during the day and evening.
6th. Aurora in the evening—not brilliant
7th. Fine.
8th. Warm and spring-like.
9th. Very pleasant.
10th. A well-defined halo round the moon from 8 to 10 P. M.
11th and 12th. Very fine.
13th. Fine.
14th. Very light rain in the morning. Cloudy in the afternoon.
15th. Occasional mist and rain.
16th. Very warm.
17th. Misty and raw.
18th. Raw and unpleasant. Mist, snow, and rain together.
19th. Raw and cold.
20th. Cloudy and raw in the morning. Clouds broken in the afternoon. Clear in the evening.
21st. Very fine.
22d. Fine.
23d. Pretty heavy rain in the afternoon.
24th. Air warm and damp.
25th. Air damp.
26th. Misty.
27th. Rain at intervals. Thunder in the evening.
28th and 29th. Pleasant.
30th. Rainy afternoon and evening. Air raw.

May, 1843.

DAYS.	BAROMETER At 6 A. M.	At 1 P. M.	At 10 P. M.	THERMOMETER At 6 A. M.	At 1 P. M.	At 10 P. M.	Daily mean.	WINDS At 6 A. M.	At 1 P. M.	At 10 P. M.	WEATHER At 6 A. M.	At 1 P. M.	At 10 P. M.	RAIN AND SNOW
1	29.50	29.54	29.72	52	62	52	55.3	S. E. 5	S. W. 2	W'ly 2	Rain	1	2	1.60
2	29.89	29.90	30.04	46	58	46	50.0	N. W. 1	N. W. 1	N. W. 1	1	2	0	
3	30.07	30.11	30.13	42	54	45	47.0	N. E. 1	S'ly 2	S'ly 1	3	10	10	
4	30.11	30.02	30.02	42	64	44	50.0	N. E. 1	S. E'ly 1	S. E'ly	0	0	0	
5	30.12	30.15	30.12	48	52	44	48.0	N. E'ly 2	N. E. 2	S'ly 1	10	1	8	
6	30.14	30.09	30.02	45	57	45	49.0	N. E. 1	N. E. 1	S'ly 1	10	2	5	
S 7	29.89	29.80	29.71	53	57	56	55.3	S. W. 1	S. W. 1	S. W. 1	10	Rain	10	1.50
8	29.65	29.58	29.66	56	70	53	59.7	S. W. 2	S. W. 2	N. W. 2	10	8	0	
9	29.71	...	29.98	53	...	47	...	N. W. 2	...	N. E.	0	...	5	
10	30.04	30.09	30.06	44	65	49	52.7	N. E. 2	N. E. 2	N. E. 1	0	0	5	
11	29.96	29.89	29.79	45	63	48	52.0	N. E. 1	N. E. 2	N. E. 3	9	10	7	
12	29.71	29.70	29.75	44	72	49	55.0	N. 1	N. E. 2	N. E. 1	0	0	0	
13	29.79	29.75	29.75	47	63	51	53.7	E'ly 2	E'ly 2	S'ly 1	5	0	5	
S 14	29.74	29.70	29.69	51	67	56	58.0	S'ly 1	S. W. 1	S'ly 1	9	0	3	
15	29.69	29.60	29.57	54	67	58	59.7	S. E'ly 1	S. E'ly 2	S'ly 1	0	0	2	
16	29.59	29.58	29.61	56	75	63	64.7	W'ly 1	N. W. 2	S. W. 1	4	0	0	
17	29.74	29.74	29.90	60	64	47	57.0	W'ly 1	S. W. 3	N. W. 2	5	9	0	
18	...	...	29.99	44	...	46	...	N. W. 2	...	N. W. 1	0	...	0	
19	29.99	...	...	44	...	53	...	N. W. 1	...	S. W. 1	0	0	0	
20	29.79	29.71	29.59	50	65	52	55.7	N. E. 1	N. E. 2	N'ly 2	7	9	8	
S 21	29.47	29.41	29.41	50	67	53	56.7	N'ly 2	N. W. 2	N. W. 1	8	6	4	
22	29.51	...	29.60	52	...	56	...	S. W'ly	...	S'ly	0	...	3	
23	29.60	29.53	29.50	54	67	58	59.7	S. E. 3	S. E. 2	S'ly 2	Rain	6	1	0.40
24	29.44	29.41	29.49	54	65	53	57.3	N. W. 3	N. W. 4	N. W. 2	3	4	0	
25	29.54	29.58	29.48	51	64	54	56.3	N. W. 2	N. W. 2	N. E. 1	0	5	10	
26	29.78	29.83	29.85	52	66	53	57.0	N. E. 1	N. E. 1	N. E. 1	5	8	10	
27	29.81	29.79	29.75	50	51	46	49.0	S. E. 1	E.	N. E. 1	Rain	Rain	Rain	
S 28	29.71	29.68	29.63	50	61	55	55.3	W'ly 1	W. 1	W. 1	10	10	0	
29	29.61	29.56	29.53	51	58	50	53.0	N. 2	N. E. 1	N. E. 1	10	10	10	
[illegible]	[illegible]	[illegible]	[illegible]	[illegible]	[illegible]	[illegible]	[illegible]	[illegible]	[illegible]	[illegible]	0	[illegible]	0	
31	...	29.39	29.51	...	62	46	...	S. W.	N. W.	N. W.	Rain	10	0	
Means	29.76	29.72	29.74	49.7	63.1	50.9	...	1.6	1.7	1.2	5.4	4.7	4.2	3.50
									1.5			4.8		

REDUCED TO SEA LEVEL.							
Max.	30.32	30.33	30.31	60	75	63	64.7
Min.	29.62	29.57	29.59	42	51	44	47.0
Mean	29.94	29.89	29.92				
Range	0.70	0.76	0.72	18	24	19	17.7
Mean of month	29.917			...	...	...	54.6
Extreme range	0.76			...	...	...	33.0

Prevailing winds from some point between—	Days.
N. & E.	11
E. & S.	5
S. & W.	5
W. & N.	10

	Days.
Clear	7
Variable / Cloudy	} 20
Rain fell on	4

REMARKS.

1st. Rain in the morning. Pleasant in the afternoon.
2d. Very fine.
3d. Pleasant.
4th. Fine
5th and 6th. Pleasant.
7th. Heavy showers and frequent thunder during the day.
8th and 9th. Pleasant.
10th. An unusually bright bow, with prismatic colors, appeared for some time about the sun between noon and 2 P. M. A fog bow also appeared about the moon in the evening, the air being hazy.
11th. Variable.
12th. Very fine.
13th, 14th, and 15th. Fine.
16th. Very fine.
17th to 20th. Fine.
21st and 22d. Pleasant.
23d. Fine shower in the morning.
24th. Fine.
25th and 26th. Pleasant.
27th. Very moderate rain most of the day.
28th and 29th. Cloudy.
30th. Pleasant.
31st. Variable.

June, 1843.

DAYS.	BAROMETER, REDUCED TO 32° F. At 6 A. M.	At 1 P. M.	At 10 P. M.	THERMOMETER. At 6 A. M.	At 1 P. M.	At 10 P. M.	Daily mean.	WINDS. (DIRECTION AND FORCE.) At 6 A. M.	At 1 P. M.	At 10 P. M.	WEATHER. (TENTHS CLOUDY.) At 6 A. M.	At 1 P. M.	At 10 P. M.	RAIN AND SNOW IN INCHES OF WATER.
1	...	...	...	44	...	45	...	N. W. 2	N. W. 2	N. W. 1	10	5	0	
2	29.93	29.89	29.86	41	62	48	50.3	N. W. 2	N. W. 2	S. W. 1	0	2	0	
3	29.72	29.59	29.63	52	68	58	59.3	S. W. 2	S. W. 3	S. W. 2	10	7	0	
S 4	29.74	29.68	29.61	53	70	56	59.7	N. W. 2	E'ly 2	S'ly 1	2	0	Foggy	
5	29.55	29.51	29.55	58	72	53	61.0	S'ly 1	S. E'ly 2	N. E. 2	4	3	10	
6	29.59	29.64	29.73	52	60	52	54.7	N'ly 1	N. E. 1	N. E. 2	10	10	8	0.25
7	29.89	29.91	30.00	48	66	57	57.0	N. W. 2	N. W. 2	N. W. 2	0	0	5	
8	29.99	29.98	29.92	55	66	58	59.7	N. W. 1	S. W. 2	S. W. 1	0	10	Shower	
9	29.64	29.60	29.65	57	67	53	59.0	S. W. 1	N. E. 1	N. W. 1	10	10	10	
10	29.55	29.44	29.46	57	82	65	68.0	S. W. 2	S. W. 3	S. W. 1	0	0	2	
S 11	29.44	29.56	29.74	67	57	56	60.0	S. W. 3	N. E. 2	N. E. 1	5	Rain	Misty	0.80
12	29.85	29.88	29.81	53	75	60	62.7	N. W. 2	N. W. 2	S. W. 1	0	0	0	
13	29.72	29.66	29.53	55	68	60	61.0	S. W. 3	S. W. 3	S. W. 2	0	2	0	
14	29.45	29.33	29.38	62	77	63	67.3	S. W. 2	W'ly 1	S. W. 1	10	2	0	
15	29.53	29.59	29.68	57	73	58	62.7	N. W. 2	W'ly 3	W'ly 1	0	0	0	
16	29.69	29.61	29.60	56	60	52	56.0	S. W. 2	S. W. 1	N'ly 1	5	Rain	0	0.82
17	29.71	29.79	29.79	52	63	58	57.7	N. W. 2	N. W. 1	N. W. 1	8	5	0	
S 18	29.80	29.81	29.83	57	72	61	63.3	N. W. 2	N. W. 2	N. W. 2	0	0	0	
19	29.95	29.96	30.01	56	74	62	64.0	N. W. 1	N. W. 1	N. W. 2	0	0	0	
20	30.07	30.07	30.02	58	77	62	65.7	W'ly 1	S. W. 2	W'ly	0	0	0	
21	30.02	29.98	29.91	62	77	64	67.7	S. W. 2	S. W. 2	S. W. 2	0	0	0	
22	29.85	29.75	29.71	66	85	68	73.0	W. 2	S. W. 2	W. 1	0	8	0	
23	29.68	29.66	29.63	68	87	72	75.7	W. 1	W'ly 2	W'ly 2	0	0	3	
24	29.62	29.52	29.48	68	87	73	76.0	W'ly 1	S. W. 3	S. W. 1	0	1	2	
S 25	29.57	29.60	29.70	69	81	67	72.3	N. W. 2	N. W. 3	N. W. 1	5	5	1	
26	29.72	29.79	29.78	62	77	65	68.0	S. E'ly 1	S. E'ly 2	S'ly 1	3	5	2	
27	29.77	29.70	29.69	64	82	73	73.0	S'ly 2	S'ly 2	S'ly 2	3	1	0	
28	29.68	29.66	29.61	71	84	73	76.0	S. W. 1	S. W. 3	S. W. 2	0	5	Rain	0.25
29	29.57	29.51	29.53	70	83	74	75.7	S. W. 1	S. W. 2	S. W. 1	8	Shower	5	
30	29.58	29.61	29.66	71	86	71	76.0	N. W. 2	N. W. 2	S'ly 1	0	3	0	
Means	29.72	29.70	29.71	58.7	73.7	61.2	...	1.7	2.1	1.3	3.1	3.8	2.9	2.12
									1.7			3.3		
REDUCED TO SEA LEVEL.														
Max.	30.25	30.25	30.20	71	87	74	76.0	Prevailing winds from some point between—		Days.			Days.	
Min.	29.62	29.51	29.56	41	57	45	50.3	N. & E.		3	Clear		13	
Mean	29.90	29.87	29.89					E. & S.		4	Variable . . .		} 8	
Range	0.63	0.74	0.64	30	30	29	25.7	S. & W.		13	Cloudy			
Mean of month	29.887			...	...	...	64.5	W. & N.		10	Rain fell on . .		9	
Extreme range	0.74			...	...	...	46.0							

REMARKS.

1st. Raw and cold.
2d. Clear. At 6 A. M., thermometer 41°; at sunrise, probably as low as 38° or 39°. Frost in some places in the vicinity.
3d. Cloudy in the morning. Thunder, with copious shower in the afternoon.
4th. Pleasant.
5th. Thunder and sprinkling of rain in the afternoon, and wind came to N. E. from 3 to 4 P. M.
6th. Showers in evening.
7th. Fine.
8th. Pleasant.
9th. Thunder and lightning in the evening, with sprinkling of rain.
10th. Appearances of rain, with lightning, in the afternoon and evening.
11th. Heavy showers at intervals. From 9 to 10 A. M., wind changed from S. W. to N. E., passing to S. E., E., &c. Temperature suddenly fell, and rain from 10 to 11 P. M.
12th and 13th. Fine.
14th. Fine. Shower at sunset.
15th. Fine.
16th. Rain in the afternoon.
17th. Cool, but pleasant.
18th. Fine.
19th. Very fine.
20th and 21st. Fine.
22d and 23d. Very clear and hot.
24th. Very clear and hot. Fresh breeze in the afternoon.
25th and 26th. Fine.
27th. Very hot. Brisk breeze in the afternoon.
28th. Very sultry and hot in the morning. Sprinkling of rain began at 8 P. M., and continued.
29th. Occasional sprinkling in the morning. Fine shower from 1 to 2 P. M.
30th. Very hot; burning sun.

July, 1843.

DAYS.	Barometer At 6 A. M.	At 1 P. M.	At 10 P. M.	Thermometer At 6 A. M.	At 1 P. M.	At 10 P. M.	Daily mean.	Winds At 6 A. M.	At 1 P. M.	At 10 P. M.	Weather At 6 A. M.	At 1 P. M.	At 10 P. M.	Rain and Snow
1	29.69	29.68	29.70	71	85	75	77.0	S. W. 1	S'ly 2	S. E. 1	5	2	4	
S 2	29.62	29.52	29.50	71	84	74	76.3	S. E. 2	S. E. 3	W'ly 1	7	8	10	
3	29.56	29.67	29.83	65	78	64	69.0	N. W. 2	N. W. 1	N. W. 1	6	0	0	
4	29.87	29.87	29.79	54	72	65	63.7	N. W. 1	W'ly 2	S. W. 3	0	2	6	
5	29.65	29.69	...	65	62	...	...	S. W. 2	W'ly 2	...	10	10, Shr.	...	0.28
6	29.76	29.71	29.72	55	75	63	64.3	N. W. 2	N. W. 2	N. W. 1	0	0	1	
7	29.70	29.63	29.53	60	72	66	66.0	N. W. 1	S. W. 3	S. W. 2	2	10	4	
8	29.60	29.58	29.60	62	81	66	69.7	W'ly 2	W'ly 3	W'ly	0	0	5	
S 9	29.68	29.68	29.68	63	82	67	70.7	N. W. 2	W'ly 1	W'ly	0	1	1	
10	29.57	29.62	29.58	64	79	66	69.7	W'ly 2	S. W. 4	S. W. 1	0	10	5	
11	29.68	29.74	29.81	64	73	64	67.0	N'ly 2	E'ly 1	N. E. 1	6	10	6	
12	29.92	29.95	30.06	59	78	62	66.3	N. E'ly 1	N. E. 1	N. E. 1	4	3	0	
13	30.10	30.10	30.09	57	75	64	65.3	N. E. 1	S'ly 1	S'ly 1	2	1	5	
14	30.06	29.98	29.91	62	77	63	67.3	S. W. 1	S'ly 3	S'ly 1	0	2	3	
15	29.83	29.79	29.79	62	79	63	68.0	S. E'ly	S. E. 2	E'ly 1	7	4	0	
S 16	29.81	29.78	29.81	57	80	62	66.3	N. E. 1	N. E. 1	N. E. 1	10	2	5	
17	29.84	29.83	29.78	62	72	64	66.0	N. E'ly 1	S'ly	S. W'ly	6	10	Rain	
18	29.59	29.58	29.54	67	78	72	72.3	S. W. 2	S. W'ly 2	S. W. 0	10	6	0	
19	29.54	29.55	29.58	70	83	70	74.3	N. W. 2	W'ly 2	N. E. 2	0	0	2	
20	29.64	29.68	29.72	59	74	58	63.7	N. W. 2	N. W'ly 3	N. W. 1	0	0	0	
21	29.73	29.73	29.74	55	79	65	66.3	N. W. 2	N. W. 3	N. W. 2	0	0	0	
22	29.75	29.74	29.74	60	76	68	68.0	N. W. 2	N. W. 2	N. W. 1	0	0	0	
S 23	29.73	29.67	29.64	68	89	73	76.7	N. W. 1	W'ly 2	S. W. 1	0	0	0	
24	29.55	29.48	29.60	68	89	70	75.7	N. W. 2	N. W. 3	N. W. 2	2	1	6	
25	29.72	29.74	29.86	56	77	64	65.7	N. W. 2	W'ly 3	N. W. 1	0	0	0	
26	29.89	29.84	29.75	63	80	71	71.3	N. W. 1	W'ly 2	N. W. 2	2	1	0	
27	29.78	29.77	29.88	68	86	70	74.7	N. W. 1	S'ly 2	S. W. 1	0	0	0	
28	29.88	...	29.64	67	...	71	...	S. W. 1	...	S. W. 3	7	10, Shr.	10	0.10
29	29.54	29.56	29.61	70	86	74	76.7	S. W. 2	S. W. 2	W'ly 1	9	10	0	
S 30	29.69	29.68	29.71	64	57	57	59.3	N. E. 2	N. E. 2	N. E. 2	10	Rain	Rain	1.45
31	29.71	29.72	29.76	57	66	62	61.7	N. E. 1	W'ly 1	N. W. 1	Rain	10	10	
Means	29.73	29.72	29.73	62.7	77.5	66.5	...	1.6	2.1	1.2	3.7	3.9	3.4	1.83
									1.6			3.7		
REDUCED TO SEA LEVEL.														
Max.	30.28	30.28	30.27	71	89	75	77.0	Prevailing winds from some point between—		Days			Days.	
Min.	29.72	29.66	29.68	54	57	57	59.3	N. & E.		4	Clear		14	
Mean	29.90	29.89	29.90					E. & S.		5	Variable . . .		} 8	
Range	0.56	0.62	0.59	17	32	18	17.7	S. & W.		9	Cloudy			
Mean of month	29.897			...	...	...	68.9	W. & N.		13	Rain fell on . .		9	
Extreme range	0.62			...	...	...	35.0							

2d. Clear after 12 o'clock last night. Towards morning, clouds and lightning, and thunder at a distance. Afterwards it cleared off, without any rain, and remained clear till 5 P. M., when clouds appeared in the west, followed by a light shower. Cloudy till 10 P. M.
3d and 4th. In general, fine.
5th. Showery.
6th. In general, fine.
7th. Pleasant.
8th. Fine. Light shower from 9 to 10 P. M.
9th. Pleasant.
10th. Sprinkling of rain at 6 P. M.
11th. Clouds occasionally general and heavy, with sprinkling of rain.
12th, 13th, and 14th. Pleasant.
15th. Light shower from 3 to 4 A. M. Fine during the day.
16th. Fine.
17th. Cloudy, with appearances of rain. Sprinkling in the evening.
18th. Cloudy in the morning. Very sultry in the afternoon, with a burning sun.
19th to 22d. Fine.
23d. Fine; fresh breeze. Very clear and burning sun.
24th. Gust of wind at 4 P. M., with appearances of rain. Showers in the vicinity, but none here.
25th. Fine. Aurora—not very bright.
26th and 27th. Fine.
28th. Cloudy at sunrise, with appearances of rain. Light shower at 2 P. M.
29th. Thunder, with sprinkling of rain. Fine showers a few miles to the south of us.
30th. Begun to rain moderately from 8 to 9 A. M. Rain increased, and continued heavy at intervals till 2 P. M. Rain again from 9 to 10 P. M.
31st. Light rain during a part of the morning.

August, 1843.

Days.	Barometer, reduced to 32° F. At 6 A. M.	At 1 P. M.	At 10 P. M.	Thermometer. At 6 A. M.	At 1 P. M.	At 10 P. M.	Daily mean.	Winds. (Direction and Force.) At 6 A. M.	At 1 P. M.	At 10 P. M.	Weather. (Tenths Cloudy.) At 6 A. M.	At 1 P. M.	At 10 P. M.	Rain and Snow in Inches of Water.	Remarks.
1	29.77	29.72	29.70	61	74	61	65.3	N'ly 2	N'ly 2	N'ly	10	8	5		1st. Pleasant, though cloudy.
2	29.76	29.76	29.79	60	74	63	65.7	E'ly 1	S'ly 2	S'ly	7	6	3		2d, 3d, and 4th. Pleasant.
3	29.87	29.90	30.00	62	74	63	66.3	N'ly 1	N. W'ly 1	S'ly 1	10	4	0		
4	30.06	30.04	30.08	60	77	64	67.0	W'ly 1	S. E'ly 2	S'ly 1	4	1	0		
5	30.14	30.11	30.08	62	80	67	69.7	S'ly 1	S'ly 2	E'ly 1	0	9	10		5th. Fine in the morning. Cloudy in the afternoon. Rain during the night.
S 6	29.88	29.83	29.81	59	64	59	60.7	E'ly 3	N. E'ly 2	N. E. 2	Rain	Misty	Misty	1.33	6th. Light rain at intervals, and mist.
7	29.86	29.84	29.81	58	74	65	65.7	S'ly 1	S'ly 1	S'ly 1	10	5	10		
8	29.79	29.73	29.75	66	77	69	70.7	S'ly 1	S'ly 1	S'ly	10	10, Shr.	10	0.25	8th. Fine shower at 4 P. M.
9	29.80	29.82	29.83	67	74	67	69.3	N. W. 1	S'ly 1	S. W'ly	Rain	Rain	8		9th. Warm, and air very damp.
10	29.82	29.79	29.71	66	72	64	67.3	W'ly 2	S. W'ly 2	N. E. 1	10	10	Rain	} 20.5	10th. Occasional light showers. Heavy rain during the night.
11	29.59	29.56	29.59	63	67	64	64.7	N. E'ly 2	N. E. 2	N. W. 2	Rain	Rain	9		11th. Occasional showers.
12	29.61	29.62	29.68	66	79	67	70.7	N. E'ly 2	S. W'ly 3	N. W.	10	7	0		12th. Heavy clouds, but no rain.
S 13	29.71	29.70	29.70	67	80	68	71.7	N. W. 1	S. W'ly 3	S. W. 1	2	3	0		13th. Sun very hot.
14	29.70	29.64	29.58	68	80	70	72.7	S. W. 1	S. W. 3	S. W. 1	0	0	0		14th. Very sultry.
15	29.62	29.61	29.70	72	80	69	73.7	W'ly 1	N. W. 2	N. W. 1	10	0	0		15th. Very hot sun. Light shower at sunrise.
16	29.72	29.72	29.77	62	75	67	68.0	N. W. 1	N. W. 1	S. W.	0	0	0		
17	29.78	29.77	29.77	62	80	68	70.0	S. W.	S. W.	S. W.	2	2	0		
18	29.78	29.76	29.79	66	80	78	74.7	S. W.	S. W.	S'ly	1	3	0		
19	29.80	29.80	29.79	72	81	74	75.7	S. W.	S'ly	S'ly	3	2	4		19th. At 6 P. M., a dead calm.
S 20	29.68	29.63	29.77	68	75	72	71.7	N. E.	N'ly	N'ly	10	10	10	} 2.00	20th. Light shower a little before sunrise, continuing, from time to time, till 10 A. M.
21	29.86	29.87	29.92	69	80	67	72.0	S. E.	S. E.	E'ly	10	6	10		21st. Light misty showers in the afternoon.
22	29.91	29.83	29.80	64	78	70	70.7	N. E.	S. E.	N. E.	10	7	10		22d. Showery.
23	29.75	29.74	29.74	70	79	72	73.7	S. E.	S. W.	S. W.	8	9	7		23d. Showers from noon to 4 P. M.
24	29.74	29.77	29.81	68	78	70	72.0	W'ly	N. W.	N. W.	9	7	0		
25	29.85	29.91	29.92	64	78	74	72.0	N. W.	N. E.	E'ly	0	3	0		25th and 26th. Pleasant.
26	29.98	29.89	29.87	66	77	68	70.3	S. W.	S. W.	S. W.	Foggy	4	0		
S 27	29.88	29.86	29.84	66	81	72	73.0	S. W.	S'ly	S. W.	0	3	0		27th. Very hot.
28	29.85	29.83	29.88	72	77	63	70.7	S. W.	S. W.	N. E.	5	Shower	10	0.60	28th. Heavy showers, with thunder, from 2 to 4 P. M.
29	29.98	...	...	62	...	64	...	N. E.	...	N. E.	10	...	0		
30	29.88	29.77	29.75	66	78	70	71.3	S. W. 2	S. W.	S. W.	10	3	0		30th. Very hot sun.
31	29.74	29.68	29.77	68	82	67	72.3	S. W. 1	S. W. 2	N. W. 3	0	0	0		31st. Very hot during the day. Thunder, with sprinkling of rain, in the evening, and cooler.
Means	29.81	29.78	29.80	65.2	76.8	67.6	...	1.3	1.8	1.4	6.8	5.7	4.1	6.23	
REDUCED TO SEA LEVEL.									1.5			5.5			
Max.	30.32	30.29	30.26	72	82	78	75.7	Prevailing winds from some point between—		Days.			Days.		
Min.	29.77	29.74	29.76	58	64	59	60.7	N. & E.		4	Clear		9		
Mean	29.98	29.95	29.97					E. & S.		8	Variable		} 11		
Range	0.55	0.55	0.50	14	18	19	15.0	S. & W.		14	Cloudy				
Mean of month	29.967			...	...	...	69.9	W. & N.		5	Rain fell on		11		
Extreme range	0.58			...	...	...	24.0								

September, 1843.

Days.	Barometer At 6 A. M.	At 1 P. M.	At 10 P. M.	Thermometer At 6 A. M.	At 1 P. M.	At 10 P. M.	Daily mean.	Winds At 6 A. M.	At 1 P. M.	At 10 P. M.	Weather At 6 A. M.	At 1 P. M.	At 10 P. M.	Rain.	Remarks.
1	29.93	29.92	29.92	63	65	60	62.7	N. E. 2	N. E. 1	N. E. 1	10	10	10		1st. Cool, with appearances of rain.
2	29.84	29.74	29.69	58	75	69	67.3	S'ly 1	S. W. 1	S. W. 1	10	3	1		2d. Warm.
S 3	29.69	29.56	29.63	70	83	71	74.7	S'ly 1	S. W. 2	S'ly	10	2	Foggy		3d. Very burning sun at mid-day.
4	29.56	29.47	29.56	70	83	74	75.7	W'ly 0	W'ly 1	W'ly 1	10	6	6		4th. Very sultry. Thunder, with appearances of rain, towards evening.
5	29.71	...	29.92	68	...	64	...	N. W. 3	...	N. E. 2	4	...	10		5th to 8th. Pleasant.
6	29.98	...	29.99	58	...	60	...	N. E. 2	...	N. E. 1	2	...	2		
7	29.98	29.99	29.95	58	70	60	62.7	N. E. 1	N. E. 2	N. E. 2	8	10	10		
8	29.87	...	29.68	60	...	58	...	N. E. 2	...	N. E. 2	10	...	0		
9	29.76	29.69	29.55	56	65	53	58.0	N. W. 2	N. W. 2	N. W.	0	0	0		9th to 12th. Very cool.
S 10	29.94	29.92	29.90	49	64	54	55.7	N. W. 1	N. W. 3	W'ly 1	6	8	5		
11	29.85	29.80	29.85	52	62	50	54.7	N. E. 1	N. E. 2	N. E. 1	9	1	7		
12	29.87	29.90	29.97	47	60	47	51.3	N. E. 2	N. E. 3	N. E. 1	10	2	0		
13	30.05	30.07	30.09	43	62	49	51.3	N'ly 1	N'ly 2	N. E. 1	0	0	0		13th. White frost this morning in many places in the vicinity.
14	30.11	30.12	30.11	42	66	54	54.0	N. E. 2	N. E. 2	N. E. 1	0	5	10		14th. Frost in the vicinity; none on the hill.
15	29.90	29.79	29.72	56	70	70	65.3	S. E. 2	S. E. 3	S. W'ly 1	Rain	Rain	4	0.40	15th. Moderate rain at intervals.
16	29.74	29.74	29.74	66	78	62	68.7	S'ly 1	S. E. 2	W'ly 1	8	2	0		16th. Very warm and sultry.
S 17	29.81	29.80	29.80	60	75	66	67.0	W'ly 1	S. W. 3	S. W. 3	0	0	0		17th. Very pleasant.
18	29.79	29.77	29.81	67	77	71	71.7	S. W. 1	S. W. 2	S. W. 1	9	0	0		18th. Very warm.
19	29.92	29.94	30.08	67	75	62	68.0	N'ly 1	N. E. 2	N. E. 1	0	0	0		19th and 20th. Pleasant.
20	30.16	30.14	30.05	56	71	61	62.7	N. E'ly 2	N. E. 2	N. E. 2	0	0	5		
21	29.85	29.68	29.52	61	76	75	70.7	S. W. 1	S. W. 3	S. W. 2	0	0	2		21st. Very sultry.
22	29.77	29.76	29.81	53	65	54	57.3	N. W. 2	N. W. 2	N. W. 1	0	0	0		22d and 23d. Very fine.
23	29.80	29.71	29.64	50	69	62	60.3	N. W. 1	S. W'ly 2	S. W.	0	0	0		
S 24	29.59	29.52	29.59	64	83	72	73.0	S. W'ly 2	W'ly 2	W'ly 1	0	0	0		24th. Very hot sun.
25	29.68	29.63	29.54	58	64	60	60.7	N. E. 2	N. E. 1	N. E. 1	10	10	Rain	1.80	25th. Heavy shower, with lightning, from 7 to 9 P. M.
26	29.51	29.56	29.65	60	61	49	56.7	N'ly 1	N'ly 1	N'ly 2	10	10	Rain		26th. Cool.
27	29.76	29.80	29.89	44	53	40	45.7	N. W'ly 2	N'ly 1	N. W. 0	2	4	0		27th. Cooler. Aurora considerably bright in the evening and through the night.
28	29.92	29.95	29.99	36	57	47	46.7	N. W. 1	N. W. 2	W'ly 1	0	5	2		28th. First appearances of White frost on the College green; only light.
29	29.90	29.80	29.84	41	63	51	51.7	N. W. 1	W'ly 1	S. W.	0	0	0		29th and 30th. Very fine.
30	29.90	29.87	29.85	46	64	51	53.7	W'ly 1	W'ly 1	W'ly	0	0	0		
Means	29.80	29.79	29.81	56.0	68.7	59.2	...	1.4	1.9	1.3	4.6	3.1	3.5	2.20	
REDUCED TO SEA LEVEL.									1.5			3.7			
Max.	30.34	30.32	30.29	70	83	75	68.7	Prevailing winds from some point between—		Days.			Days.		
Min.	29.69	29.65	29.70	36	53	40	45.7	N. & E.		12	Clear		12		
Mean	29.98	29.96	29.99					E. & S.		2	Variable		} 15		
Range	0.65	0.67	0.59	34	30	35	23.0	S. & W.		8	Cloudy				
Mean of month	20.977			...	...	...	61.3	W. & N.		8	Rain fell on		3		
Extreme range	0.69			...	...	...	47.0								

October, 1843.

DAYS.	BAROMETER, REDUCED TO 32° F. Sunrise.	At 1 P. M.	At 10 P. M.	THERMOMETER. Sunrise.	At 1 P. M.	At 10 P. M.	Daily mean.	WINDS. (DIRECTION AND FORCE.) Sunrise.	At 1 P. M.	At 10 P. M.	WEATHER. (TENTHS CLOUDY.) Sunrise.	At 1 P. M.	At 10 P. M.	RAIN AND SNOW IN INCHES OF WATER.
S 1	29.81	29.79	29.69	52	54	56	54.0	N. E. 1	S. E'ly 1	E'ly 2	Rain	Rain	Rain	1.25
2	29.49	29.41	29.40	62	72	58	64.0	N. W. 1	N. W. 2	W'ly 0	Misty	0	0	
3	29.34	29.27	29.30	52	65	51	56.0	W'ly 1	S. W. 2	S. W.	0	0	0	
4	29.35	29.36	29.56	47	55	46	49.3	S. W. 1	W'ly 3	N. W. 1	0	10	0	
5	29.70	29.69	29.70	43	55	49	49.0	N. W. 3	N. W. 3	N. W. 1	0	0	2	
6	29.73	29.65	29.66	49	62	56	55.7	N. W. 1	W'ly 1	W'ly 1	5	2	10	
7	29.74	29.73	29.78	51	54	50	51.7	N. E. 1	N. E. 1	N. E. 1	10	Rain	Rain	} 2.00
S 8	29.69	29.52	29.41	50	58	62	56.7	E'ly 1	S. E. 5	S'ly 4	Rain	Rain	Misty	
9	29.39	29.44	29.43	46	60	44	50.0	N. W. 2	N. W. 1	N. W. 2	2	8	0	
10	29.40	29.39	...	42	59	46	49.0	N. W. 1	N. W. 2	N. W. 1	8	5	0	
11	29.59	29.60	29.70	44	61	48	51.0	N. W. 1	N. W. 2	N. W. 0	0	0	0	
12	29.73	29.69	29.68	42	60	54	52.0	N. W. 1	N. E. 2	S. E'ly 1	0	0	Misty	
13	29.65	29.63	29.62	46	59	46	50.3	N. W. 1	N. W. 1	N. W. 0	2	0	0	
14	29.70	29.69	29.95	39	52	40	43.7	N. W. 2	N. W. 2	N. W. 2	4	10	0	
S 15	30.02	29.99	29.95	35	53	48	45.3	N. W. 1	S. W. 3	S. W. 0	8	10	10	
16	29.78	29.68	29.61	50	59	52	53.7	S. E. 1	S. W.	S. W. 1	Rain	5	10	1.15
17	29.65	29.51	29.61	42	52	41	45.0	N. W. 1	N. W. 2	N. W. 2	0	7	0	
18	29.69	29.62	29.62	38	55	49	47.3	N. W. 1	N. W. 2	S. W. 1	0	0	8	
19	29.49	29.69	29.94	49	52	41	47.3	S. W. 2	N. W. 3	N. W. 2	Rain	0	0	0.35
20	30.05	29.88	29.78	36	58	56	50.0	N. W. 1	S. W. 4	S. W. 3	0	0	0	
21	29.63	29.52	29.55	55	67	58	60.0	S. W. 2	S. W. 4	S. W. 1	0	0	5	
S 22	29.54	29.48	29.58	57	69	43	56.3	S. W. 1	S. W. 3	N. E. 3	10	3	10	
23	29.52	29.52	29.72	41	43	37	40.3	N. E. 1	N. W. 2	N. W. 2	Rain	8	0	
24	29.84	29.79	29.82	34	52	39	41.7	N. W. 0	N. W. 1	N. W. 0	0	0	0	
25	29.80	29.71	29.75	42	53	49	48.0	S'ly 1	S. W. 1	S. W. 1	10	Rain	0	
26	29.83	29.79	29.78	44	45	42	43.7	S. W. 1	N'ly 2	N. E. 1	10	10	10	
27	29.60	29.49	29.38	42	52	55	49.7	N. E. 2	E'ly	S'ly 1	Rain	Misty	Rain	1.70
28	29.69	29.78	29.88	42	45	39	42.0	N. W. 1	N. W. 1	N. W. 2	10	10	0	
S 29	29.88	29.84	29.89	38	46	40	41.3	N. W. 1	N. W. 1	N. W. 1	Misty	10	0	
30	29.94	29.89	29.88	38	56	47	47.0	N. W. 1	S. E'ly 2	S. W'ly 1	0	10	0	
31	29.99	30.00	30.14	32	43	32	35.7	N. W. 2	N. W. 2	N. W. 1	0	0	0	
Means	29.69	29.64	29.69	44.4	55.7	47.6	...	1.2	2.1	1.3	5.1	5.1	3.7	6.45
REDUCED TO SEA LEVEL.									1.5			4.6		
Max.	30.23	30.18	30.32	62	72	62	64.0	Prevailing winds from some point between—		Days.			Days.	
Min.	29.52	29.45	29.48	32	43	32	35.7							
Mean	29.87	29.81	29.87											
Range	0.71	0.73	0.84	30	29	30	28.3	N. & E.		5	Clear		10	
								E. & S.		2	Variable		} 15	
Mean of month 29.850				...	...	...	49.2	S. & W.		8	Cloudy			
Extreme range 0.87				...	...	...	40.0	W. & N.		16	Rain fell on		6	

REMARKS.

1st. Moderate rain nearly all day. Wind ligh about E. S. E.
2d. Very fine after 10 A. M.
3d. Very fine.
4th. Blustering at mid-day.
5th. Fine.
6th. Mild and pleasant.
7th. Very moderate but steady rain in the after noon.
8th. Moderate rain in the morning; wind E'ly Heavy wind S. E. in the afternoon, with rain in creased. Wind began to lull at 8 P. M.
9th and 10th. Fine.
11th. Very fine.
12th. Very fine through the day. Heavy mist approaching to rain in the evening.
13th, 14th, and 15th. Fine.
16th. Very heavy rain at 5 A. M., and after.
17th. Pleasant.
18th. Mild and pleasant.
19th. Fine after 10 A. M.
20th and 21st. Fine.
22d. Very mild. Wind changed from S. W. t N. E. late in the afternoon.
23d. Cool.
24th. Pleasant.
25th. Sprinkling of rain from 1 to 2 P. M. Clea evening.
26th. Pleasant.
27th. Rain in the morning, wind N. E. Rai again in the evening, wind S'ly, and warm.
28th. Clear in the evening.
29th. Cloudy during the day. Clear and plea sant in the evening.
31st. Very pleasant.

November, 1843.

DAYS.	BAROMETER Sunrise.	At 1 P. M.	At 10 P. M.	THERMOMETER Sunrise.	At 1 P. M.	At 10 P. M.	Daily mean.	WINDS Sunrise.	At 1 P. M.	At 10 P. M.	WEATHER Sunrise.	At 1 P. M.	At 10 P. M.	RAIN AND SNOW
1	30.26	30.21	30.13	26	44	39	36.3	N. W. 1	N. W. 1	N. E. 1	0	7	10	
2	29.63	29.47	29.59	50	52	41	47.7	S. E. 2	N. W. 2	N. W. 0	Rain	2	0	0.90
3	29.65	29.67	29.80	38	45	34	39.0	W'ly 3	N. W. 3	N. W. 2	0	0	0	
4	29.90	29.85	29.93	28	38	27	31.0	N. W. 1	N. W. 1	N. W. 2	0	0	0	
S 5	29.95	29.92	29.94	26	34	28	29.3	N. W. 2	N. W. 2	N. W. 2	1	0	0	
6	30.01	29.95	29.96	24	39	30	31.0	N. W. 2	N. E. 2	N'ly 0	0	0	0	
7	29.82	29.70	29.65	26	40	32	32.7	N. W. 1	S. W'ly 2	S W'ly 1	0	10	Snow	
8	29.61	29.61	29.77	26	36	30	30.7	N. W. 1	N. W. 1	N. W. 1	0	10	0	
9	29.91	29.90	29.91	26	40	35	33.7	N. W. 1	N. W.	W'ly	0	2	5	
10	29.82	29.74	29.74	32	40	37	36.3	N. E. 1	N. E. 1	N. E. 1	10	Misty	Misty	
11	29.69	29.46	29.22	36	40	37	37.7	W'ly 1	N. E. 1	N. E. 1	Foggy	Rain	Rain	
12	29.55	29.65	29.86	36	35	29	33.3	W'ly 2	W'ly 4	N. W. 1	0	5	0	
S 13	29.87	29.83	29.81	24	37	32	31.0	W'ly 1	W'ly 1	S. W. 1	0	10	Snow	
14	29.93	30.04	30.16	28	34	28	30.0	N. W. 1	N. W. 1	N. W. 1	3	10	0	
15	30.24	30.21	30.18	23	41	41	35.0	N. W. 1	S. W. 1	E'ly 2	0	10	10	
16	30.05	29.96	29.98	44	51	49	48.0	S'ly 1	S'ly 1	S'ly	Rain	Misty	Misty	0.15
17	30.05	30.02	29.94	45	53	47	48.3	W'ly 1	W'ly 1	E'ly 1	Foggy	2	10	
18	...	29.65	29.68	...	63	49	...	...	W'ly 1	W'ly	0	0	0	
S 19	29.78	...	29.85	41	...	40	...	N. W. 1	...	S. W'ly	0	...	10	
20	29.96	29.96	30.00	40	46	37	41.0	N. W. 1	N. W. 1	N. W. 0	0	0	0	
21	29.76	29.39	29.30	42	48	43	44.3	S. E. 2	S. E. 1	W'ly	10	Rain	0	0.30
22	29.40	29.39	29.59	38	42	40	40.0	N. W. 2	N. W. 3	N. W. 2	0	3	2	
23	29.74	29.70	29.73	33	48	43	41.3	N. W. 1	N. W. 2	W'ly 1	0	10	10	
24	29.59	29.51	29.63	48	58	50	52.0	S'ly 1	S'ly 1	S'ly 0	Rain	Misty	Foggy	
25	29.74	29.78	29.91	40	45	34	39.7	N. W. 1	N. W. 2	N. W. 1	0	0	0	
S 26	29.91	29.76	29.59	82	45	40	39.0	N. W. 2	N. W. 1	W'ly 1	0	0	10	
27	29.81	29.81	29.90	22	30	24	25.3	N. W. 1	N. W. 2	N. W. 2	0	0	0	
28	29.88	29.80	29.74	23	40	34	32.3	N. W. 1	N. W. 2	S. W. 1	0	0	2	
29	29.64	...	...	30	65	26	40.3	N. W. 2	...	...	0	...	...	
30	29.89	...	...	26	...	...	...	...	N. E.	...	10	...	...	
Means	29.83	29.78	29.80	32.9	43.9	36.4	...	1.3	1.5	1.1	2.8	4.9	4.6	1.35
REDUCED TO SEA LEVEL.									1.3			4.1		
Max.	30.44	30.39	30.36	50	65	50	52.0	Prevailing winds from some point between—		Days.			Days.	
Min.	29.58	29.57	29.40	22	30	24	25.3							
Mean	30.01	29.96	29.98											
Range	0.86	0.82	0.96	28	35	26	26.7	N. & E.		4	Clear		12	
								E. & S.		2	Variable		} 11	
Mean of month 29.983				...	...	...	37.7	S. & W.		6	Cloudy			
Extreme range 1.04				...	...	...	43.0	W. & N.		18	Rain fell on		7	

1st. Variable.
2d. Rain in the morning. Cleared from noon t 1 P. M.
3d and 4th. Pleasant.
5th and 6th. Cool, but very fine.
7th. Cloudy in the afternoon. Gentle snow in the evening.
8th. Ground covered lightly with snow in the morning. Raw day. Clear and pleasant in the evening.
9th. Fine.
10th. Some rain and hail in the morning. Misty in the afternoon.
11th. Foggy in the morning. Moderate rain in the afternoon.
12th. Very blustering.
13th. Rather raw.
14th. Evening very clear.
15th. Appearances of rain in the evening.
16th. Misty, with occasional light rain.
17th. Appearances of an easterly storm at night.
18th. Very pleasant.
19th. Very fine.
20th. Fine.
21st. Rain and blustering.
22d. Squall of snow, and gusty from 10 to 11 A. M.
23d and 24th. Variable, but mild.
25th, 26th, and 27th. Fine.
28th. Pleasant.
29th. Light snow in the evening.
30th. Pleasant for the most part.

December, 1843.

DAYS.	BAROMETER, REDUCED TO 32° F. Sunrise.	At 1 P. M.	At 10 P. M.	THERMOMETER. Sunrise.	At 1 P. M.	At 10 P. M.	Daily mean.	WINDS. (DIRECTION AND FORCE.) Sunrise.	At 1 P. M.	At 10 P. M.	WEATHER. (TENTHS CLOUDY.) Sunrise.	At 1 P. M.	At 10 P. M.	RAIN AND SNOW IN INCHES OF WATER.
1	30.10	...	...	20	...	...	...	N. W. 1	...	...	10	...	...	
2	29.71	...	...	28	...	26	...	N'ly 1	...	N. W.	10	...	0	
S 3	29.87	29.88	29.94	20	38	28	28.7	N. W. 1	S. W. 1	N. W. 1	0	0	0	
4	29.91	29.81	29.66	26	39	40	35.0	N. W. 1	S. W. 2	S. W. 3	0	2	8	
5	29.61	29.60	29.84	36	41	25	34.0	S. W. 1	N. W. 2	N. W. 4	0	3	10	
6	30.08	30.06	30.02	16	31	29	25.3	N. W. 1	S'ly 1	S'ly	0	2	10	
7	29.80	29.48	29.20	31	30	28	29.7	E'ly 1	N. E. 2	N. E'ly 2	Snow	Snow	Snow	1.00
8	29.61	29.62	29.63	26	36	33	31.7	N. W. 2	N. W. 2	N. W. 1	0	0	0	
9	29.51	29.43	29.44	30	37	30	32.3	S. W. 1	S. W. 1	N. W. 1	Snow	Snow	5	
S 10	29.61	29.65	29.89	30	35	24	29.7	N. W. 2	N. W. 2	N. W. 1	2	0	0	
11	29.66	29.64	29.66	28	42	34	34.7	S. W. 2	S. W. 2	S. W. 1	6	3	9	
12	29.61	29.60	29.79	30	36	22	29.3	W. 1	W'ly 1	N. W. 3	7	3	0	
13	30.17	30.27	30.39	9	21	13	14.3	N. W. 2	N. W. 2	N. W. 2	0	0	0	
14	30.37	30.21	30.22	15	34	35	28.0	S. W. 2	S. W. 2	S. W. 2	0	0	10	
15	30.21	30.14	30.21	33	44	36	37.7	S. W. 1	S. W. 1	S. W.	9	0	10	
16	30.20	30.04	29.98	35	38	33	35.3	S. W. 1	E'ly 1	N. E. 3	Snow	Misty	Misty	} 0.33
S 17	29.80	29.73	29.80	32	28	24	28.0	N. E. 2	N'ly 2	N'ly 2	Rain	Misty	Misty	}
18	29.90	29.90	29.90	26	30	28	28.0	N. W. 1	N. W.	N. W.	10	Misty	10	
19	29.97	30.00	29.98	24	33	28	28.3	N. W. 1	N. W.	N. W. 1	0	10	10	
20	29.88	29.82	29.85	32	38	34	34.7	N. W. 1	W'ly 1	W'ly	0	2	10	
21	30.00	29.97	29.92	31	41	34	35.1	N. W. 1	N. W.	N. W. 1	0	5	7	
22	...	29.69	29.67	34	41	36	37.0	W'ly	W'ly 1	W'ly	10	10	10	
23	29.79	29.83	29.83	36	37	30	34.3	N. E. 2	N. E. 2	N. E. 0	10	10	Snow	0.20
S 24	29.79	29.74	29.72	31	40	35	35.3	N. E. 1	N'ly 1	W'ly	10	5	10	
25	29.79	...	...	32	...	38	...	N. W. 1	...	W'ly 1	0	...	10	
26	29.98	29.98	29.91	33	39	34	35.3	N. E'ly 1	N. E'ly 2	E'ly 2	10	10	10	} 1.50
27	29.60	29.56	29.65	33	32	32	32.3	N. E. 2	N'ly 3	N'ly	Snow	10	10	}
28	29.60	29.59	29.49	34	41	32	35.7	N'ly	N'ly	N. E.	10	10	5	
29	29.48	29.34	29.36	31	35	23	29.7	N. W. 2	N. W. 4	N. W. 3	3	2	2	
30	29.29	29.25	29.29	18	25	22	21.7	N. W. 2	N. W. 3	N. W. 3	0	0	5	
S 31	29.37	29.41	29.61	24	33	27	28.0	N. W. 2	N. W. 3	N. W. 2	0	3	4	
Means	29.81	29.76	29.78	27.9	35.5	29.8	...	1.4	1.8	1.9	5.1	5.0	6.8	3.03
								1.7			5.8			
REDUCED TO SEA LEVEL.														
Max.	30.55	30.45	30.57	36	44	40	37.7	Prevailing winds from some point between— Days.			Days.			
Min.	29.47	29.48	29.38	9	21	13	14.3	N. & E. 7			Clear 6			
Mean	29.99	29.94	29.96					E. & S. 1			Variable . . . } 17			
Range	1.08	1.02	1.19	27	23	27	23.4	S. & W. 8			Cloudy . . . . }			
Mean of month	29.963			...	...	...	31.1	W. & N. 15			Rain or snow fell on 8			
Extreme range	1.19			...	...	...	35.0							

REMARKS.

1st. Light snow from 10 A. M. till night.
2d. Pleasant for the most part.
3d. Very pleasant.
4th. Pleasant.
5th. Cold and blustering in the evening.
6th. Cold, but not unpleasant.
7th. Steady snow all day; rather moist in the afternoon. Seven or eight inches of moist snow.
8th. Very fine.
9th. Small amount of light snow in the morning.
10th. Fine.
11th. Mild.
12th. Wind came to N. W., with blustering.
13th. Cold, but not unpleasant.
14th. Mild. Cloudy in the evening.
15th. Mild.
16th. Snow, light rain, and mist.
17th. Rain and mist. Ground and trees covered with sleet.
18th. Light snow in the afternoon.
19th, 20th, and 21st. Mild.
22d. Sprinkling of rain in the afternoon.
23d. Mild.
24th. Two and a half or three inches of light snow.
25th. Very mild.
26th. Occasional appearances of snow in the air. Snow during the night.
27th. Seven or eight inches of damp snow on the ground.
28th. Very mild.
29th. Blustering and cold in the evening.
30th. Blustering and severe.
31st. More moderate.

January, 1844.

DAYS.	BAROMETER Sunrise.	At 1 P. M.	At 10 P. M.	THERMOMETER Sunrise.	At 1 P. M.	At 10 P. M.	Daily mean.	WINDS Sunrise.	At 1 P. M.	At 10 P. M.	WEATHER Sunrise.	At 1 P. M.	At 10 P. M.	RAIN AND SNOW
1	29.72	...	29.80	26	...	28	...	N. W. 1	...	N. W.	0	...	0	
2	29.87	29.85	29.83	23	39	27	29.7	N. W. 2	N. W. 1	S. W. 1	0	4	8	
3	29.78	29.50	29.14	30	37	36	34.3	N. E. 1	S. E'ly 1	E'ly 1	Snow	Rain	Foggy	1.00
4	29.40	29.34	29.29	32	...	32	...	N. W. 2	...	N. E.	2	...	10	
5	29.55	29.60	29.75	17	18	14	16.3	N. N. W. 2	N. W. 3	N. W. 1	10	0	0	
6	29.89	29.91	29.95	14	25	18	19.0	N. W. 1	N. W. 2	N. W. 1	0	0	0	
S 7	29.82	29.60	29.47	22	40	36	32.7	S. W. 1	S. W. 1	S. W. 1	10	10	3	
8	29.66	29.74	29.93	23	23	11	19.0	N. W. 2	N. W. 3	N. W. 1	0	0	0	
9	30.03	29.94	29.76	5	16	10	10.3	N. W. 0	N. W. 0	N. E. 2	0	10	Snow	0.62
10	29.68	29.55	29.75	14	32	22	22.7	N'ly 2	W'ly 2	N. W. 1	10	0	0	
11	30.14	30.14	30.22	9	17	6	10.7	N. W. 3	N. W. 2	N. W. 1	0	0	0	
12	30.09	29.89	29.60	5	31	34	23.3	S. W'ly 1	S. W. 1	S. E'ly	2	4	Misty	
13	28.97	28.86	29.38	41	40	30	37.0	S. W. 3	W'ly 3	N. W. 4	10	5	0	
S 14	29.81	29.87	29.95	22	26	18	22.0	N. W. 2	N. W. 2	N. W. 1	0	0	0	
15	30.09	30.06	30.07	14	27	28	23.0	N. W. 1	N. W. 1	N. E'ly	0	0	5	
16	29.88	29.66	29.39	30	39	38	35.7	E'ly 2	E'ly 2	E'ly 2	Snow	Rain	Rain	} 2.50
17	29.40	28.93	29.14	36	46	34	38.7	N. E'ly 1	E'ly 2	S. W. 5	Fog, r'n	Rain	3	}
18	29.31	29.46	29.64	30	33	27	30.0	S. W'ly 3	S. W'ly 2	N. W.	4	2	0	
19	29.73	29.84	29.94	25	24	14	21.0	N. W. 2	N. W. 3	N. W. 1	0	0	0	
20	30.02	30.04	30.08	5	14	6	8.3	N. W. 2	N. W. 3	N. W. 1	0	0	0	
S 21	30.03	29.96	29.92	3	15	14	10.7	N. W. 1	N. W. 1	N. W. 0	0	2	0	
22	29.96	29.98	30.06	12	22	16	16.7	N. W. 1	N. W. 1	N. W. 0	10, Sn.	0	0	
23	29.84	...	29.40	22	...	40	...	E'ly 1	...	S. W. 1	Snow	...	10	0.20
24	29.44	29.43	29.43	30	41	32	34.3	S. W. 0	S. W. 1	S. W. 2	0	0	8	
25	29.45	29.40	29.46	22	18	7	15.7	N. W. 2	N. W. 3	N. W. 3	6	3	0	
26	29.58	29.57	29.73	—1	6	2	2.3	N. W. 2	N. W. 1	N. W. 1	0	0	0	
27	29.81	29.80	29.93	2	10	4	5.3	N. W. 2	N. W. 2	N. W. 1	5	0	0	
S 28	30.04	30.00	29.99	2	15	9	8.7	N. W. 1	N'ly 1	N. E. 1	0	3	Hazy	
[illegible]	[illegible]	29.80	29.80	4	6	1	4.3	N. W. 3	N. W. 3	N. W. 2	0	0	0	
30	29.73	29.63	29.62	1	15	10	[illegible]	[illegible]	[illegible]	[illegible]	[illegible]	[illegible]	[illegible]	
31	29.76	29.79	29.93	3	7	5	5.0	N. W. 3	N. W. 3	N. W. 0	0	0	0	
Means	29.75	29.62	29.72	16.9	24.5	19.7	...	1.7	1.9	1.4	3.6	2.9	3.4	4.32
								1.7			3.3			
REDUCED TO SEA LEVEL.														
Max.	30.32	30.32	30.40	41	46	38	38.7	Prevailing winds from some point between— Days.			Days.			
Min.	29.49	29.52	29.32	—1	6	1	2.3	N. & E. 1			Clear 14			
Mean	29.93	29.80	29.90					E. & S. 3			Variable . . . } 9			
Range	0.83	0.80	1.08	42	40	37	36.4	S. & W. 6			Cloudy . . . . }			
Mean of month	29.877			...	...	...	20.4	W. & N. 21			Rain or snow fell on 8			
Extreme range	1.08			...	...	...	45.0							

1st. Generally clear and pleasant.
2d. Very mild.
3d. Rain and snow till near sundown.
4th. Pleasant.
5th. Very severe out.
6th. Fine.
7th. Cloudy, with occasional appearances of snow. Flurry of snow during the night.
8th. Cold and severe.
9th. Air charged with fine snow in the afternoon; began to fall pretty fast at 8 P. M.
10th. Four or five inches of compact snow fell during the night of the 9th. Day pleasant.
11th. Cold, but not severe.
12th. Fine.
13th. Very blustering. Occasional dashes of rain in the morning. Wind high and blustering in the evening.
14th. Pleasant.
15th. Mild and pleasant.
16th. Moderate rain at intervals.
17th. Steady rain for the most part during the day. Wind passing from N. E. to E., S. E., S., and S. W., with increasing violence. Barometer fell rapidly; at 7 P. M., it stood at 28.85, and commenced rising very soon.
18th. Pleasant. Ground more than half bare.
19th. Pleasant.
20th. Severe cold, wind being brisk.
21st. Cold.
22d. Flurry of snow from 7 to 9 A. M.
23d. Light snow at sunrise. Wind changed gradually from E. to S. E. and S. W., and snow changed to moderate rain.
24th. Mild and pleasant as spring. Ground nearly all bare.
25th. Grew cold all day.
26th and 27th. Very cold, but not very severe to be out.
[illegible]
General haze, with a very bright and distinct halo round the moon.
29th and 30th. Very severe out.
31st. Wind very cutting and severe; rather the most severe of the last six days to be out.

February, 1844.

DAYS.	BAROMETER, REDUCED TO 32° F. Sunrise.	At 1 P. M.	At 10 P. M.	THERMOMETER. Sunrise.	At 1 P. M.	At 10 P. M.	Daily mean.	WINDS. (DIRECTION AND FORCE.) Sunrise.	At 1 P. M.	At 10 P. M.	WEATHER. (TENTHS CLOUDY.) Sunrise.	At 1 P. M.	At 10 P. M.	RAIN AND SNOW IN INCHES OF WATER.
1	30.09	30.07	30.01	10	27	24	20.3	N. W. 0	N. W. 1	S. W. 1	0	0	8	
2	29.91	29.91	29.96	28	34	29	30.3	E'ly 1	E'ly 1	N. E.	Snow	Snow	10	0.30
3	29.94	29.92	29.98	27	31	24	27.3	N'ly	N. W. 2	N. W. 0	10	10	0	
S 4	29.97	29.93	29.94	18	27	22	22.3	N. W. 2	N. W. 2	N. E. 1	0	0	3	
5	29.91	29.85	29.85	24	32	32	29.3	N'ly 1	N'ly 2	N'ly 1	10	Snow	Misty	} 0.25
6	29.72	29.65	29.63	29	36	32	32.3	N. E. 1	N. E. 1	N'ly	Misty	Misty	10	
7	29.66	29.62	29.56	24	40	32	32.0	W'ly 1	W'ly	N. W.	0	0	0	
8	29.46	29.27	29.40	27	34	24	28.3	N. E'ly 1	N. E. 2	N. W. 1	10	Snow	0	
9	29.50	29.47	29.57	20	30	11	20.3	N. W. 2	N. W. 2	N. W. 2	0	5	0	
10	29.72	29.70	29.78	7	20	18	15.0	N. W. 2	N. W. 2	W'ly 1	0	0	0	
S 11	29.94	29.96	29.97	10	25	20	18.3	N. W. 1	N. W. 2	W'ly 2	0	0	0	
12	30.07	30.11	30.22	10	33	20	21.0	N. W. 2	N. W. 2	N. W. 1	2	0	0	
13	30.13	30.01	29.88	16	38	34	29.3	N. W. 1	S. W. 2	S. W. 1	0	10	0	
14	29.81	29.81	29.94	29	36	24	29.7	W'ly 1	W'ly 2	N. W. 2	0	2	0	
15	30.01	29.99	29.79	16	37	31	28.0	N. W. 1	S. W. 1	S. E. 1	0	8	10	
16	29.50	29.58	29.55	31	40	30	33.7	N. W. 1	W'ly 1	N. W. 2	10	0	0	0.40
17	29.62	29.61	29.70	26	39	28	31.0	W'ly 1	W'ly 1	W'ly 1	5	6	0	
S 18	29.84	29.87	30.00	13	17	14	14.7	N. W. 1	N. W. 3	N. W. 2	0	0	0	
19	29.95	29.90	29.94	18	41	31	30.0	S. W. 1	S. W. 1	S. W. 1	2	4	0	
20	29.00	29.79	29.79	27	47	40	38.0	S. W. 1	S. W. 1	S. W. 1	0	0	0	
21	29.69	29.60	29.65	34	49	34	39.0	S. W. 1	S. W. 1	N. E. 2	0	0	10	
22	29.60	29.54	29.64	34	45	37	38.7	W'ly 2	W'ly 2	S. W. 1	2	0	0	
23	29.67	...	...	30	...	33	...	N. W. 1	...	N. E. 3	2	...	10	
24	29.74	29.80	29.90	28	22	16	22.0	E'ly 3	N. E. 3	N'ly 1	10	4	0	
S 25	30.03	30.06	30.09	16	29	25	23.3	N. 2	N. 1	N. W. 1	0	0	0	
26	30.11	30.03	29.96	20	39	30	29.7	W'ly 0	S. E. 2	S'ly 0	0	0	0	
27	29.77	29.66	29.70	32	38	30	33.3	S. W. 1	S. W. 1	S. W. 1	10	10	Snow	}
28	29.70	29.84	30.06	32	34	30	32.0	N. E. 4	N'ly 3	N. W. 2	Snow	Snow	0	} 1.00
29	30.02	30.00	29.95	28	41	35	34.7	N. W. 2	S. W. 1	S. E'ly 1	0	10	10	}
Means	29.83	29.80	29.84	22.9	34.6	27.2	...	1.3	1.6	1.3	3.5	4.3	3 1	1.95
									1.4			3.6		
REDUCED TO SEA LEVEL.														
Max.	30.31	30.29	30.40	34	49	37	39.0							
Min.	29.64	29.45	29.58	7	17	11	14.7							
Mean	30.01	29.98	30.02											
Range	0.67	0.84	0.82	27	32	26	24.3							
Mean of month	30.003			...	...	...	28.2							
Extreme range	0.95			...	...	...	42.0							

Prevailing winds from some point between— Days.
N. & E. 6
E. & S. 1
S. & W. 9
W. & N. 13

Days.
Clear 11
Variable . . . } 15
Cloudy . . . . }
Rain or snow fell on 6

REMARKS.

1st. Thick haze in the evening. Halo around the moon; moon wading in snow.
2d. Fine snow during nearly the whole day—about three inches deep.
3d. Mild, cloudy day, and very clear and mild in the evening.
4th. Mild and pleasant.
5th. But little accumulation of snow during the day. About two inches of moist snow and some sleet during the night.
6th. Misty all day.
7th. Very mild and pleasant.
8th. Flurry of snow occasionally.
9th. Grew cold fast in the evening.
10th to 14th. Pleasant.
15th. Pleasant. About three inches of snow fell during the night.
16th to 21st. Pleasant.
22d and 23d. Very fine.
24th. Very raw and unpleasant.
25th. Pleasant.
26th. Very pleasant.
27th. Sprinkling of rain occasionally. Commenced snowing in the evening, and continued during the night.
28th. Very driving snow-storm, continued till past noon. Clear in the evening.
29th. Mild.

March, 1844.

DAYS.	BAROMETER. At 6 A. M.	At 1 P. M.	At 10 P. M.	THERMOMETER. At 6 A. M.	At 1 P. M.	At 10 P. M.	Daily mean.	WINDS. At 6 A. M.	At 1 P. M.	At 10 P. M.	WEATHER. At 6 A. M.	At 1 P. M.	At 10 P. M.	RAIN AND SNOW.
1	29.90	29.87	29.80	37	49	37	41.0	S. W. 1	S. W. 0	S. W. 1	8	10	8	
2	29.69	29.59	29.55	38	45	39	40.7	S. W. 1	S. W. 1	S. W. 1	10	10	10	
S 3	29.70	29.70	29.65	38	49	36	41.0	S. W. 1	S. W. 1	S. W'ly 1	10	8	Foggy	
4	29.43	29.52	29.83	32	33	21	28.3	N. E. 2	N. 3	N. W. 3	Snow	Snow	0	0.75
5	30.03	30.05	30.10	12	24	20	18.7	N. W. 2	N. W. 2	N. W. 1	0	0	0	
6	30.17	30.15	30.22	23	40	32	31.7	N. W. 1	N. W. 2	N. W. 1	0	0	2	
7	30.24	30.26	30.24	24	44	34	34.0	S'ly 2	S'ly 2	S. W. 1	0	0	0	
8	30.14	29.99	29.77	32	43	46	40.3	S. W. 1	S. W. 1	S'ly 3	0	Misty	Rain	0.25
9	...	...	29.54	45	46	39	43.3	S. W. 1	W'ly 1	N. W. 1	10	10	6	
S 10	29.71	29.74	29.83	33	41	35	36.3	N. 2	N. E. 2	N'ly 1	6	0	0	
11	30.00	29.99	30.09	32	50	38	40.0	N. W. 1	N. W. 1	N. W. 1	0	0	0	
12	30.16	30.17	30.10	35	47	38	40.0	S. E. 1	S. E. 3	S. E'ly 2	5	8	10	
13	29.90	29.76	29.66	42	46	44	44.0	S. E. 3	S. E. 3	S. E. 2	10	Rain	Rain	0.75
14	29.69	29.70	29.86	42	50	40	44.0	N. W. 2	N. W. 2	N.E. 1	5	0	10	
15	29.96	29.97	29.90	32	37	32	33.7	N. E. 2	N. E. 2	N. E. 2	10	10	Hail	}
16	29.71	29.46	29.28	34	35	34	34.3	N. E. 2	N. E. 2	N. E. 2	Rain	Rain	Rain	} 2.00
S 17	29.15	29.21	29.42	34	40	37	37.0	N'ly 1	N. W. 1	N. W. 1	Rain	0	3	}
18	29.36	29.43	29.53	39	44	34	39.0	S. W. 2	S. W. 4	W'ly 3	0	2	10	
19	29.66	29.80	29.94	22	31	27	26.7	W. 3	W'ly 3	W'ly 1	5	0	0	
20	29.85	29.82	29.56	34	47	44	41.7	S. W. 2	S. W. 3	S. W. 2	2	10	10	
21	29.60	29.60	29.54	36	33	30	33.0	N. 2	N. E'ly 2	N. E. 3	10	Snow	Snow	} 0.50
22	29.46	29.36	29.48	26	32	32	30.0	N. E. 2	N'ly 2	N. W. 1	Sleet	Snow	5	}
23	29.57	29.57	29.60	26	31	28	28.3	N'ly 1	N. E. 2	N. W. 2	10	10	0	
S 24	29.73	29.73	29.73	23	40	36	33.0	N. W. 1	N. W. 2	N. W. 1	0	0	2	
25	29.60	29.50	29.85	40	53	40	44.3	S. W. 1	S. W. 2	W'ly 2	5	0	0	
26	29.89	29.79	29.81	35	57	46	46.0	S. W. 1	S. W. 1	N. W. 1	3	5	6	
27	29.95	30.06	30.11	41	40	31	37.3	N. E. 2	N. E. 3	N. E. 3	10	10	10	
28	29.91	...	29.61	32	...	36	...	N. E. 2	...	W'ly 1	10	...	10	
29	29.65	29.76	29.98	37	50	40	42.3	E'ly 1	N'ly	N. E.	0	10	10	
30	29.77	29.65	29.72	34	36	26	32.0	N. E.	N. E.	N. E.	Sleet	10	10	0.50
S 31	29.91	30.09	30.25	22	36	28	28.7	N'ly 2	N. E'ly	N. E. 3	10	0	0	
Means	29.78	29.77	29.79	32.6	41.6	34.8	...	1.6	1.9	1.7	6.1	5.8	6.0	4.75
									1.7			6.0		
REDUCED TO SEA LEVEL.														
Max.	30.42	30.44	30.42	45	57	46	46.0							
Min.	29.33	29.39	29.46	12	24	20	18.7							
Mean	29.96	29.95	29.97											
Range	1.09	1.05	0.96	33	33	26	25.3							
Mean of month	29.960			...	...	...	36.3							
Extreme range	1.11			...	...	...	45.0							

Prevailing winds from some point between— Days.
N. & E. 12
E. & S. 2
S. & W. 11
W. & N. 6

Days.
Clear 7
Variable . . . } 12
Cloudy . . . . }
Rain or snow fell on 21

REMARKS.

1st, 2d, and 3d. Mild.
4th. Damp snow from N. E. and N., with driving wind, from about 5 A. M. till 3 P. M. Snow about three or four inches deep. Clear and blustering in the evening.
5th. Blustering.
6th. Pleasant.
7th. Very pleasant.
8th and 9th. Mild.
10th. Very pleasant.
11th. Very fine.
12th. Air raw.
13th. Rain in the afternoon, and until 9½ in the evening.
14th. Pleasant.
15th. Appearances of storm. Began to snow and hail moderately between 9 and 10 P. M.
16th. Very moderate rain during the greater part of the day and evening.
17th. Moderate rain at sunrise. Snow from 9 A. M. to noon. Barometer began to rise from 9 to 10 A. M.; lowest 29.18. Cleared from 1 to 2 P. M.
18th. Pleasant in the morning. Cloudy towards night. Flurry of snow from 6 to 7 P. M. Wind very brisk at S. W.
19th. Very raw, cold, searching wind.
20th. Wind brisk and damp. Sprinkling of rain in the afternoon.
21st. Snowed moderately in the afternoon and evening, without much accumulation.
22d. Fine snow and mist till from 4 to 5 P. M. Sun came out from 5 to 6 P. M.
23d. Wind cold and raw.
24th, 25th, and 26th. Very pleasant.
27th. Air very raw.
28th. Mist through the day. Shower in the evening.
30th. It snowed or hailed in the morning. Towards evening, it snowed a small sprinkle.
31st. Snowed and hailed last night two or three inches, and lightened and thundered. Cleared off to-day about 10 A. M.

April, 1844.

DAYS.	BAROMETER, REDUCED TO 32° F. At 6 A. M.	At 1 P. M.	At 10 P. M.	THERMOMETER. At 6 A. M.	At 1 P. M.	At 10 P. M.	Daily mean.	WINDS. (DIRECTION AND FORCE.) At 6 A. M.	At 1 P. M.	At 10 P. M.	WEATHER. (TENTHS CLOUDY.) At 6 A. M.	At 1 P. M.	At 10 P. M.	RAIN AND SNOW IN INCHES OF WATER.
1	30.39	30.48	30.54	25	42	27	31.3	N'ly 1	N. E. 1	N'ly 1	2	8	0	
2	30.60	30.50	30.43	23	36	30	29.7	N'ly 1	N. E. 2	N. E. 1	0	0	0	
3	30.39	30.05	29.96	25	54	47	42.0	N'ly 1	W'ly	W'ly	0	0	2	
4	29.77	29.67	29.66	46	68	64	59.3	N. W.	S. W. 4	S. W.	3	1	8	
5	29.79	29.90	30.10	46	60	43	49.7	N'ly 2	N. W.	N. W.	2	6	0	
6	30.23	30.31	30.33	34	61	43	46.0	N'ly	E'ly 2	E'ly	0	5	10	
S 7	30.35	30.28	30.17	41	50	43	44.7	S. E'ly	S'ly	S'ly	7	9	10	
8	29.99	29.83	29.73	43	59	52	51.3	S'ly 1	S. E.	S'ly	10	2	1	
9	29.72	29.72	29.78	48	64	52	54.7	S. E'ly 1	N'ly	N'ly	10	10	0	} 0.50
10	29.91	29.89	29.88	42	63	58	51.0	N. W.	S'ly 3	W'ly	0	0	0	
11	29.92	29.94	29.97	48	72	49	56.3	N'ly	N. E.	S'ly	0	4	0	
12	30.07	30.09	30.12	43	64	48	51.7	N. E.	E'ly	S'ly	2	0	0	
13	30.06	29.97	29.68	42	66	54	54.0	S. W.	S'ly	S'ly	0	2	0	
S 14	29.55	29.77	29.71	52	78	65	65.0	S. W. 1	S'ly 1	S'ly 1	0	0	0	
15	29.71	29.82	29.91	58	60	45	54.3	S. E'ly 1	N. E. 2	N. E. 2	6	10	10	
16	29.90	29.76	29.70	45	63	49	52.3	N. E. 1	S. E'ly 2	S'ly 1	5	3	10	
17	29.62	29.63	29.82	55	68	45	56.0	S'ly 1	W'ly 2	N. W. 3	7	2	1	
18	30.08	30.07	30.10	35	52	35	40.7	N. E. 2	N. E. 2	N'ly	3	0	0	
19	30.11	30.09	30.04	30	58	44	44.0	N. W. 1	W'ly 1	S'ly 1	0	0	0	
20	29.97	29.92	29.89	44	62	47	51.0	N. E. 2	N. E'ly 1	N. E. 1	10	2	10	
S 21	29.84	29.81	29.76	46	57	45	49.3	E'ly 1	E'ly 2	E'ly 1	Foggy	Rain	Rain	0.10
22	29.76	29.83	29.99	50	67	52	56.3	N'ly 1	N'ly 1	S. W'ly 0	10	5	2	
23	30.07	30.04	30.03	52	65	45	54.0	E'ly 1	S. E. 2	E'ly 2	10	0	10	
24	29.91	29.72	29.53	47	65	56	56.0	S. W. 1	S. W. 3	S. W. 2	Rain	10	Rain	0.07
25	29.63	29.70	29.78	54	66	55	58.3	N. W. 2	N. W. 3	N. W. 1	2	3	10	
26	29.59	29.52	29.65	57	63	46	55.3	S. W. 3	S. W. 2	N. E. 2	10	10	10	
27	29.95	30.01	29.99	40	59	43	47.3	N. E. 3	N. E. 2	S. E. 1	2	7	10	
S 28	29.87	29.79	29.70	43	62	50	51.7	S. W. 1	S. W. 1	S. W. 1	5	5	0	
29	29.79	29.82	29.94	47	65	46	52.7	N. W. 2	N. W. 2	N. W. 0	0	0	0	
30	30.04	30.01	29.99	42	60	49	50.3	N. W. 1	S. E. 3	S.	0	5	5	
Means	29.95	29.93	29.94	43.3	60.1	47.6	...	1.3	1.9	1.2	4.2	4.0	4.3	0.67
									1.3			4.2		
REDUCED TO SEA LEVEL.								Prevailing winds from some point between—		Days.			Days.	
Max.	30.78	30.68	30.72	58	78	65	65.0	N. & E.		13	Clear		10	
Min.	29.73	29.70	29.71	23	36	27	29.7	E. & S.		3	Variable		} 15	
Mean	30.13	30.11	30.12					S. & W.		7	Cloudy			
Range	1.05	0.98	1.01	35	42	38	35.3	W. & N.		7	Rain fell on		5	
Mean of month	30.120			...	...	...	50.6							
Extreme range	1.08			...	...	...	55.0							

REMARKS.

1st and 2d. Raw, cold wind.
3d. Growing more mild.
4th. Very warm during the day after 9 A. M.
5th. Hazy in the forenoon. Rather dim northern light in the evening.
8th. Foggy in the morning. In the evening, wind perfectly calm, and lightning in the north.
9th. Foggy at sunrise. Began to rain moderately at 7 A. M., and continued till 10½ A. M. Cleared off at 3 P. M.
10th. Warm and mild, and not much air stirring.
11th. Hazy at 1 P. M.; warm.
12th. Clear warm day. Wind turned to the S. about 2 P. M., but a little chilly.
13th. Very fine and very warm.
14th. Oppressively warm.
15th. Wind came to N. E. at from 9 to 10 A. M. Sprinkling of rain in the afternoon.
16th, 17th, 18th. Fine.
19th. Black frost. Ice formed in shallow open vessels three-eighths of an inch in thickness.
20th. Pleasant.
21st. Very moderate rain beginning at 11 to 12 A. M.
22d. Fine in the afternoon. Cherry-tree in front of the house has one cluster of blossoms.
23d. Air very raw. Fog in the evening.
24th. Rained moderately from 7 to 8 A. M. Also moderate rain with thunder, from 7½ to 9 P. M.
25th. Pleasant.
26th. Frequent sprinkling of rain during the day.
27th. Cool.
28th. Light clouds.
29th. Very fine.
30th. Black frost in some places in the vicinity.

May, 1844.

DAYS.	Barometer At 6 A. M.	At 1 P. M.	At 10 P. M.	Thermometer At 6 A. M.	At 1 P. M.	At 10 P. M.	Daily mean.	Winds At 6 A. M.	At 1 P. M.	At 10 P. M.	Weather At 6 A. M.	At 1 P. M.	At 10 P. M.	Rain and snow
1	29.83	29.80	...	54	75	...	...	S. 3	S. 5	...	5	0	...	
2	29.69	29.63	29.63	60	75	62	65.7	S. W.	S. W.	S. W. 2	0	5	10	
3	29.65	29.60	29.58	57	67	58	60.7	S. W. 2	S. W. 2	W'ly 1	5	10	4	
4	29.56	29.54	29.53	55	71	52	59.3	N. E'ly 1	E'ly 2	N. E. 2	3	2	10	
S 5	29.62	29.63	29.69	53	69	57	59.7	W'ly 2	W'ly 3	S. W. 1	0	6	2	
6	29.69	29.57	29.32	52	72	57	60.3	S. W. 2	S. E. 3	S. W. 1	0	2	Rain	0.15
7	29.34	29.36	29.61	53	65	56	58.0	S. W. 3	W'ly 6	N. W. 4	2	2	0	
8	29.83	29.74	29.56	52	75	62	63.0	N. W. 2	S. W. 5	S. W. 3	4	8	3	
9	29.74	29.73	29.90	52	67	52	57.0	N. W. 2	N. W. 3	N. W. 2	0	0	0	
10	30.10	30.09	30.10	47	67	51	55.0	N. W. 1	S. E'ly 2	S. E'ly 1	0	0	10	
11	29.93	29.73	29.59	51	52	52	51.7	S'ly 2	S. E'ly 2	S'ly 1	10	Rain	10	0.12
S 12	29.36	29.36	29.61	63	66	54	61.0	W'ly 2	N. W'ly 4	N. W. 3	10	6	2	
13	29.80	29.89	29.93	44	64	55	54.3	N. W. 2	N. W. 2	S'ly	0	0	4	
14	29.96	29.93	29.97	51	53	49	51.0	S'ly 1	S. E'ly 1	W'ly	Rain	10	8	
15	29.97	29.90	...	48	68	53	56.3	N. W. 1	N. W. 1	S'ly	3	0	2	} 0.50
16	29.70	29.63	29.62	53	56	56	55.0	S. W. 1	S. W. 1	W'ly 1	10	Rain	6	
17	29.57	29.78	29.90	56	57	52	55.0	S. E. 2	N. E. 4	N. E. 2	Rain	10	8	
18	29.79	29.65	29.74	52	52	52	52.0	S. E. 1	S. E. 1	N. W. 2	10	Rain	0	0.50
S 19	29.84	29.87	29.90	50	64	58	57.3	N. W. 2	W'ly 3	W'ly 1	2	1	5	
20	29.89	29.73	29.56	51	56	56	54.3	E'ly 1	S. E'ly 2	S. E'ly 1	10	Misty	10	
21	29.49	29.67	29.87	56	62	49	55.7	W'ly 1	W'ly 3	N. W. 1	10, Sh'r	10	0	0.30
22	30.06	30.05	30.06	39	64	48	50.3	N. W. 2	N. E'ly 2	S'ly 0	3	4	0	
23	30.07	30.09	30.07	42	64	55	53.7	S. E. 1	S. E. 3	S'ly 2	0	0	0	
24	30.06	29.98	29.97	52	77	64	64.3	S. W. 1	S. E'ly 1	S'ly 2	0	0	0	
25	29.84	29.72	29.75	55	82	51	62.7	S. W. 2	S. W. 2	N. E. 2	4	2	10	
S 26	29.72	29.66	29.63	46	65	56	55.7	N. E. 2	N. E. 1	S. E'ly	10, Mist	6	10	
27	29.57	29.55	29.56	59	79	66	68.0	S. W. 1	S. W'ly 3	W'ly	10, Sh'r	10	Hazy	0.10
28	29.55	29.50	29.53	62	82	65	69.7	S'ly 1	S'ly 1	W'ly 2	Foggy	6	3	
29	29.61	29.62	29.70	61	72	56	66.3	N. W. 2	W'ly 2	N. W. 1	0	2	0	
30	[illegible]	[illegible]	[illegible]	[illegible]	[illegible]	[illegible]	[illegible]	[illegible]	[illegible]	[illegible]	[illegible]	[illegible]	[illegible]	
31	29.57	29.51	29.58	58	66	62	62.0	S. E'ly 2	S'ly 2	S'ly 1	Rain	Rain	10	0.28
Means	29.75	29.72	29.73	52.9	66.9	55.8	...	1.7	2.5	1.4	4.9	5.0	5.2	1.95
									1.9			5.0		
REDUCED TO SEA LEVEL.								Prevailing winds from some point between—		Days.			Days.	
Max.	30.28	30.27	30.28	63	82	66	69.7	N. & E.		5	Clear		7	
Min.	29.52	29.54	29.50	39	52	48	50.3	E. & S.		9	Variable		} 9	
Mean	29.93	29.90	29.91					S. & W.		10	Cloudy			
Range	0.76	0.73	0.78	24	30	18	19.4	W. & N.		7	Rain fell on		15	
Mean of month	29.913			...	...	...	58.5							
Extreme range	0.78			...	...	...	43.0							

1st. Cloudy. Wind strong at S. W.
2d. Cloudy. Wind strong at S. W. Sprinkling in the afternoon.
3d. Sprinkling of rain from 7 to 8 P. M., with lightning.
4th and 5th. Pleasant.
6th. Moderate rain in the evening, with thunder and lightning.
7th and 8th. Very blustering.
9th. Very transparent air.
10th. Pleasant.
11th. Moderate rain in the morning.
12th. Dash of rain at 8 P. M. Wind very brisk at N. W.
13th. Pleasant.
14th. Moderate rain from 8 to 10 A. M., then mist.
15th. Fine.
16th. Light showers in the morning.
17th. At 6 A. M., wind S. E.; soon came to N. E. Showers early in the morning. Barometer began to rise on the change of wind.
18th. Moderate rain in the morning.
19th. Pleasant.
20th. Mist, with occasional sprinkling of rain
21st. Showers from 4 to 5 A. M. Clouds dispersed towards night.
22d and 23d. Pleasant. Frost in several places in the vicinity in the mornings.
24th. Very pleasant.
25th. Very hot till about 6 P. M., when a thundergust came up, with a light shower, and wind changed from W'ly to N. E., and became cooler immediately.
26th. Raw air.
27th. Shower at 3 to 4 A. M.
28th. Heavy dashes of rain at 3 P. M.
29th. Fine.
30th. Fine. Appearances of rain in the evening.
[illegible]

DAYS.	BAROMETER, REDUCED TO 32° F. At 6 A. M.	At 1 P. M.	At 10 P. M.	THERMOMETER. At 6 A. M.	At 1 P. M.	At 10 P. M.	Daily mean.	WINDS. (DIRECTION AND FORCE.) At 6 A. M.	At 1 P. M.	At 10 P. M.	WEATHER. (TENTHS CLOUDY.) At 6 A. M.	At 1 P. M.	At 10 P. M.	RAIN AND SNOW IN INCHES OF WATER	REMARKS.
June, 1844.															
1	29.78	29.79	29.79	62	73	57	64.0	W'ly 1	W'ly 1	S'ly 1	10	0	0		1st. Very pleasant.
S 2	29.67	29.65	29.68	60	79	59	66.0	S. W. 3	S. W'ly 2	S. W'ly 1	0	8	Sho'ry	0.20	2d. Very sultry in the morning. Showers in the evening.
3	29.73	29.76	29.82	55	66	55	58.7	N. E. 1	N. E. 1	N. E. 1	10	8	0		3d. Variable. Sun out in the afternoon.
4	29.86	29.90	29.90	50	66	52	56.0	N. E. 1	S. E. 2	S'ly 0	5	3	0		4th. Evening very clear.
5	29.87	29.81	29.79	54	68	56	59.3	W'ly 1	W'ly 3	S'ly 1	8	3	0		5th. Pleasant.
6	29.73	29.67	29.65	56	71	61	62.7	S. W. 2	S'ly 3	W'ly 1	0	10	0		6th. Appearances of rain in the afternoon.
7	29.70	29.64	29.55	61	70	64	65.0	S. W'ly 1	S. W. 1	S'ly 1	5	10	Rain		7th. Rain at 9½ P. M. for a short time.
8	29.74	29.79	29.83	56	68	56	60.0	N. W. 3	N. W. 2	N. W. 1	0	0	0		8th. Very pleasant.
S 9	29.80	...	29.51	58	...	65	...	S. W. 2	...	S. W. 2	10	Shower	10	0.15	9th. Light shower, with thunder, from 4 to 5 P. M.
10	29.56	29.57	29.69	56	72	55	61.0	W'ly 2	W'ly 3	N. W. 4	0	0	0		10th. Pleasant.
11	29.82	29.87	30.01	48	67	53	56.0	N. W. 4	N. W. 2	N. W. 0	0	0	0		11th. Uncomfortably cold.
12	30.12	30.09	30.10	48	69	53	56.7	N. W. 1	S'ly 2	S'ly 1	0	0	0		12th. Faint aurora at 10 P. M.
13	30.07	30.01	29.97	52	67	55	58.0	S'ly 1	S. E. 3	S. W. 1	6	5	7		13th. Air raw. Ground excessively dry.
14	29.92	29.92	29.92	55	68	53	58.7	S. W. 1	N. W. 1	N. E. 2	10	7	10		14th. Appearances of rain in the evening.
15	30.10	30.09	30.09	50	67	55	57.3	N. E. 1	N. E. 2	E'ly 1	3	0	0		15th and 16th. Pleasant.
S 16	29.99	29.89	29.83	54	76	62	64.0	W'ly 2	W'ly 2	S. W. 1	0	0	0		
17	29.79	29.75	29.72	55	76	64	65.0	W'ly 2	S. W. 2	S. W. 1	0	7	10		17th. Sprinkling of rain from 7 to 8 P. M.
18	29.69	29.65	29.63	63	76	65	68.0	S. W. 2	S. W. 2	S. W. 1	10	10	0		18th. Light showers in the morning; little more than enough to lay the dust.
19	29.66	29.62	29.57	65	85	66	72.0	S. W. 1	S. W. 3	S. W. 3	3	1	10		19th. Appearances of rain.
20	29.57	29.56	29.60	67	82	68	72.3	S. W. 2	S. W. 2	N. W. 1	2	0	0		20th and 21st. Fine.
21	29.63	29.63	29.68	67	76	59	67.3	N. W. 1	N. W. 2	N. E. 2	4	3	4		
22	29.59	29.54	29.56	59	61	61	60.3	N. E. 2	N. E. 2	N. W. 1	Rain	10	8	0.80	22d. Rain from 7 to 11 A. M.
S 23	29.62	29.65	29.70	60	77	66	67.7	N. W. 2	N. W. 3	N. W. 1	0	0	0		23d. Very fine.
24	29.67	29.62	29.63	63	78	68	69.7	N. W. 2	N. W. 3	S. W. 3	0	0	7		24th and 25th. Pleasant.
25	29.63	29.60	29.59	68	85	71	74.7	S. W. 2	S. W. 3	S. W. 2	5	3	4		
26	29.64	29.65	29.69	71	88	73	77.3	S. W. 1	W'ly 2	W'ly 1	3	5	7		26th. Very hot. Thunder and sprinkling at 7 P. M.; shower to north.
27	29.68	29.65	29.67	68	89	70	75.7	S. W. 2	S. W. 3	S. W. 2	3	2	5		27th. Very hot.
28	29.66	29.54	29.62	71	86	71	76.0	S. W. 2	W'ly 3	W'ly 2	2	3	0		28th. Fine.
29	29.66	29.73	29.88	61	73	58	64.0	N. W. 2	N. W. 3	N. W. 1	0	0	0		29th. Very pleasant.
S 30	29.96	29.96	29.91	58	74	58	63.3	N. E. 1	E'ly 2	S. E'ly	0	6	5		30th. Pleasant.
Means	29.76	29.74	29.75	59.0	74.2	61.0	...	1.7	2.2	1.4	3.6	3.8	3.6	1.15	
REDUCED TO SEA LEVEL.									1.8			3.7			
Max.	30.30	30.27	30.28	71	89	73	77.3	Prevailing winds from some point between—		Days.			Days.		
Min.	29.74	29.72	29.69	48	61	52	56.0	N. & E.		3	Clear		9		
Mean	29.94	29.92	29.93					E. & S.		3	Variable	}	14		
Range	0.56	0.55	0.59	23	28	21	21.3	S. & W.		16	Cloudy	}			
Mean of month	29.930			...	...	...	64.7	W. & N.		8	Rain fell on		7		
Extreme range	0.61			...	...	...	41.0								
July, 1844.															
	At 6 A. M.	At 1 P. M.	At 10 P. M.	At 6 A. M.	At 1 P. M.	At 10 P. M.	Daily mean.	At 6 A. M.	At 1 P. M.	At 10 P. M.	At 6 A. M.	At 1 P. M.	At 10 P. M.		
1	29.78	29.63	29.57	61	68	68	65.7	S. W. 2	S. W. 2	S. W. 1	10	Rain	5		1st. Sprinkling of rain from 2 to 3 P. M.
2	29.56	29.58	29.56	68	84	69	73.7	W'ly 2	W'ly 2	W'ly 1	0	0	2		2d. Fine.
3	29.51	29.48	...	64	78	...	...	S. W. 2	S. W. 1	...	Rain	9	...		
4	...	...	...	...	...	...	...	...	...	...	...	...	...		
5	...	...	...	...	...	...	...	...	...	...	...	...	...		
6	...	...	29.42	...	...	70	...	...	...	S. W. 2	...	...	8		6th. Light shower at 10 P. M., with thunder.
S 7	29.56	29.58	29.68	64	78	63	68.3	N'ly 1	N'ly 1	N'ly 1	0	4	0		7th and 8th. Fine.
8	29.74	29.74	29.78	54	75	63	64.0	N'ly 2	W'ly 3	W'ly 1	0	3	0		
9	29.76	29.68	29.63	60	83	69	70.7	N. W'ly 1	W'ly 3	S. W. 3	0	2	7		9th. Wind very blustering from 3 to 5 or 6 P. M.
10	29.58	29.45	29.37	69	80	68	72.3	S. W. 2	S. W.	S. W. 2	10	7	8		10th. Cloudy, with appearance of rain.
11	29.48	29.40	29.50	67	78	60	68.3	S. W. 2	E'ly 2	N. E'ly 2	0	7, Shr.	10	0.56	11th. Very hot sun in the morning. Shower from 5 to 7 P. M.
12	29.62	29.68	29.78	61	74	61	65.3	N. E. 1	N. E. 2	N. E. 2	10	10	10		12th. Cool, with appearances of rain.
13	29.82	29.81	29.79	62	74	67	67.7	S. E. 1	S. E. 1	S. W. 1	10	10	10		
S 14	29.68	29.64	29.58	68	81	70	73.0	S. W. 1	S. W. 2	S. W. 1	10	6	7		14th. Sprinkling of rain from 6 to 7 P. M., with thunder.
15	29.62	29.60	29.64	68	84	68	73.3	W'ly 1	S. W. 1	S. W. 1	6	7	10		15th. Very warm.
16	29.60	29.48	29.50	63	59	60	60.7	E'ly 1	N'ly 2	N'ly	Rain	Rain	7	1.70	16th. Began to rain moderately at 6 A. M., and rained steadily till after 2 P. M. Some stars appeared in the evening.
17	29.59	29.60	29.67	57	80	68	68.3	N. W. 1	N. W. 1	N. W. 1	0	0	0		17th, 18th, and 19th. Very fine.
18	29.70	29.71	29.68	63	78	66	69.0	N'ly 1	N. E. 1	S. E'ly 0	0	3	0		
19	29.62	29.55	29.50	64	81	68	71.0	S. W. 1	S'ly 3	S'ly 2	5	2	Rain	} 0.70	
20	29.48	29.49	29.53	65	74	65	68.0	S. W. 1	N. E. 1	N. W. 1	10	Rain	0	}	20th. Copious showers.
S 21	29.68	29.70	29.78	64	81	69	71.3	N. W. 2	N. E. 2	S'ly 2	4	4	0		21st and 22d. Pleasant.
22	29.85	29.82	29.80	63	80	69	70.7	S. W. 1	S'ly 2	S. W. 2	0	2	7		
23	29.78	29.69	29.66	68	80	70	72.7	S. W. 1	S. W. 2	S. W. 1	7	8	4		23d and 24th. Very sultry.
24	29.68	29.65	29.68	66	77	66	69.7	N. E. 2	E'ly 1	E'ly 1	0	0	5		
25	29.68	...	29.69	61	...	58	...	N. E. 1	...	N. E.	10	...	Rain	0.47	25th. Rain at intervals.
26	29.72	...	29.71	58	...	59	...	N. E. 2	...	W'ly 1	10	...	0		26th. Pleasant.
27	29.82	29.82	29.85	56	74	60	63.3	N. E'ly 1	N. W. 1	N'ly	10	2	0		27th to 30th. Very fine.
S 28	29.93	29.93	29.98	60	78	63	67.0	S. W. 1	S. W. 2	S. W. 1	0	3	0		
29	29.98	29.93	29.92	62	76	64	67.3	S. W. 1	S. W. 2	S. W. 2	0	2	3		
30	29.88	29.81	29.82	63	78	64	68.3	S. W. 2	S. W. 3	S. W. 2	5	5	2		
31	29.78	29.76	29.70	64	79	66	69.7	S. W. 3	S'ly 3	S'ly 3	8	Rain	10	1.00	31st. Moderate rain at intervals.
Means	29.69	29.66	29.67	63.0	77.4	65.5	...	1.5	1.8	1.5	5.2	5.3	4.8	4.42	
REDUCED TO SEA LEVEL.									1.6			5.1			
Max.	30.16	30.11	30.16	69	84	70	73.7	Prevailing winds from some point between—		Days.			Days.		
Min.	29.66	29.58	29.55	56	59	58	60.7	N. & E.		9	Clear		7		
Mean	29.87	29.84	29.85					E. & S.		2	Variable	}	15		
Range	0.50	0.53	0.61	13	25	12	13.0	S. & W.		14	Cloudy	}			
Mean of month	29.853			...	...	...	68.6	W. & N.		4	Rain fell on		7		
Extreme range	0.61			...	...	...	26.0				(2 days omitted.)				

August, 1844.

DAYS.	BAROMETER, REDUCED TO 32° F. At 6 A. M.	At 1 P. M.	At 10 P. M.	THERMOMETER. At 6 A. M.	At 1 P. M.	At 10 P. M.	Daily mean.	WINDS. (DIRECTION AND FORCE.) At 6 A. M.	At 1 P. M.	At 10 P. M.	WEATHER. (TENTHS CLOUDY.) At 6 A. M.	At 1 P. M.	At 10 P. M.	RAIN AND SNOW IN INCHES OF WATER.
1	29.68	29.67	29.68	65	78	72	71.7	S'ly 2	S. W. 2	S'ly	Rain	8	10	
2	29.71	29.72	29.77	73	82	71	75.0	S'ly 1	S. W. 2	S. W. 1	10	5	10	
3	29.77	29.75	29.67	67	84	68	73.0	N. E. 2	S'ly 1	S'ly	10	8	Misty	
S 4	29.49	29.44	29.46	70	73	67	70.0	S. W. 2	S. W. 2	S. W.	10	10	2	
5	29.60	29.60	29.64	58	74	63	65.0	N. W. 2	N. W. 2	N. W. 1	0	2	0	
6	29.63	29.61	29.61	58	73	64	65.0	N. W. 1	S. W. 2	S. W. 0	0	0	0	
7	29.63	29.64	29.72	64	78	66	69.3	N. W. 1	S. W. 2	S. W. 1	0	2	0	
8	29.75	29.73	29.74	64	78	69	70.3	S. W. 3	S. W. 3	S. W. 1	0	1	0	
9	29.69	29.58	29.56	68	81	75	74.7	S. W. 2	S. W. 4	S. W. 4	2	9	10	
10	29.50	29.52	29.57	74	81	70	75.0	W'ly 2	W'ly 2	W'ly 2	7	0	10	
S 11	29.62	29.60	29.65	62	74	60	65.3	N. W. 2	N. W. 2	N. W. 2	3	8	0	
12	29.73	29.73	29.79	55	72	57	61.3	N. W. 2	N. W. 2	N. W. 1	0	3	0	
13	29.86	29.85	29.88	54	74	61	63.0	N. W. 2	S. W. 3	S. W. 1	0	2	0	
14	...	...	29.96	...	...	62	...	...	...	N. W. 1	...	Rain	6	0.73
15	29.96	29.94	29.91	56	75	62	64.3	N. W. 2	S. E. 2	E'ly	0	10	10	
16	29.89	29.84	29.78	57	80	64	67.0	W'ly 1	S'ly 2	S'ly 1	3	2	0	
17	29.69	29.59	29.61	64	80	72	72.0	S. W. 2	S. W. 2	S. W. 1	4	1	0	
S 18	29.72	29.77	29.84	64	80	67	70.3	N. W. 2	N. E. 2	S. W. 2	0	2	0	
19	29.88	29.87	29.83	64	78	70	70.7	S. W. 2	S. E. 3	S'ly 2	2	8	10	
20	29.73	...	...	70	...	...	...	S. W. 1	...	...	10	...	...	
21	...	...	29.88	...	...	58	...	...	...	N. W. 2	...	...	0	
22	29.92	29.81	29.69	53	72	58	61.0	N. E. 2	E'ly 2	S. E. 2	3	2	Rain	} 0.38
23	29.50	29.30	29.32	60	77	65	67.3	S. E. 3	S'ly 1	N. E. 2	Misty	10	Misty	
24	29.36	...	...	57	...	...	...	N. E. 2	...	...	10	...	...	
S 25	...	...	...	...	...	...	...	...	...	...	...	...	...	
26	...	...	...	...	...	...	...	...	...	...	...	...	...	
27	...	...	...	...	...	...	...	...	...	...	...	...	...	
28	...	...	...	...	...	...	...	...	...	...	...	...	...	
29	...	...	29.64	...	...	61	...	...	...	S. W. 1	...	...	2	
30	29.71	29.70	29.68	56	74	63	64.3	W'ly 1	N. W. 2	N. W. 1	0	2	0	
31	29.81	29.81	29.84	58	73	65	65.3	N. W. 1	N. W. 2	W. 1	0	6	6	
Means	29.70	29.68	29.71	62.1	76.9	65.2	...	1.8	2.1	1.4	3.9	4.8	4.1	1.11
									1.8			4.2		
REDUCED TO SEA LEVEL.														
Max.	30.14	30.12	30.14	74	84	75	75.0							
Min.	29.54	29.48	29.50	53	72	57	61.0							
Mean	29.88	29.86	20.89											
Range	0.60	0.64	0.64	21	12	18	14.0							
Mean of month	29.877			...	...	...	68.1							
Extreme range	0.66			...	...	...	31.0							

Prevailing winds from some point between— Days.
N. & E. 3
E. & S. 4
S. & W. 13
W. & N. 7

Days.
Clear 7
Variable . . . } 13
Cloudy . . . . }
Rain fell on . . 7
(4 days omitted.)

REMARKS.

1st. Light showers in the morning.
2d. Very sultry. Sprinkling of rain in the afternoon.
3d. Very sultry. Mist in the evening.
4th. Showery from 9 to 12 A. M. Cloudy in the afternoon; very sultry.
5th. Very pleasant.
6th. Very pleasant. Clouds from 4 to 6 P. M., with appearances of a shower.
7th and 8th. Very fine.
9th. Air very damp, with appearances of rain.
10th. Very damp and sultry. Sprinkling of rain from 6 to 7 P. M.
11th, 12th, and 13th. Very fine.
14th. Copious showers at intervals.
15th and 16th. Pleasant.
17th and 18th. Very warm.
19th. Warm and sultry. Air very damp in the afternoon.
20th. Very warm and sultry. Sudden change to cooler during the night.
21st. Very pleasant.
22d. Strong indication of rain in the afternoon. Commenced raining from 7 to 8 P. M.
23d. Showers in the morning. Hot sun at intervals in the afternoon. Clouds and mist in the evening, with wind N. E.
29th. Pleasant. Morning cool.
30th and 31st. Pleasant.

September, 1844.

DAYS.	BAROMETER. Sunrise.	At 1 P. M.	At 10 P. M.	THERMOMETER. Sunrise.	At 1 P. M.	At 10 P. M.	Daily mean.	WINDS. Sunrise.	At 1 P. M.	At 10 P. M.	WEATHER. Sunrise.	At 1 P. M.	At 10 P. M.	RAIN AND SNOW.
S 1	29.88	29.88	29.88	63	65	64	64.0	E'ly 2	E'ly 2	S. W'ly 1	10	Rain	7	0.90
2	29.88	29.78	29.67	64	76	68	69.3	S. W. 1	S. W. 3	S. W. 2	4	5	10	
3	29.62	...	...	68	...	...	...	S. W. 1	...	...	Rain	...	...	0.33
4	...	...	...	...	...	...	...	...	...	...	...	...	...	
5	30.03	...	30.10	50	...	52	...	N. W. 3	...	N. E.	0	...	0	
6	30.16	30.15	30.11	48	68	53	56.3	N. E. 1	N. E. 1	N. E. 1	0	0	0	
7	30.07	29.99	29.94	48	73	59	60.0	N. E. 1	N. E. 2	N. E. 1	0	0	0	
S 8	29.90	29.84	29.82	55	76	60	63.7	N. W. 1	N. W. 1	S. W. 1	0	2	0	
9	29.79	29.75	29.78	56	78	63	65.7	S. W. 1	S. E'ly 2	S'ly 1	0	2	0	
10	29.78	29.78	29.81	59	80	64	67.7	W'ly 1	W'ly 3	S. W'ly	6	2	0	
11	29.83	29.83	29.85	58	77	65	66.7	W'ly 1	S. W. 3	W'ly	0	5	8	
12	29.85	29.84	29.82	58	69	59	62.0	E'ly 2	E'ly 1	E'ly 2	10	10	10	
13	29.79	29.79	29.78	58	65	58	60.3	N. E. 3	N. E. 3	N. E. 3	10	10	9	
14	29.79	29.73	29.73	56	71	59	62.0	N. 3	N. E'ly 3	N'ly 3	8	8	0	
S 15	29.74	29.75	29.78	58	79	64	67.0	N. W. 2	N. W. 3	N. E. 1	2	2	0	
16	29.79	29.76	29.75	59	79	66	68.0	N. W'ly 1	N. W. 2	N. W. 1	0	0	0	
17	29.81	29.81	29.75	61	68	54	61.0	N. E. 3	N. E. 4	N. E. 2	4	0	0	
18	29.76	29.64	29.62	53	76	62	63.7	N. W. 2	W'ly 1	N. W. 0	5	3	0	
19	29.74	29.78	29.79	57	76	59	64.0	N. W. 1	N. W. 1	S. E. 2	3	0	0	
20	29.82	29.81	29.77	57	79	64	66.7	S. W. 1	S. W. 2	S. W. 2	0	0	0	
21	29.76	29.73	29.70	59	78	67	68.0	S. W. 2	S. W. 4	S. W. 3	6	2	6	
S 22	29.70	29.72	29.80	63	56	50	56.3	N. W. 2	N. E. 2	N. W. 1	10	Rain	0	
23	29.89	29.89	29.94	43	59	47	49.7	N. 2	N. E. 2	N. E. 0	0	0	0	
24	29.97	29.92	29.94	43	64	54	53.7	N. W. 1	E'ly 2	S. E. 3	0	2	0	
25	29.94	29.87	29.89	54	62	55	57.0	N. W. 1	S. W. 2	S. W. 2	10	10	10	
26	29.89	29.90	29.95	49	49	44	47.3	N. E. 2	N'ly 2	N. W. 0	Rain	10	0	1.00
27	30.01	29.97	30.00	41	56	42	46.3	N. W. 1	N. W. 1	N. W. 2	0	4	0	
28	29.95	29.80	29.68	33	56	47	45.3	N'ly 2	N. E. 2	N. E. 2	0	10	10	
[illegible]	[illegible]	[illegible]	[illegible]	[illegible]	[illegible]	[illegible]	[illegible]	[illegible]	[illegible]	[illegible]	Rain	Rain	Misty	0.60
30	29.50	29.55	29.84	43	61	52	52.0	N. W. 1	W'ly 3	N. W. 1	0	1	3	
Means	29.82	29.78	29.80	53.8	68.5	57.0	...	1.7	2.2	1.6	4.4	4.0	2.8	2.83
									1.8			3.7		
REDUCED TO SEA LEVEL.														
Max.	30.34	30.33	30.29	68	80	68	69.3							
Min.	29.48	29.13	29.17	33	54	42	45.3							
Mean	30.00	29.96	29.98											
Range	0.86	1.20	1.12	35	26	26	24.0							
Mean of month	29.980			...	...	...	59.8							
Extreme range	1.21			...	...	...	47.0							

Prevailing winds from some point between— Days.
N. & E. 11
E. & S. 3
S. & W. 7
W. & N. 8

Days.
Clear 10
Variable . . . } 12
Cloudy . . . . }
Rain fell on . . 7
(1 day omitted.)

REMARKS.

1st. Pretty steady rain from 10 A. M. to 3 or 4 P. M.
2d. Cloudy, and air damp. Rain during the night.
3d, 4th, and 5th. Very pleasant.
6th, 7th, and 8th. Very fine.
9th. Halo about the sun very extraordinary. See my notice of it published in the Providence Journal of Sept. 14th.
10th and 11th. Pleasant.
12th. Appearances of rain.
14th. Cloudy and cool.
15th. Very pleasant. Hot sun.
16th. Pleasant. Sun very hot.
17th. Pleasant. Rather cool.
18th to 21st. Pleasant.
22d. Two or three heavy dashes of rain in the afternoon.
23d and 24th. Pleasant, though cool. Slight frost in the vicinity.
25th. Occasional sprinkling of rain in the afternoon, and rain during the night.
26th. Rain continued moderately till 12 or 1 o'clock. Very clear and still in the evening.
27th. Pleasant. Cool towards night.
28th. First appearance of white frost in the College yard—only slight. Wind light N'ly. Barometer falling. Wind soon came more towards N. E., continued light during the day, but increased in the evening. Began to rain moderately at 10 P. M.
29th. Rain. Wind heavy N. E; at noon, hauled more to E., and somewhat abated; from 1 to 2 P. M., came round to S. W., clouds broken and sun out, wind rather light. In the course of the afternoon, wind came to W'ly and increased in strength, with rain. At 10 P. M., wind rather heavy at N. W'ly, with mist. At 6 P. M., baro- [illegible] began to rise from 6 to 7 P. M.; at 9½ P. M., was at 29.09.
30th. Pleasant.

October, 1844.

DAYS.	Barometer, reduced to 32° F. Sunrise.	At 1 P. M.	At 10 P. M.	Thermometer. Sunrise.	At 1 P. M.	At 10 P. M.	Daily mean.	Winds (Direction and Force.) Sunrise.	At 1 P. M.	At 10 P. M.	Weather (Tenths Cloudy.) Sunrise.	At 1 P. M.	At 10 P. M.	Rain and Snow in Inches of Water.
1	30.10	30.09	30.13	37	55	43	46.0	N. W. 2	N. W. 2	N. W. 1	0	0	0	
2	30.16	30.10	30.04	37	59	46	47.3	N. W. 1	S'ly 2	S'ly 1	0	0	1	
3	29.91	29.78	29.67	45	58	57	53.3	S. E'ly 1	E'ly 2	E'ly 2	3	10	Rain	} 1.42
4	29.39	29.28	29.29	58	60	54	57.3	S. E. 2	W'ly 1	...	Rain	9	0	
5	29.34	29.36	29.64	48	60	52	53.3	S. W. 2	S. W. 3	N. W.	3	8	0	
S 6	29.65	29.63	29.54	47	59	49	51.7	N. W.	N. E.	N. E.	8	8	10, R'n	0.60
7	29.55	29.63	29.77	44	54	48	48.7	N. W. 2	N. W. 2	N. W. 1	10	10	3	
8	29.84	29.80	29.78	45	57	46	49.3	N. W. 1	S. W. 3	S. W. 1	8	2	0	
9	29.69	29.63	29.73	48	66	52	55.3	W'ly 2	W'ly 1	W'ly 0	9	2	0	
10	29.69	29.53	29.52	45	68	58	57.0	W'ly 1	S. W. 3	S. W. 1	0	0	0	
11	29.69	29.73	29.84	49	52	44	48.3	N. E. 2	N. E. 2	N. W. 2	10	10	0	
12	30.00	30.01	30.07	39	51	41	43.7	N. W. 2	N. E. 2	N. E. 1	0	3	0	
S 13	30.13	30.09	30.01	44	54	48	48.7	N. W. 0	S. E'ly 2	S'ly 1	0	1	8	
14	29.88	29.76	29.61	44	57	53	51.3	S. W. 1	S. W. 3	S. W. 2	5	Rain	Rain	} 0.58
15	29.31	29.09	29.13	56	59	53	56.0	S. W. 1	S. W. 1	W'ly 2	10	Rain	10	
16	29.41	29.51	29.80	49	58	48	51.7	W'ly 2	W'ly 2	W'ly 1	3	0	0	
17	30.01	29.99	29.96	41	59	55	51.7	W'ly	S. E'ly 3	S. W. 3	0	10	10	
18	29.90	29.85	29.72	58	64	60	60.7	S. W. 1	S. W. 2	S. W. 2	10	Rain	Spr'ling	} 1.28
19	29.44	29.53	29.74	65	58	48	57.0	S. W. 6	W. 3	N. W. 1	Rain	9	0	
S 20	30.00	30.06	30.22	38	49	38	41.7	N. W. 3	N. W. 2	N. W. 1	0	0	0	
21	30.30	30.30	30.24	33	54	46	41.0	N'ly 1	E'ly 1	S. E'ly 1	0	10	10	
22	30.30	30.14	30.12	46	57	44	49.0	N. E. 1	N. E. 3	...	8	2	0	
23	30.14	30.12	30.13	39	57	44	46.0	N. E. 1	E'ly 1	E'ly	0	0	0	
24	30.19	30.13	30.13	40	60	47	49.0	N. E. 1	E'ly 1	S. E'ly 1	0	0	2	
25	30.09	29.98	29.94	48	62	53	54.3	N. E. 1	S. E'ly 1	S'ly 1	10	6	6	
26	29.89	...	29.73	50	...	55	...	S. W. 1	...	S. E'ly	0	...	10	
S 27	29.69	29.65	29.64	52	52	48	50.7	N. E.	N. E.	N. E.	10	10	10	
28	29.60	29.53	29.53	42	44	46	44.0	N. E. 4	N. E. 4	E'ly	10	10	Misty	} 1.92
29	29.33	29.21	29.39	49	50	48	49.0	N. E. 2	N'ly 1	W'ly 3	Rain	Misty	10	
30	29.57	29.61	29.69	38	48	40	42.0	N. W. 1	N. W. 2	N. W. 1	0	8	5	
31	29.69	29.72	29.86	36	45	36	39.0	N. W. 1	N. W. 2	N. W. 2	10	10	0	
Means	29.80	29.76	29.79	45.5	56.2	48.4	...	1.6	2.0	1.3	5.1	5.7	4.4	5.80
									1.6			5.1		
REDUCED TO SEA LEVEL.														
Max.	30.48	30.48	30.42	65	68	60	60.7							
Min.	29.49	29.27	29.31	33	44	38	39.0							
Mean	29.98	29.94	29.97											
Range	0.99	1.21	1.11	32	24	22	21.7							
Mean of month	29.963			...	...	...	49.8							
Extreme range	1.21			...	...	...	35.0							

Prevailing winds from some point between— Days.
- N. & E. 7
- E. & S. 5
- S. & W. 13
- W. & N. 6

Days.
- Clear 8
- Variable . . . } 15
- Cloudy . . . . }
- Rain fell on . . 8

REMARKS.

1st. Pleasant.
2d. Light white frost in the College yard.
3d. Began to rain moderately from 2 to 3 P. M., and continued during the night.
4th. Rain in the morning, wind S. E., heavy showers. Clouds became broken from noon to 1 P. M., and sun appeared.
5th. Pleasant.
6th. Cloudy in the afternoon; wind N. E. Rain during the night.
7th. Cloudy.
8th, 9th, and 10th. Pleasant.
11th. Cloudy, with appearances of rain. Clear in the evening.
12th. Pleasant.
13th. Pleasant. Copious white frost in the College yard this morning.
14th. Began to rain quite moderately from 1 to 2 P. M.; increased in the evening.
15th. Rain and drizzle.
16th. Very pleasant.
17th. Cloudy in the afternoon and evening, with appearances of rain.
18th. Rain at intervals through the day. Very high wind and stormy during the night.
19th. Storm in the morning. Barometer began to rise at 8 A. M. Clear in the evening.
20th. A splendid day, without a cloud. Very brilliant aurora, continuing from 9 P. M. through the night. A luminous bow, of a few degrees in height, spanned 60° or 70° of the horizon, from which brilliant corruscations shot up towards the zenith to the height of 60° or 70°. What was unusual and very striking, was the rapid horizontal movement of what seemed to be dense masses of light. The bow seemed to heave and swell like the ocean, and thick masses of light beneath the bows moved rapidly backwards and forwards in a horizontal direction. The whole scene underwent unusually rapid and brilliant transformations.
21st. Cloudy, with appearances of rain.
22d to 25th. Pleasant.
28th. Rain during the night.
29th. Rain in the morning, pretty heavy.

November, 1844.

DAYS.	Barometer Sunrise.	At 1 P. M.	At 10 P. M.	Thermometer Sunrise.	At 1 P. M.	At 10 P. M.	Daily mean.	Winds Sunrise.	At 1 P. M.	At 10 P. M.	Weather Sunrise.	At 1 P. M.	At 10 P. M.	Rain and Snow
1	29.95	29.90	29.90	33	49	40	40.7	N. W. 1	S. W. 1	S. W. 1	0	0	1	
2	29.90	...	29.98	38	...	46	...	N. W. 1	...	S. W. 1	9	...	0	
S 3	29.89	...	...	39	55	48	47.3	N. W. 1	S. E'ly 1	...	0	0	Hazy	
4	29.71	29.68	29.61	48	51	48	49.0	N. E. 1	N. E. 1	N. E. 2	Rain	Misty	Rain	} 1.62
5	29.40	...	29.28	42	...	42	...	N. W. 2	...	N. W. 2	Misty	...	0	
6	29.29	29.29	29.31	38	44	38	40.0	W'ly 3	W'ly 4	N. W. 4	0	10	3	
7	29.42	29.42	29.40	35	58	49	47.3	N. W. 2	W. 2	S. W. 1	1	3	0	
8	29.40	29.42	29.54	44	58	45	50.7	S. W. 1	S. W. 1	N. W. 1	3	0	2	
9	29.69	...	29.81	39	...	41	...	W'ly 1	...	S. W. 1	0	...	2	
S 10	29.95	29.89	29.68	34	51	49	44.7	N. W. 1	S'ly 1	S. W. 1	0	10	10	
11	29.69	...	29.74	46	...	46	...	S. W. 1	...	N'ly	1	Shower	10	0.27
12	29.73	29.70	29.60	44	50	52	48.7	N. E. 1	N. E. 2	E'ly 1	Misty	Misty	Rain	0.08
13	29.48	29.51	29.68	61	47	41	49.7	W'ly 1	N. W. 1	N. W. 2	Misty	Rain	8	
14	29.71	29.75	29.91	34	42	35	37.0	N. W. 2	N. W. 4	N. W.	0	0	1	
15	30.02	30.00	29.96	31	45	36	37.3	N. W. 1	N. W. 1	N. W. 1	0	0	2	
16	29.96	29.92	29.96	33	50	38	40.3	N. W. 1	N. W.	N. W.	0	0	2	
S 17	30.00	29.91	29.72	35	49	36	40.0	N. W. 1	S. W. 1	S. W.	0	0	9	
18	29.50	29.47	29.61	51	45	34	43.3	S. W. 2	S. W. 2	N. W. 3	Rain	10	0	
19	29.93	29.93	29.96	26	37	31	31.3	N. W. 2	N. W. 2	N. W. 0	0	0	0	
20	29.90	29.81	29.81	31	44	38	31.7	W'ly 1	S. W. 2	S. W. 1	9	10	6	
21	29.91	...	29.89	32	...	40	...	N. W. 1	E'ly 1	S. W. 1	0	...	5	
22	29.82	29.84	29.59	41	48	46	45.0	N. E. 1	N. E. 1	E'ly 1	Misty	Misty	Rain	} 1.00
23	29.29	29.21	29.25	45	49	47	47.0	N'ly 1	N'ly 1	N'ly 2	Misty	6	0	
S 24	29.29	29.29	29.40	40	39	30	36.3	N. W. 2	N. W. 3	N. W. 3	2	3	8	
25	29.52	29.56	29.76	25	29	24	26.0	N. W. 3	N. W. 3	N. W. 3	0	0	0	
26	29.93	29.84	29.45	18	31	35	31.3	N. W. 2	N. W. 2	S. W. 3	6	10	R'n, sn.	
27	29.68	29.75	30.00	33	34	22	29.7	N'ly 2	W'ly 2	N. W. 2	2	3	2	
28	30.03	29.92	29.74	15	19	19	17.7	N. W. 1	N'ly 2	N. E. 2	6	Snow	Snow	0.33
29	29.75	29.80	29.92	22	31	24	25.7	N'ly 2	N. W. 1	N. W. 1	10	10	0	
30	29.98	29.94	29.87	18	37	37	30.7	N. W. 1	S. W. 1	S. W. 1	0	3	10	
Means	29.73	29.70	29.70	35.9	43.7	38.3	...	1.5	1.7	1.6	4.0	5.3	4.7	3.30
									1.6			4.7		
REDUCED TO SEA LEVEL.														
Max.	30.21	30.18	30.18	61	58	52	50.7							
Min.	29.47	29.39	29.43	15	19	19	17.7							
Mean	29.91	29.88	29.88											
Range	0.74	0.79	0.75	46	39	33	33.0							
Mean of month	29.890			...	...	...	39.3							
Extreme range	0.82			...	...	...	46.0							

Prevailing winds from some point between— Days.
- N. & E. 4
- E. & S. 2
- S. & W. 11
- W. & N. 13

Days.
- Clear 10
- Variable . . . } 11
- Cloudy . . . . }
- Rain or snow fell on 9

REMARKS.

1st, 2d, and 3d. Very fine.
4th. Rain and mist. Heavy rain during the night.
5th. Pleasant.
6th. Very blustering.
7th. Pleasant.
8th and 9th. Very pleasant.
10th. Pleasant.
11th. Heavy thundershower from 2 to 3 P. M.
12th. Misty through the day. Moderate rain in the evening. During the night, wind came round to S. and S. W., and grew warm.
13th. Misty and light rain occasionally.
14th. Blustering.
15th. Pleasant
16th. Very pleasant.
17th. Pleasant.
18th. Light rain in the morning. Grew cold during the day.
19th. Very pleasant, though cool.
20th. Variable.
21st. Pleasant.
22d. Misty through the day. Rain in the evening and through the night.
23d. Occasional rain in the morning. Clear in the evening.
24th. Blustering. Total eclipse of the moon in the evening.
25th. Wind cutting and severe.
26th. Cloudy in the afternoon; wind S.W. Very moderate snow and rain in the evening.
27th. Cold and wintery.
28th. Commenced snowing at 1 P. M. Wind at N'ly and then N. E.
29th. From two to three inches of dry snow on the ground in the morning. Cloudy and raw through the day. Clear and still in the evening.

December, 1844.

Days.	Barometer, reduced to 32° F. Sun-rise.	At 1 P. M.	At 10 P. M.	Thermometer. Sun-rise.	At 1 P. M.	At 10 P. M.	Daily mean.	Winds. (Direction and Force.) Sunrise.	At 1 P. M.	At 10 P. M.	Weather. (Tenths Cloudy.) Sun-rise.	At 1 P. M.	At 10 P. M.	Rain and Snow in Inches of Water.
S 1	29.64	29.72	29.91	46	36	32	38.0	S. W. 2	N'ly 1	N'ly 1	Misty	R'n, m't	5	0.15
2	30.02	30.12	30.24	24	37	31	30.7	N. W. 1	N. W. 1	N. W. 2	0	0	8	
3	30.30	30.24	30.09	32	37	34	34.3	N. E. 1	N. E. 2	N. E. 2	10	10	10	·
4	29.80	29.59	29.59	38	38	38	38.0	N. E. 3	N. E. 3	N. E. 2	Rain	Misty	10	0.50
5	29.83	29.89	30.02	40	43	35	39.3	N'ly 1	N. W. 1	N'ly 1	10	8	3	
6	30.09	30.06	30.03	33	45	41	39.7	N'ly 1	N. E. 1	N. E. 1	10	8	10	
7	29.69	29.40	29.18	42	56	54	54.0	N. E'ly 1	S'ly 1	S. W. 3	Foggy	10, R'n	0	0.27
S 8	29.50	29.74	29.85	31	30	24	28.3	N. W. 4	N. W. 4	N. W. 2	0	0	0	
9	30.07	29.96	29.87	22	33	28	27.7	N. W. 1	S. W. 2	N. W. 1	0	3	0	
10	...	...	29.99	...	...	24	...	...	...	N. W. 1	...	...	0	
11	29.98	29.91	29.69	21	25	22	22.7	N'ly 2	N. E. 3	N. E. 4	10	10	Snow	0.33
12	29.63	29.68	29.74	24	34	22	26.7	N. W. 2	N. W. 1	N. W. 1	10	10	10	
13	29.71	29.70	29.50	20	37	33	30.0	N'ly 1	E'ly 1	E'ly	10	10	Rain, 6	
14	29.43	29.37	29.39	32	38	34	34.7	N. W. 1	W'ly 1	W'ly 1	10	5	0	
S 15	29.40	...	29.40	30	...	32	...	W'ly 1	...	W'ly	0	...	3	
16	29.41	29.36	29.33	25	33	26	28.0	N. W. 1	S. W'ly	N. W.	0	2	0	
17	29.37	29.40	29.45	22	26	22	23.3	N. W. 1	N. W. 2	N. W. 2	0	2	0	
18	29.53	29.60	29.74	20	22	19	20.3	N. W. 1	N. W. 3	N. W. 2	3	0	6	
19	29.71	29.68	29.69	24	33	29	28.7	W'ly 1	W'ly 1	W'ly 1	5	3	10	
20	29.67	29.80	29.82	22	29	18	23.0	N. W. 2	N. W. 2	N. W. 1	0	0	0	
21	29.82	29.76	29.65	14	31	32	24.7	N. W. 1	S. W. 2	E'ly 2	0	4	Snow	
S 22	29.54	29.46	29.36	39	47	46	44.0	S'ly 1	S'ly 2	S'ly 1	5	Rain	8	} 0.75
23	28.99	28.80	28.61	44	45	36	41.7	E'ly 1	S'ly 0	W'ly 3	Foggy	Foggy	9	
24	29.19	29.49	29.71	28	35	34	32.3	N. W. 3	N. W. 3	W'ly 1	2	0	0	
25	29.81	29.83	29.74	30	44	39	37.7	S. W. 2	S. W. 3	S. W. 1	3	4	2	
26	29.71	29.67	29.53	43	51	44	46.0	S. W. 3	S. W. 2	S'ly 1	8	3	7	
27	29.49	29.46	29.35	44	34	26	34.7	N'ly 1	N. E. 2	N. E. 2	10	Rain	Snow	} 0.75
28	29.36	29.45	29.64	20	24	16	20.0	N'ly 2	N. W. 2	N. W. 1	Snow	8	0	
S 29	29.76	29.79	29.91	12	29	25	22.0	N. W. 1	W'ly 2	N. W. 1	0	0	0	
30	29.82	29.45	29.51	22	42	40	34.7	S. W'ly 1	S. W. 2	N'ly 2	10	3	0	
31	29.64	29.71	29.80	36	37	28	33.7	W'ly 1	W'ly 3	N. W.	0	0	0	
Means	29.66	29.66	29.65	29.3	37.0	32.0	...	1.5	1.8	1.6	5.5	5.5	4.6	2.75
									1.6			5.2		
REDUCED TO SEA LEVEL.								Prevailing winds from some point between—		Days.			Days.	
Max.	30.48	30.42	30.42	46	56	54	54.0	N. & E.		6	Clear		9	
Min.	29.17	28.98	28.79	12	22	16	20.0	E. & S.		1	Variable		} 12	
Mean	29.84	29.84	29.83					S. & W.		7	Cloudy			
Range	1.31	1.44	1.63	34	34	38	34.0	W. & N.		17	Rain or snow fell on		10	
Mean of month	29.837			...	...	...	32.8							
Extreme range	1.69			...	...	...	44.0							

Remarks.

1st. Wind S W. and warm at sunrise; soon came to N'ly, and grew colder. Mixed rain, snow, and hail at intervals in the afternoon.
2d. Very pleasant.
3d. Appearances of storm. Flurry of snow in the evening.
4th. Moderate rain in the morning.
5th. Cloudy, but mild. Frost out of the ground.
6th. Very mild.
7th. Copious showers in the afternoon; wind brisk S'ly and S. W. Cleared in evening; wind more to W'ly.
8th. Very blustering, wind cutting.
9th. Eclipse of the sun; began at 3h. 45 m. 12 s. P. M., mean time.
10th. Very pleasant.
11th. Very raw and cold. Began to snow about sunset.
12th. Three or four inches of dry snow on the ground at sunrise. Very much drifted.
13th. Mild. Sprinkling of rain in the afternoon.
14th. Mild.
15th and 16th. Pleasant.
17th. Cold. Flurry of snow during the night.
18th. Cold. Pretty severe wind.
19th. Pleasant.
20th. Very fine.
21st. Pleasant. Began to snow very moderately at about 9 P. M.
22d. Very mild. Dashes of rain from noon to 1 P. M.; also, rain during the night.
23d. Very calm, and dense fog in the morning. Dark, dense fog in the afternoon, with dashes of rain. Wind freshened at S. W. towards sunset; high and blustering during the night, and hauled round to N. W. Barometer continued falling till 10½ P. M., when it became stationary at 28.71, and soon began to rise; at midnight, stood at 28.76.
24th. At sunrise, barometer 29.10; weather blustering, which continued during the day, but mild in the evening.
25th and 26th. Mild and pleasant.
27th. Moderate rain in the morning. Snow in the afternoon and evening.
28th. In the morning, the ground covered with six or seven inches of compact snow, and a good deal drifted.
29th. Pleasant.
30th. Mild.

January, 1845.

Days.	Barometer Sun-rise.	At 1 P. M.	At 10 P. M.	Thermometer Sun-rise.	At 1 P. M.	At 10 P. M.	Daily mean.	Winds Sunrise.	At 1 P. M.	At 10 P. M.	Weather Sun-rise.	At 1 P. M.	At 10 P. M.	Rain and Snow in Inches of Water.
1	29.49	29.55	29.55	38	44	37	39.7	S'ly	N. W.	N. W.	10	0	0	
2	29.73	...	29.92	26	...	23	...	N. W.	...	N. W.	0	...	0	
3	30.05	30.00	29.79	17	32	35	28.0	N. W. 2	E'ly 1	S. E'ly 2	0	5	10	
4	29.51	29.61	29.70	40	42	39	40.3	S. W'ly 2	W'ly 3	W'ly 1	9	0	10	
S 5	29.54	29.41	29.52	38	43	38	39.7	N. W. 1	W'ly 2	W'ly 1	7	0	10	
6	29.79	29.82	29.82	30	31	30	30.3	N. E. 1	N. E. 2	N. E. 3	10	10	Snow	} 1.00
7	29.57	29.39	29.39	32	38	34	34.7	N. E. 2	N. E. 2	N. E. 1	Rain	Misty	Misty	
8	29.69	29.69	29.81	31	37	29	32.3	N. W. 1	W'ly 2	W'ly 2	8	10	0	
9	29.89	29.75	29.72	26	38	36	33.3	N. W'ly 1	S. W. 1	N. W. 2	6	Rain	0	
10	29.69	29.68	29.71	38	36	30	34.7	N. W. 2	N. W. 2	N. W. 1	2	3	0	
11	29.63	29.56	29.52	28	36	28	30.7	N. W. 1	N. W. 1	N. W. 2	10	0	0	
S 12	29.42	29.41	29.49	26	32	26	28.0	N. W. 2	N. W. 1	N. W. 1	10	2	0	
13	29.54	29.40	29.41	26	27	18	23.7	N. W. 1	E'ly 2	N. E. 3	8	Snow	Snow	0.20
14	29.76	29.85	29.95	12	25	14	17.0	N. W. 1	N. W. 1	N. W.	3	0	0	
15	30.08	29.96	29.97	18	42	39	33.0	N. E. 2	S. W. 2	S. W. 1	Snow	10	10	
16	29.94	29.95	29.95	37	33	32	34.0	S. W. 1	N. E. 2	N. E. 2	Rain	Rain	Rain	} 0.50
17	29.80	29.75	29.45	30	37	30	32.3	N. E. 1	N. E. 1	N. E. 1	Misty	Misty	Rain	
18	29.47	29.64	30.10	34	26	9	23.0	N'ly 2	N. W. 2	N. W. 2	10	0	0	
S 19	30.23	30.26	30.21	7	16	20	14.3	N. W. 1	N. W. 1	N. W. 1	0	0	10	
20	30.05	29.95	29.86	23	34	30	29.0	N. W'ly 1	N. W. 1	N'ly 2	10	Misty	Misty	
21	29.61	29.42	29.51	29	30	26	28.3	N. E. 2	N. E'ly 2	N'ly 1	Misty	Misty	10	
22	29.65	29.75	30.00	28	32	25	28.3	N'ly 2	N. W. 2	N. W. 1	3	2	0	
23	29.21	30.24	30.26	20	34	26	26.7	N. W. 1	N. W. 1	N. W. 1	0	0	0	
24	30.09	29.92	29.59	27	40	44	37.0	N. W. 1	S. E. 1	S. E. 4	10	Rain	Rain	} 1.50
25	29.22	29.12	29.14	49	50	41	46.7	S. E. 4	S. W. 2	N. E'ly 2	Rain	4	Rain	
S 26	29.39	29.49	29.69	40	37	32	36.3	N. W. 2	N. W. 2	N. W. 2	10	8	10	
27	29.86	29.85	29.89	28	41	35	34.7	N. W. 2	N. W. 2	N. W. 1	0	0	0	
28	29.90	29.82	29.73	31	41	36	36.0	N. W. 2	S. W. 2	S. W. 2	0	5	10	
29	29.60	29.63	29.74	37	39	32	36.0	S. W. 1	N. W. 3	N. W. 2	Foggy	0	0	
30	29.74	29.70	29.75	29	28	19	25.3	N. W. 1	N. W. 3	N. W. 2	0	4	0	
31	29.71	29.64	29.84	13	21	8	14.0	N'ly	N. W. 2	N. W. 3	0	0	0	
Means	29.70	29.71	29.74	28.6	34.4	30.7	...	1.5	1.7	1.8	6.3	4.8	5.2	3.20
									1.7			5.4		
REDUCED TO SEA LEVEL.								Prevailing winds from some point between—		Days.			Days.	
Max.	30.41	30.44	30.44	49	50	44	46.7	N. & E.		6	Clear		7	
Min.	29.39	29.30	29.32	7	16	8	14.0	E. & S.		2	Variable		} 14	
Mean	29.88	29.89	29.92					S. & W.		5	Cloudy			
Range	1.02	1.14	1.12	42	34	36	32.7	W. & N.		18	Rain or snow fell on		10	
Mean of month	29.897			...	...	...	30.7							
Extreme range	1.14			...	...	...	43.0							

Remarks.

6th. Began to snow about 9 P. M. Five or six inches of damp snow fell during the night, and it then turned to rain.
7th. Moderate rain in the morning, with mist.
8th. Evening very clear and mild.
9th. Cloudy and sprinkling of rain and snow in the morning; wind S. W. Evening clear; wind N. W., and brilliant aurora with corruscations or needles.
10th, 11th, and 12th. Very fine.
13th. Cloudy. Began to snow very gently from 10 to 11 A. M; wind S. W. Wind came to E'ly and N. E., and increased in the evening.
14th. Two or three inches of light snow on the ground.
15th. Mild. Ground covered with light snow.
16th. Moderate rain at intervals through the day.
17th. Rain and mist in the morning. Rain in the evening.
18th. Grew cold fast towards night. The trees loaded with ice.
19th. Cold.
20th. Rather raw.
21st. Mist nearly all day, which froze as it fell. Snow towards evening. Trees heavily loaded with ice.
22d. Pleasant. Cloudless night.
23d. Very fine.
24th. Wind came to S. E'ly in the morning. Moderate rain in the afternoon. Heavy wind and rain in the evening. Ground quite bare of snow.
25th. Rainy.
26th. Variable.
27th. Very fine. Evening clear and mild.
28th. Very mild. Foggy towards night.
29th. Very fine.
30th Blustering in the afternoon and colder.
31st. Very cold and very severe in the evening.

February, 1845.

DAYS.	Barometer, reduced to 32° F. Sunrise.	At 1 P. M.	At 10 P. M.	Thermometer. Sunrise.	At 1 P. M.	At 10 P. M.	Daily mean.	Winds. (Direction and Force.) Sunrise.	At 1 P. M.	At 10 P. M.	Weather. (Tenths Cloudy.) Sunrise.	At 1 P. M.	At 10 P. M.	Rain and Snow in Inches of Water.
1	29.98	29.97	29.98	3	13	7	7.7	N. W. 3	N. W. 2	N. W. 2	0	0	0	
S 2	30.06	30.01	30.04	2	13	7	[illegible].3	N. W. 2	N. W. [illegible]	N. W. 2	[illegible]	0	0	
3	30.15	30.12	30.06	2	20	15	1 .3	N. W. 2	N. W.	N. W.		0	2	
4	29.88	29.59	28.97	15	24	27	2 .0	N. E. 2	N. E.	N. E. 4	1	Snow	Snow	1.00
5	28.71	28.70	28.82	28	32	18	2 .0	S. W. 2	S. W.	W'ly 2	1	10	0	
6	29.07	29.18	29.42	13	18	10	1 .7	N. W. 2	N. W.	N. W.		0	10	
7	29.54	29.63	29.76	5	16	16	1 .3	N. W. 2	N. W.	N. W.		0	0	
8	29.85	29.81	29.86	12	25	16	1 .7	S. W. 1	S. W.	N. W.		6	9	
S 9	29.86	29.80	29.79	12	24	14	1 .7	N. W. 1	N. W.	N. W.		0	0	
10	29.84	29.81	29.77	9	24	20	1 .7	N. W. 1	N. W.	S. W.		0	2	
11	29.60	29.60	29.60	27	38	33	3 .7	S. E'ly 2	S. E'ly	S. E'ly	Snow	10	10	0.10
12	29.42	29.25	29.53	36	44	32	3 .3	S. W. 1	S. W.	W'ly	Foggy	10	0	
13	30.04	30.07	30.21	8	13	6	.0	N. W. 3	N. W.	N. W.	0	0	0	
14	30.26	30.31	30.17	6	26	28	2 .0	N'ly 1	N'ly	N. E'ly	10	10	Snow	0.75
15	29.98	29.93	29.89	30	33	33	3 .0	N. E'ly 1	N. E'ly	N. E'ly	Misty	Misty	Rain	
S 16	29.69	29.59	29.56	44	45	36	4 .7	S. W. 2	S. W.	S. W.	Misty	Rain	0	
17	29.62	29.57	29.63	34	44	37	3 .3	S. W. 1	S. W.	S. W.	5	0	8	
18	29.72	29.73	29.83	31	41	32	3 .7	N. W. 1	N. W.	N. W.	0	0	0	
19	30.00	29.99	30.03	31	44	34	3 .3	N. W. 1	S. W.	S. W.	0	8	3	
20	29.89	29.85	29.82	34	45	41	4 .0	S'ly 1	S'ly	S. W.	10	5	5	
21	29.74	29.71	29.67	41	50	39	4 .3	S'ly 1	S'ly	S'ly	Foggy	5	Foggy	
22	29.75	29.73	29.86	37	51	40	4 .7	S'ly 0	N. W.	N. W.	Foggy	2	10	0.85
S 23	29.82	29.61	29.39	38	43	46	4 .3	N. E. 2	S. E.	S. E'ly	Misty	Rain	Rain	
24	29.50	29.53	29.61	37	47	39	4 .0	N. W. 2	N. W.	N. W. 1	0	0	0	
25	29.69	29.64	29.61	37	52	40	4 .0	N. W. 2	S. E'ly	S. W. 1	0	0	0	
26	29.50	29.46	29.51	36	53	36	4 .7	S'ly 1	S. E'ly	N. W. 2	0	3	0	
27	29.61	29.56	29.54	30	45	35	3 .7	N. W. 2	N. W.	N. W. 2	0	5	10	
28	29.57	29.55	29.65	30	37	28	3 .7	N. W. 2	N. W.	N. W. 2	2	8	0	
Means	29.72	29.69	29.70	23.9	34.3	27.3	...	1.6	1.6	1.4	4.5	4.4	4.6	2.70
									1.5			4.5		
REDUCED TO SEA LEVEL.														
Max.	30.44	30.49	30.39	41	53	46	43.3							
Min.	28.89	28.88	29.00	2	13	6	7.3							
Mean	29.90	29.87	29.88											
Range	1.55	1.61	1.39	39	40	40	36.0							
Mean of month	29.883			...	...	...	28.5							
Extreme range	1.61			...	...	...	51.0							

Prevailing winds from some point between— Days.
N. & E. 3
E. & S. 4
S. & W. 8
W. & N. 13

Days.
Clear 11
Variable . . . } 8
Cloudy . . . . }
Rain or snow fell on 9

REMARKS.

2d. Cold, but fine.
3d. Cold, but fine. Ground continues bare of snow.
4th. Began to snow at 8 or 9 A. M. Storm increased in violence all day. Wind very heavy in the evening N. E. and then E'ly. During the night, wind came round to S. W., and the storm ceased.
5th. Snow badly drifted, equal, perhaps, to ten inches on the level, hard packed. Flurry of snow during the night.
6th. Appearances of further storm at 10 P. M.
7th. Cold morning, but fine.
8th and 9th. Fine.
10th. Very pleasant.
11th From one to two inches of light snow in the morning. Flurry of snow in the evening.
12th. Moderate rain in the morning. Clear in the evening.
13th. Very clear and very cold.
14th. Began to snow moderately at 2 P. M., and continued through the afternoon.
15th. Mist and fog during the day. Heavy dashes of rain in the evening.
16th. Mist, with occasional light rain. Clear and very pleasant in the evening.
17th. Very mild and pleasant.
18th and 19th. Very fine.
20th. Mild.
21st. Very mild.
22d. Pleasant.
23d. Heavy thundershower at 2 P. M.; wind W'ly. Wind came again to E'ly, with rain.
24th. Very fine.
25th. Very fine. Aurora in the evening.
26th. Very fine. Gust of wind, with dashes of rain, at 9 P. M. Cleared soon.
27th and 28th. Pleasant.

March, 1845.

DAYS.	Barometer Sunrise.	At 1 P. M.	At 10 P. M.	Thermometer Sunrise.	At 1 P. M.	At 10 P. M.	Daily mean	Winds Sunrise.	At 1 P. M.	At 10 P. M.	Weather Sunrise.	At 1 P. M.	At 10 P. M.	Rain and Snow
1	29.65	29.61	29.69	27	48	34	36.3	N. E. 2	W'ly	W.	10	5	0	
S 2	29.85	29.78	29.67	30	44	37	37.0	S. E.	S'ly	S'ly	10	10	10	
3	29.28	29.39	29.83	50	46	32	42.7	S. W.	N. W.	N. W. 2	10	5	0	
4	30.06	30.02	29.99	28	44	36	36.0	N. W.	N. E. 2	N. E. 1	0	5	8	
5	29.56	29.10	...	35	52	...	...	E'ly 2	S'ly 4	...	Rain	Rain	...	1.33
6	29.71	29.86	29.99	38	47	36	40.3	N. W. 2	N. W. 3	N. W.	0	0	0	
7	29.99	29.94	29.95	31	53	34	39.3	N. E. 1	S'ly 2	N. E. 2	0	0	2	
8	29.84	29.75	29.70	36	43	39	39.3	N. E. 1	N. W. 1	S'ly 1	Foggy	10	2	
S 9	29.59	29.59	29.74	41	36	36	37.7	N. E. 1	N. E. 2	N. W. 1	Misty	Rain	3	0.25
10	29.87	29.79	29.69	33	44	31	36.0	N'ly 1	N. E. 2	N. E. 2	10	10	Snow	
11	29.56	29.72	29.93	28	27	20	25.0	N. E. 2	N. E. 3	N. W. 1	Snow	Snow	0	0.75
12	30.08	30.06	30.03	15	38	27	26.7	N. W. 1	E'ly 1	N. W. 1	0	0	0	
13	30.02	29.99	30.00	25	46	35	35.3	N. W. 1	S. W. 1	S. W.	0	2	3	
14	29.83	29.60	29.35	34	38	37	36 3	E'ly 2	E'ly 2	E'ly 1	Snow	Rain	Misty	1.00
15	29.44	29.49	29.58	34	35	25	34.7	N. W. 2	N. W. 4	N. W. 1	10	0	0	
S 16	29.45	29.33	29.33	24	32	24	26.7	N. W. 2	W'ly 3	N. W. 1	0	10	2	
17	29.20	29.14	29.22	25	40	30	31.7	S. W. 1	S. W. 2	W'ly 1	3	7	3	
18	29.31	29.31	29.30	28	39	34	33.7	W'ly 1	W'ly 2	E'ly 2	0	5	10	
19	29.44	29.43	29.46	24	30	26	26.7	N. W. 1	W'ly 3	W'ly 2	0	5	5	
20	29.43	29.40	29.53	24	35	32	30.3	W'ly 2	W'ly 3	N. W. 3	0	9	10	
21	29.61	29.62	29.77	28	30	22	26.7	N. W. 3	N. W. 3	N. W. 1	3	0	0	
22	29.82	29.78	29.81	20	39	34	31.0	N. W. 3	N. W. 2	N. W. 1	0	0	0	
S 23	29.81	29.79	29.63	32	50	42	41.3	N. W. 1	S. W. 2	S. W. 3	0	3	10	0.20
24	29.52	29.56	29.64	38	47	39	41.3	S. W. 1	S. W. 2	W'ly 2	10	7	10	
25	29.75	29.81	29.99	36	40	31	35.7	N. W. 2	N. W. 4	N. W. 1	5	0	0	
26	30.16	30.09	30.01	26	41	37	34.7	N. W. 1	S'ly 2	S'ly 2	0	0	10	
27	29.83	29.78	29.88	40	62	45	49.0	S. W. 2	S. W. 2	S. W. 1	10	2	0	
28	29.81	29.78	30.05	41	70	39	50.0	S. E. 1	S. E'ly 1	N. E. 2	7	6	10	
29	30.10	30.08	30.00	38	51	41	40.0	N. E. 1	N. E. 1	E'ly 1	Foggy	10	Foggy	
S 30	30.04	29.99	30.08	41	59	47	49.0	S. E. 2	W'ly 3	S. W. 1	Hazy	0	0	
31	30.15	30.08	29.94	44	63	50	52.3	N'ly 1	S. W. 2	S. E. 1	Foggy	2	2	
Means	29.79	29.70	29.76	32.1	44.0	34.4	...	1.5	2.3	1.5	5.4	5.0	4.3	3.53
									1.8			4.9		
REDUCED TO SEA LEVEL.														
Max.	30.34	30.27	30.26	50	70	50	52.3							
Min.	29.38	29.28	29.40	15	27	20	26.7							
Mean	29.91	29.88	29.94											
Range	0.96	0.99	0.86	35	43	30	25.6							
Mean of month	29.910			...	...	...	36.8							
Extreme range	1.06			...	...	...	55.0							

Prevailing winds from some point between— Days.
N. & E. 5
E. & S. 5
S. & W. 9
W. & N. 12

Days.
Clear 7
Variable . . . } 16
Cloudy . . . . }
Rain or snow fell on 8

REMARKS.

3d. Squall of rain from N. W. at 11 A. M. Clear in the afternoon, with wind blustering from N. W.
4th. Very mild.
5th. Rain and heavy wind in the morning. Clear in the evening.
6th. Very pleasant.
7th. Pleasant.
8th. Mild.
9th. Moderate rain in the morning.
10th. Began to snow moderately at 5 P. M.; wind E'ly.
11th. Snowed fast from early in the morning to 2 P. M., seven or eight inches, rather damp. Clear in the evening.
12th. Pleasant overhead.
13th. Very pleasant.
14th. Moderate rain all day.
15th. Pleasant. Cool in the evening.
16th. Raw and cold.
17th. Extraordinary halos about the sun were seen this morning at 7 o'clock.
18th. Raw towards night, with some snow. Flurry of snow in the night.
19th. Ground covered with snow. Cold and blustering.
20th. Very blustering and raw.
21st. Very blustering and uncomfortable.
22d. Pleasant. Evening perfectly clear and transparent.
23d. Pleasant in the morning. Wind raw in the afternoon. Appearances of rain in the evening. Showers during the night.
24th. Pleasant.
25th. Blustering. Very clear evening.
26th. Raw in the afternoon.
27th. Very fine, mild, and warm.
28th. Very warm from 10 A. M. to 3 P. M. Wind came to N. E. from 3 to 4 P. M., and grew cool fast.
29th. Rather raw.
30th and 31st. Very pleasant.

April, 1845.

DAYS.	BAROMETER, REDUCED TO 32° F. At 6 A. M.	At 1 P. M.	At 10 P. M.	THERMOMETER. At 6 A. M.	At 1 P. M.	At 10 P. M.	Daily mean.	WINDS. (DIRECTION AND FORCE.) At 6 A. M.	At 1 P. M.	At 10 P. M.	WEATHER. (TENTHS CLOUDY.) At 6 A. M.	At 1 P. M.	At 10 P. M.	RAIN AND SNOW IN INCHES OF WATER.
1	29.61	29.43	29.49	51	55	...	...	S. W. 1	S'ly 2	...	10	Rain	...	0.48
2	29.55	29.64	29.62	...	52	45	...	...	S. W. 2	S. W. 2	...	10	10	
3	29.70	29.74	29.81	38	42	32	37.3	W'ly 2	N. W. 4	N. W. 1	2	0	0	
4	29.47	29.28	29.48	34	59	41	44.7	S. E. 3	W'ly 3	N. W. 1	10	0	0	
5	29.64	29.61	29.74	32	43	35	36.7	N. W. 2	N. W. 3	N'ly 2	0	5	6	
S 6	29.76	29.73	29.73	30	45	34	36.3	N. E. 1	S. E. 2	S. E. 1	10	5	0	
7	29.74	29.70	29.61	38	49	40	42.3	S. W. 2	S. W. 2	S. W. 2	10	9	5	
8	29.50	29.44	29.41	33	34	30	32.3	N'ly 1	N. W. 2	N. W. 4	10	10	0	
9	29.56	29.73	29.74	30	42	35	35.7	N. W. 3	N. W. 3	N. W. 1	5	0	0	
10	29.50	29.34	29.36	40	41	46	42.3	S. W. 2	S. W.	S. W. 1	10	Rain	0	
11	29.42	29.46	29.66	36	44	32	37.3	N. W. 2	N. W. 2	N. W. 2	0	10	0	
12	29.74	29.76	29.66	31	40	...	...	N. W. 2	N. W. 1	...	0	...	...	
S 13	29.70	29.42	29.36	38	52	44	44.7	S. W. 2	S'ly 2	S. W. 4	...	...	...	
14	29.74	29.75	29.77	44	54	44	47.3	N. W. 1	N. W. 1	N. W. 2	...	...	...	
15	29.78	29.72	29.77	44	62	44	50.0	N. W. 1	N. W. 2	N. W. 1	...	...	...	
16	29.62	29.61	29.77	42	52	37	44.7	E. 1	S. E. 2	N. E. 2	...	...	Rain	} 1.10
17	29.80	29.85	29.95	37	37	37	37.0	N. E. 2	N. E. 3	N. E. 2	Rain	Misty	10	}
18	30.02	30.02	30.02	38	52	40	43.3	N. E. 2	N. E. 2	N. E.	10	10	10, Shr.	0.40
19	29.89	29.78	29.75	38	55	39	44.0	N. E. 1	S'ly 1	N. E. 1	Misty	10	10	0.22
S 20	29.74	29.73	29.77	38	47	37	40.7	N. E. 1	N. E. 1	N. E. 2	10	10	10	
21	29.73	29.71	29.69	38	50	48	45.3	N. E. 2	N. E. 3	N'ly 2	10	10	10	
22	29.74	29.79	29.82	44	61	46	50.3	N. W. 2	N. E. 3	N. E. 2	0	0	0	
23	29.88	29.83	29.82	43	61	44	49.3	N. W. 2	S. E. 2	S'ly 1	0	0	0	
24	29.80	29.79	29.66	46	72	51	56.3	S'ly 2	S'ly 2	S'ly 2	5	2	2	
25	29.78	29.78	29.77	53	59	49	53.7	E'ly 1	N. E. 2	S'ly 2	5	8	10, Shr.	0.14
26	29.73	29.78	29.84	40	55	41	45.3	N. E. 2	N. E. 2	N. E. 2	10	10	10	
S 27	29.73	29.80	29.65	43	58	52	51.0	S. E'ly 2	S'ly 2	S'ly 1	Foggy	10	10	
28	29.71	29.72	29.82	52	71	54	59.0	N'ly 1	N. W. 2	S. W. 1	6	2	10	
29	29.79	29.92	30.06	52	...	38	...	N'ly 2	...	N. E. 1	8	...	0	
30	30.15	30.10	30.04	36	59	44	46.3	N. E. 1	S. E. 3	S. E. 1	0	3	5	
Means	29.72	29.70	29.72	39.7	51.6	42.1	...	1.7	2.2	1.7	6.0	6.0	5.1	2.34
								1.9			5.7			
REDUCED TO SEA LEVEL.														
Max.	30.33	30.28	30.24	52	72	54	59.0							
Min.	29.60	29.46	29.54	30	34	30	32.3							
Mean	29.90	29.88	29.90											
Range	0.73	0.82	0.70	22	38	24	26.7							
Mean of month	29.893			...	...	...	44.6							
Extreme range	0.87			...	...	...	42.0							

Prevailing winds from some point between— Days.
N. & E. 9
E. & S. 6
S. & W. 6
W. & N. 9

Days.
Clear 6
Variable . . . } 9
Cloudy . . . . }
Rain fell on . . 11
(4 days omitted.)

REMARKS.

1st. Heavy shower at 2 P. M.
2d. Dashes of rain in the evening.
3d. Very blustering. Light fall of snow during the night.
4th. Ground covered with snow in the morning, which soon disappeared.
5th. Rather blustering.
6th. Raw and cold.
7th. Raw and unpleasant. Some dashes of rain, mixed with hail, in the morning. Flurry of snow during the night.
8th. Ground covered with snow in the morning. Air full of snow during a large part of the day, which, with a strong wind, has been truly wintry.
9th. More pleasant.
10th. Very light showers. Clear in the evening.
11th. Variable. Dashes of rain in the afternoon; wind at N. W. Very clear in the evening.
16th. Rain during the night.
17th. Rain in the morning. Cloudy in the afternoon.
18th. Cloudy, with some mist. Showers during the night.
19th. Mild. Showers during the night.
20th. Rather raw.
21st. Variable.
22d, 23d, and 24th. Very pleasant.
25th. Very pleasant. Shower, with thunder, during the night.
26th. Rather raw.
27th. Rather milder. Fog and appearances of rain.
28th. Very pleasant.
29th. Wind came from N'ly to N. E., and grew cooler from 8 to 10 A. M.
30th. Pleasant.

May, 1845.

DAYS.	BAROMETER At 6 A. M.	At 1 P. M.	At 10 P. M.	THERMOMETER At 6 A. M.	At 1 P. M.	At 10 P. M.	Daily mean.	WINDS At 6 A. M.	At 1 P. M.	At 10 P. M.	WEATHER At 6 A. M.	At 1 P. M.	At 10 P. M.	RAIN AND SNOW
1	...	...	29.56	...	...	51	...	...	...	S'ly	...	...	8	
2	29.53	...	29.81	55	...	51	...	N. W. 2	...	W'ly 2	4	...	0	
3	29.83	29.79	29.78	44	70	54	56.0	N. W. 2	W'ly 3	S. W. 2	0	0	9	
S 4	29.75	29.70	29.60	55	65	60	60.0	S. W. 2	S. W. 3	S. W. 3	10	2	10	
5	29.64	29.71	29.79	59	59	50	56.0	S. W. 2	W'ly 3	W'ly 1	10	10	5	
6	29.85	29.80	29.66	41	61	47	49.7	N. W. 1	S. E. 2	S'ly 1	3	1	2	
7	29.50	29.45	29.49	46	67	59	57.3	S. W. 2	S'ly 3	S'ly 2	Rain	3	10	
8	29.64	29.72	29.83	37	46	41	41.3	N. W. 2	N. E. 3	N. W. 1	Rain	10	0	
9	29.87	29.86	30.05	37	54	41	44.0	N. W. 1	N. W. 2	N. E. 1	2	3	0	
10	30.22	30.19	30.13	37	59	44	46.7	N. E. 1	S. E. 2	S'ly 3	0	0	0	
S 11	29.96	29.86	29.79	46	77	68	63.7	S. W. 2	S. W. 2	S. W. 3	0	0	2	
12	29.80	29.75	29.74	63	89	72	74.7	S. W. 1	S. W. 3	W'ly 2	0	3	2	
13	29.85	29.84	29.82	50	74	57	60.3	N. E. 2	N. E. 2	E'ly	0	6	Hazy	
14	29.72	29.63	29.49	60	70	59	63.0	S. W. 2	S'ly 2	S'ly 2	5	5	10	
15	29.39	29.35	29.50	57	67	47	57.0	S. W. 2	S'ly 2	N. W. 2	Rain	10	10	0.25
16	29.61	29.70	29.74	39	41	43	41.0	N. E'ly 2	N. E. 2	N. E. 3	Rain	Rain	10	}
17	29.72	29.65	29.65	41	42	42	41.7	N. E. 4	N. E. 5	N. E. 4	10	Rain	Rain	} 1.30
S 18	29.54	29.53	29.49	43	52	50	48.3	N. E. 3	N'ly 2	S'ly 1	Rain	10	10	}
19	29.55	29.56	29.60	52	75	57	61.3	S. W. 1	W'ly 3	W'ly 2	10	3	4, Sh'r	0.13
20	29.64	29.63	29.65	54	64	53	57.0	S. W. 2	S. E. 2	W'ly 2	3	10	8, Sh'r	0.12
21	29.71	29.71	29.79	52	66	54	57.3	W'ly 1	W'ly 3	W'ly 1	7	2	0	
22	29.79	29.75	29.63	53	64	52	56.3	W'ly 2	S'ly 3	S'ly 2	2	10	Rain	0.95
23	29.63	29.64	29.64	47	64	52	54.3	N. E. 2	W'ly 2	S. W. 1	10	9	9	
24	29.60	29.54	29.62	48	61	46	51.7	N. W. 1	N'ly 2	N. W. 3	0	5	0	
S 25	29.63	29.59	29.63	40	44	44	42.7	N. W. 2	W'ly 2	N. W. 1	0	Rain	0	0.05
26	29.60	29.44	29.51	45	63	58	55.3	W'ly 3	W'ly 4	W'ly 2	5	2	Shower	0.05
27	29.71	29.70	29.71	52	67	56	58.3	W'ly 2	S. W. 2	S'ly 2	0	0	0	
28	29.76	29.63	29.63	58	73	57	62.7	S. W. 2	S. W. 4	S. W. 2	2	0	0	
29	29.65	29.53	29.64	58	64	47	56.3	S. W. 2	S. W. 2	N. W. 2	10	Rain	10	
[illegible]	[illegible]	[illegible]	[illegible]	[illegible]	[illegible]	[illegible]	[illegible]	[illegible]	[illegible]	[illegible]	[illegible]	[illegible]	[illegible]	
31	30.02	29.99	29.93	42	64	49	51.7	N. W. 1	N. W. 1	S. W.	0	0	0	
Means	29.71	29.69	29.70	48.5	62.6	51.7	...	1.9	2.5	2.0	5.0	5.0	5.0	2.75
								2.1			5.0			
REDUCED TO SEA LEVEL.														
Max.	30.40	30.37	30.31	63	89	72	74.7							
Min.	29.57	29.53	29.67	37	41	41	41.0							
Mean	29.89	29.87	29.88											
Range	0.83	0.84	0.64	26	48	31	33.7							
Mean of month	29.880			...	...	...	54.3							
Extreme range	0.87			...	...	...	52.0							

Prevailing winds from some point between— Days.
N. & E. 6
E. & S. 3
S. & W. 15
W. & N. 7

Days.
Clear 7
Variable . . . } 12
Cloudy . . . . }
Rain fell on . . 17

REMARKS.

1st, 2d, and 3d. Pleasant.
4th. Appearances of rain this evening.
5th. Mild, with appearances of rain.
6th. Pleasant. The sun rose eclipsed. The eclipse, by observation, ended at 5 h. 14 m. 52 s. A. M., mean time. The atmosphere was quite clear.
7th. Pleasant. Sprinkling of rain at sunrise. Cleared in the morning.
8th. Air very raw and cold in the morning, with sprinkling of rain mixed with snow. Cleared about 3 P. M. The transit of Mercury occurred this day, beginning about 11 h. 34 m. A. M.—not observed in consequence of clouds. Observed ending—third contact, 6 h. 1 m. 44 s.; fourth and last contact, 6 h. 5 m. 14 s., mean time at Providence. Observed with a four-foot refractor. Air clear.
9th. White frost in the College yard—not very copious.
10th. White frost. Air raw and cool in the evening.
11th. Very warm; the ground very dry.
12th. Excessively hot for the season.
13th. Warm. Very dry, and no signs of rain.
14th. Some indications of rain.
15th. Light showers at sunrise, with thunder. Occasional sprinkling.
24th. Light frost in some places in the vicinity.
25th. Showery and cold. Snowed briskly for fifteen or twenty minutes between 10 and 11 A. M.
26th. Light shower at 9 P. M.
27th. Very pleasant.
28th. Very blustering and dusty.
29th. Occasional dashes of rain.
[illegible]

June, 1845.

DAYS.	BAROMETER, REDUCED TO 32° F. At 6 A. M.	At 1 P. M.	At 10 P. M.	THERMOMETER. At 6 A. M.	At 1 P. M.	At 10 P. M.	Daily mean.	WINDS. (DIRECTION AND FORCE.) At 6 A. M.	At 1 P. M.	At 10 P. M.	WEATHER. (TENTHS CLOUDY.) At 6 A. M.	At 1 P. M.	At 10 P. M.	RAIN AND SNOW IN INCHES OF WATER.
S 1	29.91	29.85	29.83	53	67	58	59.3	S. W.	S. W.	S. W.	0	0	0	
2	29.84	29.82	29.88	54	79	62	65.0	S. W.	W'ly 3	S. W. 2	Hazy	0	0	
3	29.90	29.85	29.84	57	80	62	66.3	S. W. 2	S. W. 2	S. W. 2	0	0	0	
4	29.81	29.77	29.74	59	80	62	67.0	S. W. 1	S. W. 2	S. W. 2	2	0	0	
5	29.68	29.59	29.67	60	81	65	68.7	S. W. 2	S. W. 3	N. W. 1	2	2	0	
6	29.83	29.78	29.75	57	73	60	63.3	N. W. 1	S. W. 2	N. W. 2	6	7	5	
7	29.82	29.83	29.81	53	70	59	60.7	N. W. 1	N. W.	S. W. 2	0	0	0	
S 8	29.75	29.70	29.65	60	83	66	69.7	S. W. 2	S. W. 1	S. W. 1	5	0	0	
9	29.63	29.60	29.67	72	90	71	77.7	S. W. 2	W'ly 3	S. W. 1	0	0	0	
10	29.73	29.75	29.69	67	84	74	75.0	W'ly 1	S. W. 3	S. W. 2	2	2	8	
11	29.58	29.50	29.65	65	65	56	62.0	S'ly 2	N. W. 2	N. W. 1	Rain	10	0	0.48
12	29.68	29.60	29.54	56	71	61	62.7	N. W. 1	S. W. 3	S. W. 2	0	5	10, Sh'r	0.58
13	29.44	29.46	29.59	61	83	65	69.7	N. W. 2	N. W. 2	S. W. 1	4	2	0	
14	29.56	29.52	29.68	65	62	63	63.3	S. W. 1	N. E. 2	W'ly 2	10	Rain	2	0.12
S 15	29.88	29.89	29.86	58	72	59	63.0	N. W. 2	N. W. 2	S. W. 2	0	0	5	
16	29.75	29.68	29.62	62	82	66	70.0	S. W. 2	W'ly 2	S. W. 2	Sh'r, 10	2	5, Sh'r	0.20
17	29.61	29.69	29.83	60	67	55	60.7	N. W. 1	N. W. 3	N. W. 3	10	0	0	
18	29.93	29.94	29.94	55	72	58	61.7	N. W. 2	N. W. 2	W'ly 1	0	3	3	
19	29.96	29.94	29.94	58	72	57	62.3	W'ly 2	W'ly 1	S. W. 1	10	0	0	
20	29.95	29.84	29.79	57	72	59	62.7	S. W. 1	S. E. 3	S. W. 2	10	0	3	
21	29.59	29.51	29.59	60	72	59	63.7	S. W. 1	S. W. 2	N. E. 1	Foggy	Shower	3	0.30
S 22	29.65	29.69	29.64	56	71	59	62.0	N'ly 1	N. W. 2	S'ly 1	0	0	0	
23	29.54	29.53	29.54	59	67	62	62.7	S. W. 1	S. W. 1	S. W.	Sh'r, 0	10	2	0.12
24	29.54	29.50	29.48	63	83	65	70.3	S. W. 2	S. W. 3	S. W. 2	0	3	5, Sh'r	0.35
25	29.56	29.56	29.60	61	74	61	65.3	N'ly 2	N. W. 2	N. W. 2	0	3	0	
26	29.68	29.64	29.63	54	73	62	63.0	N. W. 1	S. W. 2	S. W. 1	0	0	0	
27	29.63	29.61	29.65	56	75	63	64.7	N. W. 1	W'ly 3	N. W. 1	0	0	0	
28	29.65	29.60	29.52	55	79	61	65.0	S. W. 1	S. W. 1	S'ly 1	3	5	Rain	0.17
S 29	29.59	29.59	29.69	57	68	52	59.0	N. E. 1	E'ly 2	N. E. 1	3	2	3	
30	29.70	29.73	29.73	52	58	50	53.3	N. E. 3	N. E. 3	N. E. 2	10	10	Rain	
Means	29.71	29.68	29.70	58.7	74.2	61.1	...	1.5	2.2	1.6	3.9	2.9	1.9	2.32
								1.8			2.9			
REDUCED TO SEA LEVEL.								Prevailing winds from some point between— Days.			Days.			
Max.	30.14	30.12	30.12	72	90	71	77.7	N. & E. 3			Clear 10			
Min.	29.62	29.64	29.66	52	58	50	53.3	E. & S. 1			Variable . . . } 11			
Mean	29.89	29.86	29.88					S. & W. 17			Cloudy . . . . }			
Range	0.52	0.48	0.46	20	32	21	24.4	W. & N. 9			Rain fell on . . 9			
Mean of month	29.877			...	...	...	64.7							
Extreme range	0.52			...	...	...	40.0							

REMARKS.

1st to 4th. Very fine.

5th. Appearances of thunder and rain in the afternoon. Ground dry.

6th. A good deal of haze.

7th. Very fine.

8th. Very hot sun. Thunder, and appearances of rain at the S. W., at 7 A. M.

9th. Very hot, and fresh wind at W'ly.

10th. Very hot.

11th. Fine rain in the morning. Clear in the evening.

12th. Appearances of rain in evening. Thunder-shower during the night.

13th. Very fine.

14th. Light showers in the morning.

15th. Morning cloudless and very transparent. Halo about the moon in the evening.

16th. Very fine. Saw the comet this evening, at 9½ o'clock, in the N W., quite conspicuous and bright in the telescope, but not visible to the naked eye. Thundershower in the night.

17th. Very fine. Evening very clear. Comet visible to the naked eye.

18th. Very fine. Comet not visible on account of haze.

19th. Sprinkling of rain from 7 to 8 A. M. Clear in the afternoon. Comet visible, but diminished in brightness.

20th. Very fine.

21st. Showery from 10 A. M. to 1 P. M. Smart shower from 4 to 5 P. M.

22d. Very fine.

23d. Sprinkling of rain in the morning, with shower before noon.

24th. Fine shower from 7 to 8 P. M.

25th. Very fine evening, very clear. The comet distinctly visible, being about 1° N. and W. of the star Nu in the Crab (ν Cancri), observed from 9½ to 10 P. M. This is the first good evening since the 19th.

26th. Fine. The comet visible this evening. Air clear.

27th. Fine. The comet again visible, but quite faint.

28th. Commenced raining very moderately from 7 to 8 P. M.

29th. Fine, but cool.

30th. Very cold for the season. Moderate rain in the evening.

July, 1845.

DAYS.	BAROMETER At 6 A. M.	At 1 P. M.	At 10 P. M.	THERMOMETER At 6 A. M.	At 1 P. M.	At 10 P. M.	Daily mean.	WINDS At 6 A. M.	At 1 P. M.	At 10 P. M.	WEATHER At 6 A. M.	At 1 P. M.	At 10 P. M.	RAIN
1	29.71	29.73	29.75	49	62	54	55.0	N. E. 2	N. E. 1	E'ly 1	Misty	7	2	0.32
2	29.80	29.72	29.67	56	61	63	60.0	S'ly 1	S'ly	S'ly 3	10	10	10, R'n	} 1.20
3	29.59	29.48	29.50	63	67	63	64.3	S'ly 1	S. W. 1	S'ly 1	Misty	Misty	Rain	}
4	29.55	29.59	29.61	56	70	62	62.7	N. W. 1	N. W. 1	N. W. 1	0	5	3	
5	29.71	29.68	29.72	56	72	60	62.7	N. W. 1	N. W. 2	W'ly	0	3	0	
S 6	29.78	29.80	29.70	69	79	68	72.0	W'ly	W'ly	S. W.	2	2	0	
7	29.78	29.57	29.56	67	86	75	76.0	W'ly	S. W. 2	W'ly	0	1	2	
8	29.58	29.56	29.56	69	86	70	75.0	N. W. 1	N. W. 2	N. W. 1	0	2	0	
9	29.70	...	29.75	61	...	63	69.0	N. W. 2	...	N. W. 1	0	...	0	
10	29.86	29.82	29.78	56	78	65	66.3	N. W. 1	N. W. 2	W'ly 2	0	0	0	
11	29.68	29.62	29.56	63	86	74	74.3	W'ly 1	W'ly 2	S. W. 1	0	0	3	
12	29.65	29.49	29.41	72	89	76	79.0	S. W. 1	S. W. 2	S. W. 2	0	0	0	
S 13	29.48	29.51	29.52	67	83	65	71.7	N. E. 2	N. E. 1	S. W. 1	0	0	2	
14	29.48	29.41	29.49	62	88	69	73.0	S. W'ly 1	S. W. 1	S. W. 1	2	3	5, Sh'r	0.33
15	29.50	29.48	29.53	70	84	74	76.0	S. W. 1	S. W. 3	S. W. 1	2	1	5	
16	29.56	29.56	29.56	72	89	73	78.0	N. E'ly	N. E'ly	S'ly 2	2	2	Foggy	
17	29.51	29.46	29.50	72	83	74	76.3	S'ly 1	S. W'ly 3	W'ly 1	Foggy	2	0	
18	29.57	29.60	29.60	74	83	69	75.3	N. W. 2	N. W. 3	N. W. 2	0	0	0	
19	29.83	29.82	29.81	60	76	67	67.7	N. W. 2	N. W. 1	S. W. 2	0	6	7	
S 20	29.78	29.72	29.68	62	75	67	68.0	S'ly 2	S'ly 3	S'ly 2	2	5	8	
21	29.59	29.54	29.51	70	87	74	77.0	S'ly 3	S. W. 3	S. W. 2	3	3	0	
22	29.47	29.36	29.41	70	82	68	73.3	S. W. 2	S. W. 3	N. W. 1	Rain	2	0	0.35
23	29.43	29.43	29.50	63	75	60	66.0	N. W. 2	N. W. 3	N. W. 2	0	3	0	
24	29.51	...	29.56	55	...	60	...	N. W. 2	...	N. W. 2	0	...	0	
25	29.59	29.59	29.59	54	72	60	62.0	N. W. 1	N. W. 2	N. W. 1	3	2	0	
26	29.59	29.55	29.54	60	78	64	67.3	N. W'ly	S. W. 3	W'ly	0	5	0	
S 27	29.45	29.37	29.37	60	63	56	59.7	N. E. 2	E'ly 3	N'ly 1	10, R'n	8	0	0.33
28	29.34	29.31	29.39	58	75	60	64.3	N. W. 1	S. W. 2	N. W. 1	0	3	0	
29	...	29.44	29.44	...	72	66	...	...	W'ly	S. W.	...	5	10	
30	29.41	29.39	29.41	67	78	67	70.7	S. W.	S. W.	S'ly	10	8	10, R'n	0.57
31	29.40	29.51	29.57	68	76	64	69.3	W'ly	W'ly	N. W.	10	5	0	
Means	29.59	29.56	29.57	63.5	77.8	66.1	...	1.5	2.1	1.5	3.2	3.6	2.8	3.10
								1.7			3.2			
REDUCED TO SEA LEVEL.								Prevailing winds from some point between— Days.			Days.			
Max.	30.04	30.00	29.99	74	89	75	79.0	N. & E. 4			Clear 12			
Min.	29.52	29.49	29.55	49	61	54	55.0	E. & S. 1			Variable . . . } 13			
Mean	29.77	29.74	29.75					S. & W. 14			Cloudy . . . . }			
Range	0.52	0.51	0.44	25	28	21	24.0	W. & N. 12			Rain fell on . . 6			
Mean of month	29.753			...	...	...	69.1							
Extreme range	0.55			...	...	...	40.0							

REMARKS.

2d. Appearances of rain.

3d. Heavy thundershower from 5 to 6 P. M. Rain continued in the evening.

4th. Very fine.

5th and 6th. Pleasant.

7th. Very warm sun.

8th. Very hot sun, with fine breeze at mid-day.

9th. Very fine and cooler.

10th. Very fine.

11th and 12th. Very hot sun.

13th. Weather still hot.

14th. Shower at 4 P. M., with heavy thunder and wind.

15th. Very warm.

16th. Appearance of thunder-clouds in the afternoon, but no rain.

17th. Sprinkling of rain, with thunder, at 5 P. M.

18th. Very fine. Dew-point at 50° at 2 P. M.

19th. Fine.

20th. Air damp. Appearances of rain.

21st. Very hot. Dew-point 67° at 2 P. M.

22d. Thundershower at 4 A. M. Dew-point 60° at 2 P. M.

23d. Very fine. Dew-point 52° at 2 P. M. Abundance of lightning low down in the N. and E. during the evening.

24th. Very fine.

25th. Very fine. Pleasantly cool.

26th. Sprinkling of rain in the afternoon.

27th. Dew-point 53°, thermometer 60°, and raining moderately at 9 A. M., which continued till 2 P. M., at which time the lower clouds were passing briskly from the N. E., while the upper ones were passing slowly from the west.

28th. Thunder and appearances of rain in the afternoon.

August, 1845.

Days.	Barometer, reduced to 32° F. At 6 A. M.	At 1 P. M.	At 10 P. M.	Thermometer. At 6 A. M.	At 1 P. M.	At 10 P. M.	Daily mean.	Winds. (Direction and Force.) At 6 A. M.	At 1 P. M.	At 10 P. M.	Weather. (Tenths Cloudy.) At 6 A. M.	At 1 P. M.	At 10 P. M.	Rain and Snow in Inches of Water.
1	29.86	29.86	29.93	64	78	62	68.0	N. W.	N. W.	W.	0	1	0	
2	...	...	29.93	...	...	67	...	...	...	S'ly	...	...	5	
S 3	29.90	29.90	29.88	62	74	64	66.7	S. W. 1	S. W. 1	S'ly 1	10	7	0	
4	29.89	29.84	29.82	62	81	69	70.7	N. W. 1	W'ly 2	W'ly 1	0	0	0	
5	29.83	29.81	29.81	64	83	71	72.7	W'ly 1	S. W. 2	S'ly	0	4	0	
6	29.82	29.81	29.80	67	80	68	71.7	S. W. 1	S. W. 2	S'ly 1	7	0	0	
7	29.77	29.77	29.74	66	77	69	70.7	N. E. 1	S'ly 1	S'ly 1	Foggy	8	0	
8	29.73	29.72	29.72	66	80	68	71.3	S'ly 1	S. E'ly 2	S. W. 1	3	1	0	
9	29.73	...	...	69	...	...	...	S. W. 1	...	...	8	...	...	
S 10	...	...	...	...	...	...	...	...	...	...	...	...	...	
11	...	...	...	...	...	...	...	...	...	...	...	...	...	2.50
12	...	...	...	...	...	...	...	...	...	...	...	...	...	
13	...	...	...	...	...	...	...	...	...	...	...	...	...	
14	...	...	...	...	...	...	...	...	...	...	...	...	...	
15	...	...	...	...	...	...	...	...	...	...	...	...	...	
16	...	...	...	...	...	...	...	...	...	...	...	...	...	
S 17	...	...	...	...	...	...	...	...	...	...	...	...	...	
18	...	...	...	...	...	...	...	...	...	...	...	...	...	
19	...	...	...	...	...	...	...	...	...	...	...	...	...	
20	...	...	...	...	...	...	...	...	...	...	...	...	...	
21	...	...	...	...	...	...	...	...	...	...	...	...	...	1.46
22	...	...	...	...	...	...	...	...	...	...	...	...	...	1.30
23	...	...	29.70	...	...	73	..	...	...	S. W. 2	...	...	8	0.15
S 24	29.71	29.68	29.66	73	85	72	76.7	W'ly 1	N. W. 1	N. W. 1	9	2	0	
25	29.71	29.71	29.69	66	79	67	70.7	N. W. 2	N. W. 2	S. W. 1	0	0	0	
26	29.64	29.63	29.70	67	82	68	72.3	S. W. 1	N. W. 1	N. E. 1	0	2	4	
27	29.68	29.59	29.68	70	77	55	67.3	E'ly 1	S'ly 1	N. E. 2	8	10	Rain	0.22
28	29.82	29.90	30.05	55	67	53	58.3	N. E. 2	N. E. 2	N. E. 1	2	4	0	
29	30.06	...	29.92	47	67	56	56.7	N. E. 1	...	N. E'ly	0	...	2	
30	...	29.60	29.60	56	72	63	63.7	...	S'ly	W'ly 1	5	10	0	
31	29.60	29.59	29.64	58	74	61	64.3	N. W. 2	N. W. 2	N. W. 2	0	0	0	
Means	29.78	29.74	29.78	63.2	77.1	65.1	...	1.2	1.6	1.2	3.9	3.6	1.7	5.63
									1.3			3.1		
REDUCED TO SEA LEVEL.														
Max.	30.24	30.08	30.23	73	85	73	76.7	Prevailing winds from some point between—		Days.			Days.	
Min.	29.78	29.77	29.78	47	67	53	56.7	N. & E.		2	Clear		6	
Mean	29.96	29.92	29.96					E. & S.		3	Variable		} 7	
Range	0.46	0.31	0.45	26	18	20	20.0	S. & W.		7	Cloudy			
Mean of month	29.947			...	...	...	68.4	W .& N.		6	Rain fell on		5	
Extreme range	0.47			...	...	...	38.0				(13 days omitted.)			

REMARKS.

1st, 2d, and 3d. Fine.

4th. Very fine.

5th and 6th. Very warm sun.

7th. Fine. Sprinkling of rain at 5 P. M.

8th. Very burning sun.

11th. Heavy rain nearly all day.

21st. Began to rain about 5 A. M.

22d. Appearances of frost in many places in the vicinity. Grape-vine in my garden was slightly touched with frost.

23d. Showery in the afternoon.

24th. Very hot and sultry.

25th. Fine. Extraordinary meteor at 7 h. 50 m. P. M. This meteor was seen by many persons. It was followed by a report resembling the sound of a cannon, accompanied with a prolonged rumbling. The interval of time between the light and the report was probably (*i. e.*, from the best information I can collect) one minute, or from 1 m. to 1 m. 25 or 30 sec. I did not see it myself. It passed south of the zenith towards the east, and was seen in Norwich, New Haven, Slatersville, and various other places.

26th. Very warm.

27th. At about 3 P. M., wind came to N. E., with moderate rain, and a sudden fall of temperature.

28th. Quite cool.

29th. Fine.

30th. Appearances of rain.

31st. Very fine.

September, 1845.

Days.	Barometer. At 6 A. M.	At 1 P. M.	At 10 P. M.	Thermometer. At 6 A. M.	At 1 P. M.	At 10 P. M.	Daily mean	Winds. At 6 A. M.	At 1 P. M.	At 10 P. M.	Weather. At 6 A. M.	At 1 P. M.	At 10 P. M.	Rain and Snow in Inches of Water.
1	29.74	29.70	29.65	52	68	63	61.0	N. W. 1	E'ly 2	S. W. 1	0	0	10	
2	29.55	...	29.36	66	...	68	...	S'ly 2	...	S. W. 1	8	Rain	5	} 0.30
3	29.29	...	...	68	...	64	...	S. W. 1	...	S. W.	Rain	...	0	
4	...	...	29.40	...	...	68	...	...	...	S. W.	...	...	Rain	
5	29.45	29.45	29.48	60	72	60	64.0	N. W. 1	W'ly	W'ly 1	0	3	6	
6	29.55	29.59	29.66	55	69	56	60.0	N. W. 2	N. W. 2	N. W. 1	0	2	0	
S 7	29.56	...	29.39	60	...	64	...	S. W. 2	...	S. W. 2	10	...	Rain	
8	29.61	29.71	29.87	52	62	50	54.7	N. W. 2	N. W. 2	N. W. 1	0	0	0	
9	29.90	29.82	29.60	45	58	53	52.0	N. W. 1	S. W'ly 2	E'ly 1	5	10	10	
10	29.66	29.62	29.71	49	70	56	58.3	N. W. 2	W'ly 2	W'ly 1	2	2	0	
11	29.81	29.81	29.86	50	66	53	56.3	N. W. 1	N. W. 2	N. W. 1	0	2	3	
12	30.00	29.97	30.03	46	63	49	52.7	N. W. 2	N. W. 2	N. W. 1	0	0	0	
13	30.10	30.04	29.99	43	61	52	52.0	N. W. 1	E'ly 1	S. E'ly 1	0	8	6	
S 14	29.83	29.59	29.54	55	60	61	58.7	S'ly 3	S. W'ly 4	S'ly 1	Rain	Rain	10	0.27
15	29.50	...	29.54	61	...	62	...	S'ly 1	...	S'ly 2	2	...	0	
16	29.74	...	...	50	...	51	...	N. W. 1	...	W'ly	0	...	2	
17	30.00	29.93	29.88	45	69	57	57.0	N. W. 1	S. W. 1	S. W. 1	0	10	0	
18	...	29.78	29.60	60	76	65	67.0	S. W. 1	S. W. 3	S. W. 2	0	0	2	
19	29.58	29.62	29.68	64	72	57	64.3	S. W. 2	S. W. 2	S. W. 1	0	0	3	
20	29.69	29.58	29.48	51	71	66	62.7	S. W. 1	S. W. 3	S. W. 3	8, Sh'r	4	0	
S 21	29.38	29.42	29.50	66	54	48	56.0	S. W. 2	N. W. 2	N. W. 1	Rain	Rain	5	0.56
22	29.72	29.70	29.81	44	58	46	49.3	N. W. 1	N. W. 2	N. W. 1	0	0	0	
23	29.90	29.80	29.64	39	60	51	50.0	N'ly 2	E'ly 2	N. E. 2	0	6	Rain	0.50
24	29.59	29.60	29.68	50	53	51	51.3	N. E. 1	N. E. 2	N'ly 1	10	Misty	9	
25	29.72	29.71	29.74	48	62	50	53.3	N. W.	N. W. 2	N. W. 1	0	0	0	
26	29.79	29.78	29.78	48	63	50	53.7	N. W. 1	S. W. 2	S. W. 1	8	0	3	
27	29.89	29.90	29.97	48	61	55	54.7	S'ly 1	S. E. 1	S'ly 1	5	Rain	10	
S 28	30.04	30.02	30.00	50	63	54	55.7	S. W. 1	S. E. 2	S. W. 1	0	2	0	
29	30.02	29.97	29.94	52	68	54	58.0	S. W. 1	S. W. 2	S. W. 1	0	2	0	
30	29.88	29.81	29.77	52	69	62	61.0	S. W. 2	S. W. 3	S. W. 2	3	2	2	
Means	29.73	29.74	29.70	52.7	64.5	56.5	...	1.4	1.9	1.3	3.1	3.7	3.0	1.63
									1.5			3.6		
REDUCED TO SEA LEVEL.														
Max.	30.28	30.22	30.21	68	76	68	67.0	Prevailing winds from some point between—		Days			Days	
Min.	29.47	29.60	29.52	39	53	46	49.3	N. & E.		2	Clear		12	
Mean	29.91	29.92	29.88					E. & S.		4	Variable		} 10	
Range	0.81	0.62	0.69	29	23	22	18.7	S. & W.		14	Cloudy			
Mean of month	29.903			...	...	...	57.9	W. & N.		10	Rain fell on		8	
Extreme range	0.81			...	...	...	37.0							

REMARKS.

1st. Pleasant.

2d. Showery.

3d. Shower at sunrise. Very pleasant during the day.

4th. Pleasant. Clear in the morning, very hot sun. Cloudy in the afternoon. Rain in the evening for a short time.

5th. Very pleasant.

6th. Very fine.

7th. Very heavy wind during the middle of the day, and specially from 2 to 3 P. M. Shower, with lightning, in the evening.

8th. Very fine and cool.

9th. Appearances of rain. Frost this morning in some places in the vicinity.

10th and 11th. Very fine.

12th. Very fine. Evening very clear.

13th. Pleasant.

14th. Wind pretty high with light showers.

15th and 16th. Fine.

17th. Very fine. Evening splendid.

18th. Very fine.

19th. Fine.

20th. Light showers from 7 to 10 A. M.

21st. Moderate rain nearly all day.

22d. Fine.

23d. Began to rain from 8 to 9 P. M.

24th. Cool.

25th. Fine.

26th. Very fine.

27th. Pleasant.

28th, 29th, and 30th. Very fine.

October, 1845.

DAYS.	BAROMETER, REDUCED TO 32° F. Sun-rise.	At 1 P. M.	At 10 P. M.	THERMOMETER. Sun-rise.	At 1 P. M.	At 10 P. M.	Daily mean.	WINDS. (DIRECTION AND FORCE.) Sunrise.	At 1 P. M.	At 10 P. M.	WEATHER. (TENTHS CLOUDY.) Sun-rise.	At 1 P. M.	At 10 P. M.	RAIN AND SNOW IN INCHES OF WATER.
1	29.58	29.48	29.50	63	70	58	63.7	S. E. 2	N. W. 1	N. W. 1	Rain	9	0	0.80
2	29.65	29.78	29.88	50	68	53	57.0	N. W. 1	N. W.	N. W.	0	2	0	
3	29.93	29.90	29.94	49	67	56	57.3	S. W. 1	S. W. 2	S. W. 1	0	0	5	
4	29.92	29.91	29.80	52	66	56	58.0	S. E'ly 1	E'ly 1	N. E. 2	3	7	Rain	} 1.30
S 5	29.70	29.58	29.56	...	63	52	...	...	N. W.	N. E.	...	Rain	Rain	
6	29.69	29.82	29.93	52	53	50	51.7	N. E. 1	N. E. 2	N. E. 2	Misty	Misty	10	
7	30.01	30.00	30.01	48	55	51	51.3	N. E. 1	N. E. 1	N. E. 1	10	10	Misty	
8	29.95	29.90	29.87	50	65	56	57.0	N. E. 1	S. W. 2	S. W. 1	9	5	3	
9	29.78	29.68	29.64	55	62	60	59.0	S. W. 1	S'ly	S. W. 1	9	Rain	Foggy	0.50
10	29.76	29.73	29.78	54	67	55	58.7	S. E. 1	S. W. 2	S. W. 1	6	4	10	
11	29.74	29.72	29.69	55	66	63	61.3	S. E'ly 1	S. E. 2	S. W. 1	10	10	8	
S 12	29.58	29.52	29.48	65	72	66	67.7	S. W'ly 3	S. W. 3	S'ly 3	6	Misty	Rain	0.80
13	29.78	29.88	30.08	54	59	46	53.0	N. W. 2	N. W. 2	N. W. 1	4	7	0	
14	30.12	30.02	29.94	42	61	49	50.7	N. W. 1	W'ly 1	S. W. 1	2	6	6	
15	29.90	29.89	29.99	49	55	41	48.3	N. W. 1	S. W. 2	N. W. 2	9	5	0	
16	30.23	30.17	30.15	32	46	37	38.3	N. W. 1	N. W. 2	N. W. 1	0	0	2	
17	30.13	30.08	30.04	32	...	42	...	N. W. 1	...	W'ly 1	0	...	0	
18	30.08	30.01	29.98	37	58	46	47.0	W'ly 1	S'ly 2	S. W. 1	0	0	0	
S 19	29.91	29.78	29.78	48	65	56	56.3	S. W. 1	S. W. 2	S. W.	0	2	5	
20	29.90	29.92	29.94	52	52	44	49.3	W'ly 1	N. E. 2	N. E. 2	10	5	10	
21	29.99	30.01	30.19	38	39	28	35.0	N. E. 2	N. 3	N. W. 2	10	8	0	
22	30.28	30.25	30.24	23	40	31	31.3	N. W. 2	N. W. 2	N. W. 1	0	0	0	
23	30.23	30.17	30.10	26	46	33	35.0	N. W. 1	S'ly 2	S'ly 1	0	0	0	
24	30.00	29.91	29.95	28	54	42	41.3	S. W. 1	S'ly 1	S'ly 1	0	3	0	
25	30.10	30.10	30.15	35	47	34	38.7	N. W. 2	N. E. 2	N.E. 1	0	6	0	
S 26	30.16	30.10	30.10	32	51	43	42.0	N. E'ly 1	S'ly 2	S. W. 1	6	3	2	
27	30.06	29.96	29.94	43	60	48	50.3	S. W. 1	S. W. 1	S. W. 1	Foggy	2	2	
28	29.92	29.87	29.82	50	65	52	55.7	S. W. 1	S. W. 1	S. W. 1	0	0	0	
29	...	29.74	29.70	52	68	52	57.3	S. W. 1	S. W. 2	W'ly 1	0	0	0	
30	29.64	29.64	29.80	52	60	48	53.3	N. W. 1	N. W. 1	N. W.	0	6	0	
31	29.91	29.92	29.81	46	53	51	55.0	S. E.	E'ly 1	E'ly 2	10	10	10	
Means	29.91	29.88	29.89	45.5	58.4	48.4	...	1.2	1.9	1.3	4.5	5.0	3.8	3.40
									1.4			4.4		
REDUCED TO SEA LEVEL.								Prevailing winds from some point between— Days.					Days.	
Max.	30.46	30.43	30.42	65	72	66	67.7	N. & E. 5			Clear 10			
Min.	29.76	29.66	29.66	26	39	28	31.3	E. & S. 4			Variable . . . } 15			
Mean	30.09	30.05	30.07					S. & W. 13			Cloudy . . . . }			
Range	0.70	0.77	0.76	39	33	38	36.4	W. & N. 9			Rain fell on . . 6			
Mean of month	30.070			...	...	...	50.8							
Extreme range	0.80			...	...	...	46.0							

REMARKS.

1st. Rain in the morning.
2d and 3d. Pleasant.
4th. Began to rain at 8 P. M.
5th. Rainy.
6th. Mist and clouds.
7th. Mist.
8th. Pleasant.
9th. Heavy rain from 11 to 12 A. M.
10th. Warm and damp.
11th. Rained moderately at intervals in the afternoon.
12th. Showery in the afternoon and evening.
13th, 14th, and 15th. Pleasant.
16th. Very pleasant. First white frost in the College yard. No frost in the garden to injure the most delicate plant till this morning.
17th, 18th, and 19th. Very fine.
20th. Raw wind.
21st. Very cold and raw.
22d. Clear and fine, but cold.
23d. Very pleasant.
24th and 25th. Fine.
26th. Rather raw.
27th. Pleasant.
28th. Very pleasant.
29th. Very fine.
30th. Pleasant.
31st. Appearances of rain in the afternoon and evening.

November, 1845.

DAYS.	Barometer Sun-rise.	At 1 P. M.	At 10 P. M.	Thermometer Sun-rise.	At 1 P. M.	At 10 P. M.	Daily mean.	Winds Sunrise.	At 1 P. M.	At 10 P. M.	Weather Sun-rise.	At 1 P. M.	At 10 P. M.	Rain and Snow
1	29.63	29.51	29.49	52	65	54	57.0	W'ly 1	W'ly 1	S. W'ly	4	2	10	
S 2	29.45	29.38	29.38	53	52	51	52.0	S. E. 1	N. E. 1	N. E.	Rain	Rain	Rain	1.72
3	29.44	29.39	29.40	56	62	57	58.3	S'ly 1	S. W. 1	S. E. 1	Misty	10	Rain	0.63
4	29.41	29.42	29.30	57	63	52	57.3	S. W. 1	S. W. 1	W'ly	Misty	6	R'n, h'ze	0.40
5	29.46	29.45	29.58	42	49	44	45.0	S. W. 3	S. W. 4	S. W. 3	2	3	8	
6	29.58	29.56	29.51	36	53	37	42.0	S. W. 2	S. W. 1	N. W. 1	2	10	8	
7	29.54	29.53	29.55	37	51	39	42.3	N. W. 1	S. W. 1	W'ly 1	0	2	0	
8	29.56	29.49	29.39	36	46	46	42.7	N. W. 1	N. W. 1	N. E. 2	0	10	Rain	0.95
S 9	29.09	29.05	28.93	52	50	42	48.0	S. W. 1	S. W. 1	W'ly 1	10	10	Rain	0.88
10	28.76	29.04	29.43	36	42	37	38.3	N. W. 4	N. W. 3	N. W. 2	10	2	0	
11	29.58	29.60	29.69	36	51	44	43.7	N. W. 1	S. W. 1	S. W. 1	0	2	Hazy	
12	29.74	29.74	29.82	41	42	32	38.3	S. W. 1	N. W. 1	N. W. 1	10	2	0	
13	29.80	29.75	29.64	26	46	43	38.3	N. W. 1	S. W. 2	S. W. 1	0	0	2	
14	29.49	29.37	29.39	42	55	44	47.0	W'ly 1	S. W. 2	N. W. 2	3	4	0	
15	29.56	29.57	29.71	36	42	32	36.7	N. W. 2	N. W. 2	N. W. 1	0	0	2	
S 16	29.58	29.41	29.39	34	50	46	43.3	S. W. 2	S. W. 2	S. W. 1	5	2	0	
17	29.69	29.71	29.79	40	52	46	46.0	S. W. 1	S. W. 2	S. W. 1	0	Hazy	Hazy	} 0.15
18	29.82	29.79	29.74	46	55	49	50.0	S. W. 1	S. W. 1	S. W. 1	Misty	8	Foggy	
19	...	29.48	29.52	48	56	46	50.0	S. W. 1	S. W. 2	S. W. 1	Foggy	6	0	
20	29.54	29.44	29.38	42	55	46	47.7	N. W. 1	N. W. 3	N. W. 1	2	10	0	
21	29.29	29.29	29.47	48	48	36	44.0	S. W. 2	N. W. 3	N. W. 2	Rain	6	0	
22	29.69	29.69	29.76	32	42	37	37.0	N. W. 2	N. W. 2	N. W. 1	0	0	0	
S 23	29.50	29.27	29.39	48	55	42	48.3	S. W. 3	S. W'ly 3	W'ly 1	Rain	Rain	0	0.50
24	29.80	29.84	30.06	30	33	23	28.7	N. W. 2	N. W. 2	N. W. 1	0	0	0	
25	30.21	30.12	30.12	19	36	35	30.0	N. W. 1	S. W. 1	W'ly 2	0	10	0, Haze	
26	30.15	30.11	30.01	34	45	41	40.0	W. 1	S. W. 1	S. W. 1	3	6	2	
27	29.52	29.09	29.26	49	56	40	48.3	S. E. 2	S'ly 3	W'ly 2	Rain	Rain	10	3.85
28	29.59	29.62	30.06	22	26	20	22.7	N. W. 2	N. W. 2	N. W. 1	0	0	0	
29	30.26	30.32	30.36	15	26	24	21.7	N. W. 1	S. W. 1	N. E. 1	2.	0	3	
S 30	30.27	30.16	30.06	24	37	32	31.0	N. E. 1	N. E. 1	N. E. 1	10	10	Rain	
Means	29.62	29.57	29.65	39.0	48.0	40.6	...	1.5	1.7	1.3	4.8	5.2	4.8	9.08
									1.5			4.9		
REDUCED TO SEA LEVEL.								Prevailing winds from some point between— Days.					Days.	
Max.	30.45	30.50	30.54	57	65	57	58.3	N. & E. 2			Clear 7			
Min.	29.04	29.22	29.11	15	26	23	21.7	E. & S. 1			Variable . . . } 15			
Mean	29.80	29.75	29.83					S. & W. 18			Cloudy . . . . }			
Range	1.41	1.28	1.43	42	39	34	36.6	W. & N. 9			Rain fell on . . 8			
Mean of month	29.793			...	...	...	42.5							
Extreme range	1.50			...	...	...	50.0							

REMARKS.

1st. Pleasant.
2d. Rain nearly all day and last night.
3d. Moderate rain in the afternoon and evening.
4th. Thundershower in the evening.
5th. Blustering. Evening overcast.
6th. Pleasant.
7th. Very pleasant.
8th. Began to rain moderately from 4 to 5 P. M.
9th. Unpleasant.
10th. Air quite thick with snow at 8 A. M., and first frost of the season this morning.
11th. Very fine. Halo about the moon in the evening, appearing through thick haze.
12th. Fine in the afternoon. Evening very clear and still.
13th. Fine. Eclipse of the moon began at 6 h. 25 m. 45 s. P. M., Providence mean time, as nearly as I could judge. End not observed.
14th, 15th, and 16th. Very fine.
17th. Pleasant.
18th. Very thick mist and fog in the morning, and thick fog in the evening.
19th. Very fine.
20th. Fine.
21st. Sprinkling of rain at sunrise, which ceased soon.
22d. Fine.
23d. Sprinkling of rain in the morning, with heavy thunder. Shower from noon to 2 P. M. Clear in the evening.
24th. Fine.
25th. Clear and very calm at sunrise.
26th. Fine.
27th. Began to rain very moderately from 5 to 6 A. M.; wind a little S. of E. Wind hauled more to S. E. and rain increased. Front 10 A. M. to 1 P. M., the rain was violent, with wind heavy and hauling more S'ly. At 3 P. M., wind W'ly and abated, and rain nearly over. The barometer had then fallen to 29.16, and began to rise at about 3½ P. M. The amount of rain was extraordinary, being 3.85 inches.
28th and 29th. Fine.
30th. Snow in the afternoon so as to cover the ground. Moderate rain in the evening.

December, 1845.

Days.	Barometer, reduced to 32° F. Sunrise.	At 1 P. M.	At 10 P. M.	Thermometer. Sunrise.	At 1 P. M.	At 10 P. M.	Daily mean.	Winds (Direction and Force.) Sunrise.	At 1 P. M.	At 10 P. M.	Weather (Tenths Cloudy.) Sunrise.	At 1 P. M.	At 10 P. M.	Rain and Snow in Inches of Water.
1	29.76	29.43	29.17	36	49	43	42.7	N. E. 2	N. E. 2	W'ly 2	Misty	Rain	8	1.50
2	29.42	29.61	29.90	23	26	16	21.7	N. W. 3	N. W. 3	N. W. 3	0	0	0	
3	30.10	30.13	30.16	13	20	16	16.3	N. W. 1	N. W. 1	N'ly 2	0	10	10	
4	29.93	29.63	29.40	18	33	26	25.7	N'ly 2	N. E. 1	N. E. 2	Snow	Rain	R'n, h'l	1.25
5	29.26	29.42	29.66	30	28	22	26.7	W'ly 2	W'ly 3	W'ly 3	2	0	0	
6	29.85	29.90	30.02	19	26	18	21.0	N. W. 2	N. W. 3	N. W. 1	0	0	0	
S 7	30.11	30.16	30.11	16	20	16	17.3	N. W. 2	N. W. 2	N. W. 1	0	0	0	
8	29.94	29.84	29.70	25	32	30	29.0	S. W'ly 1	S. W. 2	E'ly 1	10	10	Snow	} 0.33
9	29.45	29.37	29.38	31	35	32	32.7	N'ly 1	W'ly 1	N. W.	Misty	10	3	
10	29.48	29.56	29.70	32	29	19	26.7	W'ly 1	N. W. 3	N. W. 1	3	1	0	
11	29.90	29.94	30.11	18	18	8	14.7	N. W. 1	N. W. 2	N. W. 2	0	7	0	
12	30.22	30.21	30.30	7	15	9	10.3	N. W. 1	N. W. 1	N. W. 1	0	0	0	
13	30.34	30.29	30.26	7	25	18	16.7	N. W. 2	W'ly 1	E'ly 1	0	0	3	
S 14	30.11	29.95	29.72	23	35	39	32.3	N. E. 1	N. E'ly 1	E'ly 1	10	R'n, h'l	Misty	
15	29.35	29.07	29.06	38	36	34	36.0	N. E. 2	N. W'ly 3	N. W. 4	Rain	Misty	10	
16	28.97	29.07	29.41	32	29	23	27.7	N. 4	N. 4	N. W. 4	10	10	0	
17	29.70	29.75	29.78	23	37	31	30.3	N. W. 2	N. W. 2	N. W. 1	0	0	7	
18	29.73	29.63	29.58	32	43	38	37.7	S'ly 1	S'ly 1	S'ly 1	10	10	10	
19	29.53	29.53	29.69	35	37	26	32.7	S'ly 1	S. W. 1	N. W. 1	8	10	10	
20	29.76	29.65	29.56	20	20	17	19.0	N. E'ly 1	N'ly 1	N. E. 3	10	10	Snow	} 0.15
S 21	29.55	29.55	29.62	16	19	13	16.0	N. W. 1	N. W. 2	N. W. 2	8	0	0	
22	29.72	29.73	29.85	15	23	17	18.3	W'ly 1	W'ly 2	W'ly 1	0	0	8	
23	29.99	30.02	30.13	13	27	19	19.7	N. W. 1	W'ly 2	W'ly 1	0	2	0	
24	30.24	30.18	30.14	12	28	24	21.3	E'ly 1	E'ly 1	N. E'ly 1	8	10	10	
25	29.96	29.74	29.80	24	33	24	27.0	N. E'ly 2	N. E'ly 1	N. E'ly	Snow	Misty	Snow	} 0.25
26	29.85	29.83	29.85	23	23	22	22.7	N. E'ly 2	N'ly 3	N. W'ly 2	Snow	Snow	Snow	
27	29.87	29.77	29.69	15	22	22	19.7	N. W. 1	N. W. 2	W'ly 1	0	0	8	
S 28	29.67	29.68	29.76	22	33	30	28.3	N. W. 1	W'ly 2	W'ly 1	3	10	10	
29	29.70	29.60	29.56	27	40	28	31.7	W'ly 1	S'ly 2	W'ly 2	4	3	2	
30	29.56	29.55	29.64	32	38	28	32.7	N. W'ly 1	N. W. 2	N. W. 2	0	3	10	
31	29.77	29.90	30.06	18	22	12	17.3	N. W. 2	N. W. 3	N. W. 1	0	0	0	
Means	29.76	29.73	29.76	22.4	29.1	23.2	...	1.5	1.9	1.7	4.9	5.7	5.6	3.48
									1.7			5.4		
REDUCED TO SEA LEVEL.														
Max.	30.52	30.47	30.48	38	49	43	42.7							
Min.	29.15	29.25	29.24	7	15	8	10.3							
Mean	29.94	29.91	29.94											
Range	1.37	1.22	1.24	31	34	35	32.4							
Mean of month	29.930			...	...	...	24.9							
Extreme range	1.37			...	...	...	42.0							

Prevailing winds from some point between— Days.
N. & E. 7
E. & S. 0
S. & W. 4
W. & N. 20

Days.
Clear 11
Variable . . . . } 13
Cloudy . . . . }
Rain or snow fell on 7

REMARKS.

1st. Heavy rain at intervals. Clouds broken and stars visible at 9½ P. M.
2d. Wind brisk and the cold piercing.
3d. Appearances of snow in the evening.
4th. Snowing at 5 A. M. Snow continued till towards noon; then mist and rain from S'Ely. In the evening, rain, with some hail, from N. E.
5th. Very clear in the evening.
6th. Rather blustering through the day. Evening very fine.
7th. Very fine for winter.
8th. Light snow in the evening.
9th. Mist in the morning. Clouds broken in the afternoon.
10th. Fine. Evening very clear.
11th. Cold.
12th. Cold, but not severe.
13th. At 10 P. M., wind E'ly, clouds from S'ly.
14th. Flurry of snow from 9 to 11 A. M., then hail and rain in small quantity.
15th. Very blustering in the evening; barometer falling.
16th. At 7 A. M., barometer 29.09; at 7½ A. M., 29.07, and began to rise before 8 A. M. Wind a little W. of N., and abating in strength, but still blustering through the day and evening.
17th. Fine.
18th. Very mild.
19th. Air very raw.
20th. Commenced snowing moderately from 2 to 3 P. M.
21st. Cold, but not severe. Ground covered with about 2 inches of light snow.
22d and 23d. Fine.
24th. Appearances of snow in the afternoon.
25th. Light snow at intervals.
26th. Light snow through the day, from three to four inches deep.
27th. Pleasant.
28th. Mild.
29th. Very fine.
30th. Appearances of storm in the evening.
31st. Pleasant, but cold.

January, 1846.

Days.	Barometer Sunrise.	At 1 P. M.	At 10 P. M.	Thermometer Sunrise.	At 1 P. M.	At 10 P. M.	Daily mean.	Winds Sunrise.	At 1 P. M.	At 10 P. M.	Weather Sunrise.	At 1 P. M.	At 10 P. M.	Rain and Snow in Inches of Water.
1	30.15	30.20	29.96	8	25	27	20.0	N. W. 1	S. W. 1	S. E'ly	0	8	10	
2	29.53	29.20	29.08	39	43	42	41.3	S'ly 1	S. E'ly 3	S'ly 1	Rain	Rain	8	0.92
3	29.18	29.32	29.47	36	35	33	34.7	N. W. 2	N. W. 2	N. W. 2	8	4	2	
S 4	29.44	29.44	29.70	30	36	30	32.0	N. W. 2	N. W. 2	W'ly 1	0	0	0	
5	29.91	29.95	30.05	22	37	27	28.7	N. W. 1	N. W. 1	W'ly 1	0	0	0	
6	30.16	30.16	30.14	22	36	31	29.7	N. W.	N. W.	N. W.	1	3	8	
7	29.80	29.47	29.40	33	35	34	34.0	N. E. 2	N'ly 2	N'ly 2	Rain	10	Misty	
8	29.42	29.40	29.51	34	41	37	37.3	W'ly 1	W'ly 2	W'ly 2	Misty	2	8	
9	29.60	29.58	29.52	33	37	35	35.0	W'ly 2	W'ly 3	W'ly 2	3	1	10	
10	29.55	29.47	29.52	28	30	31	29.7	W'ly 1	W'ly 2	W'ly 1	2	5	7	
S 11	29.45	29.40	29.40	30	35	30	31.7	S. W. 1	S. W. 1	N. W. 1	9	10	8	
12	29.41	29.42	29.56	28	35	29	30.7	N. W. 1	N. W. 1	N. W. 1	10	8	10	
13	29.75	29.76	29.89	26	29	18	24.3	N. W. 1	N. W. 2	N. W.	3	2	0	
14	29.90	29.80	29.76	18	34	28	26.7	W. 1	S. W. 2	S. W.	0	10	0	
15	29.80	29.80	29.71	27	41	34	34.0	S. W. 1	S. W. 2	S. W. 1	0	2	2	
16	29.50	29.38	...	30	39	...	...	S'ly 1	N. E. 2	...	10	10	Snow	
17	29.50	29.40	29.36	31	34	20	28.3	N. E. 1	N. E. 2	N. E. 2	Snow	Snow	Snow	0.75
S 18	29.62	29.72	29.84	4	5	2	3.7	N. W. 3	N. W. 2	N. W. 1	9	0	0	
19	29.93	29.81	29.93	—1	10	9	6.0	N. W. 2	N. W. 3	N. W. 3	0	0	0	
20	30.06	29.97	29.88	4	21	15	13.3	N. W. 2	N. W. 2	N. W. 1	0	3	Hazy	
21	29.71	29.50	29.40	18	28	22	22.7	W'ly 1	S. E'ly 1	N. E. 3	10	10	Snow	
22	29.65	29.62	29.75	6	6	14	8.7	N. W. 3	N. W. 3	N. W. 2	0	0	0	
23	29.99	29.96	29.94	14	26	18	19.3	N. W. 2	N. W. 2	N. W. 2	0	0	0	
24	29.87	29.76	29.63	14	30	28	24.0	N. W. 1	N. W. 2	N. W. 3	0	0	5	
S 25	29.37	29.40	29.57	29	42	34	35.0	S. W. 2	S. W. 2	N. W. 1	0	0	0	
26	29.62	29.50	29.39	31	37	33	33.7	W'ly 1	S. W. 1	S. W. 1	10	10	2	
27	29.52	29.60	29.69	24	28	17	23.0	N'ly 1	N. E. 2	N. W. 1	Snow	3	0	0.15
28	29.62	29.56	29.55	16	33	26	25.0	N. W. 1	N. W. 1	N. W. 2	5	10	2	
29	29.97	29.95	29.96	17	33	28	26.0	N. W. 1	N. W. 1	E'ly 2	0	3	10	
30	29.78	29.56	29.45	33	47	42	40.7	W'ly 1	S. W. 3	S. W. 2	10	3	Rain	
31	29.39	29.47	29.86	46	42	22	36.7	S. W. 1	N. E'ly	N. W. 3	10	10	0	
Means	29.68	29.63	29.66	23.0	31.9	26.5	...	1.4	1.9	1.7	4.8	4.7	5.0	1.82
									1.7			4.8		
REDUCED TO SEA LEVEL.														
Max.	30.34	30.38	30.32	46	47	42	41.3							
Min.	29.36	29.38	29.26	—1	5	2	3.7							
Mean	29.86	29.81	29.84											
Range	0.98	1.00	1.06	47	42	40	37.6							
Mean of month	29.837			...	...	...	27.3							
Extreme range	1.12			...	...	...	48.0							

Prevailing winds from some point between— Days.
N. & E. 6
E. & S. 2
S. & W. 10
W. & N. 13

Days
Clear 9
Variable . . . . } 13
Cloudy . . . . }
Rain or snow fell on 9

REMARKS.

1st. Morning cold, but calm.
2d. Rainy through the day. Clouds broken in the evening.
3d. Pleasant.
4th, 5th, and 6th. Very fine.
7th. Ground covered with snow at sunrise, and raining.
8th and 9th. Mild.
10th. Pleasant.
11th. Mild and pleasant.
12th. Still mild.
13th, 14th, and 15th. Mild and pleasant.
16th. Appearances of storm through the day. Began to snow moderately at 9 P. M.
17th. Snowed moderately all day. Grew colder in the evening.
18th. At sunrise, six or seven inches of snow, badly drifted, the wind severe, air full of driving snow, and the thermometer nearly down to zero.
19th. Very severe.
20th. Pleasant.
21st. Began to snow from 7 to 8 P. M.; ceased at 10 P. M., being only a flurry, and cleared cold.
22d. Very cold and severe.
23d. Pleasant.
24th and 25th. Fine.
26th. Sprinkling of rain from 5 to 7 P. M.
27th. Light snow one inch and a half deep.
28th. Bright diffused aurora in the evening.
29th. Appearances of storm in the evening.
30th. Commenced raining very moderately in the evening.
31st. Flurry of snow at sunset, and grew colder.

February, 1846.

DAYS.	BAROMETER, REDUCED TO 32° F. Sunrise.	At 1 P. M.	At 10 P. M.	THERMOMETER. Sunrise.	At 1 P. M.	At 10 P. M.	Daily mean.	WINDS. (DIRECTION AND FORCE.) Sunrise.	At 1 P. M.	At 10 P. M.	WEATHER. (TENTHS CLOUDY.) Sunrise.	At 1 P. M.	At 10 P. M.	RAIN AND SNOW IN INCHES OF WATER.
S 1	30.05	30.10	30.11	14	16	16	15.3	N'ly 2	N'ly 2	N. W. 1	Snow	10	10	
2	30.10	30.08	30.06	18	32	28	26.0	N. W. 1	N. E'ly 1	W'ly	10	10	8	
3	29.92	29.85	29.80	32	35	32	33.0	S. W. 1	S. W. 2	S. W. 2	10	10	10	
4	29.75	29.79	29.61	32	37	28	32.3	N. W. 2	N. W. 2	W'ly	5	0	3	
5	29.60	29.49	29.56	34	44	34	37.3	S. W. 1	S. W. 2	N. W. 2	5	2	2	
6	29.85	29.81	29.84	28	37	30	31.7	N. W. 2	N. W. 2	N. W. 1	0	2	Hazy	
7	29.66	29.47	29.27	29	38	32	33.0	E'ly 1	E'ly 2	N. E. 2	10	10	Snow	0.25
S 8	29.20	29.29	29.55	31	23	12	22.0	N. W. 2	N. W. 3	N. W. 2	10	0	0	
9	29.71	29.64	29.80	8	26	11	15.0	N. W. 1	W'ly 2	N. W. 3	0	0	0	
10	29.97	29.87	29.86	6	20	22	16.0	N. W. 2	N. W. 3	N. W. 1	0	0	10	
11	29.72	29.58	29.48	21	23	18	20.7	N. E. 1	N. E. 2	N. E.	10	Snow	Snow	
12	29.67	29.74	29.81	8	20	9	12.3	N. E'ly	N. W. 2	N. W. 1	10	0	0	
13	29.82	29.74	29.80	7	26	19	17.3	N. W. 1	W'ly 3	N. W. 1	0	3	0	
14	29.88	29.83	29.79	11	27	25	21.0	N. W. 1	N. W. 1	N. W. 1	0	2	Hazy	
S 15	29.25	29.07	29.40	24	26	12	20.7	N. E. 5	N. E. 5	N'ly 3	Snow	Snow	10	1.50
16	29.68	29.70	29.73	16	29	23	22.7	N. W. 1	N. W. 1	S. W. 1	9	1	Snow	
17	29.78	29.76	29.86	16	36	25	25.7	N. W. 1	W'ly 1	S. E'ly 1	3	7	10	
18	29.88	29.90	29.98	18	23	12	17.7	N. W. 1	N. W. 2	N. W. 2	6	0	0	
19	30.05	29.97	29.95	8	23	16	15.7	N. W. 1	N. W. 1	N'ly 1	0	0	0	
20	29.63	29.11	28.85	18	26	32	25.3	N. E. 2	E. N. E. 4	S. E'ly 1	10	Snow	10	0.33
21	29.26	29.28	29.48	25	33	26	28.0	N. W. 1	W'ly 2	W'ly 1	2	0	0	
S 22	29.48	29.45	29.49	25	37	24	28.7	S. W. 1	S. W. 1	N. W. 1	8	5	0	
23	29.62	29.60	29.64	20	29	22	23.7	W'ly 1	N. W. 2	N. W. 2	3	0	0	
24	29.77	29.78	29.90	14	26	17	19.0	N. W. 1	N. W. 3	N. W. 1	0	0	0	
25	29.94	29.90	29.90	16	29	17	20.7	N. W. 1	N. W. 1	N. W. 1	8	10	Hazy	
26	29.93	29.91	30.02	9	12	2	7.7	N. W. 1	N. W. 3	N. W. 2	0	5	0	
27	30.13	30.07	30.03	—2	11	10	6.3	N. W. 2	N. W. 2	N. W. 1	0	0	10	
28	29.98	29.91	29.84	8	18	13	13.0	N. W. 1	N. W. 1	N'ly 2	Snow	10	Snow	
Means	29.76	29.70	29.73	17.6	27.2	20.3	...	1.4	2.1	1.5	5.3	4.1	6.0	2.08
REDUCED TO SEA LEVEL.									1.7			5.1		
Max.	30.31	30.28	30.29	34	44	34	37.3	Prevailing winds from some point between—		Days.			Days.	
Min.	29.38	29.25	29.03	—2	11	2	6.3	N. & E.		5	Clear		7	
Mean	29.94	29.88	29.91					E. & S.		0	Variable		} 14	
Range	0.93	1.03	1.26	36	33	32	31.0	S. & W.		4	Cloudy			
Mean of month	29.910			...	...	...	21.7	W. & N.		18	Rain or snow fell on		9	
Extreme range	1.28			...	...	...	46.0							

REMARKS.

6th. Bright halo about the moon in the evening.
7th. Began to snow moderately from 4 to 5 P. M. Wind rather light N. E.
8th. About one inch of wet snow on the ground. Grew cold towards night.
9th. Cold, but fine for winter.
10th. Clouded over in the evening, with appearances of storm.
11th. Ground covered with snow, there having been a flurry during the night. Snow in the afternoon and all night.
12th. At sunrise, four or five inches of light snow, and still snowing, but ceased before 9 A. M. Clear in the afternoon and evening.
13th. Fine.
14th. Very fine. Hazy in the evening. Some stars out.
15th. Began to snow about 4 A. M.; wind heavy at N. E. or N. E. by E. Snow continued all day, with wind very heavy. Clouds broken and stars out in the evening. Snow deep and badly drifted. The barometer fell to 29.17 at 2 P. M., and began to rise about 3 P. M., with wind hauling more to north. Snow in the woods from twelve to fifteen inches deep, and rather damp.
16th. Began to snow very gently between 9 and 10 P. M.; wind light S. W.
17th. Very mild. Flurry of snow last night.
18th. Very fine.
19th. The sky somewhat obscured by haze in the evening.
20th. Began to snow about 10 A. M. Storm violent from noon to 2 P. M. Wind gradually hauled to S. E., and snow turned to rain, from 5 to 6 P. M. Rain ceased at 9½ P. M.; barometer 28.95, and at 10 P. M., 29.00; continued to rise.
21st to 24th. Very fine.
25th. Aurora this evening. Bright diffused light without streamers.
26th. Severe searching cold.
27th. Coldest morning of the winter thus far. Appearances of snow in the evening.
28th. Frequent flurries of snow.

March, 1846.

DAYS.	BAROMETER Sunrise.	At 1 P. M.	At 10 P. M.	THERMOMETER Sunrise.	At 1 P. M.	At 10 P. M.	Daily mean.	WINDS Sunrise.	At 1 P. M.	At 10 P. M.	WEATHER Sunrise.	At 1 P. M.	At 10 P. M.	RAIN AND SNOW
S 1	29.95	30.02	30.07	8	21	13	14.0	N. W. 2	N. E. 2	N. E. 1	5	0	0	
2	30.03	30.01	30.05	9	24	14	15.7	N'ly 1	N. E. 3	N'ly 2	10	10	6	
3	30.12	30.11	30.10	12	28	20	20.0	N. W. 2	N. W. 2	N. W. 1	0	0	0	
4	29.98	29.80	29.59	15	40	32	29.0	N. W. 2	S. W. 2	S. W. 3	0	2	5	
5	29.47	29.47	29.57	34	42	33	36.3	S. W. 2	W'ly 3	N. W. 2	7	2	0	
6	29.60	29.55	29.57	28	40	28	32.0	N. W. 1	W'ly 1	N. W. 2	5	10	3	
7	29.75	29.73	29.74	17	33	27	25.7	N. W. 2	N. W. 2	N. W. 1	0	0	8	
S 8	29.53	29.53	29.60	29	41	34	34.7	S'ly 1	S'ly 1	S'ly 1	Snow	5	Rain	1.40
9	29.77	29.81	29.86	31	37	32	33.3	N. W. 1	N. W. 3	N. W. 1	2	0	1	
10	29.95	29.94	30.02	30	40	30	33.3	N. W. 1	N. W. 1	N. W. 1	0	0	0	
11	30.10	30.10	30.10	25	44	32	33.7	N. W. 1	N. W. 2	S'ly 1	0	0	0	
12	30.05	29.96	29.94	30	50	40	40.0	S. W'ly 1	S. W. 2	S. W. 2	0	0	2	
13	29.86	29.78	29.64	38	57	45	46.7	S. W. 1	S. W. 2	S. W. 3	8	10	10	
14	29.38	29.13	29.19	44	45	40	43.0	S'ly 2	S'ly 1	W'ly 3	Rain	Misty	5	
S 15	29.42	29.39	29.47	33	48	36	39.0	S. W'ly 2	S. W'ly 3	S. W. 2	0	3	2	
16	29.35	29.25	29.25	34	33	33	33.3	N'ly 1	N. E. 2	N'ly 4	Misty	Rain	Rain	0.10
17	29.36	29.41	29.60	29	39	29	32.3	N. W. 3	N. W. 3	N. W. 3	10	2	0	
18	29.65	29.64	29.66	27	39	30	32.0	N. W. 2	N. W. 2	N. W. 1	0	2	0	
19	29.54	29.46	29.53	30	49	40	39.7	N. W. 2	N'ly 3	N'ly 1	0	10	Hazy	
20	29.60	29.57	29.64	38	57	47	47.3	N. W. 1	N. W. 2	N. E. 1	10	2	10	
21	29.59	29.59	29.72	40	50	36	42.0	W'ly 1	N. W. 1	N. W. 3	8	10	3	
S 22	29.88	29.87	29.95	30	46	36	37.3	N. W. 3	N. W. 2	N. W. 1	0	0	0	
23	29.97	29.89	29.84	30	51	36	39.0	N. W. 1	N. E. 1	S. W. 1	0	0	3	
24	29.77	29.73	29.69	36	38	36	36.7	S. W. 2	S'ly 2	E'ly 2	10	Misty	Rain	} 1.36
25	29.55	29.37	29.39	38	48	46	44.0	E'ly 1	S. E. 4	E'ly 1	Misty	Rain	10	
26	29.33	29.30	29.31	43	44	42	43.0	N'ly 1	N. E. 1	N. W. 1	Misty	Misty	10	
27	29.40	29.40	29.46	42	50	39	43.7	N. W. 1	S. E'ly 2	S. W. 1	10	2	0	
28	29.53	29.53	29.60	36	50	40	42.0	S. W. 1	S. W. 2	S. W. 1	0	10	3	
S 29	29.68	29.69	29.76	35	46	40	40.3	N. W. 1	W'ly 2	W'ly 1	0	3	5	
30	29.84	29.84	29.92	34	45	36	38.3	N. E. 1	N. W. 3	N. W. 2	5	3	0	
31	29.97	29.94	30.00	30	47	35	37.3	N. W. 2	N. W. 2	N. W. 1	0	4	3	
Means	29.71	29.67	29.71	30.2	42.6	34.1	...	1.5	2.1	1.6	4.5	4.5	4.2	2.86
REDUCED TO SEA LEVEL.									1.7			4.4		
Max.	30.30	30.29	30.28	44	57	47	47.3	Prevailing winds from some point between—		Days.			Days.	
Min.	29.51	29.31	29.37	8	21	13	14.0	N. & E.		5	Clear		10	
Mean	29.89	29.85	29.89					E. & S.		5	Variable		} 13	
Range	0.79	0.98	0.91	36	36	34	33.3	S. & W.		9	Cloudy			
Mean of month	29.877			...	...	...	35.6	W. & N.		12	Rain or snow fell on		8	
Extreme range	0.99			...	...	...	49.0							

REMARKS.

1st. Very fine. A half inch of dry, fresh-fallen snow on the ground in the morning.
2d. Raw and cold, with the air full of snow. Partly clear in the evening.
3d, 4th, and 5th. Very fine.
6th. Cloudy. Wind came more to N. W., and cleared in the evening.
7th. Fine.
8th. Snowed gently from 7 to 10 A. M. Sprinkling of rain in the evening.
9th, 10th, and 11th. Very fine.
12th. Very fine. Observed the double comet (Biela's) this evening.
13th. Dashes of rain in the evening, which continued all night.
14th. Rain nearly all day. Partly clear in the evening, with wind blustering at about N. W. Barometer fell to 29.17 at 7 P. M., and soon commenced rising.
15th. Very fine.
16th. Moderate rain and mist during the day.
17th. Very blustering.
18th. Very fine. Biela's comet showed well this evening, but not double, so far as I observed.
19th. Very fine.
20th. Very mild. Appearances of rain in the evening.
21st. Shower from 10 to 11 A. M. Comet appeared well to-night; the companion barely visible with a power of one hundred.
22d. Very fine. Evening very clear. Comet visible, but not the companion.
23d. Very fine.
24th. Rain very moderate in the evening.
25th. Rain at intervals
26th. Thundershower at 3 A. M.
27th. Cleared in the morning and very pleasant.
28th. Variable.
29th. Pleasant.
30th and 31st. Fine.

April, 1846.

DAYS.	Barometer, reduced to 32° F. At 6 A. M.	At 1 P. M.	At 10 P. M.	Thermometer. At 6 A. M.	At 1 P. M.	At 10 P. M.	Daily mean.	Winds (Direction and Force.) At 6 A. M.	At 1 P. M.	At 10 P. M.	Weather (Tenths Cloudy.) At 6 A. M.	At 1 P. M.	At 10 P. M.	Rain and Snow in Inches of Water.
1	30.08	30.05	30.09	29	44	33	35.3	N. W. 2	N. W. 2	N. W. 2	0	0	0	
2	30.14	30.05	30.09	28	46	36	36.7	N. W. 1	N. W. 2	N. W. 1	0	0	0	
3	30.12	30.13	30.19	29	43	34	35.3	N. W. 1	E'ly	N. W. 1	0	2	0	
4	30.27	30.28	30.30	30	42	32	34.7	N. W. 1	N. E'ly	N. W. 1	0	0	0	
S 5	30.31	30.26	30.23	28	50	40	39.3	N. W. 1	S. E. 2	S'ly 2	0	0	Hazy	
6	30.18	30.15	30.21	34	66	47	49.0	S. W. 1	S. W. 1	S. W. 1	6	Hazy	0	
7	30.22	30.10	30.02	40	55	44	46.3	N. W. 1	S. E. 3	S'ly 2	0	3	Hazy	
8	29.89	29.78	29.95	42	55	44	47.0	S. W. 2	S. W. 2	N. W. 1	10	10	Hazy	
9	30.17	30.15	30.15	34	52	37	41.0	N. W. 1	S'ly 2	S'ly 1	0	0	Hazy	
10	30.09	29.93	29.88	32	54	44	43.3	S. W.	S'ly 2	S'ly 1	3	2	Hazy	
11	29.69	29.57	29.44	46	60	51	52.3	S. W. 1	S'ly 3	S. W. 2	10	10	5	
S 12	29.59	29.45	29.31	45	47	46	46.0	N'ly 1	W'ly 1	N. W. 1	Rain	10	9	0.20
13	29.39	29.34	29.49	31	47	31	36.3	N. W. 2	N. W. 2	N. W. 2	0	5	3	
14	29.70	29.71	29.74	28	43	36	35.7	N. W. 2	N. W. 2	N. W. 2	0	0	0	
15	29.52	29.65	29.95	38	42	32	37.3	S. W. 3	N. W. 2	N. W. 2	Rain	2	0	0.25
16	30.14	30.10	30.10	32	46	33	37.0	N. W. 1	S. E. 2	S'ly 1	0	0	0	
17	30.06	29.95	29.94	38	57	46	47.0	S. W. 2	S. W. 2	S. W. 1	0	0	0	
18	29.92	29.84	29.79	48	62	52	54.0	S. W. 1	S'ly 2	S. W. 3	Hazy	2	0	
S 19	29.69	29.70	29.87	52	64	48	54.7	S. W. 1	N. W. 2	N. W. 1	10	1	0	
20	30.04	30.02	29.88	42	63	52	52.3	N. W. 1	W'ly 1	S. W. 2	0	0	5	
21	29.79	29.66	29.78	53	76	64	64.3	S. W. 1	W. 2	S. W. 1	5	0	0	
22	29.88	29.86	29.78	46	62	45	51.0	N. E. 2	S. E. 0	N'ly 1	10	10	0	
23	29.76	29.73	29.68	46	75	54	58.3	N. W. 1	W'ly 1	S. W. 1	3	8	Rain	
24	29.56	29.42	29.42	52	75	62	63.0	S. W. 1	S'ly 1	S. W. 1	Hazy	Hazy	Rain	
25	29.69	29.69	29.73	38	47	38	41.0	N. E. 2	N. E. 1	S'ly 1	2	0	0	
S 26	29.69	29.57	29.50	36	55	48	46.3	S. E'ly 1	S'ly 2	S'ly 1	0	0	2	
27	29.59	29.56	29.61	44	65	44	51.0	N. W. 1	N. W. 2	S'ly 2	0	0	0	
28	29.68	29.68	29.74	40	67	47	51.3	S'ly 1	S. E. 1	S'ly 1	0	0	0	
29	29.74	29.71	29.65	42	60	49	50.3	N. E. 1	S'ly 2	S'ly 1	0	10	Rain	1.30
30	29.43	29.40	29.49	51	57	50	52.7	S. E. 1	S. W. 2	N. W. 1	Rain	9	0	
Means	29.87	29.82	29.83	39.1	55.8	44.0	...	1.3	1.7	1.4	3.5	3.5	3.5	1.75
									1.5			3.5		
REDUCED TO SEA LEVEL.														
Max.	30.49	30.28	30.48	53	76	64	64.3	Prevailing winds from some point between—		Days.			Days.	
Min.	29.57	29.52	29.49	28	42	31	34.7	N. & E.		2	Clear		15	
Mean	30.05	30.00	30.01					E. & S.		7	Variable		} 9	
Range	0.92	0.76	0.99	25	34	33	29.6	S. & W.		11	Cloudy			
Mean of month	30.020			...	...	...	46.3	W. & N.		10	Rain fell on		6	
Extreme range	1.00			...	...	...	48.0							

REMARKS.

1st. Fine.
2d. Very fine.
3d and 4th. Fine, but cool.
5th. Pleasant.
6th and 7th. Very fine.
8th. Halo about the moon in the evening.
9th. Halo about the moon.
10th. Pleasant.
11th. Appearances of rain during the day.
12th. Light showers.
13th. Snow and rain in the afternoon. Cleared at 10 to 11 P. M.
14th. Snow on the ground in the morning.
15th. Blustering.
16th. Beautiful aurora, with streamers, at 10 P. M.
17th, 18th, and 19th. Very fine.
20th. Fine.
21st. Very fine and very warm for the season.
22d. Cloudy till evening, then very clear.
23d. Warm and damp. Sprinkling of rain at 10 P. M.
24th. Sprinkling of rain at 9 to 10 P. M.
25th. Very fine. Large eclipse of the sun; began at 11 h. 11 m. 40.5 s. A. M., ended at 1 h. 51 m. 20 s. P. M., mean solar time; duration 2 h. 39 m. 39.5 s.
26th. Very fine.
27th and 28th Fine.
29th. Sprinkling of rain began at 6 P. M. Rain during the night.
30th. Rain in the morning. Clear in the evening.

May, 1846.

DAYS.	Barometer At 6 A. M.	At 1 P. M.	At 10 P. M.	Thermometer At 6 A. M.	At 1 P. M.	At 10 P. M.	Daily mean.	Winds At 6 A. M.	At 1 P. M.	At 10 P. M.	Weather At 6 A. M.	At 1 P. M.	At 10 P. M.	Rain and Snow in Inches of Water.
1	29.51	29.50	29.49	46	56	52	51.3	S. E. 1	S. E. 2	S'ly 1	Hazy	10	Rain	0.55
2	29.44	29.39	29.48	44	55	50	49.7	N'ly 1	N. E. 1	N. E. 1	Misty	10	2	
S 3	29.55	29.59	29.70	50	65	52	55.7	S. W. 1	S. E. 1	S'ly 1	Foggy	10	2	
4	29.79	29.75	29.75	45	65	51	53.7	S'ly 1	S'ly 2	S'ly 1	Foggy	2	0	
5	29.77	29.70	29.64	47	65	58	56.7	S'ly 1	S. E'ly 2	S'ly 1	0	0	5	
6	29.69	29.75	29.77	52	51	43	48.7	N. E. 2	N. E. 2	N. E. 1	10	10	10	
7	29.82	29.81	29.81	37	62	46	48.3	N. E. 1	E'ly 2	N. E. 2	0	5	10	
8	29.82	29.78	29.78	43	67	51	53.7	N. E. 1	N. E. 1	N. E. 1	Rain	7	10	
9	29.74	29.65	29.50	49	62	54	55.0	N. E. 1	S. E. 1	S. E. 1	Foggy	Foggy	Rain	} 0.80
S 10	29.24	29.11	29.00	56	62	54	57.3	S. E. 1	S. E. 1	S'ly 1	Rain	10	10	
11	29.07	29.13	29.26	44	48	40	44.0	N. W. 3	N. W. 2	N. W. 2	0	10	8	
12	29.34	...	29.56	39	...	49	...	N. W. 2	...	N. W. 1	2	...	0	
13	29.79	29.78	29.78	43	62	51	52.0	N. W. 2	S'ly 3	S'ly 2	0	2	2	
14	29.89	29.91	29.90	55	71	53	59.7	S. W. 3	S. W. 3	S. W. 2	0	4	2	
15	29.91	29.88	29.88	57	69	54	60.0	S. W. 2	S. W. 2	S. W. 2	10	10	10	
16	29.91	29.93	29.93	55	69	57	60.3	S. W. 1	S. W. 2	S'ly 1	6	7	10	
S 17	29.92	29.88	29.81	57	70	60	62.3	S. E. 1	S. W. 1	S. W. 1	Rain	10	10	0.67
18	29.68	29.51	29.61	60	73	47	60.0	S. W. 2	S. W. 3	N. W. 2	6	4	Rain	0.50
19	29.71	29.68	29.68	38	52	43	44.3	N'ly 2	N. W. 2	N. W. 1	0	0	0	
20	29.65	29.48	29.51	40	60	50	50.0	N. W. 1	W'ly 3	S. W. 2	0	0	10	
21	29.67	29.75	29.87	43	52	45	46.7	N. W. 2	W'ly 2	N. W. 1	0	0	0	
22	29.99	29.96	29.96	41	61	48	50.0	N. W. 1	S. W. 2	S. W. 1	0	2	0	
23	29.89	29.81	29.73	48	54	52	51.3	S. W. 1	S. E.	S. W. 1	4	Misty	Rain	1.43
S 24	29.77	29.74	29.78	55	67	56	59.3	N. W. 1	N. E. 1	N. E. 1	10	3	10	
25	29.80	29.71	29.67	47	63	53	54.3	N. E. 1	S. W. 1	E'ly 1	Foggy	10	Foggy	
26	29.64	29.59	29.64	52	71	55	59.3	E'ly 1	N. E. 1	E'ly 1	Foggy	1	Foggy	
27	29.66	29.61	29.59	52	58	53	54.3	E'ly 1	E'ly 1	E'ly 1	10	Rain	Rain	0.30
28	29.54	29.53	29.52	51	60	50	53.7	E'ly 1	E'ly 1	E'ly 1	10	10	Misty	
29	29.53	29.56	29.60	48	55	48	50.3	N. E'ly 1	N. E. 1	N. E. 1	Misty	10	10	
30	[illegible]	[illegible]	[illegible]	47	52	48	49.0	N. E. 1	N. E. 1	N. E. 2	10	Rain	10	} 0.33
S 31	29.72	29.72	[illegible]	[illegible]	[illegible]	[illegible]	[illegible]	[illegible]	[illegible]	[illegible]	10	Rain	10	
Means	29.68	29.66	29.67	48.0	61.0	50.7	...	1.3	1.7	1.3	6.6	6.6	7.1	4.58
									1.4			6.8		
REDUCED TO SEA LEVEL.														
Max.	30.17	30.14	30.14	60	73	58	62.3	Prevailing winds from some point between—		Days.			Days.	
Min.	29.25	29.20	29.18	37	48	40	44.0	N. & E.		11	Clear		5	
Mean	29.86	29.83	29.85					E. & S.		8	Variable		} 15	
Range	0.92	0.85	0.96	23	25	18	18.3	S. & W.		7	Cloudy			
Mean of month	29.847			...	...	...	53.3	W. & N.		5	Rain fell on		11	
Extreme range	0.99			...	...	...	36.0							

REMARKS.

1st. Rain in the afternoon, with thunder.
2d. Mild. Evening pleasant.
3d. Mild.
4th and 5th. Very fine.
6th. Appearances of rain at 10 P. M.; clouds from N. W.
7th. Rather raw.
8th. Occultation of Spica Virginis at 8 h. 41 m. 51 s., mean solar time.
9th. Fine showers in the evening.
10th. Heavy thundershower from 5 to 6 A. M.
11th. Very blustering.
12th. Cold for the season.
13th. Pleasant.
14th. Very windy.
15th. Appearances of rain.
16th. Sprinkling of rain from noon to 1 P. M.
17th. Fine showers in the morning.
18th. Fine shower from 6 to 7 P. M., with lightning.
19th. Very cool. Aurora in the evening with faint streamers.
20th. Sprinkling of rain in the evening.
21st. Cool and very clear.
22d. Fine, but cool.
23d. Heavy thundershowers from 7 to 10 P. M.
24th. Pleasant.
25th. Fog and appearances of rain.
26th. Warm and damp air.
27th. Light showers.
28th. Occasional light showers, with mist.
29th. Mist and fog.
30th. Light rain occasionally.
31st. Light showers.

June, 1846.

DAYS.	BAROMETER, REDUCED TO 32° F. At 6 A. M.	At 1 P. M.	At 10 P. M.	THERMOMETER. At 6 A. M.	At 1 P. M.	At 10 P. M.	Daily mean.	WINDS. (DIRECTION AND FORCE.) At 6 A. M.	At 1 P. M.	At 10 P. M.	WEATHER. (TENTHS CLOUDY.) At 6 A. M.	At 1 P. M.	At 10 P. M.	RAIN AND SNOW IN INCHES OF WATER.
1	...	...	...	52	73	58	61.0	N. E. 1	S'ly 1	S'ly 1	10	9	10	
2	...	...	...	56	70	61	62.3	S'ly 1	S. E. 2	S'ly 1	Foggy	9	10	
3	...	...	...	62	75	63	66.7	W'ly 2	W'ly 2	S. W. 2	3	0	0	
4	...	...	...	63	83	64	70.0	S. W. 2	S. W. 2	S. W. 3	0	2	8	
5	...	...	...	65	80	66	70.3	S. W. 2	S. W. 3	S. W. 2	5	10	8	
6	...	...	...	63	72	56	63.7	N. W. 2	N. W. 2	N. W. 1	10	0	0	
S 7	...	...	...	53	68	56	59.0	N. W. 2	N. W. 2	W'ly 1	0	0	0	
8	...	...	...	54	69	57	60.0	N. W. 1	E'ly 1	S. W'ly	0	5	3	
9	...	...	...	51	69	54	58.0	N'ly 1	N. E. 1	S. W. 1	0	3	5	
10	...	...	...	51	74	57	60.7	N. W. 1	S. E. 2	S. W.	3	3	2	
11	...	...	...	57	79	61	65.7	S. W. 1	S. W. 1	N. E. 2	2	6	10	
12	...	...	...	56	64	49	56.3	N. E. 2	N. E. 2	N. E. 2	10	2	0	
13	...	...	...	45	70	54	56.3	N. E. 1	S. E. 2	S'ly 1	0	3	0	
S 14	...	...	...	52	72	60	61.3	S. W. 1	S. W. 2	S. W. 1	6	2	0	
15	...	...	...	63	73	64	66.7	S. W. 1	S. W. 2	S. W. 1	2	3	Sh'r, 7	0.35
16	...	...	...	58	67	54	59.7	S. W. 2	N. E. 2	N. E. 2	3	0	0	
17	...	...	...	52	72	54	59.3	N. E. 1	S. E. 2	...	2	2	0	
18	...	...	...	...	...	...	...	...	...	...	...	...	...	
19	...	...	...	...	77	64	...	...	S. W. 1	S. W. 1	...	3	Rain	
20	...	...	...	63	67	54	61.3	S. W.	N. E'ly 1	N. E. 1	5	10	Sh'r, 5	0.40
S 21	...	...	...	53	62	53	56.0	N. E. 2	N. E. 1	N. E. 1	10	10	6	
22	...	...	...	49	55	50	51.3	N. W. 1	W'ly 2	N. W. 1	8	10	5	
23	...	...	...	46	54	50	50.0	N'ly 1	N. E. 1	N. E. 1	10	Misty	Rain	0.25
24	...	...	...	48	65	53	55.3	N. E. 1	N'ly 1	N'ly 1	10	7	10	
25	...	...	...	50	66	52	56.0	N. E. 1	N. E. 2	N. E. 1	3	5	3	
26	...	...	...	52	62	51	55.0	N. E. 1	N. E. 2	N. E. 2	Rain	5	Rain	}
27	...	...	...	51	64	54	56.3	N. E. 1	N. E. 2	N'ly 1	10	6	0	}
S 28	...	...	...	57	70	61	62.7	N. W. 1	N. W. 1	S. W. 1	8	4	10	} 0.40
29	...	...	...	61	73	62	65.3	W'ly 1	S. W. 1	S. W. 1	Rain	5	0	}
30	...	...	...	62	73	62	65.7	S. W. 1	S'ly 1	S. E'ly 1	Foggy	2	Foggy	}
Means	...	...	...	55.2	69.6	57.0	...	1.3	1.6	1.3	5.6	4.8	5.0	1.30
									1.4			5.1		
REDUCED TO SEA LEVEL.								Prevailing winds from some point between—		Days.			Days.	
Max.	...	...	...	65	83	66	70.3	N. & E.		10	Clear		6	
Min.	...	...	...	45	54	49	50.0	E. & S.		6	Variable		} 13	
Mean	...	...	...					S. & W.		9	Cloudy		}	
Range	...	...	...	20	29	17	20.3	W. & N.		5	Rain fell on		10	
Mean of month			...	...	...	...	60.6				(1 day omitted.)			
Extreme range			...	...	...	...	38.0							

REMARKS.

Barometer injured; *i. e.*, air got into the sealed end by being moved.
1st. Warm. Sun appeared occasionally.
2d. Warm and damp. Sprinkling of rain in the afternoon.
3d. Very fine.
4th. Warm and fine.
5th. Very sultry. Slight sprinkling at noon.
6th. Fine.
7th to 10th. Very fine.
11th. Fine.
12th. Variable. Wind at sunset rather fresh at N. E.; clouds at the same time moving from S. of W.
13th. Pleasant.
14th. Very fine. Hot sun. Ground dry.
15th. Thundershower at from 6 to 7 P. M.
16th. Air rather raw.
17th and 18th. Pleasant.
19th. Light showers at sunrise; also, from 8 to 9 P. M., with some thunder.
20th. Fine shower at 7 P. M.
21st. Occasional sprinkling of rain.
22d. Very cool for the solstice.
23d. Very cool, with occasional light rain.
24th and 25th. Still cool.
26th. Mist, and occasional rain.
27th. Clear and mild in the evening.
28th. More pleasant. Showers during the night.
29th. Rained moderately at sunrise.
30th. Sunny and pleasant at mid-day.

July, 1846.

DAYS.	Barometer At 6 A. M.	At 1 P. M.	At 10 P. M.	Thermometer At 6 A. M.	At 1 P. M.	At 10 P. M.	Daily mean.	Winds At 6 A. M.	At 1 P. M.	At 10 P. M.	Weather At 6 A. M.	At 1 P. M.	At 10 P. M.	Rain and snow
1	...	...	...	61	65	63	63.0	E'ly 2	E'ly 1	E'ly 1	Rain	Rain	Foggy	0.16
2	...	...	...	63	78	67	69.3	E'ly 1	S. W. 2	W'ly 1	10	5	6	
3	...	...	...	63	76	...	...	E'ly 1	E'ly 1	...	5	6	...	
4	...	...	...	...	...	...	...	...	...	...	...	...	...	
S 5	...	...	...	...	...	...	...	...	...	...	...	...	...	
6	...	...	...	...	...	...	...	...	...	...	...	...	...	
7	...	...	...	64	77	64	68.3	W'ly 2	W'ly 2	N. W. 1	5	3	2	
8	...	...	...	58	76	64	66.0	N. W'ly 1	W'ly 2	N. W. 1	2	3	5	
9	...	...	29.65	60	79	66	68.3	N'ly 1	N. W. 2	N. W. 1	2	2	3	
10	29.69	29.68	29.65	67	91	76	78.0	N. W. 1	N. W. 2	S. W. 2	2	5	3	
11	29.68	29.67	29.68	75	92	69	78.7	W'ly 1	W'ly 3	N. W. 2	2	5	Shower	0.28
S 12	29.60	29.56	29.58	71	86	71	76.0	S. W'ly 1	S. W'ly 3	N. W. 2	3	3	0	
13	29.69	29.70	29.71	64	82	66	70.7	N. W. 1	W'ly 3	N. W. 2	0	3	3	
14	29.68	29.67	29.69	64	71	62	65.7	S. W. 1	N. W. 2	N. W. 2	5	3	0	
15	29.78	29.80	29.92	54	72	55	60.3	N. W. 2	N. W. 2	N. W. 1	0	2	0	
16	30.06	30.05	30.15	50	72	56	59.3	N. W. 1	N. W. 1	N. E. 1	0	5	0	
17	30.22	30.21	30.15	58	64	54	58.7	N. E. 2	N. E. 1	N. E. 1	10	10	10	
18	30.06	30.00	30.00	53	59	58	56.7	N. E. 1	N. E. 1	N. E. 1	10	Misty	10	
S 19	29.90	29.91	29.90	58	67	61	62.0	N. E. 1	N. E. 1	N. E. 1	Misty	10	10	
20	29.88	29.85	29.85	58	74	63	65.0	N. E. 1	N. E. 1	S. W. 1	10	4	0	
21	29.90	29.90	29.93	63	75	67	68.3	S. W. 1	S. W. 2	S. W. 1	10	3	7	
22	29.93	29.88	29.83	66	70	64	66.7	S. W. 1	S. W. 1	S. W. 1	Shower	Rain	10	} 1.00
23	29.59	29.50	29.53	64	76	67	69.0	S. W. 1	N. W.	W'ly	Rain	5	0	}
24	29.56	29.53	29.53	64	80	66	70.0	N. W. 1	S'ly 2	S. W. 1	0	8	0	
25	29.55	29.68	29.82	65	62	55	60.7	S. W. 2	N. E. 2	N. E. 2	Foggy	10	10	
S 26	29.89	29.90	29.91	60	70	60	63.3	N. E. 2	N. E. 1	S'ly 1	10	7	10	
27	29.93	29.90	29.91	60	72	59	63.7	S'ly 1	S. W. 1	S. W. 1	Rain	5	0	
28	29.92	29.86	29.68	58	74	61	64.3	N. W. 1	S. W. 2	W'ly	Foggy	0	0	
29	29.59	29.64	29.71	62	81	68	70.3	S. W'ly 2	S. W. 2	W'ly 1	8	6	2	
30	29.67	29.60	29.73	72	87	76	78.3	S. W. 2	S. W. 3	W. 2	Foggy	3	5	
31	29.67	29.66	29.68	76	88	76	80.0	S'ly 4	S. W. 2	S. W. 1	10	2	8	
Means	29.79	29.78	29.79	62.5	75.6	64.2	...	1.4	1.8	1.3	6.4	5.1	4.2	1.44
									1.5			5.2		
REDUCED TO SEA LEVEL.								Prevailing winds from some point between—		Days.			Days.	
Max.	30.40	30.39	30.33	76	92	76	80.0	N. & E.		6	Clear		4	
Min.	29.73	29.68	29.71	50	59	54	56.7	E. & S.		2	Variable		} 13	
Mean	29.96	29.95	29.96					S. & W.		10	Cloudy		}	
Range	0.67	0.71	0.62	26	33	22	23.3	W. & N.		10	Rain fell on		11	
Mean of month			29.957	...	...	...	67.4				(3 days omitted.)			
Extreme range			0.72	...	...	...	42.0							

REMARKS.

1st. Light rain at intervals, and foggy.
2d. Pleasant.
3d, 4th, and 5th. Warm and sultry.
8th. Pleasant. Clearer sunlight than any day in three weeks.
9th. Very fine.
10th. Very hot.
11th. Thundershower from 8 to 9 P. M.
12th. Sprinkling of rain at 5 P. M.
13th. Fine.
14th. Shower from 8 to 10 P. M. Evening beautifully clear.
15th and 16th. Very fine.
17th. Sprinkling of rain in the afternoon.
18th. Cold. Clouds, with occasional sprinkling. Some rain during the night.
19th. Little warmer, with occasional mist.
20th. Pleasant. Evening very clear.
21st. Warm and damp.
22d. Fine showers in the morning.
23d. Heavy rain in the morning.
24th. Fine.
25th. Quite cool. Misty.
26th. Sprinkling of rain in the evening.
27th. Rain at sunrise. Sun out a large part of the day.
28th, 29th, and 30th. Fine.
31st. Fog in the morning. Thunder, with sprinkling of rain at 6 P. M.

August, 1846.

DAYS.	BAROMETER, REDUCED TO 32° F. At 6 A. M.	At 1 P. M.	At 10 P. M.	THERMOMETER. At 6 A. M.	At 1 P. M.	At 10 P. M.	Daily mean.	WINDS. (DIRECTION AND FORCE.) At 6 A. M.	At 1 P. M.	At 10 P. M.	WEATHER. (TENTHS CLOUDY.) At 6 A. M.	At 1 P. M.	At 10 P. M.	RAIN AND SNOW IN INCHES OF WATER.
1	29.71	29.77	29.78	72	75	66	71.0	N. W. 3	N. E. 2	N. E. 1	8	10	10	
S 2	29.85	29.88	29.95	65	79	64	69.3	N. W. 2	N. E. 2	N. E. 1	3	0	0	
3	30.03	30.04	30.03	59	83	65	69.0	N. E. 1	N. E. 1	S'ly 1	0	0	0	
4	29.98	...	29.77	63	...	73	...	S'ly 1	...	S'ly	0	...	0	
5	29.84	29.80	29.69	72	93	78	81.0	W'ly 1	W'ly 1	S. W. 1	0	0	0	
6	29.72	29.70	29.76	74	91	77	80.7	W'ly 1	W'ly 2	N. W. 1	0	5	0	
7	29.85	29.90	...	70	84	...	...	N'ly 2	N. W. 2	...	0	3	...	
8	29.96	29.89	29.87	72	80	69	73.7	N. W. 1	S. E. 4	N. E.	6	2	Shower	0.35
S 9	29.80	29.79	29.82	68	84	70	74.0	N. E.	S. W.	S. 4	1	...	...	
10	29.78	29.59	29.64	68	78	65	70.3	N. E.	N. E. 1	N. W'ly 1	10	10	Shower	0.45
11	29.77	29.82	29.86	63	75	64	67.3	N. E. 1	N. E. 1	N'ly 1	3	0	0	
12	29.88	29.87	29.82	63	79	68	70.0	S. W. 1	S. W. 2	S. W. 1	0	2	0	
13	29.77	29.60	29.60	70	84	74	70.0	S. W. 1	S. W. 2	S. W. 1	0	0	0	
14	29.68	29.62	29.62	74	89	73	78.7	S. W. 1	S. W. 2	S'ly 1	0	6	0	0.10
15	29.67	29.66	...	72	81	...	...	S'ly 1	W'ly 1	...	Foggy	3	...	0.58
S 16	...	...	...	...	...	...	...	...	...	...	...	...	...	
17	...	...	...	...	...	...	...	...	...	...	...	...	...	
18	...	...	...	...	...	...	...	...	...	...	...	...	...	
19	...	...	...	...	...	...	...	...	...	...	...	...	...	
20	...	...	...	...	...	...	...	...	...	...	...	...	...	
21	...	...	...	...	...	...	...	...	...	...	...	...	...	
22	...	...	29.69	...	...	67	...	...	...	S. W.	...	...	10	
S 23	29.65	29.64	29.66	68	71	66	68.3	S. W. 1	N. W. 1	N. W. 1	Rain	Rain	4	0.45
24	29.89	29.93	29.96	60	74	60	64.7	N. E. 1	N. E. 1	N. E. 1	5	5	0	
25	30.04	30.03	30.02	58	72	58	62.7	N. E. 1	S. E'ly 1	N. E. 1	3	10	Rain	} 0.80
26	29.99	29.95	29.94	55	59	58	57.3	N. E. 1	N. E. 1	N. E. 1	Rain	Rain	10	
27	29.94	29.94	29.94	60	74	67	67.0	N. E. 1	W'ly 1	S. W. 1	10	8	2	
28	29.98	29.98	29.97	66	79	68	71.0	N'ly	W'ly 1	W'ly 1	Foggy	5	5	
29	29.96	29.89	29.84	70	81	73	74.7	S'ly	S'ly 1	S'ly 1	Foggy	10	8	
S 30	29.79	...	...	71	...	...	...	W'ly	...	...	5	...	...	
31	...	29.82	29.81	...	82	71	...	...	W'ly 1	S. W'ly	...	0	0	
Means	29.84	29.82	29.82	66.6	79.4	67.9	...	1.2	1.5	1.1	4.5	4.7	3.4	2.73
									1.3			4.2		
REDUCED TO SEA LEVEL.														
Max.	30.22	30.22	30.21	74	93	78	81.0							
Min.	29.83	29.77	29.80	55	59	58	57.3							
Mean	30.01	29.99	29.99											
Range	0.39	0.45	0.41	19	34	20	23.7							
Mean of month	29.997			...	...	...	71.3							
Extreme range	0.45			...	...	...	38.0							

Prevailing winds from some point between— Days.
N. & E. 7
E. & S. 2
S. & W. 12
W. & N. 4

Days.
Clear 10
Variable . . . } 6
Cloudy . . . . }
Rain fell on . . 9
(6 days omitted.)

REMARKS.

4th. Hot sun.
5th. Excessively hot.
6th. The heat slightly abated. A good deal of haze in the atmosphere.
8th. Quite warm. Hazy; whole sky slightly clouded. From 8 to 10 P. M., rained fast.
9th. Clear and pleasant. From 8 to 9 P. M., light rain.
10th. Fine shower from 7 to 9 P. M.
11th and 12th. Very fine.
13th. Very warm.
14th. Thundershower at 3 to 4 P. M.
15th. Copious shower at 2 P. M., with thunder.
22d. Sprinkling of rain in the afternoon.
23d. Rain in the morning.
24th. Aurora at the north—rather bright, without streamers.
25th. Moderate rain in the evening.
26th. Moderate rain through the day.
28th. Fine.
29th. Warm and close.
31st. Very warm.

September, 1846.

DAYS.	BAROMETER At 6 A. M.	At 1 P. M.	At 10 P. M.	THERMOMETER At 6 A. M.	At 1 P. M.	At 10 P. M.	Daily mean.	WINDS At 6 A. M.	At 1 P. M.	At 10 P. M.	WEATHER At 6 A. M.	At 1 P. M.	At 10 P. M.	RAIN AND SNOW
1	29.83	...	29.77	67	...	74	...	S. W. 1	...	S. W.	Hazy	...	0	
2	29.87	29.87	29.87	72	86	71	76.3	N. W.	S. W.	S. W.	0	0	0	
3	29.84	29.77	29.78	71	85	75	77.0	S. W. 1	S. W'ly 2	S. W. 2	Hazy	3	3	
4	29.77	29.74	29.76	75	85	75	78.3	S. W. 2	S. W. 2	S. W. 3	8	5	3	
5	29.82	29.81	29.90	75	87	77	79.7	S. W. 2	S. W'ly 3	W'ly 2	10	3	0	
S 6	29.96	29.96	29.96	76	87	79	80.7	N. W. 1	S. W. 2	W'ly 1	0	2	0	
7	29.96	29.91	29.86	74	90	75	79.7	S. W. 1	S. W. 3	S. W. 1	Hazy	2	1	
8	29.76	29.70	29.77	72	87	69	76.0	S. W. 1	S. W. 2	N. E. 2	0	4	Shower	1.37
9	29.98	30.04	30.08	59	62	48	56.3	N. E. 3	N. E. 3	N. W.	2	2	0	
10	30.25	30.27	30.26	50	67	55	57.3	N. E. 1	N. E. 2	N. E. 1	0	1	3	
11	30.19	30.08	29.97	55	77	66	66.0	N. E. 1	N. E. 1	S'ly 1	1	7	0	
12	29.88	29.76	29.69	69	79	73	73.7	S'ly 1	S. W. 2	S. W. 1	Foggy	3	8, Shr.	0.96
S 13	29.72	29.73	29.83	67	83	72	74.0	N. W. 1	N'ly 1	S. W. 1	0	0	0	
14	29.72	29.60	29.52	65	77	72	71.3	N. W. 1	S. E'ly	S. W. 1	0	5	0	
15	29.43	29.50	29.75	72	73	54	66.3	S. W. 1	N. W. 4	N. W. 2	0	0	0	
16	29.81	29.84	29.88	48	65	52	55.0	N. W.	N. W. 2	N. W. 1	0	0	0	
17	29.89	29.85	29.78	47	71	58	58.7	N. W. 1	S. W. 2	S. W. 1	0	5	3	
18	29.69	29.61	29.64	53	69	60	60.7	E'ly 1	E'ly 2	N. E. 2	3	10	10	
19	29.80	29.88	29.92	50	70	63	61.0	N'ly 1	W'ly 1	W'ly 1	0	0	0	
S 20	30.01	30.00	29.95	55	75	62	64.0	N. W. 1	S. E'ly 2	S. E'ly 1	0	8	0	
21	29.89	29.78	29.80	57	67	62	62.0	S. W. 1	S. W. 1	N. W. 1	Foggy	Rain	0	
22	29.95	29.98	29.96	55	64	52	57.0	N. E. 1	N'ly 1	N. W. 1	10	5	0	
23	30.00	29.94	29.91	47	69	56	57.3	N. W. 1	N. W. 1	N. W. 1	0	0	0	
24	29.90	29.84	29.86	55	73	63	63.7	N. W. 1	S. W. 2	S. W. 1	0	0	7	
25	29.89	...	29.71	59	...	64	...	E'ly 1	...	N. E. 1	10	...	10	
26	29.52	29.58	29.72	66	67	54	62.3	S. W. 2	N. W. 2	N. W. 1	4	10	10	
S 27	29.76	29.74	29.71	47	64	55	55.3	N. W. 1	N. W. 1	S. E'ly	4	3	Rain	
28	29.76	29.93	30.00	46	62	48	52.0	N. W. 1	N. W. 2	N'ly 1	0	0	0	
[illegible]	[illegible]	[illegible]	[illegible]	[illegible]	[illegible]	[illegible]	[illegible]	[illegible] 1	[illegible]	[illegible] 1	0	[illegible]	[illegible]	
30	29.76	29.63	29.60	57	77	62	65.3	S. W. 1	S. W. 2	S. W. 1	3	2	0	
Means	29.86	29.83	29.84	60.5	74.5	63.5	...	1.2	1.9	1.3	3.6	3.4	2.8	2.33
									1.5			3.3		
REDUCED TO SEA LEVEL.														
Max.	30.43	30.45	30.44	76	90	79	80.7							
Min.	29.61	29.68	29.70	45	62	48	52.0							
Mean	30.04	30.00	30.02											
Range	0.82	0.77	0.74	31	28	31	28.7							
Mean of month	30.020			...	...	...	66.2							
Extreme range	0.84			...	...	...	45.0							

Prevailing winds from some point between— Days.
N. & E. 6
E. & S. 2
S. & W. 14
W. & N. 8

Days.
Clear 11
Variable . . . } 13
Cloudy . . . . }
Rain fell on . . 6

REMARKS.

1st. Very warm.
2d, 3d, and 4th. Very hot.
5th, 6th, and 7th. Excessively hot.
8th. Heavy shower from 6 to 8 P. M.
9th. Fine.
10th. Fine and cool.
11th. Very fine.
12th. Lightning in the west at 10 P. M. Tempest and rain from 10 to 12 P. M.
13th. Very warm.
14th. Fine.
15th. Gust, and change of weather to cooler from 11 to 12 A. M.
16th. Very fine.
17th. Fine.
18th. Appearances of rain.
19th. Very fine.
20th. Fine. Cloudy at mid-day.
21st. Sprinkling of rain at intervals. Evening clear, with an aurora in the north, somewhat bright, with streamers.
22d. Light showers in the morning. Evening clear.
23d. Very fine. Brilliant aurora at 10 P. M., without streamers.
24th. Fine.
25th. Appearances of rain.
26th. Showers at 9 A. M.
27th. Light shower at from 8 to 9 P. M.
28th and 29th. Very fine.
30th. Fine.

October, 1846. New Moon, 20d. 2h. 36m. A. M.

Days.	Barometer, reduced to 32° F. Sunrise.	At 1 P. M.	At 10 P. M.	Thermometer. Sunrise.	At 1 P. M.	At 10 P. M.	Daily mean.	Winds (Direction and Force.) Sunrise.	At 1 P. M.	At 10 P. M.	Weather (Tenths Cloudy.) Sunrise.	At 1 P. M.	At 10 P. M.	Rain and Snow in Inches of Water.
1	29.62	29.59	29.76	57	75	56	62.7	S. W. 1	S. W.	N. E. 2	2	Hazy	10	
2	29.82	29.79	29.75	50	56	54	53.3	N. E. 2	N. E. 1	N. E. 1	10	10	Misty	
3	29.76	29.69	29.84	48	56	46	50.0	N'ly 2	N. E. 2	N'ly 1	2	5	0	
S 4	29.93	29.90	29.95	38	58	48	48.0	N. E. 2	N. E'ly 1	N. E. 2	0	5	8	
5	29.97	29.93	29.97	48	58	52	52.7	N. E. 1	S'ly 1	S. W. 1	10	Misty	0	
6	30.05	30.05	30.06	50	68	55	57.7	S. W'ly 1	W'ly 1	W'ly 1	0	0	0	
7	30.08	30.08	29.98	55	74	60	63.0	W'ly 1	W'ly 2	W'ly 1	Foggy	0	0	
8	30.07	30.05	30.11	60	79	63	67.3	W'ly 1	W'ly 1	N. E. 1	0	0	0	
9	30.08	29.88	29.82	55	75	65	65.0	N. E. 1	S. W. 2	N. E. 2	Foggy	0	10	
10	30.05	30.10	30.22	43	52	40	45.0	N. W. 2	N. W. 3	N. W. 2	0	0	0	
S 11	30.28	30.31	30.27	35	53	42	43.3	N. W. 2	N. E. 1	N. E'ly 1	0	0	0	
12	30.23	30.13	30.09	35	61	53	49.7	W'ly 1	S. W. 2	S. W. 1	0	2	0	
13	29.89	29.66	29.28	54	65	65	61.3	S. E. 1	S. E. 3	S. E. 5	10	Rain	Rain	} 0.90
14	29.59	29.55	29.54	55	62	56	57.7	N. W. 1	S. W. 1	N. W. 1	0	Rain	8	
15	29.73	29.72	29.88	43	60	49	50.7	N. W. 1	N. W. 1	N. W. 1	0	0	0	
16	30.09	30.04	29.94	42	63	57	54.0	N. W. 1	S. W. 2	S. W. 2	0	8	0	
17	29.88	29.82	29.81	57	71	57	61.7	S. W. 2	S. W. 2	S. W. 1	3	7	10	
S 18	29.71	29.64	29.75	43	44	41	42.7	N. E. 2	N. E. 2	N. E. 2	Misty	Misty	Misty	
19	29.94	29.98	30.05	38	48	38	41.3	N'ly 2	N. W. 1	N. W. 1	10	5	0	
20	30.10	30.03	29.99	30	53	44	42.3	N. W. 1	S. E. 1	S. E'ly 1	5	10	10	
21	29.95	29.89	29.99	42	56	44	47.3	N. W. 1	N. W. 1	N. W. 1	3	3	0	
22	30.02	29.85	29.75	35	53	43	43.7	N. W. 1	S. W. 2	N. W. 2	0	10	0	
23	29.95	29.85	29.79	28	41	40	36.3	N. W. 1	W'ly 2	W'ly 1	0	2	10	
24	29.64	29.61	29.82	43	57	42	47.3	S. W. 2	S. W. 2	W'ly 1	10	1	0	
S 25	29.94	30.00	30.18	34	51	40	41.7	N. W. 1	N. W. 2	N. W. 1	0	0	0	
26	30.36	30.28	30.15	32	51	51	44.7	E'ly 1	S. E'ly 2	S'ly 2	0	0	10	
27	29.98	29.81	29.70	57	67	60	61.3	S'ly 2	S. W'ly 3	S. W. 2	10	10	10	
28	29.62	29.58	29.61	50	47	38	45.0	N'ly 2	N'ly 2	W'ly 1	10	Misty	Rain	0.65
29	29.79	29.83	29.97	32	47	38	39.0	N. W. 1	N. W. 2	N. W. 1	6	0	0	
30	30.12	30.15	30.30	38	52	38	42.7	W'ly 1	W'ly 1	N. E. 2	7	10	Rain	0.30
31	30.39	30.44	30.48	30	48	45	41.0	N. E. 2	N. E. 2	N. E. 2	10	10	10	
Means	29.96	29.91	29.93	43.8	58.1	49.0	...	1.4	1.7	1.5	4.0	5.1	5.0	1.85
									1.5			4.7		
REDUCED TO SEA LEVEL.								Prevailing winds from some point between—		Days.			Days.	
Max.	30.57	30.62	30.66	60	79	65	67.3	N. & E.		7	Clear		8	
Min.	29.77	29.73	29.46	28	41	38	41.7	E. & S.		4	Variable		} 15	
Mean	30.14	30.08	30.11					S. & W.		12	Cloudy			
Range	0.80	0.89	1.20	32	38	27	25.6	W. & N.		8	Rain fell on		8	
Mean of month	30.110			...	...	...	50.3							
Extreme range	1.20			...	...	...	51.0							

Remarks.

1st. Wind came suddenly to N. E. about 8 P. M., and blew briskly.
2d. Mist, with occasional dashes of rain.
3d. Very clear in the evening.
4th. Cool in the morning, but no frost in this immediate vicinity.
5th. Fine evening.
6th. Pleasant.
7th. Very fine.
8th. Fine, and very warm.
9th. Lightning and sprinkling of rain from 9 to 10 P. M.
10th and 11th. Very fine.
12th. First slight appearance of white frost in the College yard.
13th. Wind very heavy at S. E. in the afternoon and evening, with moderate rain.
14th. Light showers in the afternoon.
15th and 16th. Fine.
17th. Appearances of rain.
18th. Mist, with some rain.
19th. Fine.
20th. Black frost. Ice formed in shallow vessels of water.
21st. Fine.
22d. Showers from 6 to 7 P. M. Clear at 9 P. M.
23d. Appearances of storm.
24th. Pleasant.
25th. Very fine.
26th. Appearances of storm in the evening.
27th. Appearances of rain.
28th. Light shower at 3 A. M. Showers in the morning and evening.
29th. Ground covered with snow this morning. Evening clear.
30th. Moderate rain in the afternoon and evening.
31st. Air rather raw.

November, 1846. New Moon, 18d. 5h. 52m. P. M.

Days.	Barometer Sunrise.	At 1 P. M.	At 10 P. M.	Thermometer Sunrise.	At 1 P. M.	At 10 P. M.	Daily mean.	Winds Sunrise.	At 1 P. M.	At 10 P. M.	Weather Sunrise.	At 1 P. M.	At 10 P. M.	Rain and Snow
S 1	30.48	30.42	30.39	44	54	45	47.7	N. E. 2	N. E. 2	N. E. 1	10	10	8	
2	30.28	30.20	30.18	47	64	50	53.7	N. E'ly 1	N. E'ly 1	S. E. 1	10	8	Hazy	
3	30.11	30.04	30.03	53	66	59	59.3	N. E. 1	S. E'ly 2	S'ly 1	Misty	9	Hazy	
4	29.96	29.94	30.06	58	61	51	56.7	S'ly 1	S. W. 2	N. E. 2	Foggy	Misty	10	
5	30.14	30.20	30.20	40	56	46	47.3	N. W. 1	N. E. 2	E'ly 1	2	2	3	
6	30.23	30.21	30.19	43	55	42	46.7	N. E. 1	N. E. 2	N. E. 1	10	10	Hazy	
7	30.19	30.12	30.11	41	59	46	48.7	N. E. 1	N. E. 1	N. E. 1	3	9	5	
S 8	30.08	30.04	30.04	42	59	50	50.3	N. E. 1	N. E. 1	N. E. 1	10	10	10	
9	29.96	29.91	29.91	47	55	49	50.3	N. E. 1	N. E. 1	N. E. 2	Rain	Rain	Misty	1.15
10	29.93	29.90	29.92	48	52	56	52.0	N'ly 1	N. E. 1	N. E. 1	Misty	Misty	Misty	
11	29.90	29.83	29.82	50	54	52	52.0	N. E. 1	N. E. 1	N. E. 1	Misty	Misty	10	
12	29.83	29.84	29.94	48	48	45	47.0	N. E. 2	N. E. 3	N. E. 3	Rain	Misty	Misty	0.35
13	29.98	29.95	29.95	44	46	44	44.7	N. E. 3	N. E. 3	N. E. 3	10	10	8	
14	29.95	29.95	29.99	44	47	45	45.3	N. E. 2	N. E. 2	N. E. 2	10	10	10	
S 15	29.99	29.95	29.98	45	53	47	48.3	N. E. 2	N. E. 2	N. E. 2	10	10	10	
16	29.90	29.92	29.98	46	42	44	44.0	N. E. 2	N. E. 2	N'ly 2	10	Rain	5	0.60
17	30.04	30.01	30.04	38	52	41	43.7	N'ly 1	N. E. 1	N. E. 2	0	0	2	
18	30.08	30.08	29.96	41	48	42	43.7	N. E. 1	S. E. 2	S. 2	Misty	0	0	
19	29.83	29.69	29.34	44	57	56	52.3	S. 0	S'ly 2	S. E'ly 4	Misty	10	Rain	0.72
20	29.08	29.19	29.45	46	57	40	47.7	W' 3	W'ly 3	N. W. 3	5	7	Hazy	
21	29.69	29.69	29.71	38	49	38	41.7	N. 1	N. W. 1	N. W. 1	2	0	0	
S 22	29.64	29.49	29.31	36	53	45	44.7	S. 1	S. W. 2	S. W. 1	3	1	5	
23	29.15	29.30	29.60	36	44	33	37.7	N. 2	N. W. 3	N. W. 3	Rain	5	0	0.20
24	29.57	29.51	29.54	32	43	36	37.0	N. 1	N. W. 2	N. W. 2	3	0	0	
25	29.41	29.10	28.47	35	33	30	32.7	N'ly 1	N. E. 1	N'ly 3	Snow	Snow	Snow	1.10
26	29.05	29.28	29.47	22	29	26	25.7	N. W. 3	N. W. 4	N. W. 3	10	8	0	
27	29.72	29.80	29.88	28	33	30	30.3	W'ly 3	W' 2	W'ly 1	2	10	10	
28	29.75	29.71	29.81	38	46	37	40.3	S. W. 1	S. 1	W'ly 1	10	2	2	
S 29	29.79	29.68	29.68	38	42	36	38.7	S'ly 1	N'ly 1	N. W. 1	Rain	3	0	0.50
30	29.70	29.79	29.89	34	34	26	31.3	W'ly 1	N. W. 3	N. W. 3	2	7	5	
Means	29.85	29.82	29.86	41.5	49.7	42.9	...	1.4	1.9	1.8	7.7	6.9	6.4	4.62
									1.7			7.0		
REDUCED TO SEA LEVEL.								Prevailing winds from some point between—		Days.			Days.	
Max.	30.66	30.60	30.57	58	66	59	59.3	N. & E.		16	Clear		4	
Min.	20.23	29.28	28.65	22	29	26	25.7	E. & S.		3	Variable		} 18	
Mean	30.03	30.00	30.04					S. & W.		3	Cloudy			
Range	1.43	1.32	1.92	36	37	33	33.6	W. & N.		8	Rain or snow fell on		8	
Mean of month	30.023			...	...	...	44.7							
Extreme range	2.01			...	...	...	44.0							

Remarks.

1st. Rather raw.
2d. Pleasant.
3d. Mild.
4th. Moderate rain at intervals in the afternoon.
5th. Bright halo about the moon at 10 P. M.; continued all night.
6th. Bright halo about the moon at 10 P. M.
7th. Pleasant.
8th. Halo about the moon at 4 A. M. Appearances of rain in the afternoon.
9th. Rainy.
10th and 11th. Clouds and mist.
12th. Clouds and mist, with rain.
13th. Clouds and mist, some stars visible in the evening.
14th. Sun appeared once or twice in the morning.
15th. Clouds continue. One or two glimpses of the stars only.
16th. Rain in the morning. Wind came to the N. W., and partly clear in the evening.
17th. Very fine.
18th. Foggy in the morning.
19th. Foggy in the morning. Rain in the evening, with very blustering wind at a little E. of S. At 9 P. M., barometer 29.46, and falling; at 10 P. M., barometer 29.31, wind as before.
20th. Very blustering.
21st. Pleasant.
22d. Copious white frost. Pleasant.
23d. Rain in the morning; blustering. Very clear in the evening, with strong wind.
24th. Fine.
25th. Wind light N. E., with very gentle snow. Barometer falling. Wind increased during the morning; snow also increased, mixed with rain. Wind very strong from 5 to 7 P. M., with barometer falling rapidly. At 8 P. M., barometer 28.70; at 8½ P. M., 28.66; at 9 P. M., 28.57; at 10 P. M., 28.57, wind N'ly, and snow; at 10½ P. M., 28.60, having began to show an upward tendency soon after 10 P. M.
26th. Very blustering. Evening very clear.
27th. Pleasant.
28th. Very fine.
29th. Moderate rain in the morning. Clear in the evening.
30th. Fine.

December, 1846. New Moon, 18d. 7h. 34m. A. M.

Days.	Barometer, reduced to 32° F. Sunrise.	At 1 P. M.	At 10 P. M.	Thermometer. Sunrise.	At 1 P. M.	At 10 P. M.	Daily mean.	Winds (Direction and Force.) Sunrise.	At 1 P. M.	At 10 P. M.	Weather (Tenths Cloudy.) Sunrise.	At 1 P. M.	At 10 P. M.	Rain and Snow in Inches of Water
1	30.04	30.05	30.15	24	32	25	27.0	N. W. 1	N. W. 3	N. W. 1	3	0	0, Hazy	
2	30.24	30.20	29.96	24	33	36	31.0	N. W. 1	S'ly 1	E'ly 1	10	Hail	Rain	} 0.68
3	29.57	29.48	29.60	53	55	38	48.7	S'ly 3	W'ly 2	W'ly 1	Rain	9	0	
4	29.76	29.80	29.90	33	37	35	35.0	N. W. 2	N. W. 2	N. W. 2	3	2	9	
5	30.19	30.16	30.23	28	35	28	30.3	N. W. 1	N. W. 2	N. W. 2	0	0	2	
S 6	30.26	30.30	30.33	23	30	23	25.3	N. W. 1	N. W. 2	N. W. 1	0	0	0	
7	30.30	30.17	29.99	18	35	37	30.0	N. W. 1	W'ly 1	E'ly 2	0	9	10	
8	29.60	29.50	29.51	43	49	44	45.3	E'ly 1	S. W. 1	W'ly 1	Misty	Misty	10	} 0.72
9	29.50	29.62	29.89	36	40	30	35.3	N'ly 1	N'ly 2	N. W. 1	R'n, sn.	0	0	
10	29.95	29.85	29.54	24	38	34	32.0	N. W. 1	S. E'ly 1	E'ly 2	0	10	Snow	1.00
11	29.49	29.51	29.66	33	36	22	30.3	N'ly 1	N. W. 1	N. W. 2	Snow	9	0	
12	29.70	29.69	29.70	17	22	17	18.7	N. W. 1	N. W. 2	N. W. 2	0	0	0	
S 13	29.69	29.64	29.70	18	25	21	21.3	N. W. 1	N. W. 2	N. W. 2	0	0	0	
14	29.76	29.76	29.78	15	22	18	18.3	N. W. 1	N. W. 2	N. W. 1	0	0	0	
15	29.76	29.73	29.81	14	21	13	16.0	N. W. 1	N. W. 2	N. W. 1	0	0	0	
16	29.90	29.90	29.93	10	24	16	16.7	N. W. 1	N. W. 1	N. W. 1	0	2	0	
17	29.91	29.74	29.31	12	27	32	23.7	N. E. 1	N. E. 2	N. E. 4	10	10	Rain	0.75
18	29.15	29.09	29.14	33	35	35	34.3	N. E. 2	N'ly 2	N'ly 1	Misty	10	10	
19	29.21	29.19	29.28	25	37	34	32.0	N. W. 1	W'ly 2	W'ly 2	0	7	10	
S 20	29.40	29.48	29.64	30	35	27	30.7	N. W. 1	W'ly 2	W'ly 1	10	10	0	
21	29.71	29.77	29.98	24	31	25	26.7	W'ly 1	W'ly 2	N. W. 2	8	0	0	
22	30.09	30.12	30.12	18	31	29	26.0	W'ly 1	S. W'ly 1	W'ly 1	0	Snow	10	
23	30.15	30.19	30.21	18	27	19	21.3	N. W. 1	N. W. 1	N. W. 1	2	0	0	
24	30.21	30.12	29.91	14	29	32	25.0	N. W. 1	N. W. 1	S. W. 2	0	0	10	
25	29.72	29.48	29.41	33	40	33	35.3	S'ly 1	S. W. 1	N'ly 3	5	10	Rain	
26	29.83	29.90	29.91	20	25	24	23.0	N. W. 2	N. W. 2	W'ly 2	2	0	Hazy	
S 27	29.57	29.39	29.33	38	43	44	41.7	S. W. 1	S. W. 1	S. W. 3	10	10	5	
28	29.44	29.38	29.42	42	44	42	42.7	S. W. 1	S. W. 1	N'ly 1	10	10	10	
29	29.93	30.10	30.16	24	31	25	26.7	N. W. 1	N. W. 1	N. W. 1	0	0	8	
30	...	29.57	29.75	...	44	35	...	...	S. 2	N. W. 1	...	Rain	0	
31	29.86	...	29.82	40	...	42	...	N. W. 1	...	S. W.	5	...	Rain	
Means	29.80	29.76	29.78	26.1	33.8	29.5	...	1.3	1.6	1.6	4.2	4.2	5.0	3.15
								1.5			4.5			
REDUCED TO SEA LEVEL.														
Max.	30.48	30.48	30.51	53	55	44	48.7							
Min.	29.33	29.27	29.32	10	21	13	16.0							
Mean	29.98	29.94	29.96											
Range	1.15	1.21	1.19	43	34	31	32.7							
Mean of month 29.960				...	...	...	29.8							
Extreme range 1.24				...	...	...	45.0							

Prevailing winds from some point between— Days.
N. & E. 2
E. & S. 1
S. & W. 9
W. & N. 19

Days.
Clear 10
Variable . . . } 11
Cloudy . . . . }
Rain or snow fell on 10

Remarks.

1st. Halo about the moon at 9 P. M.
2d. Halo and mist in the afternoon. Moderate rain in the evening.
3d. Rain in the morning. Clear in the evening.
4th and 5th. Pleasant.
6th. Very fine.
7th. Appearances of storm in the evening.
8th. Mist. Rain during the night, commencing at 10 o'clock.
9th. Snow and rain in the morning. Clear in the evening.
10th. Began to snow at 6 P. M.; wind about E. by N.
11th. Ground covered with heavy damp snow, about one foot deep on the level.
12th. Cold, but very clear.
13th to 16th. Fine.
17th. Began to snow at 3 P. M.; wind brisk at N. E. Rain in the evening, with wind much increased and heavy at the same point.
18th. Mist in the morning. Sprinkling of rain in the evening.
19th. Mild.
20th. Clear in the evening.
21st. Fine.
22d. Light scattering of snow at 2 P. M.
23d. Fine.
24th. Appearances of rain; wind S. W., increasing at 10 P. M.
25th. Moderate rain began at 4 P. M.; wind S. W.
26th. Fine.
27th. Halo about the moon in the evening.
28th. Mild.
29th. Very fine.
30th. Rain from 10 A. M. to 4 P. M.
31st. Sprinkling of rain in the evening.

January, 1847. New Moon, 16d. 7h. 37m. P. M.

Days.	Barometer Sunrise.	At 1 P. M.	At 10 P. M.	Thermometer Sunrise.	At 1 P. M.	At 10 P. M.	Daily mean.	Winds Sunrise.	At 1 P. M.	At 10 P. M.	Weather Sunrise.	At 1 P. M.	At 10 P. M.	Rain and Snow in Inches of Water
1	29.71	29.79	29.84	44	...	44	...	S. W. 1	...	N'ly 1	9	...	10	
2	29.79	29.86	29.98	36	39	36	37.0	N'ly 1	N'ly 1	W'ly 1	Misty	Misty	Foggy	
S 3	30.04	30.05	30.17	37	42	32	37.0	N. W. 1	N. W. 1	N. W. 1	10	8	0	
4	30.25	30.21	29.94	29	39	36	34.7	N. E. 1	N. E. 2	E'ly 2	10	10	Rain	
5	29.35	29.53	29.69	48	50	42	46.7	W'ly 3	W'ly 3	W'ly 3	Rain	0	0	
6	29.85	29.85	29.83	36	47	35	39.3	W'ly 1	S. W. 1	S'ly 1	0	0	0	
7	29.60	29.36	29.01	30	43	45	39.3	N. E. 1	N. E. 1	S'ly 1	Foggy	Rain	10	
8	29.60	29.73	30.03	22	27	19	22.7	W'ly 3	N. W. 3	N. W. 2	0	0	0	
9	30.19	30.15	30.15	14	25	26	21.7	N. W. 2	S. W. 1	S. W. 1	0	8	10	
S 10	30.11	30.07	30.05	28	31	26	28.3	S. W. 1	S. W. 1	S. W. 1	10	Snow	10	
11	29.86	29.69	29.79	22	25	20	22.3	N. E. 1	N'ly 2	N. W. 1	Snow	9	2	0.65
12	30.03	30.07	30.24	14	21	16	17.0	N. W. 1	W'ly 2	N. W. 1	0	0	0	
13	30.30	30.20	29.99	14	31	31	25.3	N. W. 1	S. W. 1	S. W. 1	0	10	Hazy	
14	29.81	29.69	29.70	31	47	37	38.3	S. W. 2	S. W. 1	W'ly 1	10	10	0	
15	29.90	29.76	29.59	37	44	40	40.3	S. W. 1	E'ly 2	E'ly	10	10	Foggy	
16	29.47	29.39	29.70	40	50	34	41.3	S. W. 1	S. W. 1	N. W. 3	10	9	0	
S 17	30.20	30.21	30.34	16	22	14	17.3	N. W. 1	N. W. 1	N. W. 2	0	0	0	
18	30.22	30.19	29.54	20	35	42	32.3	S'ly 1	S. W. 1	S. W. 1	10	Snow	Rain	0.20
19	29.63	29.70	30.14	37	35	19	30.3	N. W. 2	N. W. 2	N. W. 2	8	3	5	
20	30.31	30.30	30.20	14	23	19	18.7	N. W. 1	N. W. 1	N. W. 1	8	2	2	
21	29.95	29.79	29.84	15	27	16	19.3	N. W. 1	N. W. 1	N. W. 2	2	5	0	
22	30.00	29.97	30.00	7	19	15	13.7	N. W. 2	N. W. 2	N. W. 2	0	0	0	
23	29.77	29.61	29.75	20	35	29	28.0	S. W. 1	S. W. 3	W'ly 1	0	0	2	
S 24	29.84	29.71	29.88	27	43	34	34.7	S. W. 1	S. W. 2	W'ly 1	3	4	1	
25	30.26	30.15	30.20	20	31	23	24.7	N. E'ly 1	N'ly 1	N. E. 1	2	0	0	
26	30.16	30.56	29.67	25	37	41	34.3	N. E. 1	S. E. 2	S'ly 1	10	10	10, R'n	
27	29.73	29.86	29.99	33	29	14	25.3	N'ly 2	N. W. 2	N. W. 3	10	0	0	
28	30.31	30.30	30.30	8	25	21	18.0	N. W. 2	N. W. 2	N. W. 1	0	0	0	
29	30.06	29.90	29.34	26	41	[illegible]	[illegible]	W'ly 2	W'ly 1	S. E. 3	5	10	Rain	1.28
30	28.76	28.96	29.34	36	32	22	30.0	N. W. 1	N. W. 3	N. W. 5	10	5	3	
S 31	29.58	29.65	29.76	12	21	16	16.3	N. W. 2	N. W. 2	N. W.	2	0	2	
Means	29.92	29.88	29.87	25.7	33.9	28.5	...	1.4	1.6	1.6	5.8	4.9	4.1	2.13
								1.5			4.9			
REDUCED TO SEA LEVEL.														
Max.	30.49	30.74	30.52	48	50	45	46.7							
Min.	28.94	29.14	20.10	7	19	14	13.7							
Mean	30.10	30.06	30.05											
Range	1.55	1.60	1.33	41	31	31	33.0							
Mean of month 30.070				...	...	...	29.4							
Extreme range 1.80				...	...	...	43.0							

Prevailing winds from some point between— Days.
N. & E. 3
E. & S. 2
S. & W. 12
W. & N. 14

Days.
Clear 9
Variable . . . } 13
Cloudy . . . . }
Rain or snow fell on 9

Remarks.

1st. Very mild and pleasant.
2d. Mist and fog.
3d. Mild. Evening very fine and clear.
4th. Snow began at 7 A. M., turned to rain at 9 A. M.
5th. Dashes of rain at sunrise. Very clear in the evening.
6th. Very fine. Frost in most places entirely out of the ground.
7th. Began to rain from noon to 1 P. M. At 6 P. M., wind S. W'ly, very blustering, barometer falling. At 6½ P. M., barometer 29.10; at 7 P. M., 29.07; at 7½ P. M., 29.08; at 8 P. M., 29 09; at 10 P. M., 29.12, and the wind entirely ceased.
8th. Cold, but fine.
9th. Haze and gathering clouds in the evening.
10th. The ground covered with snow.
11th. Began to snow at 4 to 5 A. M., and continued nearly all day. Cleared from 9 to 10 P. M. Seven to eight inches of light dry snow fell.
12th. Fine.
13th. Moderate in the afternoon.
14th. Appearances of storm through the day. Very clear in the evening.
15th. Thick fog in the evening.
16th. Light rain in the morning. Clear in the evening and very blustering; wind N. W.
17th. Fine.
18th. Commenced snowing at 11 A. M., but soon turned to moderate rain, which continued during the afternoon and evening.
19th. Rather blustering.
20th. At 7 A. M., barometer 30.41; at 10 A. M., 30.47; at 2 P. M., 30.41.
21st. Evening very clear and cold.
22d. Cold, but fine for winter.
23d. Very blustering.
24th. Very fine in the evening.
25th. Very fine.
26th. Light showers in the evening.
27th. Very cold evening.
28th. Very fine.
29th. Rain in the afternoon and evening.

February, 1847. New Moon, 15d. 6h. 18m. A. M.

Days.	Barometer, reduced to 32° F. Sunrise.	At 1 P. M.	At 10 P. M.	Thermometer. Sunrise.	At 1 P. M.	At 10 P. M.	Daily mean.	Winds. (Direction and Force.) Sunrise.	At 1 P. M.	At 10 P. M.	Weather. (Tenths Cloudy.) Sunrise.	At 1 P. M.	At 10 P. M.	Rain and Snow in Inches of Water.
1	29.83	29.86	29.97	13	30	23	22.0	N. W.	N. E'ly	N. E.	5	10	10	
2	30.16	30.14	30.12	27	49	36	37.3	N. E.	S. E'ly	S. E. 1	9	10	9	
3	29.92	29.69	29.03	40	47	43	43.3	S. E.	S. E. 3	S'ly 2	10	Rain	5	0.96
4	29.11	29.25	29.45	28	23	15	22.0	N. W. 2	N. W. 2	N. W. 2	Snow	0	10	
5	29.56	29.54	29.58	10	25	25	20.0	N. W. 1	N. W. 2	N. W. 1	3	0	8	
6	29.70	29.62	29.65	25	41	30	32.0	N. W.	N. W. 1	N. 1	9	7	3	
S 7	29.70	29.61	29.55	25	41	31	32.3	N. W. 1	N. W. 1	S. W. 1	0	2	2	
8	29.48	29.49	29.59	32	41	34	35.7	N. W. 1	N. W. 1	W'ly 1	2	7	10	
9	29.45	29.45	29.65	39	51	40	43.3	S. W. 3	W'ly 2	N'ly 1	8	10	10	
10	29.73	29.71	29.71	32	36	34	34.0	N. E'ly 1	N. E. 1	N'ly 1	Snow	Misty	10	
11	29.72	29.70	29.79	30	37	24	30.3	N. W. 1	N. W. 2	N. W. 1	3	7	0	
12	29.83	29.76	29.79	20	31	24	25.0	N. W. 1	S. W'ly 2	N. W. 2	6	7	0	
13	29.90	29.84	29.85	17	29	21	22.3	N. W. 1	W'ly 2	N. W. 1	0	10	0	
S 14	29.87	29.86	29.86	24	33	29	28.7	W'ly 1	W'ly 2	N'ly 1	3	10	3	
15	29.75	29.74	30.03	34	45	28	35.7	S. W'ly 2	W'ly 1	N. W. 2	Snow	7	3	
16	30.30	30.33	30.04	17	27	26	23.3	N'ly 1	N. E. 2	N. E. 2	7	10	Snow	
17	29.76	29.77	29.94	26	41	32	33.0	E'ly 1	N. W. 1	W'ly 2	Misty	5	10	
18	30.12	30.11	30.09	26	41	33	33.3	N. W. 1	S. E'ly 1	S'ly 1	2	8	10	
19	30.06	30.05	30.11	28	35	31	31.3	N. E. 1	E'ly 1	S'ly 1	Snow	10	10	
20	30.17	30.15	30.16	32	33	31	32.0	W'ly 1	E'ly 1	E'ly	10	10	10	1.75
S 21	30.10	29.90	29.79	22	27	26	25.0	N. E. 2	N. E. 2	N. E. 1	Snow	Snow	Snow	
22	29.71	29.57	29.55	17	27	17	20.3	N. E. 1	N. E. 1	N. E. 3	10	Snow	Snow	
23	29.78	29.90	30.07	9	20	15	14.7	N. W. 1	N. W. 2	N. W. 1	5	0	0	
24	30.18	30.18	30.16	6	29	16	17.0	N. W. 1	N. W. 1	S. W'ly 1	0	0	Hazy	
25	30.09	30.00	30.04	20	28	23	23.7	W'ly 1	S'ly 1	N. E'ly 1	10	10	10	
26	30.14	30.17	30.17	11	32	23	22.0	N'ly 1	N. W. 1	W'ly 1	0	0	Hazy	
27	30.12	29.80	29.19	23	34	39	32.0	N. E. 1	S. E'ly 2	S. E. 3	10	Sn., h'l	Rain	
S 28	29.06	29.16	29.20	37	38	33	36.0	W'ly 2	W'ly 2	W'ly 2	8	10	0	
Means	29.83	29.80	29.79	23.9	34.7	27.9	...	1.3	1.6	1.4	6.5	7.1	6.9	2.71
								1.4			6.8			
REDUCED TO SEA LEVEL.														
Max.	30.48	30.33	30.35	40	57	43	43.3							
Min.	29.24	29.34	29.21	6	20	15	14.7							
Mean	30.01	29.98	29.97											
Range	1.24	0.99	1.14	34	31	28	28.6							
Mean of month	29.986			...	...	...	28.8							
Extreme range	1.27			...	...	...	45.0							

Prevailing winds from some point between— Days.
N. & E. 7
E. & S. 5
S. & W. 0
W. & N. 16

Days.
Clear 4
Variable . . . } 16
Cloudy . . . . }
Rain or snow fell on 8

REMARKS.

1st. Cold.

2d. Mild.

3d. Wind light S. E'ly in the morning. Began to rain moderately at 10½ A. M.; rain continued during afternoon, and wind increased in strength, with barometer falling rapidly. At 7 P. M., wind increased to a gale; barometer 29.24. At 7½ P. M., barometer 29.17; at 8 P. M., 29.10; at 8½ P. M., 29.14; at 9 P. M., 29.14, wind S'ly and much abated, and rain heavy. At 10 P. M., wind still more abated, and barometer 29.14; rain ceased, and the clouds rapidly dispersing; stars out in various directions. At 10½ P. M., barometer still 29.14; nearly all clear overhead.

4th. Blustering and severe. Flurry of snow during the night.

7th. Very fine. Flurry of snow, one inch deep, during the night.

8th. Pleasant.

9th. Very mild.

10th. Light snow in the morning. Mist in the afternoon. One and a half to two inches of moist snow fell.

11th. Evening very clear.

12th. Pleasant.

13th. Evening very clear.

14th. Haze all around the horizon in the evening.

15th. Flurry of snow at sunrise.

16th. Began to snow at about 7 P. M.

17th. At sunrise, about one inch and a half of moist snow on the ground, which nearly all disappeared during the day.

18th. Very mild. Two inches of light snow during the night.

19th and 20th. Very mild.

21st. Snow during the day; wind light N. E. At 9 P. M., snowing quite moderately. Snow six to eight inches deep.

22d. Snow ceased for awhile in the morning, but soon returned, and the storm increased in violence. Barometer at 4 P. M. was 29.60, and began to rise before 9 P. M. Snow about one foot deep.

23d, 24th, and 25th. Pleasant.

26th. Very pleasant.

27th. Steady rain in the afternoon and evening.

28th. Pleasant.

March, 1847. New Moon, 16d. 4h. 3m. P. M.

Days.	Barometer Sunrise.	At 1 P. M.	At 10 P. M.	Thermometer Sunrise.	At 1 P. M.	At 10 P. M.	Daily mean.	Winds Sunrise.	At 1 P. M.	At 10 P. M.	Weather Sunrise.	At 1 P. M.	At 10 P. M.	Rain and Snow in Inches of Water.
1	29.36	29.41	29.61	26	29	25	26.7	W'ly 2	W'ly 3	N. W. 2	5	2	2	
2	29.76	29.79	29.91	25	28	24	25.7	N. W. 1	N. W. 2	N. W. 1	3	0	0	
3	30.01	30.03	29.99	20	34	33	29.0	N. W. 1	W'ly 2	S. W'ly 1	0	0	10	
4	29.92	29.93	29.94	32	...	29	...	S. W'ly 1	...	N'ly 1	10	...	0	
5	30.06	30.10	30.18	26	38	33	32.3	N. W. 1	N. E. 1	N. E. 1	0	2	0	
6	30.30	30.30	30.26	25	42	33	33.3	W'ly 1	W'ly 1	W'ly 1	2	0	2	
S 7	30.20	30.02	29.87	29	41	38	36.0	W'ly 1	S. E'ly 1	S. E'ly 1	3	10	Misty	
8	29.80	29.80	29.92	44	52	38	44.7	W'ly 1	W'ly 1	W'ly 2	10	4	0	
9	30.08	30.08	30.06	32	37	32	33.7	N. W. 1	W'ly 1	N'ly 1	2	10	10	
10	29.90	29.87	29.75	33	37	35	35.0	S. W. 2	S. W. 2	N. W. 3	10	Rain	0	
11	29.87	29.80	29.77	24	29	24	25.7	N. W. 2	N. W. 2	N. W. 1	3	6	Hazy	
12	29.72	29.68	29.70	17	29	24	23.3	N. W. 1	N. W. 2	W'ly 2	0	0	0	
13	29.70	29.65	29.74	20	30	24	24.7	N. W. 2	N. W. 2	N. W. 1	10	0	0	
S 14	29.80	29.74	29.83	17	33	28	26.0	N. W. 2	N. W. 2	N. W. 1	0	0	0	
15	29.87	29.86	29.86	22	40	29	30.3	W'ly 1	W'ly 2	W'ly 1	0	3	0	
16	29.90	29.84	29.90	18	29	21	22.7	N. W. 1	N. W. 2	N. W. 2	0	2	0	
17	30.01	29.98	30.04	19	34	29	27.3	N. W. 2	N. W. 2	N. W. 2	0	5	0	
18	30.07	29.96	29.91	27	45	33	35.0	N. W. 1	S. E. 2	S'ly 1	0	3	3	
19	29.96	29.99	30.06	26	42	33	33.7	N. W. 1	N. W. 1	N. W. 1	6	2	0	
20	30.10	30.02	29.89	30	45	39	38.0	N. W. 1	S. E'ly 2	S. E. 3	0	2	10	
S 21	29.69	29.73	29.82	47	50	41	46.0	S. W. 2	S. W. 1	N. E. 2	10	Rain	Misty	0.33
22	29.79	29.71	29.70	34	35	32	33.7	N. E. 3	N. E. 4	N. E. 1	Misty	Misty	Rain	
23	29.72	29.71	29.64	29	35	35	33.0	N. 2	N. E. 2	N. E. 1	10	Misty	10	
24	29.51	...	29.74	35	...	35	...	N'ly 1	...	W'ly	Rain	...	0	0.10
25	29.84	29.81	29.70	31	50	41	40.7	N. W. 1	S. W. 2	S'ly 1	0	3	0	
26	29.74	29.81	29.14	37	52	49	46.0	E'ly 1	S. E'ly 1	S. E. 3	8	10	Rain	
27	28.43	28.59	29.23	37	37	29	34.3	S. E'ly 3	N. W. 3	N. W. 2	Misty	10	10	
S 28	29.57	29.66	29.80	24	34	27	28.3	N. W. 2	N. W. 2	N. W. 2	0	0	0	
29	29.74	29.52	29.50	27	35	32	31.3	W'ly 1	S. W. 2	N. W. 1	9	Snow	5	
30	29.73	29.76	29.77	23	39	33	31.7	N. W. 1	N. W. 2	S'ly 2	2	0	7	
31	29.61	29.72	29.85	24	35	25	28.0	N. E. 2	N'ly 1	N. W. 1	Snow	10	0	
Means	29.80	29.80	29.81	27.7	37.8	31.7	...	1.5	1.9	1.5	4.7	4.5	3.9	3.17
								1.6			4.4			
REDUCED TO SEA LEVEL.														
Max.	30.48	30.48	30.44	47	52	49	46.0							
Min.	28.61	28.77	29.32	17	28	21	22.7							
Mean	29.98	29.98	29.99											
Range	1.87	1.71	1.12	30	24	28	23.3							
Mean of month	29.983			...	...	...	32.4							
Extreme range	1.87			...	...	...	35.0							

Prevailing winds from some point between— Days.
N. & E. 3
E. & S. 4
S. & W. 4
W. & N. 20

Days.
Clear 12
Variable . . . } 9
Cloudy . . . . }
Rain or snow fell on 10

1st. Blustering.

2d. Rather blustering. Evening very fine.

3d and 4th. Pleasant.

5th. Very fine.

6th. Splendid day.

7th. Mist, with appearances of rain.

8th. Very clear in the evening.

9th. Air very raw and disagreeable.

10th. A little rain during the day. Very clear in the evening.

11th. Very raw and unpleasant.

12th. Fine, but cold.

13th. Fine.

14th. Very fine, though cool.

15th. Fine.

16th. Flurry of snow from N. W. at sunset, then clear.

17th. Very fine.

18th. Flurry of snow from 5 to 7 P. M.

19th. Very fine. During the evening a brilliant aurora, extending from N. W. round to N. E. and somewhat beyond, with coruscations shooting up, and Merry Dancers running in splendid profusion quite across the heavens from north to south.

20th. Pleasant during the day. Appearances of storm in the evening.

21st. Moderate rain at intervals.

22d. Cold and wet; rain and drizzle.

23d. Rain and drizzle.

24th. Small amount of rain and snow in the morning. Very clear in the evening.

25th. Very fine.

26th. Sprinkling of rain in the afternoon. Rain and wind increased in the evening.

27th. At 7½ A. M., barometer 28.53; wind strong S. E'ly. At 8½ A. M., barometer 28.50; at 9 A. M., 28.46; at 10 A. M., 28.46; at 11 A. M., 28.54, wind W'ly 3, rain and snow; at noon, 28.60, wind N. W'ly; at 1 P. M., 28.70; at 2 P. M., 28.80; at 6 P. M., 29.10. At 9 A. M., the barometer was lower than at any time since the commencement of my Diary in Dec. 1831.

28th. Cold and blustering.

29th. Very raw and chilly in the morning, the air full of snow. Evening mild.

30th. Pleasant.

31st. Snow in the morning, seven or eight inches deep. Clear in the evening.

Note.—Rain-gauge defective. Amount of rain in this month taken from the record of Z. Allen.

April, 1847. New Moon, 15d. 1h. 14m. A. M.

Days.	Barometer, reduced to 32° F. At 6 A. M.	At 1 P. M.	At 10 P. M.	Thermometer. At 6 A. M.	At 1 P. M.	At 10 P. M.	Daily mean	Winds (Direction and Force.) At 6 A. M.	At 1 P. M.	At 10 P. M.	Weather (Tenths Cloudy.) At 6 A. M.	At 1 P. M.	At 10 P. M.	Rain and Snow in Inches of Water.
1	30.11	30.10	30.07	15	33	26	24.7	N. W. 1	N. W. 2	W'ly 1	0	2	0	
2	29.91	29.70	29.73	31	42	34	35.7	S'ly 3	S'ly 1	N. W. 1	Snow	Misty	10	
3	29.77	29.76	29.84	36	46	38	40.0	S. W. 1	S. W'ly 1	W'ly 1	7	5	0	
S 4	29.84	29.65	29.58	39	43	35	39.0	N'ly 1	S'ly 2	N. E. 2	10	10	10	
5	29.78	29.86	29.98	32	47	38	39.0	N. W. 1	N. E. 2	N. W. 1	5	2	0	
6	30.00	29.94	29.78	35	43	39	39.0	S. W'ly 1	S. W. 2	S'ly 1	5	10	Rain	
7	29.62	29.62	29.78	38	54	45	45.7	N. W'ly 1	N. W'ly 2	N. W. 2	7	6	8	
8	29.89	29.65	29.65	41	44	44	43.0	N. W. 1	W'ly	W'ly	0	4	4	
9	29.39	29.51	29.70	50	55	42	49.0	N. W. 1	N. W. 2	N. W. 1	Sh'r, 7	2	0	
10	29.59	29.41	29.47	37	60	44	47.0	W'ly 2	S. W'ly 4	N. W. 1	0	7	0	
S 11	29.64	29.63	29.77	35	43	32	36.7	N. W. 1	N. W. 3	N. W. 1	0	5	0	
12	29.81	29.57	29.67	33	51	48	44.0	S. W'ly 1	S. W. 2	N. W. 2	9	5	10	
13	29.81	29.86	29.96	42	48	36	42.0	W'ly 1	N'ly 1	N. W. 1	10	0	0	
14	29.98	29.99	29.96	32	52	39	41.0	N. W. 1	S. W. 3	N. W.	0	0	0	
15	29.81	29.65	29.66	32	59	41	44.0	S.	S. W.	N. W.	9	10	10	
16	29.74	29.78	29.82	30	44	39	37.7	N. W.	N. W. 2	N. W.	0	4	0	
17	29.79	29.70	29.69	39	50	41	43.3	S. W. 2	S. W. 3	S. W. 1	8	10	Rain	
S 18	29.84	29.85	30.21	28	41	29	32.7	N. W. 2	N. W. 3	N. W. 2	0	3	0	
19	30.30	30.25	30.20	26	47	36	36.3	N. W. 2	S. W. 2	S. W. 1	0	7	5	
20	30.17	30.13	30.09	31	56	46	44.3	S. W'ly 1	S. W. 2	S. W. 2	2	4	10	
21	29.99	29.82	29.82	46	69	57	57.3	S. W. 1	S. W. 2	S. W. 1	Misty	9	8	
22	29.84	29.77	29.85	56	82	55	64.3	S. W. 1	S. W. 3	N. E. 2	3	2	10	
23	...	29.89	30.06	42	38	36	38.7	N. E. 2	N. E. 2	N. E. 3	Misty	Rain	9	
24	...	30.11	30.12	...	42	32	...	...	N. E.	N. E.	...	7	0	
S 25	30.19	30.11	30.01	30	44	36	36.7	N. W.	S.	S.	0	3	0, Haze	
26	29.87	29.68	29.57	34	65	53	50.7	S. W.	S. W.	S. W.	0	5	10	
27	29.40	29.81	29.44	46	70	44	53.3	S. E. 2	N. W. 4	N. W. 3	7	9	0	
28	29.68	29.69	29.69	33	52	43	42.7	W. 2	N. W. 2	S. W. 2	0	0	3	
29	29.50	29.34	29.31	49	63	53	55.0	S. W. 1	S. W. 1	S. W. 1	10	10	10, R'n	0.15
30	29.45	29.42	29.54	45	65	45	51.7	N. W. 1	S. W. 1	N. W. 3	0	3	9	
Means	29.81	29.76	29.80	36.6	51.6	40.8	...	1.3	2.1	1.6	4.4	5.5	4.8	1.72
									1.7			4.9		
REDUCED TO SEA LEVEL.														
Max.	30.48	30.43	30.39	56	82	57	64.3							
Min.	29.57	29.49	29.49	15	33	26	24.7							
Mean	29.99	29.94	29.98											
Range	0.91	0.94	0.90	41	49	31	39.6							
Mean of month	29.970			...	...	...	43.0							
Extreme range	0.99			...	...	...	67.0							

Prevailing winds from some point between— Days.
N. & E. 3
E. & S. 0
S. & W. 14
W. & N. 13

Days.
Clear 7
Variable . . . } 14
Cloudy . . . . }
Rain fell on . . 9

Remarks.

1st. Snow about six inches deep on the ground. Thermometer 15° at sunrise. Large portions of the cove froze over last night. The day pleasant.
2d. Snow fell in the morning about two inches deep.
3d. Very fine.
4th. Mist, and occasional sprinkling of rain.
5th. Very fine.
6th. Rain in the evening, with thunder and lightning.
7th and 8th. Pleasant.
9th. Shower from 4 to 5 A. M. The day very blustering.
10th. Very blustering. Dashes of rain during the day.
11th. Cool, and rather blustering.
12th. Variable.
13th. Fine.
17th. Small quantity of rain in the evening.
18th. Very blustering and cold for the season.
19th. Thermometer at sunrise stood at 24°: the ground frozen quite hard. Air raw and chilly through the day.
20th. Pleasant.
21st. Very warm and sultry. Observed a full-grown, active grasshopper in the street—rara avis.
22d. Summer heat and sultry. Wind changed from S. W. to N. E. from about 7 to 9 P. M.
23d. Mist at sunrise. Commenced raining moderately from 8 to 9 A. M. Rain, hail, and snow from 4 to 5 P. M., the snow falling in scattered flakes of extraordinary size, many of them being fully an inch in diameter.
24th. Cold and blustering.
25th. Chilly.
27th. Cold and blustering in the afternoon.
28th. More pleasant at sunrise, a great deal of ice, and the ground frozen.
29th. Light showers in the afternoon.

NOTE.—Rain-gauge defective. Amount of rain in this month taken from the record of Z. Allen.

May, 1847. New Moon, 14d. 10h. 15m. A. M.

Days.	Barometer At 6 A. M.	At 1 P. M.	At 10 P. M.	Thermometer At 6 A. M.	At 1 P. M.	At 10 P. M.	Daily mean.	Winds At 6 A. M.	At 1 P. M.	At 10 P. M.	Weather At 6 A. M.	At 1 P. M.	At 10 P. M.	Rain and Snow
1	29.76	29.71	29.82	35	55	48	46.0	N. W. 2	N. W. 1	N. W. 1	0	2	5	
S 2	29.92	29.91	29.69	44	45	39	42.7	S'ly 1	E'ly 2	N. E. 1	10	Rain	Rain	1.20
3	29.74	29.72	29.89	38	58	47	47.7	W'ly 1	W'ly 2	W'ly 1	3	5	0	
4	29.96	30.02	29.98	48	60	47	51.7	N. W. 1	N. W.	W'ly 1	0	2	0	
5	30.00	30.02	30.03	45	68	48	53.7	N'ly 1	N. W. 1	S. W. 1	0	2	0	
6	29.97	29.92	29.88	47	71	49	55.7	W'ly 1	E'ly 1	S. E'ly 1	0	2	0	
7	29.74	29.57	29.45	43	62	46	50.3	N. E. 2	N. E. 2	N. E. 3	0	10	Misty	
8	29.30	29.26	29.40	44	55	52	50.3	N. E. 2	N. E. 2	N'ly 1	Misty	10	10	
S 9	29.57	29.64	29.75	55	70	54	59.7	W'ly 1	S'ly 2	S'ly 1	3	2	0	
10	29.80	29.75	29.76	53	73	57	61.0	S'ly 1	S'ly 1	S'ly 1	4	0	Foggy	
11	29.73	29.67	29.66	55	76	60	63.7	S'ly 1	S. E'ly 1	S. W. 1	Foggy	3	0	
12	29.70	29.72	29.79	50	55	45	50.0	N. E. 2	N. E. 2	N. E. 2	Misty	10	10	
13	29.78	29.80	29.80	45	47	45	45.7	N. E. 3	N. E. 2	N. E. 3	10	10	5	
14	29.83	29.85	29.86	40	49	44	44.3	N. E. 3	N. E. 2	N. W. 2	Misty	10	0	
15	29.83	29.85	29.88	41	57	43	47.0	N. E. 2	N. E. 3	N. E. 2	0	4	0	
S 16	29.88	29.86	29.86	42	60	45	49.0	N. E. 3	N. E. 3	N. E. 2	0	0	0	
17	29.88	29.74	29.71	44	65	47	52.0	N. E. 2	N. E. 2	N. E. 1	0	0	2	
18	29.56	29.51	29.53	51	55	53	53.0	N'ly 1	N. W. 1	N'ly 1	10	Rain	10	0.25
19	29.59	29.62	29.69	50	71	56	59.0	N. W. 1	S'ly 2	Calm	0	3	1	
20	29.76	29.75	29.83	48	70	51	56.3	N. E. 1	N. E. 2	N. E. 1	0	0	0	
21	29.87	29.80	29.85	46	72	48	55.3	N. E. 1	S'ly 2	S. E'ly 1	0	4	Foggy	
22	29.79	29.75	29.76	47	56	54	52.3	S'ly 1	S'ly 1	S'ly 1	Foggy	10	10	
S 23	29.81	29.80	29.88	58	63	58	59.7	S. W. 1	S. W. 2	S'ly	9	5	Foggy	
24	29.85	29.80	29.72	57	67	63	62.3	S. E'ly 1	S. W. 1	S. E'ly 2	Misty	10	Shower	0.30
25	29.67	29.63	29.66	63	75	65	67.7	S. W. 1	S. W. 2	S. W. 1	10	5	0	
26	29.64	29.66	29.81	55	74	58	62.3	S. W. 1	S. W. 1	N. W. 2	4	Shower	8	
27	29.98	29.95	29.97	50	71	54	58.3	N'ly 1	S. E'ly 2	S. W. 2	2	5	7	
28	29.89	29.82	29.79	51	74	64	63.0	S. W. 1	S. E'ly 2	S. W. 1	1	0	0	
29	29.77	29.67	29.58	57	76	61	64.7	N'ly 1	S. E'ly 1	W'ly 1	3	0	8	
S 30	29.75	29.85	29.95	46	53	47	48.7	N. E. 2	N. E. 2	N. E. 1	Rain	10	3	0.27
31	29.97	29.97	29.90	44	61	48	51.0	N. E'ly 1	S. W. 2	E'ly 1	3	10	Rain	
Means	29.81	29.79	29.81	48.1	63.3	51.5	...	1.4	1.7	1.4	4.3	5.3	4.8	2.02
									1.5			4.8		
REDUCED TO SEA LEVEL.														
Max.	30.21	30.23	30.24	63	76	65	67.7							
Min.	29.51	29.47	29.61	35	45	43	42.7							
Mean	29.99	29.96	29.99											
Range	0.70	0.76	0.63	28	31	22	25.0							
Mean of month	29.980			...	...	...	54.3							
Extreme range	0.77			...	...	...	41.0							

Prevailing winds from some point between— Days.
N. & E. 10
E. & S. 7
S. & W. 9
W. & N. 5

Days.
Clear 12
Variable . . . } 13
Cloudy . . . . }
Rain fell on . . 6

Remarks.

1st. Pleasant.
2d. Moderate rain from 10 A. M.
3d. Pleasant.
4th. Fine.
5th and 6th. Very fine.
7th. Morning very cool. Began to mist at 4 P. M.
8th. Mist, and occasional light rain.
9th, 10th, and 11th. Very fine.
12th. Mist and clouds, but no rain.
13th. Cold and blustering.
14th. Cool, with occasional mist. Wind came to N. W. from 7 to 8 P. M.
15th. Fine, but cool. Aurora in the evening, with faint streamers.
16th. Fine.
17th. Pleasant.
18th. Gentle rain from N. W'ly and N'ly most of the day.
19th and 20th. Very fine.
21st. Pleasant.
22d. Fog, and appearances of rain.
23d. Pleasant.
24th. Occasional mist during the day. Shower in the evening, and again during the night.
25th. Very fine.
26th. Halo around the moon in the evening.
27th. Pleasant.
28th. Very fine.
29th. Hot sun. Lightning at the north in the evening.
30th. Light rain in the morning. Cool.
31st. Rain in the evening.

NOTE.—On the 1st of May, I commenced observations with a standard cistern barometer (with an ivory point and adjusting screw), made by J. H. Temple, Boston. The Vernier reads to the 1-100 of an inch, and the readings have been uniformly taken at the lowest ring of the meniscus formed at the top of the tube. The thickness of the meniscus is very nearly 3-100 of an inch; hence, all the readings of this month must be increased by that amount. The means and the reductions to sea level are corrected. The readings will hereafter be to the top of the meniscus.

June, 1847. New Moon, 12d. 7h. 44m. P. M.

DAYS.	BAROMETER, REDUCED TO 32° F. At 6 A. M.	At 1 P. M.	At 10 P. M.	THERMOMETER. At 6 A. M.	At 1 P. M.	At 10 P. M.	Daily mean.	WINDS. (DIRECTION AND FORCE.) At 6 A. M.	At 1 P. M.	At 10 P. M.	WEATHER. (TENTHS CLOUDY.) At 6 A. M.	At 1 P. M.	At 10 P. M.	RAIN AND SNOW IN INCHES OF WATER.
1	29.77	29.69	29.58	51	62	60	57.7	N'ly 1	N'ly 1	E'ly 1	Misty	Misty	10, Sh'r	1.10
2	29.57	29.60	29.75	59	74	60	64.3	N. W. 1	N. W. 2	Calm	10	3	0	
3	29.83	29.77	29.74	56	73	62	63.7	N. W. 1	S. W. 2	S'ly 1	4	3	Shower	} 1.13
4	29.56	29.45	29.57	59	72	66	65.7	S. E. 2	S. W. 2	W'ly 1	Rain	10	3	
5	29.68	29.67	29.76	65	72	57	64.7	N. W. 1	W. 1	N. W. 2	0	7	0	
S 6	29.84	29.78	29.81	54	74	61	63.0	N. W. 1	N. W'ly 2	Calm	2	4	0	
7	29.88	29.88	29.93	54	78	60	64.0	N. W. 1	N'ly 1	S'ly 2	0	2	0	
8	30.02	29.98	30.00	60	78	66	68.0	S'ly 1	S'ly 1	S'ly 1	Hazy	6	10	
9	30.01	29.95	29.86	61	65	62	62.7	S'ly 1	S'ly 2	S. W. 2	10	Rain	2	
10	29.75	29.71	29.68	63	80	64	69.0	S. W. 2	S. W. 3	S. W. 2	5	0	0	
11	29.64	29.56	29.51	65	77	65	69.0	S. W. 3	S. W. 3	S. W. 2	10	8	Rain	0.35
12	29.48	29.46	29.60	65	74	57	65.3	S. W. 1	N. W. 2	N. W. 1	8	0	6	
S 13	29.58	29.56	29.45	58	77	62	65.7	N. W. 1	S'ly 3	S. W. 2	0	2	Rain	0.47
14	29.34	29.22	29.25	60	71	58	63.0	S. W. 1	S. W. 2	N. W. 2	8	Sh'r, 5	5	0.28
15	29.31	29.40	29.56	50	60	50	53.3	N. W. 2	W. 2	N. W. 1	3	8	0	
16	...	...	29.79	49	...	60	...	N. W. 1	N. W. 2	N. W. 1	0	2	0	
17	29.88	29.86	29.98	54	75	58	62.3	N. W. 1	N'ly 2	Calm	0	2	0	
18	30.09	30.03	30.06	57	77	61	65.0	N. E. 1	N. E. 2	S'ly 1	0	1	2	
19	30.06	...	29.93	58	...	59	...	S. W. 1	...	S. W. 1	5	...	Rain	
S 20	29.83	29.81	29.80	62	65	56	61.0	S'ly 2	S'ly 3	S'ly 1	10	10	Misty	} 1.60
21	29.67	29.75	29.86	60	63	61	61.3	S'ly 2	N. W. 1	E'ly	Rain	10	8	
22	29.94	29.89	29.85	57	68	65	...	N. E. 1	E'ly 1	S'ly 1	Foggy	Rain	Rain	0.45
23	29.86	29.84	29.88	61	75	69	68.3	N. W. 1	W'ly 2	W'ly 1	10	4	3	
24	29.96	29.92	29.88	62	82	68	70.7	N. W. 1	W'ly 1	W'ly 1	0	2	0	
25	29.84	29.84	29.79	67	86	75	76.0	N. W. 1	W'ly 1	W'ly 1	0	0	2	
26	29.81	29.74	29.75	70	86	72	76.0	W'ly 1	N. W. 1	N. W. 1	0	4	Sh'r, 0	
S 27	29.74	29.72	29.70	70	87	76	77.7	N. W. 1	N. W. 1	W'ly 1	0	1	0	
28	29.70	29.65	29.65	72	90	73	78.3	N. W. 1	N'ly 1	W'ly 1	0	5	Sh'r, 9	0.10
29	29.61	29.62	29.66	72	68	65	68.3	S'ly 1	N. E. 1	N. E. 2	5	Rain	10	0.90
30	29.71	29.73	29.75	62	65	60	62.3	N. E. 1	N. E. 1	N. E. 1	Rain	10	2	0.60
Means	29.76	29.72	29.75	60.4	74.1	62.9	...	1.2	1.7	1.2	4.8	4.9	4.4	6.98
									1.4			4.7		
REDUCED TO SEA LEVEL.								Prevailing winds from some point between—		Days.			Days.	
Max.	30.27	30.21	30.24	72	90	76	78.3							
Min.	29.49	29.40	29.43	49	60	50	53.3							
Mean	29.94	29.89	29.93											
Range	0.76	0.81	0.81	23	30	26	25.0	N. & E.		5	Clear		8	
								E. & S.		1	Variable		} 7	
Mean of month			29.920	...	...	...	65.8	S. & W.		11	Cloudy			
Extreme range			0.87	...	...	...	41.0	W. & N.		13	Rain fell on		15	

REMARKS.

1st. Rain during the preceding night, and occasional showers this morning. Some stars out in the evening. Thundershower during the night.
2d. Pleasant.
3d. Sprinkling of rain in the evening.
4th. Showery in the morning.
5th and 6th. Fine.
7th. Very fine.
8th. Fine.
9th. Light showers in the morning, just enough to lay the dust.
10th. Very fine.
11th. Air very damp. Began to rain moderately from 8 to 9 P. M.
12th. Very fine. Aurora in the evening—quite brilliant at 10 o'clock.
13th. Began to rain from 8 to 9 P. M.
14th. Fine shower from the S. W. Thunder in the afternoon. From 4 to 5 P. M., wind came to N. W., and grew cool.
15th. Very cool and blustering.
16th. Frost in some places in the vicinity this morning.
17th. Very fine. Gust and sprinkling of rain from 4 to 5 P. M.
18th. Very fine.
19th. Rained very gently in the evening.
20th. Sprinkling of rain in the afternoon and evening. Rain during the night.
21st. Moderate rain in the morning.
22d. Drizzle. Showers in the evening.
23d. Fine in the afternoon.
24th. Very fine.
25th. Very fine and warm.
26th. Warm. Light showers at 7 P. M.
27th. Very warm sun.
28th. Light shower, with thunder, from 5 to 6 P. M.
29th. Morning very hot. Thundershower from noon to 1 P. M., with showers till 4 P. M.
30th. Moderate rain in the morning. Clear in the evening.

July, 1847. New Moon, 12d. 6h. 30m. A. M.

DAYS.	BAROMETER At 6 A. M.	At 1 P. M.	At 10 P. M.	THERMOMETER At 6 A. M.	At 1 P. M.	At 10 P. M.	Daily mean.	WINDS At 6 A. M.	At 1 P. M.	At 10 P. M.	WEATHER At 6 A. M.	At 1 P. M.	At 10 P. M.	RAIN AND SNOW
1	29.79	29.80	29.86	59	70	60	63.0	N. E. 2	N. E. 3	N. E. 2	6	10	10	
2	29.88	29.89	29.92	59	69	62	63.3	N. E. 2	N. E. 2	N. E. 1	6	10	9	
3	29.92	29.88	29.88	58	76	63	65.7	N'ly 1	N. E. 2	Calm	3	0	0	
S 4	29.83	29.80	29.80	65	84	73	74.0	W'ly 1	N. W. 1	Calm	6	1	0	
5	29.79	29.76	29.79	73	90	77	80.0	W'ly 1	N. W. 1	N. W. 1	0	0	0	
6	29.84	29.82	29.83	69	84	73	75.3	N'ly 1	N. E. 1	S'ly 1	Hazy	10	Hazy	
7	29.83	29.78	29.83	67	87	73	75.7	S'ly 1	N. W'ly 2	E'ly 1	Hazy	Hazy	0	
8	29.86	29.84	29.87	70	86	72	76.0	E'ly 1	E'ly	S'ly 1	Hazy	0	6	
9	29.85	29.82	29.83	70	85	70	75.0	S'ly 1	S'ly 1	S'ly 1	Hazy	0	0	
10	29.81	29.76	29.79	67	83	73	74.3	S'ly 1	S. E'ly 2	S'ly 1	8	5	7	
S 11	29.79	29.79	29.80	72	83	73	76.0	S'ly 1	S'ly 2	S'ly 1	Foggy	8	10	
12	29.77	29.73	29.67	70	81	73	74.7	S'ly 2	S'ly 2	S'ly 1	10	3	2	
13	29.57	29.57	29.55	73	83	72	76.0	S'ly 1	S. W'ly 1	N'ly	Foggy	Shower	0	0.08
14	29.64	29.70	29.77	63	79	65	69.0	N. W. 1	N. E. 2	N. E. 2	5	0	0	
15	29.76	29.76	29.82	62	79	63	68.0	N. W. 1	S. E'ly 2	N. E. 1	0	3	0	
16	29.87	29.88	29.93	62	79	70	70.3	N. E'ly 1	W'ly 1	W'ly 1	2	3	0	
17	29.97	29.90	29.87	65	83	73	73.7	W'ly 2	S. W. 3	S. W. 2	0	0	0	
S 18	29.92	29.91	29.97	74	88	68	76.7	W'ly 1	W'ly 2	N. E. 1	0	5	10	
19	29.94	29.89	29.89	70	93	76	79.7	S'ly 1	S. W. 2	S. W. 2	10	1	0	
20	29.91	29.82	29.81	75	91	77	81.0	S. W'ly 2	S. W. 2	S. W. 2	0	1	0	
21	29.86	29.81	29.79	73	87	77	79.0	S. W. 2	S. W. 3	S. W. 2	0	1	10	0.60
22	29.79	...	29.83	75	...	73	78.0	S. W. 2	...	N. E'ly	8	...	Rain	
23	29.93	29.94	30.01	73	83	72	76.0	W'ly 1	W'ly 2	S. W. 1	5	6	3	
24	29.03	30.01	29.96	68	83	70	73.7	N. W. 1	S. E'ly 2	Calm	0	0	0	
S 25	29.91	29.80	29.65	70	81	73	74.7	S. W. 2	S. W. 2	S. W. 1	10	9	Rain	
26	29.57	29.45	29.62	74	89	69	77.3	S. W. 2	S. W. 3	N'ly 2	10	4	Shower	0.40
27	29.73	29.79	29.80	55	63	55	57.7	N'ly 2	N. E. 2	Calm	2	4	0	
28	29.84	29.82	29.90	53	71	59	61.0	N. E. 1	N. W. 2	Calm	0	5	0	
29	29.94	29.93	29.93	55	72	58	61.7	N. W. 1	N. W. 2	Calm	0	0	0	
30	29.90	29.89	29.79	52	73	66	63.7	N. E. 1	S. E. 1	S. E. 2	3	10	Rain	} 1.20
31	29.66	29.66	29.75	70	80	71	73.7	S. E. 2	S. W. 2	S. W. 1	Rain	6	0	
Means	29.80	29.81	29.82	66.5	81.3	69.3	...	1.4	1.9	1.4	5.3	4.0	3.8	2.28
									1.6			4.4		
REDUCED TO SEA LEVEL.								Prevailing winds from some point between—		Days.			Days.	
Max.	30.15	30.19	30.19	75	93	77	81.0							
Min.	29.21	29.63	29.73	52	63	55	57.7							
Mean	29.97	29.98	29.99											
Range	0.94	0.56	0.46	23	30	22	23.3	N. & E.		9	Clear		10	
								E. & S.		3	Variable		} 15	
Mean of month			29.980	...	...	...	72.4	S. & W.		13	Cloudy			
Extreme range			0.98	...	...	...	41.0	W. & N.		6	Rain fell on		6	

REMARKS.

1st. Cool for the season.
2d. Cool; occasional sunshine.
3d. Fine.
4th. Very hot.
5th. Very hot air, light.
6th. Thick haze all day; very sultry.
7th. Very warm and sultry, and hazy. Scarcely a breath of air.
8th. Very warm.
9th. Very warm; hazy through the day. Aurora in the evening.
10th. Very warm.
12th. Very warm, with fresh breeze.
13th. Gust from 2 to 3 P. M., with thunder and light rain.
14th to 17th. Fine.
18th. Morning very hot and sultry. Thunder from noon to 1 P. M. Wind came to N. E., and grew cooler immediately.
19th. Very hot.
20th. Very hot, with a fine breeze.
21st. Appearances of rain in the evening.
22d. Fine rain from 6 to 9 P. M., with thunder.
23d. Very warm.
24th. Very fine.
25th. Air very damp and close. Sprinkling of rain at 11 A. M. and 9 P. M.
26th. Shower and gust at 4 P. M.
27th. Very cool.
28th. Cool in the morning. Thermometer at sunrise 51° to 52°. Day fine.
29th. Very fine, but cool.
30th. Commenced raining very moderately at 6 P. M., and continued through the night.
31st. Rained moderately at intervals till 9 A. M. Clear and very warm in the afternoon.

August, 1847. New Moon, 10d. 7h. 20m. P. M.

Days.	Barometer, reduced to 32° F. At 6 A. M.	At 1 P. M.	At 10 P. M.	Thermometer. At 6 A. M.	At 1 P. M.	At 10 P. M.	Daily mean.	Winds. (Direction and Force.) At 6 A. M.	At 1 P. M.	At 10 P. M.	Weather. (Tenths Cloudy.) At 6 A. M.	At 1 P. M.	At 10 P. M.	Rain and Snow in Inches of Water.	Remarks.
S 1	29.85	29.81	29.81	72	80	70	74.0	S. W. 1	S. W. 1	S. W. 1	10	Spr'ling	Rain		1st. Sprinkling of rain at intervals.
2	29.79	29.80	29.87	70	81	68	73.0	N'ly 1	N. W. 3	W. 1	10	1	0		2d. Very fine.
3	29.91	29.83	...	62	79	...	...	N. W. 1	N. 1	...	3	2	...		
4	...	...	...	...	...	...	...	...	...	...	...	...	...		
5	...	...	...	...	...	...	...	...	...	...	...	...	...		
6	...	...	...	...	...	...	...	...	...	N. E.	...	...	Rain		
7	...	...	...	...	...	...	...	...	...	...	...	...	...		
S 8	...	...	...	...	...	...	...	...	...	N. E.	...	...	Rain	4.85	
9	...	...	...	...	...	...	...	...	...	...	...	...	...		
10	...	...	...	...	...	...	...	...	E'ly	...	...	...	Rain		
11	...	...	29.96	...	...	74	...	...	...	S. W. 2	...	...	0		11th. Fine.
12	29.91	29.84	29.85	72	86	73	73.7	S. W. 1	W'ly 1	N. W. 1	9	6	0		12th. Sprinkling of rain in the afternoon. Very clear in the evening.
13	29.88	29.86	29.87	68	85	71	74.7	N. W. 1	N. W. 1	Calm	0	2	0		13th and 14th. Fine.
14	29.88	29.87	29.86	71	80	72	74.3	S. E. 1	S. E. 1	Calm	Foggy	2	Hazy		
S 15	29.89	29.91	29.88	63	72	66	67.0	N. E. 2	E'ly 2	N. E. 2	10	10	10		15th. Appearances of rain in the evening.
16	29.88	29.78	29.75	63	73	66	67.3	N. E. 2	N. E. 2	N. E. 2	10	5	0		16th. Evening very clear.
17	29.75	29.59	29.57	57	76	67	66.7	N. E. 1	S. E.	S. E.	10	5	5		17th. Pleasant.
18	29.45	29.41	29.46	70	81	66	72.3	S'ly	S. W.	N. W.	Rain	5	Shower	0.65	18th. Fine shower in the afternoon.
19	29.53	...	29.72	59	...	58	...	N. W.	...	N. W. 1	0	...	0		19th to 23d. Very fine.
20	29.80	29.72	29.76	53	78	62	62.7	N. W. 1	S. W. 2	S. W. 1	0	0	0		
21	...	...	29.70	59	...	67	...	N. W. 1	...	S. W.	0	...	0		
S 22	29.69	29.76	29.77	62	78	66	68.7	W'ly 1	W'ly 1	S. W. 1	5	0	0		
23	29.86	29.84	29.87	57	73	62	64.0	N. W. 1	N. E. 1	N. W. 1	0	0	2		
24	29.97	30.01	30.07	58	72	60	63.3	N. W. 1	N. W. 2	Calm	0	0	0		24th. Very fine. Splendid evening.
25	30.17	30.10	30.08	58	74	62	64.7	N. W. 1	N. W. 1	W'ly 1	0	2	6		25th. Very fine.
26	30.00	...	...	57	...	...	...	N. W. 1	...	...	9	...	...		26th. Sprinkling of rain in the afternoon.
27	...	...	29.85	...	...	66	...	...	...	S. W. 1	...	...	0		27th. Fine.
28	29.88	29.90	29.83	69	74	68	70.3	S. W. 1	S. E.	S. W. 1	Foggy	10	10		28th. Appearances of rain.
S 29	29.80	29.80	29.91	70	77	71	72.7	S. W. 1	S. W. 1	N. W. 1	10	2	2		29th. Very sultry. Sprinkling of rain from cumulus clouds in the afternoon.
30	29.99	29.88	29.89	62	78	64	68.0	N. W. 1	N. W. 1	S. E'ly 1	0	2	Foggy		30th and 31st. Fine.
31	29.86	...	29.84	68	...	71	...	S. W. 1	...	S. W. 1	Foggy	...	5		
Means	29.84	29.82	29.83	63.6	77.3	66.8	...	1.1	1.4	1.2	5.7	3.6	3.2	5.50	
								1.2			4.1				
Reduced to sea level.								Prevailing winds from some point between— Days.			Days.				
Max.	30.35	30.28	30.26	72	86	74	74.7	N. & E. 2			Clear 8				
Min.	29.63	29.59	29.66	53	72	58	62.7	E. & S. 2			Variable . . . } Cloudy . . . . } 6				
Mean	30.01	29.99	30.00					S. & W. 9			Rain fell on . . 10				
Range	0.72	0.69	0.60	19	14	16	12.0	W. & N. 11			(7 days omitted.)				
Mean of month	30.000			...	...	...	69.2								
Extreme range	0.76			...	...	...	33.0								

September, 1847. New Moon, 9d. 10h. 39m. A. M.

Days.	Barometer At 6 A. M.	At 1 P. M.	At 10 P. M.	Thermometer At 6 A. M.	At 1 P. M.	At 10 P. M.	Daily mean.	Winds At 6 A. M.	At 1 P. M.	At 10 P. M.	Weather At 6 A. M.	At 1 P. M.	At 10 P. M.	Rain and Snow in Inches of Water.	Remarks.
1	29.83	...	29.83	71	...	71	...	N. W. 1	...	N. W. 1	2	...	0		1st. Very fine.
2	29.85	...	29.83	70	...	71	...	S. W. 1	...	S. W.	Foggy	...	2		2d. Very warm. Thunder in the afternoon, but no rain.
3	29.87	29.79	29.78	72	83	72	75.7	S. W. 1	S. W. 1	S. W. 1	10	8	9		3d. Very sultry.
4	29.81	29.78	29.87	72	86	74	77.3	S. W. 2	S'ly 2	S. W. 1	10	5	10		4th. Very hot and sultry.
S 5	29.86	29.81	29.75	72	83	74	76.3	S. W. 2	S. W. 3	S. W. 3	10	5	3		5th. Wind very fresh and air damp. Clouds abundant, but no rain.
6	29.74	29.75	29.92	72	78	67	72.3	S. W. 2	N. W. 1	N. W. 1	Rain	5	6	0.57	6th. Very warm.
7	30.06	30.03	30.05	56	74	60	63.3	N. E. 1	N. E. 2	N. E. 1	2	6	10		7th. Pleasant.
8	30.04	29.97	29.93	60	73	71	68.0	N. E. 1	N. E. 1	S. E. 1	10	Misty	Misty		8th. Misty, with appearances of rain.
9	29.87	29.81	29.85	72	82	64	72.7	S'ly 1	S. W. 2	N. E. 1	Misty	5	Rain		9th. Shower at 5 A. M. From 8 to 9 P. M., the wind came to N. E., and it rained.
10	29.95	30.01	30.06	56	58	59	57.7	N. E. 2	N. E. 2	N. E. 2	Rain	Rain	10	2.43	10th. Copious rain during the day.
11	...	...	30.03	...	...	59	...	...	...	N. E. 1	Misty	Misty	Misty		11th. Heavy mist.
S 12	29.95	29.87	29.78	59	65	61	61.7	N. E. 2	N. E. 2	N. E. 1	Misty	10	10		12th. Mist.
13	...	29.43	29.50	60	62	63	61.7	N. E. 1	N. E. 2	N. W. 1	Rain	Rain	5	2.45	13th. Steady rain and very brisk wind all the morning till 2 P. M. Mostly clear in the evening.
14	29.69	29.65	29.76	57	71	53	60.3	N. W. 1	N. W. 1	N. W. 1	0	0	0		14th. Shower at 5 P. M. Evening very clear and cool.
15	29.89	29.80	29.88	47	61	51	53.0	N. W. 1	N'ly 2	N. W. 2	0	0	0		15th. Very clear in the evening.
16	29.89	29.79	29.83	43	65	52	53.3	N. W. 1	N. W. 1	S. W. 1	0	0	0		16th. Very fine. Auroral display of red light from 9½ to 10½ P. M; white streamers shooting up through diffused red light.
17	29.89	29.79	29.87	47	66	56	56.3	S. W. 1	S. E. 1	S'ly 1	0	0	0		17th. Very fine.
18	...	...	29.91	...	...	54	...	...	...	N. E. 1	...	...	0		18th. Fine.
S 19	29.89	29.80	29.71	50	64	58	57.3	N. E. 1	E'ly 2	N. E. 2	3	10	0		19th. Appearances of storm in the evening.
20	29.61	29.50	29.51	54	54	51	53.0	N. E. 2	N. E. 2	N. E. 1	10	Rain	Rain	1.05	20th. Rain nearly all day.
21	29.48	29.49	29.64	51	66	56	57.7	N'ly 1	N. W. 2	N. W. 1	9	3	0		21st. Fine.
22	29.81	29.80	29.89	53	68	54	58.3	N. W. 2	N. W. 2	N. W. 1	0	0	0		22d. Very fine.
23	29.88	29.81	29.80	49	72	59	60.0	N. W. 1	N. W. 2	S. W. 1	0	0	2		23d. Bright halo about the moon.
24	29.92	29.83	29.86	54	62	57	57.7	N. E. 1	N. E. 1	N. E. 1	10	10	10		24th. Appearances of storm in the evening.
25	29.83	29.75	29.66	54	68	54	58.7	N. E. 2	N. E. 2	N. E. 3	10	Rain	Rain	0.90	25th. Moderate rain in the afternoon.
S 26	29.69	29.70	29.72	52	55	52	53.0	N. E. 2	N. E. 3	N. E. 2	10	10	Misty		26th. Mist and appearances of rain.
27	29.70	29.66	29.66	53	58	55	55.3	N. E. 2	N. E. 2	N. E. 1	10	Misty	10		27th. Frequent mists.
28	29.50	29.45	29.47	58	68	60	62.0	S. W. 1	S. W. 1	S. W. 1	Misty	10	8		28th. Mild and misty.
29	29.48	29.48	29.60	50	63	55	56.0	N. W. 1	N. W. 1	Calm	2	2	0		29th. Fine aurora in the evening, with brilliant coruscations.
30	29.61	29.59	29.67	53	63	51	55.7	W'ly 1	N'ly 1	N. W. 1	5	2	0	0.05	30th. Sprinkling of rain in the morning. Evening clear.
Means	29.80	29.74	29.79	59.7	68.0	59.8	...	1.4	1.7	1.3	6.4	5.9	5.1	8.35	
								1.5			5.5				
Reduced to sea level.								Prevailing winds from some point between— Days.			Days.				
Max.	30.24	30.21	30.24	72	86	74	77.3	N. & E. 13			Clear 9				
Min.	29.66	29.61	29.65	43	54	51	53.0	E. & S. 1			Variable . . . } Cloudy . . . . } 13				
Mean	29.98	29.91	29.97					S. & W. 6			Rain fell on . . . 8				
Range	0.58	0.60	0.59	29	32	23	24.3	W. & N. 10							
Mean of month	29.953			...	...	...	62.5								
Extreme range	0.63			...	...	...	43.0								

October, 1847. New Moon, 9d. 3h. 58m. A. M.

Days.	Barometer, reduced to 32° F. At 6 A. M.	At 1 P. M.	At 10 P. M.	Thermometer. At 6 A. M.	At 1 P. M.	At 10 P. M.	Daily mean.	Winds. (Direction and Force.) At 6 A. M.	At 1 P. M.	At 10 P. M.	Weather. (Tenths Cloudy.) At 6 A. M.	At 1 P. M.	At 10 P. M.	Rain and Snow in Inches of Water.
1	29.60	29.47	29.66	48	65	51	54.7	W'ly 1	S. W. 2	N. W. 1	7	10	0	
2	...	...	29.90	43	...	50	...	N. W. 1	N. W. 1	N. W. 1	2	2	0	
S 3	30.02	30.03	30.09	44	61	48	51.0	N. W. 1	N. W. 2	N. E. 2	0	3	0	
4	30.01	29.92	29.84	43	60	49	50.7	N'ly 2	N. E. 2	N. E. 1	0	0	0	
5	29.72	29.65	29.70	45	65	57	55.7	N. E. 1	N. E. 2	E'ly 1	0	3	2	
6	29.80	29.83	29.89	54	70	56	60.0	N. E. 1	N. E. 1	N. E. 1	4	10	3	
7	30.03	29.93	29.87	51	62	52	55.0	N. E. 1	N. E. 2	N. E. 1	10	5	0	
8	29.70	29.49	29.23	51	63	59	57.7	N. E. 2	N. E. 2	E'ly	10	10	Rain	0.75
9	29.10	29.13	29.35	53	60	51	54.7	N. W. 1	N. W. 3	N. W. 1	9	2	0	
S 10	29.34	29.41	29.58	52	63	50	55.0	W'ly 3	W'ly 2	N. W. 2	0	0	0	
11	29.65	29.64	29.87	43	57	41	47.0	W'ly 1	W'ly 2	N. W. 1	0	2	0	
12	29.89	29.84	29.50	38	57	53	49.3	N. W. 1	S'ly 2	S. E. 4	0	2	Rain	
13	29.24	29.32	29.41	61	53	48	54.0	S. W. 2	N. W. 2	N. W. 1	10	Rain	10	
14	...	29.61	29.72	38	54	44	45.3	N. W. 1	N. W. 1	N. W. 1	0	0	2	
15	...	...	30.18	...	...	40	...	...	...	N. E. 1	...	...	0	
16	30.21	30.17	30.16	34	54	50	46.0	N. W. 1	S'ly 2	S'ly 1	0	8	10	
S 17	30.10	30.02	30.03	44	64	56	54.7	S. W. 1	S. W. 2	S. W. 1	3	6	9	
18	30.08	29.99	29.94	44	63	54	53.7	W'ly 1	S. W'ly 2	S'ly 1	Foggy	0	Foggy	
19	29.84	29.78	29.89	62	71	57	63.3	S. W. 2	S. W. 2	W'ly 1	7	7	8	
20	29.94	29.89	30.02	52	58	45	51.7	N. E. 1	N. E. 1	Calm	10	0	0	
21	30.14	30.04	30.08	40	60	51	50.3	N'ly 1	S'ly 1	S. W. 1	0	0	10	1.20 (12th–29th)
22	29.99	29.83	29.75	50	64	58	57.3	S. W. 1	S. W. 3	S. W. 2	10	8	8	
23	29.69	...	30.11	54	...	44	...	N. 1	...	N. W.	Rain	...	0	
S 24	30.12	30.04	29.88	38	56	51	48.3	N. E. 1	S. E. 2	S. E. 1	5	10	Rain	
25	29.66	29.50	29.67	60	64	51	58.3	S. E. 3	W.	N. W. 1	5	10, Sh'r	0	
26	30.09	30.03	30.28	37	42	30	36.3	N. W. 2	N. W. 2	N. W. 1	0	1	0	
27	30.46	30.37	30.42	22	39	30	30.3	N. W. 1	N. W. 1	N. W. 1	0	0	0	
28	30.51	30.51	30.52	24	38	30	30.7	N'ly 1	N'ly 1	N'ly	0	0	0	
29	30.47	30.33	30.24	27	52	38	39.0	Calm	S. W. 2	S. W. 1	0	2	0	
30	30.27	30.21	30.28	33	56	40	43.0	W'ly 1	W'ly 1	E'ly 1	0	0	0	
S 31	30.29	30.20	30.12	40	56	46	47.3	N. E. 1	N. E. 1	S'ly 1	5	2	0	
Means	29.93	29.86	29.91	44.2	58.1	47.7	...	1.3	1.7	1.2	3.7	3.9	3.3	1.95
								1.4			3.6			
REDUCED TO SEA LEVEL.														
Max.	30.69	30.69	30.70	62	71	59	63.3							
Min.	29.28	29.31	29.41	22	38	30	30.3							
Mean	30.11	30.04	30.09											
Range	1.41	1.38	1.29	40	33	29	33.0							
Mean of month 30.080				...	...	...	50.0							
Extreme range 1.42				...	...	...	49.0							

Prevailing winds from some point between—	Days.		Days.
N. & E.	8	Clear	13
E. & S.	1	Variable }	12
S. & W.	9	Cloudy }	
W. & N.	13	Rain fell on	6

REMARKS.

1st. Evening very clear.
2d. Fine.
3d and 4th. Very fine.
5th. Fine.
6th. Variable.
7th. Pleasant.
8th. Began to rain moderately from 5 to 6 P. M
9th. Blustering.
10th. Blustering, but warm sun. Evening very clear.
11th. Fine. Very clear in the evening.
12th. First white frost in the College yard, being light in patches. Began to rain moderately at [illegible] P. M.; wind fresh at S. E.
13th. Occasional showers in morning. Clouds broken in the evening.
14th. Very fine.
16th. Thick white frost.
17th and 18th. Fine.
19th. Very mild.
20th. Very splendid evening.
21st. Very mild.
22d. Variable.
23d. Rain in the morning.
24th. Showery in the evening.
25th. Heavy shower from noon to 2 P. M. Very clear in the evening.
26th to 31st. Very fine.

November, 1847. New Moon, 7d. 10h. 3m. P. M.

Days.	Barometer Sunrise.	At 1 P. M.	At 10 P. M.	Thermometer Sunrise.	At 1 P. M.	At 10 P. M.	Daily mean.	Winds Sunrise.	At 1 P. M.	At 10 P. M.	Weather Sunrise.	At 1 P. M.	At 10 P. M.	Rain and Snow
1	30.07	29.99	29.97	42	63	54	53.0	S'ly 1	S'ly 1	S'ly 1	Foggy	3	6	
2	29.91	29.81	29.75	45	66	51	54.0	E'ly 1	E'ly 1	E'ly 1	2	0	0	
3	29.70	29.58	29.58	44	67	54	55.0	N. W. 1	S'ly 1	S'ly 1	0	0	0	
4	29.50	29.44	29.50	51	72	52	58.3	S'ly 1	W'ly 1	W'ly 1	0	5	2	
5	29.56	29.54	29.65	52	62	43	52.3	N. E. 1	W'ly 2	N. W. 2	10	0	0	
6	...	...	29.90	...	...	42	...	...	...	N. W. 2	...	...	5	
S 7	30.12	30.06	30.13	33	49	42	41.3	N. W. 1	N. E. 1	E'ly 1	0	5	5	
8	30.05	29.93	29.78	43	58	58	53.0	N. E. 1	S. W. 2	S. W. 2	10	10	10	
9	29.78	29.68	29.72	57	65	59	60.3	S. W. 1	S. W. 2	S. W. 1	10	10	5	
10	29.87	29.81	29.93	56	55	44	51.7	W'ly 1	N. W. 2	N. W. 2	10	4	9	
11	30.01	29.96	30.06	37	44	37	39.3	N. W. 1	N. W. 2	N. W. 1	0	10	5	
12	30.12	29.98	29.96	35	45	41	40.3	W'ly 2	W'ly 1	S. W. 1	5	5	10	
13	29.95	29.93	30.01	40	47	40	42.3	W'ly 1	W'ly 1	W'ly 1	10	10	10	
S 14	29.72	29.37	29.43	44	52	42	46.0	E'ly 2	N. E. 1	N. W.	Rain	10	5	1.00
15	29.39	29.46	29.66	40	47	40	42.3	W'ly 1	N. W. 2	N. W. 2	3	7	0	
16	29.91	29.97	29.96	38	44	38	40.0	N. W. 1	N. W. 1	W'ly 1	10	0	8	
17	29.93	29.85	29.89	44	62	50	52.0	S. W. 2	S. W. 1	S. W. 1	5	10	3	
18	29.90	29.74	29.64	44	64	55	54.3	S. W. 1	S. W. 1	S. W. 1	4	5	6	
19	29.59	29.59	29.79	54	53	41	49.3	S. W. 1	W'ly 1	N. W. 2	Rain	Rain	10	0.62
20	30.09	...	30.28	32	...	37	...	N. 1	...	N'ly 1	10	...	10	
S 21	30.25	30.19	30.19	35	48	41	41.3	N. E'ly 1	S'ly 1	S. W. 1	10	10	10	
22	30.19	30.15	30.12	35	54	53	47.3	S. W. 1	S. W. 1	S. W. 1	10	5	10	
23	30.09	30.08	29.98	54	55	55	54.7	S. W. 1	S. W. 1	S. W. 1	Misty	Misty	Misty	
24	29.84	29.68	29.48	56	64	61	60.3	S'ly 1	S'ly 2	S'ly 2	Foggy	Rain	Rain	
25	29.49	...	29.48	58	...	54	...	S. W. 1	...	W'ly	10	10	4	4.10
26	29.65	29.70	29.84	44	47	35	42.0	W'ly 1	N. W. 1	N. W. 1	0	2	0	
27	...	...	29.86	32	...	32	...	N. W. 2	...	N'ly	6	...	10	
S 28	29.80	29.75	29.77	30	40	34	34.7	W. 1	W.	N. 1	7	5	10	
29	30.08	30.06	30.27	22	24	11	19.0	N. 3	N. W. 2	N. W. 2	4	0	0	
30	30.49	30.45	30.50	8	24	20	17.3	N. W. 1	N. E. 1	N. E. 1	0	0	0	
Means	29.89	29.83	29.87	41.6	52.7	43.9	...	1.2	1.4	1.3	6.3	5.8	5.7	5.72
								1.3			5.9			
REDUCED TO SEA LEVEL.														
Max.	30.67	30.63	30.68	58	72	61	60.3							
Min.	29.57	29.55	29.61	8	24	11	17.3							
Mean	30.07	30.01	30.05											
Range	1.10	1.08	1.07	50	48	50	43.0							
Mean of month 30.043				...	...	...	46.1							
Extreme range 1.13				...	...	...	64.0							

Prevailing winds from some point between—	Days.		Days.
N. & E.	3	Clear	6
E. & S.	2	Variable }	21
S. & W.	13	Cloudy }	
W. & N.	12	Rain fell on	3

REMARKS.

1st and 2d. Fine.
3d and 4th. Very fine.
5th. Fine.
6th. Blustering.
7th. Fine.
8th. Appearances of rain.
9th. Very mild.
10th and 11th. Pleasant.
12th. At 7 P. M., halo about the moon in the S. W.; the air filled with condensing vapor. Soon clouds spread over the heavens, with appearances of storm. From 9 to 10 P. M., the clouds seemed to be lighted up with the aurora in patches.
13th. Stars visible occasionally in the evening, but no meteors.
14th. Began to rain about 5 A. M.; wind nearly east. Rain ceased from 11 to 12 A. M.
15th. Evening clear.
16th. Fine.
17th. Pleasant.
18th. Very mild.
19th. Began to rain at about 5 A. M., and continued moderately till noon.
20th. Weather raw and disagreeable.
21st. Air rather raw.
23d. Mist and fog all day.
24th. Mist and light showers through the day. Heavy rain, with high wind, in the evening.
25th. Very mild.
26th. Fine. Evening very clear. Appearances of aurora, not very bright.
27th. Cool.
28th. Cool and raw.
29th. Very sharp cold, with severe wind.
30th. Very cold.

December, 1847. New Moon, 7[d.] 3[h.] 22[m.] P. M.

Days.	Barometer, reduced to 32° F. Sunrise.	At 1 P. M.	At 10 P. M.	Thermometer. Sunrise.	At 1 P. M.	At 10 P. M.	Daily mean.	Winds. (Direction and Force.) Sunrise.	At 1 P. M.	At 10 P. M.	Weather. (Tenths Cloudy.) Sunrise.	At 1 P. M.	At 10 P. M.	Rain and Snow in Inches of Water.
1	30.41	30.27	30.12	26	43	44	37.7	N. E. 1	S'ly 1	S. E'ly 1	10	9	10	
2	29.82	29.68	29.63	51	61	58	56.7	S. W. 3	S. W. 4	S. W. 3	Rain	Rain	Rain	1.40
3	29.51	29.38	29.31	53	47	43	47.7	S'ly 1	N. E. 2	N. E. 1	Foggy	Rain	Rain	1.25
4	29.70	29.88	29.92	33	38	29	33.3	N. W. 1	W. 1	N. W.	0	0	0	
S 5	29.90	29.77	...	26	44	37	35.7	N. W. 1	N. W. 1	N. E. 1	2	10	Rain	0.15
6	29.74	29.78	30.01	33	38	29	33.3	N. W. 1	N. W. 1	N. W. 1	7	2	0	
7	30.24	30.24	30.38	25	38	34	32.3	N. W. 1	S'ly 1	Calm	2	0	0	
8	30.36	30.29	30.27	32	47	40	39.7	S'ly 1	S. W. 2	S. W. 1	0	2	0	
9	30.23	30.13	30.03	43	59	53	51.7	S. W. 1	S. W. 2	S'ly 2	0	6	8	
10	29.95	29.88	29.92	58	62	58	59.3	S. W. 2	S. W. 3	S. W. 2	10	10	10	
11	29.77	29.83	30.17	60	64	42	55.3	S. W. 3	S. W. 2	N. W. 1	10	10	0	
S 12	30.31	30.26	30.12	33	51	45	43.0	N. W. 1	E'ly 1	E'ly 1	0	3	Misty	0.20
13	29.95	29.85	29.85	48	65	53	55.3	S. W. 1	S. W. 2	S'ly 1	10	4	Foggy	
14	29.78	29.74	29.71	47	59	57	54.3	S'ly 1	S'ly 1	S'ly 1	Foggy	Misty	Rain	0.80
15	29.63	29.64	29.94	53	63	43	53.0	S'ly 1	N. W. 1	N. E. 3	Foggy	Misty	Rain	
16	30.08	30.20	29.91	32	34	32	32.7	N. E. 1	N. E. 3	N. E. 3	3	10	Hail	
17	29.81	29.69	29.65	36	40	32	36.0	N. E. 3	N. E. 2	N. E. 3	Rain	Misty	Sn., r'n	1.45
18	29.69	29.73	29.80	23	32	23	26.0	N. E. 2	N'ly 1	N. W. 1	Snow	9	2	
S 19	29.66	29.57	29.73	29	42	34	35.0	N. 2	N. W. 1	N. 1	7	3	10	⎫
20	29.89	29.88	29.99	31	34	27	30.7	N. W. 1	N. W. 1	N. W. 1	8	10	8	⎪
21	30.00	29.87	29.76	19	21	20	20.0	N. W. 1	N. W. 1	N. W. 1	3	10	10	⎪
22	29.42	29.41	29.36	17	21	18	18.7	N. W. 1	N'ly 1	N'ly 1	10	Snow	10	⎪
23	29.44	...	29.38	17	...	28	...	N. W. 1	...	S. W. 2	0	...	10	⎪
24	29.28	29.37	29.60	32	37	24	31.0	S. W. 2	W'ly 1	N. W. 1	6	2	2	⎬ 0.72
25	29.69	29.67	29.53	29	37	23	29.7	N. W. 2	N. W. 1	N. E. 2	10	5	Snow	⎪
S 26	29.51	29.65	29.88	20	22	11	17.7	N'ly 2	N. W. 2	N. W. 2	Snow	0	0	⎪
27	30.32	30.27	30.33	9	17	16	14.0	N. W. 1	N. W. 2	N. 1	0	0	10	⎪
28	30.27	30.10	30.12	19	33	35	29.0	N. W. 1	S. W. 1	S. W. 1	10	10	2	⎪
29	30.18	30.10	30.15	32	45	40	39.0	S. W. 1	S. W. 2	W'ly 1	2	2	0	⎭
30	30.14	30.09	30.07	36	52	42	43.3	S. W. 1	S. W. 1	S'ly 1	2	3	Foggy	
31	30.05	29.96	29.98	43	50	47	46.7	S'ly 1	S'ly 1	S'ly 1	Foggy	Foggy	Foggy	
Means	29.89	29.87	29.89	33.7	43.2	36.0	...	1.4	1.5	1.4	6.2	6.3	6.9	5.97
								1.4			6.5			
REDUCED TO SEA LEVEL.								Prevailing winds from some point between— Days.			Days.			
Max.	30.59	30.47	30.56	58	65	58	59.3	N. & E. 4			Clear 5			
Min.	29.46	29.55	29.49	9	17	11	14.0	E. & S. 2			Variable . . . ⎫ 14			
Mean	30.07	30.05	30.07					S. & W. 11			Cloudy . . . . ⎭			
Range	1.13	0.92	1.07	49	48	47	45.3	W. & N. 14			Rain or snow fell on 12			
Mean of month	30.063			...	...	...	37.6							
Extreme range	1.13			...	...	...	56.0							

Remarks.

1st. Appearances of storm.
2d. Rain through the day, sometimes brisk.
3d. Moderate rain nearly all day.
4th. Fine.
5th. Rain and unpleasant. Began to rain from 9 to 10 P. M.
6th. Fine.
7th, 8th, and 9th. Very fine.
10th. Very warm.
11th. Dashes of rain. Wind very fresh S. W. Evening clear and calm.
12th. Very pleasant in the morning. Mist and appearances of storm in the evening.
13th. Variable.
14th. Thick mist and fog during the day. Rain in the evening.
15th. Wind came to N. W. in the morning. Air very soft and spring-like. Wind changed to N. E. in the afternoon, and freshened. Heavy mist mixed with rain in the evening.
16th. Rain during the day, the wind increasing. Began to hail briskly from 9 to 10 P. M.
17th. Very tempestuous during the night.
18th. Stormy in the morning. Pretty clear in the evening.
19th. Rather raw.
20th and 21st. Indications of storm in the evening.
22d. Light, gentle snow in the afternoon.
23d. Appearances of storm in the evening. An inch and a half of snow during the night.
24th. Flurry of snow from 4 to 5 P. M.
25th. Light snow in the afternoon—nearly three inches.
26th. Severe cold in the afternoon, and the snow blowing furiously.
27th. Very cold.
28th. Much moderated.
29th. Mild.
30th. Very mild.
31st. Thick fog, with occasional sprinkling of rain.

January, 1848. New Moon, 6[d.] 6[h.] 59[m.] A. M.

Days.	Barometer Sunrise.	At 1 P. M.	At 10 P. M.	Thermometer Sunrise.	At 1 P. M.	At 10 P. M.	Daily mean.	Winds Sunrise.	At 1 P. M.	At 10 P. M.	Weather Sunrise.	At 1 P. M.	At 10 P. M.	Rain and Snow
1	29.88	29.75	29.61	46	52	54	50.7	S'ly 1	S'ly 1	S. W. 2	Foggy	Foggy	10, Sh'r	0.45
S 2	29.43	29.46	29.66	55	45	38	49.3	S. W. 2	N. W. 2	N. W. 1	10	10	6	
3	30.03	29.92	29.92	32	43	33	36.0	N. W. 1	N. E. 2	N. E.	0	0	0	
4	29.71	29.68	29.97	33	44	34	37.0	S. W.	S. W. 2	N. W. 1	7	10	0	
5	30.09	29.87	29.38	26	33	43	34.0	N. W. 1	S'ly 2	S. W. 3	8	10	10	
6	29.53	29.61	29.72	24	25	20	23.0	N. W. 2	N. W. 3	. W. 2	0	0	10	
7	29.85	29.83	29.99	12	21	16	16.3	N. W. 1	N. W. 1	N. W. 1	0	0	6	
8	29.98	29.83	29.67	16	30	33	26.3	N. W. 1	N. E. 1	N. E. 1	3	10	Snow	
S 9	28.97	29.17	29.62	48	43	18	36.3	S. W. 3	W'ly 2	N. W. 3	Rain	0	0	1.25
10	29.97	30.00	30.21	6	10	0	5.3	N. W. 2	N. W. 2	N. W. 2	0	0	0	
11	30.34	30.26	30.02	—4	14	24	11.3	N. W. 1	S. W. 1	S. W. 2	0	3	10	
12	30.19	30.20	30.35	21	31	21	24.3	W'ly 1	W'ly 1	W'ly 1	0	0	0	
13	30.40	30.34	30.24	18	31	33	27.3	N. E'ly 1	N. E'ly 1	N. E. 1	9	10	M't, r'n	
14	30.19	30.15	30.16	33	45	40	39.3	Calm	N'ly 1	N'ly 1	Misty	10	Misty	
15	30.10	29.94	29.84	45	51	45	47.0	S'ly 1	S'ly 1	S'ly 1	Rain	Rain	Foggy	0.62
S 16	30.01	30.02	30.13	45	44	35	41.3	N'ly 1	N. W. 2	. W. 1	9	0	4	
17	29.94	29.88	30.03	33	43	31	35.7	N'ly 1	N. W. 2	. W. 1	10	2	0	
18	29.81	29.63	29.97	26	44	20	30.0	S'ly 1	S. W. 2	. W. 3	0	10	0	
19	30.29	30.27	30.41	10	17	16	14.3	N. W. 2	N. W. 2	. W. 1	0	0	0	
20	30.25	30.09	30.06	15	35	33	27.7	S. W'ly 1	S. W. 2	W. 2	2	0	6	
21	29.91	29.69	29.60	33	46	39	39.3	S. W. 1	S. W. 2	N. W. 1	0	2	2	
22	29.85	29.84	29.89	30	35	30	31.7	N. W. 1	W'ly 1	N. W. 1	8	2	10	
S 23	30.03	30.03	30.25	27	30	23	26.7	N. E. 1	N. E. 2	N'ly 1	10	10	0	
24	30.45	30.43	30.47	15	32	28	25.0	N. W. 1	E'ly 1	E'ly 1	0	0	0	
25	30.37	30.22	30.12	31	46	40	39.0	S. W'ly 1	...	S'ly 1	10	...	Hazy	
26	30.10	29.97	29.88	37	51	45	47.7	S. W. 1	E'ly 1	N. E. 1	10	10	10	
27	29.73	29.41	29.35	40	45	39	41.3	N. E. 1	N. E'ly 1	N. E'ly 2	Rain	Rain	10	2.50
28	29.39	29.33	29.39	37	48	39	41.3	W'ly 1	W'ly 1	W'ly 1	5	3	10	
29	[illegible]	[illegible]	29.70	[illegible]	[illegible]	[illegible]	[illegible]	W'ly 1	N'ly 3	N'ly 2	9	Snow	10	
S 30	29.88	29.85	29.91	29	37	32	32.7	N. W. 1	N. W. 1	N. W. 1	0	0	2	
31	29.85	29.69	29.57	30	42	36	36.0	N. W. 1	S'ly 1	S'ly 1	5	5	10	
Means	29.95	29.86	29.91	28.7	36.9	31.4	...	1.2	1.6	1.4	5.4	4.9	5.4	4.82
								1.4			5.2			
REDUCED TO SEA LEVEL.								Prevailing winds from some point between— Days.			Days.			
Max.	30.63	30.61	30.65	55	52	54	50.7	N. & E. 7			Clear 7			
Min.	29.57	29.35	29.53	—4	10	0	5.3	E. & S. 1			Variable . . . ⎫ 17			
Mean	30.13	30.04	30.09					S. & W. 10			Cloudy . . . . ⎭			
Range	1.06	1.26	1.12	59	42	54	45.4	W. & N. 13			Rain or snow fell on 7			
Mean of month	30.087			...	...	...	32.3							
Extreme range	1.30			...	...	...	59.0							

Remarks.

1st. Thick fog all day; little wind. Frost out of the ground in most places. Some rain during the night.
2d. Sprinkling of rain in the afternoon. Partially clear in the evening.
3d. Fine.
4th. Pleasant.
5th. Appearances of storm in the evening. Occasional dashes of rain.
6th. Cold and blustering.
7th. Pleasant.
8th. Began to snow very moderately at 4 P. M. Rain during the night.
9th. Very blustering.
10th. Very cold. Wind piercing through the day.
11th. Thermometer 4° below zero. Wind moderate at N. W.; came to S W. during the morning. Evening cloudy, wind brisk; appearances of storm.
12th. Very fine.
13th. Mist and rain in the evening. Ground covered with ice.
14th. Ground covered with sleet in the morning.
15th. Light rain at intervals.
16th. Halo about the moon.
17th. Evening very clear and mild.
18th. Snow squall at 3 P. M., when the wind changed suddenly from S. W. to N. W., and grew colder.
19th. Cold, but not unpleasant.
20th. Very pleasant.
21st. Fine.
22d. Very pleasant.
23d. Cloudy during the day. Very clear in the evening.
24th. Very fine.
25th and 26th. Very mild.
27th. Heavy rain.
28th. Very mild. Frost nearly out of the ground in warm places.
29th. Began to snow from 9 to 10 A. M.; about two inches of damp snow fell. Mostly clear at sunset. Cloudy in the evening.
30th. Very fine. Wet under foot.
31st. Very mild.

February, 1848. New Moon, 4d. 8h. 34m. P. M.

Days.	Barometer, reduced to 32° F: Sunrise.	At 1 P. M.	At 10 P. M.	Thermometer: Sunrise.	At 1 P. M.	At 10 P. M.	Daily mean.	Winds (Direction and Force): Sunrise.	At 1 P. M.	At 10 P. M.	Weather (Tenths Cloudy): Sunrise.	At 1 P. M.	At 10 P. M.	Rain and Snow in Inches of Water.
1	29.18	29.25	29.46	30	32	45	36.0	N'ly 3	N. W. 1	N. W. 1	Snow	10	0	
2	29.58	29.60	29.70	22	32	25	26.3	N. W. 1	N. W. 1	N. W. 1	0	0	0	
3	29.77	29.70	29.78	20	39	30	29.7	N. W. 1	N. W. 1	N. W. 1	0	2	0	
4	29.68	29.48	29.23	25	38	30	31.0	N. E. 1	E'ly 1	N. E. 5	10	Sn., r'n	Snow	
5	28.91	28.60	28.78	30	32	29	30.3	N. W. 3	N. W. 1	N. W. 1	10	10	0	2.95
S 6	28.89	28.94	29.13	26	30	26	27.3	N. W. 1	N. W. 1	N. W. 1	Snow	Snow	5	
7	29.32	29.34	29.47	24	29	23	25.3	W'ly 1	N. W. 2	N. W. 1	5	2	7	
8	29.53	29.63	29.72	17	29	17	21.0	N. W. 1	N. W. 1	N. W. 1	0	0	0	
9	29.83	29.77	29.65	13	27	22	20.7	N. W. 1	N. W. 1	N. W. 1	0	0	8	
10	29.59	29.60	29.82	27	33	14	24.7	W'ly 1	N. W'ly 2	N. W. 1	3	3	0	
11	29.99	29.93	30.02	2	15	11	9.3	N. W'ly 2	N. W. 2	N. W. 1	0	0	0	
12	30.07	30.00	30.02	6	24	18	16.0	N. W. 1	W'ly 1	N'ly 2	0	0	Hazy	
S 13	29.94	29.83	29.87	19	27	20	22.0	N'ly 2	N. W. 2	N. W. 1	10	0	0	
14	29.80	29.70	29.67	16	37	24	25.7	N. W. 1	N. W. 1	N. W. 1	0	5	2	
15	29.73	29.70	29.73	20	33	25	26.0	N. W. 1	N. W. 1	N. W. 1	0	0	0	
16	29.82	29.73	29.79	21	34	24	26.3	N. W. 1	N. W. 2	N. W. 1	0	0	0	
17	29.80	29.71	29.78	20	35	26	27.0	N. W. 1	N. W. 1	N. W. 0	0	0	0	
18	29.98	29.93	29.96	21	35	26	27.3	N. W. 1	N. W. 1	N. W. 0	0	0	0	
19	29.92	29.78	29.70	22	43	34	33.0	N. W. 1	N. W. 1	N. W. 1	0	2	3	
S 20	29.59	29.46	29.34	35	37	33	35.0	S. W. 1	N. E. 1	N. E. 1	Rain	Rain	Misty	}
21	29.38	29.45	29.76	38	47	38	41.0	W'ly 1	N. W. 2	N. W. 2	2	3	0	} 0.65
22	29.92	29.91	29.78	37	38	35	36.7	N'ly 1	E'ly 1	E'ly 1	10	Snow	Misty	}
23	29.66	29.69	29.80	33	44	36	37.7	W'ly 1	W'ly 2	N. W. 1	10	0	0	
24	29.91	29.92	29.97	32	33	25	30.0	W'ly 1	N. W. 2	N. W. 1	10	10	0	
25	30.15	30.14	30.19	15	19	15	16.3	N'ly 2	N. W. 2	N. W. 1	0	0	0	
26	30.15	29.96	29.84	11	30	25	22.0	N. W. 1	S'ly 1	S. W. 1	0	3	0	
S 27	29.77	29.68	29.84	27	38	28	31.0	S. W. 1	S. W. 1	W'ly 1	2	1	0	
28	29.97	29.87	29.64	14	38	32	28.0	N. W. 1	S. W. 1	S'ly 2	0	10	Snow	0.20
29	29.26	29.19	29.37	36	36	25	32.3	S. W. 2	N. W. 3	N. W. 2	9	3	6	
Means	29.69	29.64	29.68	22.7	33.2	26.2	...	1.3	1.4	1.2	3.8	3.6	2.8	3.80
									1.3			3.4		
REDUCED TO SEA LEVEL.														
Max.	30.33	30.32	30.37	38	47	45	41.0							
Min.	29.07	28.98	28.96	2	15	11	9.3							
Mean	29.87	29.82	29.86											
Range	1.26	1.34	1.41	36	32	34	31.7							
Mean of month	29.850			...	...	...	27.4							
Extreme range	1.41			...	...	...	45.0							

Prevailing winds from some point between— Days.
N. & E. 3
E. & S. 0
S. & W. 3
W. & N. 23

Days.
Clear 15
Variable . . . } 7
Cloudy . . . . }
Rain or snow fell on 7

REMARKS.

1st. Snowing at 5 A. M., which continued till from 1 to 2 P. M.—about four inches of damp snow. Very clear in the evening.
2d and 3d. Very fine.
4th. Began to rain and snow at 3 P. M. Storm increased, and snowed fast in the evening.
5th. From six to eight inches of damp snow during the night. At 7 P. M., barom. 28.87. At 9 P. M., barom. 28.84; ther. 50°; wind light at N. W., and clear; exter. ther. 29°. At 10 P. M., barom. 28.84; at 11 P. M., 28.84.
6th. Light snow during a large part of the day—one inch, perhaps, in depth.
7th. Pleasant.
8th. Very fine. Aurora in the evening.
9th and 10th. Fine.
11th. Very fine.
12th. Pleasant.
13th. Rather raw.
14th to 19th. Very fine.
20th. Very moderate rain at N. E.
21st. Beautiful aurora, which appeared in diffused light of considerable brightness early in the evening. Between 9 and 10 o'clock, it became brilliantly red, with occasional white streamers shooting up through it, the heavens at the time being without a cloud, except low in the south, the air very clear, and the moon but little past the full.
22d. Snow in the afternoon—from two to three inches, quite damp.
23d. Brilliant auroral streamers from 7 to 9 P. M.
24th. Diffused aurora in the evening.
25th and 26th. Fine.
27th. Fine. Evening very clear.
28th. Began to snow very moderately from 4 to 6 P. M.
29th. Flurry of snow at from 1 to 2 P. M.

March, 1848. New Moon, 5d. 8h. 9m. A. M.

Days.	Barometer: Sunrise.	At 1 P. M.	At 10 P. M.	Thermometer: Sunrise.	At 1 P. M.	At 10 P. M.	Daily mean.	Winds: Sunrise.	At 1 P. M.	At 10 P. M.	Weather: Sunrise.	At 1 P. M.	At 10 P. M.	Rain and Snow in Inches of Water.
1	29.51	29.58	29.85	19	25	19	21.0	N. W. 4	N. W. 3	W. 3	0	0	0	
2	30.16	30.15	30.14	15	28	25	22.7	N. W. 1	N. W. 1	N. E. 1	0	8	5	
3	29.77	29.63	29.55	22	31	28	27.0	N. E. 2	...	N. W. 1	Snow	...	0	0.50
4	29.91	29.94	29.90	21	29	25	25.0	N. W. 1	N. W. 1	N. W. 1	0	0	0	
S 5	29.71	29.70	29.79	29	29	18	25.3	W'ly 1	N. W. 3	N. W. 2	10	0	0	
6	29.86	29.75	29.81	16	30	27	24.3	N'ly 2	W'ly 2	N. W. 1	5	4	0	
7	30.00	29.94	29.98	27	45	37	36.3	S. W. 1	S. W.	S. W. 1	2	3	2	
8	29.62	29.71	29.74	35	52	47	44.7	S. W. 1	S. W. 2	W'ly 1	3	1	0	
9	29.80	29.79	29.61	48	44	38	43.3	S. W. 1	N. W. 1	N. E. 2	10	Rain	Rain	
10	29.38	29.25	29.44	35	37	30	34.0	N. E. 2	N. E. 1	N. W. 3	Rain	10	8	1.50
11	29.73	29.73	29.91	21	33	29	27.7	N. W. 2	N. W. 2	N. W. 1	0	0	0	
S 12	30.15	30.05	29.79	24	33	40	32.3	N. W. 1	S'ly 2	S'ly 1	0	10	Rain	0.15
13	29.71	29.60	29.76	40	50	30	40.0	S. W'ly 1	S. W.	W. 2	10	10	0	
14	29.82	29.66	29.74	20	27	17	21.3	N. W. 1	N. W. 2	N. W. 2	0	4	0	
15	29.80	29.77	29.92	8	19	13	13.3	N. W. 2	N. W. 2	N. W. 2	0	3	0	
16	30.07	29.99	29.95	8	19	15	14.0	N. W. 1	N. W. 2	N. W. 2	0	0	0	
17	29.74	29.61	29.54	11	22	25	19.3	N. W. 2	...	N'ly 2	0	...	10	
18	29.61	29.58	29.71	25	43	28	32.0	N'ly 1	S. E'ly 1	W'ly 1	10	8	2	
S 19	29.90	29.89	29.81	27	45	37	36.3	N. W. 1	S. E. 1	S'ly 1	3	0	10	
20	29.90	29.87	29.73	35	55	43	44.3	N. W. 1	N. W. 1	S. W. 1	0	2	10	
21	29.46	29.42	29.58	43	57	41	47.0	S. W. 1	S. W. 2	W'ly 2	0	6	1	
22	29.70	29.71	29.77	36	52	42	43.3	N. W. 1	N. W. 1	E'ly 1	0	0	3	
23	29.88	29.88	29.93	37	37	31	35.0	N. E. 2	N. E. 2	N. E. 1	10	Snow	0	
24	30.09	30.04	30.09	25	38	31	31.3	N'ly 2	N'ly 2	N. E. 1	0	0	0	
25	30.15	30.03	29.95	29	47	36	37.3	N'ly 1	N. E'ly 1	N. E. 1	0	0	0	
S 26	29.83	29.75	29.72	36	52	44	44.0	N. W. 1	S'ly 1	S'ly 1	2	3	10	
27	29.71	29.70	29.75	42	53	48	47.7	S. W. 1	S. W. 1	S. W. 1	10	10	10	
28	29.83	29.87	29.83	40	41	40	40.3	N'ly 1	N. E. 1	N. E. 1	10	Misty	Rain	0.25
29	29.79	29.78	29.97	40	59	46	48.3	N'ly 1	N. W. 2	W'ly 1	10	5	0	
30	30.01	30.05	30.06	42	62	48	50.7	N. W. 1	S'ly 1	S'ly	0	0	0	
31	30.02	29.88	29.72	46	64	55	55.0	S. W'ly 1	S. W. 2	S. W. 3	6	10	2	
Means	29.82	29.78	29.81	29.1	40.6	33.3	...	1.4	1.5	1.5	3.9	4.1	3.5	2.40
									1.5			3.8		
REDUCED TO SEA LEVEL.														
Max.	30.34	30.33	30.32	48	64	55	55.0							
Min.	29.56	29.43	29.62	8	19	13	13.3							
Mean	30.00	29.96	29.99											
Range	0.78	0.90	0.70	40	45	42	41.7							
Mean of month	29.983			...	...	...	34.3							
Extreme range	0.91			...	...	...	56.0							

Prevailing winds from some point between— Days.
N. & E. 6
E. & S. 1
S. & W. 9
W. & N. 15

Days.
Clear 11
Variable . . . } 12
Cloudy . . . . }
Rain or snow fell on 8

REMARKS.

1st. Very blustering and severe.
2d. Began to snow very moderately at 8 P. M.
3d. Snow in the morning—about six or seven inches, rather damp.
4th. Very fine.
5th. Very blustering.
6th. Flurry of snow from 10 to 11 A. M., and very blustering.
7th and 8th. Very fine.
9th. Showery in the morning. Steady rain in the afternoon and evening.
10th. Rainy.
11th. Very pleasant, though cool.
12th. Air very raw. Began to rain between 8 and 9 P. M.
13th. Rather raw.
14th. Very raw and cold in the afternoon.
15th. Very cold day.
16th. Very cold.
17th. Still raw and cold.
18th. Fine.
19th. Sprinkling of rain in the evening.
20th. Mild and spring-like.
21st and 22d. Very fine.
23d. Snow and rain for a short time to-day.
24th. Quite cold. Aurora in the evening not very bright.
25th. Fine.
26th. Appearances of storm in the evening.
27th. Appearances of rain in the evening.
28th. Rain in the evening; wind light N. E.
29th and 30th. Very fine.
31st. Blustering, and streets very dusty.

April, 1848. New Moon, 3d. 5h. 53m. P. M.

DAYS.	Barometer, reduced to 32° F. At 6 A. M.	At 1 P. M.	At 10 P. M.	Thermometer. At 6 A. M.	At 1 P. M.	At 10 P. M.	Daily mean.	Winds. (Direction and Force.) At 6 A. M.	At 1 P. M.	At 10 P. M.	Weather. (Tenths Cloudy.) At 6 A. M.	At 1 P. M.	At 10 P. M.	Rain and Snow in Inches of Water.
1	29.54	29.76	29.96	55	43	38	45.3	S. W. 3	N. W. 2	N. W. 2	10	Rain	0	
S 2	30.11	30.13	30.22	32	47	35	38.0	N. W. 2	N. W. 2	N. W. 1	0	3	0	
3	30.43	30.49	30.49	28	48	38	38.0	N. E. 2	N. E. 2	S'ly 1	0	1	8	
4	30.46	30.34	29.99	38	44	38	40.0	S'ly 1	S. W. 2	S. W. 2	10	10	10	
5	29.81	29.79	29.89	48	60	40	49.3	S'ly 1	W'ly 1	N. 2	9	4	0	
6	29.88	29.76	29.75	32	52	41	41.7	N. W. 2	N. W. 2	N. W. 1	1	0	0	
7	29.75	29.72	29.83	35	51	38	41.3	N. W. 1	N'ly 3	N'ly 1	0	0	0	
8	29.79	29.76	29.78	35	58	47	46.7	N. W. 1	N. W. 1	S'ly 1	0	0	0	
S 9	29.83	29.73	29.71	38	66	48	50.7	N. W. 1	N. W. 1	S'ly 1	0	0	0	
10	29.77	29.65	29.67	45	68	56	56.3	N. W. 1	S'ly 2	N. W. 1	0	0	2	
11	29.73	29.79	29.95	43	59	40	47.3	N. W. 1	N. E. 1	N. W. 1	0	0	0	
12	30.01	29.81	29.68	40	57	40	45.7	N. E. 1	N. E. 1	...	10	10	...	
13	29.57	29.45	29.51	40	55	41	46.3	S'ly 1	S'ly 1	N. W. 1	10	10	Shower	} 0.45
14	29.54	29.57	29.66	36	51	37	40.7	N. W. 1	...	W'ly 1	0	...	5	
15	29.70	29.68	29.71	35	56	46	45.7	N. W. 1	S'ly 1	S'ly 1	2	0	0	
S 16	29.76	29.71	29.75	42	66	43	50.3	N. W. 1	W'ly 1	N. E. 1	0	5	0	
17	29.83	29.90	29.99	40	64	41	48.3	...	...	N'ly 1	...	...	0	
18	30.13	30.00	29.97	34	55	44	44.3	N. W. 2	S'ly 2	E'ly 1	0	10	10	
19	29.94	29.95	29.94	34	33	28	31.7	N. E. 3	N. E. 3	N. W. 1	Sn., h'l	Snow	2	0.50
20	29.98	29.96	29.92	28	45	40	37.7	N. W. 2	N. W. 1	S'ly 2	0	0	0	
21	29.88	29.85	29.89	41	65	53	53.0	W'ly 1	N'ly 2	W'ly 1	5	0	0	
22	29.82	29.65	29.68	52	65	55	57.3	S. W. 1	S. W. 2	N'ly 2	3	0	10	
S 23	29.79	29.67	29.52	55	63	51	56.3	N. E'ly 1	S. E. 2	S. E. 2	5	0	10	
24	29.43	29.45	29.71	53	56	41	50.0	N. E. 2	N. W. 2	N. W. 1	5	0	0	
25	29.86	29.86	29.96	38	57	43	46.0	W'ly 2	W'ly 1	S. W.	0	5	0	
26	29.90	29.92	29.92	45	59	48	50.7	S'ly 2	S'ly 1	...	10	8	...	
27	29.91	29.91	30.15	48	59	47	51.3	N. E.	N. E.	N. E. 1	10	2	0	
28	30.19	30.15	30.02	44	57	44	48.3	S. E. 1	S'ly 2	S'ly 2	5	3	9	
29	29.88	29.62	29.87	45	69	47	53.7	S'ly 2	S. W. 3	W'ly 1	10	10	5	
S 30	30.04	29.96	30.02	43	61	50	51.3	N. W. 1	N. W. 1	W'ly 1	3	0	0	
Means	29.88	29.83	29.87	40.7	56.3	43.3	...	1.1	1.7	1.2	4.1	3.6	2.8	0.95
								1.3			3.5			
REDUCED TO SEA LEVEL.														
Max.	30.64	30.67	30.67	55	69	56	57.3	Prevailing winds from some point between—		Days.			Days.	
Min.	29.61	29.63	29.69	28	33	28	31.7	N. & E.		5	Clear		15	
Mean	30.06	30.01	30.05					E. & S.		1	Variable }		9	
Range	1.03	1.04	0.98	27	36	28	25.6	S. & W.		7	Cloudy }			
Mean of month	30.030			...	...	...	46.8	W. & N.		17	Rain or snow fell on		6	
Extreme range	1.06			...	...	...	41.0							

REMARKS.

1st. Rained moderately from 9 A. M. till noon.
2d. Fine, though cool.
3d. Raw air. Ground frozen pretty hard in the morning.
4th. Appearances of rain.
5th. Fine.
6th. Fine. Aurora in the evening.
7th. Fine.
8th, 9th, and 10th. Very fine.
11th. Fine.
12th. Variable.
13th. Moderate rain from 5 to 8 P. M.
14th. Showery from 5 to 8 P. M., and quite cold. Wind N. E.
15th. Very fine.
16th. Sprinkling of rain between 1 and 3 P. M. Evening very fine.
17th. Very fine.
18th. Cool.
19th. Snow and rain most of the day. Ground white with snow in the afternoon. Cleared in the evening.
20th. Pleasant.
21st and 22d. Very fine.
23d. Pleasant.
24th. Fine.
25th. Pleasant.
26th. Rather cool. Sprinkling in the morning.
27th. Rather cool.
28th. Rather raw.
29th. Appearances of rain in the morning.
30th. Very fine.

May, 1848. New Moon, 3d. 2h. 7m. A. M.

DAYS.	Barometer At 6 A. M.	At 1 P. M.	At 10 P. M.	Thermometer At 6 A. M.	At 1 P. M.	At 10 P. M.	Daily mean	Winds At 6 A. M.	At 1 P. M.	At 10 P. M.	Weather At 6 A. M.	At 1 P. M.	At 10 P. M.	Rain and Snow in Inches of Water.
1	30.07	29.98	29.89	42	65	52	53.0	N. W. 1	S. E'ly 2	S'ly 2	0	5	10	
2	29.71	29.64	29.45	53	65	45	54.3	S'ly 1	S'ly 1	N. E. 2	10	10	Rain	} 2.10
3	29.27	29.34	29.47	46	55	52	51.0	N. E. 1	N'ly 1	N. W. 1	Rain	Misty	5	
4	29.66	29.62	29.88	50	71	57	59.3	W. 1	N'ly 2	N. W. 1	0	0	2	
5	29.84	29.79	29.73	53	61	55	56.3	S'ly 1	S. E'ly 1	S'ly 1	8	10	10	
6	29.71	29.61	29.68	53	71	58	60.7	N. E. 1	N. E. 1	N. E. 1	Foggy	4	10	
S 7	29.58	29.46	29.47	57	71	64	64.0	S. E. 1	S. E. 2	W'ly 1	Foggy	2	5	
8	29.55	29.58	29.64	55	74	59	62.7	N. W. 2	N. W. 2	W'ly 1	0	0	8	
9	29.65	29.57	29.76	53	66	52	57.0	N. E. 2	N. E. 2	N. E. 1	10	5	6	
10	29.75	29.69	29.62	52	70	54	58.7	S'ly 1	S. E'ly 3	S'ly 1	0	8	10	
11	29.11	29.02	29.40	48	52	48	49.3	N. E. 3	N. W. 3	N. W. 1	Rain	5	2	0.75
12	29.45	29.44	29.51	48	66	52	55.3	N. W. 1	N. W. 2	N. E'ly 1	2	8	10	
13	29.54	29.54	29.60	48	66	52	55.3	...	...	S'ly	...	...	10	
S 14	29.61	29.57	29.74	52	57	49	52.7	S. W. 1	W'ly 3	W'ly 1	3	6	3	
15	29.90	29.84	29.85	46	68	56	56.7	S. W. 1	S. W. 2	S. W. 2	2	3	Hazy	
16	...	29.70	29.74	53	70	64	62.3	...	S. W. 2	S. W. 1	...	10	10	
17	29.81	29.73	29.75	62	71	59	64.0	S. W. 1	S. W. 1	S. W. 1	10	3	0	
18	29.61	29.73	29.77	57	83	70	70.0	S. W. 1	N. W. 2	W'ly 1	2	0	0	
19	29.81	29.73	29.69	61	88	69	72.7	N. W. 1	S. W. 2	W'ly 2	0	0	5	
20	29.67	29.58	...	66	...	...	66.0	S. W. 1	...	...	8	...	...	
S 21	...	...	...	...	...	...	...	...	...	...	...	...	...	
22	29.56	29.57	29.60	53	52	49	51.3	N. E. 2	N. E. 2	N. E. 2	Misty	Rain	Misty	0.85
23	29.75	29.75	29.79	48	69	53	51.7	N. E. 1	N. E. 1	N. E. 1	10	10	2	
24	29.82	29.77	29.75	52	62	52	55.3	N. E. 1	N. E. 1	N. E. 1	Misty	10	Misty	
25	29.82	29.77	29.75	51	67	63	60.3	N. E. 1	S. E. 2	S'ly	10	2	2	
26	29.69	29.68	29.78	62	68	63	64.3	S. E. 1	S. E. 1	E'ly 1	8	Rain	0	
27	29.92	29.94	29.97	56	67	53	62.0	N. E. 2	N. E. 2	N. E. 1	10	2	10	
S 28	30.05	30.02	30.03	54	68	58	60.0	N. E. 1	S. E'ly 1	S'ly 1	10	2	5	
29	30.02	29.94	29.87	55	70	60	61.7	S'ly 1	...	S'ly 1	10	...	3	
[illegible]	[illegible]	[illegible]	[illegible]	[illegible]	[illegible]	[illegible]	[illegible]	[illegible]	[illegible]	[illegible]	[illegible]	[illegible]	[illegible]	[illegible]
31	29.35	29.39	29.58	57	64	47	56.0	N. W. 1	N. W. 2	N. W. 1	3	9	0	
Means	29.68	29.65	29.69	53.5	67.0	56.1	...	1.2	1.8	1.2	6.4	6.1	5.9	5.00
								1.4			6.1			
REDUCED TO SEA LEVEL.														
Max.	30.25	30.20	30.21	66	88	70	72.7	Prevailing winds from some point between—		Days.			Days.	
Min.	29.29	29.20	29.50	42	52	46	49.3	N. & E.		8	Clear		5	
Mean	29.86	29.83	29.87					E. & S.		8	Variable }		14	
Range	0.96	1.00	0.71	24	36	25	23.4	S. & W.		8	Cloudy }			
Mean of month	29.853			...	...	...	58.9	W. & N.		5	Rain fell on		10	
Extreme range	1.05			...	...	...	46.0				(2 days omitted.)			

REMARKS.

1st. Slight appearances of white frost in the College yard.
2d. Pleasant. Appearances of rain in the evening; rain.
3d. A little rain during the preceding night. Rain began between 8 and 9 P. M., and continued through the night; heavy at intervals.
4th. Very fine.
5th. Sprinkling of rain in the morning.
6th. Fog and mist in the morning. Pleasant in the afternoon.
7th. Sprinkling of rain from 6 to 7 P. M., with lightning.
8th. Fine.
9th. Rather cool.
10th. Variable, with appearances of rain in the evening.
11th. At sunrise, wind heavy N. E., with rain. At 6 A. M., barom. 29.20, and falling; at 11 A. M., 28.44; at 1 P. M., 29.13, with wind strong at N. W. Clear in the evening.
12th. Pleasant.
13th. Sprinkling of rain from 1 to 2 P. M.
14th. Air raw for the season.
15th. Bright halo about the moon.
16th. Air damp.
17th. Fine.
18th. Very fine.
19th and 20th. Very hot.
21st. Rain in the evening, with thunder.
22d. Moderate rain by spells.
23d. Very cool.
24th. Misty and cool.
25th. Very fine.
26th. Light showers from 1 to 2 P. M.
27th. Warm sun at mid-day. Cool evening.
28th. Pleasant.
29th. Very fine.
30th. Rain during the day. Clear in the evening.
31st. Grew quite cool after 3 P. M. Aurora in the evening, rather bright and low down.

June, 1848. New Moon, 1d. 9h. 31m. A. M., and 30d. 5h. 11m. P. M.

Days	Barometer, reduced to 32° F. At 6 A. M.	At 1 P. M.	At 10 P. M.	Thermometer At 6 A. M.	At 1 P. M.	At 10 P. M.	Daily mean	Winds (Direction and Force) At 6 A. M.	At 1 P. M.	At 10 P. M.	Weather (Tenths Cloudy) At 6 A. M.	At 1 P. M.	At 10 P. M.	Rain and Snow in Inches of Water
1	29.68	29.55	29.68	44	59	57	53.3	N. W. 2	N. W. 2	N. W. 1	0	8	0	
2	29.72	29.72	29.70	48	70	58	58.7	N. W. 1	N. W. 2	N. W. 1	0	2	0	
3	29.65	29.58	29.58	54	83	71	69.3	N. W. 1	N. W. 1	N'ly 1	0	3	5	
S. 4	29.60	29.72	29.66	57	79	62	66.0	N. E. 2	N. E. 1	S'ly 1	0	2	0	
5	29.69	29.68	29.63	56	64	54	58.0	N. E'ly 1	E'ly 1	E'ly 1	Foggy	Rain	Rain	0.35
6	29.48	29.57	29.63	52	63	54	56.3	N. E. 2	N. E. 2	N'ly 1	Foggy	10	5	
7	29.53	29.62	29.69	54	61	53	56.0	N. E. 2	N. E. 2	N. E. 1	10	10	Rain	
8	29.74	29.64	29.59	54	58	58	56.7	N. E. 2	N. E. 2	N. E. 2	10	Misty	10	
9	29.59	29.56	29.68	58	70	55	61.0	N'ly 2	N. W. 2	N'ly 1	5	8	5	
10	29.66	29.65	29.66	60	76	64	66.7	S'ly 1	S. W. 2	S. W. 1	5	8	5	
S 11	29.65	29.54	29.68	62	80	63	68.3	W'ly 1	W'ly 2	N. W. 1	2	0	0	
12	29.71	29.64	29.67	53	63	50	55.3	N. W. 1	N. W. 3	N. W. 2	0	0	0	
13	29.62	29.53	29.58	46	61	54	53.7	N. W. 2	N. W. 2	N. W. 1	6	2	0	
14	29.58	29.50	29.62	53	74	61	62.7	N. W. 2	N. W. 2	N. W. 1	0	8	2	
15	29.63	29.62	29.62	60	80	65	68.3	N. W. 1	N. W. 1	S. W. 1	2	5	5	
16	29.61	29.56	29.61	69	91	78	79.3	W'ly 1	W'ly 2	W'ly 1	0	2	2	
17	29.72	29.69	29.72	65	84	69	72.7	N. E. 1	S. E'ly 2	S. E. 1	0	0	2	
S 18	29.74	29.72	29.75	68	81	72	73.7	S. E. 1	S. E. 2	S. W. 2	0	3	5	
19	29.75	29.71	29.71	72	85	70	75.7	S. W. 2	S. W. 2	S'ly 2	8	8	10	
20	29.64	29.62	29.57	67	75	67	69.7	S. W. 1	S. W. 2	S. W. 2	Rain	10	10	0.55
21	29.51	29.51	29.27	68	85	68	73.7	S. W. 1	S. W. 2	N. W'ly 1	10	7	0	
22	29.64	29.70	29.71	65	81	66	70.7	N. W. 1	W'ly 1	S. W. 1	3	8	0	
23	29.76	29.62	29.49	67	78	72	72.3	S. W. 1	S. E. 2	W'ly 1	10	8	Rain	
24	29.54	29.61	29.70	68	77	66	70.3	N. W. 2	...	N. W. 2	8	...	0	
S 25	29.76	29.74	29.68	50	79	65	64.7	N. W. 1	W'ly 2	N. W. 1	0	3	1	
26	29.89	29.91	29.92	63	77	63	67.7	W. 1	S. E'ly 2	S'ly	0	2	0	
27	29.93	29.90	29.76	63	80	65	69.3	S. W. 2	S. W. 2	S. W. 1	4	7	2	
28	29.77	29.68	29.75	68	89	74	77.0	S. W. 2	S. W. 1	S'ly 1	5	8	10	
29	29.77	29.76	29.81	72	77	67	72.0	S. W. 1	N. E. 2	N. E'ly 1	5	10	2	
30	29.22	29.72	29.78	62	73	62	65.7	N. E. 1	N. E. 2	N. E. 1	Rain	10	10	2.90
Means	29.66	29.65	29.66	59.9	75.1	63.4	...	1.4	1.8	1.2	4.4	5.4	4.0	3.80
									1.5			4.6		
REDUCED TO SEA LEVEL.														
Max.	30.11	30.09	29.99	72	91	78	79.3							
Min.	29.40	29.68	29.45	44	58	50	53.3							
Mean	29.84	29.83	29.84											
Range	0.71	0.41	0.54	28	33	28	26.0							
Mean of month	29.837			...	...	...	66.1							
Extreme range	0.71			...	...	...	47.0							

Prevailing winds from some point between— Days.
N. & E. 7
E. & S. 3
S. & W. 7
W. & N. 13

Days.
Clear 10
Variable . . . } 14
Cloudy . . . . }
Rain fell on . . . 6

REMARKS.

1st. Very cool.
2d. Very fine.
3d. Very warm.
4th. Fine.
5th. Moderate rain in the afternoon.
6th. Variable.
7th. Occasional light rain and cool.
8th. Mist occasionally.
9th. Cool.
10th. Pleasant.
11th. Very fine.
12th. Very cool for the season.
13th. Very fine, but cool.
14th and 15th. Fine.
16th. Extremely hot.
17th. Very fine.
18th. Very fine. Sun very hot from 2 to 4 P. M.
19th. Very hot. Appearances of rain in the evening.
20th. Rain in the morning, and occasionally through the day.
21st. Thunder from 5 to 6 P. M., but no rain.
22d. Fine.
23d. Thunder and shower at 8 P. M.
24th. Very fine.
25th. Fine.
26th. Very fine.
27th. Fine.
28th. Very hot. Thunder and lightning at 10 P. M., with a dash of rain.
29th. Very warm in the morning. Wind came to N. E. from noon to 1 P. M., and grew cooler.
30th. Rained steadily and copiously in the morning.

July, 1848. New Moon, 30d. 2h. 17m. A. M.

Days	Barometer At 6 A. M.	At 1 P. M.	At 10 P. M.	Thermometer At 6 A. M.	At 1 P. M.	At 10 P. M.	Daily mean	Winds At 6 A. M.	At 1 P. M.	At 10 P. M.	Weather At 6 A. M.	At 1 P. M.	At 10 P. M.	Rain and Snow in Inches of Water
1	29.73	29.70	29.71	61	76	62	66.3	E'ly 1	S. E'ly 1	N. E. 1	10	10	Rain	} 0.25
S 2	29.77	29.70	29.64	60	74	62	65.3	N. E. 1	N. E. 1	N. E. 1	10	10	10	}
3	29.40	29.32	29.35	61	72	65	66.0	N. E. 1	S. E'ly 1	W'ly 1	10	10	0	
4	29.54	29.57	29.68	62	74	60	65.3	W'ly 1	N. W. 2	N. W. 1	0	4	0	
5	29.72	29.67	29.60	58	78	61	65.7	N. W. 1	N. W. 1	N. W.	0	1	10	0.60
6	29.58	29.57	29.66	57	74	59	60.0	N. W. 1	N. W. 1	N. E. 1	2	10	0	
7	29.70	29.79	29.90	57	62	55	58.0	N. E. 2	N. E. 3	N. E. 1	Misty	10	10	
8	30.04	30.04	30.09	55	74	58	62.3	N. E. 1	N. E. 1	N. E. 1	2	3	2	
S. 9	30.09	30.04	29.99	55	74	62	63.7	S'ly 1	S. W. 2	S. W. 1	3	9	Rain	0.50
10	29.97	29.92	29.92	62	73	67	67.3	S. W'ly 1	S. W. 1	S. W. 1	8	6	0	
11	29.98	29.97	29.96	62	83	72	72.3	S'ly 1	S'ly 2	Calm	10	3	2	
12	30.01	29.96	29.93	72	80	69	73.7	S. W. 1	S. E'ly 2	S'ly 1	2	0	8	
13	29.92	29.82	29.79	71	80	71	74.0	S. W. 1	S. E'ly 1	S'ly 1	10	10	10	
14	29.66	29.58	29.53	72	82	72	75.3	S. W. 1	S'ly 1	S. W. 1	Rain	10	10	0.25
15	29.55	29.53	29.53	70	80	76	75.3	N. W. 1	...	N. W. 1	0	...	0	
S 16	29.56	29.47	29.55	63	77	61	67.0	N. W. 1	N. W.	N. W. 1	0	0	0	
17	29.59	29.72	29.78	55	76	63	64.7	N. W. 1	N. W. 1	N. W. 1	0	2	0	
18	29.77	29.85	29.89	61	82	66	69.7	N. W. 1	N. W. 2	...	0	3	...	
19	29.89	29.86	29.89	63	84	69	72.0	N. W. 1	S. W. 1	S. W. 1	0	2	2	
20	29.86	29.82	29.82	66	86	69	73.7	S. W. 1	S. W. 1	S. W. 1	0	0	0	
21	29.80	29.78	29.82	69	87	70	75.3	S. W. 1	S. W. 2	S. W. 1	0	0	0	
22	29.79	29.67	29.74	71	85	74	76.7	S. W. 1	S. W. 3	S. W. 1	10	3	0	
S 23	29.73	29.70	29.74	75	84	74	77.7	S. W. 2	S. W. 3	S. W. 1	10	10	7	
24	29.72	29.68	29.79	72	82	71	75.0	S. W. 1	N. W.	W'ly 2	3	3	10	
25	29.82	29.81	29.86	70	86	71	75.7	S. W. 1	S. W. 2	S. W. 1	0	3	0	
26	29.85	29.81	29.81	71	90	75	78.7	S. W. 1	S. W. 1	S. W. 1	5	5	10	
27	29.80	29.72	29.75	76	86	76	79.3	S. W. 2	S. W. 5	S. W. 7	10	10	10	0.20
28	29.81	29.83	29.89	72	80	66	72.7	N. W. 1	...	N. W.	9	...	0	
29	29.93	29.90	29.92	65	71	66	67.3	N. W. 1	N. W.	N. W.	5	10	10	
S 30	29.91	29.88	29.91	55	80	62	65.7	S. E. 1	S. E. 1	S. E. 1	3	4	0	
31	29.78	29.64	29.54	65	76	70	70.3	E. 1	S. E. 1	S. E. 1	Rain	10	Foggy	0.05
Means	29.79	29.75	29.77	64.6	79.0	66.9	...	1.1	1.7	1.0	4.9	5.5	4.7	1.85
									1.3			5.0		
REDUCED TO SEA LEVEL.														
Max.	30.27	30.22	30.27	76	90	76	79.3							
Min.	29.67	29.50	29.53	55	62	55	58.0							
Mean	29.97	29.93	29.95											
Range	0.60	0.72	0.74	21	28	21	21.3							
Mean of month	29.950			...	...	...	70.2							
Extreme range	0.77			...	...	...	35.0							

Prevailing winds from some point between— Days
N. & E. 8
E. & S. 6
S. & W. 12
W. & N. 10

Days
Clear 9
Variable . . . } 17
Cloudy . . . . }
Rain fell on . . . 5

REMARKS.

1st. Moderate rain at 9 P. M.
2d. Cool and damp.
3d. Moderate rain in the morning. Clear in the evening.
4th. Very fine.
5th. Copious showers from 6 to 7 P. M., with thunder and lightning.
6th. Fine.
7th. Very cold mist most of the day. Fire and overcoats comfortable, almost necessary.
8th. Cool.
9th. Began to rain moderately at sunset.
10th. Pleasant.
11th. Very brilliant aurora from 9 to 10 P. M., needles shooting from N. W. round to N. E. up to a point a little south of the zenith, and, I judged, a little also to the east. Merry Dancers at the same time ran rapidly over the heavens from north to south. The diffused light in the upper region was occasionally pink.
12th. Fine.
13th. Air very damp.
15th. Fine.
16th to 19th. Very fine.
20th and 21st. Very fine and very warm.
22d. Appearances of rain in the morning.
23d. Very warm and sultry.
24th. Fine. Shower to the north.
25th. Very fine.
26th. Very hot.
27th. Sultry; appearances of rain.
28th. Cool and damp in the morning.
29th. Cool; appearances of rain. Showers to the south.
30th. Very fine indeed.
31st. Rainy.

August, 1848. New Moon, 28d. 1h. 53m. P. M.

Days.	Barometer, reduced to 32° F. At 6 A. M.	At 1 P. M.	At 10 P. M.	Thermometer. At 6 A. M.	At 1 P. M.	At 10 P. M.	Daily mean.	Winds. (Direction and Force.) At 6 A. M.	At 1 P. M.	At 10 P. M.	(Force)	Weather. (Tenths Cloudy.) At 6 A. M.	At 1 P. M.	At 10 P. M.	Rain and Snow in Inches of Water.
1	29.51	29.62	29.74	69	81	67	72.3	N. W. 1	N. W. 2	N. W.	1	7	8	0	
2	29.84	29.89	29.95	62	78	67	69.0	N. W. 2	N. W. 2	N. W.	1	0	5	0	
3	30.05	30.02	30.03	64	79	79	74.0	N. W. 1	S. 3	S. R.	1	4	6	8	
4	29.89	29.85	29.84	65	78	69	67.3	S. E. 1	...	S. W.	1	Foggy	...	10, Sh'r	
5	29.67	29.59	29.66	70	84	71	75.0	S. W. 2	S. W. 3	S. W.		10	5	2	
S 6	29.68	29.70	29.78	68	80	68	72.0	N. W. 1	W'ly	N. W.	1	0	2	0	
7	29.92	29.93	29.98	62	82	67	70.3	N. W. 1	N. W. 1	N. W.	1	0	2	0	
8	30.00	29.97	30.00	67	83	70	73.3	N. W. 1	N. W. 1	N. W.	1	0	3	0	
9	29.99	29.91	30.21	68	85	70	74.3	N. W. 1	S. W. 1	S. W.	1	0	6	4	
10	29.75	29.84	29.83	66	84	68	72.7	S. W. 1	S. W. 2	S. W.	1	0	0	0	
11	29.76	29.86	29.94	67	84	73	74.7	W'ly 1	W'ly 1	S. W.	1	0	0	7	
12	29.99	29.99	30.03	76	84	72	77.3	S. W. 1	S. W. 1	S. W.	1	9	2	10	
S 13	30.03	30.01	30.02	70	85	77	77.3	S. E'ly 1	S. E. 1	S. E'ly		10	5	Sh'r, 5	
14	29.95	29.96	30.00	74	82	73	76.3	S. E'ly	S. W. 1	W'ly	1	5	Shower	3	0.33
15	30.03	30.03	30.00	74	86	74	78.0	S. W. 1	S. W.	S. W.	1	3	2	0	
16	29.97	29.91	29.87	74	85	75	78.0	S. W. 1	S. W. 1	S. W.	1	10	3	0	
17	29.84	29.77	...	75	87	...	81.0	S. W. 1	S. W. 2	...		8	3	0	
18	29.61	29.51	...	...	...	...	...	...	...	...		Rain	Rain	...	3.20
19	29.56	29.61	...	...	...	...	...	...	...	...		...	...	...	
S 20	...	...	...	...	...	...	...	...	...	...		...	...	...	
21	29.81	29.80	...	...	...	...	...	...	...	...		...	...	...	
22	29.87	29.87	...	...	...	...	...	...	...	...		...	...	...	
23	29.91	29.92	...	...	...	...	...	...	...	...		...	...	...	
24	29.95	29.84	...	...	...	...	...	...	...	...		...	...	...	
25	29.99	30.04	...	...	...	...	...	...	...	...		...	...	...	
26	30.15	30.11	...	...	...	...	...	...	...	...		...	...	...	
S 27	30.12	...	...	...	...	...	...	...	...	...		...	...	...	
28	29.90	29.76	...	...	...	...	...	...	...	...		...	...	Rain	0.20
29	29.54	29.58	...	...	...	...	...	...	...	...		...	...	...	
30	29.73	29.69	...	...	...	...	...	...	...	...		...	...	...	
31	29.58	29.54	29.55	...	84	67	75.7	...	N. E. 1	N. E.	1	...	...	...	
Means	29.85	29.83	29.90	74.8	82.8	71.0	...	1.1	1.6	1.0		4.7	4.0	3.3	3.73
									1.2				4.0		
REDUCED TO SEA LEVEL.															
Max.	30.33	30.29	30.39	75	87	77	81.0								
Min.	29.69	29.69	29.73	62	78	67	67.8								
Mean	30.03	30.01	30.08												
Range	0.64	0.60	0.66	13	9	10	13.7								
Mean of month	30.040			...	...	...	76.2								
Extreme range	0.70			...	...	...	25.0								

Prevailing winds from some point between— Days.
N. & E. 1
E. & S. 3
S. & W. 9
W. & N. 5

Days.
Clear 6
Variable . . . } 7
Cloudy . . . . }
Rain fell on . . 5
(13 days omitted.)

Remarks.

1st. Fine.
2d. Cool, but very fine.
3d. Warm. Appearances of a thunderstorm at 5 P. M.
4th. Fine. Shower in the night.
5th. Fine.
6th. Very fine.
7th to 10th. Very fine. Very hot sun.
11th. Very hot sun.
12th. Very hot. Thin fog-clouds in the evening.
13th. Very hot. Two light showers in the afternoon.
14th. Frequent showers, with intervals of bright sunshine between them.
15th. Very fine and very hot.
16th and 17th. Very fine.
18th. Very heavy rain.
19th. Variable.
21st to 27th. Clear.
28th. Cloudy, with light rain in the evening.
29th, 30th, and 31st. Fair.

Note.—The entries from the 18th to the 31st, inclusive, are taken from the barometric record of Mr. George Boker, and reduced 9-100 of an inch—that being found by comparison to be the mean difference in the readings. Mr. B.'s observations are made at 9 A. M. and 3 P. M.

September, 1848. New Moon, 27d. 4h. 27m. A. M.

Days.	Barometer At 6 A. M.	At 1 P. M.	At 10 P. M.	Thermometer At 6 A. M.	At 1 P. M.	At 10 P. M.	Daily mean.	Winds At 6 A. M.	At 1 P. M.	At 10 P. M.	(Force)	Weather At 6 A. M.	At 1 P. M.	At 10 P. M.	Rain and Snow in Inches of Water.
1	29.54	29.50	29.54	67	83	68	72.7	W'ly 1	W'ly 2	N. W.	2	3	6	0	
2	29.60	29.58	29.62	63	76	67	68.7	N. W. 2	N. W. 2	N. W.	1	0	4	10	
S 3	29.75	29.74	29.78	63	75	64	67.3	N. W. 2	N'ly 2	N. W.	1	2	7	0	
4	29.79	29.73	29.71	61	79	69	69.7	N. W. 1	N. W. 1	N. W.	1	0	4	6	
5	29.76	29.71	29.68	63	80	69	70.7	N. W. 1	...	N. W.	1	5	...	9	
6	29.73	29.74	29.79	70	79	61	70.0	N'ly 1	...	N. W.	1	9	...	0	
7	29.81	29.81	29.85	53	68	56	59.0	N. W. 1	...	N. W.	1	0	...	0	
8	29.91	29.80	29.78	56	71	57	61.3	N. W. 1	N. E'ly 2	S'ly	1	0	0	3	
9	29.74	29.70	29.69	57	73	65	65.0	S'ly 1	...	S'ly	1	6	...	6	
S 10	29.85	29.83	29.87	57	70	60	62.3	N. E'ly 1	N. E'ly 1	S'ly	1	10	10	0	
11	29.89	29.82	29.78	59	80	66	68.3	S'ly 1	S. W. 2	S. W.	1	Foggy	5	1	
12	29.76	29.82	29.98	65	64	50	59.7	N'ly 1	N'ly 1	...		10	Shower	...	
13	30.07	30.02	30.10	42	59	50	50.3	N'ly 1	N. W. 2	N. E.	1	0	0	0	
14	30.06	29.95	29.78	42	60	57	53.0	N'ly 1	E'ly 2	S. E'ly	3	0	10	10	
15	29.39	29.23	29.43	64	76	52	64.0	S. W. 2	S. W. 2	N. W.		Misty	5	0	
16	29.60	29.60	29.68	44	61	48	51.0	N. W. 1	N. W. 1	N. W.	1	0	10	0	
S 17	29.80	29.76	29.71	42	65	54	53.7	N. W. 1	S. E'ly 1	N. W.	1	0	3	0	
18	29.54	29.67	29.84	52	71	56	59.7	N'ly 1	...	N. W.	1	Rain	...	0	1.90
19	29.99	29.95	29.92	51	71	57	59.7	N. W. 1	S. E. 2	N. W.	1	0	3	0	
20	29.84	29.74	29.65	59	73	68	66.7	S. W. 2	S. W. 2	S. W.	1	0	9	10	
21	29.69	29.69	29.78	57	70	58	61.7	N'ly 1	N'ly 1	N'ly	1	8	8	8	
22	29.75	29.68	29.67	50	53	45	49.3	N'ly 1	N'ly 2	N'ly	1	Rain	0	0	0.25
23	29.69	29.65	29.66	41	50	45	45.3	N. W. 1	...	N. W.	1	0	...	0	
S 24	29.65	29.63	29.71	49	64	54	55.7	W'ly 1	W'ly 2	N. W.	1	0	5	0	
25	29.74	29.73	29.67	50	63	59	60.7	W'ly 1	S. W. 1	S. W.	1	Rain	5	2	0.30
26	29.74	29.74	29.88	51	60	41	50.7	N. W. 1	N. W. 2	N. W.	2	2	0	0	
27	29.86	29.74	29.59	34	54	42	43.3	N. W. 1	N. E. 2	N. E.	1	0	4	2	
28	29.48	29.44	29.57	36	62	47	48.7	N. E'ly 1	W'ly 1	W'ly	1	2	2	2	
29	29.62	29.60	29.65	45	67	63	58.3	S. W. 1	S. W. 2	S. W.	1	10	10	8	
30	29.70	29.73	29.79	62	75	66	67.7	S. W. 1	...	S. W.	1	5	...	10	
Means	29.74	29.71	29.74	53.5	68.4	57.1	...	1.1	1.7	1.1		4.1	4.8	3.0	2.45
									1.3				5.5		
REDUCED TO SEA LEVEL.															
Max.	30.25	30.20	30.28	70	83	69	72.7								
Min.	29.57	29.41	29.61	34	50	41	43.3								
Mean	29.92	29.89	29.92												
Range	0.68	0.79	0.67	36	33	28	29.4								
Mean of month	29.910			...	...	...	59.7								
Extreme range	0.87			...	...	...	49.0								

Prevailing winds from some point between— Days.
N. & E. 6
E. & S. 2
S. & W. 6
W. & N. 16

Days.
Clear 9
Variable . . . } 15
Cloudy . . . . }
Rain fell on . . 6

Remarks.

1st. Fine. Light shower at noon.
2d, 3d, and 4th. Very fine.
5th. Fine.
6th, 7th, and 8th. Very fine.
9th. Very fine. Sprinkling of rain at 5 and 9 P. M.
10th. Cloudy all day. Clear in the evening.
11th. Very pleasant.
12th. Variable. Dashes of rain from the N. W. Became very cool in the afternoon, with heavy clouds. Clear in the evening. Total eclipse of the moon observed.
13th. Very cool. Evening very clear.
14th. Appearances of storm in the evening with occasional rain.
15th. Occasional light rain in morning. Very clear in the evening.
16th and 17th. Pleasant.
18th. Rain.
19th. Fine.
20th. Mist, and appearances of rain in the evening.
21st. Pleasant.
22d. Very fine.
23d. Very fine, but cool for the season.
24th. Very fine.
25th Pleasant.
26th. Fine.
27th. Very fine. Frost in some places in the vicinity.
28th. First appearance of white frost in the College yard. Air dry, and frost not copious.
29th. Mild, with appearances of rain.
30th. Variable. Very warm.

October, 1848. New Moon, 26d. 9h. 38m. P. M.

Days.	Barometer, reduced to 32° F. At 6 A. M.	At 1 P. M.	At 10 P. M.	Thermometer. At 6 A. M.	At 1 P. M.	At 10 P. M.	Daily mean.	Winds. (Direction and Force.) At 6 A. M.	At 1 P. M.	At 10 P. M.	Weather. (Tenths Cloudy.) At 6 A. M.	At 1 P. M.	At 10 P. M.	Rain and Snow in Inches of Water.
S 1	29.93	29.97	30.01	66	70	66	67.3	S. W. 1	...	S. W. 1	10	...	Rain	
2	30.19	30.19	30.24	58	51	50	53.0	N. E. 2	N. E. 2	N. E. 2	Rain	Rain	10	3.30
3	30.23	30.19	30.08	51	54	52	52.3	N. E. 2	N. E. 1	N. E. 1	Misty	Rain	Rain	
4	29.95	29.89	29.84	53	56	54	54.3	N'ly 1	N'ly 1	N. W. 1	Misty	Misty	10	
5	29.87	29.88	29.94	54	67	54	58.3	N. W. 1	N. W. 2	N. W. 1	10	8	0	
6	30.11	30.04	30.13	48	62	49	53.0	N. W. 3	N. E. 1	...	0	0	...	
7	30.13	30.00	29.91	44	66	54	54.7	N. W. 1	S'ly 2	S. W. 1	0	0	2	
S 8	29.81	29.79	30.08	56	64	43	54.3	W'ly 1	N. W. 1	N. W. 2	10, Sh'r	3	0	
9	30.12	30.01	29.88	36	55	45	45.3	N. W. 1	E'ly 1	E'ly 1	0	0	0	
10	29.69	29.63	29.79	52	57	47	52.0	S. W'ly 2	W'ly 1	N. W. 1	8	Rain	0	
11	29.95	29.92	29.90	35	53	40	42.7	N. W. 1	N. W. 2	N. W. 1	0	0	0	
12	29.83	29.75	29.92	36	63	48	49.0	N. W. 1	W'ly 2	N. W. 1	0	0	0	
13	30.08	30.04	30.02	36	54	38	42.7	N. W. 1	N. W. 1	N. E'ly	0	0	2	
14	29.97	29.80	29.67	33	52	42	42.3	N. E. 1	...	S. W. 1	7	...	0	
S 15	29.61	29.64	29.76	43	63	47	51.0	N. W. 1	N. W. 1	N. W. 1	0	0	0	
16	29.75	29.65	29.63	41	68	61	56.7	N. W. 1	S'ly 1	S. W. 3	0	8	10	
17	29.65	29.63	29.64	62	75	61	66.0	S'ly 1	S'ly 1	S'ly 1	10	8	Rain	0.15
18	29.61	29.55	29.35	59	58	61	59.3	E'ly 1	N. E. 1	N. E. 1	10	Rain	Rain	}
19	29.27	29.24	29.39	53	59	52	54.7	S. E. 1	S'ly 1	W'ly 1	Misty	Misty	10	} 0.50
20	29.48	29.44	29.57	45	55	42	50.7	N. W. 1	N. W. 1	N. W. 1	0	7	0	
21	29.67	29.59	29.66	38	55	43	45.3	N. W. 1	W'ly 1	N. W. 1	2	10	0	
S 22	29.67	29.60	29.63	35	51	41	42.3	N'ly 1	N. W. 1	N. W. 1	2	0	0	
23	29.69	29.56	29.72	35	51	42	42.7	N. W. 1	N. W. 2	N. W. 1	0	0	0	
24	29.74	29.62	29.55	40	55	55	50.0	N'ly 1	E'ly 1	S'ly 1	10	Rain	Misty	0.10
25	29.78	29.76	29.83	47	57	43	49.0	N. W. 1	N. W. 1	N. W. 1	0	0	0	
26	29.80	29.81	29.68	37	53	42	44.0	N. E'ly 1	S'ly 1	S. W. 1	10	10	2	
27	29.54	29.49	29.51	37	53	40	43.3	N'ly 1	N. W'ly 1	N'ly 1	3	6	0	
28	29.68	29.64	29.63	34	53	45	44.0	N. W. 1	...	S. W'ly 1	0	...	2	
S 29	29.60	29.58	29.59	50	63	59	57.3	S'ly 1	S. W. 2	S. W. 1	10	Rain	10	
30	29.67	29.60	29.54	58	64	57	59.7	S. W. 1	E'ly 1	E'ly 0	10	Misty	7	
31	29.58	29.57	29.60	55	59	54	56.0	S. W'ly 1	S. W. 1	S. W. 1	Foggy	Misty	Foggy	
Means	29.80	29.74	29.76	46.0	58.6	49.2	...	1.2	1.2	1.0	5.2	5.7	4.2	4.05
									1.1			5.0		

REDUCED TO SEA LEVEL.							
Max.	30.41	30.37	30.42	66	75	66	67.3
Min.	29.45	29.42	29.53	33	51	38	42.3
Mean	29.98	29.92	29.94				
Range	0.96	0.95	0.89	33	24	28	25.0
Mean of month	29.947			...	...	...	51.3
Extreme range	1.00			...	...	...	42.0

Prevailing winds from some point between—	Days.
N. & E.	7
E. & S.	2
S. & W.	8
W. & N.	14

	Days.
Clear	10
Variable } Cloudy }	11
Rain fell on	10

Remarks.

1st. Moderate rain in the evening.
2d. Heavy shower in the morning, and rain and mist in the afternoon. Rain again in the night.
3d. Moderate nearly all day and in the evening.
4th. Mist in morning. Stars out in the evening.
5th. Evening very clear.
6th. Very fine.
7th. Slight appearances of white frost in the College yard.
8th. Light shower at 7 A. M.; wind westerly. Clouds soon passed away. Grew cooler in the afternoon. Very clear in the evening.
9th. Very fine.
10th. Variable Light shower from 1 to 2 P. M.
11th and 12th. Very fine.
13th. Bright and well-defined halo about the moon, having about 22° radius.
14th and 15th. Very fine.
16th. Appearances of rain.
17th. Began to rain moderately at 9 P. M.
18th. Rained moderately at intervals.
19th. Mist, with occasional sprinkling of rain.
20th. Very fine.
21st and 22d. Pleasant.
23d. Aurora in the evening.
24th. Drizzle and mist mixed with some rain.
25th. Aurora in the evening; quite bright coruscations, rising occasionally to the height of 40°.
26th. Mild.
27th. Pleasant.
28th. Very fine.
29th. Occasional light showers.
30th and 31st. Mist and fog.

November, 1848. New Moon, 25d. 4h. 21m. P. M.

Days.	Barometer Sunrise.	At 1 P. M.	At 10 P. M.	Thermometer Sunrise.	At 1 P. M.	At 10 P. M.	Daily mean.	Winds Sunrise.	At 1 P. M.	At 10 P. M.	Weather Sunrise.	At 1 P. M.	At 10 P. M.	Rain and Snow in Inches of Water.
1	29.72	29.64	29.62	44	54	40	46.0	N. W. 1	N. W. 1	N. W. 1	9	0	0	
2	29.77	29.80	30.01	35	50	37	40.7	N. W. 1	N. W. 1	N. W. 1	0	0	0	
3	30.20	30.21	30.28	36	50	37	41.0	N. W. 1	N. W. 3	N. W. 1	0	4	0	
4	30.15	30.04	29.96	37	52	50	46.3	...	...	N. E. 1	...	...	Rain	
S 5	29.74	29.39	29.45	53	58	42	51.1	S. E'ly 3	S. E. 3	N. W. 1	Misty	Rain	0	1.80
6	29.64	29.61	29.70	34	48	39	40.3	N. W. 1	N. W. 1	N. W. 1	0	0	1	
7	29.71	29.68	29.88	35	46	35	38.7	N. W. 1	N. W. 1	N. W. 1	5	3	0	
8	30.05	29.98	29.98	28	44	34	35.3	N. W. 1	N. W. 1	N. W. 1	0	3	7	
9	29.86	29.82	30.01	34	44	28	35.3	S. E. 1	N. W. 1	N. W. 1	Snow	7	0	0.10
10	30.13	30.11	30.24	22	30	20	24.0	N. W. 1	N. W. 1	N. W. 1	0	2	0	
11	30.35	30.29	30.24	13	33	29	25.0	N. W. 2	N. W. 1	W'ly 1	0	0	5	
S 12	30.21	30.15	30.23	34	39	36	36.3	E'ly 1	N. E. 1	N. E. 1	10	Misty	Rain	0.40
13	30.11	30.10	30.16	35	39	27	33.7	W'ly 1	N. W'ly 3	N. W. 1	10	2	0	
14	30.14	30.06	29.96	24	42	31	32.3	N. E. 1	S. W. 1	S'ly 1	0	3	5	
15	29.78	29.68	29.73	34	49	38	40.3	S. W. 1	S. W. 1	N. W. 1	10	7	0	
16	29.82	29.68	29.73	31	48	44	41.0	N. W. 1	S. W. 1	S. W. 1	0	2	Hazy	
17	29.77	29.77	29.89	45	48	39	44.0	S. W. 1	S. W. 2	W'ly 1	10	5	10	
18	29.95	29.92	30.03	37	40	31	36.0	W'ly	W'ly 1	N'ly 1	10	8	0	
S 19	30.03	29.98	29.75	28	35	32	31.7	N'ly 2	N'ly 2	N. E. 2	8	10	Snow	}
20	29.43	29.41	29.55	32	32	31	31.7	N. E'ly 3	N. W. 2	N. W. 2	Snow	Misty	10	} 1.00
21	29.70	29.66	29.70	28	40	32	33.3	N. W. 1	N. W. 1	N. W. 1	0	0	0	
22	29.77	29.72	29.78	30	43	31	34.7	N. W. 1	N. W. 1	N. W. 1	0	2	0	
23	29.84	29.77	29.80	31	43	33	35.7	W'ly 1	E'ly 1	W'ly 1	10	0	0	
24	29.85	29.69	29.46	31	45	48	41.3	S'ly 1	S'ly 1	S'ly 1	Foggy	Foggy	Rain	0.50
25	29.24	29.25	29.43	54	55	42	50.3	S. W. 1	W'ly 1	W'ly 1	10	2	0	
S 26	29.51	29.50	29.71	35	46	34	38.3	W'ly 1	W'ly 1	N. W. 1	0	4	0	
27	29.99	30.00	30.12	34	36	25	31.7	N'ly 1	N. W. 1	N. W. 1	10	2	0	
28	30.19	30.05	30.08	24	37	32	31.0	N. W. 1	N. W. 1	N. W. 1	0	1	0	
29	30.03	29.92	29.92	34	47	40	40.3	S. W. 1	S. W. 1	S. W. 1	0	2	2	
30	29.78	29.75	29.90	46	56	41	47.7	S. W. 1	S. W. 2	W'ly 1	4	6	0	
Means	29.88	29.82	29.88	33.9	44.3	35.3	...	1.2	1.3	1.1	5.0	4.0	3.0	3.80
									1.2			4.0		

REDUCED TO SEA LEVEL.							
Max.	30.53	30.47	30.46	54	58	50	51.0
Min.	29.42	29.43	29.61	13	30	25	24.0
Mean	30.06	30.00	30.06				
Range	1.11	1.04	0.85	41	28	25	27.0
Mean of month	30.040			...	...	...	37.8
Extreme range	1.11			...	...	...	45.0

Prevailing winds from some point between—	Days.
N. & E.	3
E. & S.	1
S. & W.	8
W. & N.	18

	Days.
Clear	12
Variable } Cloudy }	11
Rain or snow fell on	7

Remarks.

1st. Fine.
2d and 3d. Very fine.
4th. Sprinkling of rain in the evening. First frost to injure dahlias, and not much.
5th. Mist and moderate rain in the morning. Heavy rain, and strong wind at S. E. in the afternoon. Cleared from 6 to 7 P. M. Evening very clear.
6th and 7th. Very fine.
8th. Severe black frost this morning; the first for the season on this hill. Day very fine.
9th. Flurry of snow this morning; ground white in some places. Transit of Mercury in the morning, beginning at 6 h. 17 m., and ending at 11 h. 41 m.; not seen at all, by reason of clouds.
10th. Cold, but pleasant.
11th. Very cold morning.
12th. Ground white with snow in some places this morning, and snow in the air. Mist all day. Rain in the evening.
15th. Cloudy in the morning. Very fine in the evening.
16th. Pleasant.
17th. Mild.
18th. Mild. Grew cool in the evening.
19th. Wind N'ly and N. E., raw. Began to snow from 8 to 9 P. M., and continued through the night, with heavy wind and heavy fall of snow for the season—being six or eight inches on the level.
20th. Storm raging with considerable violence at sunrise, and snow much drifted. The average on the level would be, perhaps, eight or nine inches, and very damp.
21st. Very fine. Aurora very brilliant from 7 to 8 P. M., extending from N. N. W. to N. E. Coruscations sprang from the horizon, and shot up to the height of 30°. The light continued through the evening, but with diminished brilliancy.
22d and 23d. Very fine.
24th. Foggy. Rain in the evening.
25th. Pleasant.
26th. Pleasant. Aurora quite bright at 10 P. M.
27th. Fine. Evening very clear. Faint aurora
28th. Very fine.
29th. Pleasant.
30th. Very fine.

December, 1848. New Moon, 25[d.] 11[h.] 14[m.] A. M.

DAYS.	Barometer, reduced to 32° F. Sunrise.	At 1 P. M.	At 10 P. M.	Thermometer. Sunrise.	At 1 P. M.	At 10 P. M.	Daily mean.	Winds (Direction and Force.) Sunrise.	At 1 P. M.	At 10 P. M.	Weather (Tenths Cloudy.) Sunrise.	At 1 P. M.	At 10 P. M.	Rain and Snow in Inches of Water
1	30.09	30.02	30.04	32	44	37	37.7	W. 1	N. W. 1	E'ly 1	4	2	10	
2	29.80	29.49	29.61	40	55	46	47.0	E'ly 1	S. E. 3	W'ly 1	Misty	Misty	0	0.25
S 3	29.81	29.80	30.00	40	46	36	40.7	W'ly 1	W'ly 2	W'ly 1	0	0	0	
4	30.00	30.01	30.16	40	56	45	47.0	S. W'ly 1	W'ly 1	W'ly 1	10	7	10	
5	30.22	30.15	30.16	39	49	40	42.7	N. E'ly 1	N. E. 1	N. E. 1	10	10	Misty	
6	30.04	29.95	30.02	40	40	34	38.0	N. E. 1	N. E. 1	N'ly 1	10	Misty	Misty	
7	30.03	29.92	29.91	34	35	33	34.0	N. E. 1	N. E. 1	N'ly 1	Rain	Rain	Misty	0.10
8	29.78	29.69	29.83	35	59	55	49.7	W'ly 1	S. W. 1	S. W. 1	Misty	10	7	
9	30.01	30.02	29.98	43	49	40	44.0	N. W. 1	N. W. 1	N. E. 1	2	5	8	
S 10	29.90	29.69	29.49	40	47	56	47.7	E'ly 1	S'ly 1	S'ly 1	10	Rain	Rain	0.40
11	29.58	29.64	29.82	44	47	35	42.0	N. W. 1	N. W. 1	N. W. 1	7	3	4	
12	29.89	29.94	30.01	32	38	30	33.3	N'ly 1	N'ly 1	N. W. 1	10	10	0	
13	30.09	30.11	30.15	30	43	40	37.7	N'ly 1	E'ly 1	E'ly 1	8	10	10	
14	30.03	29.99	29.78	40	50	46	45.3	N. E. 1	E'ly 1	S'ly 1	10	10	Foggy	
15	29.65	29.62	29.94	46	51	35	44.0	S. W. 1	S. W. 1	N. W. 1	Foggy	Rain	0	} 0.45
16	30.07	29.97	29.75	28	47	47	40.7	N. W. 1	S. E'ly 1	S'ly 1	0	10	Rain	
S 17	29.63	29.66	29.69	47	53	42	47.3	W'ly 1	W'ly 1	N. W. 1	0	0	2	
18	29.72	29.81	29.83	45	53	39	45.7	N. W. 1	N. W. 1	N. W. 1	0	0	0	
19	29.68	29.55	29.66	45	62	52	53.0	S'ly 1	S. W. 1	S. W. 1	Foggy	2	4	
20	29.93	29.97	29.87	40	43	35	39.3	N. W. 1	N. E. 1	N. E. 1	9	10	10	
21	29.77	29.72	29.96	35	31	24	30.0	N. E. 1	N'ly 1	N. 3	Sn., r'n	10	Snow	
22	30.01	29.78	29.64	16	25	12	17.7	N. 1	N'ly 2	N'ly 3	Snow	Snow	Snow	0.76
23	30.11	30.11	30.23	11	18	10	12.7	N. W. 1	N. W. 1	N. W. 1	0	0	0	
S 24	30.19	30.06	29.73	12	27	40	26.3	N. W. 1	N. W. 1	S. W. 1	8	10	Rain	} 0.50
25	29.71	29.64	29.52	40	42	40	40.7	S. W. 1	S. W. 1	W'ly 2	10	Rain	2	
26	29.87	30.00	30.30	32	33	24	29.7	W'ly 3	W'ly 3	N. W. 1	0	2	0	
27	30.37	30.15	29.50	20	21	34	25.0	N'ly 1	N. E. 1	S. E'ly	10	Snow	Snow	0.50
28	29.50	29.86	30.03	28	34	22	28.0	N. W. 1	N. W. 2	N. W. 1	0	0	0	
29	30.08	29.96	29.71	24	27	30	27.0	N. W. 1	N. E'ly 1	N. E'ly 1	10	Snow	Snow	
30	29.49	29.31	29.51	28	32	30	30.0	N'ly 1	N'ly 1	N. W. 1	Snow	Snow	0	0.87
S 31	29.69	29.78	29.97	29	37	30	32.0	N. W. 1	N. W. 2	N. W. 1	0	0	0	
Means	29.90	29.85	29.86	34.0	41.8	36.0	...	1.1	1.2	1.2	6.6	6.8	5.7	3.83
								1.2			6.4			
REDUCED TO SEA LEVEL.								Prevailing winds from some point between— Days.			Days.			
Max.	30.55	30.33	30.48	47	62	56	53.9							
Min.	29.67	29.49	29.67	11	18	10	12.7							
Mean	30.08	30.03	30.04					N. & E. 9			Clear 7			
Range	0.88	0.84	0.81	36	44	46	40.3	E. & S. 5			Variable . . . } 10			
Mean of month	30.050			...	...	...	37.3	S. & W. 5			Cloudy . . . . }			
Extreme range	1.06			...	...	...	52.0	W. & N. 12			Rain or snow fell on 14			

REMARKS.

1st. Thick haze in the evening, deepening into clouds.
2d. Rain in the afternoon, with wind S. E., S'ly, and S. W. Cleared from 7 to 8 P. M., with wind W'ly.
3d and 4th. Very fine.
5th. Mist in the afternoon, and appearances of rain.
6th. Mist, approaching to rain.
7th. Rain and heavy mist.
8th. Very mild in evening; wind light N. E., with clouds passing from S. W'ly.
9th. Occasional rain and mist in the afternoon. Rain increased in the evening.
10th. Halo about the moon at 10 P. M.
11th. Variable.
12th. Air very raw. Evening clear.
13th. Mild for the season.
14th. Very mild.
15th. Moderate rain at intervals in the morning. Very clear in the evening.
16th. Rain in the evening.
17th. Clear, mild, and pleasant as May. Aurora in the evening.
18th. Very fine.
19th. Pleasant.
20th. Scattered snow-flakes falling at sunset. Moderate rain at 10 P. M.
21st. Snow in the afternoon.
22d. Severe snow all day, without intermission.
23d. Snow nine or ten inches deep, and somewhat drifted. Aurora brilliant, with streamers.
24th. Air filled with fine needles of snow in the afternoon. Rain in the evening.
25th. Moderate rain and fog all day. Cleared from 11 to 12 P. M.
26th. Very fine.
27th. Began to snow moderately at 2 P. M. Some rain during the night.
28th. Very fine.
29th. Began to snow moderately at 10 A. M., and continued through the day and evening.
30th. Snowed moderately till 3 P. M. Cleared in the evening, five or six inches of damp snow having fallen.
31st. Very fine.

January, 1849. New Moon, 24[d.] 4[h.] 55[m.] A. M.

DAYS.	Barometer Sunrise.	At 1 P. M.	At 10 P. M.	Thermometer Sunrise.	At 1 P. M.	At 10 P. M.	Daily mean.	Winds Sunrise.	At 1 P. M.	At 10 P. M.	Weather Sunrise.	At 1 P. M.	At 10 P. M.	Rain and Snow
1	30.07	30.01	29.76	20	33	27	26.7	N. W. 1	N. W. 1	N. W. 1	0	7	10	
2	29.66	29.71	29.68	10	11	0	7.0	N. W. 2	N. W. 2	N. W. 2	0	0	0	
3	29.59	29.53	29.56	2	18	14	11.3	N. W. 1	N. W. 2	N. 2	0	0	0	
4	29.56	29.44	29.36	15	20	16	17.0	N. W. 3	W'ly 2	N. W. 1	9	7	0	
5	29.23	29.22	29.31	19	17	18	18.0	W'ly 2	N. W. 2	W'ly 2	0	5	6	
6	29.46	29.63	29.74	20	25	18	21.0	N. W. 1	N. W. 2	N. W. 1	0	0	0	
S 7	29.91	29.93	30.01	10	18	11	13.0	N. W. 1	N. W. 1	N. W. 1	0	5	0	
8	30.02	29.94	29.88	14	32	29	25.0	N'ly 1	N'ly 1	W'ly	10	10	10	
9	29.80	29.67	29.60	28	31	24	27.7	N'ly 1	N. E. 1	N. E. 2	10	5	10	
10	29.73	29.78	29.91	8	12	3	7.7	N. W. 2	N. W. 2	N. W. 2	4	0	2	
11	30.13	30.11	30.26	—4	9	6	3.7	N. W. 1	N. W. 2	N. W. 1	0	0	0	
12	30.46	30.43	30.43	3	20	17	13.3	N. W. 1	N. W. 1	N. W. 1	0	0	2	
13	30.26	30.09	29.93	24	39	38	33.7	S. W. 2	S. W. 2	S. W. 1	8	10	Misty	
S 14	29.71	29.73	29.92	42	46	41	43.0	S. W. 2	W'ly 2	W'ly 1	Rain	5	0	} 0.50
15	29.97	29.72	29.43	35	36	42	37.7	S. W. 1	S. E'ly 1	W'ly 3	10	Misty	8	
16	29.83	29.88	30.02	29	32	27	29.3	W'ly 2	N. W. 2	N. W. 1	4	0	0	
17	29.82	29.56	29.66	32	43	31	35.3	S. W'ly 2	S. W. 3	N. W. 3	10	9	0	
18	30.10	30.10	30.33	14	14	11	13.0	N. W. 2	N. W. 3	N. W. 1	0	0	0	
19	30.58	30.53	30.51	5	13	10	6.0	N. W. 1	N. W. 2	N. W. 1	0	0	0	
20	30.38	30.16	29.94	12	33	35	26.7	S. W. 1	S. W. 2	S. W. 1	1	0	Rain	
S 21	29.96	29.87	29.97	28	38	33	33.0	N. W. 1	N. W. 1	N. W. 1	1	4	10	
22	30.09	29.99	29.91	16	21	18	18.3	N. W. 1	N. W. 2	N. W. 1	3	1	0	
23	29.90	29.97	30.01	23	34	26	27.7	N. W. 1	W'ly 2	W'ly 1	1	3	0	
24	30.01	29.97	29.98	26	45	40	37.0	W'ly 1	S. W. 2	S. W. 1	0	7	10	
25	29.99	29.89	29.78	39	42	43	41.3	S. W. 1	S. W. 1	S. W. 2	10	Rain	Rain	0.10
26	29.49	29.39	29.60	45	53	40	46.0	S. W. 2	S. W. 2	N. W. 2	Rain	8	0	
27	30.02	30.07	30.18	24	31	23	26.0	N. W. 2	N. W. 2	N. W. 1	0	0	2	
S 28	30.37	30.29	30.20	16	29	30	25.0	N. W. 1	N. W. 1	S. W. 1	6	1	10	
29	29.97	29.79	29.64	34	45	42	40.3	S. W. 1	S. W. 1	S. W. 1	10	10	10	
30	[illegible]	[illegible]	[illegible]	[illegible]	[illegible]	[illegible]	[illegible]	[illegible] 1	N'ly 2	N'ly 3	Rain	10	10	0.20
31	30.10	30.22	30.33	12	18	10	13.3	N'ly 2	N. W. 2	N. W. 2	6	0	0	
Means	29.93	29.88	29.89	20.7	29.0	23.9	...	1.4	1.7	1.5	4.2	4.1	4.2	0.80
								1.5			4.2			
REDUCED TO SEA LEVEL.								Prevailing winds from some point between— Days.			Days.			
Max.	30.76	30.71	30.69	45	53	43	46.0							
Min.	29.41	29.40	29.49	—4	9	0	0.0							
Mean	30.11	30.05	30.07					N. & E. 1			Clear 12			
Range	1.35	1.31	1.20	49	44	43	40.0	E. & S. 0			Variable . . . } 12			
Mean of month	30.080			...	...	...	24.5	S. & W. 9			Cloudy . . . . }			
Extreme range	1.36			...	...	...	57.0	W. & N. 21			Rain or snow fell on 7			

REMARKS.

1st. Pleasant. Appearances of storm in the evening.
2d. Clear, but very cold.
3d. Very fine, but cold; wind piercing.
4th. Fine, but cold.
5th. Flurry of snow at 11 A. M., and grew cooler.
6th. Fine. Evening splendid.
7th. Very fine.
8th. Very mild in the afternoon, with some appearances of storm.
9th. Appearances of storm in the evening.
10th. Very cold in the evening; wind brisk.
11th. Thermometer 4° below zero at sunrise. Very cold, but otherwise pleasant.
12th. Pleasant.
13th. The air chilly and raw. Appearances of rain in the evening.
14th. Light rain and mist early in the morning. Cloudy through the day. Clear at 10 P.M. Aurora in the north, not very bright.
15th. Moderate rain from S. E. in the afternoon. Wind came to westward from 8 to 9 P. M, and stars appeared.
16th. Fine.
17th. Sprinkling of rain in the morning; wind S. W. Evening clear, with wind very brisk at N. W.
18th. Fine.
19th. At 9½ A. M., the barometer stood at 30.63. Cold, but pleasant.
20th. Grew cloudy towards evening. Began to rain and mist moderately from 8 to 9 P. M.
21st. Clear. A light dusting of snow on the ground in the morning.
22d. Pleasant.
23d. Pleasant. Evening very clear.
24th. Very mild.
25th. Began to rain very moderately from 10 to 11 A. M. [illegible] but little. [illegible] in the evening.
26th. Light rain early in the morning. Very blustering from 10 to 12 P. M.
27th. Fine.
28th. Pleasant. In the evening, cloudy and appearances of storm.
29th. Very mild.
30th. Wind changed from S. W. to N. W. from 7 to 8 A. M. Grew quite cold towards evening.
31st. Pleasant.

February, 1849. New Moon, 22d. 8h. 21m. A. M.

DAYS.	BAROMETER, REDUCED TO 32° F. Sun-rise.	At 1 P. M.	At 10 P. M.	THERMOMETER. Sun-rise.	At 1 P. M.	At 10 P. M.	Daily mean.	WINDS. (DIRECTION AND FORCE.) Sunrise.	At 1 P. M.	At 10 P. M.	WEATHER. (TENTHS CLOUDY.) Sun-rise.	At 1 P. M.	At 10 P. M.	RAIN AND SNOW IN INCHES OF WATER.
1	30.00	29.60	29.69	18	37	38	31.0	N'ly 1	N. E. 1	W'ly 1	10	Snow	10	
2	29.73	29.62	29.57	35	33	32	33.3	W'ly 1	W'ly 1	W'ly 1	10	...	5	
3	29.59	29.83	30.01	28	28	19	25.0	W'ly 1	N. W. 3	N. W. 1	2	0	0	
S 4	30.05	29.84	29.84	15	32	28	25.0	N. W. 3	W'ly 2	S. W. 1	0	2	5	
5	29.65	29.57	29.68	31	32	26	29.7	N. E. 1	N. E. 1	N'ly	Snow	Snow	Hazy	} 0.40
6	29.75	29.76	29.63	13	34	20	22.3	N'ly 1	E'ly 1	N. E. 1	5	10	Snow	}
7	29.65	29.66	29.99	11	30	10	17.0	N. W. 1	N. W. 1	N. W. 3	0	0	0	
8	30.03	29.91	29.52	3	23	29	18.3	N. W. 1	S. W. 2	S. W. 2	0	5	Snow	
9	29.31	29.40	29.59	29	27	17	17.7	S. W. 2	W'ly 2	N. W. 2	2	0	4	
10	29.90	29.89	29.83	6	16	21	14.3	N. W. 1	N. W. 2	W'ly 1	0	0	10	
S 11	29.65	29.59	29.74	34	45	21	33.3	S. W. 1	W'ly 1	N. E. 2	10	6	10	
12	29.72	29.63	29.56	15	9	6	10.0	N. E. 2	N. E. 3	N. E. 3	10	Snow	10	
13	29.75	29.69	29.81	6	18	10	11.3	N. W. 1	N. W. 1	N. W. 1	3	2	0	
14	29.82	29.79	29.79	10	20	18	16.0	N. W. 1	N. W. 1	N. W. 2	10	0	5	
15	29.83	29.80	29.82	3	16	6	8.3	N. W. 1	N. W. 1	N. W. 1	0	0	0	
16	29.89	29.85	29.88	—1	16	5	6.7	N. W. 1	N. W. 1	N. W. 1	2	0	0	
17	29.88	29.84	29.86	7	16	12	11.7	N'ly 2	N'ly 2	N. W'ly 3	10	10	5	
S 18	29.90	29.89	30.03	9	18	10	12.3	N'ly 3	N'ly 2	N. W. 1	10	10	0	
19	30.31	30.30	30.45	2	14	4	6.7	N. W. 1	N. W. 1	N. W. 1	0	0	0	
20	30.55	30.47	30.43	1	27	16	14.7	N. W. 1	N. E. 1	N. E. 1	5	10	10	
21	30.46	30.45	30.49	14	31	26	25.7	N. E. 1	N. E. 1	N. E. 1	10	5	10	
22	30.47	30.35	30.34	25	33	27	28.3	N. E. 1	N. E. 2	N. E. 3	10	10	10	
23	30.17	30.15	30.14	27	35	31	31.0	N. E. 3	N. E. 2	N. E. 1	10	10	0	
24	30.11	30.05	29.89	28	42	35	35.0	N'ly 1	N. E. 1	N. E. 1	0	0	10	
S 25	29.92	29.92	30.04	34	36	33	34.3	E'ly 2	E'ly 1	N. E'ly 2	10	Snow	M't, sn.	}
26	30.16	30.20	30.32	34	37	33	34.7	N. E. 3	N. E. 3	N. E. 3	10	Snow	Misty	}
27	30.47	30.51	30.57	33	36	32	33.7	N. E. 2	N. E. 2	N. E. 2	10	10	Snow	} 0.20
28	30.46	30.53	30.40	32	37	33	34.0	N. E. 1	N. E. 2	N. E. 1	10	10	Misty	}
Means	29.97	29.93	29.96	17.9	27.8	21.3	...	1.5	1.6	1.6	6.0	5.5	6.2	0.60
								1.6			5.9			
REDUCED TO SEA LEVEL.														
Max.	30.73	30.71	30.75	35	45	38	34.0	Prevailing winds from some point between—		Days.			Days.	
Min.	29.49	29.58	29.70	—1	9	4	6.7							
Mean	30.15	30.11	30.14					N. & E.		14	Clear		7	
Range	1.24	1.13	1.05	36	36	34	27.3	E. & S.		0	Variable }		11	
Mean of month	30.133			...	...	...	22.4	S. & W.		1	Cloudy }			
Extreme range	1.26			...	...	...	46.0	W. & N.		13	Rain or snow fell on		10	

REMARKS.

1st. Began to snow from 7 to 8 A. M., and snowed very fast till 11 or 12 o'clock, the snow growing quite damp, and being seven or eight inches deep. Scarcely any wind, but vanes pointing E'ly.

2d. Began to snow moderately from 9 to 10 A. M., and continued till 1 P. M.

3d. Pleasant.

4th. Pleasant. Bright corona around the moon at 9 P. M., of brilliant prismatic colors.

5th. Began to snow moderately about 6 A. M., and continued till 2 to 3 P. M.

6th. Light snow floating in the air during the day. Light fall of snow in the evening.

7th. Fine.

8th. Began to snow moderately from 7 to 8 P. M. Barometer falling pretty fast.

9th. An inch of fresh snow on the ground this morning. Grew cold towards night, with the wind very severe.

10th. Cold. Appearances of snow in the evening.

11th. Very mild in the morning. Wind changed to N. E. from 3 to 4 P. M., and grew cooler immediately.

12th. Began to snow from noon to 1 P. M., and ceased from 7 to 8 P. M. At 9 P. M., the sky was quite cleared, but clouded over before 11 P. M. The wind piercing and cold.

13th. Fine.

14th. Flurry of snow in the evening for a short time.

15th. Fine.

16th. At sunrise, ther. 1° below zero; at 8 A. M., it stood at zero; wind very light, and morning pleasant. Aurora in the evening.

17th. Flurry of snow from 5 to 6 P. M. Clear before midnight.

18th. Raw and cold.

19th. Fine, but cold. Aurora quite brilliant.

20th. Very raw and cold to the feelings.

21st. Very mild.

22d. Appearance of storm in the evening.

23d. Evening very mild and very clear.

24th. Very mild.

25th. Began to snow gently from 11 to 12 A. M.; continued through the day, with some mist.

26th. Snow and mist; the snow melting as it fell, and small in amount.

27th. Flurry of snow at 10 P. M.

28th. Air full of snow in the morning. Mist in the evening.

March, 1849. New Moon, 24d. 8h. 57m. A. M.

DAYS.	Barometer Sun-rise.	At 1 P. M.	At 10 P. M.	Thermometer Sun-rise.	At 1 P. M.	At 10 P. M.	Daily mean.	Winds Sunrise.	At 1 P. M.	At 10 P. M.	Weather Sun-rise.	At 1 P. M.	At 10 P. M.	Rain and snow
1	30.19	29.99	30.02	36	46	38	40.0	S. W. 1	S. W. 1	N. W. 1	10	10	0	
2	30.11	30.09	30.11	27	35	28	30.0	N. E. 2	N. E. 2	N. E. 2	2	7	10	
3	30.12	30.10	30.19	25	32	27	28.0	N. E. 2	N. E. 2	N. E. 2	10	10	10	
S 4	30.32	30.29	30.32	18	33	23	24.7	N'ly 1	N. E. 2	N. E. 1	0	5	0	
5	30.33	30.29	30.30	17	34	25	25.3	N. E. 1	N. E. 2	N. E. 1	0	0	0	
6	30.36	30.29	30.18	24	40	33	32.3	N. E'ly 1	E'ly 2	E'ly 2	3	2	10	
7	29.94	29.72	29.62	33	37	32	34.0	S. E. 2	S. E. 2	N. W. 1	Sprinl'g	Rain	5	0.20
8	29.63	29.57	29.68	31	38	31	33.3	N. W. 2	N. W. 3	N. W. 2	0	5	0	
9	29.64	29.51	29.53	30	34	28	30.7	N. W. 2	N. W. 3	N. W. 2	6	2	0	
10	29.47	29.37	29.41	24	35	29	29.3	N. W. 2	N. W. 3	N. W. 1	0	0	0	
S 11	29.51	29.40	29.50	26	39	32	32.3	N. W. 1	N. W. 2	N. W. 1	0	0	0	
12	29.59	29.69	29.74	26	44	39	36.3	N. W. 1	N. W. 2	N. W. 1	0	0	10	
13	29.72	29.75	29.80	33	50	41	41.3	W'ly 1	S. W. 2	S. W. 1	3	4	3	
14	29.96	30.02	30.10	31	41	34	35.3	N. E. 1	S. E. 2	E'ly 2	10	10	10	
15	30.04	29.98	29.73	33	41	35	36.3	E'ly 1	S. E'ly 2	E'ly 1	10	Misty	Rain	0.55
16	29.70	29.69	29.71	34	46	32	37.3	N. 1	N. W. 1	N. W. 1	10	10	0	
17	29.69	29.51	29.67	32	58	45	45.0	N. 1	S. W. 3	S. W. 1	0	2	10	
S 18	29.68	29.62	29.79	35	48	33	38.7	N. W. 1	N. W. 1	N. W. 2	5	10	0	
19	29.91	30.00	30.08	27	38	30	31.7	N. W. 1	N. W. 3	N. W. 1	0	0	0	
20	30.05	29.90	29.78	34	53	45	44.0	S. W. 2	S. W. 3	S. W. 3	0	5	Rain	}
21	29.56	29.47	29.25	45	53	52	50.0	S'ly 4	S. W'ly 4	S. W'ly 2	Rain	Rain	Rain	}
22	29.50	29.83	30.14	34	43	31	39.3	N. W. 2	N. W. 2	N. W. 0	R'n, sn.	1	0	} 3.12
23	30.31	30.31	30.26	25	43	34	34.0	N. E. 1	S'ly 2	S. E'ly 1	0	4	0	}
24	30.22	30.09	30.12	34	51	45	43.3	S'ly 1	S'ly 2	S'ly 1	8	6	10	
S 25	30.02	29.92	29.77	42	50	46	46.0	S. E'ly 1	S. E'ly 2	S. E'ly 3	10	10	Misty	
26	29.77	29.76	29.77	38	37	33	36.0	N. E'ly 1	N. E'ly 1	N. E'ly 1	Rain	Rain	R'n, h'l	}
27	29.73	29.68	29.65	31	35	38	34.7	N. E'ly 2	N. E. 3	N. E. 3½	Misty	Rain	Misty	}
28	29.54	29.65	29.85	38	44	40	40.7	N. E. 3½	N. E. 2	N. E. 2	Rain	Misty	Misty	} 2.12
29	29.85	29.83	29.80	41	47	43	43.7	N. E. 2	N. E. 2	N. E. 2	Misty	Rain	Misty	}
30	29.77	29.74	29.71	42	50	45	45.7	N. E. 2	N'ly 2	N. E'ly 1	Rain	10	10	}
31	29.69	29.60	29.66	45	62	45	50.7	N'ly 1	N. W. 1	N. W. 1	10	9	0	
Means	29.87	29.83	29.85	32.0	43.1	36.0	...	1.5	2.2	1.5	5.7	6.2	5.4	5.99
								1.7			5.8			
REDUCED TO SEA LEVEL.														
Max.	30.54	30.49	30.50	45	62	52	50.7	Prevailing winds from some point between—		Days.			Days.	
Min.	29.55	29.56	29.43	17	32	23	24.7							
Mean	30.05	30.01	30.03					N. & E.		12	Clear		7	
Range	0.89	0.94	1.07	28	30	29	26.0	E. & S.		4	Variable }		15	
Mean of month	30.030			...	...	...	37.0	S. & W.		5	Cloudy }			
Extreme range	1.11			...	...	...	45.0	W. & N.		10	Rain or snow fell on		9	

REMARKS.

1st. Very mild. Evening clear.

2d. Appearances of storm in the evening, the moon shining very dimly through deep haze thickening into clouds.

3d. Appearances of storm in the evening.

4th. Pleasant.

5th. Very fine.

6th. Appearances of storm in the evening.

7th. Rain very moderate and light during most of the day. Wind came to N.W. from 7 to 8 P.M., and at 11 P. M. quite clear.

8th. Fine. Large eclipse of the moon: began at 6 h. 40 m. 15 s. P. M., mean solar time; ended at 9 h. 40 m. 20 s. P. M.; duration, 3 h. 5 s. Clear.

9th and 10th. Very fine.

11th. Very fine; nearly without a cloud.

12th. Fine. Appearances of rain in evening.

13th. Haze in the evening.

14th. Indications of storm.

15th. Began to rain about 3 P. M., and rained rather briskly till 7 P. M., with wind light at E. S. E. nearly.

16th. Changeable. Thick fog at 6 P. M.

17th. Very mild and spring-like.

18th. Pleasant. Aurora in the evening, quite bright, but no streamers.

19th. Very chilly to the feelings. Evening fine.

20th. Began to sprinkle at 10 P. M.

21st. Rained quite moderately in the morning; wind pretty heavy at about S. S. W. In the afternoon, the rain increased. In the evening, rain and wind both heavy. At 10 P. M., wind began to lull, and rain slackened. Barometer at 29.35, without any indications of rising.

22d. At sunrise, therm. 34°, barom. 29.58 and rising. At 9 A. M., barom. 29.77. Day and evening very fine.

23d. Fine.

24th. Very mild.

25th. Mist during the afternoon.

26th. Rain and mist during the day; wind light at a little N. of E. Rain and hail in the evening.

27th. At sunrise, the ground partly covered with snow. Heavy storm in the afternoon and evening. Amount of rain moderate.

28th. Heavy rain in the morning.

29th. Rain and mist, by turns, all day.

30th. Occasional rain and mist. Between noon and 1 P. M., the sun was discernible, but showery in afternoon. In the evening, occasional glimpses of the stars were seen.

31st. Weather mild, and evening clear.

April, 1849. New Moon, 22d. 6h. 46m. P. M.

DAYS.	BAROMETER, REDUCED TO 32° F. At 6 A. M.	At 1 P. M.	At 10 P. M.	THERMOMETER. At 6 A. M.	At 1 P. M.	At 10 P. M.	Daily mean.	WINDS. (DIRECTION AND FORCE.) At 6 A. M.	At 1 P. M.	At 10 P. M.	WEATHER. (TENTHS CLOUDY.) At 6 A. M.	At 1 P. M.	At 10 P. M.	RAIN AND SNOW IN INCHES OF WATER.
S 1	29.69	29.66	29.81	39	46	32	39.0	N. W. 2	N. W. 2	N. W. 1	2	0	0	
2	29.75	29.72	29.83	31	43	34	36.0	N. W. 1	N. W. 2	N. W. 1	3	3	0	
3	29.88	29.80	29.81	31	61	49	47.0	W'ly 1	W'ly 1	W'ly 1	0	0	5	
4	29.81	29.75	29.71	45	59	46	50.0	S. W. 1	S. E. 1	S. E'ly 1	8	8	10	
5	29.62	29.48	29.72	46	55	45	48.7	S'ly 1	S. W. 2	N. W. 2	Foggy	Misty	0	
6	29.84	30.01	30.00	37	55	44	45.3	N. W. 1	N. W. 1	N. W. 1	0	0	0	
7	30.13	29.97	29.77	43	55	55	51.0	N. W. 1	S'ly 2	S'ly 1	2	2	4	
S 8	29.76	29.78	29.96	54	61	45	53.3	N. W. 2	N. W. 2	N. W. 2	0	3	5	
9	30.02	29.98	29.98	38	55	41	44.7	N'ly 1	N. E'ly 1	S'ly 1	0	0	0	
10	29.93	29.80	29.58	39	47	44	43.3	S'ly 1	S'ly 2	S. E'ly 1	1	Rain	Rain	0.22
11	29.50	29.53	29.71	41	53	41	45.0	N'ly 1	N. W. 2	N. W. 3	10	2	0	
12	29.82	29.77	29.89	35	56	42	44.3	N. W. 2	N. W. 2	N. W. 1	0	0	0	
13	29.88	29.71	29.55	40	56	53	49.7	N. W. 2	S. E'ly 1	S. W'ly 1	10	10	10	
14	29.49	29.46	29.57	44	44	26	38.0	N'ly 2	N. W. 2	N. W. 1	2	4	0	
S 15	29.52	29.39	29.42	24	35	28	29.0	N. W. 3	N. W. 3	N. W. 2	3	2	0	
16	29.37	29.34	29.50	24	36	35	31.7	W'ly 2	W'ly 2	W'ly 1	2	10	10	
17	29.59	29.54	29.56	32	52	38	40.7	W'ly 1	W'ly 1	S. W'ly 1	8	0	0	
18	29.55	29.48	29.23	38	58	43	46.3	S. E. 1	S. E. 2	N. E. 3	2	10	Rain	1.05
19	29.17	29.15	29.37	36	55	36	42.3	S. W. 1	S. E'ly 1	N'ly 1	3	5	0	
20	29.52	29.52	29.69	36	59	35	43.3	N. W. 1	W'ly 1	N. W. 1	0	2	Sh'r, 0	0.10
21	29.76	29.81	29.90	32	48	38	39.3	N. W. 1	N. W. 1	N. W. 1	0	0	0	
S 22	29.93	29.87	29.89	40	46	40	42.0	N. W. 1	S. E. 1	S. E. 2	9	10	10, Sh'r	
23	29.99	29.99	29.80	38	54	42	44.7	N. W. 1	S. W. 1	S'ly 3	3	4	10	
24	29.62	29.77	29.86	51	60	48	53.0	W'ly 2	W'ly 2	W'ly 1	10	5	1	
25	29.95	29.95	29.97	42	65	47	51.3	N. W. 1	W'ly 1	N. W. 1	2	5	0	
26	29.96	30.01	30.16	47	63	42	50.7	N. W. 2	N. E. 2	N. E. 1	8	6	9	
27	30.24	30.23	30.21	39	59	38	45.3	N. E. 2	N. E. 1	N. W. 1	9	3	1	
28	30.09	29.85	29.68	38	56	54	49.3	E. 1	S. E. 2	S. E. 1	10	Foggy	Rain	0.25
S 29	29.70	29.71	29.90	55	64	49	56.0	W'ly 1	N. W. 1	N. W. 1	10	2	0	
30	30.10	30.10	29.91	39	55	45	46.3	N. E. 1	S. E. 2	S. E'ly 1	0	0	Hazy	
Means	29.77	29.74	29.78	39.1	50.4	41.8	...	1.4	1.6	1.3	4.2	4.2	5.0	1.62
								1.4			4.5			
REDUCED TO SEA LEVEL.								Prevailing winds from some point between— Days.			Days.			
Max.	30.42	30.41	30.34	55	65	55	56.0							
Min.	29.35	29.33	29.41	24	35	32	29.0							
Mean	29.95	29.92	29.94					N. & E. 3			Clear 9			
Range	1.07	1.08	0.93	31	30	23	27.0	E. & S. 6			Variable . . . } 14			
Mean of month	29.937			...	...	...	43.7	S. & W. 6			Cloudy . . . . }			
Extreme range	1.09			...	...	...	41.0	W. & N. 15			Rain fell on . . 7			

REMARKS.

1st. Very pleasant.
2d and 3d. Very fine.
4th. Pleasant. Very thick haze and clouds in the evening. Wind S. E'ly, while the clouds passed from W'ly.
5th. Occasional sprinkling and mist in morning. Cleared from 5 to 6 P. M., with wind at N. W.
6th. Pleasant.
7th. Variable.
8th. Pleasant.
9th. Fine.
10th. Sprinkling of rain in afternoon. Heavy shower in the evening.
11th. Very fine.
12th. Fine.
13th. Sprinkling of rain from 6 to 7 P. M.
14th. Very chilly and severe. Appearances of snow at 2 P. M. and towards sunset. Evening clear and cold.
15th. The ground at sunrise was frozen more than an inch in depth. Wind through the day very cold and piercing.
16th. Very cold and uncomfortable. From 1 to 2 P. M., wet clothes froze in the wind.
17th. Pleasant.
18th. Began to rain at about 8 P. M., with wind very fresh at N. E.
19th. Flurry of snow from 8 to 9 A. M. Sprinkling of rain at 3 P. M. Very clear in evening.
20th. Brisk shower from 5 to 6 P. M. Clear at 10½ P. M. Saw the "Telescopic Comet" visible about 10° N. W. of Arcturus.
21st. Very fine. Saw the comet again.
22d. Very damp. Very light showers in the afternoon.
23d. Chilly wind, and appearance of storm in the evening.
24th. Very fine. The comet barely discernible by the naked eye, when its position is previously known.
25th. Very fine. Clear at 11 P. M.. The comet distinctly visible to the naked eye.
26th. Pleasant.
27th. Very fine. The comet again seen by the naked eye.
28th. Shower in the afternoon.
29th. Very fine.
30th. Pleasant.

May, 1849. New Moon, 22d. 2h. 28m. A. M.

DAYS.	BAROMETER At 6 A. M.	At 1 P. M.	At 10 P. M.	THERMOMETER At 6 A. M.	At 1 P. M.	At 10 P. M.	Da'ly mean.	WINDS At 6 A. M.	At 1 P. M.	At 10 P. M.	WEATHER At 6 A. M.	At 1 P. M.	At 10 P. M.	RAIN AND SNOW
1	29.87	29.79	29.94	54	77	57	62.7	S. W. 1	S. W. 2	N. W. 1	10	4	5	
2	30.10	30.13	30.21	44	56	44	48.0	N. W. 1	N. W. 1	N. W. 1	0	0	0	
3	30.35	30.23	30.15	39	62	48	49.7	N. W. 2	S'ly 2	S'ly 2	0	4	10	
4	29.92	29.77	29.84	50	76	62	62.7	W'ly 2	W'ly 1	W'ly 1	10	5	5	
5	30.01	30.09	30.15	48	49	44	47.0	N. E. 2	N. E. 2	E'ly 1	Rain	Rain	10	0.25
S 6	30.14	30.08	29.99	44	55	41	46.7	N. E. 1	N. E. 2	E'ly 1	10	Sh'r, 10	Sprin'lg	
7	29.93	29.81	29.84	41	66	48	51.7	N. E. 1	S. E'ly 2	S'ly 2	10	8	10	
8	29.77	29.73	29.70	47	59	47	51.0	S. W'ly 1	S. W. 1	S. E'ly 2	10	10	10	
9	29.70	29.78	29.87	44	50	44	46.0	N. E. 1	N. E. 1	N. E. 1	Misty	Rain	7	0.23
10	29.88	29.82	29.80	46	64	45	51.7	N. E. 1	S. W'ly 1	S'ly 1	8	5	2	
11	29.76	29.68	29.72	41	61	40	47.3	N. E. 1	N. E. 1	N. E. 1	Misty	5	0	
12	29.76	29.73	29.76	40	66	47	47.7	N.N.E. 1	N.W'ly 1	N. W. 1	0	7	0	
S 13	29.76	29.65	29.42	51	53	53	52.3	S. W. 1	S. W. 1	S. W'ly 3	8	Rain	Rain	1.50
14	29.25	29.24	29.29	50	63	48	53.7	N. W. 2	S. W. 2	N. E. 1	4	10	0	
15	29.36	29.45	29.60	48	59	47	51.3	N. W. 1	N. W. 2	N. W. 1	8	6	0	0.35
16	29.69	29.72	29.83	45	65	48	52.7	N. W. 2	N. W. 2	S. E'ly 1	0	6	1	
17	29.86	29.86	29.92	45	68	51	54.7	N. W. 1	S'ly 2	S. W. 1	0	3	2	
18	29.88	29.85	29.85	48	70	50	59.3	N. E. 1	N. E. 2	N. E. 1	6	4	0	
19	29.86	29.84	29.93	50	71	54	58.3	N. W. 1	N. W. 1	N. W. 1	0	1	0	
S 20	29.97	29.91	29.87	54	76	58	62.7	N. W. 1	S. W. 3	S. W. 3	0	3	5	
21	29.85	29.73	29.89	57	82	48	62.3	S. W. 2	S. W. 2	N. W. 3	3	4	2	
22	29.90	29.81	29.67	50	72	59	60.3	N. E. 1	N. E. 1	S. W. 2	10	8	5	
23	29.50	29.40	29.49	59	79	64	67.3	S. W. 2	S. E'ly 2	W'ly 2	5	6	8, Sh'r	0.05
24	29.70	29.79	29.91	50	51	44	48.3	N. E. 2	N. E. 2	N. E. 2	Misty	10	10	
25	29.94	29.91	29.83	42	49	44	45.0	N. E. 1	N. E.	N. E. 1	Rain	Rain	10	0.34
26	29.89	29.87	29.89	45	65	50	53.3	N. E. 1	N'ly 2	N. W. 1	10	3	0	
S 27	29.89	29.88	29.90	52	75	57	61.3	W'ly 1	S. W. 1	S. W. 1	4	8	9	
28	29.93	29.95	30.00	40	73	55	59.0	N. E. 1	S. E. 2	S'ly 2	0	4	8	
29	30.04	30.02	30.05	52	72	53	59.0	N. E. 2	N. E. 2	N. E. 3	Rain	10	10	
30	30.03	29.98	29.99	53	61	52	55.3	N. E. 2	N. E. 1	N. E. 2	Misty	Misty	Misty	
31	29.96	29.92	29.89	51	53	51	51.7	N. E. 1	N. E. 1	N. E. 1	Misty	Rain	10	0.71
Means	29.85	29.82	29.84	48.0	64.5	50.1	...	1.3	1.6	1.5	6.3	6.6	5.5	3.43
								1.5			6.1			
REDUCED TO SEA LEVEL.								Prevailing winds from some point between— Days.			Days.			
Max.	30.53	30.41	30.39	59	82	64	67.3							
Min.	29.43	29.42	29.47	39	49	40	45.0							
Mean	30.03	30.00	30.02					N. & E. 11			Clear 3			
Range	1.10	0.99	0.92	20	33	24	22.3	E. & S. 3			Variable . . . } 22			
Mean of month	30.017			...	...	...	54.2	S. & W. 11			Cloudy . . . . }			
Extreme range	1.11			...	...	...	43.0	W. & N. 6			Rain fell on . . 6			

REMARKS.

1st. Pleasant.
2d. Very fine. Comet visible in the telescope, in presence of the moon ten days' old; its motion very rapid.
3d. Pleasant. Appearances of rain in evening.
4th. Sprinkling of rain from 8 to 9 A. M., and from 5 to 6 P. M.
5th. Very moderate. Rain during most of day.
6th. Sprinkling of rain at intervals through day.
7th. Cool morning.
8th. Raw and cold for the season.
9th. Mist and drizzle most of the day. Partly clear at 10 P. M.
10th. Pleasant.
11th. Variable day. Very clear evening.
12th. Ther. fell to 38° last night. Pleasant day. Aurora from 10 to 11 P. M., low and quite bright, without coruscations.
13th. Began to rain moderately about 11 A. M.; continued through P. M.—sometimes briskly.
14th. At 3 P. M., there was a shower of hail, which continued not more than 4 or 5 minutes, but in that time the quantity which fell was very extraordinary. In the space of one minute from the commencement, the ground was white with it, and at the end of the shower it might be scraped up anywhere in the garden by the handful. The hailstones were not ice, but compact balls of snow, flattened on one, two, or three, and sometimes four, sides, so as to present a somewhat angular appearance. Very many of the balls were ⅜ of an inch, while some were very nearly ½ inch, in diameter. All that I particularly examined, which was a large number, were so soft as to be crushed between the fingers, or have their form changed. In the largest-sized balls, I observed that they were softer in the centre than at the surface. These large balls were intermixed with many smaller ones of different structure, and evidently formed under different circumstances, many of them being light, soft balls of snow. When wet by the rain which followed, they were all readily formed into massive snow-balls. The hail was very restricted in its extent in one direction—that is, from north to south. In the southerly part of the city, there was none at all. In Charlesfield Street, less than a quarter of a mile south of this spot, none was observed. It extended in a northerly direction about two miles, and easterly, so far as I can learn, about seven miles. It came from a distance at the west. It has been reported from New Haven.

June, 1849. New Moon, 20d. 9h. 10m. A. M.

Days.	Barometer, reduced to 32° F. At 6 A. M.	At 1 P. M.	At 10 P. M.	Thermometer. At 6 A. M.	At 1 P. M.	At 10 P. M.	Daily mean.	Winds. (Direction and Force.) At 6 A. M.	At 1 P. M.	At 10 P. M.	Weather. (Tenths Cloudy.) At 6 A. M.	At 1 P. M.	At 10 P. M.	Rain and Snow in Inches of Water.
1	29.86	29.86	29.96	53	71	56	60.0	N. W. 2	N. E. 2	N. E. 2	7	5	10	
2	29.96	29.89	29.85	57	69	60	62.0	S. E. 1	S'ly 2	S'ly 2	9	2	10	
S 3	29.82	29.72	29.72	64	72	64	66.7	N. E. 1	S. E. 1	S'ly 1	Foggy	10	Foggy	
4	29.65	29.53	29.58	63	78	65	68.7	S'ly 1	S'ly 1	N. W. 1	Foggy	1	Sh'r, 5	0.37
5	29.69	29.71	29.78	55	70	59	61.3	N. W. 2	N. W. 8	N. W. 1	0	1	0	
6	29.85	29.75	29.75	54	77	58	63.0	N. W. 1	N. W. 2	N. W. 1	0	0	3	
7	29.75	29.64	29.59	55	74	61	63.3	N. W. 1	S'ly 2	S. W. 1	3	5	5	
8	29.52	29.54	29.61	61	54	48	54.3	S. W. 1	N. E. 2	N'ly 1	8	Rain	2	0.08
9	29.68	29.68	29.71	51	73	58	60.7	N. W. 1	S. E'ly 2	S'ly 1	3	4	10	
S 10	29.72	29.81	29.92	59	69	52	60.0	E'ly 2	E'ly 1	N. E. 2	10	9	2	
11	30.06	30.08	30.12	48	69	51	56.0	N. E. 1	N. E. 2	N. E. 1	3	2	0	
12	30.14	30.16	30.16	47	70	54	57.0	N'ly 1	N. E. 2	N. E. 1	0	0	Hazy	
13	30.16	30.08	30.08	49	76	59	61.3	N. W. 2	S. W. 2	S'ly 2	3	2	10	
14	30.08	30.04	30.01	57	78	61	65.3	S. W. 2	S. W. 3	S'ly 1	5	5	0	
15	29.94	29.84	29.75	60	75	64	66.3	S. W. 2	S. W.	S'ly	7	...	0	
16	29.73	29.65	29.76	63	76	68	69.0	S'ly 2	S. W. 2	N. W. 1	5	10	0	0.46
S 17	29.95	30.00	30.02	66	81	62	69.7	N. W. 1	E'ly 3	S. E. 1	0	5	0	
18	30.08	30.06	30.06	62	82	69	71.0	N. W. 2	S'ly 2	S. W. 2	0	5	2	
19	30.01	29.92	29.91	67	90	73	76.7	S. W. 2	W'ly 3	S. W. 1	0	2	0	
20	29.87	29.83	29.82	71	92	73	78.7	W'ly 1	N. W. 2	S. E'ly 1	3	2	0	
21	29.87	29.84	29.83	75	97	76	82.7	N. W. 1	N. W. 1	S'ly 1	0	0	0	
22	29.83	29.79	29.74	75	97	79	83.7	N. W. 1	N. W. 2	S'ly 1	0	2	0	
23	29.72	29.65	29.66	76	94	73	81.0	N. W. 1	N. W. 2	N. W. 1	3	5	0	
S 24	29.69	29.64	29.54	70	86	72	76.0	N. W. 1	S. 3	S. E'ly 2	8	5	Rain	0.07
25	29.51	29.51	29.60	68	85	69	74.0	W. 1	N. W. 2	N. W. 1	0	0	0	
26	29.62	29.58	29.72	66	87	68	73.7	N. W. 2	N. W. 2	N. W. 2	0	1	0	
27	29.75	29.72	29.73	60	85	72	72.3	N. W. 1	N. W. 2	N. W. 1	3	2	5	
28	29.78	29.80	29.76	61	66	60	62.3	N. E. 1	N. E. 1	N. E. 1	5	Rain	10	} 0.25
29	29.60	29.58	29.66	57	61	56	58.0	N. E. 1	N'ly 2	N'ly 2	Rain	10	9	
30	29.70	29.62	29.56	55	85	68	69.3	N. W. 1	W'ly 3	S. W. 2	10	5	0	
Means	29.82	29.78	29.80	60.8	78.0	63.6	...	1.3	2.0	1.3	4.2	4.1	3.4	1.23
								1.5			3.9			
REDUCED TO SEA LEVEL.								Prevailing winds from some point between—		Days.			Days.	
Max.	30.34	30.34	30.34	76	97	79	83.7	N. & E.		8	Clear		13	
Min.	29.69	29.69	29.72	47	54	48	54.3	E. & S.		5	Variable		} 9	
Mean	30.00	29.96	29.98					S. & W.		8	Cloudy			
Range	0.65	0.65	0.62	29	43	31	29.4	W. & N.		9	Rain fell on		8	
Mean of month	29.980			...	...	...	67.5							
Extreme range	0.65			...	...	...	50.0							

Remarks.

1st. Pleasant.
2d. Air raw at night.
3d. Foggy. Light shower from noon to 1 P. M.
4th. Copious thundershower from 6½ to 8 P. M.
5th, 6th, and 7th. Very fine.
8th. Light rain, with mist, from 10 A. M. to 3 P. M.
9th. Pleasant.
10th. Sun out occasionally in the afternoon.
11th. Pleasant, but cool.
12th. Fine.
13th. Pleasant.
14th. Pleasant. Evening clear and very mild.
15th. Appearances of rain. Light mist at 8 P. M.
16th. Morning very sultry. Heavy thundershower in the afternoon.
17th. Very fine.
18th. Very hot sun.
19th. Intensely hot.
20th. Intensely hot. Air fresh in the evening from S'ly.
21st. Heat extreme.
22d. Heat unabated.
23d. Very warm, but a good air. Dashes of rain, with thunder, at 9 A. M.
24th. Rather cooler. Showery in the evening so as to lay the dust.
25th. Fine.
26th. A beautiful meteor was seen at 15 to 20 minutes past 8 P. M., passing the meridian plane 10° or 12° below Polaris, making with it a small angle, the meteor passing from the east to the west side. The light was very brilliant, being white tinged with blue. When it burst, it separated into several reddish fragments. Its course was seen through about 10° of the great circle. It was seen by several persons. The daylight was still strong. It very much resembled a brilliant rocket.
27th. Pleasant.
28th. Sprinkling of rain; little more than enough to lay the dust.
29th. Rain and damp. Kindled a fire to make the house comfortable.

July, 1849. New Moon, 19d. 4h. 7m. P. M.

Days.	Barometer At 6 A. M.	At 1 P. M.	At 10 P. M.	Thermometer At 6 A. M.	At 1 P. M.	At 10 P. M.	Daily mean.	Winds At 6 A. M.	At 1 P. M.	At 10 P. M.	Weather At 6 A. M.	At 1 P. M.	At 10 P. M.	Rain and Snow in Inches of Water.
S 1	29.57	29.57	29.67	67	76	60	67.3	N. W. 2	N. W. 3	N. W. 1	0	2	0	
2	29.72	29.76	29.85	53	69	56	59.3	N. E. 2	N. E. 3	N. W. 1	2	10, Sh'r	7	0.20
3	29.90	29.95	30.01	51	69	56	58.7	N. 2	N'ly 2	N'ly 1	0	8, Sh'r	0	
4	30.05	...	30.03	52	...	56	54.0	N'ly 1	...	N'ly 1	9	...	10	
5	29.99	20.96	29.96	59	68	62	63.0	N. E. 1	E'ly 2	N. E. 1	Rain	10	Misty	
6	29.95	29.93	29.96	61	81	65	69.0	N'ly 1	N. W. 2	W'ly 2	10	4	5	
7	29.96	29.93	29.93	65	84	68	72.3	S. W. 2	S. W. 2	S. W. 2	10	10, Sh'r	8	0.32
S 8	29.90	29.90	30.01	72	84	70	75.3	S. W. 1	S. W. 2	S. W. 1	8	5	10	
9	29.93	29.95	29.98	67	81	69	72.3	N. E. 1	E'ly 2	E'ly 2	Foggy	6	Misty	
10	29.99	29.96	29.96	70	84	70	74.7	S'ly 2	S. W. 2	S. W. 2	Foggy	5	0	
11	30.00	29.95	29.99	72	91	78	80.3	W'ly 1	W'ly 2	W'ly 1	5	0	0	
12	29.99	29.92	29.85	75	94	80	83.0	W'ly 2	W'ly 3	W'ly 1	0	0	0	
13	29.82	29.74	29.66	80	97	82	86.3	W'ly 2	N. W. 3	W'ly 1	0	0	0	
14	29.62	29.64	29.84	79	81	64	74.0	W'ly 1	N. W. 2	N. E. 2	0	10	2	
S 15	29.95	29.94	30.01	56	74	60	63.3	N. E. 2	N. E. 3	N'ly 2	0	2	0	
16	30.03	...	29.91	56	...	65	60.5	N. W. 2	...	N. W. 1	0	...	10	
17	29.86	29.84	29.87	59	86	68	71.0	W'ly 1	W'ly 3	S. W. 1	2	1	0	
18	29.91	29.90	29.95	66	85	67	72.7	S. W. 2	S. W. 3	S. W. 1	2	0	0	
19	29.97	29.94	29.95	69	83	69	73.7	S. W. 1	S. E. 3	S'ly 2	7	0	0	
20	29.94	29.84	29.79	69	90	74	77.7	S. W. 1	S. W. 3	S. W. 2	8	0	3	
21	29.61	29.52	29.56	74	77	68	73.0	S. W. 3	S. W. 2	S. W. 2	Rain	10	Rain	1.18
S 22	29.63	29.69	29.83	67	84	69	73.3	N. W. 1	N. W. 2	N. W. 1	6	2	0	
23	29.89	29.93	30.02	62	82	65	69.7	N. by E. 2	S'ly 2	N. E'ly 1	4	1	0	
24	30.08	30.06	30.07	63	83	65	70.3	E'ly 1	E'ly 2	S'ly 1	Foggy	0	0	
25	30.10	30.00	29.97	63	83	69	71.7	E'ly 1	E'ly 2	E'ly 1	3	3	10	
26	29.91	29.80	29.76	65	81	74	73.3	S. E. 2	S. W. 3	S'ly 1	10	Misty	Rain	
27	29.74	29.74	29.80	70	87	69	75.3	N. W. 2	N. W. 3	N. W. 2	0	2	2	
28	29.88	29.85	29.83	65	82	62	69.7	N. W. 1	E'ly 1	E'ly 1	4	10	0	
S 29	29.86	29.83	29.83	63	81	66	70.0	N'ly 1	S'ly 2	S'ly	4	0	0	
30	29.84	29.81	29.83	63	83	71	72.3	S. W. 2	S'ly 3	S. W. 2	2	2	0	
31	29.77	29.74	29.79	74	87	72	77.7	S. W. 2	S. W. 3	N. W. 2	10	3	Rain	0.30
Means	29.88	29.85	29.89	65.4	82.3	67.4	...	2.2	2.5	1.4	5.0	4.0	3.8	2.00
								2.0			4.3			
REDUCED TO SEA LEVEL.								Prevailing winds from some point between—		Days.			Days.	
Max.	30.28	30.24	30.25	80	97	82	86.3	N. & E.		8	Clear		12	
Min.	29.75	29.70	29.74	51	68	56	54.0	E. & S.		3	Variable		} 12	
Mean	30.06	30.03	30.07					S. & W.		10	Cloudy			
Range	0.53	0.54	0.51	29	29	26	32.3	W. & N.		10	Rain fell on		7	
Mean of month	30.053			...	...	...	71.7							
Extreme range	0.58			...	...	...	46.0							

Remarks.

1st. Very fine.
2d. Shower of rain and hail at 3 P. M.
3d. Damp and unpleasant; showery. Evening beautifully clear.
4th. Very pleasant.
5th. Cool for the season. Mist at intervals.
6th. Fine.
7th. Showery in the afternoon and evening; amount of rain small.
8th. Thunder, with appearances of rain, in the afternoon.
9th. Air very damp. Sprinkling of rain several times, so as to wet the surface of the ground.
10th. Very sultry and damp. Evening clear.
11th. Very hot, and air damp.
12th. Heat very intense; breeze fresh. This night the hottest so far.
13th. At 8 A. M., the thermometer in the shade, with a fresh current of air, stood at 86°; at 10 A. M., 90°; at 1 P. M., 97°; and at 3½ P. M., at 100° in the shade, but somewhat affected by local reflection.
14th. Warm in the morning. Light shower at 2½ P. M.; wind came to N. E., and air became much cooler.

Dew-point—
15th. 7 A. M. 43°; 2 P. M. 42°.
16th. 7 " 45; 2 " 45; 9 to 10 P.M., cl'dy.
17th. 7 " 52; 1 " 46.
18th. 7 " 59; 1 " 56; 7 P. M. 56°.
19th. 7 " 62; 1 " 64; 10 " 65.
20th. 7 " 65; 1 " 58; 7 " 65.
21st. 7 " 68; 1 " 68; 10 " 65.
Heavy shower, with thunder, in the evening.
22d. 7 A. M. 60°; 1 P. M. 54°; 10 P. M. 54°.
23d. 7 " 54; 1 " 60; 7 " 62.
24th. 7 " 60; 1 " 60.
25th. 7 " 58; 1 " 59; 7 " 62.
26th. 7 " 63; 1 " ..; 7 " 69.
Began to rain at 10 P. M.
27th. 7 " 59; 1 " 61. Evening fine.
28th. 7 " 53; 1 " 53. Evening fine.
29th. 7 " 53; 1 " 57; 7 P. M. 62°.
30th. 7 " 62; 1 " 69. Evening fine.
31st. 7 " 69; 1 " 72. Sh'r at 4 P. M.

Note.—The 13th of this month was the hottest day since the beginning of my Register in December, 1831. The mean of four observations—viz., at 6 A. M., 1 P. M., 3½ P. M., and 10 P. M.—is 90°.

August, 1849. New Moon, 18d. 0h. 24m. A. M.

DAYS.	BAROMETER, REDUCED TO 32° F At 6 A. M.	At 1 P. M.	At 10 P. M.	THERMOMETER. At 6 A. M.	At 1 P. M.	At 10 P. M.	Daily mean.	WINDS. (DIRECTION AND FORCE.) At 6 A. M.	At 1 P. M.	At 10 P. M.	WEATHER. (TENTHS CLOUDY.) At 6 A. M.	At 1 P. M.	At 10 P. M.	RAIN AND SNOW IN INCHES OF WATER.
1	29.88	29.89	29.89	60	69	59	62.7	N. E. 2	N. E. 1	N. E.	Rain	10	0	0.20
2	29.96	29.94	29.98	59	80	62	67.0	E'ly 1	N. E. 1	0	4	2	0	
3	30.00	29.96	29.94	59	80	65	67.3	0	S. by E. 2	N. W. 1	0	0	0	
4	29.89	29.83	29.84	60	80	66	68.7	W'ly 1	S. E'ly 2	S'ly 1	0	1	Rain	0.20
S 5	29.84	29.85	29.87	64	83	67	71.3	N. W. 1	N. W. 1	S. E'ly	1	3	5	
6	29.83	29.77	29.73	69	76	71	72.0	S. E. 1	S'ly 1	S. W. 2	10	Rain	Shower	
7	29.71	29.71	29.76	67	82	67	72.0	W'ly 1	N. W. 2	N. W. 1	4	3	0	
8	29.84	29.78	29.83	64	81	67	70.7	N. W. 1	N. W. 2	S. W. 1	0	3	0	
9	29.84	29.77	29.76	64	77	68	69.7	S. W. 1	S. S. E. 3	S'ly 2	Foggy	2	10	
10	29.67	29.67	29.79	72	72	69	71.0	S. E. 3	S. E. 2	S. E. 1	10	Rain	10	} 1.80
11	29.69	29.71	29.75	67	80	71	72.7	S. E. 1	N. E. 1	E'ly 1	Sh'r, 10	8	2	
S 12	29.77	29.80	29.77	70	74	64	69.3	E. 1	N. E. 3	N. 2	8	10	Rain, 9	0.56
13	29.76	29.78	29.74	64	77	70	70.3	W. 1	S. 3	S. 0	3	2	0	
14	29.66	29.56	29.50	67	76	68	70.3	S. E. 1	S. E. 4	S. W. 2	9	5	8	0.17
15	29.45	29.48	29.59	63	76	63	67.3	N. W. 2	N. W. 5	N. W. 1	0	3	0	
16	29.64	29.68	29.74	56	78	68	67.3	N. W. 3	N. 1	W. 0	0	0	0	
17	29.78	29.81	29.84	62	82	73	69.0	W. 1	S'ly 4	S. W. 1	4	3	1	
18	29.84	29.87	29.88	70	77	72	73.0	S. W. 1	S. 3	Calm	9	2	0	
S 19	29.88	29.87	29.87	62	78	71	70.3	N. 2	N. E. 2	E'ly 1	2	5	0	0.20
20	29.89	29.89	29.87	66	77	68	70.3	N. E. 2	E. 2	E. 1	10	6	0	
21	29.86	29.81	29.77	64	75	70	69.7	S. W. 1	S. E. 4	S. W. 1	3	5	1	
22	29.80	29.79	29.77	70	80	73	74.3	N. W. 1	N. W. 5	N. W. 0	3	5	1	
23	29.73	29.64	29.52	68	71	66	68.3	W. 1	S. E. 1	N. E. 4	10	10	10, Sh'r	0.26
24	29.69	29.75	29.81	64	78	64	68.7	N. 4	N. E. 4	N. W. 1	9	1	0	
25	29.83	29.85	29.86	60	82	70	70.7	N. W. 1	N. W. 2	N. W. 2	0	0	0	
S 26	29.91	29.93	29.96	65	84	70	73.0	W. 1	S. W. 3	S. W. 1	0	0	0	
27	29.97	29.95	29.98	66	83	70	72.0	S. W. 2	S. W. 3	S. W. 1	3	1	0	
28	29.97	29.96	29.99	70	82	...	76.0	S. W. 1	S. W. 2	S. W. 1	5	10	10	
29	30.00	29.97	29.98	72	81	70	74.3	S. W. 1	S. W. 2	S'ly 1	10	10	6	
30	29.98	29.92	29.91	69	82	68	73.0	S. W'ly 1	S. W. 2	S. W. 1	10	1	10	
31	29.84	29.72	29.71	70	83	72	75.0	S. W. 2	S'ly 2	S. W. 1	10	8	10	
Means	29.82	29.80	29.81	65.3	78.6	68.0	...	1.4	2.4	1.2	5.4	4.4	3.7	3.39
									1.7			4.5		
REDUCED TO SEA LEVEL.								Prevailing winds from some point between—		Days.			Days.	
Max.	30.18	30.15	30.17	72	84	73	76.0							
Min.	29.63	29.66	29.68	56	69	59	62.7							
Mean	30.00	29.98	29.99					N. & E.		3	Clear		10	
Range	0.55	0.49	0.45	16	15	14	13.3	E. & S.		10	Variable		} 13	
Mean of month	29.990			...	...	...	70.6	S. & W.		10	Cloudy			
Extreme range	0.55			...	...	...	28.0	W. & N.		8	Rain fell on		8	

REMARKS.

1st. Evening very fine and mild.
2d. Very fine. Evening perfectly calm and cloudless.
3d. Very fine. At 9 P. M., wind very light from N. W.
4th. Began to rain from 9½ to 10 P. M., with lightning in the west.
5th. Wind came to S. S. E. from 3 to 4 P. M.
6th. Light showers through the day and evening.
7th. Evening very clear, and refreshingly cool.
8th. Very fine.
9th. Air very damp in the evening, with indications of rain.
10th. Began to rain about 9 A. M., and rained nearly all day.
11th. Very heavy showers, with thunder, at 1 and 3 A. M. Amount of rain at 1 P. M., 1.8 inch.
12th. Began to rain at 2½ P. M., and rained steadily but moderately till 7½ P. M.
13th. Foggy this morning till 9 A. M.
14th. Light showers after 4 P. M. till 7 P. M.
15th. Clear morning.
16th, 17th, and 18th. Pleasant.
19th. At 6 A. M., wind from north; low, scudding fog-clouds coming from that direction; higher up, a few clouds passing from the east; still higher, a few clouds passing from the west. At 7 A. M., the thermometer rose to 64°. At 1 P. M., light showers.
20th. Cloudy and foggy at 6 A. M. Cleared off about 10 A. M. Cloudy again at noon.
21st. At 6 A. M., clouds from S. W.
23d. Began to rain very moderately in the morning, and continued till 1 P. M. Light showers in the afternoon and evening.
24th. Pleasant.
25th. Very clear day.
26th. Very clear.
27th. Fog-clouds in the morning.
28th. Sultry, with some appearances of rain.
29th. Warm and sultry.
30th. Clear the larger part of the day, and air pleasant.
31st. Some mist in the evening.

NOTE.—In the morning, the mean dew-point has been 4°.4 below the mean temperature; and at 1 P. M., 16°.4 below.

September, 1849. New Moon, 16d. 10h. 54m. A. M.

DAYS.	Barometer At 6 A. M.	At 1 P. M.	At 10 P. M.	Thermometer At 6 A. M.	At 1 P. M.	At 10 P. M.	Daily mean.	Winds At 6 A. M.	At 1 P. M.	At 10 P. M.	Weather At 6 A. M.	At 1 P. M.	At 10 P. M.	Rain
1	29.74	29.74	29.76	53	66	56	58.3	N. E. 2	N. E. 2	N. E. 1	Rain	9	2	0.78
S 2	29.89	29.96	29.97	52	66	53	57.0	N. by W 1	N. W. 2	N. W. 2	0	0	0	
3	30.10	30.11	30.16	46	70	52	56.0	N. by W 1	N. W. 1	S. W. 1	0	0	0	
4	30.16	30.11	30.11	50	69	60	59.7	S. W. 1	S. W. 3	S. W. 1	0	5	10	
5	30.07	30.01	29.94	62	79	64	68.3	S. W. 1	S. W.	S. W. 1	Rain	...	0	} 1.00
6	29.85	29.80	29.64	60	79	69	69.3	S. W. 2	S. E. 3	S. E. 2	2	6	Rain	
7	29.56	29.63	29.84	71	82	58	70.3	S. W. 2	S. W. 2	N. W. 1	10	9	Sh'r, 0	
8	29.94	29.94	29.93	50	66	54	56.7	N. by W 2	N. W. 2	N. W. 1	0	0	0	
S 9	30.01	30.06	30.14	50	66	56	57.3	N. W. 2	N'ly 2	N. W. 1	0	0	0	
10	30.20	30.19	30.20	49	70	56	58.3	N. W. 1	N. E. 1	N. E. 1	0	0	0	
11	30.23	30.21	30.24	52	70	57	59.7	N. by E. 2	N. E. 2	N. E. 1	0	3	0	
12	30.22	30.14	30.10	51	71	57	59.7	N. E'ly 1	S. E. 2	N. E. 1	2	0	0	
13	30.08	30.03	30.08	57	76	60	64.3	S. E'ly 1	S. E'ly 1	S'ly 1	0	0	0	
14	30.14	30.12	30.09	57	72	64	64.3	N. E. 1	N. E. 1	S. E'ly 1	10, Fog	4	10	
15	29.93	29.82	29.96	59	72	63	64.7	S. by E. 1	S. W. 2	N. W. 2	9	10, Sh'r	0	
S 16	29.96	29.86	29.81	60	74	65	66.3	N. E. 1	S. W. 2	S. W. 1	6	10	0	
17	29.68	29.67	29.68	65	72	67	68.0	S. W. 2	S. W. 2	S. W. 1	3	10	Sh'r, 0	
18	29.79	29.79	29.97	61	71	53	61.7	N. W. 1	N. W. 2	N. W. 2	0	1	0	
19	30.10	30.09	30.10	48	60	48	52.0	N. W. 1	N. W. 1	N. W. 1	0	1	1	
20	30.06	30.00	29.93	48	64	50	54.0	N. E. 1	E'ly 1	N. E. 1	10	2	0	
21	29.87	29.87	29.88	50	65	52	55.7	N. E. 1	N. E. 3	N. E. 1	5	6	0	
22	29.81	29.69	29.53	51	71	59	60.3	N. E. 2	S. E. 2	S. E. 1	10	9	Rain	
S 23	29.32	29.29	29.38	63	71	51	61.7	S. W. 1	W'ly 3	W'ly 3	Rain	5	0	0.25
24	29.41	29.44	29.51	48	70	49	55.7	W'ly 2	W'ly 3	W'ly 1	0	2	0	
25	29.60	29.57	29.57	50	73	59	60.7	W'ly 1	W'ly 2	S. W. 2	0	2	0	
26	29.46	29.40	29.49	59	76	59	61.3	S. W. 2	S. W. 3	W'ly 3	2	2	Sh'r, 10	0.65
27	29.66	29.66	29.81	51	61	46	52.7	N. W. 1	N. W. 3	N. W. 1	9	2	0	
28	29.79	29.73	29.78	46	72	62	60.0	N. W. 1	S. W. 2	S. W. 1	0	0	0	
29	[illegible]	[illegible]	[illegible]	[illegible]	[illegible]	[illegible]	[illegible]	[illegible]	[illegible]	[illegible]	[illegible]	[illegible]	[illegible]	
S 30	29.67	29.64	29.55	53	57	53	54.3	N. E. 1	N. E. 1	N. E. 1	9	10	Rain	0.46
Means	29.87	29.84	29.86	54.2	70.1	57.1	...	1.3	2.0	1.3	3.1	3.5	2.7	3.14
									1.5			3.2		
REDUCED TO SEA LEVEL.								Prevailing winds from some point between—		Days.			Days.	
Max.	30.41	30.39	30.42	71	82	69	70.3							
Min.	29.50	29.47	29.56	46	60	46	52.0							
Mean	30.05	30.02	30.04					N. & E.		8	Clear		13	
Range	0.91	0.92	0.86	25	22	23	18.3	E. & S.		3	Variable		} 7	
Mean of month	30.037			...	...	...	60.5	S. & W.		11	Cloudy			
Extreme range	0.95			...	...	...	36.0	W. & N.		8	Rain fell on		10	

1st. Fine rain in the morning. Evening clear and fine.
2d. Very clear. Scarcely a cloud during the day.
3d. At sunrise, thermometer 44°. Day very fine.
4th. Very fine.
5th. Rain in the morning. Pleasant in the afternoon.
6th. Began to rain moderately at 8 P. M.
7th. Light showers at 3 P. M.
8th to 11th. Very fine.
12th. Very fine. Faint aurora at 10 P. M.; low faint streamers.
13th. Very fine.
14th. At 7 A. M., the thermometer stood at 61°, while the dew-point was 60°.
15th. Wind came to S. W. early in the morning Light showers at 2 P. M. Evening very clear, with wind at N. W.
16th. Air damp and rather raw. Clouds prevailed.
17th. Very damp and sultry. Sprinkling of rain at 2 h. 45 m. P. M.
18th. Very fine. Aurora in the evening, with faint streamers.
19th. Very fine.
20th. Evening very clear.
21st. Clouds prevailed through the day. Evening clear.
22d. Began to rain at 10½ P. M.
23d. Showery in the morning. Evening very clear.
24th and 25th. Very fine.
26th. Appearances of rain in evening. Heavy shower from 10½ to 11 P. M.
27th. Fine. Evening very clear.
28th. Fine.
29th. Pleasant.
[illegible] during the night equal to .46 inch.

October, 1849. New Moon, 16d. 0h. 10m. A. M.

Days.	Barometer, reduced to 32° F. Sunrise.	At 1 P. M.	At 10 P. M.	Thermometer. Sunrise.	At 1 P. M.	At 10 P. M.	Daily mean.	Winds (Direction and Force.) Sunrise.	At 1 P. M.	At 10 P. M.	Weather (Tenths Cloudy.) Sunrise.	At 1 P. M.	At 10 P. M.	Rain and Snow in Inches of Water.
1	29.46	29.38	29.53	51	52	44	49.0	N. E. 2	N. E. 3	N'ly 3	Rain	Rain	10	0.90
2	29.61	29.73	29.83	40	55	48	47.7	N. W. 2	N. W. 2	N. E'ly 1	2	4	9	
3	29.88	29.84	29.88	45	59	47	50.3	N. E. 1	N. E. 1	N. E. 1	5	2	0	
4	29.80	29.69	29.71	45	54	51	50.0	N. E. 1	N. E. 1	N'ly 1	10	Rain	Rain	} 0.50
5	29.76	29.76	29.83	48	56	51	51.7	N. E. 1	N. E. 1	N. E. 1	Rain	10	10	
6	29.83	29.72	29.57	46	55	49	50.0	N. E. 1	N. E. 1	N. E. 2	10	Rain	Rain	} 2.75
S 7	29.19	29.09	29.26	49	51	49	49.7	N. E. 3	N. E. 3	N. E. 2	Rain	10	Rain	
8	29.56	29.66	29.85	42	50	47	46.3	N. W'ly 1	N. W. 1	N. W. 1	10	10	10	
9	29.91	29.92	29.91	41	54	50	48.3	...	N. W. 1	N. E. 1	...	10	10	
10	29.86	29.76	29.63	48	54	53	51.7	N. E. 2	N. E. 1	N. E. 1	10	Rain	Rain	} 0.75
11	29.35	29.19	29.21	55	57	46	52.7	S. E. 1	S. W. 3	W'ly 3	Rain	9	8	
12	29.45	29.48	29.62	46	61	50	52.3	W'ly 2	W'ly 2	W'ly 1	5	5	5	
13	29.66	29.64	29.77	44	57	45	48.7	N. W. 2	N. E. 2	N. E. 2	2	3	0	
S 14	29.92	29.99	30.10	38	49	40	42.3	N. by E. 2	N. E. 2	N. E. 1	0	0	0	
15	30.16	30.09	30.08	35	55	45	45.0	N. by W 1	S. E'ly 2	S. E'ly	0	2	2	
16	30.08	30.01	30.06	45	62	54	53.7	S'ly 2	S'ly 3	S'ly 2	4	2	9	
17	30.00	29.94	29.93	55	67	60	60.7	S'ly 1	S'ly 2	S'ly 1	Foggy	10	10	
18	29.99	29.99	30.03	57	60	52	56.3	N. W. 1	N. W. 2	N. W. 1	9	10	10	
19	30.09	30.05	30.06	48	59	48	51.7	N. E. 1	N. E. 1	N. E. 1	9, Sh'r	10	6	
20	30.09	30.04	30.07	40	56	44	46.7	N. E. 1	N. E. 1	N. E. 1	2	0	0	
S 21	30.08	30.01	29.85	41	59	60	53.3	N'ly 1	E'ly 1	S. E. 1	10	8	Rain	} 0.50
22	29.44	29.33	29.33	63	66	62	63.7	S'ly 1	S. W. 2	S. W'ly 2	Misty	Misty	2	
23	29.54	29.45	29.40	50	65	53	56.0	W'ly 1	S. W. 2	S. W. 1	0	0	0	
24	29.46	29.54	29.82	46	54	46	48.7	W'ly 2	N. W. 2	N. W. 1	0	7	0	
25	29.92	29.84	29.96	46	54	46	48.7	N. W. 1	W'ly 2	N. W. 1	2	5	2	
26	30.16	30.15	30.14	41	56	43	46.7	N. E. 1	S'ly 2	S'ly 1	0	0	0	
27	30.07	30.01	29.99	47	60	48	51.7	S'ly 1	...	N. W. 1	10	...	0	
S 28	30.08	30.06	30.03	48	60	54	54.0	N. E. 1	S'ly 5	S. E. 1	0	10	Foggy	
29	29.91	29.72	29.34	57	65	64	62.0	S. E. 1	S. E. 2	S. E. 4	Foggy	10	Rain	1.15
30	29.33	29.45	29.60	51	62	41	51.3	N. W. 1	...	N. W. 2	10	...	0	
31	29.76	29.77	29.98	36	45	32	37.7	W'ly 1	N. W. 2	N. W. 2	7	6	0	
Means	29.79	29.75	29.81	46.6	57.1	49.1	...	1.3	2.0	1.5	6.2	7.0	5.6	6.55
								1.6			6.2			
REDUCED TO SEA LEVEL.														
Max.	30.34	30.33	30.32	63	67	62	63.7							
Min.	29.37	29.27	29.39	35	45	32	37.7							
Mean	25.97	29.93	29.99											
Range	0.97	1.06	0.93	28	22	30	26.0							
Mean of month	29.963			...	...	...	50.9							
Extreme range	1.07			...	...	...	35.0							

Prevailing winds from some point between— Days.

- N. & E. 11
- E. & S. 7
- S. & W. 5
- W. & N. 8

Days.

- Clear 6
- Variable . . . } 16
- Cloudy . . . . }
- Rain fell on . . 9

Remarks.

1st. Steady rain through the day.

2d. Thermometer 38° at sunrise. At 10 P. M., wind N. E., while the clouds were passing from the west.

3d Clouds prevailed through the day. Clear evening.

4th. Began to rain moderately at 8 A. M. Rainy through the day.

5th. Moderate rain at intervals in the morning.

6th. Began to rain moderately at 5 P. M. Steady rain continued. From 11 P. M. to 1 or 2 in the morning, rain and wind very heavy.

7th. Heavy rain, with thunder, from 7 to 8 A. M. Moderate rain at intervals during the day.

8th. Clouds thin, but no sun. Appearances of storm in the evening.

9th. Clouds thin, but no sun.

10th. Mist and rain in afternoon and evening.

11th. Evening very blustering.

12th. Mild, with many clouds.

13th. Very clear evening, with slight show of the aurora quite low down in the north.

14th. Very cool. Aurora late in the evening.

15th. First white frost in the College yard—quite copious. Thermometer in the garden 33°.

16th. Mild.

17th. Sun out at intervals. Stars appeared occasionally in the evening, but were, for the most part, concealed by clouds.

18th. Clouds thin. Sun occasionally seen.

19th. Clouds rather thin. Sprinkling of rain at 5 A. M.

20th. Very fine.

21st. Clouds prevailed. Began to rain very gently at 9½ P. M.

22d. Mostly clear in the evening.

23d. Very fine.

24th. Evening very clear.

25th. Pleasant.

26th. Fine.

27th. Pleasant.

28th. Clear in the morning. Evening raw and damp.

29th. Began to rain moderately at 7 P. M., but heavy at intervals, with high wind.

30th. Clouds prevailed during the day. Very clear in the evening, with appearances of aurora, notwithstanding the presence of the moon nearly full.

31st. Clouds prevailed during the day. Evening very clear.

November, 1849. New Moon, 14d. 4h. 5m. P. M.

Days.	Barometer Sunrise.	At 1 P. M.	At 10 P. M.	Thermometer Sunrise.	At 1 P. M.	At 10 P. M.	Daily mean.	Winds Sunrise.	At 1 P. M.	At 10 P. M.	Weather Sunrise.	At 1 P. M.	At 10 P. M.	Rain and Snow in Inches of Water.
1	30.05	29.97	29.97	27	39	31	32.3	N. W. 1	N. W. 2	N. W. 1	3	3	0	
2	29.95	29.85	29.77	30	42	35	35.7	N. W. 1	N. W.	N. W. 1	4	...	0	
3	29.72	29.71	29.73	32	50	50	44.0	W'ly 1	S. W.	S'ly 1	5	...	2	
S 4	29.85	29.85	29.93	50	67	54	57.0	S'ly 1	N. W. 2	N. E. 1	5	2	10	
5	29.96	29.88	29.89	44	58	52	51.3	N. E. 1	S. E. 2	S. E. 1	Hazy	10	Rain	
6	29.99	29.95	29.94	50	55	52	52.3	N. E. 1	N. E. 1	E'ly 1	Misty	10	10	
7	29.85	29.75	29.75	52	61	56	56.3	S'ly 1	S'ly 1	S'ly 1	10	Misty	10	
8	29.75	29.66	29.57	53	65	61	59.7	S'ly 1	S. E'ly 1	E'ly 3	10	10	Shower	} 1.62
9	29.49	29.48	29.53	61	64	56	60.3	S. E'ly 3	E'ly 2	E'ly 2	Rain	9	Rain	
10	29.56	29.56	29.61	53	59	45	52.3	S'ly 1	S'ly 1	W'ly 1	Foggy	10	0	
S 11	29.64	29.62	29.65	46	54	47	49.0	N. W. 2	N. W. 1	N. W. 2	8	8	10	
12	29.68	29.68	29.78	45	57	44	48.7	N. W. 2	N. W. 2	N. W. 1	3	2	0	
13	29.80	29.79	29.79	44	55	44	47.7	N. W. 2	N. W. 2	N. W. 1	2	4	0	
14	29.79	29.71	29.78	43	64	47	51.3	W'ly 1	W'ly 1	N. W. 1	2	0	0	
15	29.97	29.96	30.07	39	44	36	39.7	N'ly 1	N. E'ly 1	N. E. 1	0	0	0	
16	30.15	30.10	30.10	31	49	39	39.7	N. W. 1	N. W. 1	N. W. 1	0	0	2	
17	30.04	29.96	29.90	33	53	42	42.7	N. W. 1	S. W'ly 1	Calm	0	2	0	
S 18	29.84	29.77	29.71	40	55	46	47.0	Calm	N. E. 1	N. E. 2	3	10	7	
19	29.67	29.46	29.38	45	48	46	46.3	N. E. 3	N. E. 3	N. E. 3	10	Rain	Rain	} 0.80
20	29.37	29.37	29.43	42	47	43	44.0	N. E. 2	N'ly 2	N'ly 1	Rain	10	10	
21	29.57	29.57	29.69	42	52	43	45.7	N by W. 2	N. W. 2	N. W. 1	7	2	0	
22	29.83	29.79	29.81	42	54	44	46.7	N. W. 1	S. W. 1	S. W. 1	0	0	5	
23	29.88	29.84	29.91	45	58	49	50.7	S. W. 1	S. W. 1	S. W. 1	10	0	2	
24	30.03	29.98	30.02	45	58	50	51.0	N. W. 1	S. W. 1	Calm	5	10	Rain	
S 25	30.01	29.84	29.70	49	57	58	54.7	E'ly 2	E'ly 1	S'ly 2	10	10	10	
26	29.63	29.58	29.58	58	62	50	56.7	S. W. 2	W'ly 2	W'ly 1	5	10	5	
27	29.66	29.65	29.76	39	47	40	42.0	W'ly 2	N. W. 2	N. W. 1	0	0	0	
28	29.81	29.75	29.83	36	45	36	39.0	W. 2	W'ly 1	N. W. 1	0	8	5	
29	29.73	29.60	29.49	31	40	36	35.7	N. W. 1	W'ly 1	W'ly 1	0	3	10	
30	29.53	29.52	29.64	34	45	36	38.3	W'ly 2	W'ly 2	N. W. 1	3	5	0	
Means	29.79	29.74	29.76	42.7	53.5	46.2	...	1.5	1.5	1.3	4.5	5.7	4.9	2.42
								1.4			5.0			
REDUCED TO SEA LEVEL.														
Max.	30.33	30.28	30.28	61	67	61	60.3							
Min.	29.55	29.55	29.56	27	39	31	32.3							
Mean	29.97	29.92	29.94											
Range	0.78	0.73	0.72	34	28	30	28.0							
Mean of month	29.943			...	...	...	47.5							
Extreme range	0.78			...	...	...	40.0							

Prevailing winds from some point between— Days.

- N. & E. 5
- E. & S. 4
- S. & W. 8
- W. & N. 13

Days.

- Clear 12
- Variable . . . } 12
- Cloudy . . . . }
- Rain fell on . . 6

Remarks.

1st. Thermometer in the garden 26°. Evening clear.

2d. Fine. Evening very clear.

3d. Hazy during the day. Sun red.

4th. Very hazy. The sun of a deep red hue.

5th. Light rain in the afternoon and evening.

6th. Mist frequent during the day.

7th. Cloudy, with occasional mist.

8th. Heavy dashes of rain from 5 to 6 P. M.; wind fresh from easterly.

9th. Heavy showers in the morning. Nearly clear at 7 P. M. Rain again between 8 and 10 P. M.

10th. Fog in the morning. Evening clear.

11th. Clouds prevailed. Sun only occasionally seen.

12th. Fine. Evening very mild and clear.

13th to 17th. Very fine.

18th. Cloudy the greater part of the day.

19th. Began to rain from 9 to 10 A. M., and continued through the day and night.

20th. Moderate rain in the morning.

21st. Pleasant. Evening very clear.

22d. Pleasant. Evening much overcast with clouds.

23d Very fine.

24th. Began to rain very gently from 5 to 6 P. M.

25th. Appearances of rain. Wind very fresh at S. W. in the night.

26th. Very mild.

27th. Aurora quite bright from 4 to 5 A. M. Very fine through the day. Evening transparently clear.

28th. Pleasant.

29th. Appearances of storm.

30th. Pleasant. Evening very clear.

December, 1849. New Moon, 14d. 10h. 30m. A. M.

Days.	Barometer, reduced to 32° F. Sunrise.	At 1 P. M.	At 10 P. M.	Thermometer. Sunrise.	At 1 P. M.	At 10 P. M.	Daily mean.	Winds (Direction and Force.) Sunrise.	At 1 P. M.	At 10 P. M.	Weather (Tenths Cloudy.) Sunrise.	At 1 P. M.	At 10 P. M.	Rain and Snow in Inches of Water
1	29.45	29.39	29.58	37	52	28	39.0	S. W. 1	N. W. 3	N. W. 1	4	5	0	
S 2	29.92	30.15	30.13	15	29	28	24.0	N. W. 3	N. W. 1	N. E. 1	0	7	10	} 0.80
3	29.86	29.66	29.58	34	49	40	41.0	N. E. 3	N. E. 2	N. E. 2	Rain	Rain	Rain	
4	29.68	29.70	29.66	32	35	35	34.0	N. W. 2	N. W. 2	N. W.	10	10	10	
5	29.59	29.49	29.55	35	40	34	36.3	W. 1	S. W. 2	N. W. 1	10	Rain	0	
6	29.53	29.40	29.52	35	44	30	36.3	W'ly 1	W. by S. 2	N. W. 2	9	8	0	
7	29.77	29.80	29.92	27	30	24	27.0	N. W. 2	N. W. 3	N. W. 3	0	0	0	
8	30.08	29.90	29.99	24	31	29	28.0	N. W. 2	N. W. 1	N. W. 1	5	7	2	
S 9	29.97	29.86	29.59	23	30	30	27.7	N. W. 1	N'ly 1	N. E. 1	9	Hail	0	
10	29.69	29.70	29.76	34	40	35	36.3	W. 1	W'ly 1	N. E. 1	10	10	Snow	
11	29.79	29.81	30.02	31	32	21	28.0	N. W. 1	N. W. 3	N. W. 2	10	0	0	
12	30.14	30.21	30.14	17	27	20	21.3	N. W. 2	N. W. 3	N. W. 2	0	0	0	
13	30.07	29.97	29.89	22	35	30	29.0	W. N. W. 1	W. N. W. 2	W'ly 1	2	5	10	
14	29.83	29.78	29.85	24	38	31	31.0	N. W. 1	E'ly 1	N. E. 1	0	0	0	
15	30.19	30.08	30.14	25	41	33	33.0	N. E. 1	N. E. 1	N. E. 1	0	9	5	
S 16	29.99	29.80	29.59	39	43	47	43.0	S. E. 1	S. E. 1	S'ly 1	Misty	Rain	10	0.45
17	29.64	29.69	29.87	40	45	32	39.0	W'ly 1	N. W. 2	N. W. 3	2	4	0	
18	30.05	30.05	30.19	24	32	23	26.3	N. W. 1	N. W. 2	N. W. 1	0	0	0	
19	30.33	30.21	29.93	19	34	37	30.0	N. E'ly 1	S. E. 1	S. E'ly 3	0	10	Snow	0.27
20	29.73	29.57	29.41	43	55	50	49.3	S'ly 1	S'ly	S. W.	10	10	Sh'r, 10	0.10
21	29.67	29.78	29.94	36	41	29	35.3	N. W. 2	N. W. 1	N. W. 2	0	0	0	
22	29.80	29.41	28.85	28	37	41	35.3	N. E. 1	E'ly 3	S. W. 3	10	Rain	10	1.10
S 23	29.20	29.39	29.51	29	36	33	32.7	N. W. 3	W'ly 2	W'ly 2	5	1	5	
24	29.53	29.39	29.28	32	37	33	34.0	N. E. 1	E'ly 1	N'ly 1	10	Rain	10	
25	29.31	29.39	29.65	26	20	7	17.7	N. W'ly 1	N. W. 3	N. W. 2	Snow	4	0	
26	30.10	30.01	29.91	7	17	22	15.3	N. W. 2	N. W. 2	W'ly 2	0	0	10, Sn.	
27	29.88	29.87	29.95	21	31	28	26.7	N. W. 1	N. W. 1	N. W. 1	0	0	1	
28	30.13	30.17	30.09	23	31	29	27.7	N. W. 1	N. W. 1	W'ly 1	0	2	10	
29	29.94	29.71	29.58	29	42	36	34.0	N. E. 1	Calm	W'ly	Snow	Misty	10	} 0.80
S 30	29.86	29.91	29.98	25	30	26	27.0	N. W. 1	N. W. 1	N. W. 1	0	0	10	
31	29.85	29.86	30.00	21	21	20	20.7	N. E. 2	N. W. 2	N. W. 1	Snow	0	10	
Means	29.83	29.78	29.78	27.6	35.6	30.4	...	1.5	1.8	1.6	5.0	5.2	4.9	3.52
									1.6			5.0		
Reduced to sea level.														
Max.	30.51	30.39	30.37	43	55	50	49.3							
Min.	29.38	29.57	29.03	7	17	7	15.3							
Mean	30.01	29.96	29.96											
Range	1.13	0.82	1.34	36	38	43	34.0							
Mean of month	29.977			...	...	...	31.2							
Extreme range	1.48			...	...	...	48.0							

Prevailing winds from some point between— Days.
N. & E. 6
E. & S. 2
S. & W. 2
W. & N. 21

Days.
Clear 8
Variable . . . } 8
Cloudy . . . . }
Rain or snow fell on 15

Remarks.

1st. Variable.
2d. Very cold and raw, with appearances of storm.
3d. Ground covered with snow about a half inch deep at sunrise, with hail and rain falling at the time, and wind fresh at N. E. At noon, the snow had disappeared. First snow of the season.
4th. Cloudy.
5th. Raw air at sunrise. Sprinkling of rain from 11 A. M. to 1 P. M.
6th. Flurry of snow from 8 to 9 P. M. Cleared, and grew much colder.
7th. Fine.
8th. Cool, but not unpleasant.
9th. Occasional mist and sleet in the afternoon and evening.
10th. Began to snow moderately from 10 to 11 P. M.
11th. Ground covered with snow an inch deep. Clear in the afternoon and evening.
12th. Very fine, but cool.
13th. Pleasant. Appearances of storm in the evening.
14th. Mild. 15th. Pleasant.
16th. Mist in morning. Brisk rain from 11 to 12 A. M. Light rain and mist in the afternoon.
17th. Pleasant. Blustering in the evening.
18th. Fine.
19th. Began to snow moderately at 7 P. M., and ceased about 10 P. M.
20th. Snow disappeared. Shower at 5 to 6 P. M.
21st. Fine. Faint fog-bow about moon at 9 P. M.
22d. Began to hail and rain from 1 to 2 P. M.; wind light E'ly. Wind and storm increased. At 6 P. M., wind heavy, and barom. fallen to 29.02. At 8 P. M., wind hauled to S. W.; barom. 28.95. From 10 to 11 P. M., barom. stationary at 28.94. Clouds broken, and the moon out at intervals.
23d. Pleasant. Light flurry of snow on the ground in the morning.
24th. Flurry of snow on the ground at sunrise. Moderate rain and snow from 11 A. M. to 3 P. M.
25th. Snowing at sunrise; wind light at N. W. Snow soon ceased. Evening cold; piercing wind.
26th. Cold. Appearances of storm in evening.
27th. Ground this morning covered with snow from 1 to 2 inches deep. The day pleasant.
28th. Appearances of snow in the evening.
29th. Began to snow moderately about sunrise, and continued with some mist.
30th. Day very fine. Appearances of snow in the evening.
31st. Snowing at sunrise, which ceased about 10 A. M. Then clear, and again cloudy.

January, 1850. New Moon, 13d. 6h. 11m. A. M.

Days.	Barometer Sunrise.	At 2 P. M.	At 10 P. M.	Thermometer Sunrise.	At 2 P. M.	At 10 P. M.	Daily mean.	Winds Sunrise.	At 2 P. M.	At 10 P. M.	Weather Sunrise.	At 2 P. M.	At 10 P. M.	Rain and Snow
1	30.11	30.03	30.03	9	24	19	17.3	N. W. 2	...	N. W. 1	0	8	0	
2	30.09	30.00	30.01	19	30	26	25.0	N. W. 1	...	S. W. 1	5	...	Snow	
3	29.95	29.86	29.64	26	35	30	30.3	S. W. 1	N. E. 1	N. E. 1	10	10	Snow	
4	29.64	29.66	29.75	29	37	28	31.3	N. W. 1	N'ly 1	N. W. 2	10	10	5	
5	29.84	29.86	29.99	18	30	21	23.0	N. W. 1	N. W. 2	N. W. 2	0	0	0	
S 6	30.19	30.22	30.28	16	28	21	21.7	N. W. 2	N. W. 2	N. W. 2	0	0	0	
7	30.21	30.07	29.73	20	35	34	29.7	N. W. 1	N. E. 1	E'ly 2	10	10	Rain	} 0.52
8	29.60	29.87	30.04	30	32	31	31.0	N. E. 2	N. E. 1	N. E. 1	Snow	10	Snow	
9	30.06	29.90	29.79	25	33	36	31.3	N. E. 1	N. E. 1	W'ly 2	10	10	0	
10	29.97	30.05	30.09	33	33	19	28.3	N. W. 1	N. W. 2	N. W. 2	2	2	0	
11	29.94	29.65	29.25	23	38	46	35.7	N. E. 1	S. E. 2	S. E. 3	10	Rain	Rain	1.18
12	29.20	29.32	29.61	41	49	37	42.3	S. W. 1	N. W. 1	N. W. 3	10	6	0	
S 13	29.91	30.00	30.13	28	32	27	29.0	N. W. 2	N. W. 2	N. W. 2	2	0	5	
14	30.10	30.12	30.27	16	23	22	20.3	N. W. 3	N. by E. 3	N'ly 3	10	8	0	
15	30.22	30.11	30.01	22	33	30	28.3	N. W. 2	...	N. W. 2	0	...	3	
16	29.89	29.76	29.89	32	37	29	32.7	W'ly 2	N. W. 2	N. W. 1	Snow	0	0	
17	29.92	29.84	29.76	24	39	36	33.0	N. W. 1	N. W. 1	S. E. 1	2	10	10	
18	29.64	29.44	29.31	34	39	32	35.0	E'ly 1	N. E. 1	N. E. 2	Foggy	Foggy	Snow	1.00
19	29.74	29.84	30.02	24	29	22	25.0	N. W. 2	N. W. 3	N. W. 1	0	0	0	
S 20	30.10	30.03	30.03	20	31	23	24.7	N. W. 1	N. W. 2	N. W. 1	0	0	2	
21	30.01	29.93	29.64	26	38	35	33.0	N'ly 1	S. E'ly 1	E'ly 2	10	10	Rain	} 2.10
22	29.11	29.04	29.71	40	36	35	37.0	E. by S. 2	N. W. 3	N. W. 3	Rain	10	2	
23	29.98	30.06	30.20	29	38	31	32.7	N. W. 2	N. W. 1	N. W. 1	0	0	0	
24	30.31	30.26	30.20	25	41	35	33.7	N. W. 1	N. W. 1	S. W. 2	0	10	10	
25	29.88	29.68	29.83	35	51	39	41.7	S. E. 1	S. W. 1	S. W. 1	Rain	9	6	0.30
26	29.86	29.77	29.73	37	46	36	39.7	N. W. 1	S. W. 1	S. W. 1	9	4	Hazy	
S 27	29.55	29.46	29.63	39	50	39	42.7	S'ly 2	S. W. 1	N. W. 1	Misty	9	0	
28	29.77	29.70	29.37	31	43	32	35.3	N. W. 1	E'ly 2	N. E. 2	2	10	Snow	0.50
29	29.64	29.77	30.00	28	31	23	27.3	N'ly 1	N. W. 2	N. W. 1	10	0	0	
30	[illegible]	[illegible]	[illegible]	[illegible]	[illegible]	[illegible]	[illegible]	[illegible]	[illegible]	[illegible]	0	0	0	
31	30.42	30.27	30.01	13	33	35	27.0	N. W. 1	S'ly 2	S. W. 2	0	2	9	
Means	29.91	29.87	29.90	26.1	35.5	29.8		1.4	1.6	1.7	5.5	5.8	4.6	5.00
									1.6			5.3		
Reduced to sea level.														
Max.	30.60	30.45	30.54	41	51	46	42.7							
Min.	29.29	29.22	29.43	9	24	16	17.3							
Mean	30.09	30.05	30.06											
Range	1.31	1.23	1.11	32	27	30	25.4							
Mean of month	30.067			...	...	...	30.5							
Extreme range	1.38			...	...	...	42.0							

Prevailing winds from some point between Days.
N. & E. 7
E. & S. 2
S. & W. 4
W. & N. 18

Days.
Clear 9
Variable . . . } 10
Cloudy . . . . }
Rain or snow fell on 12

Remarks.

1st. Very fine.
2d. Pleasant. Dusting of snow in evening.
3d. Another dusting of snow this evening.
4th. Mild.
5th and 6th. Very fine.
7th. Mild. Flurry of snow during the night.
8th. Light snow at sunrise and at 9 P. M.
9th. Occasional flurries of snow, with mist late in the afternoon. Cleared from 8 to 9 P. M.
10th. Pleasant.
11th. Began to rain moderately from noon to 1 P. M., and increased. Pretty heavy in evening. Barometer fell with considerable rapidity.
12th. The snow and ice have nearly all disappeared. Very mild and pleasant.
13th. Pleasant for the season.
14th. Very raw. Clouds general, but thin.
15th. Pleasant.
16th. Flurry of snow from 7 to 8 A. M.
17th. Appearances of storm in the evening.
18th. Began to rain and snow from 2 to 3 P. M. Soon changed to snow, which fell fast till between 10 and 11 P. M. At 10 P. M., barom. 29.38. At 11 P. M., clouds broken. At 11½ P. M., mostly clear, and barom. at 29.50.
19th. About six inches of damp snow on the ground this morning, giving by the gauge nearly one inch of water. Aurora, not very bright, noticed at 11½ P. M.
20th. Pleasant.
21st. Random snow in the air in the afternoon. Mist and rain at 5 P. M., with wind E. N. E., which became moderate rain, and continued through the evening.
22d. Barom. at sunrise 29.18; wind rather fresh at about E. by S., and raining moderately. At 9 A. M., bar. 29.15; still raining. At 11 A. M., bar. 29.08; foggy, and wind light N. W. At 1 P. M., bar. 29.12; wind blustering at N. W., and rain [illegible]
23d. Very fine.
24th. Pleasant. Cloudy in the afternoon. Some flakes of snow in the evening.
25th. Moderate rain from 5 to 10 A. M.
26th. Pleasant. Halo about moon in evening.
27th. Wind came to W'ly, and clouds dispersed from 2 to 3 P. M.
28th. Began to snow and hail moderately at 2½ P. M.; wind light E'ly.
29th. About five inches of moist snow on the ground this morning.
30th. Very fine.
31st. Pleasant.

February, 1850. New Moon, 12d. 1h. 21m. A. M.

DAYS.	BAROMETER, REDUCED TO 32° F. Sunrise.	At 2 P. M.	At 10 P. M.	THERMOMETER. Sunrise.	At 2 P. M.	At 10 P. M.	Daily mean.	WINDS. (DIRECTION AND FORCE.) Sunrise.	At 2 P. M.	At 10 P. M.	WEATHER. (TENTHS CLOUDY.) Sunrise.	At 2 P. M.	At 10 P. M.	RAIN AND SNOW IN INCHES OF WATER.
1	30.06	30.00	30.06	30	43	32	35.0	W'ly 1	W'ly 1	N. W. 1	5	0	0	
2	29.94	29.89	29.73	30	34	32	32.0	W'ly 1	S. E'ly 1	E'ly 1	10	Rain	10	} 0.65
S 3	28.97	29.22	29.65	49	39	23	37.0	S. W. 3	N. W. 2	N. W. 2	Rain	2	3	
4	30.04	29.98	30.09	12	21	17	16.7	N. W. 2	N. W. 2	N. W. 1	0	2	2	
5	30.28	30.28	30.45	10	15	6	10.3	N. W. 2	N. W. 3	N. W. 1	0	2	0	
6	30.50	30.52	30.46	0	15	14	9.7	N. W. 1	N. W. 1	N. W. 1	0	0	0	
7	30.35	30.20	30.18	18	33	25	25.3	Var.	S. W. 1	Calm	9	Snow	0	
8	30.10	30.01	29.84	19	37	37	31.0	S. W'ly 1	S. W'ly 1	S. W. 1	9	Snow	10	
9	29.75	29.64	29.46	39	46	45	43.3	S. W. 1	S'ly 1	S'ly 2	Foggy	Misty	Rain	1.45
S 10	29.06	29.08	29.35	46	52	36	44.7	S'ly 1	W. by S. 2	W'ly 1	F'g, sh'r	2	0	
11	29.50	29.48	29.60	32	42	36	36.7	W. by S. 1	W'ly 2	W'ly 2	0	6	9	
12	29.76	29.75	29.87	34	39	30	34.3	N. W. 2	W.N.W. 2	N. W. 1	3	0	0	
13	29.96	29.95	29.86	25	36	30	30.3	N. W. 1	N. W. 1	S. W. 1	0	0	0	
14	29.67	29.47	28.96	28	41	43	37.3	N. E. 1	E. N. E. 2	S. W'ly 2	3	10, R'n	4	1.28
15	28.91	28.90	29.24	36	44	30	36.7	S. W. 1	W'ly 1	N. W. 3	9	10	0	
16	29.51	29.69	29.84	20	30	26	25.3	N. W. 1	N. W. 2	N. W. 1	0	0	0	
S 17	29.85	29.76	29.72	24	41	35	33.3	S. W. 1	S. W. 2	W'ly 2	0	0	0	
18	29.64	29.50	29.39	31	50	36	39.0	S. W. 1	S'ly 1	S. E'ly 1	0	6	7	
19	29.19	29.14	29.33	32	43	31	35.3	N'ly 1	N'ly 2	N. W. 4	10	9	0	
20	29.52	29.61	29.55	24	39	37	33.3	N. W. 2	W N W. 2	S. W. 2	0	0	10	
21	29.30	29.37	29.64	40	50	37	42.3	W'ly 2	W'ly 3	N. W. 2	0	0	0	
22	29.84	29.94	30.10	25	28	22	25.0	N. W. 3	N. W. 3	N. W. 1	3	0	0	
23	30.17	30.08	30.03	14	34	26	24.7	N. W. 1	W.S.W. 1	N. W. 1	0	0	0	
S 24	29.98	29.86	29.67	23	38	34	31.7	W N W 1	S'ly 1	S. W. 1	0	0	Hazy	
25	29.27	29.24	29.47	36	47	38	40.3	S. W. 2	S. W. 2	N. W. 1	10	10	2	
26	29.56	29.48	29.54	31	51	40	40.7	S. W. 1	S. W. 2	S. W. 1	2	0	1	
27	29.63	29.66	29.87	37	46	32	38.3	N. W. 1	W N.W. 2	W'ly 1	1	0	0	
28	29.98	29.88	29.65	22	37	33	30.7	N. W. 2	S'ly 1	S. E'ly 2	2	2	Snow	
Means	29.72	29.70	29.74	27.4	38.2	30.8	...	1.4	1.7	1.5	3.8	4.0	3.1	3.38
									1.5			3.6		
REDUCED TO SEA LEVEL.														
Max.	30.68	30.70	30.64	49	52	45	44.7	Prevailing winds from some point between—		Days.			Days.	
Min.	29.09	29.08	29.14	0	15	6	9.7	N. & E.		1	Clear		14	
Mean	29.90	29.88	29.92					E. & S.		3	Variable		} 7	
Range	1.59	1.62	1.50	49	37	39	35.0	S. & W.		8	Cloudy			
Mean of month	29.900			...	...	...	32.2	W. & N.		16	Rain or snow fell on		7	
Extreme range	1.62			...	...	...	52.0							

REMARKS.

1st. Very fine for the season.
2d. Moderate rain at intervals in the morning.
3d. At sunrise, wind strong S. W.; moderate rain; bar. 29.06. Bar. began to rise at 8½ A. M.; at 9 A. M., stood at 29.10, with wind W'ly and clouds broken; continued to rise, and sun out at noon.
4th. Fine.
5th. Very cold; wind piercing.
6th. At sunrise, ther. at zero; wind light N. W.; bar. 30.56. At 11 A. M., bar. 30.66; cold, but not unpleasant. At 1 P. M., bar. 30.58.
7th. Scattering flakes of snow at 9 A. M.; wind light S. W. Snow continued till about 2 P. M.
8th. Snow flakes falling from 11 A. M. to 3 P. M.
9th. Moderate rain about 3 P. M., continuing through evening and night; wind heavy at S'ly.
10th. Rain ceased about 6 A. M.; wind abated. From 7 to 8 A. M., light rain; wind S. by W.; bar. 29.13; foggy. At 9 A. M., bar. 29.14; at 11 A. M., 29.16, wind light S. W. Cleared about noon.
11th. Pleasant. 12th. Very fine.
13th. Fine. Light patches of haze in evening.
14th. At sunrise, pleasant; wind light N. E'ly; light, thin clouds in different parts of sky. At 9 A. M., overcast; wind increased. At 2½ P. M., began to rain moderately; wind fresh at about E. N. E. From 5 to 8 P. M., rain copious; nearly ceased by 8¾ P. M., and wind much abated; bar. 29.03. At 9 P. M., calm and stars out; bar. 29.03. At 9½ P. M., mostly clear; wind light W'ly; bar. 29.03. At 10 P. M., bar. 29.05; wind W'ly, fresh and rather gusty. At 11 P. M., bar. 29.05.
15th. At 5 A. M., mostly clear. At sunrise, bar. 28.99; clouds broken. At 9 A. M., bar. 29.03; at 10 A. M., 29.03; at 1 P. M., 29.00. At 2 P. M., flurry of snow. At 5 P. M., bar. 29.06; wind N. W'ly. At 6 P. M., bar. 29.13; wind fresh at N. W. Frost quite out of the ground in many places.
16th, 17th, and 18th. Very fine.
19th. Clouds general, but thin. Cleared from 7 to 8 P. M. Wind very blustering in evening.
20th. Pleasant. 21st. Fine.
22d. Blustering. Evening very fine.
23d. Very fine.
24th. Very fine. Evening hazy, with light clouds. Halo about the moon.
25th. Mild. Evening very fine.
26th and 27th. Very fine.
28th. Pleasant in morning. Wind S'ly and air very raw in afternoon. Began to snow at 10 P. M. Very little frost in ground for the last fortnight.

March, 1850. New Moon, 13d. 6h. 9m. P. M.

DAYS.	BAROMETER At 6 A. M.	At 2 P. M.	At 10 P. M.	THERMOMETER At 6 A. M.	At 2 P. M.	At 10 P. M.	Daily mean.	WINDS At 6 A. M.	At 2 P. M.	At 10 P. M.	WEATHER At 6 A. M.	At 2 P. M.	At 10 P. M.	RAIN AND SNOW
1	28.89	28.80	29.18	40	50	39	43.0	Var.	W N W 3	W'ly 3	Rain	2	9	1.37
2	29.48	29.53	29.53	29	41	34	34.7	N. W. 1	N. W. 2	S. W. 2	0	0	0	
S 3	29.59	29.57	29.73	36	22	15	24.3	N. E. 2	N. E. 2	N. W. 1	10	Snow	0	
4	29.94	29.97	30.01	11	24	22	19.0	N. W. 1	N. W. 2	N. W. 1	0	0	0	
5	30.03	30.07	30.00	23	34	28	28.3	N. W. 1	N. W. 2	W'ly 1	6	0	0	
6	29.87	29.76	29.44	27	43	38	36.0	S. W. 1	S. W. 1	S. W. 2	5	Rain	Rain	1.60
7	28.86	28.94	29.19	38	41	36	38.3	N. W. 1	N. W. 2	N. W'ly 3	F'g, m't	10	6	
8	29.38	29.51	29.78	33	39	30	34.0	N. W. 2	N. W. 3	N. W. 3	4	9	0	
9	29.88	29.90	29.88	25	41	36	34.0	N. W. 1	N. W. 1	W'ly 1	0	2	10	
S 10	29.71	29.62	29.71	34	46	33	37.7	S. E'ly 1	W'ly 1	N. W. 1	10	7	3	
11	29.82	29.87	29.92	25	35	29	29.7	N. W. 2	N. W. 3	N. W. 1	2	0	0	
12	29.89	29.96	30.04	30	36	31	32.3	E'ly 1	N. 2	N. E'ly 1	Snow	7	0	
13	30.05	29.90	29.65	34	52	51	45.7	S. by W. 1	S. W. 3	S. W. 3	2	3	Rain	} 0.52
14	29.55	29.38	29.49	51	58	49	52.7	S. W. 2	S. W. 1	S. W. 2	Rain	10	0	
15	29.60	29.76	29.90	39	51	36	42.0	N. W. 2	N. W. 2	N. W. 1	0	3	0	
16	29.98	29.97	30.10	32	50	37	39.7	N. W. 2	N. 2	E'ly 2	5	9	10	
S 17	30.11	30.03	29.93	36	42	35	37.7	E. N. E. 1	S. E'ly 2	S. E'ly 1	10	10	10	
18	29.78	29.67	29.63	33	33	32	32.7	E'ly 2	E. N. E. 2	N. E. 2	10	Snow	Snow	0.25
19	29.73	29.82	30.01	29	30	24	27.7	N. E. 2	N. 2	N. W. 3	10	3	0	
20	30.12	30.14	30.04	17	25	21	21.0	N. W. 3	N. W. 3	N. W. 2	0	0	0	
21	29.97	29.79	29.63	19	36	32	29.0	N. W. 2	N. W. 2	N. W. 2	0	0	3	
22	29.64	29.60	29.60	25	43	36	34.7	W. 2	N. W. 2	N. W. 1	0	0	9	
23	29.54	29.31	29.36	35	35	28	32.7	N. E. 1	N. E. 2	N'ly 2	10	Snow	7	1.00
S 24	29.46	29.47	29.50	27	37	29	31.0	N. W. 1	N. W. 2	N. W. 1	0	0	0	
25	29.51	29.44	29.48	23	34	28	28.3	W'ly 1	N. W. 3	N. W. 3	0	3	0	
26	29.52	29.51	29.60	23	35	30	29.3	W S.W. 1	W. 3	N. W. 1	0	0	0	
27	29.65	29.67	29.61	30	40	34	34.7	N. W. 2	W'ly 1	N. W. 1	9	10	10	
28	29.44	29.33	29.46	28	36	30	31.3	N. 1	N. by E. 1	N. W'ly 1	Snow	Snow	7	0.45
29	29.58	29.65	29.72	26	43	32	33.7	N. W. 1	S. W. 1	W'ly 1	2	0	0	
30	29.81	29.81	29.88	32	47	36	38.3	N. W. 2	N. W. 2	W'ly 1	0	0	0	
S 31	29.88	29.77	29.78	34	49	38	40.3	N'ly 1	N. E. 1	N'ly 1	10	8	0	
Means	29.69	29.66	29.70	29.8	39.0	32.6	...	1.5	2.0	1.6	5.0	5.0	3.7	5.19
									1.7			4.6		
REDUCED TO SEA LEVEL.														
Max.	30.30	30.32	30.28	40	58	51	52.7	Prevailing winds from some point between—		Days.			Days.	
Min.	29.04	28.98	29.36	11	22	15	19.0	N. & E.		5	Clear		12	
Mean	29.87	29.84	29.88					E. & S.		1	Variable		} 9	
Range	1.26	1.34	0.92	29	36	36	33.7	S. & W.		3	Cloudy			
Mean of month	29.863			...	...	...	34.0	W. & N.		22	Rain or snow fell on		10	
Extreme range	1.34			...	...	...	47.0							

REMARKS.

1st. At sunrise, foggy and moderate rain; quite calm. During night, wind heavy S. E. and E'ly, with snow and rain. At 7 A. M., bar. 28.96; at 8½ A. M., 28.92; wind light and variable, mostly from N. At 10 A. M., bar. 28.90; wind light but steady at N. W. At 1 P. M., wind blustering at about W. N. W. At 2½ P. M., barom. indicates upward movement; at 3 P. M., 28.95; at 6 P. M., 29.08. Aurora seen through broken clouds in the north.
2d. Very fine.
3d. Began to snow moderately at 9 A. M. At 10 A. M., barometer 29.75. Evening very clear. The ground scarcely covered with snow.
4th. Faint aurora observed from 9 to 11 P. M.
5th. Very fine.
6th. Began to rain moderately at 2 P. M.
7th. At 6 A. M., bar. 28.92; wind light N. W.; fog and mist. At 10 P. M., stars out and misty.
8th. Raw and blustering. Evening very clear.
9th. Fine. Began to be overcast about 8 P. M.
10th. Light flurry of snow on ground this morning. At 9 A. M., flurry of snow. Pleasant P. M.; half clear; wind light S. E. At 9 P. M., flurry of snow; wind W'ly. At 10 P. M., clear; wind N. W.
11th. Rather blustering. Evening very fine till 10 o'clock; quite hazy at 11 P. M.
12th. At 6 A. M., light snow, which continued till 9 A. M.—about one inch. Evening clear.
13th. Began to rain from 8 to 9 P. M.; wind S. W.
14th. Moderate rain in morning. In evening, clouds and lightning low down in the N. W.; else very clear.
15th. Very fine. 16th. Pleasant.
17th. Air raw and chilly.
18th. Moderate snow all day, melting as it fell.
19th. One or two inches of snow on the ground, which disappeared in the morning.
20th. Piercing cold wind.
21st. More pleasant. 22d. Pleasant.
23d. Damp snow fell from 7 A. M. till 8 or 9 P. M. Seven or eight inches deep, notwithstanding the melting underneath. At 9 P. M., clouds broken.
24th. About eight inches of damp snow on the ground; largest quantity at one time this winter.
25th. Wind cold and piercing.
26th. More pleasant.
27th. Clouds thin through the day.
28th. At sunrise, snow nearly two inches deep, and snowing. Snow continued through the day. At 9 P. M., clouds broken and moon out.
29th. Pleasant.
30th. Very fine. Snow nearly disappeared.
31st. Pleasant. Aurora quite bright in evening.

April, 1850. New Moon, 12d. 7h. 39m. P. M.

Days.	Barometer, reduced to 32° F. At 6 A. M.	At 2 P. M.	At 10 P. M.	Thermometer. At 6 A. M.	At 2 P. M.	At 10 P. M.	Daily mean.	Winds. (Direction and Force.) At 6 A. M.	At 2 P. M.	At 10 P. M.	Weather. (Tenths Cloudy.) At 6 A. M.	At 2 P. M.	At 10 P. M.	Rain and Snow in Inches of Water.
1	29.91	29.95	30.02	34	54	41	43.0	N. W. 1	N. W. 1	N. W. 1	0	0	0	
2	30.02	29.91	29.91	38	64	48	50.0	S. W. 1	S. W. 1	S. W. 1	0	0	3	
3	29.83	29.68	29.48	49	66	50	55.0	S. W. 2	S. W. 2	S. E'ly 2	0	9	10	
4	29.11	28.95	29.37	50	45	32	42.3	N. E. 2	N. E. 2	N'ly 3	Rain	Rain	Misty	1.90
5	29.57	29.65	29.48	31	36	32	33.0	N. 1	N. E. 2	N. E. 2	Misty	10	Snow	} 0.50
6	29.45	29.47	29.56	31	33	31	31.7	N. E. 3	N. E. 2	N. W. 1	Snow	Sn., r'n	9	
S 7	29.58	29.58	29.64	30	48	39	39.0	N. W. 1	N. W. 2	N. W. 1	0	0	0	
8	29.61	29.49	29.61	37	57	35	43.0	S. W. 2	S. W. 3	N. W. 3	4	10	6	
9	29.73	...	29.84	25	...	29	...	N. W. 2	...	N. W. 2	0	...	0	
10	29.87	29.77	29.85	29	43	32	34.7	N. W. 1	N. W. 2	N. W. 1	9	0	0	
11	29.89	29.77	29.79	29	51	33	37.7	N. W. 2	S. E. 2	S. E. 1	0	0	0	
12	29.80	29.78	29.75	35	44	34	37.7	E. 2	S. E. 2	S. E. 2	Snow	10	2	0.10
13	29.63	29.35	29.10	34	44	35	37.7	E'ly 1	E'ly 3	W. 2	5	Rain	0	0.45
S 14	29.25	29.36	29.49	32	37	30	33.0	W'ly 3	W'ly 3	W'ly 3	5	8	0	
15	29.62	29.66	29.79	30	38	32	33.3	N. W. 4	N. W. 4	N. W. 2	0	2	0	
16	29.72	29.72	29.84	33	38	29	33.3	N. W. 3	N. W. 3	N. W. 2	0	0	0	
17	29.87	29.80	29.94	26	41	28	31.7	N. W. 2	N. W. 2	N. W. 2	0	0	5	
18	30.01	30.05	30.06	26	44	34	34.7	N. W. 2	N. 2	N. E. 1	0	1	1	
19	30.02	29.85	29.78	36	54	41	43.7	W'ly 1	S. W. 3	S. W. 2	3	10	7	
20	29.87	29.81	29.89	40	60	38	46.0	N. W. 1	E'ly 2	N. W. 1	0	8	8	
S 21	29.99	30.02	30.07	40	55	39	44.7	E'ly 1	E'ly 1	E'ly 1	2	5	0	
22	30.02	29.93	29.74	42	49	52	47.7	S. W. 2	S'ly 2	S'ly 2	10	10, R'n	10	
23	29.56	29.58	29.83	53	57	40	50.0	S'ly 1	S'ly 2	N. W. 3	Misty	Misty	0	
24	30.05	29.96	29.88	33	50	42	41.7	N. W. 2	N. W. 2	S. W. 1	0	0	0	
25	29.85	29.77	29.78	43	69	54	55.3	W. 2	W. by S. 3	S. W. 2	1	4	5	
26	29.78	29.72	29.73	56	69	54	59.7	S. W. 1	S'ly 2	S'ly 1	10	10	10	
27	29.80	29.79	29.78	53	61	51	55.0	S'ly 1	S'ly 2	S'ly 1	Foggy	10	10	
S 28	29.77	29.78	29.75	53	59	50	54.0	S'ly 2	S'ly 2	S'ly 2	Foggy	5	Foggy	
29	29.45	29.25	29.62	51	63	51	55.0	S. by E. 2	S. W. 3	N. W. 3	Rain	7	2	1.72
30	29.93	29.95	29.91	42	67	51	53.3	N. W. 1	S. W. 2	S. W. 2	0	0	0	
Means	29.75	29.70	29.75	38.0	51.6	39.6	...	1.7	2.3	1.8	4.3	5.5	3.9	4.67
									1.9			4.6		
REDUCED TO SEA LEVEL.								Prevailing winds from some point between— Days.			Days.			
Max.	30.23	30.23	30.25	56	69	54	59.7	N. & E. 3			Clear 12			
Min.	29.29	29.13	29.37	25	33	28	31.7	E. & S. 6			Variable . . . } 9			
Mean	29.93	29.88	29.93					S. & W. 11			Cloudy . . . . }			
Range	0.94	1.10	0.88	31	36	26	28.0	W. & N. 10			Rain or snow fell on 9			
Mean of month	29.913			...	...	...	43.1							
Extreme range	1.12			...	...	...	44.0							

Remarks.

1st and 2d. Very fine.
3d. Very mild. Appearances of rain in the evening.
4th. Rain all day. From 5 to 6 P. M., rain and snow.
5th. Mist and occasional snow. Air very raw.
6th. Began to snow last evening at 10 o'clock, and continued all night and through this day moderately, and with occasional mixture of rain. About four inches of snow on the ground this morning. Clouds broken, and wind at N. W. in the evening. Bright aurora under the clouds at the north, which continued all night.
7th. Very fine. Snow nearly all disappeared during the day. Aurora again this evening, but not very bright.
8th. Pleasant in the morning. Very blustering in the evening.
9th. Cold and uncomfortable.
10th. Very fine.
11th. Air raw.
12th. Snowed moderately, melting as it fell, from about 5 to 10 A. M.
13th. Very changeable. Rained from about 1 to 4 P. M. Snowed from 4 to 5 P. M., melting as it fell.
14th. Very windy. A fall of snow in afternoon.
15th. Very cold and blustering.
16th. Flurry of snow for a few minutes at 8 P. M. Wind piercing from N. W. all day, and the cold severe.
17th. More pleasant, but still cold.
18th. Pleasant. Evening mild.
19th. Mild.
20th and 21st. Pleasant.
22d. Sprinkling of rain in the afternoon.
23d. Wind came to N. W. about 5 P. M. Evening clear and very gusty.
24th. Very pleasant.
25th. Very spring-like.
26th. Clouds general all day, but thin.
27th. Clouds thin, and occasional fog.
28th. Heavy fog in the evening.
29th. Heavy rain in the morning. Cleared from 1 to 2 P. M. Very gusty in the afternoon.
30th. Very fine.

May, 1850. New Moon, 11d. 6h. 1m. P. M.

Days.	Barometer At 6 A. M.	At 2 P. M.	At 10 P. M.	Thermometer At 6 A. M.	At 2 P. M.	At 10 P. M.	Daily mean.	Winds At 6 A. M.	At 2 P. M.	At 10 P. M.	Weather At 6 A. M.	At 2 P. M.	At 10 P. M.	Rain
1	29.77	29.70	29.92	51	57	42	50.0	S. W. 2	W'ly 3	N. W. 1	0	10	0	
2	29.92	29.92	29.96	39	53	44	45.3	N. W. 2	N. W. 2	N. W. 1	0	8	0	
3	30.03	29.89	29.88	44	63	50	52.3	N. W. 1	N. W. 2	S. W. 2	0	0	2	
4	29.76	29.68	29.71	50	60	46	52.0	S. W. 1	S. W. 1	N. E. 2	5	10	Rain	
S 5	29.77	29.76	29.70	45	48	55	49.3	N. E. 2	N. E. 2	E'ly 1	Misty	Rain	Misty	
6	29.69	29.62	29.60	55	62	56	57.7	S. E. 2	S. W'ly 2	S. W. 1	Rain	Foggy	9	2.22
7	29.71	29.79	29.91	45	64	51	53.3	N. W. 1	N. W. 1	N. W. 1	0	0	0	
8	29.95	29.89	29.81	45	65	51	53.7	N. W. 1	S. E'ly 2	S. E'ly 1	1	6	2	
9	29.51	29.25	29.39	52	54	46	50.7	S. E. 3	S. by W. 3	N. W. 1	Rain	Rain	0	1.10
10	29.59	29.57	29.66	42	58	45	48.3	N. W. 2	N. W. 3	W'ly 1	0	5	0	
11	29.69	29.63	29.66	42	55	44	47.0	N. W. 1	S. E'ly 2	S'ly 1	2	10	3	
S 12	29.67	29.58	29.63	41	61	49	50.3	N. W. 2	N. W. 2	N. W. 1	5	8	0	
13	29.60	29.62	29.69	52	76	57	61.7	W. by S. 2	W. by S. 3	S. W. 1	1	8	2	
14	29.76	29.78	29.78	51	66	54	57.0	N. E. 2	N. E. 2	S. E. 1	3	9	10	
15	29.72	29.57	29.33	54	59	49	54.0	S. E. 2	E'ly 2	N. E. 2	10	Rain	Misty	} 0.12
16	29.22	29.17	29.22	48	62	54	54.7	N.N.E. 2	N.N.E. 2	N. W. 2	Misty	10	2	
17	29.22	29.18	29.20	54	73	57	61.3	W'ly 2	S. W. 2	S. W. 2	2	10	8	
18	29.35	29.44	29.66	47	67	44	52.7	N. W. 2	N. W. 3	N. W. 1	3	2	0	
S 19	29.76	29.73	29.71	47	65	49	53.7	N. W. 2	N. W. 2	S. W. 1	0	3	0	
20	29.88	29.85	29.86	49	58	48	51.7	S. E. 2	S. E. 2	N. W. 2	3	8	Rain	0.50
21	29.90	29.93	29.98	48	53	46	49.0	S. E'ly 2	N. W. 1	W'ly 1	Rain	10	5	
22	30.03	30.04	30.04	42	63	47	50.7	N. W. 1	S. W. 2	S'ly 1	5	3	5	0.18
23	30.02	30.04	29.98	45	55	46	48.7	N. W. 2	N. E. 2	N. E. 2	Rain	10	10	
24	29.91	29.89	30.01	45	65	47	52.3	N. 2	S. E'ly 2	S'ly 1	5	4	2	
25	30.04	30.04	30.07	46	57	48	50.3	N. E. 2	N. E. 2	N. E. 2	10	10	Rain	
S 26	29.98	29.92	29.79	48	54	47	49.7	N. E. 2	N. E. 2	N'ly 1	Misty	10	Rain	} 0.73
27	29.61	29.49	29.47	46	54	61	53.7	N'ly 2	N'ly 2	N. W. 2	Rain	Rain	10	
28	29.49	29.63	29.73	61	61	50	57.3	N. W. 2	N. E. 3	N. E. 2	2	10	10	
29	29.70	29.62	29.61	51	62	52	56.0	N. W. 1	S. E'ly 2	S. E. 1	8	2	10, Sh'r	
[illegible]	[illegible]	[illegible]	[illegible]	[illegible]	[illegible]	[illegible]	[illegible]	[illegible]	[illegible]	[illegible]	[illegible]	[illegible]	Misty	[illegible]
31	29.71	29.72	29.80	46	58	46	50.0	N. E. 1	N. E. 2	N. E. 2	10	10	7	
Means	29.73	29.70	29.72	47.7	60.0	49.3	...	1.7	2.1	1.4	5.1	7.6	5.4	5.00
									1.7			6.0		
REDUCED TO SEA LEVEL.								Prevailing winds from some point between— Days.			Days.			
Max.	30.22	30.22	30.25	61	76	61	61.7	N. & E. 10			Clear 5			
Min.	29.40	29.35	29.38	39	48	42	45.3	E. & S. 5			Variable . . . } 8			
Mean	29.91	29.87	29.90					S. & W. 6			Cloudy . . . . }			
Range	0.82	0.87	0.87	22	28	19	16.4	W. & N. 10			Rain fell on . . 18			
Mean of month	29.893			...	...	...	52.3							
Extreme range	0.90			...	...	...	37.0							

Remarks.

1st. Squally from 1 to 3 P. M. Evening very pleasant.
2d. Pleasant.
3d. Very fine.
4th. Sprinkling at intervals in the afternoon. Very moderate rain in the evening.
5th. Mist and showers through the day.
6th. Heavy rain in the morning. Fog and mist in the afternoon.
7th. Very fine. In the evening, aurora quite bright from N. W. round to N. E., but without any streamers.
8th. Pleasant.
9th. Rain in the morning; heavy wind at S. E. and then S'ly. Cleared from 4 to 6 P. M. Evening fine.
10th. Pleasant.
11th. Air raw and chilly.
12th. Air raw. Aurora in the evening from 10° to 15° high, without streamers.
13th. Very pleasant in the morning. Heavy gusts of wind, with dashes of rain, in the afternoon.
14th. Pleasant.
15th. Moderate rain nearly all day.
16th. Mist, and occasional showers. Cleared about 9 P. M.
17th. Sprinkling of rain at 3 P. M. Heavy thunder, with rain, from 7 to 8 P. M.
18th. Fine.
19th. Very fine.
20th. Dashing rain at 1 P. M. Thunder and rain at 8 P. M., the rain continuing moderate till 9½ P. M.
21st. Showery through the day.
22d. Pleasant.
23d. Sprinkling and light showers: quite cool.
24th. Pleasant.
[illegible] with mist and a light shower in the evening.
26th. Thundershower from 8 to 9 P. M.
27th. Heavy thundershower from 5 to 6 A. M. Showery during the day.
28th. Very warm till 10 A. M., when the wind changed from N. W'ly to N. E., and the air immediately became cooler. Occasional light showers.
29th. Sprinkling of rain at 6 A. M.; wind N. W.
30th. Rain and mist. Weather very uncomfortable.
31st. Sun out occasionally. Light shower at 7 P. M.

June, 1850. New Moon, 10d. 2h. 11m. A. M.

Days.	Barometer, reduced to 32° F. At 6 A. M.	At 2 P. M.	At 10 P. M.	Thermometer. At 6 A. M.	At 2 P. M.	At 10 P. M.	Daily mean.	Winds. (Direction and Force.) At 6 A. M.	At 2 P. M.	At 10 P. M.	Weather. (Tenths Cloudy.) At 6 A. M.	At 2 P. M.	At 10 P. M.	Rain and Snow in Inches of Water.
1	29.80	29.75	29.74	46	59	45	50.0	N. E. 2	N. E. 2	N. E. 1	10	10	3	
S 2	29.74	29.70	29.75	47	74	55	58.7	N'ly 1	N. by E. 2	N. W'ly 1	2	7	5, Spr.	
3	29.82	29.82	29.87	54	74	54	60.7	N. W. 2	N. W. 2	S. W'ly 1	3	5	0, Spr.	
4	29.98	30.01	30.09	55	72	59	62.0	N. by E. 2	N. E. 2	N. W'ly 1	3	0	2	
5	30.14	30.11	30.14	56	82	59	65.7	N'ly 1	N. by E. 2	S. W. 1	0	0	0	
6	30.14	30.06	30.07	58	72	58	62.7	S. by W. 2	S. by E. 3	S'ly 1	1	2	0	
7	29.99	29.88	29.82	58	73	60	63.7	S'ly 1	S. E'ly 2	S'ly 1	1	1	0	
8	29.69	29.58	29.63	59	78	64	67.0	S'ly 2	S. E'ly 2	S'ly 1	3	8	10, Spr.	
S 9	29.57	29.52	29.55	64	82	66	70.7	N. W. 1	N. W. 1	S. W'ly 1	10	3	8	
10	29.44	29.25	29.43	63	76	55	64.7	S. W. 2	S. W. 2	N. W. 2	Rain	7, Spr.	0	1.00
11	29.67	29.77	29.89	51	64	54	56.3	N. W. 3	N. W. 2	N. W. 1	8	9	0	
12	29.88	29.82	29.73	53	79	58	63.3	N. W. 1	S. W. 3	W'ly 2	2	6	0	
13	29.69	29.63	29.67	63	85	66	71.3	S. W. 2	S. W. 3	S. W. 1	5	1	0	
14	29.67	29.66	29.70	64	84	69	72.3	S. W. 2	S. W. 2	S. W. 1	4	3	0	
15	29.74	29.73	29.78	63	80	62	71.7	S'ly 1	N'ly 2	N. W. 2	Spr., 7	2	8	
S 16	29.95	29.96	29.96	58	73	57	62.7	N. E. 2	N. E. 1	S'ly 1	0	0	0	
17	29.97	29.93	29.93	54	72	57	61.0	S. W'ly 1	S. W. 2	S. W. 1	1	0	0	
18	29.92	29.86	29.88	59	88	65	70.7	S. W. 1	S. W. 2	S. W. 2	0	0	5	
19	29.89	29.81	29.79	67	89	75	77.0	S. W. 2	S. by E. 1	S. W. 2	5	3	6	
20	29.79	29.73	29.71	75	93	73	80.3	S. W. 1	S. W. 2	N. W. 1	3	5	10, Sh'r	0.10
21	29.78	29.78	29.91	70	86	66	74.0	N. W. 2	N'ly 2	S'ly 1	2	4	2	
22	30.03	29.98	29.96	65	75	60	66.7	S'ly 1	S'ly 2	S'ly 2	5	...	10	
S 23	29.82	29.74	29.72	63	70	64	65.7	E. by S. 2	E'ly 1	W'ly 1	Rain	10	10	0.40
24	29.73	29.73	29.75	62	79	65	68.7	N'ly 1	N. W. 2	S'ly 1	10	3	0	
25	29.77	29.74	29.81	62	77	61	66.7	N. W. 1	N. W. 1	N. W. 1	0	3	0, Sh'r	0.10
26	29.80	29.83	29.73	62	78	66	68.7	N. W. 2	N. W. 3	N. W. 2	0	2	5	
27	29.78	29.76	29.75	64	84	68	72.0	S. W. 3	S. W. 2	S. W. 2	8	4	10	
28	29.72	29.71	29.72	65	80	70	71.7	E'ly 1	S'ly 1	S'ly 1	Misty	10	Misty	
29	29.65	29.57	29.64	65	87	75	75.7	S'ly 1	S. W. 2	S. W. 1	10, Sh'r	5	2	1.00
S 30	29.64	29.62	29.63	75	89	72	78.7	S. W. 1	S. W. 3	N. W. 0	8	5	0	
Means	29.81	29.77	29.79	60.7	78.3	62.6	...	1.6	2.0	1.2	4.7	4.1	3.2	2.60
REDUCED TO SEA LEVEL.								1.6			4.0			
Max.	30.32	30.29	30.32	75	93	75	80.3	Prevailing winds from some point between—		Days.			Days.	
Min.	29.62	29.43	29.61	46	59	45	50.0	N. & E.		3	Clear		7	
Mean	29.99	29.94	29.97					E. & S.		5	Variable		} 14	
Range	0.70	0.86	0.71	29	34	30	30.3	S. & W.		12	Cloudy			
Mean of month	29.967			...	...	...	67.2	W. & N.		10	Rain fell on		9	
Extreme range	0.89			...	...	...	48.0							

REMARKS.

1st. Very cool. Sun out occasionally in the afternoon. Evening mostly clear.
2d. Pleasant. Sprinkling of rain about 6 P. M.
3d. Sprinkling of rain at 4 P. M., and again, with thunder, from 6 to 7 P. M.
4th. Pleasant.
5th, 6th, and 7th. Very fine.
8th. Light shower, with thunder, at 3 P. M.
9th. Very hot sun at mid-day.
10th. Heavy rain in the morning. Sun out from 1 to 2 P. M. Heavy showers from 3 to 5 P. M. Evening very clear and cool.
11th. Dashes of rain at 1 P. M. Evening clear.
12th. Pleasant. Evening very fine.
13th. Sun very hot.
14th. Very fine.
15th. Sprinkling of rain at 8 A. M.
16th, 17th, and 18th. Very fine.
19th. Very hot.
20th. At 2 P. M., the thermometer stood at 93°. At 3 h. 20 m. P. M., the wind changed from S. W. to N. W., and was quite gusty, accompanied with thunder. At 4 P. M., sprinkling of rain. At 4½ P. M., the thermometer had fallen to 78°, being 15° in two hours. Light thundershower from 8 to 9 P. M.
21st. Fine.
22d. Pleasant. Appearances of rain in the evening.
23d. Fine showers in the morning. Sun out occasionally in the afternoon.
24th. Very fine.
25th. Pleasant. Brisk shower from 5 to 6 P. M.
26th and 27th. Pleasant.
28th. Occasional mist, with appearances of rain.
29th. Very heavy rain about 2 o'clock this morning.
30th. Very warm. Evening clear and very still.

July, 1850. New Moon, 9d. 9h. 19m. A. M.

Days.	Barometer At 6 A. M.	At 2 P. M.	At 10 P. M.	Thermometer At 6 A. M.	At 2 P. M.	At 10 P. M.	Daily mean.	Winds At 6 A. M.	At 2 P. M.	At 10 P. M.	Weather At 6 A. M.	At 2 P. M.	At 10 P. M.	Rain and Snow
1	29.65	29.63	29.73	72	85	64	73.7	S. W. 2	N. E. 2	N. E. 2	5	7, Sh'r	10	
2	29.77	29.78	29.84	61	71	61	64.3	N. E. 2	N. E. 2	N. E. 2	10	10	10	
3	29.82	29.78	29.75	61	66	64	63.7	N. E. 2	E'ly 2	E'ly 1	10	Rain	10	0.15
4	29.75	29.73	29.74	63	79	70	70.7	W'ly 1	S. E. 2	S'ly 2	10	8	0	
5	29.69	29.60	29.53	70	91	78	79.7	S'ly 1	W'ly 2	W'ly 1	10, Sh'r	3	Shower	
6	29.50	29.50	29.62	72	84	67	74.3	N. W. 2	N. W. 2	N. W. 1	3	2	0	0.35
S 7	29.74	29.72	29.71	65	81	66	70.7	N. W. 2	N. W. 3	N. W. 2	0	6	0	
8	29.73	29.74	29.78	67	80	65	70.7	N. W. 2	N. W. 2	N. W. 1	0	2	0	
9	29.81	29.82	29.88	59	81	61	67.0	N. W. 1	N. W. 2	E'ly 1	0	4	0	
10	29.96	29.98	30.01	56	79	62	65.7	N. E. 1	N. E. 1	N. E. 1	0	2	0	
11	30.02	29.98	29.96	56	76	58	63.3	N'ly 1	N. E. 2	N. E. 1	0	0	0	
12	29.95	29.88	29.88	56	76	63	65.0	N'ly 1	S. E. 2	S. W. 1	0	1	2	
13	29.89	29.85	29.84	64	80	64	69.3	S. W. 2	S'ly 2	E'ly 2	5	6	0	
S 14	29.86	29.84	29.85	70	80	73	74.3	S. W. 2	S. W. 3	S. W. 2	9	10	10	
15	29.88	29.85	29.92	73	88	75	78.7	S. W. 2	S. W. 3	S. W. 1	10	5	10	
16	29.97	29.96	29.99	74	89	74	79.0	S. W. 2	S. W. 2	S. W. 2	9	8	10	
17	29.99	29.96	29.94	74	88	76	79.3	S. W. 2	S. W. 2	S. W. 1	8	7	10	
18	29.91	29.83	29.83	75	85	74	78.0	S. W. 2	S. W. 3	S. E'ly 1	10	3	9	
19	29.79	29.58	29.56	74	76	72	74.0	S. E. 3	S. E. 4	S. E. 3	Rain	Rain	10	1.00
20	29.58	29.61	29.73	69	77	70	72.0	S. W. 2	S. W. 2	S. W. 1	8	Rain	8	
S 21	29.76	29.74	29.76	68	84	74	75.3	S. W. 1	S'ly 2	S'ly 1	3	2	5	
22	29.76	29.79	29.86	67	83	72	74.0	N. E. 1	N. E. 2	S'ly 1	1	3, Sh'r	0	0.10
23	29.87	29.90	29.91	72	90	71	77.7	N'ly 1	N. E'ly 1	S'ly 1	2	7	1	
24	29.92	29.85	29.80	66	86	73	75.0	N'ly 1	S. E'ly 2	S. W. 2	3	2	0	
25	29.70	29.65	29.75	71	92	70	77.7	S. W. 1	W'ly 2	N. W. 2	3	4	3	
26	29.87	29.85	29.84	58	71	62	63.7	N. E. 2	N. E. 2	N. W. 2	2	7	1	
27	29.89	29.84	29.86	54	80	66	66.7	N. W. 1	S. W. 1	S'ly 1	1	4	9	
S 28	29.86	29.84	29.83	64	74	72	70.0	S'ly 2	S'ly 2	S. W. 2	Rain	10	10	} 0.75
29	29.75	29.70	29.66	74	84	75	77.7	S. W. 2	S. W. 2	S. W. 2	Rain	10	0	
30	29.70	29.67	29.67	75	88	70	77.7	S. W. 2	S. W. 2	N. E. 2	5	5	10	
31	29.75	29.76	29.83	68	86	72	75.3	N. E. 1	E'ly 2	S. E. 2	10	3	4	
Means	29.81	29.78	29.80	66.7	81.6	68.8	...	1.6	2.1	1.5	5.4	5.5	4.9	2.35
REDUCED TO SEA LEVEL.								1.7			5.3			
Max.	30.20	30.16	30.19	75	92	78	79.7	Prevailing winds from some point between—		Days.			Days.	
Min.	29.68	29.68	29.71	54	66	58	63.3	N. & E.		9	Clear		8	
Mean	29.98	29.95	29.97					E. & S.		5	Variable		} 10	
Range	0.52	0.48	0.48	21	26	20	16.4	S. & W.		12	Cloudy			
Mean of month	29.967			...	...	...	72.4	W. & N.		5	Rain fell on		13	
Extreme range	0.52			...	...	...	38.0							

REMARKS.

1st. Very hot and sultry in the morning. Light showers at 2 P. M. Wind came to N. E., and grew cooler fast.
2d. Quite cool.
3d. Commenced raining moderately at noon. Light rain and mist in the afternoon.
4th. Pleasant.
5th. Very warm. Sprinkling of rain at 7 A. M. Light shower at 9 P. M. Heavy thunder and rain about midnight.
6th to 10th. Very fine.
11th. Very fine. Aurora quite bright from 9 to 10 P. M., with faint narrow streamers shooting up nearly to the zenith.
12th. Very fine.
13th. Pleasant.
14th. Clouds thick, with appearances of rain in the evening.
15th. Very warm. Appearances of shower in the evening. The ground is becoming very dry.
16th. Very hot. Sun out at intervals. Sprinkling of rain about 7 A. M.
17th. Very warm. Sprinkling of rain several times.
18th. Very burning sun at intervals. Cloudy for the greater part of the day.
19th. Rain began very moderately between 5 and 6 A. M. Storm heavy, with rain and wind from 10 A. M. to 2 P. M. Clouds broken, with clear sky in patches at sunset.
20th. Sprinkling of rain at different times.
21st. Pleasant. Clouds abundant.
22d. Brisk shower at 1½ P. M.
23d. Very sultry.
24th. Very fine.
25th. Very hot. Sprinkling of rain from 4 to 6 P. M.
26th. Very fine.
27th. Very pleasant.
28th. Copious rain from 3 to 4 A. M.
29th. Copious rain from 3½ to 5 A. M., with thunder. Evening clear.
30th. Very sultry in the morning. Wind came round from S. W. to N. E., from 4 to 6 P. M., with thunder and sprinkling of rain.
31st. Very sultry and damp.

August, 1850. New Moon, 7d. 4h. 25m. P. M.

Days.	Barometer, reduced to 32° F. At 6 A. M.	At 2 P. M.	At 10 P. M.	Thermometer. At 6 A. M.	At 2 P. M.	At 10 P. M.	Daily mean.	Winds. (Direction and Force.) At 6 A. M.	At 2 P. M.	At 10 P. M.	Weather. (Tenths Cloudy.) At 6 A. M.	At 2 P. M.	At 10 P. M.	Rain and Snow in Inches of Water.
1	29.78	29.65	29.75	70	86	73	76.3	S. E. 2	S. W. 3	S. W. 1	Rain	9	1	} 0.50
2	29.72	29.72	29.74	71	80	72	74.3	N'ly 2	N. E. 2	S. W'ly 1	Rain	8	5	
3	29.75	29.73	29.73	68	80	72	73.3	W'ly 2	S. W. 2	S. W. 2	Foggy	Rain	5	
S 4	29.70	29.66	29.74	72	82	73	73.7	S'ly 2	S. by E. 2	S'ly 2	Rain	3	0	0.30
5	29.74	29.74	29.74	74	85	71	76.7	S'ly 2	S. W'ly 2	S. W. 2	10	9	4	
6	29.78	29.75	29.73	70	85	70	75.0	W'ly 1	S. W. 2	S. W. 2	6	5	Rain	2.25
7	29.73	29.72	29.82	68	82	69	73.0	N. W. 2	N. E. 1	N. W. 1	3	1	Sh'r, 2	0.25
8	29.90	29.87	29.86	64	76	66	68.7	N. 2	N. E. 3	S. E. 2	0	2	3	
9	29.77	29.63	29.54	64	73	70	69.0	S. W. 2	S. W. 2	S. W. 1	10	Rain	0	
10	29.48	29.55	29.65	69	80	61	70.0	W'ly 1	N. W. 2	N. W. 1	3	2	0	
S 11	29.76	29.74	29.84	56	74	59	63.0	N. W. 2	N. W. 2	N. W. 1	0	1	0	
12	29.85	29.77	29.73	54	80	70	68.0	W'ly 1	W'ly 3	S. W. 2	2	6	0	
13	29.68	29.66	29.48	68	86	72	75.3	W by S. 2	S. W. 2	S. W. 2	6	3	Rain	} 1.80
14	29.49	...	29.72	67	70	60	65.7	N'ly 2	...	N. E. 1	Rain	...	0	
15	29.72	29.76	29.82	59	63	59	60.3	N. E'ly 1	N. E. 1	N. E. 1	9	Rain	10	0.05
16	29.82	29.75	29.78	60	75	59	64.7	N. E. 1	S. W. 2	N. W. 2	8	8	0	
17	29.84	29.84	29.97	49	68	54	57.0	N. W. 2	N. W. 2	N. W. 1	0	1	0	
S 18	29.99	29.92	29.90	49	68	52	56.3	N'ly 1	N. by E. 2	N. E. 1	0	7	0	
19	29.86	29.81	29.87	49	73	60	60.7	N. by E. 1	N. E. 2	E'ly 1	0	4	3	
20	29.85	29.84	29.87	52	70	60	60.7	N'ly 1	N. E. 3	N. E. 2	2	5	9	
21	29.85	29.79	29.77	57	79	63	66.3	N. W. 3	N. W. 3	N. W. 1	0	1	0	
22	29.67	29.61	29.63	57	77	62	65.3	N. W. 3	N. W. 4	N. W. 1	0	1	0	
23	29.62	29.62	29.63	56	77	68	67.0	N. W. 2	W. 4	W'ly 2	4	5	2	
24	29.62	29.62	29.64	65	84	72	73.7	W. 1	S. W. 1	S. W. 1	0	4	2	
S 25	29.57	29.37	29.10	69	68	63	66.7	S. E. 3	E. 5	W'ly 5	10	Rain	10	2.50
26	29.38	29.40	29.47	64	83	64	70.3	W. 2	S. W. 2	N. W. 2	0	1	0	
27	29.61	29.66	29.88	59	76	58	64.3	N. W. 2	N. W. 3	N. W. 1	0	5	0	
28	29.98	30.02	30.01	52	72	61	61.7	N. W. 1	N. W. 1	S'ly 1	0	0	0	
29	30.03	30.03	30.03	56	80	66	67.3	W. 1	S. W. 1	W. 1	0	2	0	
30	30.04	30.02	29.99	59	76	66	67.0	S. W. 1	S. 3	S. W. 1	2	2	0	
31	29.97	29.94	29.89	67	72	65	68.0	S. W. 2	S. E. 3	S'ly 1	4	3	0	
Means	29.76	29.74	29.75	61.7	76.8	65.0	...	1.7	2.3	1.5	4.2	4.6	2.5	7.65
								1.8			3.8			
REDUCED TO SEA LEVEL.								Prevailing winds from some point between—	Days.				Days.	
Max.	30.22	30.21	30.21	74	86	73	76.7							
Min.	29.56	29.55	29.28	49	63	52	56.3							
Mean	29.93	29.91	29.92					N. & E.	7		Clear		11	
Range	0.46	0.46	0.93	25	23	21	20.4	E. & S.	4		Variable	}	10	
Mean of month	29.920			...	...	...	67.8	S. & W.	12		Cloudy	}		
Extreme range	0.94			...	...	...	37.0	W. & N.	8		Rain fell on		11	

Remarks.

1st. Light thundershower between 7 and 8 A. M. Shower again from 5 to 6 P. M.
2d. Rain till 9 A. M.
3d. Light shower, with thunder, at 2 P. M.
4th. Moderate rain, with thunder, from 4 to 7 A. M.
5th. Very sultry.
6th. Sun very scorching in the morning. Powerful rain, with thunder, from 3½ to 6 P. M. Light showers in the evening.
7th. Brisk shower, with thunder, from 7 to 8 P. M.
8th. Very pleasant.
9th. Sprinkling of rain at 2 P. M. Clear evening, very damp, with flashes of lightning low down in the east.
10th. Evening very clear. Forty-four shooting stars were counted from about 7¾ to 10 o'clock. The greater number moved towards the S.W. Of the above number, some ten or twelve were very bright, leaving behind them a streak of light some 10° or 15° in length, which continued not more than three seconds; some near the zenith—all pretty high up.
11th and 12th. Very fine.
13th. Began to rain moderately from 7 to 8 P. M., which was heavy at intervals during the night.
14th. Rain ceased about 7 A. M. Clear in the afternoon and evening.
15th. Light showers in the morning; quite cool.
16th. Cool; massive clouds abundant. Very clear at 10 P. M.
17th. Very cool, and air extremely dry. Dew-point 45°.
18th. Very cool. Heavy clouds at mid-day. Evening very clear.
19th. Wind, in the region of clouds, N. W.; on the ground, N. E.
20th. Variable.
21st and 22d. Very fine.
23d. Pleasant.
24th. Hazy at times.
25th. Began to rain moderately about 7 A. M. Rain increased, and was heavy through the day; ceased about 6 P. M.
26th. Fine.
27th. Very fine.
28th. Pleasant.
29th. Very pleasant.
30th. Hazy at 1 P. M.
31st. Fog-clouds in the morning. Light shower during the night.

September, 1850. New Moon, 6d. 0h. 20m. A. M.

Days.	Barometer At 6 A. M.	At 2 P. M.	At 10 P. M.	Thermometer At 6 A. M.	At 2 P. M.	At 10 P. M.	Daily mean.	Winds At 6 A. M.	At 2 P. M.	At 10 P. M.	Weather At 6 A. M.	At 2 P. M.	At 10 P. M.	Rain and Snow in Inches of Water.
S 1	29.87	29.87	30.00	70	81	68	73.0	S. 2	S. by E. 2	S'ly 1	9	3	0	
2	30.01	29.96	29.95	63	83	73	73.0	S. E. 1	S. by E. 2	S. E'ly 2	Foggy	5	10	
3	29.87	29.74	29.86	72	78	66	72.0	S'ly 2	N. W. 1	N'ly 1	10, R'n	10	0	2.00
4	29.87	...	29.84	59	...	63	...	N. W. 2	...	N. W. 1	0	...	0	
5	29.85	...	29.78	63	...	68	...	S. E'ly 1	...	S'ly 1	Foggy	...	10	
6	...	29.80	29.94	...	81	72	...	...	S. E. 2	S. W'ly	...	2	Hazy	
7	29.90	29.87	29.78	73	72	66	70.3	S. E. 2	S. E. 1	N. E. 2	10	Rain	Rain	} 2.00
S 8	29.43	29.44	29.71	65	68	63	65.3	N. E. 2	N. W. 2	N. W. 1	Rain	10	0	
9	29.80	29.78	29.80	54	71	61	62.0	N. W. 1	N. W. 2	N. W. 1	0	1	Hazy	
10	29.87	...	29.82	59	...	58	...	N. W. 1	...	S. W. 1	1	...	0	
11	29.70	29.59	29.65	59	77	53	63.0	S. W. 1	S. W. 2	N. W. 1	Foggy	5	Shower	0.25
12	29.75	29.65	29.78	51	63	48	54.0	N. W. 1	N. W. 3	N. W. 2	0	2	0	
13	29.66	29.67	29.82	45	64	48	52.3	N. W. 1	N. W. 2	N. W. 1	0	3	0	
14	29.74	29.69	29.74	46	67	52	55.0	N. W. 2	N. W. 1	N. W. 2	5	8	2	
S 15	29.75	29.76	29.89	48	64	53	55.0	N. W. 2	N. E. 1	N. E. 1	0	3	2	
16	29.96	29.95	30.01	47	65	50	54.0	N. by E. 1	N. E. 2	N'ly 1	Foggy	5	0	
17	30.05	29.93	29.92	45	65	48	52.7	N. by E. 1	N. E. 2	N. E. 1	0	0	0	
18	29.79	29.72	29.66	45	68	55	56.0	N. E. 1	N. E. 2	N. W. 1	9	3	Foggy	
19	29.66	29.59	29.56	55	72	60	62.3	N. E. 1	S. W. 1	S. W. 2	Foggy	2	8	
20	29.60	29.65	29.83	57	72	55	61.3	N. W. 1	N. W. 2	N. W. 1	2	2	1	
21	29.97	29.98	30.03	51	70	54	58.3	N. W. 2	E'ly 1	S. E'ly 1	0	2	0	
S 22	30.06	30.03	30.03	53	69	56	59.3	S. E'ly 2	S. E. 2	S. E. 1	0	0	0	
23	29.99	29.93	29.95	59	74	55	62.7	S. W. 2	S. W. 3	S. W. 1	8	0	0	
24	29.87	29.75	29.72	55	75	62	64.0	S. W. 2	S. W. 3	S. W. 2	5	8	10	
25	29.85	29.81	29.83	58	71	57	62.0	N. W. 2	N. by E. 2	N. E. 2	2	7	8	
26	29.85	29.81	29.79	53	58	55	55.3	N. E. 2	S. E. 2	E'ly 2	10, R'n	10	Misty	
27	29.75	29.65	29.56	54	58	56	56.0	N'ly 2	N'ly 1	N. W'ly 2	R'n, m't	Misty	Rain	0.75
28	29.47	29.45	29.61	60	69	61	63.3	S. W. 2	S. W. 3	N. W. 2	8	3	0	
S 29	[illegible]	[illegible]	[illegible]	[illegible]	[illegible]	[illegible]	[illegible]	[illegible]	[illegible]	[illegible]	[illegible]	[illegible]	[illegible]	
30	30.09	30.06	30.07	39	58	45	47.3	N. W. 2	N. W. 2	S. W.	0	0	0	
Means	29.89	29.77	29.80	55.4	69.9	57.5	...	1.1	1.9	1.4	5.0	4.2	4.0	5.00
								1.6			4.4			
REDUCED TO SEA LEVEL.								Prevailing winds from some point between—	Days.				Days.	
Max.	30.27	30.24	30.25	73	83	73	73.0							
Min.	29.61	29.62	29.74	39	58	44	47.3							
Mean	30.00	29.94	30.01					N. & E.	6		Clear		12	
Range	0.66	0.62	0.51	34	25	29	25.7	E. & S.	6		Variable	}	10	
Mean of month	29.983			...	...	...	60.7	S. & W.	7		Cloudy	}		
Extreme range	0.66			...	...	...	44.0	W. & N.	11		Rain fell on		8	

Remarks.

1st. Sprinkling of rain from 2 to 3 P. M.
2d. Light fog at sunrise. Sprinkling of rain at 4 P. M. Air very damp.
3d. Heavy rain from 2 to 4 A. M.; again from 9 to 12 A. M.; wind S'ly. Clouds broken at 2 P. M. Evening clear, with aurora low down, but rather bright.
4th. Very fine.
5th. Air very damp, with appearance of rain.
6th. Very fine.
7th. Began to rain moderately at 8½ A. M.; Rained heavily at intervals through the day and evening.
8th. Rain in the morning. Clouds broken at 1 P. M. Evening clear.
9th. Very fine.
10th. Aurora in evening, with faint streamers.
11th. Heavy gust of rain and wind from N. W. at 4½ P. M.
12th. Very cool.
13th and 14th. Very fine.
15th. Pleasant.
16th. Pleasant. Evening very clear and still.
17th. Very fine, but cool.
18th. Pleasant.
19th. Foggy in the morning. Air damp through the day.
20th to 23d. Very fine.
24th. Air damp. Appearances of rain in the evening.
25th. Pleasant. Wind E. of N. in the afternoon, while the clouds came from N. W.
26th. Light rain and mist during the day and evening.
27th. Light rain and mist in morning. Heavy shower, with thunder, from 10 to 11 P. M.
28th. Pleasant. Clouds heavy at times.
29th. [illegible]
30th. A very brilliant meteor was seen, at three or four minutes before 9 P. M., to pass from a point near Epsilon Persei to Atik Persei, in the left foot of which it exploded, forming a dense mass of light, which gradually spread and declined in brightness, but remained visible twenty minutes. A bright streak of light marked, for some time, the path over which it passed.

October, 1850. New Moon, 5d. 9h. 48m. A. M.

Days.	Barometer, reduced to 32° F. Sunrise.	At 2 P. M.	At 10 P. M.	Thermometer. Sunrise.	At 2 P. M.	At 10 P. M.	Daily mean.	Winds. (Direction and Force.) Sunrise.	At 2 P. M.	At 10 P. M.	Weather. (Tenths Cloudy.) Sunrise.	At 2 P. M.	At 10 P. M.	Rain and Snow in Inches of Water.
1	30.01	29.89	29.89	42	64	50	52.0	S. W. 1	S. W. 2	S. W. 1	5	0	0	0.15
2	29.72	...	29.47	47	...	49	...	S. W. 1	...	N. W. 1	10	Rain	0	
3	29.43	29.48	29.63	44	54	46	48.0	N. W. 2	N. W. 3	N. W. 2	0	2	0	
4	29.83	29.83	29.85	41	63	46	50.0	N. W. 2	N. W. 2	N. W. 1	0	0	0	
5	29.87	29.79	29.74	45	68	55	56.0	S. W. 1	S. W. 2	S. W. 1	0	0	1	
S 6	29.64	29.67	29.80	57	63	44	54.7	S. W. 1	N. W. 2	N. W. 1	10	1	1	
7	29.85	29.84	30.00	37	51	37	41.7	N. W. 2	N. W. 3	N. W. 1	0	3	0	
8	29.96	29.86	29.87	31	53	45	43.0	N. W. 1	W'ly 2	S. W. 1	0	3	Hazy	
9	29.82	29.82	29.90	43	68	53	54.7	S. W. 1	S. W. 1	S. W. 1	2	7	0	
10	30.01	30.05	30.08	53	68	54	58.3	S. W. 1	S'ly 1	S. W. 1	2	1	0	
11	29.98	29.84	29.69	52	63	57	57.3	S. E'ly 1	S. E. 2	S'ly 1	Foggy	10	2	
12	29.45	29.37	29.42	59	72	55	62.0	S. W. 2	W'ly 2	W. 3	Shower	8	8	
S 13	29.49	29.48	29.58	47	55	44	48.7	N. W. 3	N. W. 3	N. W. 1	0	3	1	
14	29.44	29.59	29.65	42	61	46	49.7	N. W. 1	W'ly 3	N. W. 1	5	0	0	
15	29.81	29.75	29.85	38	60	48	48.7	N. W. 2	N. W. 3	N. W. 1	0	1	0	
16	29.88	29.79	29.75	46	66	51	54.3	N. W. 2	W'ly 2	W'ly 1	0	0	0	
17	29.69	29.65	29.68	54	68	62	61.3	S'ly 1	S. W. 2	S. W. 1	Foggy	5	9	
18	29.69	29.56	29.49	60	64	63	62.3	S'ly 1	S. W'ly 1	S. W. 1	Rain	0	Rain	0.80
19	29.33	29.41	29.58	61	68	53	60.7	S. W'ly 1	W. by S. 1	N. W. 2	10	3	9	
S 20	29.61	29.46	29.48	42	55	45	47.3	N. W. 2	N. E. 2	N. W. 1	8	8	5	
21	29.62	29.60	29.72	43	55	43	47.0	N. W. 2	N. W. 3	N. W. 1	5	5	0	
22	29.73	29.69	29.70	43	63	54	53.3	S. W. 1	S. W. 2	S. W. 1	3	5	0	
23	29.67	29.68	29.72	57	66	59	60.7	S. W. 2	S. by E. 2	S'ly 1	9	9	8	
24	29.69	29.75	29.87	63	71	60	64.7	S. W'ly 3	S. W'ly 2	S. W. 2	10	9	10	
25	29.89	29.82	29.79	60	71	62	64.3	S'ly 1	S'ly 1	S. W'ly 1	Foggy	9	8, Sh'r	
26	29.67	29.65	29.36	63	65	60	62.7	S. W'ly 3	S. E. 2	S. W'ly 2	Rain	Rain	6	} 1.15
S 27	29.26	29.19	29.42	52	55	44	50.3	S. W. 2	S. W. 2	N. W. 3	4	Rain	0	
28	29.79	29.76	29.68	36	56	49	47.0	S. W. 2	W by N. 2	S. W. 1	0	5	5	
29	29.90	29.90	30.00	40	46	36	40.7	N. W. 2	N. W. 2	N. W. 1	0	0	0	
30	30.02	29.96	29.98	29	51	39	39.7	N. W. 1	W'ly 1	W'ly 1	0	0	0	
31	30.06	29.99	30.06	36	60	42	46.0	W'ly 1	S'ly 1	S. W'ly 1	3	0	0	
Means	29.74	29.70	29.73	47.2	61.4	50.0	...	1.6	1.6	1.3	4.7	4.1	2.9	2.10
									1.5			3.9		
REDUCED TO SEA LEVEL.														
Max.	30.24	30.23	30.26	63	72	63	64.7	Prevailing winds from some point between—		Days.			Days.	
Min.	29.44	29.37	29.54	29	46	36	39.7	N. & E.		0	Clear		10	
Mean	29.92	29.87	29.91					E. & S.		2	Variable		} 15	
Range	0.80	0.86	0.72	34	26	27	25.0	S. & W.		16	Cloudy			
Mean of month	29.900			...	...	...	52.9	W. & N.		13	Rain fell on		6	
Extreme range	0.89			...	...	...	43.0							

Remarks.

1st. Very fine. Aurora in the evening quite bright, with faint streamers rising 25° or 30°.
2d. Light rain in the afternoon. Clear in the evening. Aurora bright from 7 to 8 P. M., with streamers rising to the height of 45°.
3d, 4th, and 5th. Very fine.
6th. Mist at sunrise; wind S W. At 8 A. M., wind fresh at N. W., and clouds broken.
7th. At 11 P. M., thermometer in the garden 35°. This morning, first appearance of white frost in the College yard.
8th. Heavy frost this morning. Thermometer in the garden 29°. The first frost to injure plants in the garden.
9th. Very pleasant. Air soft, with light haze.
10th. Very fine.
11th. Thick fog at sunrise. Occasional mist.
12th. Sprinkling of rain from 5 to 6 A. M. and in the afternoon. Evening gusty.
13th. Pleasant. Air very dry.
14th. Pleasant. Evening very clear.
15th and 16th. Very fine.
17th. Heavy fog in the morning. Air damp all day.
18th. Air damp, with occasional sprinkling of rain and light showers.
19th. Pleasant.
20th. Air rather raw
21st. Evening remarkably clear.
22d. Very pleasant.
23d. Warm. Air damp.
24th. Air damp, but not raw.
25th. Occasional sprinkling of rain in the afternoon and evening.
26th. Sprinkling in the morning. Moderate but steady rain in the afternoon. At 10 P. M., clouds broken and stars appearing.
27th. Showery and gusty during the day.
28th. Pleasant.
29th. Fine, but cool.
30th. At sunrise, thermometer in garden 27°. Pools of water skimmed over with ice.
31st. Very fine.

November, 1850. New Moon, 3d. 9h. 32m. P. M.

Days.	Barometer Sunrise.	At 2 P. M.	At 10 P. M.	Thermometer Sunrise.	At 2 P. M.	At 10 P. M.	Daily mean.	Winds Sunrise.	At 2 P. M.	At 10 P. M.	Weather Sunrise.	At 2 P. M.	At 10 P. M.	Rain and Snow
1	30.08	29.99	30.06	44	63	52	53.0	S. W. 1	S. W. 1	S'ly 1	2	3	6	
2	30.08	30.05	30.10	54	64	54	57.3	S. W'ly 1	S. W. 1	S. W. 1	10	9	8	
S 3	30.05	29.98	30.03	53	62	50	55.0	S. W. 1	S'ly 1	S'ly 1	Foggy	9	Foggy	
4	30.03	29.99	30.07	48	58	47	51.0	N. E. 1	N. E. 1	N. E. 1	Foggy	2	0	
5	30.11	30.10	30.10	46	60	54	53.3	S. W'ly 1	S. by E. 2	S. W. 2	10	3	10	
6	30.02	29.89	29.85	55	60	58	57.7	S. W. 3	S. W. 2	S. W. 2	10	10	10	
7	30.03	30.06	30.00	46	47	36	43.0	N'ly 2	N. by E. 2	N. W. 1	9	1	0	
8	30.02	29.91	29.83	31	52	41	41.3	N'ly 1	S. E'ly 1	N. E. 2	5	9	Rain	
9	29.73	29.77	29.84	41	56	37	44.7	N'ly 2	N. E. 3	N. W. 1	10	2	0	
S 10	29.94	29.86	29.95	39	53	41	44.3	N. W. 1	N. W. 3	N. W. 1	1	3	0	
11	29.95	29.80	29.78	39	61	41	47.0	N. W. 1	W'ly 1	N. W. 1	0	3	2	
12	29.72	29.64	29.57	39	55	45	46.3	N. W. 2	S. W. 1	N. E. 3	9	10	10	
13	29.67	29.70	29.77	38	47	35	40.0	N'ly 2	N. E. 2	N. E. 1	2	0	0	
14	29.82	29.86	29.86	30	50	38	39.3	N. 2	N. W. 1	N. E. 2	0	0	0	
15	29.90	29.90	29.91	32	49	41	40.7	N. W'ly 1	S. E. 1	S. E'ly 1	1	0	4	
16	29.92	29.85	29.71	43	56	46	48.3	S. E. 2	S. E. 2	S. E'ly 1	10	10	Rain	1.20
S 17	29.32	29.22	29.26	46	55	42	47.7	N. E. 1	W'ly 2	S. W. 3	Misty	Misty	10	
18	29.26	29.37	29.51	37	46	36	39.7	W S. W. 3	W. by S. 3	W. 3	5	7	0	
19	29.48	29.51	29.67	38	48	36	40.7	W. S W. 4	N. W. 3	N. W. 1	3	2	0	
20	29.75	29.74	29.74	31	47	38	38.7	N. W. 1	N. W. 1	N. E. 1	2	3	10	
21	29.56	29.47	29.56	35	45	31	37.0	N. W. 1	N. W. 3	W'ly 3	10	7	0	
22	29.79	29.80	29.88	28	40	29	32.3	N. W. 1	N. W. 1	N. W. 1	0	0	0	
23	29.87	...	29.79	24	...	29	...	N. W. 1	...	E'ly 1	1	8	8	
S 24	29.71	29.61	29.61	26	33	27	28.7	N'ly 2	N. W. 2	N. W. 1	7	0	0	
25	29.73	29.73	29.83	28	43	33	34.7	N. W'ly 1	N. W. 1	N. W. 1	0	0	0	
26	29.87	29.78	29.91	34	39	37	36.7	N. E. 2	N. E. 2	N. E. 1	Rain	10	Foggy	
27	29.93	29.75	29.76	36	50	57	47.7	N. E. 1	S. E'ly 1	S. W. 2	Foggy	10	10	
28	29.87	29.98	29.93	57	39	38	44.7	N. E. 1	N. E. 2	N. E. 2	9	Misty	Misty	
29	29.82	29.80	29.70	35	42	42	39.7	N. E. 2	N. E. 2	S. E'ly 2	Misty	Misty	Foggy	0.90
30	29.67	29.70	29.76	42	52	37	43.7	N'ly 1	N'ly 1	N. W. 2	10	5	3	
Means	29.82	29.79	29.81	39.2	50.4	40.9	...	1.5	1.7	1.5	6.2	5.2	5.0	2.10
									1.5			5.5		
REDUCED TO SEA LEVEL.														
Max.	30.29	30.28	30.18	57	64	58	57.7	Prevailing winds from some point between—		Days.			Days.	
Min.	29.44	29.40	29.44	24	33	27	28.7	N. & E.		8	Clear		8	
Mean	30.00	29.97	29.99					E. & S.		4	Variable		} 18	
Range	0.85	0.88	0.74	33	31	31	29.0	S. & W.		8	Cloudy			
Mean of month	29.987			...	...	...	43.5	W. & N.		10	Rain fell on		4	
Extreme range	0.89			...	...	...	40.0							

Remarks.

1st. Pleasant.
2d. Very mild.
3d. Mild, with some appearances of rain.
4th and 5th. Pleasant.
6th. Mild. Appearances of rain in the evening.
7th. Cooler. Evening remarkably clear.
8th. Began to sprinkle at 6 P. M. Light rain; wind N. E.
9th. Day gusty. Evening still and very clear.
10th. Blustering at mid-day. Evening still and very clear.
11th. Pleasant. Evening calm; clouds at the south.
12th. From 4 to 6 P. M., the wind came round from N. W., through S. and E., to N. E., and became quite fresh.
13th Evening still and clear. No meteors were observed, though a look-out was kept up till a late hour in the evening.
14th. Very fine.
15th. Very bright fog-bow about the moon in the early part of the evening
16th. Began to rain moderately at 8 P. M. Heavy rain during the night.
17th. Misty in the morning. Clouds broken in the afternoon. Evening gusty.
24th. Pleasant, but cold.
25th. Very fine.
26th. Sprinkling of rain in the morning. Fog in the evening.
27th. Foggy in the morning. Stars out at 8 P. M. Thick clouds at 10 P. M.
28th. Cold mist in the afternoon and evening.
29th. Mist, with occasional light rain. Heavy showers in the night.
30th. Cloudy in the morning. Evening clear.

December, 1850. New Moon, 3d. 0h. 8m. P. M.

DAYS.	Barometer, reduced to 32° F. Sunrise.	At 2 P. M.	At 10 P. M.	Thermometer. Sunrise.	At 2 P. M.	At 10 P. M.	Daily mean.	Winds (Direction and Force.) Sunrise.	At 2 P. M.	At 10 P. M.	Weather (Tenths Cloudy.) Sunrise.	At 2 P. M.	At 10 P. M.	Rain and Snow in Inches of Water
S 1	29.75	29.70	29.77	32	51	40	41.0	S. W'ly 2	W'ly 2	W'ly 1	2	2	3	
2	29.86	...	29.95	31	...	36	...	N'ly 2	...	N. E. 2	9	...	7	
3	29.95	29.85	29.72	36	44	42	40.7	N. E. 1	E'ly 1	N. E. 2	10	0	Rain	0.33
4	29.86	29.93	29.96	41	52	45	46.0	N'ly 1	N. W. 1	N'ly 1	9	7	10	
5	29.95	29.81	29.85	44	44	39	42.3	N. E. 1	N. E. 1	N. E. 2	Rain	Misty	Rain	
6	30.00	30.00	29.99	34	38	31	34.3	N'ly 2	N'ly 2	N'ly 2	6	10	Snow	
7	29.73	29.48	29.11	32	37	32	33.7	N. E. 2	N. E. 2	N. E. 2	R'n, sn.	Rain	Misty	1.37
S 8	29.28	29.50	29.81	28	29	24	27.0	N. W. 3	N. W. 4	N. W. 2	0	1	0	
9	29.89	29.84	29.68	23	36	36	31.7	W'ly 2	S. W. 3	S. W. 2	0	10	10	
10	29.65	29.64	29.81	32	39	24	31.7	S. W. 2	N. W. 2	N. W. 2	5	2	0	
11	29.89	29.88	29.84	22	34	29	28.3	N. W. 2	S. W. 1	N. W. 2	7	Snow	2	
12	29.79	29.68	29.72	31	43	38	37.3	W'ly 1	W'ly 1	S'ly 1	6	10	10	
13	29.89	30.05	30.12	21	19	11	17.0	N'ly 2	N. W. 2	N. W. 1	10	0	0	
14	30.23	30.09	30.02	8	25	26	19.7	N. W. 2	S. W. 1	S. W. 2	0	2	6	
S 15	29.90	29.81	29.87	32	39	32	34.3	S. W. 1	S. W. 2	W'ly	9	10	0	
16	29.88	29.84	29.63	32	43	36	37.0	W'ly 1	S. W. 2	N'ly 2	5	10	Rain	} 0.65
17	29.37	29.45	29.68	39	40	24	34.3	N. E. 2	N. W. 2	N. W. 3	R'n, m't	10	0	
18	29.86	29.97	30.14	17	26	20	21.0	W. 2	N. W. 2	N. W. 2	0	0	0	
19	30.19	29.99	29.59	19	22	26	22.3	N. E. 1	N. E. 2	E'ly 2	10	Snow	Rain	
20	29.60	29.60	29.84	25	34	20	26.3	N. W. 1	N. W. 1	N. W. 1	10	8	0	} 0.50
21	29.84	29.64	29.72	17	36	33	28.7	N. W. 2	N. W. 2	N. W. 2	3	0	4	
S 22	29.84	29.70	29.59	31	37	31	33.0	N. W. 1	N. E. 2	N. E. 2	4	10	Snow	
23	28.69	28.52	29.77	37	28	12	25.7	N. E. 2	N'ly 1	N. W. 3	Rain	Misty	10	1.75
24	29.74	...	30.18	7	...	10	...	N. W. 3	...	N. W. 2	0	...	0	
25	30.14	...	29.61	11	...	31	...	W. 1	S. W. 2	S. W. 2	3	8	Snow	
26	29.61	29.56	29.58	27	37	30	31.3	W'ly 1	W'ly 1	W'ly 1	0	10	10	
27	29.65	29.67	29.76	24	36	28	29.3	W'ly 1	W'ly 2	W'ly 1	0	5	0	
28	29.88	...	29.79	24	...	32	...	W'ly 1	...	N. E. 2	3	...	Snow	
S 29	29.34	29.58	29.85	17	21	24	20.7	N. E. 3	N. W'ly 2	W'ly 1	Snow	10	10	1.25
30	30.09	30.20	30.33	9	17	10	12.0	N. W. 2	N. W. 1	N. W. 1	0	7	0	
31	30.28	30.20	29.76	8	20	23	17.0	N. W. 1	N'ly 1	N'ly 1	7	10	Snow	
Means	29.79	29.75	29.81	25.5	34.3	28.2	...	1.6	1.7	1.7	5.1	7.8	5.9	5.85
								1.7			6.2			
REDUCED TO SEA LEVEL.														
Max.	30.46	30.38	30.51	44	52	45	46.0							
Min.	28.77	28.70	29.29	7	17	10	12.0							
Mean	29.97	29.93	29.99											
Range	1.69	1.68	1.22	37	35	35	34.0							
Mean of month	29.963			...	...	...	29.3							
Extreme range	1.81			...	...	...	45.0							

Prevailing winds from some point between— Days.
N. & E. 8
E. & S. 0
S. & W. 7
W. & N. 16

Days.
Clear 5
Variable . . . } 12
Cloudy . . . . }
Rain or snow fell on 14

REMARKS.

1st. Very pleasant.
2d. Air very raw. Light rain from 8 to 9 A. M.
3d. Air raw. Began to rain from 4 to 5 P. M. Wind E'ly, and rather fresh.
4th. Mild.
5th. Mist and moderate rain.
6th. Hail and snow in afternoon and evening.
7th. Roofs of houses covered with snow this morning. Cold rain and mist all day.
8th. Very blustering through the day. Evening very clear, and wind moderate.
9th. Air raw, with appearances of storm in the evening.
10th. Air raw. Cloudy in the afternoon. Clear at 10 P. M., and cooler.
11th. Light snow from S. W. from 11 A. M. to 2 P. M.; ground partly covered with snow. Evening clear.
12th. Air mild. Snow during the night.
13th. Nearly two inches of snow on the ground this morning. Wind fresh and cold at N'ly.
14th. Pleasant, though cold in the morning.
15th. Cloudy during the day. Clear and pleasant in the evening.
16th. Began to rain moderately from 8 to 10 P. M. Wind N. E'ly.
17th. Moderate rain in the morning. Clear and gusty in the evening.
18th. Cold, but not unpleasant. Very clear through the day.
19th. Moderate snow from 8 A. M., with rain in the evening.
20th. Between four or five inches of wet snow on the ground. Evening clear.
21st. Pleasant.
22d. Moderate snow at 7 P. M.; wind light N. E.
23d. At 7 A. M., barom. 28.76; wind fresh N. E; raining. At 10 A. M., bar. 28.65; wind light N'ly and mist. At 1.30 P. M., bar. 28.60. At 10 P. M., clouds broken.
24th. Very cold with a piercing wind from N. W.
25th. Cloudy in the afternoon. Began to snow moderately at 8 P. M. Wind light S. W.
26th. About a half inch of fresh snow on ground.
27th. Pleasant. Evening still and very clear.
28th. Pleasant morning. Cloudy in afternoon. Wind came to N. E. about 3 P. M. Began to snow moderately at 7 P. M.
29th. At 7 A. M., wind pretty heavy N. E., and snowing. At 9 A. M., wind nearly at N.; clouds thin and broken. Seven or eight inches of compact, heavy snow fallen.
30th. Cold day. Evening still and clear.
31st. Began to snow moderately at 5 P. M.

January, 1851. New Moon, 2d. 5h. 36m. A. M.

DAYS.	Barometer Sunrise.	At 2 P. M.	At 10 P. M.	Thermometer Sunrise.	At 2 P. M.	At 10 P. M.	Daily mean.	Winds Sunrise.	At 2 P. M.	At 10 P. M.	Weather Sunrise.	At 2 P. M.	At 10 P. M.	Rain and Snow in Inches of Water
1	29.67	29.64	29.70	17	26	27	23.3	N. W. 2	W'ly 2	S. W'ly	0	5	2	
2	30.02	29.99	29.66	11	23	19	17.7	N. W'ly 1	N. W'ly 2	W'ly 1	0	4	8	
3	29.48	...	29.46	29	...	16	...	S. W'ly 2	...	N. E. 1	10	...	10	
4	29.43	29.37	29.65	14	17	11	14.0	N'ly 1	N'ly 1	N. W. 2	10	Snow	0	
S 5	29.95	29.89	29.86	4	27	27	19.3	W'ly 1	S. W'ly 2	S. W. 3	0	10	10	
6	29.86	...	29.81	31	...	27	...	S. W'ly 1	...	W'ly 1	10	...	3	
7	29.74	29.80	29.96	25	27	20	24.0	N. E'ly 1	N'ly 1	N. W. 2	Misty	Misty	0	
8	30.08	30.08	30.12	15	26	22	21.0	N. W. 2	N. W. 2	N. W. 2	0	0	10	
9	29.97	29.68	29.43	23	35	46	34.7	S. W'ly 2	N. E. 2	S'ly 2	10	Misty	Rain	0.33
10	29.44	29.44	29.50	40	45	39	41.3	W'ly 1	N. W. 2	N'ly 1	1	7	9	
11	29.61	...	29.72	32	...	31	...	N'ly 1	...	N. W. 1	2	...	0	
S 12	29.71	29.62	29.70	31	43	35	36.3	S. W. 2	S. W. 3	S. W. 1	2	2	2	
13	29.74	29.72	29.80	30	41	34	35.0	N. W. 2	N. W. 1	N. W. 1	5	0	4	
14	29.91	29.78	29.66	30	42	40	37.3	N. W. 2	S. W. 2	S. W. 3	1	5	9	
15	29.63	29.55	29.57	36	50	36	40.7	S. W. 2	S. W. 2	S. W. 1	5	6	3	
16	29.54	29.67	29.78	36	52	38	42.0	S. W. 1	N. E. 1	N. E. 2	2	0	10	
17	29.54	29.59	29.93	42	50	34	42.0	N. E. 1	W'ly 2	N. W'ly 2	Foggy	10	10	
18	30.11	30.06	30.34	26	28	15	23.0	N. W. 2	N. W. 2	N. W. 2	3	3	1	
S 19	30.57	30.48	30.46	11	24	20	18.3	N. W. 2	N. W. 2	S. E'ly 1	0	0	2	
20	30.02	29.74	29.83	34	47	35	38.7	S. S. E. 2	S. W. 2	N. W. 1	10	Rain	2	0.60
21	30.09	30.16	30.15	28	35	29	30.7	N. W. 1	N. W. 2	N. W. 1	0	0	2	
22	30.08	29.78	29.75	30	38	35	34.3	S'ly 1	S. W. 2	W'ly 2	10	Rain	10	
23	29.86	29.92	30.09	35	45	32	37.3	W. S. W. 2	W'ly 1	W'ly 1	7	2	0	
24	30.09	29.89	29.92	26	44	37	35.7	S. W. 1	S. W. 3	S. W. 1	0	2	0	
25	30.11	30.06	29.90	32	44	34	36.7	W'ly 2	S'ly 1	S. W. 1	6	5	0	
S 26	29.70	29.65	29.75	36	54	45	45.0	S. W. 1	W by S. 2	W'ly 2	5	4	2	
27	29.82	29.94	30.09	31	32	21	28.0	N. E. 1	N. E. 2	N. E. 2	10	10	0	
28	30.10	29.96	29.53	21	36	36	31.0	N. E. 2	N. E. 2	S. E. 2	8	10	Rain	} 1.00
29	28.89	28.83	29.15	45	47	14	35.3	S'ly 3	N. W. 3	N. W. 4	Rain	0	0	
30	29.49	29.69	29.96	7	8	1	5.3	N. W. 2	N. W. 3	N. W. 2	0	0	0	
31	30.11	30.29	30.53	3	10	5	6.0	N. W'ly 2	N. W. 3	N. W. 2	0	0	0	
Means	29.82	29.80	29.83	26.1	35.6	27.7	...	1.6	2.0	1.7	4.8	5.0	4.1	1.93
								1.8			4.6			
REDUCED TO SEA LEVEL.														
Max.	30.75	30.66	30.71	45	54	46	45.0							
Min.	29.07	29.01	29.33	3	8	1	5.3							
Mean	30.00	29.98	30.01											
Range	1.68	1.65	1.38	42	46	45	39.7							
Mean of month	29.997			...	...	...	29.8							
Extreme range	1.74			...	...	...	53.0							

Prevailing winds from some point between— Days.
N. & E. 5
E. & S. 0
S. & W. 13
W. & N. 13

Days.
Clear 6
Variable . . . } 19
Cloudy . . . . }
Rain or snow fell on 6

1st. Very fine.
2d. Very pleasant.
3d. Grew colder in the afternoon and evening.
4th. Air full of snow during the day.
5th. Evening thick cloudy. Wind S. W. and snow in the air.
6th. Very mild.
7th. Light mist through the day. Evening clear.
8th. Clear early in the evening; overcast at 10 o'clock.
9th. Began to mist and rain from noon to 1 P. M.; wind N. E'ly. In the evening, wind came round to S'ly, and rain increased.
10th. Very pleasant.
11th. Very mild and pleasant.
12th. Pleasant.
13th. Very pleasant.
14th. Mild. Appearances of rain in the evening.
15th. Very mild. Light haze in the evening. Halo about the moon.
16th. Hazy in the afternoon. Evening cloudy, with appearances of storm.
17th and 18th. Pleasant.
19th. Very chilly in the afternoon, with wind S. E'ly.
20th. Rain in morning. Wind varying S. E'ly to S. W., and came to N. W. towards evening and cleared.
21st. Very pleasant.
22d. Light S'ly rain and snow from 1 to 4 P. M.
23d. Very pleasant. Evening clear.
24th, 25th, and 26th. Very fine.
27th. Evening very clear.
28th. Began to rain gently at 10 P. M.
29th. At 9 A. M., barometer 28.92; at 10 A. M., 28.88 (not reduced). Wind light N. W. In the evening, wind very heavy at N. W., and the cold very severe.
30th. Cold very severe, with wind high and piercing at N. W.
31st. Cold still severe and wind heavy.

February, 1851. New Moon, 1d. 0h. 52m. A. M.

Days.	Barometer, reduced to 32° F. Sunrise.	At 2 P. M.	At 10 P. M.	Thermometer. Sunrise.	At 2 P. M.	At 10 P. M.	Daily mean.	Winds. (Direction and Force.) Sunrise.	At 2 P. M.	At 10 P. M.	Weather. (Tenths Cloudy.) Sunrise.	At 2 P. M.	At 10 P. M.	Rain and Snow in Inches of Water.
1	30.68	30.60	30.46	0	22	18	13.3	N. W. 1	S. W'ly 1	S. W'ly 2	0	3	2	
S 2	30.23	30.14	30.05	24	84	26	28.0	S. W. 2	S. W'ly 2	W'ly 1	Snow	Snow	0	
3	29.98	29.86	29.84	28	40	30	32.7	W'ly 2	W'ly 2	N. W. 1	9	0	0	
4	29.72	29.53	29.34	23	40	35	32.7	S'ly 2	S. W. 1	S. W. 2	7	Sprin'lg	10	
5	29.36	29.35	29.46	32	39	35	35.3	S. W'ly 1	W'ly 2	N. W'ly 2	4	10	8	
6	29.39	29.50	29.85	30	24	9	21.0	N. E. 2	N. W. 2	N. W. 2	Snow	5	0	
7	29.99	29.92	29.96	1	22	15	12.7	N. W. 1	W'ly 3	N. W. 1	0	5	0	
8	30.26	30.26	30.32	4	9	7	6.7	N. W. 1	N. W. 2	N. W. 2	0	1	10	
S 9	30.14	29.92	29.93	16	31	24	23.7	N. E'ly 1	N. E. 2	N. E. 1	10	Misty	Misty	
10	29.84	29.72	29.55	31	53	55	46.3	Calm	S. W. 3	S. W. 4	Foggy	10	10	
11	29.53	29.65	30.03	49	51	27	42.3	S. W. 1	N. W. 2	N. W. 2	10	9	0	
12	30.42	30.48	30.65	18	27	22	22.3	N. W. 2	N. W. 2	N. W. 1	0	0	0	
13	30.68	30.67	30.55	16	36	30	27.3	Calm	S'ly 1	S'ly 1	0	0	2	
14	30.34	30.23	30.09	36	49	46	43.7	S'ly 2	S. W. 3	S. W. 1	10	10	10	
15	29.86	29.52	29.47	43	52	53	49.3	S. W. 1	S. W. 2	S. W. 3	Rain	Rain	10	1.00
S 16	29.69	29.78	30.02	38	37	25	33.3	N. W. 1	N. W. 2	N. W. 2	10	10	0	
17	30.31	30.37	30.36	21	29	25	25.0	N. W. 2	N. W. 2	N. W. 1	0	0	0	
18	30.21	...	30.44	30	...	31	...	S. W. 2	...	N. W. 2	2	...	0	
19	30.67	30.63	30.43	21	37	29	29.0	N'ly 1	E'ly 2	S'ly 1	0	0	4	
20	30.31	30.13	30.09	30	45	43	39.3	S'ly 2	S. W. 2	S. W. 1	5	Rain	Misty	
21	30.01	29.98	29.86	42	38	35	38.3	S'ly 1	N. E. 2	N. E. 2	Rain	Rain	Rain	1.50
22	29.66	29.72	29.81	34	46	40	40.0	N'ly 2	N. W. 1	N. W. 1	10	10	0	
S 23	29.91	29.91	29.93	33	50	37	40.0	N. W. 1	N. W. 2	N. W. 1	0	3	0	
24	29.83	29.65	29.10	35	42	35	37.3	S'ly 2	S. E'ly 2	N. W'ly 3	Foggy	10	Rain	1.37
25	29.42	29.69	29.97	37	39	32	36.0	N. W. 4	N. W. 4	N. W. 2	5	0	0	
26	30.13	...	30.14	26	...	34	...	N'ly 2	...	N. E. 2	0	...	7	
27	30.08	...	29.80	30	...	41	...	E'ly 1	...	S. E'ly 2	2	...	10	
28	29.54	29.40	29.51	42	47	31	40.0	S'ly 1	W'ly 2	N. W. 2	Rain	Misty	10	
Means	30.01	29.94	29.97	27.5	37.6	31.1	...	1.5	2.0	1.7	6.1	6.2	4.4	3.87
									1.7			5.4		
REDUCED TO SEA LEVEL.								Prevailing winds from some point between—		Days.			Days.	
Max.	30.86	30.85	30.83	49	53	55	49.3							
Min.	29.54	29.53	29.28	0	9	7	6.7							
Mean	30.19	30.12	30.15					N. & E.		2	Clear		9	
Range	1.32	1.32	1.55	49	44	48	42.6	E. & S.		3	Variable }		9	
Mean of month	30.153			...	...	...	32.1	S. & W.		9	Cloudy }			
Extreme range	1.58			...	...	...	55.0	W. & N.		14	Rain or snow fell on		10	

Remarks.

1st. The barometer from 9 to 10 A. M. stood at 30.91, reduced to sea level. Weather pleasant.
2d. Sprinkling of snow in the morning; the ground barely covered. Evening clear and mild.
3d. Very pleasant.
4th. Sprinkling of rain from 2 to 3 P. M.
5th. Mild.
6th. Moist snow from 6 to 10 A. M.; the ground covered with from one to two inches of snow.
7th. Evening very clear. Faint aurora in the north.
8th. Very cold.
9th. Light mist all day, which froze as it fell.
10th. Occasional dashes of rain. Evening extremely blustering.
11th. Morning very mild, with occasional light rain. Evening clear, and much cooler.
12th. Very faint aurora this evening.
13th. At 8½ A. M., barometer 30.93, calm; at 11 A. M., 30.95, with wind light at S'ly; at noon, 30.92; at 5 P. M., 30.82, weather very fine.
14th. Occasional sprinkling of rain.
15th. Moderate rain in the morning; increased in the afternoon. In the evening, clouds thin and somewhat broken.
16th. Pleasant. Evening very clear. Frost out of the ground in many places.
17th. Very fine.
18th. Pleasant. Aurora in the north, low down but quite bright.
19th. Very fine.
20th. Sprinkling of rain at intervals during the day.
21st. Rainy day.
22d. Cloudy all day. Evening clear.
23d. Weather uncommonly mild and beautiful.
24th. Cloudy in the morning; wind light S'ly. Rain in the afternoon. Wind came round blustering at N. W. between 9 and 10 P. M.; rain still falling. Barom. began to rise at 11 P. M. Flurry of snow during the night. Frost entirely out of the ground in very many places.
25th. The ground covered with melting snow this morning. The day pleasant.
26th. Very fine.
27th. Air raw.
28th. Sprinkling of rain and mist in the morning. Flurry of snow during the night.

March, 1851. New Moon, 2d. 8h. 7m. P. M.

Days.	Barometer At 6 A. M.	At 2 P. M.	At 10 P. M.	Thermometer At 6 A. M.	At 2 P. M.	At 10 P. M.	Daily mean.	Winds At 6 A. M.	At 2 P. M.	At 10 P. M.	Weather At 6 A. M.	At 2 P. M.	At 10 P. M.	Rain and Snow
1	29.78	29.87	29.89	32	32	26	30.0	N. W. 2	N. W. 2	S. W. 1	0	0	0	
S 2	29.89	29.83	29.74	32	43	33	36.0	S'ly 1	S'ly 2	S. E'ly 1	6	10	0	
3	29.60	29.58	29.93	33	36	25	31.3	N. W. 1	N. W. 3	N. W. 2	5	5	0	
4	30.06	29.98	29.83	23	45	41	36.3	S. W. 2	S. W. 3	S. W. 1	0	7	9	
5	29.78	29.84	29.90	40	60	38	46.0	S. W. 2	N. W. 1	E'ly 1	3	4	0	
6	29.77	29.62	29.93	45	62	37	48.0	S. W. 2	S. W. 3	N. W. 2	5	10	10	
7	30.12	30.10	30.04	32	41	35	36.0	N. W. 2	E'ly 2	N. E. 2	9	10	10	
8	29.72	29.65	29.72	29	33	28	30.0	N. E. 3	N. E. 2	N. E'ly 2	Snow	10	Snow	1.00
S 9	29.75	29.78	29.87	28	37	26	30.3	N'ly 1	N. W. 2	N. W. 2	10	8	0	
10	29.81	29.77	29.94	24	49	32	35.0	W. by S. 1	S. W. 1	N. W. 1	9	9	2	
11	29.99	29.83	29.79	27	45	40	37.3	N. W. 1	S. W. 3	W'ly 2	0	3	5	
12	29.89	29.99	30.12	33	35	22	30.0	N. W. 2	N. W. 3	N. W. 1	0	0	0	
13	30.06	29.84	29.92	22	38	28	29.3	N. E. 1	S. W'ly 1	S'ly 1	8	Snow	10	
14	30.10	30.15	30.05	17	28	27	24.0	N. W. 3	N'ly 2	S. W'ly 2	3	0	1	
15	29.94	29.74	29.71	36	56	49	47.0	S. W. 1	S. W. 2	S. W. 1	Foggy	8	10	
S 16	29.77	29.81	29.79	39	33	30	34.0	N. E. 3	N. E. 3	N. E. 3	10	Hail	10	
17	29.70	29.63	29.44	30	34	31	31.7	N. E. 2	N. E. 2	N. E. 4	Snow	Hail	Snow	} 1.00
18	29.23	29.23	29.26	32	84	28	31.3	N. E. 4	N. E. 3	N. E. 2	Snow	Snow	Snow	
19	29.26	29.25	29.34	32	42	34	36.0	N. W. 1	N. W. 2	N. W. 1	10	10	10	
20	29.35	29.36	29.49	32	42	34	36.0	N. W. 1	N. W. 2	N. W. 1	Snow	9	0	
21	29.56	29.60	29.69	34	46	35	38.3	W N W 2	N. W. 2	N. W. 1	9	7	2	
22	29.74	29.76	29.82	36	49	39	41.3	N. W. 1	N'ly 2	N'ly 1	2	2	0	
S 23	29.90	29.86	29.67	35	56	42	44.3	N'ly 1	S'ly 1	S'ly 2	0	8	10	
24	29.34	29.35	29.42	35	49	46	43.3	N. E. 2	N. W. 2	N'ly 1	10	3	10	
25	29.66	29.76	30.13	40	40	31	37.0	N. W. 2	N. 2	N'ly 2	3	0	0	
26	30.29	30.20	30.08	29	48	38	38.3	N'ly 1	S'ly 2	S. W. 2	0	0	0	
27	29.99	29.83	29.80	42	65	53	53.3	S. W. 2	S. W. 2	S. W. 2	5	8	2	
28	29.68	29.67	30.02	51	64	39	51.3	S. W. 2	N. W. 3	N. W. 1	6	3	0	
29	30.20	30.24	...	32	56	...	...	N. W. 2	S'ly 2	...	0	0	...	
S 30	30.22	30.10	...	38	63	...	...	S. W. 2	S. W. 2	...	10	2	...	
31	29.95	29.86	29.95	53	73	56	60.7	S. W. 2	S. W. 2	S. W. 1	10	9	2	
Means	29.81	29.78	29.80	33.7	46.3	35.6	...	1.8	2.1	2.0	5.9	6.0	4.6	2.00
									1.9			5.5		
REDUCED TO SEA LEVEL.								Prevailing winds from some point between—		Days.			Days.	
Max.	30.47	30.42	30.31	53	73	56	60.7							
Min.	29.41	28.41	29.44	17	28	22	24.0							
Mean	29.99	29.96	29.98					N. & E.		5	Clear		7	
Range	1.06	1.01	0.87	36	45	34	36.7	E. & S.		1	Variable }		15	
Mean of month	29.977			...	...	...	38.5	S. & W.		12	Cloudy }			
Extreme range	1.06			...	...	...	56.0	W. & N.		13	Rain or snow fell on		9	

Remarks.

1st. The ground this morning was covered with snow, which disappeared during the day.
2d. Raw S'ly air.
3d and 4th. Pleasant.
5th. Mild, warm, and very spring-like.
6th. Clouds general, but thin. Very warm for the season.
7th. Appearances of storm in the evening.
8th. Moist snow in morning, five or six inches deep. Dusting of snow in the evening.
9th. The ground this morning covered with from one to two inches of fresh snow, which fell during the night.
10th. A beautiful shower of snow, with large flakes, at 10 A. M. Evening fine.
11th. Pleasant. The snow of the 8th nearly all gone.
12th. Pleasant, but cool.
13th. Light snow in the afternoon.
14th. Cold this morning. Wind during the day swung round from N. E'ly, through the E., to S'ly.
15th. Clouds pretty general, but thin.
16th. Light hail in the afternoon. Air raw and uncomfortable.
17th. Moderate snow and hail all day. Wind heavy at night.
18th. Damp snow continued falling all day, which was much drifted by the violence of the wind; equal to six or seven inches on the average.
19th. Wind light, and heavens covered with thin clouds.
20th. Air full of snow from 7 to 10 A. M., and again at 6 P. M. Clear at 10 P. M.
21st. Pleasant.
22d. Very fine. Snow of the 17th and 18th nearly all gone.
23d. Mild. Clouds prevalent, but thin.
24th. Misty from 7 to 10 A. M. Pleasant in the afternoon.
25th. Pleasant. Evening very clear.
26th and 27th. Very fine.
28th. Warm in the morning. Wind changed from S. W. to N. W., with a heavy gust, between noon and 1 P. M.
29th. Very fine.
30th. Pleasant.
31st. Pleasant, and the warmest day since the 24th of September last, being 188 days. Thermometer 73° at 1 P. M.

April, 1851. New Moon, 1d. 1h. 25m. P. M.

Days.	Barometer, reduced to 32° F. At 6 A. M.	At 2 P. M.	At 10 P. M.	Thermometer. At 6 A. M.	At 2 P. M.	At 10 P. M.	Daily mean.	Winds (Direction and Force.) At 6 A. M.	At 2 P. M.	At 10 P. M.	Weather (Tenths Cloudy.) At 6 A. M.	At 2 P. M.	At 10 P. M.	Rain and Snow in Inches of Water.
1	30.10	30.11	30.12	40	60	41	47.0	N. by E. 2	E'ly 2	S. E. 1	0	0	0	
2	30.13	29.99	29.61	35	50	49	44.9	S. W. 2	S'ly 2	S. E'ly 2	3	Sprinl'g	Rain	} 0.75
3	29.57	29.53	29.67	43	60	48	50.3	N'ly	W'ly 3	N. W. 2	Rain	2	0	
4	29.77	29.77	29.89	40	65	45	50.0	S. W. 2	S. W. 3	S. W. 2	0	5	0	
5	29.93	29.94	29.90	40	65	52	52.3	S. W. 2	S. W. 2	S. W. 1	2	3	6	
S 6	29.81	29.69	29.67	53	57	56	55.3	S. W. 2	S. W. 3	S'ly 1	10	Rain	10	1.00
7	29.87	29.89	30.03	45	58	46	49.7	N. W. 1	N. W. 2	W'ly 1	0	2	Hazy	
8	30.00	29.87	29.48	44	61	58	54.3	N. W. 2	S'ly 3	S. E'ly 3	3	8	Rain	1.60
9	29.86	30.00	30.11	43	54	43	46.7	N. W. 1	N. W. 2	Calm	1	0	0	
10	30.11	30.06	30.07	43	63	49	51.7	S. W. 2	S. W. 3	W'ly 1	0	0	5	
11	30.16	30.17	30.23	40	48	35	41.0	N. E. 2	N. E. 2	N. E'ly 1	10	9	5	
12	30.28	30.21	30.20	32	44	31	35.7	N'ly 2	N'ly 2	N'ly 1	5	5	0	
S 13	30.13	29.86	29.71	30	45	35	36.7	N'ly 2	N. W. 2	N. W. 1	0	3	0	
14	29.61	29.51	29.51	30	52	39	40.3	N. E. 2	N. E. 2	N. E. 2	0	0	Rain	
15	29.52	29.52	29.43	39	42	39	40.0	N. E. 3	N. N. W. 3	N. E. 4	Misty	Misty	Rain	
16	29.28	29.17	29.31	38	39	37	38.0	N. E. 4	N. E. 5	N. E. 4	Rain	Rain	Rain	} 2.25
17	29.35	29.41	29.43	36	37	36	36.3	N. E. 3	N. E. 3	N. E. 3	Rain	Rain	Misty	
18	29.45	29.49	29.51	36	39	38	37.7	N.N.E. 2	N.N.E. 2	N'ly 2	10	10	10	
19	29.49	29.43	29.41	40	58	39	45.7	N'ly 1	E'ly 2	S. E'ly 1	10	10	Rain	} 1.10
S 20	29.16	29.18	29.31	34	33	36	34.3	N. E. 3	N. E. 3	N'ly 2	Rain	Snow	Misty	
21	29.29	29.24	29.27	40	50	39	43.0	N. W. 1	N. W. 1	N'ly 2	9	10	Rain	
22	29.31	29.32	29.48	44	57	48	49.7	N. W. 2	N. W. 2	N. W. 2	8	0	0	
23	29.54	29.55	29.55	48	64	52	54.7	N. W. 2	N. W. 2	N. W. 1	3	0	0	
24	29.56	29.43	29.48	50	68	51	56.3	W'ly 1	S. E. 2	N. E. 1	5	9	0	
25	29.58	29.56	29.70	46	60	46	50.7	N. 2	N. W. 2	N. W. 1	0	0	0	
26	29.75	29.71	29.76	41	64	46	50.3	N. W. 1	N. W. 2	N. W. 1	0	0	0	
S 27	29.77	29.73	29.76	48	67	44	53.0	S. E'ly 1	S. E. 1	N. E. 2	5	9	5	
28	29.72	29.71	29.74	42	52	42	45.3	N. E. 2	N. E. 2	N. E. 2	9	Sprinl'g	10	
29	29.86	29.88	29.97	40	60	46	48.7	N. E. 2	N. E. 2	W'ly 1	5	7	0	
30	29.99	29.96	29.86	42	61	47	50.0	W'ly 2	S. E'ly 2	S. W. 2	0	10	Rain	1.10
Means	29.73	29.70	29.71	40.7	54.4	43.8	...	1.9	2.3	1.7	4.9	5.7	5.3	7.80
								2.0			5.3			
REDUCED TO SEA LEVEL.														
Max.	30.46	30.39	30.41	53	68	58	56.3							
Min.	29.34	29.35	29.45	30	33	31	34.3							
Mean	29.91	29.88	29.89											
Range	1.12	1.04	0.96	23	35	27	22.0							
Mean of month	29.893			...	...	...	46.3							
Extreme range	1.12			...	...	...	38.0							

Prevailing winds from some point between— Days.
N. & E. 9
E. & S. 7
S. & W. 5
W. & N. 9

Days.
Clear 9
Variable . . . } 8
Cloudy . . . . }
Rain or snow fell on 13

REMARKS.

1st. Very fine.
2d. Began to sprinkle at 1 P. M. Light rain in the evening.
3d. Light rain at 6 A. M. Nearly clear at 10 A. M. Fine afternoon and evening.
4th. Very fine.
5th. Pleasant.
6th. Heavy showers during the day; thunder occasionally from 4 to 5 P. M. Evening cloudy, but no rain.
7th. Very light haze in evening. Bow around the moon.
8th Began to rain about 6 P. M. Heavy showers in the evening.
9th and 10th. Very fine.
11th. Rather chilly.
12th. Cold and raw. Snow-flakes occasionally fell.
13th. Ground hardly frozen this morning.
14th. Ground again frozen. At 4 P. M., wind fresh S. E'ly; in the evening, N. E., and began to rain very moderately between 9 and 10 P. M.
15th. Mist and light rain through the day. In the evening, wind heavy.
16th. Wind and storm very heavy during the day. The barometer began to rise at 3 P. M., and, rising one-tenth of an inch, it became stationary at about 5½ P. M., standing at 29.36 for six or eight hours. Flakes of snow, mingled with rain, fell from 10 to 11 A. M.
17th. Storm somewhat abated, but still heavy. The amount of rain on the 16th and 17th somewhat uncertain, in consequence of one rain-gauge being blown from its place and the other leaking. It was not less than two inches, probably more.
18th. Occasional mist during the day.
19th. In the afternoon, wind high S. E'ly and very raw. Sprinkling of rain at 10 P. M.
20th. Rain, and snow in large heavy flakes which sometimes quite covered the ground.
21st. Moderate rain in afternoon and evening.
22d. Fine. Evening very clear.
23d to 26th. Very fine.
27th. Overcast, but clouds thin.
28th. Light sprinkling of rain.
29th. Pleasant.
30th. Began to rain very moderately at 4 P. M., increasing in the evening.

May, 1851. New Moon, 1d. 3h. 54m. A. M., and 30d. 8h. 39m. P. M.

Days.	Barometer At 6 A. M.	At 2 P. M.	At 10 P. M.	Thermometer At 6 A. M.	At 2 P. M.	At 10 P. M.	Daily mean.	Winds At 6 A. M.	At 2 P. M.	At 10 P. M.	Weather At 6 A. M.	At 2 P. M.	At 10 P. M.	Rain and Snow
1	29.55	29.51	29.58	48	62	42	50.7	N. W. 1	N. W. 1	N. W. 3	10	7	0	
2	29.61	29.63	29.85	40	55	41	45.3	W'ly 2	W'ly 2	N. W. 2	0	3	0	
3	29.97	29.92	29.91	38	63	49	50.0	N. W. 2	S. W. 2	S. W. 2	0	4	10	
S 4	29.77	29.71	29.68	52	64	...	...	S. W. 2	S. W. 1	S. W. 2	10	10	Rain	} 2.00
5	29.58	29.53	29.43	36	40	35	37.0	N. E. 3	N. E. 3	N. E. 3	Rain	10	Rain	
6	29.54	29.66	29.77	37	57	43	45.7	N. W. 2	N. W. 2	W. 1	2	5	3	
7	29.85	29.82	29.84	43	55	43	47.0	W. 1	S'ly 2	N. W. 1	8	10	0	
8	29.88	29.81	29.84	39	60	46	48.3	W'ly 1	S. E'ly 2	N. W'ly 1	3	9	3	
9	29.86	29.78	29.74	44	67	50	53.7	W'ly 1	S. E'ly 2	S. W. 1	5	2	8	
10	30.01	30.00	29.88	55	79	58	64.0	S. W'ly 1	N. W. 3	S. W. 1	2	8	10	
S 11	29.88	29.88	29.90	54	65	55	58.0	N. E. 1	E'ly 1	E'ly 1	Rain	10	Rain	
12	29.89	29.87	29.84	53	68	57	59.3	E'ly 2	E'ly 1	S. E'ly	10	9	10	
13	29.79	29.64	29.65	59	73	62	64.7	S. W. 2	S'ly 2	S'ly 1	10	0	6	
14	29.67	29.63	29.87	63	75	58	65.3	N. W. 2	N. W. 1	N. W. 3	10	9	6	
15	29.91	30.01	30.07	48	65	48	53.7	N'ly 2	N. W. 2	S'ly 2	3	2	0	
16	30.10	30.05	29.99	50	68	50	56.0	S. W'ly 2	S'ly 3	S'ly 1	0	1	0	
17	29.83	29.76	29.67	53	65	59	59.0	S. W. 3	S. W. 4	S. W. 1	5	Rain	0	
S 18	29.80	29.83	29.90	57	55	50	54.0	N. E. 2	N. E. 2	E'ly 1	9	Rain	0	
19	29.98	29.98	29.95	47	68	50	55.0	N'ly 2	S. E'ly 2	S'ly 2	0	0	5	
20	29.80	29.58	29.50	54	75	64	64.3	S. W. 2	S. W'ly 2	S. W'ly 2	10	9	Rain	0.15
21	29.56	29.61	29.76	63	79	61	67.7	N. W. 2	N. W. 3	E'ly 2	1	5	0	
22	29.83	29.75	29.57	56	70	60	62.0	N. E. 2	N. E. 2	S'ly 2	0	5	Rain	1.10
23	...	29.34	29.68	63	83	56	67.3	S. W. 2	S. W. 2	N. W. 3	10	5	0	
24	30.03	30.09	30.14	48	67	52	55.7	N. W. 3	N. W. 2	S'ly 1	0	0	0	
S 25	30.20	30.23	30.21	50	71	51	57.3	S. W. 1	S. W. 2	S. W. 1	0	0	0	
26	30.18	30.06	29.98	48	75	58	60.3	S. W. 2	S. W. 2	S. W. 1	0	0	0	
27	29.95	29.89	29.81	61	83	63	69.0	S. W. 2	S. W. 2	S. W. 2	3	5	Sprinl'g	
28	29.68	29.68	29.83	63	85	66	71.3	S. W. 2	S. W. 3	N. W. 2	10	2	0	
29	29.89	29.91	29.91	56	55	46	52.3	N. E'ly 2	N. E. 2	N. E. 2	8	10	Rain	} [illegible]
30	[illegible]	[illegible]	[illegible]	[illegible]	[illegible]	[illegible]	[illegible]	[illegible]	[illegible]	[illegible] 1	[illegible]	10	0	
31	29.99	29.99	30.05	46	64	51	53.7	N'ly 3	N'ly 2	N. E. 2	2	5	0	
Means	29.84	29.81	29.83	50.6	66.4	52.2	...	1.9	2.1	1.7	5.3	5.6	4.2	3.58
								1.9			5.0			
REDUCED TO SEA LEVEL.														
Max.	30.38	30.41	30.39	63	85	66	71.3							
Min.	29.72	29.52	29.61	36	40	35	37.0							
Mean	30.02	29.98	30.01											
Range	0.66	0.89	0.78	27	45	31	34.3							
Mean of month	30.003			...	...	...	56.4							
Extreme range	0.89			...	...	...	50.0							

Prevailing winds from some point between— Days.
N. & E. 8
E. & S. 2
S. & W. 14
W. & N. 7

Days.
Clear 7
Variable . . . } 10
Cloudy . . . . }
Rain fell on . . 14

REMARKS.

1st. Cloudy in the morning. Evening clear. Aurora in the north—quite bright, but without streamers.
2d. Very fine.
3d. Pleasant. Cloudy evening.
4th. Began to rain moderately at 7 P. M., increasing in the evening.
5th. Rain during the day, mixed occasionally with hail.
6th. Pleasant.
7th. Brisk shower from the west between 4 and 5 P. M. Evening still and clear. Frost in many places this morning; ice in some.
8th. Frost in many places this morning. Sprinkling of rain at 4 P. M. Evening pleasant.
9th. Pleasant during the day. Thundershower between 6 and 8 P. M. Clear at 11 P. M.
10th. Very mild and pleasant.
11th. Light rain at intervals.
12th. Mild and pleasant.
13th. Pleasant. Frequent lightning at the N. W. and N. in the evening. Severe tempest and destructive hail-storm in Worcester.
14th. Mostly cloudy. Occasional sprinkling of rain.
15th. Pleasant.
16th. Very fine.
17th. Sprinkling of rain in the afternoon.
18th. Sprinkling of rain from 1 to 2 P. M.
19th. Pleasant.
20th. Cloudy, but warm. Shower from 9 to 10 P. M.
21st. Very fine.
22d. Pleasant in the morning. Began to rain very moderately at 6 P. M. Thunder and rain in the evening. Heavy rain and thunder about midnight.
23d. Cloudy in the morning; wind fresh and [illegible] N. W., very fresh. Evening clear.
24th, 25th, and 26th. Very fine.
27th. Pleasant. Sprinkling of rain at evening.
28th. Very fine.
29th. Began to rain moderately from 2 to 3 P. M.
30th. Light rain and mist at 6 P. M. Cloudy through the day. Very clear and cool in the evening.
31st. Pleasant.

June, 1851. New Moon, 29d. 1h. 17m. A. M.

DAYS.	Barometer, reduced to 32° F. At 6 A. M.	At 2 P. M.	At 10 P. M.	Thermometer. At 6 A. M.	At 2 P. M.	At 10 P. M.	Daily mean.	Winds (Direction and Force.) At 6 A. M.	At 2 P. M.	At 10 P. M.	Weather (Tenths Cloudy.) At 6 A. M.	At 2 P. M.	At 10 P. M.	Rain and Snow in Inches of Water.
S 1	30.00	29.96	29.85	55	75	58	62.7	N. W. 2	N. E. 1	S. W. 2	3	1	Sprinl'g	
2	29.64	29.49	29.50	57	73	58	62.7	S. W. 2	S. W. 2	N. W. 3	10	4	0	
3	29.53	29.52	29.56	53	68	54	58.3	N. W. 3	N. W. 3	N. W. 2	0	5	2	
4	29.58	29.56	29.73	55	73	55	61.0	W'ly 2	W'ly 3	N. W. 1	4	3	0	
5	29.84	29.81	29.83	56	71	54	60.3	N. W. 3	N. W. 3	N. W. 1	0	0	0	
6	29.78	29.70	29.56	54	73	62	63.0	N'ly 2	N. E. 3	S. W. 1	0	0	10	
7	29.40	29.38	29.54	58	53	49	53.3	S. W. 1	N. E. 2	N. E. 3	Rain	Rain	10	0.75
S 8	29.64	29.66	29.68	48	60	51	53.0	N. E. 2	N. E. 2	S. E. 2	7	10	10	
9	29.52	29.52	29.67	51	62	52	55.0	S. E. 3	N'ly 2	N'ly 1	Rain	10	10	0.75
10	29.78	29.79	29.87	55	71	57	61.0	N. W. 3	W'ly 3	W'ly 1	2	1	0	
11	29.91	29.73	29.67	58	76	65	66.3	N. W. 2	S. W. 4	S. W. 1	0	1	Shower	
12	29.70	29.67	29.74	60	76	58	64.7	N. W. 2	N. W. 2	N. W. 2	0	2	0	
13	29.79	29.76	29.83	60	76	59	65.0	N. W. 2	N. W. 2	N. W. 1	0	2	5	
14	29.87	29.85	29.92	56	75	56	62.3	N. W. 2	N. W. 2	N. E. 2	0	3	5	
S 15	29.92	29.82	29.79	58	76	52	62.0	N. W. 1	N. W. 2	N'ly 3	0	5	Rain	
16	29.85	29.99	30.11	51	61	47	53.0	N. E. 2	N. E. 3	N. E. 1	10	5	0	
17	30.19	30.20	30.21	46	70	50	55.3	N. 2	N. E. 3	N. E. 1	0	5	0	
18	30.20	30.18	30.13	53	77	61	63.7	N'ly 1	N. W. 2	S. W'ly 2	0	3	0	
19	30.12	29.96	29.88	56	75	60	63.7	N. W. 1	S.byW. 3	S. W'ly 2	3	2	0	
20	29.82	29.77	29.78	60	80	66	68.7	S'ly 2	S. W'ly 3	S. W. 2	0	0	7	
21	29.80	29.74	29.74	67	82	66	71.7	S. W. 2	S. W. 3	S. W. 1	7	4	0	
S 22	29.71	29.67	29.65	70	79	66	71.7	S. W. 1	S. E'ly 1	S. E'ly 2	7	8	Misty	
23	29.64	29.59	29.63	70	88	67	75.0	S'ly 1	S. E'ly 2	S'ly 1	Foggy	8	Foggy	
24	29.67	29.67	29.75	56	60	58	58.0	N. E. 2	N. E. 2	N. E'ly 1	10	9	10	
25	29.76	29.71	29.75	61	83	64	69.3	W'ly 2	N.W'ly 3	N. W. 1	0	2	2	
26	29.79	29.72	29.70	64	81	68	71.0	N. W. 1	S. E'ly 2	S. E'ly 1	2	3	10	
27	29.74	29.61	29.67	70	84	67	73.7	S. W'ly 2	S. W. 2	Calm	Rain	5	0	0.40
28	29.73	29.74	29.75	63	78	68	69.7	N. E'ly 2	S. E'ly 2	S'ly 1	5	3	Hazy	
S 29	29.71	29.68	29.62	70	83	71	74.7	S. E'ly 1	S'ly 2	S'ly 1	Hazy	0	Hazy	
30	29.65	29.59	29.62	71	90	72	77.7	S'ly 1	S'ly 2	S'ly 1	Hazy	0	0	
Means	29.78	29.73	29.76	58.7	74.3	59.7	...	1.8	2.4	1.9	3.8	4.0	4.4	1.90
									2.0			4.1		

REDUCED TO SEA LEVEL.	At 6 A. M.	At 2 P. M.	At 10 P. M.	At 6 A. M.	At 2 P. M.	At 10 P. M.	Daily mean.
Max.	30.38	30.38	30.39	71	90	72	77.7
Min.	29.58	29.56	29.68	46	53	47	53.0
Mean	29.96	29.90	29.94				
Range	0.80	0.82	0.71	25	37	25	24.7
Mean of month	29.933			...	...	...	64.2
Extreme range	0.83			...	...	...	44.0

Prevailing winds from some point between— Days.
- N. & E. 8
- E. & S. 5
- S. & W. 7
- W. & N. 10

Days.
- Clear 10
- Variable . . . } 11
- Cloudy . . . . }
- Rain fell on . . 9

Remarks.

1st. Sprinkling of rain in the evening.
2d. Brisk shower between 4 and 5 P. M. Evening clear.
3d. Pleasant.
4th. Pleasant. Evening clear.
5th. Very fine From 8 to 12 P. M., bright aurora at the north, without streamers. A little before 10 P. M., a well-defined, luminous belt, from 2° to 3° in width, was observed stretching across the heavens from N. W. to S. E., reaching in either direction to within about 30° of the horizon. It had a slow motion S'ly, and disappeared in some twenty-five or thirty minutes after it was first noticed. The mid heavens being quite clear at the time, the belt was a conspicuous and beautiful object.
6th. Fine during the day. Appearances of rain in the evening.
7th. Rainy day.
8th. Raw and cold. Fires necessary to comfort.
9th. Rainy in the morning. Cloudy in the afternoon and evening.
10th. Fine.
11th. Day fine. Thunder and light shower at 10 P. M.
12th and 13th. Very fine.
14th. Pleasant in the morning. Sprinkling of rain at 3½ P. M.; again from 7 to 8 P. M., with a very perfect rainbow.
15th. Pleasant till 5 P. M. Light shower in the evening.
16th. Very cold; fires quite necessary; frost in some low places.
17th. Fine, but cold for the season; frost in some places.
18th. Very fine.
19th and 20th. Pleasant.
21st. Very fine.
22d. Pleasant; top of the ground very dry.
23d. Mist and fog, with a light shower at 3 P. M.
24th. Very cool.
25th. Very fine.
26th. Very warm.
27th. At 6 A. M., heavy thundershower, with gust of wind. Aurora quite bright in the evening.
28th. Pleasant.
29th. Warm and sultry.
30th. Extremely hot, and very damp. At 2½ P. M., thermometer 92° in the shade.

July, 1851. New Moon, 28d. 9h. 32m. P. M.

DAYS.	Barometer At 6 A. M.	At 2 P. M.	At 10 P. M.	Thermometer At 6 A. M.	At 2 P. M.	At 10 P. M.	Daily mean.	Winds At 6 A. M.	At 2 P. M.	At 10 P. M.	Weather At 6 A. M.	At 2 P. M.	At 10 P. M.	Rain and Snow in Inches of Water.
1	29.64	29.63	29.74	73	90	71	78.0	S'ly 1	S. E'ly 2	N. E'ly 2	9	3	Rain	0.85
2	29.79	29.77	29.81	65	83	68	72.0	N. W. 3	N. E'ly 2	N. E'ly 1	2	3	0	
3	29.79	29.75	29.65	63	80	68	70.3	N'ly 1	S'ly 1	S. E'ly 2	3	8	Rain	1.00
4	29.49	29.47	29.58	64	69	59	64.0	E'ly 1	E'ly 2	N. W. 2	10	Rain	0	0.60
5	29.67	...	29.72	57	...	60	...	W'ly 2	...	N. W. 1	1	...	0	
S 6	29.76	29.70	29.69	63	82	66	70.3	W'ly 2	S. W. 3	S. W. 2	1	3	5	
7	29.64	29.60	29.76	67	75	62	68.0	S. W. 3	S. W. 2	W'ly 1	10	10	2	
8	29.82	29.85	29.85	58	76	63	65.7	N. W. 2	S'ly 2	S'ly 2	2	6	8	
9	...	...	29.68	...	...	69	...	...	...	S'ly 1	...	...	9	
10	29.58	29.50	29.61	69	83	72	74.7	S. W'ly 2	S. W. 2	W'ly 1	Rain	9	10	0.62
11	29.71	29.72	29.83	70	85	67	74.0	N. W. 1	W'ly 2	W'ly 1	10	5	5	
12	29.91	29.99	29.87	62	78	65	68.3	N.W'ly 2	N.W'ly 2	N. W. 1	5	2	0	
S 13	29.84	29.78	29.81	66	79	57	67.3	W'ly 2	N. W. 2	N. E. 1	2	3	0	
14	29.82	29.82	29.76	58	74	63	65.0	N. E. 2	N. E. 2	N. E. 2	0	2	5	
15	29.70	29.69	29.61	64	83	70	72.3	N. W. 2	S. W. 3	S. W. 3	2	5	10	
16	...	...	29.61	...	...	68	...	...	...	S. W. 2	...	...	Shower	
17	29.57	...	29.52	70	...	74	...	S. W. 2	...	W'ly 1	3	...	0	
18	29.60	29.60	29.58	78	84	70	77.3	W'ly 1	W'ly 3	W'ly 1	8	0	3	
19	29.58	29.65	29.51	74	74	74	74.0	S. W. 2	S'ly 1	W'ly 1	Misty	Rain	Misty	0.85
S 20	29.53	29.53	29.71	70	81	67	72.7	N. W. 2	N. W. 2	S. W. 1	5	3	0	
21	...	29.86	29.92	...	89	68	...	...	W'ly 1	W. 1	...	8	2	
22	29.96	29.92	29.90	68	85	70	74.3	W'ly 1	W'ly 2	S. W. 1	3	6	0	
23	29.88	29.84	29.88	71	84	72	75.7	S. W. 2	W. 1	W. 1	6	4	0	
24	29.86	29.84	29.77	73	80	72	75.0	W'ly 1	W. 2	S. W. 2	Misty	Rain	10	
25	29.67	29.65	29.62	74	88	75	79.0	S. W. 2	S. W. 3	W'ly 2	10	5	Rain	0.60
26	29.53	29.42	29.42	72	80	70	74.0	S. W'ly 2	S. W. 2	W. 1	5	Shower	1	0.37
S 27	29.32	29.29	29.35	70	80	66	72.0	N. W. 3	N. W. 2	N. W. 1	0	7	0	
28	29.37	29.41	29.51	67	72	65	68.0	N. W. 1	N. W. 2	N. E. 1	0	9	5	
29	29.55	29.67	29.83	62	63	54	59.7	N. E. 2	N. E. 2	N. E. 1	Rain	10	0	0.30
30	29.88	29.88	29.94	55	72	52	59.7	N. E. 2	N. E. 2	N. E. 1	9	5	0	
31	29.96	29.93	29.94	53	70	58	60.3	N'ly 1	N. E. 2	N. E. 2	0	10	3	
Means	29.69	29.69	29.71	66.3	79.2	66.3	...	1.8	2.0	1.4	5.1	6.1	4.1	5.19
									1.7			5.1		

REDUCED TO SEA LEVEL.	At 6 A. M.	At 2 P. M.	At 10 P. M.	At 6 A. M.	At 2 P. M.	At 10 P. M.	Daily mean.
Max.	30.14	30.17	30.12	78	90	75	79.0
Min.	29.50	29.47	29.53	53	63	52	59.7
Mean	29.86	29.86	29.88				
Range	0.64	0.70	0.59	25	27	23	19.3
Mean of month	29.867			...	...	...	70.6
Extreme range	0.70			...	...	...	38.0

Prevailing winds from some point between— Days.
- N. & E. 6
- E. & S. 2
- S. & W. 14
- W. & N. 9

Days.
- Clear 5
- Variable . . . } 10
- Cloudy . . . . }
- Rain fell on . . 16

Remarks.

1st. Alternate sunshine and copious showers, with some thunder.
2d. Pleasant.
3d. Rain, with light thunder, between 10 and 11 P. M.
4th. Heavy showers at intervals, with some thunder. Evening clear and cool.
5th. Very fine.
6th. Pleasant in the morning. Light showers from 7 to 8 P. M.
7th. Dashes of rain at 5 A. M. Occasional light showers.
8th. Pleasant.
9th. Light showers from noon to 1 P. M.
10th. Light rain and thunder from 6 to 7 A. M. Heavy showers, with frequent thunder and lightning, in the afternoon; very perfect rainbow a little before sunset. Moon out in the evening.
11th and 12th. Very fine.
13th. Light showers, with thunder, at 7 P. M.
14th. Very fine.
15th. Pleasant.
16th. Appearance of rain in morning. Shower at 11 P. M.
17th. Very warm, and not much air.
18th. Pleasant, but rather sultry.
19th. Frequent showers, with a great deal of thunder and lightning. Thunder in some cases in the afternoon, very near and very heavy.
20th to 23d. Very fine.
24th. Occasional sprinkling of rain.
25th. Very sultry during the day. Thundershower from 10 to 11 P. M.
26th. Pleasant. Copious thundershower from noon to 1 P. M.
27th. Occasional light showers.
28th. Cool. Showery from 2 to 4 P. M.
29th. Rainy in the morning. Clear in the evening.
30th. Very cool. Fires quite necessary to comfort in the evening.
31st. Cold for the season. Fires quite necessary.

August, 1851. New Moon, 26d. 5h. 12m. P. M.

Days.	Barometer, reduced to 32° F. At 6 A. M.	At 2 P. M.	At 10 P. M.	Thermometer. At 6 A. M.	At 2 P. M.	At 10 P. M.	Daily mean.	Winds (Direction and Force.) At 6 A. M.	At 2 P. M.	At 10 P. M.	Weather (Tenths Cloudy.) At 6 A. M.	At 2 P. M.	At 10 P. M.	Rain and Snow in Inches of Water.
1	29.95	29.92	29.90	59	68	58	61.7	N. E. 2	N. E. 2	N. E. 1	10	10	10	
2	29.88	29.84	29.88	62	75	63	66.7	N. W. 1	S. W'ly 2	W. 2	3	5	0	
S 3	29.90	29.89	29.95	66	78	65	69.7	S. W.	S. E. 1	S'ly 1	0	4	4	
4	29.99	29.99	29.92	64	71	62	65.7	S. W. 1	S. W. 3	N. E. 2	Foggy	10	Rain	0.10
5	29.93	29.90	29.92	62	75	67	68.0	N'ly 1	S. W. 2	S. W. 1	10	4	0	
6	29.95	...	29.91	66	...	65	...	N. W. 1	...	W'ly	2	...	2	
7	29.88	29.82	29.77	67	83	70	73.3	S. W. 2	S. W. 3	S. W. 1	1	8	Rain	0.15
8	29.79	29.79	29.83	70	86	71	75.7	S. W. 1	N. W. 2	N. W. 1	2	5	0	
9	29.78	29.67	29.68	72	78	66	72.0	S. W. 1	S. W. 2	W'ly 2	Rain	10	Shower	1.25
S 10	29.74	29.77	29.79	65	74	64	67.7	N. W. 1	N. W. 2	N. W. 2	2	0	3	
11	29.83	29.75	29.77	57	79	64	66.7	N. W. 1	S. E'ly 2	S. W. 1	0	3	3	
12	29.79	29.78	29.83	66	78	66	70.0	S. W'ly 1	S. W. 2	S. W. 1	7	3	2	
13	29.84	29.76	29.77	68	86	70	74.7	S. W. 2	S. W. 2	S. W. 1	10	3	0, Sh'r	} 0.40
14	29.67	29.72	29.65	74	78	63	71.7	N. W. 1	W'ly 2	N. W. 2	Shower	10	0	}
15	29.70	29.76	29.72	60	74	65	66.3	N. W. 1	N. W. 1	N. W. 1	7	8	3	
16	29.73	...	29.78	56	...	60	...	N. W. 1	...	N. W. 2	2	...	3	
S 17	29.77	29.75	29.69	62	62	58	60.7	W'ly 2	W'ly 2	Calm	7	Rain	Misty	0.75
18	29.73	29.76	29.85	54	72	60	62.0	N'ly 2	N. W'ly 1	N'ly 1	6	8	0	
19	29.93	29.90	29.95	57	73	60	63.3	N. W. 1	N. W. 1	N. W. 2	0	6	0	
20	29.99	29.94	29.88	60	72	63	65.0	N. W. 1	S. E. 1	S'ly 2	9	10	Rain	0.50
21	29.94	29.92	29.95	60	73	64	65.7	E'ly 1	S'ly 2	W'ly 2	10	10	10	
22	29.84	29.74	29.68	67	82	72	73.7	S. E'ly 2	S. W'ly 4	W. 5	Misty	10	5	
23	29.65	29.61	29.65	74	84	69	75.7	W'ly 1	W'ly 1	W'ly 1	4	5	0	
S 24	...	29.67	29.72	...	80	66	...	...	S. W. 2	N. W. 1	...	0	0	
25	29.64	29.67	29.53	68	82	72	74.0	N. W. 2	S. W. 3	S. W'ly 1	0	5	7	
26	29.49	29.57	29.84	59	67	55	60.3	N. W. 3	N. W. 4	W'ly 3	9	2	0	0.62
27	29.98	29.95	30.01	53	70	53	58.7	W. 1	N. W. 2	N. W. 1	0	3	0	
28	30.06	30.03	30.05	62	73	59	64.7	W. 1	S. W. 2	S. W. 1	0	0	0	
29	30.06	30.06	30.03	55	79	60	64.7	N. W. 2	N. W. 2	N. W. 1	0	0	0	
30	30.02	29.98	29.96	59	82	59	66.7	N. W. 1	S. W. 2	S. W. 1	0	0	0	
S 31	29.94	29.90	29.96	62	85	70	72.3	S. W. 2	S. W. 1	S. W. 1	0	0	2	
Means	29.85	29.82	29.83	62.9	76.5	63.8	...	1.7	2.0	1.5	4.7	5.1	3.5	3.77
REDUCED TO SEA LEVEL.								1.7			4.8			
Max.	30.24	30.24	30.23	74	86	72	75.7	Prevailing winds from some point between—		Days.			Days.	
Min.	29.67	29.75	29.71	53	62	53	58.7	N. & E.		1	Clear		12	
Mean	30.02	29.99	30.00					E. & S.		3	Variable		} 10	
Range	0.57	0.49	0.52	21	24	19	17.0	S. & W.		14	Cloudy		}	
Mean of month	30.003			...	...	...	67.7	W. & N.		13	Rain fell on		9	
Extreme range	0.57			...	...	...	33.0							

Remarks.

1st. Mist in the morning.
2d. Very fine.
3d. Pleasant.
4th. Moderate rain in the afternoon; wind E'ly and N. E.
5th. Pleasant. Evening clear.
6th. Very fine.
7th. Pleasant through the day. Began to rain moderately from 7 to 8 P. M.
8th. Fine. Evening very clear and splendid.
9th. Heavy shower from 7 to 8 A. M. Thunder-shower from 7 to 8 P. M. Watched for meteors from 10 P. M. till midnight, sky mostly clear, but only four were seen.
10th, 11th, and 12th. Pleasant.
13th. Very warm and sultry. Showers in the afternoon and evening.
14th. Heavy shower in the morning, with a good deal of thunder. Cloudy in the afternoon. Evening clear.
15th and 16th. Pleasant.
17th. Moderate rain nearly all day.
18th. Cool. Appearances of rain in morning.
19th. Cool, but fine.
20th. Cool. Rain in the evening.
21st. Very damp. Appearances of rain.
22d. Damp. Shower in the afternoon, with high wind. A tornado of extreme violence passed over West Cambridge this day, between 5 and 6 P. M.
23d. Pleasant.
24th. Very fine.
25th. Appearances of rain in the evening.
26th. Rain and thunderstorm last night. To-day, high wind, cool and clear; the air very dry.
27th. Very fine. Air cool and dry.
28th, 29th, and 30th. Very fine.
31st. Fine, the sun very hot and scorching.

September, 1851. New Moon, 25d. 1h. 4m. A. M.

Days.	Barometer At 6 A. M.	At 2 P. M.	At 10 P. M.	Thermometer At 6 A. M.	At 2 P. M.	At 10 P. M.	Daily mean.	Winds At 6 A. M.	At 2 P. M.	At 10 P. M.	Weather At 6 A. M.	At 2 P. M.	At 10 P. M.	Rain and Snow in Inches of Water.
1	30.07	30.08	30.08	62	71	56	63.0	N. W. 1	N. E. 2	N. E. 1	2	1	2	
2	29.98	29.69	29.67	53	63	57	57.7	N. E. 1	S. E. 2	N. W. 2	8	Rain	10	0.60
3	29.76	29.94	29.97	57	60	54	57.0	N. E. 3	N. E. 3	N. E. 1	Misty	Misty	5	
4	29.74	...	30.05	54	...	56	...	N. E. 1	...	N. E. 1	5	...	0	
5	30.06	30.03	30.01	55	74	64	64.3	N'ly 1	S. W. 2	S'ly 1	3	0	Foggy	
6	30.00	29.94	29.94	61	83	68	70.7	S. W. 1	S. W. 1	S. W.	Foggy	3	0	
S 7	29.94	29.90	29.92	68	86	70	74.7	S. W. 1	S. W. 1	S. W. 1	0	4	0	
8	29.94	29.92	29.92	72	82	70	74.7	S. W. 1	S. W. 1	S. W. 1	6	Shower	0	
9	29.95	29.98	30.03	71	80	63	71.3	W. 1	E'ly 2	E'ly 1	0	6	8	
10	30.02	29.95	29.95	62	77	67	68.7	N'ly 1	N. E. 2	S'ly 2	0	0	2	
11	29.92	29.86	29.90	71	87	74	77.3	S. E'ly 1	S. E'ly 1	N. W'ly 1	5	3	2	
12	29.84	29.76	29.70	66	87	74	75.7	S'ly 1	S. E'ly 2	W'ly 2	2	2	5	
13	29.66	29.61	29.77	69	88	59	72.0	W'ly 2	N. W. 2	N. E. 3	0	5	Rain	0.25
S 14	29.97	29.99	30.13	48	59	47	51.3	N. E. 3	N. E. 2	N. E. 1	8	0	0	
15	30.26	30.28	30.30	40	60	47	49.0	N. 2	N'ly 2	Calm	0	0	0	
16	30.32	30.25	30.24	43	64	50	52.3	N. W. 1	N. W. 1	N. W. 1	0	0	0	
17	30.26	30.24	30.25	46	65	47	52.7	N. W. 2	N. E. 2	N. E. 1	1	0	0	
18	30.22	30.14	30.09	44	68	53	55.0	N. E. 1	E'ly 2	Calm	0	1	0	
19	30.00	29.89	29.89	52	75	57	61.3	S. E. 1	S. E. 1	S'ly 1	3	1	0	
20	29.90	29.88	29.87	57	77	64	66.0	S. W. 1	S. W. 2	S. W. 1	1	2	0	
S 21	29.85	29.81	29.97	63	81	55	66.3	S. W. 1	S. W. 1	N. E. 2	4	5	Rain	0.10
22	30.08	30.13	30.14	46	54	49	49.7	N. E. 2	N. E. 2	N. E. 1	10	10	10	
23	30.00	29.74	29.48	43	58	62	54.3	E'ly 2	S. E. 2	S. W. 2	8	10	Rain	0.40
24	29.66	29.77	30.00	49	57	40	48.7	N. W. 2	N. W. 3	N. W. 1	6	0	0	
25	30.08	30.04	29.98	35	57	42	44.7	N'ly 1	S'ly 1	E'ly 1	0	0	0	
26	29.88	29.80	29.75	42	62	55	53.0	N. W'ly 1	S. E'ly 2	S'ly 2	9	5	Sprin'le	
27	29.65	29.63	29.69	57	65	62	61.3	N. E. 1	N. E. 1	N'ly 1	Rain	10	10	0.87
S 28	29.70	29.73	29.79	57	66	62	61.7	N. E. 2	N. E. 1	N. E'ly 1	Misty	0	Misty	
29	[illegible]	[illegible]	[illegible]	[illegible]	[illegible]	[illegible]	[illegible]	[illegible]	[illegible]	[illegible]	[illegible]	[illegible]	[illegible]	[illegible]
30	29.64	29.67	29.70	57	64	57	59.3	S. W. 2	W'ly 2	N. W'ly 1	0	9	0	
Means	29.94	29.91	29.94	55.2	70.1	57.0	...	1.4	1.7	1.2	4.2	4.0	4.0	2.47
REDUCED TO SEA LEVEL.								1.4			4.1			
Max.	30.50	30.46	30.48	72	88	74	77.3	Prevailing winds from some point between—		Days.			Days.	
Min.	29.82	29.79	29.66	35	54	40	44.7	N. & E.		11	Clear		12	
Mean	30.12	30.08	30.12					E. & S.		8	Variable		} 8	
Range	0.68	0.67	0.82	37	34	34	32.6	S. & W.		6	Cloudy		}	
Mean of month	30.107			...	...	...	61.0	W. & N.		5	Rain fell on		10	
Extreme range	0.84			...	...	...	53.0							

Remarks.

1st. Very fine.
2d. Sprinkling of rain at intervals. A brisk thundershower between 6 and 7 P. M. Fires quite comfortable.
3d. Mist, with occasional sprinkling of rain.
4th. Pleasant, though cool. Evening very clear.
5th. Pleasant.
6th. Very fine. Very brilliant aurora, which continued through the night.
7th. Warm and very damp. Brilliant aurora visible this morning between 3 and 4 o'clock.
8th. Sultry. Sprinkling of rain in the morning. Clear in the afternoon and evening.
9th and 10th. Pleasant.
11th. Extremely hot and sultry at mid-day.
12th. Extremely hot. Sprinkling of rain from 8 to 9 P. M.
13th. Very hot till 4 P. M., when we had a fine shower, with light thunder. Wind came round to N. E., and grew cooler fast; showers continued. At 10 P. M., the thermometer stood at 59°, having fallen 29° in eight hours.
14th. At 6 A. M., the thermometer stood at 48°; at 9 A. M., at 52° in the shade and exposed to a current of air, having varied through 40° in sixteen hours.
15th. White frost this morning in some places in this vicinity. The day cool, but pleasant.
16th. Very fine.
17th. Very fine. Evening cool. Fires necessary.
18th. Very fine.
19th. Very fine; the top of the ground quite dry.
20th. Very pleasant; burning sun at mid-day.
21st. Wind came to N. E. from 6 to 7 P. M., with moderate rain.
22d. Cloudy, but no rain.
23d. [illegible]
24th. Air very dry and clear.
25th. Very fine.
26th. Air raw in the afternoon. Sprinkling of rain in the evening.
27th. Morning rainy. Clouds broken in the afternoon. Rain again during the night.
28th. A good deal of mist, without rain.
29th. Light rain in the morning. Remarkable aurora of red light, which was very brilliant at 7½ P. M., forming a splendid crown of light a little south of the zenith.
30th. Pleasant.

October, 1851. New Moon, 24d. 10h. 2m. A. M.

DAYS.	BAROMETER, REDUCED TO 32° F.			THERMOMETER.				WINDS. (DIRECTION AND FORCE.)			WEATHER. (TENTHS CLOUDY.)			RAIN AND SNOW IN INCHES OF WATER.
	Sunrise.	At 2 P. M.	At 10 P. M.	Sunrise.	At 2 P. M.	At 10 P. M.	Daily mean.	Sunrise.	At 2 P. M.	At 10 P. M.	Sunrise.	At 2 P. M.	At 10 P. M.	
1	...	29.79	29.90	...	60	49	...	...	N. W. 1	N. W. 1	...	3	0	
2	29.97	29.94	29.88	42	62	47	50.3	N. W. 1	N. W. 1	N. W. 1	0	0	0	
3	29.72	29.58	29.50	43	60	47	50.0	S. E. 1	S. E'ly 2	S. E. 1	1	1	6	
4	29·51	...	29.70	46	...	54	...	N. W. 1	...	N. W. 1	7	...	2	
S 5	29.76	29.79	29.91	52	60	48	53.3	N'ly 1	N'ly 1	N. W. 2	8	10	0	
6	30.00	29.95	29.97	42	61	47	50.0	N. W. 1	N. W. 1	E'ly 1	0	0	0	
7	30.00	30.00	30.00	47	65	49	53.7	N. W. 1	S'ly 1	S. E'ly 1	0	0	0	
8	30.03	30.01	30.05	48	69	54	57.0	S'ly 1	S'ly 2	S. W'ly 2	0	0	0	
9	30.16	30.13	30.21	51	70	54	58.3	S'ly 1	S. E'ly 2	S'ly 1	0	0	0	
10	30.13	30.02	29.98	48	68	52	56.0	S'ly 1	S. E'ly 2	S'ly 1	Foggy	0	0	
11	30.00	29.94	29.94	49	75	63	62.3	N'ly 1	S'ly 1	S. W'ly 2	2	5	6	
S 12	29.89	29.78	29.76	62	70	66	66.0	S'ly 1	S. E'ly 2	S. E'ly 1	10	Rain	Shower	} 0.75
13	29.63	29.45	29.54	66	70	60	65.3	S. E'ly 2	S'ly 2	W'ly 2	Misty	Misty	5	
14	29.61	29.64	29.66	48	60	49	52.3	W'ly 1	S. W'ly 3	N. W'ly 1	3	4	2	
15	29.70	29.75	29.90	46	59	43	49.3	N. W. 2	N. W. 2	N. W. 2	0	3	0	
16	30.02	30.04	30.06	36	53	41	43.3	N. W. 2	N. W. 2	W'ly 1	0	0	1	
17	30.11	30.05	30.06	34	55	42	43.7	N. W. 1	S. E'ly 2	Calm	3	5	0	
18	30.05	29.99	29.84	41	65	57	54.3	S'ly 1	S'ly 2	S. E'ly 3	2	8	10	
S 19	29.26	29.08	29.34	49	53	50	50.7	N. E. 4	N. E. 2	N. W. 2	Rain	Misty	2	1.10
20	29.60	29.62	29.75	47	60	48	51.7	N. W'ly 2	N. W. 2	N. W. 1	1	1	0	
21	29.79	29.74	29.74	47	68	62	59.0	S'ly 1	S. E'ly 2	S'ly 1	Foggy	3	10	
22	29.82	29.76	29.74	55	55	50	53.3	N. W. 1	N. W. 1	N. W. 1	10	Rain	7	0.15
23	29.77	29.79	29.98	39	51	38	42.7	N. W. 2	N. W. 4	N. W. 2	0	2	0	
24	29.87	29.78	29.70	38	55	50	47.7	N. W. 1	W'ly 3	S. W. 2	5	1	5	
25	29.72	29.49	29.40	49	63	58	56.7	S. W. 3	S. W. 3	S. W. 3	0	8	Rain	
S 26	29.41	29.42	29.29	51	53	40	48.0	W'ly 2	N. W. 1	N'ly 2	9	Rain	Rain	} 1.20
27	29.18	29.40	29.71	32	35	30	32.3	N'ly 3	N. W. 2	N. W. 1	Snow	2	0	
28	29.96	29.91	29.96	33	51	50	44.7	S. W. 2	S. W. 3	S. W. 1	9	8	10	
29	30.08	30.05	30.00	50	64	56	56.7	S. W. 2	S. W. 2	S. W. 2	9	10	10	
30	29.87	29.71	29.53	58	63	61	60.7	S'ly 3	S. E'ly 3	S. E. 3	4	Misty	Rain	
31	29.44	29.44	29.57	55	60	44	53.0	N. W. 2	N. W. 2	N. W. 1	8	4	0	
Means	29.80	29.77	29.79	46.8	60.4	50.3	...	1.6	2.0	1.5	4.7	4.6	3.7	3.20
									1.7			4.3		
REDUCED TO SEA LEVEL.														
Max.	30.34	30.31	30.39	66	75	66	66.0	Prevailing winds from some point between—		Days.				
Min.	29.36	29.26	29.47	32	35	30	42.7	N. & E.		1	Clear		11	
Mean	29.98	29.94	29.97					E. & S.		9	Variable		} 13	
Range	0.98	1.05	0.92	34	40	36	23.3	S. & W.		7	Cloudy			
Mean of month	29.963			...	...	...	52.5	W. & N.		14	Rain or snow fell on		7	
Extreme range	1.13			...	...	...	45.0							

REMARKS.

1st. Pleasant. Evening very clear.

2d. Very fine. Aurora at the north, quite distinct, but not brilliant.

3d, 4th, and 5th. Pleasant.

6th and 7th. Very fine.

8th. Very fine. Warmer at mid-day than for the last fortnight.

9th and 10th. Very fine.

11th. Pleasant.

12th. Warm. Sultry air from the S. E., with occasional light showers.

13th. Showery in the morning. Clouds broken in the evening, and partly clear. Air through the day warm and damp.

14th. Very pleasant.

15th and 16th. Very fine.

17th. Evening very still and clear.

18th. Pleasant. Appearances of rain in the evening.

19th. Rain last night and this morning. Mostly clear in the evening.

20th. Very fine. Aurora in the evening, with streamers quite bright.

21st. Very mild. Lightning at the N. W. in the evening.

22d Moderate showers through the day. Stars out in the evening.

23d. Very fine. Faint aurora in the evening.

24th. Pleasant.

25th. Pleasant in the morning. Cloudy in the afternoon. Light rain began at 9 P. M. Wind very fresh at S. W.

26th. Light rain at intervals through the day. Rain and storm increased in the evening.

27th. Snowing briskly at sunrise this morning, with fields and buildings covered with snow. Up to this day, there has been no frost on College Hill to injure the most delicate plants.

28th. The ground slightly frozen this morning; snow still remaining on the north sides of fences and buildings.

29th. Very mild.

30th. Heavy rain and wind in the evening.

31st. Pleasant.

November, 1851. New Moon, 22d. 8h. 58m. P. M.

DAYS.	BAROMETER Sunrise.	At 2 P. M.	At 10 P. M.	THERMOMETER Sunrise.	At 2 P. M.	At 10 P. M.	Daily mean.	WINDS Sunrise.	At 2 P. M.	At 10 P. M.	WEATHER Sunrise.	At 2 P. M.	At 10 P. M.	RAIN
1	29.63	29.66	29.68	40	56	45	47.0	N. W. 1	N. W. 2	N. W. 1	0	1	7	
S 2	29.50	29.31	29.21	44	56	52	50.7	N. W. 1	S. W. 1	S. W. 1	7	Rain	6	0.25
3	29.07	29.04	29.12	45	52	43	46.7	N. W. 2	N. W. 2	N. W. 2	6	10	Misty	
4	29.22	29.29	29.40	37	43	35	38.3	N. W. 2	N. W. 2	N. W. 2	5	10	7	
5	29.55	29.57	29.73	30	42	35	35.7	N. W. 2	N. W. 3	N. W. 2	0	0	7	
6	29.87	29.82	29.91	26	38	28	30.7	N. W. 2	N. W. 2	N. W. 1	0	0	0	
7	29.94	29.96	29.98	26	38	30	31.3	N. W. 2	N. W. 2	N. W. 1	0	0	0	
8	29.98	29.92	29.89	30	47	45	40.7	N. W. 2	S. W. 2	S. W. 3	0	5	10	
S 9	29.94	29.95	30.00	43	51	42	45.3	W'ly 1	N. W. 1	N. W. 2	10	8	10	
10	29.97	29.83	30.10	38	44	30	37.3	N. W. 2	N. W. 1	N. W. 1	10	Rain	0	
11	30.31	30.39	30.52	24	32	23	26.3	N. W. 1	N. W. 2	N. W. 2	0	0	6	
12	30.51	30.35	30.16	19	34	32	28.3	N. W. 1	N. W. 1	N. W. 1	0	0	5	
13	30.01	29.97	29.94	32	36	28	32.0	N. W. 1	N. W. 2	N. W. 3	8	8	2	
14	29.92	29.80	29.67	26	42	34	34.0	N. W. 1	N. W. 1	S. W. 1	9	9	Misty	
15	29.42	28.95	29.42	34	40	38	37.3	N. E. 2	N. E. 2	...	Rain	Rain	0	1.70
S 16	29.66	29.80	29.91	34	43	33	36.7	N. W. 2	N. W. 1	N. W. 1	8	2	5	
17	29.89	29.79	29.89	32	48	35	38.3	E'ly 1	S. W. 1	N. W. 1	8	5	0	
18	29.92	29.96	30.00	32	43	31	35.3	N. W. 1	N. W. 2	N. W. 1	3	8	10	
19	30.06	30.05	30.08	27	38	29	31.3	N. W. 2	N. W. 2	N. E. 1	0	4	0	
20	30.10	30.05	29.92	25	43	35	34.3	N. E'ly 1	E'ly 2	E'ly 2	1	10	10	
21	29.61	29.17	29.15	40	55	44	46.3	N. E. 2	S. E'ly 3	W'ly 3	Rain	Rain	0	2.25
22	29.31	29.45	29.61	36	45	40	40.3	W'ly 2	W'ly 2	W'ly 2	1	8	5	
S 23	29.78	29.76	29.80	33	45	40	39.3	S. W. 2	W'ly 2	W'ly 2	2	8	10	
24	29.74	29.76	29.91	31	44	32	35.7	W'ly 1	W'ly 2	N. W. 2	2	1	2	
25	29.94	29.78	29.30	28	34	33	31.7	W'ly 1	N. E'ly 1	E'ly 3	7	10	Rain	0.70
26	29.24	29.59	29.91	31	35	28	31.3	N'ly 2	N. W. 3	N. W. 1	10	2	0	
27	30.06	30.03	29.91	27	40	32	33.0	N. W. 2	N. W. 2	W'ly 1	0	1	8	
28	29.62	29.33	29.16	37	45	39	40.3	S. W. 1	S. W. 1	N. W. 3	Rain	Rain	2	0.15
29	29.40	...	29.75	37	...	31	...	W'ly 4	...	N. W. 1	6	...	0	
S 30	29.82	29.77	29.83	28	40	32	33.3	N. W. 1	N. W. 2	N. W. 2	0	3	8	
Means	29.77	29.73	29.76	32.4	43.1	35.1	...	1.6	1.8	1.7	4.4	5.6	5.0	5.05
									1.7			5.0		
REDUCED TO SEA LEVEL.														
Max.	30.69	30.57	30.70	45	56	52	50.7	Prevailing winds from some point between—		Days.				
Min.	29.25	29.13	29.30	19	32	23	26.3	N. & E.		4	Clear		8	
Mean	29.95	29.91	29.94					E. & S.		0	Variable		} 16	
Range	1.44	1.44	1.40	26	24	29	24.4	S. & W.		6	Cloudy			
Mean of month	29.933			...	...	...	36.9	W. & N.		20	Rain fell on		6	
Extreme range	1.57			...	...	...	37.0							

REMARKS.

1st. Very fine.

2d. Rain from 11 A. M. to 3 P. M.

3d. Occasional mist.

4th. Variable.

5th. Pleasant.

6th and 7th. Very fine.

8th. Appearances of rain in the evening.

9th. Mild, with appearances of rain.

10th. Showery in the afternoon. Very clear late in the evening.

11th. Cold, but fine.

12th. Very pleasant.

13th. Pleasant. Kept a look-out for meteors in the evening, but none were observed.

14th. Began to mist from 8 to 9 P. M.

15th. Heavy rain. Clouds broken at 4 P. M., and wind shifted from N. E. to N. W. Evening clear. At 3½ P. M., the barometer stood, reduced to the sea level, at 29.11, and commenced rising at 4 P. M., and continued to rise rapidly. Wind very blustering in the evening. The barometer has not fallen so low since January 29th, when it stood at 29.06.

16th. Pleasant.

17th. Light showers in the morning. Clear at 10 P. M.

18th. Pleasant.

19th. Very fine.

20th. Air chilly, with appearances of storm.

21st. Heavy rain in the morning, and moderate rain in the afternoon. The barometer reached its lowest point at 7 P. M., 29.26 (reduced), and began to rise. Clear at 10 P. M.

22d. Variable.

23d. Pleasant.

24th. Very fine.

25th. Snow commenced falling at 3 P. M. and continued till 8 P. M., when it turned to rain, with from two to three inches of snow on the ground.

26th. Cloudy at intervals in morning. Evening clear. Ground covered with snow.

27th. Pleasant overhead. Snow still remains in many places.

28th. Drizzling rain through the day. Very clear at 11 P. M.

29th. Very blustering in the morning. Evening still and clear

30th. Pleasant.

December, 1851. New Moon, 22d. 10h. 26m. A. M.

Days.	Barometer, reduced to 32° F. Sunrise.	At 2 P. M.	At 10 P. M.	Thermometer. Sunrise.	At 2 P. M.	At 10 P. M.	Daily mean.	Winds (Direction and Force.) Sunrise.	At 2 P. M.	At 10 P. M.	Weather (Tenths Cloudy.) Sunrise.	At 2 P. M.	At 10 P. M.	Rain and Snow in Inches of Water
1	29.76	29.60	29.63	24	30	27	27.0	N. W. 3	N. W. 4	N. W. 2	0	0	0	
2	29.62	29.50	29.46	23	31	24	26.0	N. W. 2	N. W. 2	N. W. 1	0	0	0	
3	29.52	29.53	29.64	19	32	24	25.0	N. W. 2	N. W. 1	N. W. 1	1	0	3	
4	29.66	29.34	29.84	27	32	26	28.3	N. W. 2	N'ly 1	N'ly 2	10	10	10	
5	29.99	30.01	30.22	27	28	19	24.7	N'ly 2	N. W. 2	N. W. 2	10	4	0	
6	30.34	30.35	30.33	14	27	23	21.3	N'ly 2	N. W. 1	N. W. 2	0	0	3	
S 7	30.24	30.17	30.01	27	32	32	30.3	N'ly 1	S'ly 1	S'ly 1	10	Snow	10	
8	29.86	29.50	29.52	34	47	42	41.0	S. W. 1	S. W. 2	W'ly 3	Rain	8	2	
9	29.76	29.75	29.87	31	38	29	32.7	N. W. 3	W'ly 4	N. W. 1	0	5	0	
10	29.40	29.53	29.36	29	37	36	34.0	N. W. 1	S. W. 3	S. W'ly 2	9	0	7	
11	29.64	29.69	29.79	19	22	18	19.7	N. W. 4	N. W. 3	N. W. 2	2	0	0	
12	29.83	29.74	29.51	17	27	39	27.7	N. W. 1	E'ly 2	S'ly 1	9	10	10	
13	29.54	29.53	29.62	27	38	20	28.3	W'ly 2	N. W'ly 1	N. W. 3	8	3	0	
S 14	29.90	29.90	29.74	11	24	23	19.3	N. W. 1	N. W. 2	S. W. 2	0	2	10	
15	29.65	29.39	29.32	31	32	26	29.7	N. E. 2	N. E. 1	N. W. 2	Snow	10	10	0.50
16	29.40	29.62	29.75	22	21	12	18.3	W'ly 2	W'ly 2	N. W. 1	0	0	0	
17	29.76	29.75	29.72	0	13	5	6.0	N. W. 1	N. W. 2	N. W. 2	0	0	0	
18	29.64	29.59	29.60	1	15	14	10.0	N. W. 2	W'ly 2	W'ly 2	0	0	0	
19	29.60	29.54	29.44	14	29	20	21.0	S. W. 2	S. W. 2	S. W. 2	0	0	0	
20	29.35	29.31	...	25	33	...	...	S. W. 1	S. W. 2	...	3	2	...	
S 21	29.91	29.88	30.05	15	28	16	19.7	W'ly 2	W'ly 3	N. W. 1	2	10	0	
22	30.11	30.05	29.94	17	25	20	20.7	E'ly 1	N. E'ly 1	N'ly 2	9	10	10	
23	29.80	29.82	30.05	17	24	14	18.3	N. E. 2	N'ly 2	N. W. 1	Snow	10	0	
24	30.03	29.97	29.62	10	26	29	21.7	N. W. 1	S. W. 1	S. W. 3	8	10	Snow	
25	29.64	29.77	29.94	27	29	9	21.7	S. W'ly 2	N. W. 3	N. E. 2	5	8	Snow	
26	30.06	30.18	30.32	—1	10	4	4.3	N. W. 2	N'ly 2	N'ly 2	1	0	0	
27	30.48	30.43	30.33	1	21	23	11.3	N. W'ly 2	N. W. 1	E'ly 1	0	10	10	
S 28	30.09	29.94	29.79	34	46	45	41.7	S. E'ly 1	S'ly 1	S'ly 2	Misty	Rain	Rain	0.87
29	29.79	29.84	29.95	43	50	37	43.3	W'ly 1	W'ly 2	N. W. 1	10	2	1	
30	30.01	29.96	29.88	33	46	44	41.0	W'ly 2	S. W. 2	S. W. 1	2	3	10	
31	29.89	29.79	29.51	43	46	50	46.3	S. W. 1	S. W. 2	S'ly 2	8	Misty	Rain	1.25
Means	29.81	29.77	29.79	21.3	30.3	25.0	...	1.7	1.9	1.7	4.7	4.7	4.5	2.62
								1.8			4.6			
REDUCED TO SEA LEVEL.														
Max.	30.66	30.61	30.51	43	50	50	46.3							
Min.	29.53	29.49	29.50	—1	10	4	4.3							
Mean	29.99	29.95	29.97											
Range	1.23	1.12	1.01	44	40	46	42.0							
Mean of month	29.970			...	...	...	25.5							
Extreme range	1.17			...	...	...	51.0							

Prevailing winds from some point between— Days.
N. & E. 3
E. & S. 2
S. & W. 8
W. & N. 18

Days.
Clear 11
Variable . . . } 12
Cloudy . . . . }
Rain or snow fell on 8

REMARKS.

1st. Very blustering, and very clear.
2d. Pleasant.
3d. Very fine.
4th. Appearances of storm in the evening.
5th. Cloudy in morning. Evening very clear and cold.
6th. Fine.
7th. Light shower of hail and snow from noon to 1 P. M.
8th. Light shower at sunrise. Clouds broken in the afternoon. Heavy dashes of rain at 8 P. M., and clear and gusty at 10 P. M.
9th. Very blustering through the day. Evening calm and very clear.
10th. Pleasant.
11th. Very cold and wind severe.
12th. Flurry of snow from 3 to 4 P. M.
13th. Mild through the day. Grew cold very fast in the evening, with severe wind.
14th. Air very raw in the afternoon, with wind S. W.
15th. Began to snow from 6 to 7 A. M., and continued till 1 P. M.; snow about four inches on the level. Snow again late in the evening.
16th. Between six and seven inches of snow on the ground this morning. Evening still and cold.
17th. Wind light, but very cold.
18th. Cold, but not unpleasant.
19th. Very fine.
20th. Pleasant.
21st. Pleasant. Evening very clear.
22d. Rather mild, with appearances of storm.
23d. About an inch of light snow on the ground this morning. Evening cold and clear.
24th. Flurry of snow in the evening.
25th. Cold in the afternoon. Flurry of snow at 10 P. M.
26th. Extremely cold.
27th. Very cold morning. Weather moderated, and appearances of storm in the evening.
28th. Light steady rain in the afternoon and evening.
29th. Very mild and pleasant.
30th. Pleasant.
31st. Commenced raining from 6 to 7 P. M.

January, 1852. New Moon, 21d. 2h. 19m. A. M.

Days.	Barometer Sunrise.	At 1 P. M.	At 10 P. M.	Thermometer Sunrise.	At 1 P. M.	At 10 P. M.	Daily mean.	Winds Sunrise.	At 1 P. M.	At 10 P. M.	Weather Sunrise.	At 1 P. M.	At 10 P. M.	Rain and Snow
1	29.58	29.69	29.84	38	42	33	37.7	N. W. 2	N. W. 2	N. W. 1	10	10	0	
2	29.94	29.89	29.86	25	31	26	27.3	N'ly 2	N. E. 2	N. E. 2	3	10	5	
3	29.88	29.77	29.73	25	30	27	27.3	N. E. 2	N. E. 2	N. E. 3	10	10	Snow	
S 4	29.59	29.46	29.36	32	32	30	31.3	N. E. 3	N. E. 2	N. E. 3	R'n, sn.	Rain	Misty	} 1.20
5	29.28	29.24	29.28	32	36	35	34.3	N. E. 2	N'ly 2	N. W. 1	Snow	10	9	}
6	29.16	28.91	28.89	32	34	31	32.3	N. E'ly 2	N. E. 3	N. E. 3	Misty	R'n, h'l	Snow	0.80
7	29.05	29.27	29.55	28	29	16	24.3	N. W. 3	N. W. 3	N. W. 3	10	8	0	
8	29.70	29.76	29.78	12	28	17	19.0	N. W. 3	N. W. 2	N. W. 1	0	2	2	
9	29.64	29.47	29.50	17	31	29	25.7	N'ly 1	N'ly 2	N'ly 1	10	10	10	
10	29.61	29.67	29.69	29	40	33	34.0	N. W'ly 1	S. W. 2	S. W. 1	10	8	10	
S 11	29.56	29.45	29.52	31	37	26	31.3	N'ly 1	N'ly 1	N. W'ly 2	Snow	10	0	
12	29.53	29.52	29.53	25	31	18	24.7	N. W'ly 2	W'ly 3	N. W. 3	8	2	10	
13	29.52	29.44	29.32	18	25	16	19.7	N. W. 2	W'ly 2	W'ly 2	7	3	10	
14	29.40	29.48	29.30	11	26	26	21.0	N. W. 2	W'ly 2	W'ly 2	0	10	0	
15	29.31	29.27	29.44	29	36	24	29.7	S. W. 2	S. W. 2	N. W. 2	9	6	Snow	
16	29.63	29.53	29.43	—2	13	20	10.3	N. W. 1	S. W. 1	S. W. 1	0	5	0	
17	29.74	29.83	30.05	19	22	10	17.0	S. W'ly 2	N. W. 3	N. W. 1	6	2	5	
S 18	30.12	29.98	29.66	11	12	6	9.7	N. W. 1	N. E. 2	N. E. 3	10	Snow	Snow	} 0.60
19	29.44	29.48	29.80	5	8	2	5.0	N. E. 3	N'ly 2	N. W. 1	Snow	Snow	0	}
20	30.20	30.17	30.13	—1	8	8	5.0	W'ly 1	W'ly 2	W'ly 2	0	0	0	
21	30.04	29.83	29.77	9	29	11	16.3	S. W. 2	S. W. 1	N. W. 1	7	10	0	
22	29.88	29.93	30.12	4	19	8	10.3	N. W. 2	N. W. 2	N. W. 1	0	2	0	
23	30.14	30.13	30.34	7	23	10	13.3	N. W. 1	W'ly 2	N. W. 2	0	10	0	
24	30.13	29.99	30.02	11	30	24	21.7	W'ly 2	W'ly 3	S. W. 1	0	0	0	
S 25	30.02	29.91	29.75	20	39	31	30.0	S. W. 1	S. W. 1	S. W'ly 1	0	0	2	
26	29.51	29.47	29.56	35	43	27	38.3	S. W. 2	S. W'ly 1	N. W. 1	10	5	0	
27	29.66	29.70	29.83	14	25	16	18.3	N. W. 2	W'ly 1	N. W. 1	0	0	0	
28	29.88	...	29.60	23	...	37	...	S. W. 1	...	S'ly 2	5	...	10	
29	29.56	29.62	29.71	38	44	37	39.7	N. W. 1	N. W. 2	N. W. 1	9	0	6	
30	[illegible]	[illegible]	[illegible]	[illegible]	[illegible]	[illegible]	[illegible]	[illegible]	[illegible]	[illegible]	[illegible]	[illegible]	10	
31	30.14	30.18	30.10	28	27	27	27.3	N. E. 2	N. E. 3	N. E. 2	Snow	Snow	Snow	0.10
Means	29.70	29.67	29.69	20.5	29.0	22.3	...	1.8	2.0	1.7	6.4	6.4	4.7	2.70
								1.8			5.8			
REDUCED TO SEA LEVEL.														
Max.	30.38	30.36	30.52	38	44	37	39.7							
Min.	29.23	29.09	29.07	2	8	2	5.0							
Mean	29.88	29.85	29.87											
Range	1.15	1.27	1.45	40	36	35	34.0							
Mean of month	29.867			...	...	...	23.9							
Extreme range	1.45			...	...	...	46.0							

Prevailing winds from some point between— Days.
N. & E. 7
E. & S. 0
S. & W. 8
W. & N. 16

Days.
Clear 7
Variable . . . } 11
Cloudy . . . . }
Rain or snow fell on 13

REMARKS.

1st. Cloudy, with occasional mist during the day. Evening very clear, and as mild as spring.
2d. Air rather raw in the afternoon.
3d. Air filled with snow during the greater part of the day.
4th. Moderate rain, hail, and mist.
5th. Snow in the morning. Clouds broken and the moon out in the evening.
6th. Rain, hail, and snow during the day. In the evening, damp heavy snow. At 11 P. M., the barometer (not reduced) stood at 28.90, being the lowest point reached since Dec. 23, 1850, when it fell to 28.60.
7th. From eight to ten inches of snow on the level this morning.
8th. Pleasant.
9th. Flurry of snow from noon to 1 P. M., and again during the night.
10th. Very mild, with appearances of storm in the evening.
11th. Light snow in air in the morning. Evening clear.
12th. Severe wind in the afternoon and evening.
13th. Pleasant. Evening cloudy and air raw.
14th. Flurry of snow during the night. This morning clear and cold.
15th. Pleasant. Flurry of snow in the evening, and wind changed from S. W. to N. W.
16th. Flurry of snow from 7 to 8 P. M. Clear and mild at 10 P. M.
17th. Severe wind at mid-day.
18th. Snow mist this morning. Snow increased during the day, and still more in the evening, the wind and cold being very severe.
19th. Snow continued to fall moderately till 2 P. M. Six or seven inches have fallen, and it is much drifted. Aurora at the north quite bright in the evening, but without streamers.
20th. Very cold.
21st. [illegible] Evening clear.
22d. Cold, but not unpleasant.
23d. Pleasant.
24th. Very pleasant.
25th. Very mild and pleasant. Aurora with streamers in evening, but not very conspicuous.
26th. Very cold.
27th. Very fine.
28th. Pleasant.
29th. Very pleasant.
30th. Appearances of storm in the evening.
31st. Snow fell at intervals during the day, from one to two inches deep on the level.

February, 1852. New Moon, 19d. 7h. 46m. P. M.

Days.	Barometer, reduced to 32° F. Sunrise.	At 1 P. M.	At 10 P. M.	Thermometer. Sunrise.	At 1 P. M.	At 10 P. M.	Daily mean.	Winds. (Direction and Force.) Sunrise.	At 1 P. M.	At 10 P. M.	Weather. (Tenths Cloudy.) Sunrise.	At 1 P. M.	At 10 P. M.	Rain and Snow in Inches of Water.
S 1	29.75	29.53	29.56	31	24	23	26.0	N. E'ly 2	N'ly 2	N'ly 2	Misty	8	Snow	0.33
2	29.54	29.62	29.73	20	30	21	23.7	N'ly 2	N. W. 2	N. W. 1	10	9	0	
3	29.80	29.79	29.82	18	30	21	23.0	N. W. 2	N. W. 1	N. W. 1	0	0	0	
4	29.76	29.61	29.57	27	38	32	32.3	S. W. 1	S. W. 2	N'ly 2	10	3	0	
5	29.60	29.56	29.63	28	50	37	38.3	S. W'ly 1	W'ly 1	W'ly 1	10	1	0	
6	29.67	29.61	29.33	32	44	38	38.0	N. W. 1	S. W. 1	S'ly 1	0	0	Sprinl'g	
7	29.36	29.44	29.61	36	44	32	37.3	S. W'ly 1	W'ly 3	W'ly 4	2	10	0	
S 8	29.85	29.92	29.99	24	30	24	26.0	N. W. 1	N. W. 2	N. W. 1	0	0	0	
9	29.97	29.89	29.91	23	39	34	32.0	N. W. 1	S. W. 3	S. W. 2	0	1	2	
10	29.97	29.95	29.80	27	44	38	36.3	S'ly 1	S'ly 2	S. W. 1	1	0	10	
11	29.48	29.33	29.21	43	50	42	45.0	S'ly 2	S'ly 3	S'ly 1	Rain	Rain	10	0.75
12	29.34	29.33	29.59	35	36	24	31.7	W. by S. 2	W. by S. 3	W'ly 3	10	7	2	
13	29.90	29.81	29.80	22	34	26	27.3	W. by N. 2	W by N. 2	S. W. 2	4	10	10	
14	29.79	29.78	29.93	24	24	17	21.7	N'ly 2	N. E. 2	N'ly 1	10	Snow	0	
S 15	30.02	29.83	29.64	11	28	28	22.3	N. W. 2	N. W'ly 1	S. W. 2	0	0	10	
16	29.29	29.21	29.36	32	32	21	28.3	W. by S. 1	W'ly 3	N. W. 2	Snow	0	0	0.30
17	29.45	29.49	29.67	13	24	18	18.3	N. W. 2	N. W. 3	N. W. 1	2	0	4	
18	29.83	29.86	30.16	17	28	9	18.0	S. W. 1	W'ly 2	N. W. 2	0	3	0	
19	30.32	30.27	30.34	2	22	8	10.7	N. W. 1	N'ly 1	N. W. 2	7	9	1	
20	30.44	30.42	30.39	4	20	12	12.0	N. W. 2	N. W. 2	N. W. 2	0	0	0	
21	30.35	30.22	29.94	7	30	29	22.0	N. W. 1	S. W'ly 2	S. W. 2	0	10	10	
S 22	29.52	29.41	29.43	26	36	32	31.3	N. E. 2	N. W'ly 2	N. W. 1	Snow	10	5	0.30
23	29.33	29.26	29.26	35	43	36	38.0	W. N. W. 1	W. N. W. 2	W'ly 1	10	4	10	
24	29.28	29.27	29.30	30	45	37	37.3	W by N. 1	W. by S. 1	S'ly 2	5	2	10	
25	29.10	28.99	29.26	36	54	36	42.0	S. W. 2	S'ly 1	N. W. 4	3	9	0	
26	29.58	29.78	29.91	24	35	24	27.7	N. W. 2	W'ly 3	N. W. 2	0	3	2	
27	30.01	30.06	30.12	17	32	28	25.7	N. W. 2	N. W. 3	N. W. 2	0	2	Hazy	
28	30.09	29.53	29.01	27	31	41	33.0	N. E. 2	S. E'ly 3	S'ly 3	Snow	Snow	Rain	1.40
S 29	29.40	29.77	29.98	25	27	21	24.3	N. W'ly 4	N. W. 3	N. W. 1	0	0	2	
Means	29.72	29.67	29.70	24.0	34.6	27.2	...	1.5	2.1	1.8	4.6	4.5	4.4	2.00
									1.8			4.5		
REDUCED TO SEA LEVEL.														
Max.	30.62	30.60	30.57	43	54	42	45.0	Prevailing winds from some point between—		Days.				
Min.	29.28	29.17	29.19	2	20	8	10.7						Days.	
Mean	29.90	29.85	29.88					N. & E.		2	Clear		8	
Range	1.34	1.43	1.38	41	34	34	34.3	E. & S.		2	Variable		} 11	
Mean of month 29.877				...	...	...	28.6	S. & W.		11	Cloudy			
Extreme range 1.45				...	...	...	52.0	W. & N.		14	Rain or snow fell on 10			

REMARKS.

1st. Mist, hail, snow, and some sunshine.
2d. Cloudy in morning. Evening very clear.
3d and 4th. Very fine.
5th. Mild and pleasant. Evening very clear.
6th. Pleasant. Light shower from 7 to 8 P. M.
7th. Pleasant in the morning. Blustering in the afternoon and evening.
8th and 9th. Very fine.
10th. Fine during the day. Evening cloudy, with indications of storm.
11th. Moderate rain through the day.
12th. Flurry of snow at 8 A. M., and again at 1 P. M. The ground nearly bare of snow.
13th. Flurry of snow from 6 to 7 P. M.
14th. Light snow in the afternoon—ground just covered. Clear at 10 P. M., and cold.
15th. Air raw in afternoon; wind S. W. Appearances of storm in the evening.
16th. Snowing at sunrise, which continued more or less till 10 A. M., when the clouds brushed away. Snow from two to three inches on the level. Evening clear and cool.
17th. Cold, but pleasant. Aurora in evening.
18th. Pleasant. Grew cold in the afternoon.
19th. At 9 A. M., barom. 30.40. Very brilliant aurora in the evening, streamers and merry dancers, exhibiting in turn red, pink, green, and white light. At 10 h. 20 m., a most beautiful crown of red and white light was formed a little south of the zenith, the wind at the time being light from the N. W., and the thermometer standing at 8°. The merry dancers seemed to spring up in every part of the heavens, with a movement for the most part towards the zenith.
20th. Cold, but pleasant.
21st. Pleasant. Cloudy in the afternoon and evening.
22d. Snow in the morning.
23d. Snowed moderately from 8 to 10 A. M.
24th. Mild and pleasant.
25th. The warmest day since Nov. 21, 1851. Thermometer 54° at 1 P. M.
26th. Pleasant.
27th. Pleasant. Thick haze in the evening.
28th. Steady snow in the morning; wind E'ly. Rain in the afternoon; wind hauling to S. E. Rain continued in evening, wind changing to S. W'ly. At 11 P. M., barometer 29.05; at midnight, 29.30; half hour later, 29.00, when it seemed to be stationary, and probably began to rise very soon.
29th. Very blustering.

March, 1852. New Moon, 20d. 1h. 34m. P. M.

Days.	Barometer. At 6 A. M.	At 1 P. M.	At 10 P. M.	Thermometer. At 6 A. M.	At 1 P. M.	At 10 P. M.	Daily mean.	Winds. At 6 A. M.	At 1 P. M.	At 10 P. M.	Weather. At 6 A. M.	At 1 P. M.	At 10 P. M.	Rain and Snow.
1	30.04	29.95	29.84	21	30	24	25.0	N. W. 2	N'ly 1	N. E'ly 2	1	10	10	
2	29.65	29.67	30.04	25	23	13	20.3	N. E. 2	N. W'ly 2	N. W. 3	Misty	Snow	0	
3	30.21	30.25	30.37	10	24	15	16.3	N. W. 2	N. W. 2	N. W. 1	0	0	0	
4	30.41	30.33	30.08	11	29	25	21.7	N. W. 2	W'ly 1	S. W'ly 2	0	5	Snow	
5	29.84	29.67	29.75	26	41	31	32.7	E'ly 1	N. W'ly 1	N. W. 1	10	10	10	
6	29.89	29.87	29.91	26	40	31	32.3	N. W. 2	N. W. 1	N. W. 1	4	5	10	
S 7	30.03	30.03	30.09	26	35	26	29.0	N. W. 2	N. W. 3	N. W. 1	0	0	0	
8	30.10	30.01	29.80	26	42	36	34.7	W'ly 1	S. W. 2	S. W. 2	5	3	10	
9	29.52	29.26	29.21	40	54	52	48.7	S. W. 2	S. W. 1	S. W'ly 3	9	9	2	
10	29.61	29.82	30.13	38	45	31	38.0	N. W. 2	N. W. 2	N. W. 2	1	2	0	
11	30.38	30.44	30.42	26	46	30	34.0	N. by W. 2	E'ly 1	S. by E. 1	0	0	0	
12	30.29	30.03	29.92	31	54	47	44.0	S. W. 2	S. W'ly 3	S. W. 2	10	9	10	
13	29.87	29.74	29.80	50	58	52	53.3	W N W 1	N'ly 1	N. W. 1	10	10	10	
S 14	29.80	29.78	29.61	44	46	36	42.0	N. W. 2	N. E. 3	N. E. 2	10	10	Rain	0.25
15	29.46	29.40	29.51	36	51	38	41.7	N. E. 2	N. W. 1	W'ly 1	10	9	3	
16	29.73	29.72	29.78	33	48	38	39.7	N. W. 2	N. W. 2	N. W. 1	0	2	0	
17	29.81	29.75	29.56	34	39	33	35.3	N. E. 2	N. E. 2	N. E. 4	10	10	Snow	
18	29.51	29.51	29.69	33	35	33	33.7	N. E. 4	N. E. 2	N'ly 2	Rain	Rain	10	1.45
19	29.83	29.72	29.81	26	35	27	29.3	N. W. 2	N. W. 2	N. W'ly 2	2	4	10	
20	29.74	29.72	29.88	20	31	22	24.3	N. W. 2	N. W. 3	N. W. 2	0	5	0	
S 21	29.94	29.84	29.57	16	32	33	27.0	N. W. 2	S. W'ly 2	S. W'ly 3	0	8	Snow	
22	29.56	29.57	29.49	31	40	35	35.3	N. W. 1	N'ly 2	S. W'ly 1	7	0	10	
23	29.22	29.02	29.14	36	44	35	38.3	S. E. 2	S. W. 1	W'ly 2	10	Rain	0	
24	29.31	29.19	29.09	32	43	35	36.7	N. W. 2	S'ly 2	S'ly 1	10	5	10	
25	29.12	29.40	29.62	32	40	33	35.0	N. E. 2	N. W. 2	N. W. 1	Snow	2	0	0.85
26	29.68	29.66	29.57	29	47	41	39.0	N. W. 1	S'ly 2	S'ly 1	2	2	10	
27	29.73	29.83	29.93	35	49	40	41.3	N. W. 2	N. E'ly 1	N. E. 2	5	10	10	
S 28	30.07	30.09	30.14	35	48	35	39.3	N. E'ly 2	N. E. 3	N. E. 2	3	0	2	
29	30.15	29.97	29.93	30	49	34	37.7	N'ly 1	E'ly 3	N. E'ly 2	3	8	9	
30	29.93	29.87	29.92	32	43	33	36.0	N. E. 2	N. E. 2	E'ly 2	10	10	10	
31	29.93	29.80	29.53	32	40	37	36.3	N. E. 2	S. E. 3	E'ly 2	10	10	Rain	1.00
Means	29.82	29.77	29.77	29.7	41.3	33.3	...	1.9	1.9	1.8	5.5	6.1	6.3	3.55
									1.9			6.0		
REDUCED TO SEA LEVEL.														
Max.	30.59	30.62	30.60	50	58	52	53.3	Prevailing winds from some point between—		Days.				
Min.	29.30	29.20	29.27	10	23	13	16.3						Days.	
Mean	30.00	29.95	29.95					N. & E.		8	Clear		7	
Range	1.29	1.42	1.33	40	35	39	37.0	E. & S.		1	Variable		} 11	
Mean of month 29.967				...	...	...	34.8	S. & W.		8	Cloudy			
Extreme range 1.42				...	...	...	48.0	W. & N.		14	Rain or snow fell on 13			

1st. Cold and raw, with indications of storm.
2d. The air full of mist. Hail and snow during the day. Clouds broken at sunset. Evening clear and cold.
3d. Very clear and cold.
4th. Very clear in the morning. Overcast in the afternoon. Snow in the evening.
5th. Half an inch of fresh snow on the ground this morning.
6th. Pleasant.
7th. Very pleasant.
8th. Pleasant through the day. Appearance of storm in the evening.
9th. Light showers from 5 to 6 A. M., and again at 6 P. M. Clouds broken in the evening, and quite clear at 11 P. M.
10th. Pleasant.
11th. Very fine.
12th. Mild. Sprinkling of rain at 6 P. M.
13th. Air damp; occasional sprinkling of rain. The warmest day since Oct. 31, 1851. Ther. 58° at 1 P. M.
14th. Began to rain moderately from 3 to 4 P. M., and continued through the evening.
15th. Cloudy in the morning. Warm sunshine from 3 to 5 P M; dashes of rain from 5 to 6 P. M. Starlight and heavy fog in the evening.
16th. Very fine.
17th. Air raw. Began to snow from 7 to 8 P. M.
18th. Rain and mist during the day.
19th. Air raw and uncomfortable.
20th. Cold and uncomfortable.
21st. Air very raw and cold. Began to snow from 9 to 10 P. M.
22d. Ground covered with snow this morning.
23d. Rain from 11½ A. M. to 2 P. M. Evening clear.
24th. Pleasant in the morning. Began to snow from 11 to 12 P. M.
25th. Snow continued till from 8 to 9 A. M.—damp, and from three to four inches deep. Clouds broken in the afternoon. Evening clear.
26th. Snow of yesterday nearly gone.
27th. Cloudy, with some appearance of storm.
28th. Very fine.
29th. Air raw. In the evening, wind N. E'ly, clouds at the same time broken and coming from the N. W.
30th. Air very raw and uncomfortable. Flakes of snow at 5 P. M.
31st. Rain in the afternoon and evening.

April, 1852. New Moon, 19d. 6h. 37m. A. M.

Days.	Barometer, reduced to 32° F. At 6 A. M.	At 1 P. M.	At 10 P. M.	Thermometer. At 6 A. M.	At 1 P. M.	At 10 P. M.	Daily mean.	Winds (Direction and Force.) At 6 A. M.	At 1 P. M.	At 10 P. M.	Weather (Tenths Cloudy.) At 6 A. M.	At 1 P. M.	At 10 P. M.	Rain and Snow in Inches of Water
1	29.60	29.74	29.77	34	52	37	41.0	N. W. 3	W. 3	E'ly 2	2	0	2	
2	29.75	29.63	29.65	37	53	35	41.7	S. W. 2	y 2	N. W'ly 2	3	10	9	
3	29.74	29.71	29.80	28	37	30	31.7	N. W. 2	W. 3	N. W. 2	0	7	0	
S 4	29.88	29.86	29.84	27	45	37	36.3	N. W. 2	E. 2	N. E'ly 2	0	4	10	
5	29.78	29.75	29.50	31	43	32	35.3	N. E. 1	N. E. 2	E'ly 4	9	10	Snow	} 1.15
6	29.30	29.31	29.38	32	35	28	31.7	N. E. 4	N'lly 3	N'ly 1	Snow	Misty	10	
7	29.62	29.67	29.69	30	46	35	37.0	N. W. 2	W. 1	N. W. 1	7	1	0	
8	29.73	29.68	29.63	32	52	42	42.0	N. W. 1	N. 'ly 2	S. W. 1	0	5	10	
9	29.44	29.41	29.49	37	34	40	37.0	N. by E. 2	N. E. 2	N. E. 1	10	Snow	10	
10	29.61	29.58	29.68	39	51	43	44.3	N. W. 2	N. W. 3	N. W. 1	3	2	3	
S 11	29.73	29.69	29.72	35	56	43	44.7	N. W. 1	N. W. 1	S'ly 1	0	0	10	
12	29.75	29.72	29.64	42	45	36	41.0	S. E'ly 2	E'ly 2	N. E. 3	10	Sprinl'g	Misty	
13	29.49	29.49	29.54	32	32	34	32.7	N. E. 3	N. E. 3	N'ly 1	R'n, h'l	Snow	5	1.65
14	29.62	29.59	29.53	36	56	40	44.0	N'ly 1	E'ly 2	E'ly 2		3	10	
15	29.43	29.16	29.00	37	38	35	36.7	E'ly 2	N. E. 2	N. E. 2	1	Rain	Misty	1.35
16	29.15	29.33	29.59	34	46	38	39.3	N. W. 3	N. W. 4	N. W. 1	0	5	0	
17	29.72	29.76	29.78	36	60	40	45.3	N. W. 1	S'ly 1	S. W'ly 1	0	0	0	
S 18	29.75	29.70	29.63	40	45	37	40.7	N. E. 2	N. E. 3	N. E. 4	Misty	10	10	
19	29.46	29.40	29.40	37	40	38	38.3	N. E. 3	N. E. 3	N. E. 3	Misty	Rain	Rain	}
20	29.31	29.28	29.04	38	40	39	39.0	N. E. 2	N. E. 2	N. E. 3	Rain	Rain	Rain	} 2.40
21	28.66	28.83	28.88	46	48	42	45.3	E. S. E. 4	S. S. E. 2	S'ly 2	Rain	Rain	10	}
22	28.88	28.93	29.08	44	55	43	47.3	S'ly 1	S. W. 2	N. W. 1	10	8	2	
23	29.12	29.16	29.31	43	56	42	47.0	N. W. 1	N. by E. 1	N'ly 2	4	8	10	
24	29.44	29.45	29.55	38	53	38	43.0	N. W. 2	N. W. 2	N. W. 2	7	8	0	
S 25	29.68	29.62	29.67	34	58	48	46.7	N. W. 2	N. W. 1	N. W. 1	2	5	7	
26	29.66	29.58	29.31	46	60	50	52.0	S. W. 1	S. W. 1	S. W. 2	5	9	Shower	0.10
27	29.35	29.34	29.51	47	57	42	48.7	S. W'ly 1	2	N. W. 3	10	2	0	
28	29.58	29.53	29.62	36	53	42	43.7	N. W. 2	N. W. 3	N. W. 1	0	5	5	
29	29.64	29.57	29.65	39	59	48	48.7	N. W. 2	N. W. 3	S. W. 1	0	0	2	
30	29.67	29.62	29.72	48	65	46	53.0	W'ly 1	S. W. 2	S. W. 1	3	0	2	
Means	29.52	29.50	29.52	37.2	49.0	39.3	...	1.9	2.2	1.8	5.4	6.1	6.2	6.65
								2.0			5.9			
REDUCED TO SEA LEVEL.								Prevailing winds from some point between— Days.			Days.			
Max.	30.06	30.04	30.02	48	65	50	53.0	N. & E. 11			Clear 6			
Min.	28.84	29.01	29.06	27	32	30	31.7	E. & S. 1			Variable . . . } 11			
Mean	29.70	29.68	29.70					S. & W. 7			Cloudy . . . . }			
Range	1.22	1.03	0.96	21	33	20	21.3	W. & N. 11			Rain or snow fell on 13			
Mean of month	29.693			...	...	...	41.8							
Extreme range	1.22			...	...	...	38.0							

Remarks.

1st. Pleasant.
2d. Pleasant A. M. Light rain from 5 to 6 P. M.
3d. Blustering and cold. Evening very clear.
4th. Pleasant in the morning. Appearances of storm in the evening.
5th. Began to snow at 9 P. M.: wind brisk at about E. N. E. At 11½ P. M., wind blew heavily.
6th. Snow continued nearly all day; damp and heavy; eight or nine inches on the level—being the deepest snow during the winter.
7th. Very pleasant. A white bow of 22° 30′ radius about the sun from 11 A. M. to noon.
8th. Pleasant day. Evening thick cloudy.
9th. Began to snow moderately at 9 A. M., and continued till noon, melting as it fell.
10th. Bow round the sun from 9 to 10½ A. M., the upper half being quite well defined and fringed with red on the inside.
11th. Very fine morning. Cloudy evening. The snow of the 5th and 6th lingers in some places.
12th. Frequent sprinkling and mist during day.
13th. Rain at 5 A. M.; turned to hail at 7 A. M., and then to snow, which continued till sunset, with pretty heavy wind at N. E., and then N. N. E. Partially clear in evening. Seven inches of snow.
14th. Pleasant. Snow melting rapidly.
15th. Rain began at 7 A. M.; continued all day.
16th. Occasional sprinkling in morning. Evening very clear. The snow of the 13th disappeared during this day.
17th Very fine. The warmest day of the season thus far. Thermometer 60° at 1 P. M.
18th. Light mist at times; air very raw and uncomfortable.
19th. Heavy storm all day.
20th. Moderate rain nearly all day.
21st. At 6 A. M., the barometer (not reduced) stood at 28.74, being the lowest since Dec. 23, 1850, with heavy wind at about E. S. E. At 8 A. M., barometer 28.60. Moderate rain nearly all day, the wind hauling to S'ly, and abating in force, in the afternoon.
22d. Light showers at intervals. Clear in the evening, and bright aurora, with streamers and merry dancers, in the north.
23d, 24th, and 25th. Pleasant.
26th. Mostly overcast. Showers, with thunder, at 10 P. M.
27th. Pleasant. Evening very clear.
28th. Pleasant.
29th. Pleasant. Fog-bow round the moon at 9½ P. M.
30th. Very fine.

May, 1852. New Moon, 18d. 10h. 7m. P. M.

Days.	Barometer At 6 A. M.	At 1 P. M.	At 10 P. M.	Thermometer At 6 A. M.	At 1 P. M.	At 10 P. M.	Daily mean.	Winds At 6 A. M.	At 1 P. M.	At 10 P. M.	Weather At 6 A. M.	At 1 P. M.	At 10 P. M.	Rain and Snow in Inches of Water
1	29.76	29.61	29.53	44	56	42	47.3	S. W. 1	S. E. 1	N. E. 2	Rain	10	Misty	
S 2	29.54	...	29.61	41	60	46	49.0	N. E. 2	...	N. W. 1	Rain	...	3	
3	29.67	29.66	29.95	48	61	39	49.3	N. W. 1	N. W. 3	N. W. 1	0	4	0	
4	30.07	30.08	30.12	37	55	46	46.0	N. W. 2	N. E. 2	N. W. 1	1	1	5	
5	30.16	30.14	30.10	46	72	51	56.3	N. W. 2	N. by E. 1	S. W. 1	0	0	2	
6	30.10	30.06	30.07	52	75	60	62.3	S'ly 1	S. W. 2	S'ly 1	0	0	0	
7	30.02	29.90	29.92	56	87	59	67.3	S. W. 2	S. W. 3	S. W. 2	1	0	0	
8	29.84	29.77	29.81	56	79	56	63.7	S. W. 2	S. W. 3	S. W. 2	Hazy	2	0	
S 9	29.76	29.71	29.69	55	76	58	63.0	S. W. 1	S. W. 2	S. W. 2	3	0	3	
10	29.69	29.71	29.78	55	72	58	61.7	N. W. 1	N. W. 2	N. W. 1	9	8	0	
11	29.90	29.94	29.94	50	73	53	58.7	N. E. 2	E'ly 2	S'ly 2	0	3	9	
12	29.87	29.75	29.80	53	53	47	51.0	S. E'ly 2	E'ly 2	N. E. 3	10	Rain	Misty	} 2.00
13	29.87	29.86	29.82	47	46	44	45.7	N. E. 3	N. E. 4	N. E. 3	Misty	Rain	Rain	}
14	29.80	29.80	29.76	43	46	44	44.3	N. E. 4	N. E. 2	N'ly 1	10	10	10	
15	29.75	29.70	29.66	47	55	50	50.7	N. W'ly 1	S. E'ly 2	S'ly 1	10	10	10	
S 16	29.68	29.66	29.69	53	70	54	59.0	N. W. 1	S. E. 2	S'ly 2	10	5	5	
17	29.66	29.58	29.49	52	63	58	57.7	S. E'ly 2	S. E'ly 3	S. W'ly 1	10	9	10	
18	29.71	29.73	29.81	50	64	51	55.0	N. W. 2	N. W. 2	N. W. 2	7	0	0	
19	29.87	29.77	29.74	50	69	50	56.3	N. W.	S. E. 2	S. E'ly 1	0	0	5	
20	29.69	29.66	29.88	52	69	48	56.3	S. W. 2	N. W. 2	N. W. 1	5	3	0	
21	30.01	29.96	29.93	46	67	50	54.3	N. W. 2	S. E. 2	S'ly 1	0	0	0	
22	29.91	29.88	29.89	54	79	58	63.7	W'ly 3	S. W'ly 2	S. W'ly 2	0	8	0	
S 23	29.85	29.76	29.73	58	70	58	62.0	S. W. 1	S. W. 2	S. W. 1	10	10	7	
24	29.74	29.67	29.60	56	65	52	57.7	N. E. 2	N. E. 2	N. E. 2	7	4	0	
25	29.50	29.54	29.73	59	74	55	62.7	N'ly 2	N. W. 3	N. W. 1	3	0	0	
26	29.80	29.74	29.70	53	73	55	60.3	N'ly 2	E'ly 2	S'ly 2	0	3	3	
27	29.50	29.54	29.40	55	63	60	59.3	S. by E.	S'ly 2	S. W. 1	Sprinl'g	10	6	
28	29.62	29.69	29.80	56	75	54	61.7	N. E. 2	S. E. 2	S. E. 1	10	3	10	
29	29.81	29.75	29.58	59	68	58	61.7	S.	S. 1	S. 1	Misty	7	Misty	
S 30	29.45	29.49	29.60	74	75	57	60.7	S. W.	N. W. 2	N. 1	7	0	0	
31	29.73	29.68	29.60	51	68	57	58.7	N. W. 3	N. W. 3	N. W.	0	0	0	
Means	29.78	29.76	29.77	51.9	67.0	52.5	...	1.9	2.2	1.5	5.2	4.1	4.1	2.00
								1.9			4.5			
REDUCED TO SEA LEVEL.								Prevailing winds from some point between— Days.			Days.			
Max.	30.34	30.32	30.30	74	87	60	68.7	N. & E. 7			Clear 12			
Min.	29.63	29.67	29.58	37	46	39	44.3	E. & S. 8			Variable . . . } 11			
Mean	29.90	29.94	29.95					S. & W. 8			Cloudy . . . . }			
Range	0.71	0.65	0.72	37	41	21	24.4	W. & N. 8			Rain fell on . . 8			
Mean of month	29.950			...	...	...	57.1							
Extreme range	0.76			...	...	...	50.0							

Remarks.

1st. Light showers from 7 to 9 A. M.
2d. Light shower early in the morning. Shower from 8 to 9 P. M. Mostly clear at 10 P. M.
3d. Pleasant.
4th. Very fine.
5th. Very fine. Warmest day since October 11, 1851.
6th. Very fine, with summer heat.
7th. The thermometer in the shade, exposed to a fresh breeze, stood at 87° at 2 P. M. Warmest day since September 13, 1851.
8th. Very fine.
9th. Very pleasant.
10th. Cloudy in the morning. Sprinkling of rain at noon. Evening very clear, with auroral streamers at the north.
11th. Pleasant.
12th. Began to rain moderately at 7 A. M., with wind S. E'ly, which soon hauled more to the E., and then N. E., with increased force and more copious rain.
13th. Rain and heavy wind through the day.
14th. Cloudy, with occasional mist.
15th. Occasional sprinkling of rain.
16th. Pleasant.
17th. Cloudy, with occasional light mist. Lightning in the evening.
18th. Pleasant. Bright aurora in the evening, but no streamers.
19th. Very fine. Bright aurora in the evening, without streamers.
20th. Very fine. Evening clear, with aurora in the north, and streamers not very bright.
21st and 22d. Very fine.
23d, Sprinkling of rain at 9 A. M. and at 3 P. M.
24th. Pleasant.
25th. Very fine.
26th. Pleasant.
27th. Sprinkling of rain from 7 to 8 A. M.
28th. Pleasant.
29th. Cloudy and misty.
30th and 31st. Very fine.

June, 1852. New Moon, 17d. 11h. 39m. A. M.

Days.	Barometer, reduced to 32° F. At 6 A. M.	At 1 P. M.	At 10 P. M.	Thermometer. At 6 A. M.	At 1 P. M.	At 10 P. M.	Daily mean.	Winds. (Direction and Force.) At 6 A. M.	At 1 P. M.	At 10 P. M.	Weather. (Tenths Cloudy.) At 6 A. M.	At 1 P. M.	At 10 P. M.	Rain and Snow in Inches of Water.
1	29.67	29.62	29.62	60	72	60	64.0	W. 1	S'ly 2	W.	0	5	8	
2	29.58	29.48	29.57	62	79	66	69.0	W. 1	S. W. 2	S. W. 1	2	4	0	
3	29.46	29.33	29.37	70	84	68	74.0	S. W.	S. W. 3	S. W. 2	10	8	4	
4	29.54	29.59	29.62	62	61	52	58.3	N. W. 1	N. W.	N. W.	9	10	7	
5	29.70	29.67	29.76	50	64	51	55.0	N. W. 3	N. W. 3	N. W.	0	0	0	
S 6	29.81	29.75	29.70	58	72	54	61.3	N. W.	S. W. 3	S. W. 3	0	3	10	
7	29.68	29.64	29.77	60	72	59	63.7	S. W. 3	S. W. 1	W. 3	7	10	5	
8	29.79	29.63	29.45	68	70	62	66.7	S.	S. 1	E. 2	10	8	Rain	0.50
9	29.38	29.45	...	65	73	...	69.0	S. W. 2	S. W. 1	...	7	8	...	
10	...	29.57	29.87	...	74	58	66.0	...	S. W. 3	W. 2	...	3	2	
11	29.95	29.96	30.04	58	68	52	59.3	N. W.	N. W. 3	N. W.	0	4	0	
12	30.01	30.08	30.10	52	70	53	58.3	N.	N. W.	N. 1	8	9	0	
S 13	30.16	30.14	30.15	62	84	59	68.3	N. W.	N'ly	N. W. 1	0	3	0	
14	30.15	30.14	30.01	62	78	65	68.3	S. W. 1	S'ly 2	S. W. 1	0	2	0	0.15
15	29.92	29.80	29.74	55	78	71	68.0	S. W. 2	W by N 2	Calm	5	2	0	
16	29.73	29.70	29.72	74	94½	74	80.7	N. W. 1	W. by N. 1	N. W'ly 2	2	3	10	
17	29.73	29.68	29.67	74	86	70	76.7	N. W'ly 1	N. W. 1	N. E'ly 1	3	8	Rain	
18	29.60	29.53	29.54	68	86	71	75.0	N. E. 1	S. W. 2	W'ly 1	10	8	0	
19	29.61	29.58	...	65	87	...	76.0	N. W. 1	S. 2	...	1	7	...	
S 20	29.62	29.58	29.65	68	81	65	71.3	S. W. 2	S. W. 2	S'ly 2	10	3	8	0.20
21	29.64	29.65	29.64	63	86	65	71.3	S. W'ly 1	S. S. E. 2	S'ly 1	1	4	0	
22	29.59	29.50	29.43	67	79	66	70.7	S. W'ly 2	S. W. 3	W'ly 2	10	2	3	0.25
23	29.60	29.61	29.64	63	75	62	66.7	N. W. 2	W'ly 3	W'ly 2	2	0	2	
24	29.65	29.58	29.42	62	72	63	65.7	S. W. 2	S. E'ly 3	S'ly 2	4	0	7	
25	29.40	29.50	29.75	62	67	57	62.0	N. W. 2	N. W. 3	N. W. 2	3	8	0	
26	29.85	29.83	29.85	56	79	60	65.0	N. W. 1	W. 2	S. W. 1	0	3	0	
S 27	29.86	29.80	29.79	65	82	65	70.7	S. W. 1	S. W. 2	S. W. 2	3	2	9	
28	29.77	29.73	29.76	66	82	68	72.0	S. W. 1	S. W. 2	S. W. 1	2	3	3	
29	29.75	29.73	29.66	66	85	64	71.7	S. W. 1	S. W. 3	S. W. 1	2	5	0	
30	29.66	29.63	29.65	68	84	69	73.7	S. W. 2	S. W. 3	W'ly 1	0	2	2	
Means	29.72	29.58	29.71	63.1	77.5	62.5	...	1.5	2.1	1.5	4.2	4.5	3.6	1.00
REDUCED TO SEA LEVEL.									1.7			4.1		
Max.	30.34	30.32	30.33	74	94½	74	80.7	Prevailing winds from some point between—		Days.			Days.	
Min.	29.56	29.51	29.55	50	61	51	55.0	N. & E.		0	Clear		8	
Mean	29.90	29.86	29.89					E. & S.		3	Variable		} 12	
Range	0.78	0.81	0.78	24	33	23	25.7	S. & W.		15	Cloudy			
Mean of month			29.883	...	...	...	67.7	W. & N.		12	Rain fell on		10	
Extreme range			0.83	...	...	...	44.5							

Remarks.

1st. Very pleasant.
2d. Pleasant. Sprinkling of rain in morning.
3d. Sultry. Light shower at noon, and in the evening accompanied with some thunder. Rainbow just before sunset.
4th. Pleasant. Light shower at noon.
5th. Very fine. Cool for the season.
6th. Pleasant. Windy.
7th. Blustering. Light shower at noon.
8th. Windy in the morning. Showers in the afternoon and during the night.
9th. Pleasant.
10th. Very pleasant.
11th. Very fine. Aurora in the evening.
12th, 13th, and 14th. Very fine.
15th. Thundershower from 8½ to 10 A. M. Aurora in the evening.
16th. Extremely hot. The mean of two thermometers in the shade, exposed to the breeze, at 1 P. M., was 94°.5—being 2°.5 higher than the highest point reached during the last summer. On the 13th of July, 1849, the same thermometer in the same place stood at 97°.
17th. Thunder and light showers in evening.
18th. Pleasant, though warm.
19th. Pleasant.
20th. Thundershower from 4 to 5 A. M.
21st. Very fine.
22d. Thundershower from 7 to 8 P. M.
23d and 24th. Pleasant.
25th. Very cool for the season.
26th. Very pleasant.
27th. Pleasant.
28th. Fine. Sun hot.
29th. Fine. Sun scorching.
30th. Warm and sultry. Thunder and sprinkling of rain at 4 P. M.

July, 1852. New Moon, 16d. 11h. 7m. P. M.

Days.	Barometer At 6 A. M.	At 1 P. M.	At 10 P. M.	Thermometer At 6 A. M.	At 1 P. M.	At 10 P. M.	Daily mean.	Winds At 6 A. M.	At 1 P. M.	At 10 P. M.	Weather At 6 A. M.	At 1 P. M.	At 10 P. M.	Rain and Snow in Inches of Water.
1	29.71	29.67	29.55	70	80	68	72.7	S. W. 1	S. W. 2	S'ly 2	10	7	Foggy	
2	29.36	29.44	29.56	70	78	59	69.0	S. W. 3	S. W. 3	N. W. 1	10	3	3	0.20
3	29.65	29.64	29.75	58	76	62	65.3	N. W. 2	N. W. 3	N. W. 1	0	0	0	
S 4	29.84	29.83	29.84	64	82	64	70.0	N. W. 2	N. W. 3	S. W. 2	0	0	2	
5	29.85	29.81	29.81	66	87	68	73.7	W'ly 2	W'ly 2	S. W. 2	1	2	2	
6	29.86	29.86	29.94	68	88	65	73.7	W by S. 2	E'ly 2	E'ly 1	4	5	0	
7	29.96	29.96	29.97	63	80	64	69.0	S. E. 2	S. E. 2	S'ly 2	2	0	8	
8	29.92	29.86	29.86	63	86	68	69.0	S. E'ly 1	S. W'ly 2	S. W. 1	6	0	0	
9	29.86	29.83	29.85	71	93	72	78.7	S. W. 2	S. W. 3	S. W. 2	0	0	0	
10	29.88	29.87	29.91	70	92	66	76.0	W by S. 1	S. W. 2	S. W. 1	0	1	0	
S 11	29.92	29.85	29.87	72	89	72	77.7	S. W. 2	S. W. 2	S. W. 2	5	0	10	
12	29.88	29.88	29.93	73	90	73	78.7	S. W. 2	S'ly 2	S. E. 2	10	3	10	
13	29.95	29.93	29.85	72	84	72	76.0	S. by E. 2	S. by E. 3	S. E'ly 2	10	5	9	
14	29.77	29.71	29.76	74	83	71	76.0	S'ly 2	S. W. 1	S. W. 1	8	8	8	
15	29.80	29.82	29.94	70	84	65	73.0	N. E'ly 2	N. E. 2	N. E. 1	2	7	0	
16	29.97	29.95	29.88	63	85	64	70.7	N. E. 2	S. W'ly 2	S. E'ly 1	5	4	6	
17	29.79	29.73	29.70	64	62	56	60.7	N. E'ly 1	N. E. 2	N. E. 1	10	Rain	10	0.70
S 18	29.75	29.81	29.97	58	77	61	65.3	N'ly 2	N. W. 1	S'ly 1	3	5	0	
19	30.09	30.07	30.06	58	79	60	65.7	N'ly 1	S. E. 2	S'ly 1	1	0	0	
20	30.03	29.92	29.86	65	90	70	75.0	S. W'ly 1	S. W'ly 2	W. 2	3	2	0	
21	29.86	29.74	29.70	74	92	74	80.0	W. 1	W. 2	W. 1	3	4	0	
22	29.76	29.57	29.59	76	95	76	82.3	N. W. 1	N. W. 1	N. W. 1	0	3	0	
23	29.65	29.61	29.71	76	90	68	78.0	N. W. 2	N. W. 2	N. W. 1	0	3	1	
24	29.77	29.76	29.80	64	80	64	69.3	N. W. 2	N. 2	S. E'ly 2	0	8	3	
S 25	29.83	29.79	29.78	64	81	66	70.3	S. E'ly 1	S. E. 2	S'ly 2	0	4	3	
26	29.66	29.58	29.59	66	70	60	65.3	S'ly 3	S'ly 3	N'ly 1	10	Rain	3	0.78
27	29.69	...	29.70	60	...	62	...	N. W. 1	...	N. W. 1	2	...	0	
28	29.79	29.83	29.82	60	81	64	68.3	N. W. 1	N. W. 2	S. W. 1	0	3	0	
29	29.76	29.61	29.54	68	86	71	75.0	S. W. 2	S. W. 3	S. W. 2	8	2	3	
30	29.38	29.30	29.37	70	87	72	76.3	S. W. 3	S. W. 3	N. W. 1	10	5	9	
31	29.45	29.47	29.63	66	84	67	72.3	N. W. 2	W'ly 3	N. W. 2	5	2	9	
Means	29.79	29.76	29.78	67.0	83.7	66.6	...	1.8	2.1	1.4	4.3	3.4	3.5	1.68
REDUCED TO SEA LEVEL.									1.8			3.7		
Max.	30.27	30.25	30.24	76	95	76	82.3	Prevailing winds from some point between—		Days.			Days.	
Min.	29.54	29.48	29.55	58	62	56	60.7	N. & E.		2	Clear		13	
Mean	29.97	29.94	29.96					E. & S.		6	Variable		} 12	
Range	0.73	0.77	0.69	18	33	20	21.6	S. & W.		13	Cloudy			
Mean of month			29.957	...	...	...	72.4	W. & N.		10	Rain fell on		6	
Extreme range			0.79	...	...	...	39.0							

Remarks.

1st. Variable, with occasional sprinkling of rain. Evening foggy.
2d. Thundershower from 1 to 2 A. M. Pleasant day.
3d. Very fine. Aurora in the evening, not very bright.
4th and 5th. Very fine.
6th. Burning sun at mid-day.
7th. Very fine.
8th. Very fine. Ground excessively dry in this vicinity.
9th. Very hot, with a fresh breeze from S. W. At 9 P. M., lightning low in the N. W. From 10 to 11 P. M., aurora at the north, not very bright.
10th. Very burning sun; top of the ground excessively parched.
11th. Very hot and sultry.
12th. Sprinkling of rain at 4½ P. M., and again at 10 P. M.
13th. Very sultry.
14th. Sprinkling of rain from 9 to 10 P. M.
15th and 16th. Pleasant.
17th. Rainy day.
18th. Pleasant.
19th. Very fine.
20th. At 6 A. M., wind light S. W'ly, and upper clouds coming from N. W. Day pleasant.
21st. Sultry.
22d. Heat very oppressive. Thermometer in the shade, at 1 P. M., stood at 95°—being higher than at any time since July 13, 1849, when it stood at 97° in the same place.
23d. Very hot.
24th. Fine; heat much abated.
25th. Pleasant. Clouds in the afternoon came from N. W. while the wind came from S'ly.
26th. Rain commenced falling moderately at 7 A. M., and continued till 6 P. M.
27th and 28th. Very fine.
29th. Pleasant.
30th Very warm and sultry.
31st. Pleasant.

August, 1852. New Moon, 15d. 8h. 50m. A. M.

DAYS.	Barometer, reduced to 32° F. At 6 A. M.	At 1 P. M.	At 10 P. M.	Thermometer. At 6 A. M.	At 1 P. M.	At 10 P. M.	Daily mean.	Winds (Direction and Force.) At 6 A. M.	At 1 P. M.	At 10 P. M.	Weather (Tenths Cloudy.) At 6 A. M.	At 1 P. M.	At 10 P. M.	Rain and Snow in Inches of Water.
S 1	29.70	29.71	29.79	63	80	63	68.7	N'ly 2	W'ly 2	W'ly 1	10	5	5	
2	29.83	29.82	29.83	60	77	58	65.0	N. W. 1	N. W. 2	N. W. 1	0	4	0	
3	29.83	...	29.79	58	...	57	...	N. W. 1	...	N. W. 1	0	...	2	
4	29.76	29.75	29.72	58	72	66	65.3	N. W. 1	S'ly 3	S'ly 2	1	Rain	10	} 1.20
5	29.51	29.64	29.69	61	68	61	63.3	N. E. 1	N'ly 1	N. W. 1	Rain	10	9	
6	29.67	29.65	29.69	58	74	61	64.3	N. E. 2	E'ly 2	N. E. 1	10	10	3	
7	29.67	29.65	29.69	60	76	60	65.3	N. E. 1	N. E. 1	N. W. 1	10	9	1	0.87
S 8	29.74	29.73	29.75	62	78	64	68.0	S. W'ly 1	S'ly 2	Calm	0	3	0	
9	29.76	29.72	29.75	65	83	67	71.7	S. W. 1	S. W. 1	S. W'ly 1	2	5	10	
10	29.76	29.76	...	66	80	...	...	S. W. 1	S. W'ly 2	...	3	6	...	0.50
11	...	...	...	...	...	...	...	...	...	...	...	...	...	
12	...	...	...	...	...	...	...	...	...	...	...	...	...	
13	...	...	...	...	...	...	...	...	...	...	...	...	...	
14	...	...	29.83	...	...	63	...	...	...	S. W. 1	...	...	0	
S 15	29.74	29.66	29.76	66	85	68	73.0	S. W. 1	S. W. 3	S. W. 1	3	2, Sh'r	0	0.25
16	29.97	29.98	30.03	57	74	57	62.7	N. W. 2	N. W. 1	S'ly 1	0	1	0	
17	30.06	30.01	29.94	58	75	59	64.0	S. E. 1	S. E. 2	E'ly 1	3	5	7	
18	29.91	...	29.84	56	...	60	...	S'ly 1	...	S. W'ly 1	0	...	0	
19	29.83	29.76	29.78	60	86	66	70.7	S'ly 1	S. W'ly 3	S. W. 1	3	2	0	
20	29.84	29.86	29.97	65	70	62	65.7	N. E. 2	N. E. 2	N. E. 2	8	6	10	
21	30.07	...	30.13	60	...	58	...	N. E. 1	...	N. E. 1	Misty	...	0	
S 22	30.17	30.15	30.16	55	76	59	63.3	N. E. 1	S. E. 1	S. E. 1	9	4	2	
23	30.17	30.13	30.09	55	74	61	63.3	S. E. 1	S. E. 2	S. E. 1	Foggy	7	0	
24	30.07	29.98	29.95	60	79	67	68.7	S'ly 1	S'ly 1	S. E. 1	8	5	0	
25	29.92	...	29.89	68	...	68	...	S'ly 2	...	...	10	...	...	
26	...	29.54	29.61	...	70	70	...	...	S. E. 2	S. 1	...	2	Rain	1.37
27	29.60	...	29.59	71	...	70	...	S. W. 1	...	S.	8	...	10	} 0.75
28	29.69	29.62	29.68	69	78	70	72.3	N. 1	S.	S. E.	5	10	Rain	
S 29	29.56	29.54	29.62	65	62	60	62.3	N. E. 2	N. E. 3	N. E. 3	Rain	Rain	Rain	2.87
30	29.71	29.79	29.86	60	64	60	61.3	N. W. 3	N. W. 3	N. W. 1	Rain	10	10	0.19
31	29.91	29.84	29.83	62	75	64	67.0	N'ly 2	N'ly	W. 1	6	10	4	
Means	29.82	29.79	29.82	61.5	75.3	62.9	...	1.3	1.9	1.2	5.8	6.2	4.3	8.00
									1.5			5.4		
REDUCED TO SEA LEVEL.														
Max.	30.35	29.33	30.34	71	86	70	73.0							
Min.	29.69	29.72	29.77	55	62	57	57.5							
Mean	30.00	29.97	30.00											
Range	0.66	0.61	0.57	16	24	13	15.5							
Mean of month	29.990			...	...	...	66.6							
Extreme range	0.66			...	...	...	31.0							

Prevailing winds from some point between— Days.
N. & E. 6
E. & S. 5
S. & W. 11
W. & N. 6

Days.
Clear 6
Variable . . . } 10
Cloudy . . . . }
Rain fell on . . 12
(3 days omitted.)

Remarks.

1st. Pleasant.
2d. Very fine. Thunder at 4 P. M., but no rain.
3d. Very fine. Ther. at sunrise stood at 54°.
4th. Sprinkling of rain at 1 P. M., and again at 7 P. M.
5th. Heavy rain last night. Rain and mist in the morning. Cloudy in the afternoon
6th. Sun out towards night; evening clear.
7th. Copious thundershower from 4 to 5 P. M.
8th. Very fine.
9th. Light shower at 2 P. M.; sprinkling of rain from 10 to 11 P. M. Lightning in the N. W. from 8 to 9 P. M.
10th. Rain from 2 to 4 P. M.
11th, 12th, and 13th. Pleasant. Rather cool and no rain.
14th. Pleasant.
15th. Pleasant. Showery from 3 to 4 P. M.
16th. Very fine. During the afternoon, the wind swung round through the N. E. and E. to S'ly.
17th. Pleasant.
18th. Very fine.
19th. Very fine, though hot.
20th. Sprinkling of rain at 4 P. M.
21st. Cloudy in the morning. Evening clear.
22d. Pleasant.
23d Air cold and raw for the season.
24th and 25th. Pleasant.
26th. Rainy.
27th. Showery.
28th. Air close and sultry. Shower in the afternoon.
29th. Cold N. E. rain storm.
30th. Storm continued, with but little rain.
31st. Very pleasant in the morning. Showery in the afternoon.

September, 1852. New Moon, 13d. 5h. 31m. P. M.

DAYS.	Barometer. At 6 A. M.	At 1 P. M.	At 10 P. M.	Thermometer. At 6 A. M.	At 1 P. M.	At 10 P. M.	Daily mean.	Winds. At 6 A. M.	At 1 P. M.	At 10 P. M.	Weather. At 6 A. M.	At 2 P. M.	At 10 P. M.	Rain.
1	29.84	29.86	29.76	62	80	69	70.3	N. W. 1	W.	N. W.	2	0	0	
2	29.81	29.75	29.77	68	81	70	73.0	N. W.	S. W. 1	W. 1	0	0	0	
3	29.74	29.66	29.74	68	80	72	73.3	S. W. 1	S. W. 3	S. W. 1	Hazy	0	8	
4	29.83	29.90	29.88	65	76	64	68.3	W'ly	N. W. 2	N. W. 1	8	6	0	
S 5	30.05	30.04	30.07	60	72	59	63.7	N. W. 2	N. W. 1	N. W.	0	0	0	
6	30.08	30.02	30.02	56	75	60	63.7	W. 1	S. W.	W. 1	0	0	0	
7	30.02	29.97	29.99	60	78	66	68.0	W'ly 1	W. 2	W. 1	0	0	0	
8	30.07	30.05	30.07	64	80	70	71.3	W.	S. W.	S. W.	0	5	0	
9	30.04	29.97	29.90	66	83	79	76.0	W.	W. 1	W.	0	0	0	
10	29.81	29.71	29.69	62	83	72	72.3	W.	W. 2	W.	5	8	9	
11	29.64	29.69	29.57	70	82	70	74.0	S. W.	S. W. 2	S. W. 1	10	8	10	
S 12	29.27	29.24	29.34	70	75	68	71.0	S. 2	S'ly 3	S. E'ly 1	Rain	10	8	1.25
13	29.36	29.45	29.70	64	66	50	60.0	N. W. 1	N. W. 3	N. W. 1	10	3	0	
14	29.87	29.84	29.86	47	68	59	58.0	N. W. 2	N. W. 2	W. 2	0	4	10	
15	29.87	29.83	29.86	60	66	59	61.7	S. W. 2	S. W. 2	S. W. 1	10	Rain	10	
16	29.98	29.95	30.01	51	65	50	55.3	N. W. 1	N. W. 1	N. W. 2	2	2	0	
17	30.10	30.05	30.08	43	62	52	52.3	N. W. 2	N. W. 1	N. W. 2	0	2	0	
18	30.11	30.07	30.08	48	65	53	55.3	N. 2	N. E. 2	N'ly 1	0	5	0	
S 19	30.06	29.96	29.95	52	70	56	59.3	N'ly 1	N. E. 1	N. E. 1	2	9	10	
20	29.90	29.86	29.89	56	74	64	64.7	S'ly 1	S. W. 1	N. W. 1	2	5	5	
21	29.88	29.82	29.77	63	75	66	68.0	S. W. 1	S. W. 2	S. W. 2	Foggy	5	9	
22	29.78	...	29.83	64	...	56	...	S. W. 1	N. W. 1	N. W. 2	5	2	0	
23	29.91	29.89	29.97	51	65	51	55.7	N. W. 2	N. W. 2	N. W. 1	0	6	0	
24	30.04	30.00	29.99	56	59	48	54.3	N. 1	N. E. 2	N. E. 1	0	10	3	
25	29.96	29.82	29.67	51	63	56	56.7	S'ly 1	S. E'ly 1	S'ly 1	8	10	10	
S 26	29.50	29.42	29.56	56	65	52	57.7	S. E. 2	W'ly 1	N. W. 2	Rain	10	0	0.15
27	29.70	29.75	29.92	48	60	48	52.0	N. W. 1	N. W'ly 2	N. W. 2	0	0	5	
28	29.87	29.82	29.79	53	68	58	59.7	E'ly 2	S. W. 3	S. W. 2	8	3	0	
29	29.86	29.90	30.01	53	62	45	53.3	N. W. 2	N'ly 2	N. W. 2	10	5	0	
30	30.12	30.08	30.09	39	54	43	45.3	N'ly 2	N. E. 2	N. E. 1	0	5	0	
Means	29.87	29.84	29.86	57.5	70.8	59.5	...	1.5	1.8	1.3	4.3	4.8	3.2	1.40
									1.5			4.1		
REDUCED TO SEA LEVEL.														
Max.	30.30	30.26	30.27	70	83	79	76.0							
Min.	29.45	29.42	29.52	39	54	43	45.3							
Mean	30.05	30.02	30.04											
Range	0.85	0.84	0.75	31	29	36	30.7							
Mean of month	30.037			...	...	...	62.6							
Extreme range	0.88			...	...	...	44.0							

Prevailing winds from some point between— Days.
N. & E. 4
E. & S. 2
S. & W. 10
W. & N. 14

Days.
Clear 13
Variable . . . } 12
Cloudy . . . . }
Rain fell on . . 5

Remarks.

1st. Very fine.
2d. Pleasant. Hot sun. No air stirring.
3d. Very fine. Good breeze during the day.
4th. Shower from 6 to 7 A. M. Day pleasant.
5th. Fine. Air rather cool.
6th and 7th. Very fine.
8th. Warm. Little air stirring. Sun hot.
9th. Very warm and sultry.
10th. Cloudy and warm.
11th. Cloudy, with occasional light showers.
12th. Rain in the morning. Showery in the afternoon. Evening clear.
13th. Rain last night. Day fine.
14th. Very fine. Cool.
15th. Cloudy, with light showers. Stars out in the evening.
16th. Very fine. Aurora in the evening, without streamers.
17th and 18th. Very fine.
19th and 20th. Pleasant.
21st. Foggy in the morning. Day pleasant.
22d and 23d. Very fine.
24th. Cool, but pleasant.
25th. Cloudy, with some appearances of storm.
26th. Light shower at 6 A. M., and again at 1 P. M. Evening very clear.
27th. Very fine.
28th. Pleasant.
29th. Light shower in the afternoon. Evening clear.
30th. Pleasant. Light frost in low grounds in the vicinity.

October, 1852. New Moon, 13d. 2h. 6m. A. M.

Days.	Barometer, reduced to 32° F. Sunrise.	At 1 P. M.	At 10 P. M.	Thermometer. Sunrise.	At 1 P. M.	At 10 P. M.	Daily mean.	Winds (Direction and Force.) Sunrise.	At 1 P. M.	At 10 P. M.	Weather (Tenths Cloudy.) Sunrise.	At 1 P. M.	At 10 P. M.	Rain and Snow in Inches of Water.
1	30.10	30.10	30.13	40	63	51	51.3	N'ly 1	N. E. 1	N. E. 1	5	8	10	
2	30.12	30.03	29.99	53	67	56	58.7	N. E. 1	S. W'ly 2	S'ly 1	8	0	0	
S 3	30.16	30.09	30.08	51	63	50	54.7	N. E. 1	N. E. 2	E'ly 1	3	2	0	
4	29.94	29.75	29.56	55	61	60	58.7	S'ly 2	S'ly 2	W'ly 1	10	Rain	2	
5	29.57	29.47	29.55	50	73	43	55.3	W'ly 2	W'ly 2	N. W. 1	3	3	0	
6	29.56	29.46	29.57	43	65	54	54.0	N. W. 1	S. W. 2	S. W. 1	5	6	2	
7	29.67	29.66	29.69	53	72	57	60.7	N. W. 1	W'ly 2	N. W. 1	3	3	0	
8	29.71	29.65	29.74	61	69	57	62.3	S. W. 1	S. W. 1	N. E. 2	10	10	Misty	
9	29.88	29.87	29.76	50	57	53	53.3	N. E. 2	N. E. 2	N. E. 2	10	10	Misty	
S 10	29.65	29.59	29.59	52	68	64	61.3	E'ly 2	S. E'ly 2	S'ly 1	Misty	Misty	Rain	0.20
11	29.69	29.79	29.90	58	67	53	59.3	N. W. 3	N. W. 3	N. W. 1	5	0	0	
12	29.94	29.85	29.83	52	67	58	59.0	Calm	S. W. 3	S. W. 2	10	2	5	
13	29.92	29.90	29.87	56	55	47	52.7	N'ly 1	N. E. 2	N. E. 1	10	10	10	
14	29.86	29.74	29.53	46	53	48	49.0	N. E. 2	N. E. 2	N. E. 3	10	10	Rain	} 1.00
15	29.45	29.46	29.67	39	50	41	43.3	N. E. 3	N. W. 2	N. W. 2	Rain	10	0	
16	29.79	29.85	30.00	36	47	36	39.7	N. W. 2	N'ly 3	N. W. 1	0	4	1	
S 17	30.10	30.00	29.92	30	51	47	42.7	N. W. 1	N. W. 2	S. W. 2	0	4	10	
18	29.89	29.76	29.53	53	66	59	59.3	S. W. 1	S. W. 2	S. W. 4	8	10	10	
19	29.61	29.68	29.97	58	62	48	56.0	N. W. 1	N. W. 3	N. E. 3	9	5	9	
20	30.04	30.08	30.05	41	44	44	43.0	N. E'ly 2	N. E'ly 2	N'ly 2	10	10	10	
21	29.94	29.79	29.67	43	48	46	45.7	N. E'ly 2	N. by E. 3	N. W. 2	10	7	0	
22	29.63	29.56	29.65	46	59	48	51.0	N'ly 2	N. by E. 2	N. W. 2	7	10	0	
23	29.79	29.75	29.75	44	60	47	50.3	N'ly 2	N N W. 3	N. W. 2	0	0	0	
S 24	29.74	29.68	29.67	45	62	51	52.7	N. W. 2	N. W. 2	N. W. 1	0	2	0	
25	29.68	29.66	29.84	51	65	48	54.7	N. W. 1	N. W. 2	N. W. 1	2	1	2	
26	30.11	30.19	30.29	38	45	34	39.0	N. W. 1	N. W. 2	N. W. 2	2	0	3	
27	30.33	30.26	30.17	31	52	46	43.0	N. W. 1	S. E'ly 2	S'ly 1	3	8	10	
28	30.05	...	29.92	51	...	53	...	S. E. 2	S'ly 2	S'ly 1	10	10	2	
29	29.85	29.75	29.90	53	71	53	59.0	S. W. 2	S. W. 2	N. E. 2	5	5	10	
30	29.90	29.82	29.70	51	54	55	53.3	N. E. 1	E'ly 2	E'ly 1	10	Misty	Rain	
S 31	29.65	29.65	29.69	48	49	46	47.7	N. E. 2	N. E. 2	N. E. 2	Rain	Rain	Misty	0.10
Means	29.85	29.80	29.81	47.7	59.5	50.1	...	1.6	2.1	1.6	6.4	6.1	5.0	1.30
									1.8			5.8		
REDUCED TO SEA LEVEL.														
Max.	30.51	30.44	30.47	61	73	64	62.3							
Min.	29.63	29.64	29.71	30	44	34	39.0							
Mean	30.03	29.98	29.99											
Range	0.88	0.80	0.76	31	29	30	23.3							
Mean of month 30.000				...	...	...	52.4							
Extreme range 0.88				...	...	...	43.0							

Prevailing winds from some point between— Days.
N. & E. 10
E. & S. 3
S. & W. 7
W. & N. 11

Days.
Clear 10
Variable . . . } 13
Cloudy . . . . }
Rain or snow fell on 8

Remarks.

1st. Pleasant. Frost this morning in the vicinity on low grounds.
2d. Very fine.
3d. Pleasant.
4th. Light shower in the morning. Nearly clear at 11 P. M.
5th and 6th. Pleasant.
7th. Very fine.
8th. Light shower at 5 A. M., and also at 7 P. M.
9th. Overcast, with occasional sunshine.
10th. Mist during the day. Light shower in the evening.
11th and 12th. Very fine.
13th. Air rather raw.
14th. Light rain in the evening.
15th. Rain in the morning, mixed at times with considerable snow; wind at N. W.
16th. Cold for the season.
17th. Heavy frost this morning, being the first of the season on College Hill. In exposed situations, the ground was slightly frozen. Sprinkling of rain from S. W. at 6 P. M.
18th. Mild, with appearances of storm in the afternoon.
19th. Auroral light conspicuous among broken clouds at the north, which was observed from 9 to 10 P. M.
20th. Overcast; occasional mist.
21st. Cloudy in the morning. Clear at 11 P. M.
22d. Cloudy for the most part during the day. Beautifully clear at 11 P. M., with the wind at N. W'ly.
23d to 26th. Very fine.
27th. Pleasant.
28th. Overcast.
29th. Very mild. Wind changed from S. W. to N. E. between 3 and 4 P. M.
30th. Mist. Light rain in the evening.
31st. Light rain and mist.

November, 1852. New Moon, 11d. 11h. 33m. A. M.

Days.	Barometer Sunrise.	At 1 P. M.	At 10 P. M.	Thermometer Sunrise.	At 1 P. M.	At 10 P. M.	Daily mean.	Winds Sunrise.	At 1 P. M.	At 10 P. M.	Weather Sunrise.	At 1 P. M.	At 10 P. M.	Rain and Snow
1	29.70	29.65	29.59	45	51	47	47.7	N'ly	N. E. 2	N. E. 2	Misty	10	Misty	
2	...	29.19	29.19	50	63	52	55.0	N. E'ly 2	S. W. 2	S. W. 1	Rain	7	5	0.70
3	29.45	29.57	29.76	50	55	47	50.7	W. by N. 2	N. W. 3	N. W. 3	0	5	5	
4	29.84	...	29.81	43	...	38	...	N. W. 2	...	N. W. 2	2	...	0	
5	29.81	29.72	29.77	41	47	37	41.7	N. W. 1	N. W. 1	N. W. 2	Sprin'le	10	3	
6	29.78	29.72	29.67	31	47	44	40.7	N. E. 2	E'ly 1	E'ly 1	6	10	10	
S 7	29.35	29.27	29.52	44	50	43	45.7	E'ly 1	N. W. 1	N. W. 2	Rain	10	10	0.30
8	29.67	29.72	29.88	38	50	41	43.0	W'ly 2	N. W. 3	N. W. 1	0	2	8	
9	29.89	29.83	29.90	37	47	40	41.3	N. E. 2	N. E'ly 2	N. E. 1	10	10	10	
10	29.90	29.89	29.99	36	46	36	39.3	N'ly 2	N. W'ly 1	N. W. 2	Misty	5	0	
11	30.08	30.03	29.99	34	45	38	39.0	N. W. 2	N. W. 1	N. W. 1	9	3	5	
12	29.77	29.49	29.57	45	51	41	45.7	S. W. 2	S. E. 3	W'ly 2	8	Rain	0	0.60
13	29.59	29.56	29.53	35	42	41	39.3	W. by S. 2	W. by S. 1	S. W. 2	2	10	10	
S 14	29.42	29.33	29.37	35	37	32	34.3	N. W'ly 2	N. W. 2	N. W. 2	5	9	4	
15	29.41	29.35	29.38	27	36	34	32.3	N. W. 1	N. W. 2	W'ly 3	2	1	2	
16	29.42	29.49	29.63	36	44	35	38.3	W by N. 2	W by N. 4	N. W'ly 2	0	1	5	
17	29.74	29.71	29.73	35	43	37	38.3	W. 2	W. by S. 3	S. W. 2	7	5	8	
18	29.68	29.69	29.75	37	43	36	38.7	N. E. 1	N. E. 2	N. E'ly 2	10	9	5	
19	29.82	29.76	29.67	35	43	35	37.7	N'ly 2	N. by E. 2	N'ly 2	10	10	8	
20	29.80	29.86	29.97	34	38	33	35.0	N. by E. 2	N. by E. 2	N. E'ly 2	9	10	9	
S 21	30.10	30.08	30.15	28	36	28	30.7	N. W. 2	N. W. 2	N. W. 1	0	0	0	
22	30.21	30.12	29.96	24	41	36	33.7	N. W. 2	E'ly 2	S. E'ly 2	5	10	Misty	
23	29.73	29.70	29.79	35	37	32	34.7	N. E. 2	N. E. 2	N'ly 3	Rain	Misty	10	0.50
24	29.92	29.81	29.76	20	29	23	24.0	N by W. 2	N. W. 3	N. W. 1	0	0	0	
25	29.82	29.83	...	26	37	...	...	N. W. 2	N. W. 2	...	2	5	...	
26	29.78	29.61	29.34	36	44	53	44.3	E'ly 2	E. by S. 1	S. E'ly 2	10	Rain	Rain	2.50
27	29.20	29.30	29.68	55	50	39	48.0	S'ly 1	W'ly 3	N. W. 1	Foggy	2	0	
S 28	29.98	30.00	30.13	33	42	33	36.0	N. W. 1	N. W. 2	N. W. 2	0	0	0	
29	30.09	30.05	30.10	34	48	39	40.3	S. W. 2	S. W. 3	N. W. 1	7	9	3	
30	30.09	30.14	30.06	34	43	35	37.3	N. W. 1	N. W. 2	N. W. 1	5	6	0	
Means	29.76	29.71	29.75	36.4	44.3	38.1	...	1.8	2.0	1.8	6.0	6.5	5.2	4.60
									1.9			5.9		
REDUCED TO SEA LEVEL.														
Max.	30.39	30.32	30.33	55	63	53	55.0							
Min.	29.38	29.37	29.37	20	29	23	24.0							
Mean	29.94	29.89	29.93											
Range	1.01	0.95	0.96	35	34	30	31.0							
Mean of month 29.920				...	...	...	39.6							
Extreme range 1.02				...	...	...	43.0							

Prevailing winds from some point between— Days.
N. & E. 7
E. & S. 2
S. & W. 5
W. & N. 16

Days.
Clear 8
Variable . . . } 14
Cloudy . . . . }
Rain fell on . . 8

Remarks.

1st. Mist, with occasional sprinkling of rain.
2d. Mist, with light rain.
3d and 4th. Pleasant.
5th. Sprinkling of rain at 7 A. M. Cloudy day. Clear at 11 P. M.
6th. Appearances of storm in the afternoon and evening.
7th. Rain in the morning. Evening clear.
8th. Pleasant.
9th. Appearances of storm in the evening.
10th. Pleasant. Faint aurora in the evening.
11th. Pleasant. Aurora quite bright at 9 P. M., partly concealed by clouds.
12th. Commenced raining between 9 and 10 A. M.; wind fresh S. E'ly. Continued to rain till between 3 and 4 P. M., when the wind came to N. W., and rain ceased. Kept a lookout for meteors in the evening, but saw none.
13th. Thick clouds in the evening.
14th. Air rather raw. Light flurry of snow about 4½ P. M.
15th. Rather cold for the season.
16th and 17th. Pleasant.
18th. Cloudy.
19th. Pleasant.
20th. Clouds, with occasional sunshine.
21st. Splendid day and evening.
22d. Appearances of storm.
23d. Rain in the morning. Mist in afternoon.
24th. Very fine.
25th. Pleasant.
26th. Rainy through the day and evening.
27th. Fog and mist in the morning. At 10 P. M., very clear.
28th. Very fine.
29th. Pleasant.
30th. Fine. Evening splendid.

December, 1852. New Moon, 10d. 10h. 23m. P. M.

Days.	Barometer, reduced to 32° F. Sunrise.	At 1 P. M.	At 10 P. M.	Thermometer. Sunrise.	At 1 P. M.	At 10 P. M.	Daily mean.	Winds (Direction and Force.) Sunrise.	At 1 P. M.	At 10 P. M.	Weather (Tenths Cloudy.) Sunrise.	At 1 P. M.	At 10 P. M.	Rain and Snow in Inches of Water
1	30.05	30.06	30.17	35	45	33	37.7	W'ly 2	N. W. 2	N. W. 1	3	3	1	
2	30.14	30.14	30.18	32	50	37	39.7	N. W. 1	N. W. 1	N. W. 1	1	1	0	
3	30.19	30.13	30.06	33	50	41	41.3	S. W. 2	S. W. 2	E'ly 2	5	7	10	
4	29.76	29.65	29.51	46	53	47	48.7	N. E. 2	N. E. 2	N. E. 1	Misty	Misty	Misty	
S 5	29.46	29.40	29.51	45	47	48	46.7	N. E. 1	N. E. 1	N. W. 2	10	10	2	
6	29.70	29.74	29.76	41	53	44	46.0	N. W. 2	S. W. 2	S. W. 1	2	5	6	
7	29.76	29.68	29.60	53	63	54	56.7	S. W. 2	S. W. 2	S'ly 1	5	1	Hazy	
8	29.51	29.62	29.77	54	56	41	50.3	N. W. 3	W. by S. 2	N. W'ly 1	5	0	0	0.30
9	29.84	29.80	29.71	35	51	45	43.7	N. W. 1	S. by E. 2	E'ly 2	2	5	10	
10	29.70	29.72	29.71	44	53	48	48.3	N'ly 1	N. W. 1	N. W. 1	10	10	10	
11	29.38	29.29	29.20	41	38	35	38.0	N. E. 3	N. E. 3	N. E. 2	Rain	Rain	Misty	1.25
S 12	29.59	29.71	29.86	33	39	33	35.0	N. W. 2	N. W. 3	N. W. 2	1	0	0	
13	29.91	29.79	29.71	30	38	34	34.0	W'ly 1	S. W. 1	W'ly 3	7	10	2	
14	30.08	30.15	30.26	28	32	21	27.0	N. W. 2	N. W. 2	N. W. 2	3	2	0	
15	30.27	30.27	30.41	16	29	22	22.3	N. W. 2	N'ly 1	N. W. 1	7	10	0	
16	30.44	30.34	30.07	19	36	34	29.7	N'ly 2	N. by E. 1	N. E'ly 2	0	10	10	
17	29.61	29.27	29.16	38	46	36	40.0	S. E. 2	N'ly 1	N. W. 1	Rain	Foggy	0	1.25
18	29.35	...	29.61	28	...	28	...	N. W. 3	...	N. W. 4	10	...	0	
S 19	29.89	29.77	29.57	25	35	32	30.7	W by N 2	N. W. 2	S. W. 2	0	10	4	
20	29.47	29.47	29.62	39	46	37	40.7	S. W. 1	W'ly 1	N'ly 2	10	8	Rain	
21	29.72	29.76	29.95	31	28	21	26.7	N. E. 2	N. E. 2	N. W. 1	Misty	Misty	4	
22	29.29	30.38	30.50	10	20	16	15.3	N. W. 2	N'ly 2	N. W. 2	0	3	7	
23	30.49	30.21	29.87	17	32	39	29.3	N. W. 2	N. E. 1	S'ly 1	2	10	Rain	}
24	...	29.58	29.58	40	53	50	47.7	S. W. 1	S. W. 2	S. W. 1	10	10	Rain	} 0.90
25	29.76	29.80	29.89	40	45	34	39.7	N. W'ly 1	N'ly 2	N. W'ly 2	9	10	9	}
S 26	29.56	29.53	29.81	36	45	36	39.0	E'ly 2	N. W. 2	W'ly 3	Misty	2	5	}
27	30.20	30.23	30.03	29	36	34	33.0	N. W. 2	E'ly 2	E'ly 2	1	9	Rain	
28	29.54	29.29	29.46	47	56	39	47.3	S. E'ly 2	S. S. W. 4	W'ly 3	Foggy	Misty	5	
29	29.83	29.88	29.99	33	38	34	35.0	W'ly 2	W. by S. 3	W'ly 2	0	10	7	
30	29.99	30.06	29.96	33	39	40	37.3	S. W. 1	S. W. 1	S'ly 1	9	10	3	
31	29.90	29.90	29.77	37	32	28	32.3	N. E. 2	N. E. 2	N. E. 2	10	Misty	10	
Means	29.81	29.82	29.81	34.5	42.8	36.1	...	1.8	1.8	1.7	6.1	6.8	5.5	3.70
								1.8			6.1			
REDUCED TO SEA LEVEL.														
Max.	30.67	30.56	30.68	54	63	54	56.7	Prevailing winds from some point between— Days.			Days.			
Min.	29.47	29.45	29.34	10	20	16	22.3	N. & E. 9			Clear 4			
Mean	29.99	30.00	29.99					E. & S. 1			Variable . . . } 13			
Range	1.20	1.11	1.34	44	43	38	34.4	S. & W. 9			Cloudy . . . . }			
Mean of month	29.997			...	...	...	37.8	W. & N. 12			Rain or snow fell on 14			
Extreme range	1.34			...	...	...	53.0							

Remarks.

1st. Very fine.
2d. Very fine and warm for the season.
3d. Pleasant.
4th. Mist, with occasional light rain.
5th. Mist during the day. Mostly clear at 10 P. M.
6th. Very mild and pleasant.
7th. Uncommonly mild and warm for the season. The warmest day since October 29th.
8th. Heavy rain at 3 A. M. Pleasant during the day.
9th. Appearances of storm in the evening.
10th. Very mild.
11th. Cold northeast rain storm.
12th. Pleasant.
13th. Began to snow moderately from 1 to 2 P. M., the snow melting as it fell. Mostly clear at 10 P. M.
14th. Cold, but fine.
15th. Very fine, though cold.
16th. Appearances of storm in the afternoon. Began to snow at 11 P. M.
17th. At sunrise, ground covered with snow, and raining, with wind at the N. E. Foggy in the afternoon. At 10 P. M., the moon shining upon a cloudless sky, and weather very mild.
18th. Cold and blustering.
19th. Rain and cold.
20th. Began to rain moderately at 9 P. M.
21st. Mist in the morning. Flurry of snow from 4 to 5 P. M. Clouds broken in the evening.
22d. Pleasant, but cold.
23d. Fine hail began to fall from 2 to 3 P. M., which was followed by snow from S. E'ly, and then by rain.
24th. Cloudy. At 10 P. M., light rain.
25th. Very mild.
26th. Mist and light rain in the morning. Evening partly clear.
27th. Light rain in the evening.
28th. Rain in the afternoon, with wind heavy at S. W'ly. Barometer began to rise from 5 to 6 P. M., and the wind came round to W'ly. Mostly clear at 10 P. M. The ground is entirely free of frost.
29th. Pleasant.
30th. Very mild.
31st. Mist and light rain in the afternoon.

January, 1853. New Moon, 9d. 10h. 45m. A. M.

Days.	Barometer Sunrise.	At 1 P. M.	At 10 P. M.	Thermometer Sunrise.	At 1 P. M.	At 10 P. M.	Daily mean.	Winds Sunrise.	At 1 P. M.	At 10 P. M.	Weather Sunrise.	At 1 P. M.	At 10 P. M.	Rain and Snow
1	29.59	29.50	29.62	28	32	34	31.3	N. E. 1	N. E. 2	N. E. 2	Foggy	Rain	Rain	1.60
S 2	29.97	30.00	30.04	24	31	30	28.3	N. 2	N. E'ly 2	N. E. 2	1	5	10	
3	29.97	29.86	29.84	30	36	30	32.0	N. E. 1	N. E. 1	N. E. 2	10	10	10	
4	29.75	29.65	29.65	28	24	20	24.0	N. E. 3	N'ly 3	N. E'ly 4	Snow	10	Snow	0.30
5	29.75	29.86	29.91	21	27	17	21.7	N. W'ly 2	N. W. 2	N. W. 2	10	2	0	
6	29.89	29.80	29.78	15	37	29	27.0	N. W. 2	S. W. 2	S. W. 1	0	10	2	
7	29.73	29.66	29.86	28	45	39	37.3	S. W'ly 1	W'ly 2	W'ly 2	0	2	1	
8	29.99	29.97	30.01	30	47	31	36.0	S. W. 2	W'ly 2	N. W'ly	0	2	0	
S 9	29.87	29.77	29.87	34	53	41	42.7	S'ly 1	S. W. 1	S. W. 1	Foggy	6	0	
10	30.01	30.03	30.02	34	45	34	37.7	N. W. 2	N. W. 2	W'ly 1	1	1	3	
11	29.95	29.94	30.07	37	48	34	39.7	S. W. 2	S. E. 1	N'ly 2	8	10	3	} 1.50
12	30.16	30.15	30.12	27	34	30	30.3	N. E. 3	N. E. 2	N. E. 4	Snow	10	10	}
13	30.01	30.00	29.96	27	20	20	22.3	N. E. 4	N. E. 4	N. E. 4	Snow	Snow	Snow	
14	29.90	29.84	29.81	23	29	31	27.7	N. E. 3	N'ly 2	N'ly 1	10	Snow	10	
15	29.75	29.60	29.56	30	36	32	32.7	N. W. 1	W'ly 2	W'ly 1	1	3	7	
S 16	29.52	29.49	29.56	20	16	8	14.7	W by N 2	N. W. 3	N. W. 4	3	8	10	
17	29.60	29.67	29.73	7	23	16	15.3	N. W. 3	N. W. 2	N. W. 1	0	0	0	
18	29.76	29.73	29.75	22	31	26	26.3	N. W. 1	N. W. 1	N. E. 2	10	10	Snow	
19	29.79	29.79	29.87	21	28	18	22.3	N. W. 2	N. W. 2	N. W. 2	5	2	0	
20	29.79	29.66	29.62	18	31	28	25.7	N. W. 2	N. W. 2	N'ly 1	2	3	10	
21	29.71	29.70	29.77	29	37	26	30.7	N. W. 1	N. W. 2	N. W. 1	5	3	0	
22	29.78	29.67	29.63	21	41	32	31.3	N. W. 1	S. W. 2	S. W. 1	2	7	6	
S 23	29.38	29.00	28.68	34	40	37	37.0	E'ly 1	E'ly 2	S. E'ly 1	10	Rain	Foggy	0.87
24	28.70	28.82	28.97	36	41	36	37.7	S. W. 2	S. W. 3	S. W. 2	10	3	10	
25	29.32	29.22	29.20	27	32	32	30.3	N. W. 1	S. 1	W. 2	8	0	Snow	
26	29.53	29.76	30.17	12	21	6	13.0	N. W. 1	W. 2	N. W. 3	0	2	0	
27	30.34	30.35	30.49	8	23	12	14.3	N. W. 1	N. W. 1	N. W. 1	0	0	0	
28	30.52	30.43	30.39	13	28	19	20.0	N. W. 1	N. W. 1	N. W.	0	0	0	
29	30.25	30.03	29.74	18	32	29	26.3	N. W.	S.	S. 1	0	0	0	
S 30	29.49	29.44	29.56	31	43	38	37.3	W. 1	W'ly 2	N. W. 2	4	5	10	
31	29.79	29.76	29.96	22	32	23	25.7	N. W. 2	N. W. 2	N. W. 2	1	10	0	
Means	29.79	29.75	29.75	24.4	33.6	27.0	...	1.7	1.9	2.0	4.9	5.2	5.2	4.27
								1.9			5.1			
REDUCED TO SEA LEVEL.														
Max.	30.70	30.61	30.67	37	53	41	42.7	Prevailing winds from some point between— Days.			Days.			
Min.	28.88	29.00	28.86	7	16	6	13.0	N. & E. 7			Clear 7			
Mean	29.97	29.93	29.93					E. & S. 2			Variable . . . } 15			
Range	1.82	1.61	1.81	30	37	35	29.7	S. & W. 8			Cloudy . . . . }			
Mean of month	29.943			...	...	...	28.3	W. & N. 14			Rain or snow fell on 9			
Extreme range	1.84			...	...	...	47.0							

Remarks.

1st. Light rain all day. Ground covered with sleet in the morning, which disappeared during the day. No frost in the ground at this time.
2d. Air raw in the afternoon, and appearances of storm in the evening.
3d. Appearances of storm.
4th. Storm, with wind very heavy at N. E'ly, in the afternoon and evening.
5th. The ground this morning partly covered with snow blown into small drifts and ridges.
6th. Pleasant.
7th. Very mild and pleasant. Very little frost in the ground.
8th. Very fine.
9th. Pleasant and mild.
10th. Very fine.
11th. Very mild and pleasant. Frost nearly all out of the ground.
12th. Began to snow at 7 A. M.; quantity which fell during the morning quite small.
13th. Snowed without intermission all day; quantity large, and much drifted.
14th Light snow occasionally; much drifted; probably nine or ten inches deep on the level.
15th. Very mild and pleasant.
16th. At sunrise, ther. 20°; fell to 16° at 8½ A. M. In the evening, wind high and cold.
17th. Morning cold, but fine.
18th. Began to snow very moderately at 7 P. M.
19th. One-half inch of fresh snow on the ground this morning. Day fine.
20th. Pleasant. Began to snow very gently from 10 to 11 P. M.
21st. A mere dusting of fresh snow last night. Day fine.
22d. Pleasant. Cloudy and haze in evening.
23d. Began to rain at 9 A. M. Showers during the day. Foggy in the evening. At 9½ P. M., the barometer stood at 28.90 (reduced); at 10 P. M., the same; at 10½ P. M., still the same.
24th. Very pleasant. Cloudy late in evening.
25th. Very pleasant morning. Cloudy and raw in afternoon. Light snow at 10 P. M.
26th. Clear and cold. Sharp wind in afternoon. Weather grew rapidly colder after 1 P. M.
27th. Still and cold. Perfectly clear.
28th. Milder than for a day or two past. Very fine.
29th. Very pleasant morning. Raw S'ly wind in the afternoon.
30th. Pleasant.
31st. Cloudy in the afternoon, till nearly 10 P. M., when the sky became clear.

February, 1853. New Moon, 8d. 0h. 25m. A. M.

Days.	Barometer, reduced to 32° F. Sunrise.	At 1 P. M.	At 10 P. M.	Thermometer. Sunrise.	At 1 P. M.	At 10 P. M.	Daily mean.	Winds (Direction and Force.) Sunrise.	At 1 P. M.	At 10 P. M.	Weather (Tenths Cloudy.) Sunrise.	At 1 P. M.	At 10 P. M.	Rain and Snow in Inches of Water.
1	30.23	30.24	30.29	15	32	29	25.3	N. W. 1	S. E. 2	E'ly 1	0	1	4	
2	30.25	30.14	30.00	31	40	40	37.0	S. E'ly 2	S'ly	S'ly 1	10	10	10	
3	29.97	29.96	30.07	41	49	39	43.0	S'ly 1	N'ly 1	N'ly 1	Foggy	10	Foggy	0.60
4	30.10	30.07	30.11	36	40	38	38.0	E'ly 2	S. E. 2	S. E'ly 1	Foggy	Foggy	Rain	
5	30.10	30.05	30.00	41	46	41	42.7	S'ly 1	S. E'ly 1	S'ly 1	Foggy	Foggy	Foggy	
S 6	29.88	29.81	29.79	46	58	49	51.0	S. byE. 1	S. by E. 2	S. W'ly 2	Foggy	Misty	Rain	2.25
7	29.78	29.72	29.76	37	38	35	36.7	N. E. 2	N. E. 2	N. W. 1	10	Rain	5	0.15
8	29.82	29.83	29.88	27	37	27	30.3	N. W. 2	N. W. 2	N. W. 1	0	2	0	
9	29.87	...	29.95	23	...	17	20.0	N. W. 1	...	N. W. 2	1	...	0	
10	29.93	29.76	29.56	16	30	32	26.0	W'ly 2	S. W. 3	S'ly 2	2	10	Snow	
11	29.50	29.48	29.53	34	41	36	37.0	S'ly 1	S'ly 1	S'ly 1	9	5	0	
12	29.71	29.83	29.96	36	39	22	32.3	W.byN. 1	N. W. 2	N. E. 2	5	0	2	
S 13	29.77	29.44	29.43	24	32	18	24.7	N. E. 2	E'ly 1	N. W. 2	Snow	Misty	2	0.40
14	29.53	29.68	30.02	20	24	14	19.3	W'ly 2	N. W'ly 4	N. W. 2	0	0	0	
15	30.20	30.18	30.11	11	27	28	22.0	N. W. 1	N. W. 2	S. W. 2	0	2	5	
16	30.01	29.70	29.42	35	37	43	38.3	S. E'ly 2	S. E. 3	S'ly 2	10	Rain	Rain	1.00
17	29.65	29.68	29.80	30	32	22	28.0	N. W. 3	N. W. 4	N. W. 2	0	0	0	
18	29.85	29.76	29.68	20	29	25	24.7	N. W. 2	N. W. 3	W'ly 2	3	10	Snow	
19	29.67	29.59	29.34	18	21	15	18.0	N. E. 2	N. E. 2	N. E. 3	10	10	10	
S 20	29.36	29.39	29.46	7	22	22	17.0	N'ly 3	N. W. 2	N. W. 1	3	0	0	
21	29.70	29.72	29.80	19	31	23	24.3	N. W. 2	N. W. 2	N. W. 1	0	0	0	
22	29.81	29.68	29.58	27	43	41	37.0	S. E'ly 2	S. E'ly 3	S. E'ly 1	4	9	10	
23	29.27	28.95	28.92	43	45	37	41.7	S. W. 1	S. W. 2	W'ly 3	Rain	Rain	5	1.35
24	29.19	29.19	29.43	25	30	18	24.3	N. W. 2	N. W. 4	N. W. 3	1	2	3	
25	29.54	29.52	29.69	20	31	24	25.0	W byN 2	N. W. 4	N. W. 2	1	1	2	
26	29.74	29.76	29.84	19	31	24	24.7	N. W. 2	N. W. 2	N. W. 1	0	3	0	
S 27	30.06	30.02	30.10	19	37	27	27.7	N. W. 2	N. W. 1	N. W. 1	0	0	0	
28	30.04	29.74	29.60	31	33	33	32.3	S. E. 2	E'ly 2	N'ly 2	10	Sn., h'l	Rain	
Means	29.80	29.73	29.75	26.8	35.4	29.2	...	1.7	2.3	1.6	5.0	5.5	5.2	5.75
								1.9			5.2			
REDUCED TO SEA LEVEL.														
Max.	30.43	30.42	30.47	46	58	49	51.0							
Min.	29.37	29.13	29.10	7	21	14	17.0							
Mean	29.98	29.91	29.93											
Range	1.06	1.29	1.37	39	37	35	34.0							
Mean of month	29.940			...	...	...	30.5							
Extreme range	1.37			...	...	...	51.0							

Prevailing winds from some point between— Days.
N. & E. 4
E. & S. 8
S. & W. 3
W. & N. 13

Days.
Clear 10
Variable . . . . } 8
Cloudy . . . . }
Rain or snow fell on 10

REMARKS.

1st. Pleasant.
2d. Mild, with appearances of storm.
3d. Heavy rain from about 3 to 5 A. M. The snow has nearly all disappeared from the ground.
4th. Foggy during the day. Light rain in the evening.
5th. Fog and fine mist all day. Wind light S. E'ly.
6th. Mist during the day. Copious rain in the evening.
7th. Moderate rain from 10 A. M. to 1 P. M. Clear at 11 P. M. Frost entirely out of the ground in most places.
8th. Very fine.
9th. Pleasant in morning. Grew cold towards night.
10th. Air very raw, with wind S'ly. Flurry of snow in the evening.
11th. Cloudy in the morning, with light mist. Evening very clear and mild.
12th. Very pleasant.
13th. Snow from 7 to 8 A. M. Light hail, mist, and rain in the afternoon. Evening clear.
14th. Wind cold and severe.
15th. Pleasant.
16th. Rain began to fall at 9 A. M., and continued through the day and evening.
17th. Very blustering.
18th. Pleasant. Flurry of snow in the evening.
19th. The ground lightly covered with snow. Raw and cold.
20th. Morning cold, with severe wind. Evening still and pleasant.
21st. Very fine. Evening splendid.
22d. Mild, with appearances of storm in the evening.
23d. Heavy rain from S. W. in the morning. At 7½ P. M., the barometer stood at 28.84; at 10 P. M., at 29.00.
24th. Very blustering and cold.
25th. Blustering.
26th. Very fine.
27th. Very fine; day and evening nearly cloudless.
28th. Snow, hail, and rain in driblets.

March, 1853. New Moon, 9d. 3h. 11m. P. M.

Days.	Barometer Sunrise.	At 1 P. M.	At 10 P. M.	Thermometer Sunrise.	At 1 P. M.	At 10 P. M.	Daily mean.	Winds Sunrise.	At 1 P. M.	At 10 P. M.	Weather Sunrise.	At 1 P. M.	At 10 P. M.	Rain and Snow
1	29.57	29.46	29.23	29	31	33	31.0	N. E. 2	N. E. 2	N. E. 3	Misty	Rain	Rain	0.80
2	29.42	29.52	29.63	29	41	36	35.3	N. W. 2	N. W'ly 2	N. W. 1	8	3	9	
3	29.63	29.55	29.61	34	37	33	34.7	N. E. 1	S. E'ly 2	N. W.	8	Rain	0	
4	29.64	29.64	29.48	27	40	33	33.3	N. W'ly 2	W byN. 3	N. E. 2	0	2	10	
5	29.13	29.32	29.64	30	33	27	30.0	N. E. 4	N. W. 4	N. W. 1	Snow	8	0	
S 6	29.74	29.67	29.80	21	36	30	29.0	N. W. 1	N. W. 2	N. E. 1	0	0	10	
7	29.83	29.80	29.77	26	39	33	32.7	N. W. 1	S. W. 1	S. W. 2	4	1	5	
8	29.61	29.79	30.03	36	46	38	40.0	S. W. 2	N. W. 1	S. W'ly 1	9	7	8	
9	29.92	29.68	29.77	38	47	40	41.7	S. E'ly 2	S. W. 2	N. W. 2	10	10	0	
10	30.17	30.26	30.31	30	41	29	33.3	N. W. 1	N. W. 1	N. E'ly 1	4	0	0	
11	30.22	30.01	29.85	31	37	34	34.0	N. E'ly 2	N. E'ly 3	N'ly 3	10	10	Rain	0.20
12	29.77	29.74	29.68	34	34	34	34.0	N. E. 3	N. E. 2	N. W'ly 1	Misty	10	10	
S 13	29.58	29.52	29.56	38	45	34	39.0	W'ly 2	N. W'ly 3	N. W. 1	7	2	0	
14	29.56	29.49	29.65	29	37	17	27.7	S. W'ly 1	S. W'ly 3	N. W. 4	0	5	0	
15	29.71	29.78	29.85	10	22	15	15.7	N. W. 3	N. W. 4	N. W. 3	0	0	0	
16	30.00	30.01	30.04	13	28	24	21.7	N. W. 3	N. W. 3	N. W. 2	0	0	0	
17	30.09	29.92	29.67	23	42	40	35.0	N. W. 1	S'ly 2	E'ly 1	0	10	Rain	} 0.35
18	29.35	28.97	29.13	40	55	39	44.7	S'ly 2	S. W. 2	N. W. 3	Misty	9	0	}
19	29.58	29.70	29.86	35	40	31	35.3	N. W. 3	N. W. 4	N. W. 1	0	2	0	
S 20	29.89	29.78	29.68	28	51	44	41.0	W'ly 2	W.byS. 2	S. W. 2	0	0	0	
21	29.52	29.42	29.43	47	62	46	51.7	S. W. 2	S. W. 2	N. W. 1	5	0	9	
22	29.40	29.34	29.37	42	60	40	47.3	W.byS. 1	W byN 2	W'ly 2	2	2	5	
23	29.36	29.35	29.42	34	53	35	40.7	W'ly 1	W.by S 2	N. W. 1	3	8	2	
24	29.46	29.50	29.64	33	45	35	37.7	N. W. 2	N. W. 3	N. W. 2	2	6	3	
25	29.77	29.67	29.68	35	46	39	40.0	N. W. 2	N. W. 2	N. W'ly 2	0	2	9	
26	29.58	29.36	29.27	40	52	41	44.3	S. W. 2	S. E'ly 2	S'ly 1	9	2	Sprin'lg	
S 27	29.25	29.32	29.57	40	49	36	41.7	N. W'ly 2	N. W. 2	N. W. 2	2	6	5	
28	29.73	29.72	29.88	32	41	37	36.7	N. W. 2	N. W. 3	N. W. 2	2	10	10	
29	29.89	29.87	29.82	37	48	38	41.0	N. W. 2	N. W. 2	N. W. 1	2	0	0	
30	29.56	29.45	29.54	42	61	49	50.7	S. W. 2	S. W. 3	N. W. 1	10	4	0	
31	29.70	29.61	29.61	39	58	48	48.3	N. W'ly 1	N. W. 2	W'ly 1	0	9	10	
Means	29.67	29.62	29.66	32.3	40.5	35.1	...	1.9	2.3	1.7	4.4	4.7	4.7	1.35
								2.0			4.6			
REDUCED TO SEA LEVEL.														
Max.	30.40	30.44	30.49	47	62	49	51.7							
Min.	29.31	29.15	29.31	10	22	15	15.7							
Mean	29.85	99.80	29.84											
Range	1.09	1.29	1.18	37	40	34	36.0							
Mean of month	29.830			...	...	...	36.0							
Extreme range	1.34			...	...	...	52.0							

Prevailing winds from some point between— Days.
N. & E. 3
E. & S. 2
S. & W. 9
W. & N. 17

Days.
Clear 7
Variable . . . . } 14
Cloudy . . . . }
Rain or snow fell on 10

1st. Moderate rain in the afternoon and evening.
2d. Mild and pleasant.
3d. Sprinkling of rain from noon to 2 P. M wind came to N. W. in the afternoon.
4th. Appearances of storm in the evening. Air very raw.
5th. Heavy fall of snow last night and this morning, commencing about midnight, and continuing till near noon. Evening clear. Snow from 8 to 10 inches deep.
6th. Pleasant.
7th. Very pleasant.
8th. Pleasant. Snow of the 5th has nearly all disappeared.
9th. Showery during the day. Bright starlight at 11 P. M.
10th. Very fine.
11th. Light snow and rain commenced falling about 5 P. M. The rain continued in the evening.
12th. Mist and clouds.
13th. Fine. Evening still and very splendid.
14th. Mild and pleasant in the morning. During the afternoon, the wind came to N. W., with distant snow squalls and grew cold fast, with violent winds which continued unabated at 11 P. M.
15th. Wind cold and severe all day. Evening very clear and cold.
16th. Pleasant, but cold.
17th. Mild and pleasant in the morning. Raw and misty in the afternoon. Rain in the evening.
18th. Moderate rain in the morning; wind S'ly. Brisk thundershower from 6 to 7 P M.
19th. Pleasant. Evening very splendid.
20th. Very fine.
21st. Very mild and pleasant.
22d. Very fine.
23d. Pleasant. Dashes of rain from 7 to 8 P. M. Very clear at 11 P. M.
24th. Blustering, and very dusty.
25th. Pleasant.
26th. Southerly air; rather raw. Sprinkling of rain at 10 P. M.
27th. Pleasant.
28th. Air raw and cold, with occasional snowflakes.
29th and 30th. Very fine.
31st. Mild and pleasant.

April, 1853. New Moon, 8d. 6h. 49m. A. M.

Days.	Barometer, reduced to 32° F. At 6 A. M.	At 1 P. M.	At 10 P. M.	Thermometer. At 6 A. M.	At 1 P. M.	At 10 P. M.	Daily mean.	Winds. (Direction and Force.) At 6 A. M.	At 1 P. M.	At 10 P. M.	Weather. (Tenths Cloudy.) At 6 A. M.	At 1 P. M.	At 10 P. M.	Rain and Snow in Inches of Water.
1	29.49	29.57	29.73	41	41	36	39.3	N. E. 2	N. E. 2	N. W. 1	Rain	10	0	0.50
2	29.94	29.94	30.01	32	50	34	38.7	N. by E. 2	N. E. 2	N. E. 1	2	2	0	
S 3	30.01	29.91	29.82	32	52	37	40.3	S. W. 2	S. W. 2	S. W. 1	0	10	Rain	
4	29.54	29.42	29.14	35	39	42	38.7	N. E. 2	N. E. 1	E'ly 1	Misty	Rain	Rain	1.50
5	28.85	28.83	29.33	49	43	40	44.0	S. W. 2	W'ly 4	N. W. 3	Rain	10	2	
6	29.43	29.31	29.46	36	53	41	43.3	S. W. 1	S. W. 1	S. W. 2	5	Rain	Rain	0.40
7	29.60	29.66	29.76	33	47	36	38.7	N. W. 1	N. W. 2	N. W. 1	0	1	0	
8	29.79	29.74	29.63	36	56	46	46.0	N. W. 1	S'ly 2	S'ly 2	3	4	0	
9	29.51	29.46	29.61	46	65	49	53.3	S. W. 4	S. W. 3	N. W. 2	Sprinl'g	3	0	
S 10	29.66	29.69	29.90	42	49	37	42.7	W by N 1	N. W. 3	N. W. 2	2	2	0	
11	30.08	30.10	30.13	32	48	38	39.3	N. W. 2	S. W'ly 2	S. W'ly 2	0	2	2	
12	30.11	29.99	29.81	36	52	45	44.3	S. W. 2	S. W. 2	S. W. 2	3	8	Rain	
13	29.72	29.71	29.65	48	61	49	52.7	S. W. 2	E'ly 1	S. E'ly 1	Rain	9	Rain	0.90
14	29.41	29.44	29.67	44	43	35	40.7	N. E. 1	N. E. 2	N. E. 2	Misty	Misty	Misty	
15	29.90	29.99	30.06	33	47	39	39.7	N. W. 2	N. W. 2	N. W. 1	0	1	0	
16	30.21	30.12	30.06	33	53	41	42.3	N. W. 1	S. E'ly 2	S'ly 2	2	6	10	
S 17	29.91	29.75	29.73	33	38	37	36.0	N. E. 1	N. E. 2	N. E'ly 2	Snow	Rain	10	0.85
18	29.81	29.82	29.89	34	47	35	35.3	N. by E. 2	N by W 2	N. W. 1	4	2	0	
19	29.90	29.79	29.81	36	61	43	46.7	S. W. 2	S. W. 2	S. W. 1	0	0	3	
20	29.81	29.65	29.68	45	49	47	47.0	S. W. 2	S. W. 2	N. W. 2	Misty	Rain	9	0.30
21	29.86	29.84	29.90	45	63	44	50.7	N. E'ly 2	E'ly 2	S'ly 2	10	2	2	
22	29.83	29.56	29.28	44	51	49	48.0	S'ly 2	S. by E. 2	S'ly 2	8	10	Rain	0.45
23	29.43	29.62	29.80	51	56	43	50.0	N. W. 3	N. W. 2	N. W. 1	2	0	1	
S 24	29.94	29.88	29.85	38	51	39	42.7	N. E'ly 2	N. E. 2	S. E'ly 1	6	10	2	
25	29.79	29.79	29.73	40	42	36	39.3	N. E. 2	N. E. 2	N. E. 2	9	Misty	Rain	0.15
26	29.76	29.78	29.88	36	53	41	43.3	N'ly 2	N. W. 2	N. E. 1	6	2	0	
27	29.98	29.96	29.97	40	60	44	48.0	S'ly 1	S'ly 2	S'ly 1	0	0	0	
28	29.96	29.89	29.91	45	61	45	50.3	S. by E. 1	S. by E. 2	S. E'ly 1	0	2	0	
29	29.86	29.74	29.74	46	67	53	55.3	S. W'ly 1	S. W. 2	S. W. 2	0	3	Hazy	
30	29.90	29.90	29.95	50	62	45	52.3	N. W. 2	N. W. 2	N. W. 2	5	0	0	
Means	29.77	29.73	29.76	39.7	52.0	41.5	...	1.6	2.0	1.6	4.9	5.3	4.4	5.05
									1.8			4.9		
REDUCED TO SEA LEVEL.								Prevailing winds from some point between—		Days.			Days.	
Max.	30.39	30.30	30.31	51	67	53	55.3	N. & E.		5	Clear		9	
Min.	29.08	29.01	29.32	32	39	34	35.3	E. & S.		6	Variable }		8	
Mean	29.95	29.91	29.94					S. & W.		12	Cloudy }			
Range	1.36	1.29	0.99	19	28	19	20.0	W. & N.		7	Rain or snow fell on		13	
Mean of month			29.933	...	...	...	44.4							
Extreme range			1.38	...	...	...	35.0							

Remarks.

1st. Moderate rain and air rather raw in the morning. Evening clear.
2d. Pleasant.
3d. Morning fine. Air raw in the afternoon. Began to rain moderately at 9 P. M. Snow and rain at midnight.
4th. Light rain and mist through the day. Heavy thundershower from 7½ to 8 P. M. Rain continued.
5th. At noon, the barometer stood at 28.87, and began to rise soon. Aurora in the evening, without streamers, but bright.
6th. Shower at 1 P. M. Thundershower, with hail, at 5 P. M., and rain in the evening. The morning was pleasant.
7th. Very fine.
8th. Very pleasant.
9th. Heavy wind at S. W., and sprinkling of rain at sunrise. Mostly clear in the afternoon and evening.
10th. Cool, and rather blustering.
11th. Pleasant.
12th. Began to rain moderately from 5 to 6 P. M.
13th. Light rain in the morning, and again in the evening.
14th. Rain from 6 to 8 P. M.
15th. Very fine.
16th. Pleasant.
17th. Snowed fast from 6 to 8 A. M.; then rain. Wind light.
18th. Pleasant. Evening very clear.
19th. Very pleasant.
20th. Very moderate rain in the morning.
21st. Pleasant.
22d. Cloudy in the morning. Mist in the afternoon. Rain in the evening, with thunder.
23d. Very fine.
24th. Cool. Air raw.
25th. Air raw, with mist. Moderate rain in the evening.
26th. Pleasant.
27th to 30th. Very fine.

May, 1853. New Moon, 7d. 10h. 58m. P. M.

Days.	Barometer At 6 A. M.	At 1 P. M.	At 10 P. M.	Thermometer At 6 A. M.	At 1 P. M.	At 10 P. M.	Daily mean	Winds At 6 A. M.	At 1 P. M.	At 10 P. M.	Weather At 6 A. M.	At 1 P. M.	At 10 P. M.	Rain
S 1	30.05	30.00	30.03	44	52	40	45.3	N. W. 2	N. W. 3	N. W. 2	0	0	0	
2	30.06	29.96	29.97	38	59	48	48.3	N. W. 2	N. W. 2	N. W. 1	0	2	0	
3	30.07	30.02	29.86	45	54	47	48.7	N. W. 2	S. E'ly 2	S'ly 2	9	10	3	
4	29.87	29.88	29.94	46	61	44	50.3	N. E'ly 1	N. E. 2	N. E. 1	5	7	0	
5	29.90	29.78	29.70	45	53	47	48.3	N. E. 2	E'ly 2	N. E. 2	10	10	Rain	1.05
6	29.57	29.60	29.75	42	50	43	45.3	N. E. 2	N. E. 2	N. E'ly 1	10	10	2	
7	29.85	29.81	29.81	42	63	45	50.0	N. E. 2	N. E. 2	S. E'ly 1	0	1	0	
S 8	29.79	29.71	29.48	46	57	51	51.3	S. E'ly 2	S. E'ly 2	E'ly 1	10	10	Rain	0.95
9	29.58	29.66	29.73	44	63	51	52.7	N. W. 2	S'ly 2	S'ly 1	9	3	0	
10	29.78	29.77	29.78	49	64	49	54.0	S. W. 1	S'ly 2	S. W'ly 2	Foggy	0	0	
11	29.73	29.74	29.86	49	71	52	57.3	S. W. 2	N. W. 2	N. W. 1	10	3	0	
12	29.92	29.84	29.79	50	67	54	57.0	N. E. 1	S'ly 2	S'ly 2	0	4	9	
13	29.86	29.86	29.96	50	59	50	53.0	N. W. 1	N. W. 2	N. W. 1	3	8	0	
14	30.00	29.95	29.97	48	69	55	57.3	N. W. 1	S. W'ly 3	N. W. 2	0	2	0	
S 15	30.02	29.95	29.95	54	76	55	61.7	S. W'ly 2	S. W. 3	S. W'ly 1	4	4	3	
16	29.86	29.77	29.78	56	78	63	65.7	S. W. 2	S. W. 3	S. W. 1	5	3	5	
17	29.82	29.81	29.81	64	87	68	73.0	S. W. 2	S. W. 3	S. W. 2	5	2	4	
18	29.78	29.86	29.78	65	62	47	58.0	S. W. 2	N. E. 2	N. E. 2	5	5	10	
19	29.51	29.46	29.46	52	55	46	51.0	W. by S. 1	N. E. 1	N. W'ly 1	Rain	Rain	5	1.15
20	29.49	29.54	29.66	45	62	47	51.3	N. W. 3	N. W. 3	N. W. 1	2	2	0	
21	29.69	29.62	29.61	49	71	56	58.7	W'ly 2	S. W. 2	S. W. 2	0	2	3	
S 22	29.62	29.58	29.66	57	74	56	62.3	S. W. 2	S. W. 3	S. W. 2	2	0	3	
23	29.69	29.64	29.75	56	76	59	63.7	S. W. 2	S. W. 3	S. W. 2	2	4	5	
24	29.79	29.80	29.75	60	75	55	63.3	S. W'ly 2	S'ly 3	N. W. 2	8	10	7	
25	29.73	29.69	29.60	59	71	55	61.7	N. E. 1	S. E'ly 2	N. E'ly 1	Rain	9	Rain	0.75
26	29.42	29.30	29.26	58	63	55	58.7	E'ly 2	S. E'ly 2	S. W. 2	Misty	Rain	Rain	1.05
27	29.49	29.58	29.70	55	77	59	63.7	N. W. 2	W'ly 2	S. W'ly 1	10	4	0	
28	29.72	29.72	29.72	60	79	62	67.0	S. W. 2	S. 2	S. W. 1	5	0	0	
S 29	29.66	29.63	29.79	62	80	61	67.7	S. W. 1	S. W. 2	S. W. 2	2	2	0	
30	29.81	29.73	29.74	61	74	64	66.3	S. W. 2	S. W. 3	S. W. 2	0	2	10	
31	[illegible]	[illegible]	[illegible]	[illegible]	[illegible]	[illegible]	[illegible]	[illegible]	[illegible]	[illegible]	10	[illegible]	0	
Means	29.78	29.75	29.76	51.7	66.7	52.6	...	1.8	2.3	1.5	5.3	4.5	3.5	4.95
									1.9			4.4		
REDUCED TO SEA LEVEL.								Prevailing winds from some point between—		Days.			Days.	
Max.	30.25	30.20	30.21	65	87	68	73.0	N. & E.		8	Clear		9	
Min.	29.60	29.48	29.44	38	50	40	45.3	E. & S.		3	Variable }		14	
Mean	29.90	29.93	29.94					S. & W.		14	Cloudy }			
Range	0.65	0.72	0.77	27	37	28	27.7	W. & N.		6	Rain fell on		8	
Mean of month			29.943	...	...	...	57.0							
Extreme range			0.81	...	...	...	49.0							

Remarks.

1st. Rather cool, but fine. Clouds of dust in the streets.
2d. Very fine. Aurora in the evening extending from N. W. to N. E., with beautiful streamers reaching nearly to the zenith.
3d. Air rather raw.
4th. Brisk showers at about 2 A. M. The day pleasant.
5th. Began to rain moderately at 9 P. M.
6th. Occasional mist through the day. Evening clear.
7th. Pleasant.
8th. At 1 P. M., wind S'ly, while the clouds came from N. W. Rain in the evening.
9th. Very fine.
10th. Pleasant.
11th. Sprinkling of rain at 6 A. M. Pleasant in the afternoon and evening.
12th. Very pleasant.
13th and 14th. Very fine.
15th. Pleasant.
16th. Pleasant. The thermometer at 1 P. M. (78°) was higher than at any time since Sept. 11th, being over eight months. Frequent lightning in the N. E at 10 P. M.
17th. From 1 to 2 P. M., the thermometer stood at 87°, placed in the shade in a brisk current of air.
18th. At 6 A. M., very warm; wind S.W. Wind came to N. E. about 10 A. M., and grew cooler.
19th. Heavy shower, with thunder, from 3 to 5 A. M. Rain at intervals during the day. Thunder in the afternoon. At 11 P. M., clear and mild.
20th. Cool and blustering.
21st. Very pleasant.
22d. Very fine.
23d. Pleasant.
24th. Sprinkling of rain at 6 P. M. Aurora in the evening.
25th. Copious rain in the morning. Rain again [illegible]
26th. Steady rain in the afternoon and evening.
27th. Pleasant.
28th and 29th. Very fine.
30th. Pleasant.
31st. Pleasant, but cool.

June, 1853. New Moon, 6d. 2h. 54m. P. M.

DAYS.	Barometer, reduced to 32° F. At 6 A. M.	At 1 P. M.	At 10 P. M.	Thermometer. At 6 A. M.	At 1 P. M.	At 10 P. M.	Daily mean.	Winds. (Direction and Force.) At 6 A. M.	At 1 P. M.	At 10 P. M.	Weather. (Tenths Cloudy.) At 6 A. M.	At 1 P. M.	At 10 P. M.	Rain and Snow in Inches of Water.
1	30.11	30.07	30.11	46	71	49	55.3	N. E. 2	N. E. 2	N. E. 1	0	3	0	
2	30.09	30.03	30.04	46	68	56	56.7	N. E. 1	S. E. 2	S. E'ly 2	0	0	10	
3	29.96	29.85	29.79	57	70	62	63.0	S. by W. 2	S. W'ly 3	S. W. 2	10	7	10	
4	29.73	...	29.95	64	...	51	...	S. W. 2	...	N. E. 1	6	...	0	0.20
S 5	29.77	29.76	29.75	54	72	56	60.7	N. E'ly 2	N. E. 2	N. E'ly 1	0	0	2	
6	29.91	29.87	29.80	52	70	54	58.7	N by W 2	S. by E. 3	S'ly 2	3	0	0	
7	29.75	29.68	29.69	55	73	62	63.3	S. W. 2	S. W. 3	S. W. 2	2	7	10	
8	29.77	29.83	29.95	62	71	56	63.0	W'ly 2	N. E. 2	S. E'ly 1	Rain	5	0	0.10
9	30.05	30.07	30.08	54	74	53	60.3	N. E. 1	E'ly 2	N. E. 1	0	2	0	
10	30.07	30.03	29.97	48	74	62	61.3	N. E'ly 1	S. E'ly 2	S'ly 2	2	0	10	
11	29.96	29.94	29.99	59	71	61	63.7	S. E'ly 1	S. E'ly 2	S'ly 1	0	5	10	
S 12	30.10	30.16	30.17	62	75	59	65.3	N. E. 2	E'ly 2	E'ly 1	10	3	9	
13	30.16	30.01	29.92	56	76	62	64.7	S. E'ly 2	S. W. 3	S. W. 2	5	6	8	
14	29.92	29.91	29.95	64	86	65	71.7	S. W'ly 2	S'ly 2	S. W'ly 2	5	2	0	
15	29.95	29.91	29.87	65	75	62	67.3	S'ly 2	S. E'ly 3	S. by E. 2	Foggy	0	2	
16	29.87	29.79	29.81	64	88	65	72.3	S. by E. 2	S. W. 3	S. W. 2	0	2	0	
17	29.74	29.67	29.66	68	84	68	73.3	S. W. 3	S. W. 3	S. W. 2	10	0	10	
18	29.67	29.65	29.68	68	82	64	71.3	S. W. 2	S. W. 2	S. W. 2	10	3	2	
S 19	29.68	29.68	29.77	66	87	70	74.3	S. W. 1	W'ly 2	W'ly 1	0	3	4	
20	29.75	29.67	29.69	69	91	78	79.3	W by N 1	S. W. 2	S. W. 1	9	5	3	
21	29.70	29.67	29.71	76	94	77	82.3	S. W. 2	W'ly 3	W'ly 2	1	1	4	
22	29.72	29.70	29.78	72	86	63	73.7	N. E'ly 1	N. E. 2	N. E. 2	5	4	3	
23	29.72	29.63	29.57	63	85	78	75.3	N. E'ly 1	N. E. 1	S'ly 1	10	2	10	
24	29.51	29.57	29.71	74	79	66	73.0	N. W. 3	W'ly 3	N. W. 2	8	1	0	
25	29.77	29.75	29.89	59	77	57	64.3	N. W. 2	N. W'ly 3	N. W. 2	0	3	0	
S 26	29.97	29.95	30.04	57	75	60	64.0	N. W. 2	N. W. 2	N. W. 1	0	4	5	
27	30.00	29.91	29.76	60	66	57	61.0	W. S. W. 3	S. W. 3	S. W. 1	10	Rain	Rain	0.60
28	29.80	29.80	29.83	57	78	60	64.3	N'ly 1	E'ly 1	S. W. 1	10	8	0	
29	29.83	29.80	29.86	61	75	65	66.7	S. W. 1	S. W. 3	S'ly 1	7	10	10	
30	29.79	29.75	29.68	66	78	71	71.7	S. W. 2	S. W. 3	W'ly 1	10	3	2	
Means	29.86	29.83	29.85	60.8	77.6	62.3	...	1.8	2.3	1.5	5.1	3.3	4.5	0.90
REDUCED TO SEA LEVEL.									1.9			4.3		
Max.	30.34	30.34	30.35	76	94	78	82.3	Prevailing winds from some point between—		Days.			Days.	
Min.	29.69	29.75	29.75	46	66	49	55.3	N. & E.		7	Clear		8	
Mean	30.04	30.01	30.03					E. & S.		5	Variable		13	
Range	0.65	0.59	0.60	30	28	29	27.0	S. & W.		14	Cloudy			
Mean of month 35.027				...	...	...	66.9	W. & N.		4	Rain fell on		9	
Extreme range 0.66				...	...	...	48.0							

REMARKS.

1st. Frost this morning in the vicinity. Aurora quite bright at 11 P. M., without streamers.
2d. Frost in the vicinity again this morning. Day pleasant.
3d. Variable. Frequent lightning in the west at 10 P. M. Heavy thunder from 11 to 12 P. M.
4th. Dashes of rain at 6 A. M. Morning warm and sultry. From 11 A. M to noon, wind changed from S. W. to N. E., with rain and sudden fall of temperature.
5th and 6th. Very fine.
7th. Pleasant. Appearances of rain in evening.
8th. Light rain early in the morning. Evening splendid.
9th. Very fine.
10th. Day pleasant. Evening cloudy.
11th. Pleasant. Evening overcast.
12th and 13th. Pleasant.
14th. Very hot sun.
15th. Very fine.
16th. At 1 P. M., thermometer stood at 88° in the shade, in a brisk current of air.
17th. Fog-clouds in the morning. Hot sun from 9 A. M. to 5 P. M. Evening mostly overcast.
18th. Sprinkling of rain last night.
19th. Sun very scorching. Vegetation beginning to show signs of drought.
20th. At 2 P. M., thermometer stood at 90° in the shade, in a fresh breeze.
21st. At 2 P. M., thermometer stood at 94° in the shade, free from the effects of reflection; at 2½ P. M., at 95° in the shade, and when freely swung in the air; at 3 P. M., at 94°; at 6 P. M., at 92°; at 10 P. M., at 77°; and at 12 P. M., at 76°. Mean of four observations—viz., at 6 A. M., 1 P. M., 2½ P. M., and 10 P. M.—85°.5; being as warm as any day on my Record of 22 years' continuance, with the exception of July 13, 1849, when the thermometer rose to 97°, with a mean of 90° for four observations at the times above mentioned.
22d. Thunder and sprinkling of rain from 5 to 6 P. M. Evening cool.
23d. Heat abated. Sprinkling of rain at 11 P. M.
24th. Pleasant. Evening cool.
25th. Fine. Evening quite cool and clear.
26th. At sunrise, thermometer 49°. At 8 A. M., dew-point 43°; at 1 P. M., 42°. Sprinkling of rain at 7 P. M.
27th. Moderate rain in afternoon and evening.
28th. Very fine.
29th. Pleasant.
30th. Sprinkling of rain from 6 to 8 P. M.

July, 1853. New Moon, 6d. 2h. 45m. A. M.

DAYS.	Barometer At 6 A. M.	At 1 P. M.	At 10 P. M.	Thermometer At 6 A. M.	At 1 P. M.	At 10 P. M.	Daily mean.	Winds At 6 A. M.	At 1 P. M.	At 10 P. M.	Weather At 6 A. M.	At 1 P. M.	At 10 P. M.	Rain
1	29.70	29.69	29.67	70	85	70	75.0	W'ly 2	N. W. 1	W'ly 1	2	8	0	
2	29.77	29.75	29.83	65	78	65	69.3	N. W. 2	N. W. 3	N. W. 1	0	0	0	
S 3	29.90	29.87	29.84	62	78	68	69.3	N. W. 1	S. W. 3	S. W. 2	0	2	7	
4	29.77	29.72	29.66	72	82	72	75.3	S. W. 2	S. W. 2	S. W. 2	10	10	2	
5	29.62	29.62	29.68	70	86	66	74.0	S. W. 1	S. W. 2	N. W. 2	4	3	6	
6	29.71	29.71	29.78	68	82	66	72.0	N. W. 3	N. W. 2	N. W. 1	2	2	0	
7	29.85	29.86	29.93	65	82	62	69.7	N. W. 1	N. W. 2	N. W. 1	0	2	0	
8	29.94	29.86	29.74	60	87	70	72.3	S. W. 1	S. W. 3	S. W. 2	0	7	0	
9	29.83	29.81	29.77	72	88	72	77.3	S. W. 2	S'ly 2	W'ly 1	3	7	Rain	0.60
S 10	29.81	29.80	29.77	72	83	72	75.7	S. W. 1	S. W. 1	S. W. 1	8	8	Rain	0.75
11	29.76	29.73	29.75	66	79	68	71.0	N. W. 1	W'ly 2	W. 1	10	5	0	
12	29.76	29.76	29.78	66	74	62	67.3	N. E'ly 2	N. E. 2	N. E. 2	9	10	3	
13	29.87	29.91	29.96	62	78	65	68.3	N. W. 2	N. W. 1	N. W. 5	0	1	6	
14	30.08	29.91	29.91	62	81	63	68.7	N. W. 1	S'ly 2	S'ly 1	0	3	0	
15	29.84	29.73	29.69	61	81	66	69.3	S. W. 1	S. W. 2	S. W. 1	0	2	0	
16	29.63	29.58	29.57	69	74	68	70.3	S. W. 3	S. W. 3	W'ly 1	10	10	5	0.40
S 17	29.62	29.64	29.79	66	80	63	69.7	N. W. 2	N. W. 2	N. W. 1	5	3	0	
18	29.94	29.91	29.94	58	80	63	67.0	N. W. 1	S. W. 2	N. W. 1	0	2	0	
19	29.97	...	29.98	63	...	65	...	S. W. 1	...	S. W. 2	2	...	6	
20	29.79	29.80	29.79	61	76	64	67.0	E'ly 2	N'ly 1	N. W. 1	Rain	5	2	0.90
21	29.79	29.75	29.79	63	79	65	69.0	N. W. 1	N. W. 1	S. W. 1	10	9	8	
22	29.81	29.80	29.83	64	81	65	70.0	S. W. 1	S. W. 2	S'ly 1	8	3	3	
23	29.82	29.78	29.75	64	68	61	64.3	S. W. 1	E'ly 1	N. E'ly 1	9	Rain	10	0.75
S 24	29.79	29.78	29.81	64	79	68	70.3	N'ly 1	S. W. 2	S. W. 1	10	3	0	
25	29.78	29.75	29.73	69	85	72	75.3	S. W. 2	S. W. 3	S. W. 2	10	5	6	
26	29.63	29.67	29.73	74	73	71	72.7	W'ly 1	S. W. 1	S. W.	Rain	Rain	10	1.90
27	29.81	29.77	29.77	62	64	61	62.3	N'ly 1	N. E. 2	N'ly 1	Rain	Rain	10	1.07
28	29.94	29.99	30.07	63	78	64	68.3	N. W. 1	W'ly 1	N. W. 1	6	8	Hazy	
29	30.08	30.05	30.00	64	76	66	68.7	W'ly 1	S. S. E. 2	S. W. 1	Hazy	Hazy	2	
30	29.96	29.99	29.86	67	78	71	72.0	W'ly 1	S. W. 1	W. 2	10	5	10	
S 31	29.80	29.75	29.79	73	84	73	76.7	S. W. 1	S. W. 1	N. W. 1	10	3	2	
Means	29.82	29.79	29.81	65.7	79.3	66.7	...	1.4	1.8	1.4	5.9	5.5	4.1	6.37
REDUCED TO SEA LEVEL.									1.5			5.2		
Max.	30.26	30.23	30.25	74	88	73	77.3	Prevailing winds from some point between—		Days.			Days.	
Min.	29.80	29.76	29.75	58	68	61	62.3	N. & E.		2	Clear		8	
Mean	30.00	29.97	29.99					E. & S.		1	Variable		13	
Range	0.46	0.47	0.50	16	20	12	15.0	S. & W.		17	Cloudy			
Mean of month 29.987				...	...	...	70.6	W. & N.		11	Rain fell on		10	
Extreme range 0.51				...	...	...	30.0							

REMARKS.

1st. Pleasant; sun hot.
2d and 3d. Very fine.
4th. Mostly overcast. Sprinkling of rain at 4 A. M.
5th and 6th. Very fine.
7th. Very fine. The ground getting very dry.
8th. Pleasant.
9th. Rain, with thunder, from 7 to 9 P. M. Sun very hot during the day, when not obscured by clouds.
10th. Sprinkling of rain from 11 A. M. to noon. Evening cloudy. Heavy thundershower at 11 P. M.
11th. Pleasant.
12th. Very pleasant.
13th. Pleasant.
14th. Pleasant. Sprinkling of rain from 4 to 5 P. M.
15th. Very fine.
16th. Moderate rain from 4 to 8 P. M.
17th. Fine. Evening very clear and cool.
18th. Very fine.
19th. Pleasant. Sprinkling of rain from 4 to 5 P. M.
20th. Heavy shower, with thunder, during the night and early in the morning. Pleasant in the afternoon and evening.
21st. Mostly cloudy.
22d. Pleasant.
23d. Began to rain very gently at 11 A. M., and continued through the afternoon and evening.
24th. Pleasant.
25th. Pleasant. Sun rather scorching at midday.
26th. Heavy rain from 7 to 9 A. M., with lightning and heavy thunder. Occasional showers during the day.
27th. Rain nearly all day.
28th. Pleasant, but cloudy.
29th. Hazy nearly all day.
30th. Very pleasant. Little or no air stirring.
31st. Pleasant. Rather sultry at noon.

August, 1853. New Moon, 4d. 6h. 47m. P. M.

Days.	Barometer, reduced to 32° F. At 6 A. M.	At 1 P. M.	At 10 P. M.	Thermometer. At 6 A. M.	At 1 P. M.	At 10 P. M.	Daily mean.	Winds. (Direction and Force.) At 6 A. M.	At 1 P. M.	At 10 P. M.	Weather. (Tenths Cloudy.) At 6 A. M.	At 1 P. M.	At 10 P. M.	Rain and Snow in Inches of Water.
1	29.84	29.82	29.78	69	83	70	74.0	N. W. 1	S.	S'ly 2	10	9	10	
2	29.61	29.66	29.75	71	76	62	69.7	W'ly 1	N'ly 2	N. E.	Rain	10	Rain	1.74
3	29.78	29.79	...	60	76	...	...	N. W. 1	S'ly 1	...	0	9	...	
4	...	...	...	...	...	...	...	...	...	...	Rain	Rain	Rain	} 3.04
5	...	...	...	...	...	...	...	...	...	...	...	...	...	
6	...	...	29.83	...	...	66	...	...	...	N. E. 2	...	...	Rain	
S 7	29.85	29.86	29.86	67	71	65	67.3	N. E. 1	N. E'ly 1	N. E. 1	Misty	10	10	
8	29.88	29.82	29.79	64	78	71	71.0	N'ly	S'ly 2	W. 4	Misty	4	Rain	
9	29.83	29.81	29.83	68	85	73	75.3	S'ly 1	S. W. 2	S'ly	0	0	3	
10	29.83	29.83	29.90	71	87	73	77.0	W'ly 1	W. 1	S'ly 1	0	1	0	
11	29.94	...	29.83	73	...	74	...	S'ly	...	S'ly 1	Hazy	...	0	
12	29.83	29.74	29.72	75	88	77	80.0	S. W. 1	S. 2	S. W. 1	9	0	0	
13	29.72	29.71	29.72	80	90	74	81.3	S. W. 1	S. W. 1	N. E. 1	0	5	2	
S 14	29.65	29.58	29.66	76	90	74	80.0	S. W. 3	S. W. 1	N. E. 1	2	1	Rain	0.40
15	29.80	29.84	29.89	66	75	62	67.7	N. E. 2	N. E. 3	N. E. 1	10	2	3	
16	29.88	29.90	29.86	64	76	64	68.0	N. E. 1	N. E. 2	N. E. 1	2	2	7	
17	29.82	29.73	29.63	64	67	62	64.3	N. E. 1	S. E'ly 1	Calm	10	Rain	10	
18	29.53	29.44	29.34	65	73	67	68.3	S'ly 1	S. W'ly 2	S. W. 2	Foggy	Rain	9	1.35
19	29.39	29.51	29.64	62	72	58	64.0	N. W. 3	N. W. 2	N. W. 1	5	2	0	
20	29.70	29.69	29.72	55	72	59	62.0	N. W. 1	N. E. 1	S. W. 1	3	6	5	
S 21	29.75	29.71	29.76	60	76	63	66.3	N. W. 1	W'ly 2	S. W. 1	0	3	1	
22	29.78	29.77	29.88	63	77	64	68.0	S. W. 1	S. W. 1	N. W. 1	6	5	5	0.45
23	29.97	29.99	29.93	54	71	57	60.7	N. W. 2	N. W. 2	N. W. 1	0	5	3	
24	29.93	29.82	29.72	59	69	68	65.3	Calm	S. W. 2	S. W. 1	Hazy	10	Misty	0.25
25	29.73	...	29.84	70	...	70	...	S. W. 1	...	N'ly 1	7	...	10	
26	30.02	30.03	30.02	62	70	61	64.3	N. W. 2	N. E. 2	N. E. 2	0	2	10	
27	...	29.76	29.68	69	75	66	70.0	S. E. 2	S. W. 3	S. W. 1	10	10	Rain	1.15
S 28	29.72	29.78	29.87	57	71	57	61.7	N. W. 2	N. W. 2	N. W. 1	5	2	0	
29	29.90	...	29.89	52	...	58	...	N. W. 1	...	S. W. 2	2	...	0	
30	29.90	29.86	29.73	58	75	62	65.0	S. W. 1	S. W. 2	S. W. 2	1	2	0	
31	29.79	29.74	29.84	64	78	69	70.3	S. W. 2	S. W. 3	S. W. 1	6	7	0	
Means	29.79	29.77	29.78	64.9	76.8	66.0	...	1.3	1.6	1.2	5.3	5.1	5.3	8.38
								1.4			5.2			
REDUCED TO SEA LEVEL.														
Max.	30.20	30.21	30.20	76	90	77	81.3							
Min.	29.57	29.62	29.52	52	67	57	55.0							
Mean	29.97	29.95	29.96											
Range	0.63	0.59	0.68	24	23	20	26.3							
Mean of month	29.960			...	...	...	69.2							
Extreme range	0.69			...	...	...	38.0							

Prevailing winds from some point between— Days.
N. & E. 7
E. & S. 2
S. & W. 17
W. & N. 2

Days.
Clear 6
Variable . . . } 12
Cloudy . . . . }
Rain fell on . . 12
(1 day omitted.)

Remarks.

1st. Sultry. Sprinkling of rain at 9 P. M.
2d. Rain last night, and this morning till 8 o'clock. Showers in the evening. Mostly clear at 11 P. M.
3d. Cool and very pleasant.
4th. Heavy rain; wind N. E.
5th. Pleasant.
6th. Cloudy in the morning. Rain after 5 P. M.
7th. Cloudy, with frequent mist.
8th. Very pleasant. Distant lightning early in the evening. Shower at 10 P. M.
9th. Pleasant in the morning. Very hot and without breeze in the afternoon.
10th. Very pleasant; hot sun.
11th. Very warm; no air stirring.
12th. Heat oppressive.
13th. Heat still oppressive
14th. Heat unabated. Thunder and rain at 7 P. M. Rain continued through the evening.
15th. Cool and pleasant.
16th. Pleasant.
17th. Rain began about noon, and continued in the afternoon.
18th. Frequent showers through the day.
19th. Evening splendid and very cool.
20th. Pleasant.
21st. Very fine.
22d. Pleasant. Fine shower at 5 P. M.
23d. Very fine.
24th. Pleasant in the morning. Cloudy in the afternoon. Sprinkling of rain.
25th. Very warm. Sprinkling of rain in the morning. Mostly cloudy through the day.
26th. Very fine. The comet clearly visible to the naked-eye at 8 P. M., in the N. W., not very high.
27th. Cloudy. Thunder and copious rain at 8 P. M.
28th. Very fine.
29th. At 5 A. M., ther. at 50°. Very fine.
30th. Very fine.
31st. Pleasant.

September, 1853. New Moon, 3d. 6h. 33m. A. M.

Days.	Barometer. Sunrise.	At 1 P. M.	At 10 P. M.	Thermometer. Sunrise.	At 1 P. M.	At 10 P. M.	Daily mean.	Winds. Sunrise.	At 1 P. M.	At 10 P. M.	Weather. Sunrise.	At 1 P. M.	At 10 P. M.	Rain and Snow in Inches of Water.
1	29.93	29.97	30.00	68	75	64	69.0	N. E. 2	N. E. 1	N. E. 1	10	9	0	
2	30.03	30.01	30.01	62	78	65	68.3	N. E. 1	S. W. 2	S'ly 2	0	0	0	
3	29.98	29.90	29.87	67	80	70	72.3	S. W. 2	S. W. 2	S. W. 1	10	2	10	
S 4	29.88	29.82	29.80	69	83	73	75.0	S. W. 1	S. W. 3	S. W. 2	8	3	2	
5	29.82	29.86	29.91	70	80	65	71.7	N. W. 1	N. E. 2	N. E. 1	0	0	3	
6	29.83	29.72	29.73	70	85	75	76.7	E'ly 1	E'ly 2	S. W. 1	Foggy	3	2	
7	29.68	...	29.67	72	...	69	...	S. W. 2	...	N. W.	3	...	8	
8	29.76	29.82	29.97	62	70	60	64.0	N. W. 3	N. W. 3	N. W. 1	4	1	0	
9	30.01	30.06	30.04	54	73	60	62.3	N'ly 2	E'ly 2	S. E'ly 1	2	10	9	
10	29.92	29.76	29.79	60	65	56	60.3	S. E'ly 1	N'ly 1	N. W. 1	Rain	10	0	0.30
S 11	29.94	29.89	29.99	50	69	51	56.7	N. W. 1	N. W. 2	N. W. 1	0	5	0	
12	30.07	30.00	29.97	45	65	51	53.7	N. W. 1	N. W. 2	S. W. 1	0	0	0	
13	30.01	29.81	29.78	50	70	58	59.3	S. W. 1	W. 2	N'ly 1	0	1	2	
14	29.77	29.72	29.58	56	74	66	65.3	N. W. 1	S. W. 2	S. W. 3	5	9	10	
15	29.22	29.24	29.28	66	76	63	68.3	S. W. 4	W'ly 3	W'ly 2	Rain	5	10	1.00
16	29.57	29.76	29.82	60	71	57	62.7	N. W. 2	N. W. 2	N. W.	5	2	2	
17	29.90	29.89	29.90	54	70	58	60.7	N. E. 1	E'ly 2	S'ly 2	8	10	10	0.65
S 18	29.84	29.83	29.87	64	72	66	67.3	S. W'ly 1	S. W. 1	S. W. 1	Misty	10	10	
19	29.88	29.87	29.87	66	76	66	69.3	S. W. 1	S. W. 2	S. W. 1	10	1	0	
20	29.80	29.76	29.73	69	77	69	71.7	S. W. 2	S. W. 3	S. W. 2	10	7	Misty	
21	29.68	29.52	29.59	64	69	62	65.0	N'ly 1	N'ly 1	N'ly 1	Rain	10	Misty	1.30
22	29.59	29.56	29.64	62	70	61	64.3	N. W. 1	N. W. 1	N. W. 1	9	10	10	
23	29.68	29.71	29.75	56	67	56	59.7	N. W. 1	N. W. 1	N. W. 1	9	9	0	
24	29.80	29.73	29.72	51	69	62	60.7	N. W. 1	S. W. 2	S. W. 1	0	1	0	
S 25	29.99	29.94	29.99	48	61	49	52.7	N. W. 2	N. W. 2	N. W. 1	2	1	0	
26	29.99	30.00	29.97	44	62	50	52.0	N. W. 1	N. W. 2	N. W. 1	0	0	0	
27	29.95	29.90	29.83	51	54	51	52.0	N. E. 1	N. E. 2	N. E. 1	10	10	10	
28	29.64	29.49	29.62	53	57	44	51.3	N. E'ly 1	N. E. 2	N. E.	Misty	Rain	Rain	0.55
29	29.78	29.83	29.92	43	54	40	45.7	N. W. 2	N. W. 2	N. W. 2	9	9	0	
[illegible]	[illegible]	[illegible]	[illegible]	[illegible]	[illegible]	[illegible]	[illegible]	[illegible]	[illegible]	[illegible]	[illegible]	[illegible]	[illegible]	
Means	29.82	29.80	29.81	58.0	70.0	59.4	...	1.5	1.9	1.3	5.8	4.9	4.3	3.80
								1.6			5.0			
REDUCED TO SEA LEVEL.														
Max.	30.25	30.24	30.22	72	85	75	76.7							
Min.	29.40	29.42	29.46	35	54	40	45.3							
Mean	30.00	29.98	29.99											
Range	0.85	0.82	0.76	37	31	35	31.4							
Mean of month	29.990			...	...	...	62.5							
Extreme range	0.85			...	...	...	50.0							

Prevailing winds from some point between— Days.
N. & E. 7
E. & S. 1
S. & W. 11
W. & N. 11

Days.
Clear 11
Variable . . . } 12
Cloudy . . . . }
Rain fell on . . 6

Remarks.

1st. Pleasant.
2d. Very fine.
3d. Warm and sultry.
4th. Sun very hot at mid-day.
5th. Very fine.
6th. Very warm and sultry.
7th. Fine, but warm.
8th. Very fine.
9th. Pleasant.
10th. Moderate rain in the morning. Evening very clear.
11th. Cool and very fine. Evening remarkably clear.
12th. White frost this morning in the vicinity. Day fine.
13th. Very fine.
14th. Sprinkling of rain at 5 P. M. Appearances of rain in the evening.
15th. Rain during the night and early this morning.
16th. Pleasant.
17th. Cloudy; occasional sprinkling of rain.
18th. Rain last night.
19th. Very fine.
20th. Warm and sultry.
21st. Heavy rain last night. Clouds, with some mist.
22d. Pleasant. Heavens mostly overcast.
23d. Pleasant.
24th, 25th, and 26th. Very fine.
27th. Cloudy, with appearances of storm.
28th. Mist, with occasional heavy showers.
29th. Mostly cloudy in the morning. Evening very fine.
[illegible]

October, 1853. New Moon, 2d. 5h. 10m. P. M.

Days.	Barometer, reduced to 32° F. Sunrise.	At 1 P. M.	At 10 P. M.	Thermometer. Sunrise.	At 1 P. M.	At 10 P. M.	Daily mean.	Winds. (Direction and Force.) Sunrise.	At 1 P. M.	At 10 P. M.	Weather. (Tenths Cloudy.) Sunrise.	At 1 P. M.	At 10 P. M.	Rain and Snow in Inches of Water.
1	29.77	29.69	29.62	44	59	55	52.7	N. W. 2	S. W'ly 1	S. W. 1	2	10	Rain	
S 2	29.55	29.48	29.59	56	64	51	57.0	S. W'ly 1	W'ly 2	N. W. 1	7	0	0	
3	29.58	29.56	29.77	42	53	42	45.7	N. W. 2	N. W. 3	N. W. 2	1	5	0	
4	29.87	29.84	29.70	36	59	50	48.3	N. W. 2	W'ly 3	S. W. 1	0	0	0	
5	29.66	29.48	29.32	50	66	52	56.0	S. W. 2	S. W. 4	S. W. 2	5	7	10	
6	29.37	29.46	29.68	50	54	40	48.0	W'ly 2	N. W. 4	N. W. 3	1	3	0	
7	29.77	29.74	29.82	35	51	38	41.3	N. W. 2	N. W. 4	N. W. 1	0	0	0	
8	29.90	29.81	29.74	37	60	46	47.7	N. W. 2	S. W. 1	S. W. 1	1	0	0	
S 9	29.62	29.56	29.51	47	66	55	56.0	S. W. 2	S. W. 2	S. W. 1	4	10	7	
10	29.47	29.52	29.57	59	65	46	56.7	S. W'ly 1	W'ly 2	N. W. 2	10	8	5	0.30
11	29.72	29.76	29.87	36	50	38	41.3	N. W. 2	N. W. 2	N. W. 2	5	5	3	
12	29.91	29.86	29.87	38	53	40	43.7	W by S. 2	S. W'ly 2	N. W. 1	1	8	0	
13	29.85	29.74	29.73	38	58	50	48.7	N. W. 1	W'ly 3	S. W'ly 1	0	9	10	
14	29.95	29.92	30.05	40	58	42	46.7	N. W. 1	N. W. 2	N. W. 2	0	0	0	
15	30.10	30.03	29.91	36	58	45	46.3	N. W. 1	S. W. 2	S. W. 1	0	0	0	
S 16	29.97	29.96	30.00	46	66	50	54.0	N by W. 2	N. E. 2	N'ly 1	0	0	0	
17	30.01	29.94	29.90	41	64	47	50.2	N. W'ly 1	S. W. 2	S. W. 1	1	0	0	
18	29.97	29.99	30.04	47	56	42	48.3	N'ly 1	N. E'ly 2	N. W. 1	2	3	0	
19	30.07	30.02	30.04	37	64	48	49.7	N. W. 1	N. W. 2	N. W. 1	0	0	0	
20	30.03	29.99	29.95	42	67	50	53.0	N. W. 1	S. W. 2	S. W'ly 1	1	0	3	
21	29.94	29.88	29.84	46	68	61	58.3	S. W'ly 1	S. W'ly 2	S. W'ly 1	5	4	10	
22	29.74	29.62	29.61	63	64	60	62.3	S'ly 2	S'ly 2	S'ly 1	Rain	Rain	10	0.40
S 23	29.61	29.57	29.72	61	68	54	61.0	S. W'ly 1	S. W'ly 1	W'ly 1	10	2	0	
24	29.73	29.58	28.99	47	47	57	50.3	N. E'ly 1	N. E. 2	S'ly 2	10	Rain	Rain	1.35
25	29.29	29.59	29.93	38	46	37	40.3	W by N. 4	W by N. 3	N. W. 2	2	2	3	
26	30.17	...	30.04	35	...	48	...	N. W. 1	...	S. W. 2	3	...	6	
27	29.84	29.81	29.79	53	60	55	56.0	S. W. 3	S. W. 3	S. W. 1	10	10	Rain	} 2.10
28	29.48	29.55	29.84	51	53	44	49.3	N. E. 3	N. E. 2	N'ly 1	Rain	10	3	
29	30.02	30.03	30.18	34	49	37	40.0	N. W. 2	N. W. 2	N. W. 1	0	1	0	
S 30	30.29	30.16	30.11	32	44	38	38.0	N. W. 1	N. E. 1	N. E. 2	2	10	10	
31	30.03	29.96	29.97	36	50	37	41.0	Nl'y 1	N. W. 2	N. W. 1	5	0	0	
Means	29.82	29.77	29.80	43.3	58.0	47.0	...	1.7	2.2	1.4	3.5	4.2	3.5	4.15
									1.8			3.7		
REDUCED TO SEA LEVEL.														
Max.	30.47	30.34	30.36	63	68	61	62.3	Prevailing winds from some point between—		Days.			Days.	
Min.	29.47	29.64	29.17	32	44	37	38.0	N. & E.		6	Clear		15	
Mean	30.00	29.95	29.98					E. & S.		0	Variable		} 9	
Range	1.00	0.70	1.19	31	24	24	24.3	S. & W.		15	Cloudy			
Mean of month 29.977				...	...	...	49.4	W. & N.		10	Rain fell on		7	
Extreme range 1.30				...	...	...	36.0							

Remarks.

1st. Pleasant.
2d. Pleasant. Evening very clear.
3d and 4th. Very fine.
5th. Pleasant, with appearances of storm in the evening.
6th. Very blustering; the air full of dust.
7th. Quite blustering. Evening very clear and still.
8th and 9th. Very fine.
10th. Thundershower at about 3 A. M.
11th. Pleasant.
12th. Very fine.
13th. Pleasant. Sprinkling of rain at 6 P. M.
14th. Very fine. Evening splendid.
15th. Very fine. First white frost on the fences about the College yard. (Last year, the first was on the 17th.)
16th to 19th. Very fine.
20th. Very fine. Fog-bow about the moon at 11 P. M., very distinct.
21st. Pleasant. Mist in the evening.
22d. Very warm and sultry, with occasional showers.
23d. Cloudy in the morning. Pleasant in the afternoon and evening.
24th. Rain in the afternoon: wind S. E., heavy. At 8 P. M., barometer 29.17 (not reduced); wind very heavy, and raining. At 9 P. M., bar. 29.13; wind slackened. At 10 P. M., bar. 29.10; wind much abated. At 11 P. M., bar. 29.09; wind moderate at S. W'ly.
25th. Very blustering.
26th. Air raw and chilly at S. W.
27th. Cloudy. Began to rain moderately from 7 to 8 P. M. Heavy rain during the night.
28th. Moderate rain this morning. Cloudy in the afternoon. Mostly clear at 10 P. M.
29th. Very fine.
30th. The first black frost on College Hill. The ground lightly frozen. Air raw and chilly, with indications of snow.
31st. Very fine.

November, 1853. New Moon, 1d. 3h. 31m. A. M., and 30d. 2h. 5m. P. M.

Days.	Barometer Sunrise.	At 1 P. M.	At 10 P. M.	Thermometer Sunrise.	At 1 P. M.	At 10 P. M.	Daily mean.	Winds Sunrise.	At 1 P. M.	At 10 P. M.	Weather Sunrise.	At 1 P. M.	At 10 P. M.	Rain and Snow
1	29.95	29.87	29.88	33	55	41	43.0	S. W. 1	S. W. 2	S. W. 2	1	0	0	
2	29.90	29.84	29.86	40	57	43	46.7	S. W. 2	S. W. 2	S. W. 2	0	1	2	
3	29.90	29.88	29.96	43	64	49	52.0	S. W. 2	S. W. 2	N'ly 2	2	10	10	
4	30.11	30.07	30.20	34	48	34	38.7	N. W. 2	N. W. 2	N. W. 2	2	0	0	
5	30.28	30.23	30.15	30	45	36	37.0	N. W. 2	S. W. 2	S. W. 2	0	10	10	
S 6	30.00	29.98	30.14	40	45	32	39.0	S. W. 2	N. W. 3	N. W. 2	10	0	0	
7	30.27	30.31	30.47	27	40	26	31.0	N. W. 1	N. W. 2	N. W. 2	0	1	3	
8	30.45	30.24	29.85	26	38	51	38.3	N. W. 2	E'ly 2	S'ly 1	10	Rain	Rain	
9	29.56	29.38	29.47	56	61	37	51.3	S. W. 4	S. W. 4	W'ly 3	10	Rain	10	1.40
10	29.79	...	30.31	33	...	29	...	N. W'ly 3	...	N. W. 2	5	...	0	
11	30.48	30.48	30.46	25	46	41	37.3	N. W. 2	S. E. 2	S'ly	0	9	10	
12	30.40	30.28	30.03	42	59	55	52.0	S'ly 1	S'ly 1	S. E'ly 1	10	10	10	
S 13	29.79	29.49	29.23	55	60	58	57.7	S. E. 2	S. E. 3	E'ly 1	10	Rain	Rain	2.50
14	29.15	29.25	29.54	48	54	39	47.0	N. W. 4	N. W. 4	N. W. 2	9	0	0	
15	29.61	29.68	29.96	40	55	43	46.0	W. by S. 2	S. W'ly 2	N. W. 1	0	1	5	
16	30.12	30.21	30.33	42	46	36	41.3	N'ly 1	N. E. 1	N. E. 1	5	10	Hazy	
17	30.37	30.35	30.18	39	45	45	43.0	N. E. 2	E'ly 2	E'ly 2	10	10	Rain	0.15
18	30.15	30.14	30.11	41	45	43	43.0	N'ly 2	N'ly 2	N. W. 2	Misty	10	10	
19	30.09	30.01	29.99	44	60	47	50.3	S. W'ly 1	S'ly 2	S'ly 1	10	2	Foggy	
S 20	29.93	29.85	29.90	50	70	46	55.3	S. W'ly 2	S. W'ly 1	N. E. 2	3	8	10	
21	29.91	29.89	29.97	44	44	42	43.3	N. E. 1	N'ly 1	N'ly 1	Rain	Misty	Misty	0.25
22	29.97	29.88	29.81	41	53	51	48.3	N'ly 1	S'ly 1	W. 2	10	10	10	
23	29.80	29.74	29.75	50	61	51	54.0	Calm	W. 1	S. W'ly 1	10	2	10	
24	29.57	29.69	30.12	52	42	21	38.3	S. W. 2	N. W. 3	N. W. 3	9	10	0	0.10
25	30.28	30.34	30.29	15	27	20	20.7	N. W. 2	N. W. 2	N. W. 1	0	0	0	
26	30.23	30.14	30.19	22	40	30	30.7	N. W. 1	S. W. 2	N. W'ly 1	5	3	0	
S 27	30.36	30.41	30.50	25	35	28	29.3	N'ly 2	N. E. 3	N. E. 2	0	0	0	
28	30.51	30.46	30.40	26	35	34	31.7	N. E. 1	N. E. 2	N. E. 2	10	10	10	
29	30.34	30.22	30.07	37	49	44	43.3	S. E'ly 1	S. E'ly 1	S'ly 1	9	10	10	
30	29.83	29.71	29.75	47	63	41	50.3	S'ly 1	S. W'ly 2	N. W. 2	Foggy	8	10	
Means	30.04	30.00	30.03	38.2	49.7	39.8	...	1.8	2.0	1.7	5.9	5.8	6.1	4.40
									1.8			5.9		
REDUCED TO SEA LEVEL.														
Max.	30.69	30.66	30.68	55	70	58	55.3	Prevailing winds from some point between—		Days.			Days.	
Min.	29.33	29.43	29.41	15	27	20	20.7	N. & E.		5	Clear		7	
Mean	30.22	30.18	30.21					E. & S.		5	Variable		} 17	
Range	1.36	1.23	1.27	40	43	38	34.6	S. & W.		10	Cloudy			
Mean of month 30.203				...	...	...	42.6	W. & N.		10	Rain fell on		6	
Extreme range 1.36				...	...	...	55.0							

Remarks.

1st and 2d. Very fine.
3d. Appearance of storm in the evening.
4th. Very fine.
5th. Pleasant.
6th. Sprinkling at 9 A. M. Afternoon and evening fine.
7th. Pleasant.
8th. Raw and cold in the morning. Began to rain from 10 A. M. to noon, with the wind cold at E'ly. Wind hauled to S'ly in the afternoon, with moderate rain and rise of temperature.
9th. Heavy rains in afternoon. Clouds broken at 11 P. M.; wind S'ly.
10th. Very pleasant.
11th. Very pleasant. Fog-bow around the moon in the evening.
12th. Mild for the season.
13th. Heavy rain in the afternoon; wind strong S. E'ly.
14th. Very blustering.
15th. Pleasant.
16th. Mild, with indications of storm.
17th. Clouds; sprinkling of rain in the evening.
18th. Morning misty.
19th. Pleasant.
20th. Very mild and warm for the season.
21st. Occasional light rain with mist.
22d. Cloudy and rain.
23d. Very mild.
24th. At 7 A. M., wind light S. W., and very warm. From 11 A. M. to noon, wind came to N. W., with brisk dashes of rain and rapid fall of thermometer. Evening very cold.
25th. Cold, but pleasant.
26th. Pleasant.
27th. Air very raw and snowy.
28th. Appearance of snow-storm.
29th. Cloudy and mild.
30th. Mild and pleasant.

December, 1853. New Moon, 30d. 0h. 58m. A. M.

Days.	Barometer, reduced to 32° F. Sunrise.	At 1 P. M.	At 10 P. M.	Thermometer. Sunrise.	At 1 P. M.	At 10 P. M.	Daily mean.	Winds (Direction and Force) Sunrise.	At 1 P. M.	At 10 P. M.	Weather (Tenths Cloudy.) Sunrise.	At 1 P. M.	At 10 P. M.	Rain and Snow in Inches of Water
1	29.74	29.68	29.78	37	40	33	36.7	W'ly 2	N. E. 2	N. E. 2	10	10	10	
2	29.83	29.80	29.84	31	38	30	33.0	N. E. 2	N. E. 2	N'ly 2	10	9	8	
3	29.79	29.77	29.76	27	35	35	32.3	N'ly 2	N'ly 2	W'ly 3	10	10	10	
S 4	29.97	29.96	30.03	20	27	20	22.3	N. W. 2	N. W. 3	N. W. 1	0	0	0	
5	30.11	30.07	30.13	15	28	20	21.0	N. W. 1	N. W. 2	N. W. 1	3	10	2	
6	30.10	29.72	29.60	24	45	44	37.7	W'ly 1	S. E'ly 3	N. W. 3	9	9	2	
7	29.77	29.83	29.95	33	41	25	33.0	N. W. 2	N. W. 2	N. W. 2	2	4	0	
8	29.99	29.96	29.96	18	35	25	26.0	N. W. 2	N. W. 2	N. W. 1	1	0	0	
9	29.94	29.91	29.86	21	40	29	30.0	N. W. 1	N. W. 2	N. W. 1	0	1	3	
10	29.79	29.74	29.76	25	46	32	34.3	N. W. 2	N. W. 2	N. E. 1	5	0	0	
S 11	29.81	29.77	29.80	29	42	34	35.0	N. E. 1	N. E. 2	N. E. 2	0	0	10	
12	29.83	29.83	29.86	34	33	32	33.0	N. E. 2	N. E. 2	N. E'ly 2	10	Misty	Misty	
13	29.86	...	29.94	31	...	28	29.5	N. E. 2	...	N'ly 1	10	...	0	
14	30.08	30.01	30.00	27	38	20	31.8	N'ly 2	N'ly 2	N'ly 2	7	8	2	
15	29.93	29.80	29.82	28	41	28	32.3	N. W. 2	N. W. 1	N'ly 1	2	0	0	
16	29.82	29.83	29.72	24	41	34	33.0	N. W. 2	N. W. 1	S. W. 1	Foggy	5	10	
17	29.60	29.44	29.05	36	44	44	41.3	S'ly 1	S. W. 1	S. W. 1	Foggy	Foggy	Rain	0.55
S 18	28.87	28.89	29.33	48	42	25	38.3	S. W. 1	W'ly 2	N. W. 3	8	8	0	
19	29.64	29.65	29.75	16	27	18	20.3	N. W. 1	W'ly 2	N. W. 2	0	0	2	
20	29.91	29.98	30.12	14	22	15	17.0	N. W. 2	N. W. 3	N. W. 1	2	0	0	
21	30.16	30.11	30.08	18	29	24	23.7	S. W'ly 1	S. W. 2	S. W. 2	6	10	10	
22	30.01	29.96	29.96	22	36	28	28.7	S. W. 2	S. W. 2	S. W. 1	5	10	5	
23	29.63	29.28	29.01	31	44	30	35.0	S. W. 1	S. E'ly 2	N. W'ly 3	10	Rain	Snow	0.85
24	29.35	29.44	29.54	19	26	23	22.7	N. W. 3	N. W. 3	N. W. 1	0	0	10	
S 25	29.59	29.61	29.67	21	25	29	25.0	N. W. 2	N. W. 2	N'ly 1	1	2	3	
26	29.45	29.17	29.05	25	35	25	28.3	S. W'ly 1	N. E. 2	N. W. 2	6	10	0	
27	29.14	29.28	29.50	28	27	16	23.7	N. W. 4	N. W. 3	N. W. 2	10	0	0	
28	29.60	29.54	29.44	14	36	30	26.7	N. W. 2	N. W. 2	N. E. 2	0	4	10	
29	28.91	28.83	29.31	21	18	4	14.3	N. E. 4	N. E. 3	N. W. 3	Snow	Snow	0	} 2.50
30	29.59	29.58	29.51	6	20	17	14.3	N. W. 2	N. W'ly 1	W'ly 1	0	10	Snow	
31	29.51	29.56	29.73	21	30	26	25.7	W'ly 1	S. W. 1	S. W. 1	10	8	10	
Means	29.72	29.66	29.70	24.6	34.4	26.8	...	1.8	2.0	1.7	5.6	5.6	4.7	3.90
								1.8			5.3			
Reduced to sea level.														
Max.	30.34	30.29	30.31	48	46	44	41.3	Prevailing winds from some point between—		Days.			Days.	
Min.	29.05	29.01	29.19	6	18	4	14.3	N. & E.		7	Clear		10	
Mean	29.90	29.84	29.88					E. & S.		0	Variable }		13	
Range	1.29	1.28	1.12	42	28	40	27.0	S. & W.		5	Cloudy }			
Mean of month	29.873			...	...	...	28.6	W. & N.		19	Rain or snow fell on		8	
Extreme range	1.35			...	...	...	44.0							

Remarks.

1st. Cool; appearances of storm in afternoon.
2d. Air raw and cold.
3d. Cloudy; appearances of storm and squalls.
4th. Cold, but pleasant. Evening still and clear.
5th. Snow-squalls from noon to 1 P. M. Evening clear and cold.
6th. Very blustering in the afternoon; wind S. W'ly; dashes of rain.
7th and 8th. Very fine.
9th. Very fine. Light fog-bow around moon.
10th. Fine. Evening splendid.
11th. Very pleasant. Thick haze in evening.
12th. Wind N. E'ly, with cold mist.
13th. Cloudy morning. Clear evening.
14th. Pleasant.
15th. Very fine and mild. Evening splendid.
16th. Pleasant.
17th. Foggy through day. Light rain in evening.
18th. Very mild morning; mostly clear from 9 to 11 A. M.; wind S. W'ly. Rain squall at ½ P. M.; wind came to N. W., and grew cold very fast. Evening clear and cold.
19th and 20th. Cold, but fine.
21st. Wind S W., and air very chilly.
22d. Mostly cloudy.
23d. Rainy day. In evening, the wind hauled from S. W. to N. W'ly, the thermometer fell, and the rain turned to snow—being the first of the season to whiten the ground.
24th. The ground dusted over with snow this morning. Blustering through the day.
25th. Pleasant.
26th. Light snow in the morning. Clear and pleasant at 10 P. M.
27th. Ground covered with snow from one to two inches deep this morning.
28th. Pleasant through the day. Appearances of storm in the evening.
29th. Great snow-storm, surpassing, in quantity of snow, violence of wind, and severity of cold, any we have had for many years. Snow badly drifted, and probably equal to sixteen or eighteen inches on the level. The barometer reached an extremely low point, standing, at 1 P. M., at 28.90 (not corrected); before 2 P. M., it began to rise. At 11 P. M., the weather clear and cold, the wind heavy at N. W., and the air perfectly thick with blowing snow. The storm commenced about midnight, and continued with violence to near sunset.
30th. Clear and cold in the morning. Began to snow again at 6 P. M.
31st. From three to four inches of fresh snow on the ground this morning.

January, 1854. New Moon, 28d. 0h. 4m. P. M.

Days.	Barometer Sunrise.	At 2 P. M.	At 10 P. M.	Thermometer Sunrise.	At 2 P. M.	At 10 P. M.	Daily mean.	Winds Sunrise.	At 2 P. M.	At 10 P. M.	Weather Sunrise.	At 2 P. M.	At 10 P. M.	Rain and Snow
S 1	29.60	29.53	29.64	31	34	26	30.3	N. E'ly 1	N. W'ly 1	N. W'ly 1	Snow	10	0	0.25
2	29.76	...	30.09	20	...	17	...	W. 1	...	N. W.	0	...	0	
3	30.27	30.18	30.04	9	27	33	23.0	W'ly 1	S. W'ly 2	S. W'ly 1	3	3	4	
4	29.97	29.89	29.89	33	45	40	39.3	S. W. 1	S. W. 1	S. W. 1	4	3	2	
5	29.96	29.96	29.85	33	43	38	38.0	S. W. 1	S. W. 1	S. W. 1	5	5	10	
6	29.66	29.61	29.90	39	43	23	34.7	S'ly 1	N. W. 2	N. W. 3	Foggy	10	5	
7	30.13	30.06	29.94	12	22	17	17.0	N. W. 2	W. by S. 2	N. W. 2	0	0	0	
S 8	29.80	29.64	29.66	18	27	20	21.7	N. W. 1	N. W'ly 1	N. W. 2	10	9	9	
9	29.79	29.88	30.00	9	17	14	13.3	N. W. 2	N. W. 2	N. W. 2	0	0	2	
10	30.09	29.97	29.97	16	37	35	29.3	N. W. 2	S. W. 2	S. W. 1	10	10	5	
11	30.07	...	30.00	18	...	24	...	N. W. 1	...	N. E. 2	5	...	Misty	
12	29.65	29.46	29.25	40	53	52	48.3	S'ly 1	S. W. 2	S. W. 3	Foggy	Rain	8	0.75
13	29.31	29.35	29.26	38	46	40	41.3	S. W. 1	S. W. 2	S. W. 1	5	3	10	
14	29.38	29.50	29.82	34	33	27	31.3	N. W. 3	N. W. 4	N. W. 2	3	4	5	
S 15	30.03	30.03	30.02	23	31	29	27.7	N. W. 1	N'ly 2	N. E. 1	1	2	Hazy	
16	29.78	29.75	29.64	32	41	39	37.3	N. E. 2	S'ly 1	S. W. 1	10	10	10	
17	29.80	29.81	30.01	38	37	30	35.0	N. W'ly 1	N'ly 2	N. W. 1	10	10	2	
18	30.09	30.06	30.05	23	26	20	23.0	N. W. 2	N. E. 2	N. E. 2	3	Snow	Snow	
19	30.16	30.10	30.04	17	31	28	25.3	N. W. 2	N. W. 1	N. W. 1	3	10	5	
20	29.69	29.51	29.42	32	34	26	30.7	N. E. 1	N. E. 1	N'ly 1	Rain	Misty	10	0.30
21	29.26	29.20	29.67	40	47	18	35.0	S'ly	S. W'ly 2	N. W. 3	Foggy	10	0	
S 22	30.10	30.14	30.19	14	21	15	16.7	N. W'ly 2	N. W'ly 2	N. W. 1	0	0	0	
23	29.90	29.91	30.25	17	22	10	16.3	N'ly 2	N. W. 3	N. W. 2	9	2	0	
24	30.23	30.00	30.10	6	24	16	15.3	S. W'ly 2	S. W. 3	S. W. 2	0	1	0	
25	30.35	30.45	30.37	6	9	8	7.7	N. W. 2	N. W'ly 2	N'ly 1	0	0	5	
26	29.84	29.58	29.53	17	35	37	29.7	N. E. 2	Calm	S. W'ly 1	Snow	10	10	0.25
27	29.60	29.56	29.68	35	35	24	31.3	N. W. 1	N. W. 2	N. W. 3	10	9	5	
28	29.96	30.08	30.34	14	14	3	10.3	N. W. 2	N. by W. 3	N. W. 2	0	0	0	
S 29	30.47	30.42	30.45	—6	9	2½	1.8	N. W. 1	N. W. 2	N. W. 1	0	0	0	
30	30.39	30.21	29.93	2	22	23	15.7	N. W. 1	N. W'ly 1	N. E. 1	10	10	Snow	0.25
31	[illegible]	[illegible]	[illegible]	[illegible]	[illegible]	[illegible]	[illegible]	[illegible]	[illegible]	[illegible]	[illegible]	[illegible]	[illegible]	
Means	29.90	29.84	29.89	23.1	31.2	24.8	...	1.5	1.8	1.6	5.5	5.7	5.1	1.80
								1.6			5.5			
Reduced to sea level.														
Max.	30.65	30.63	30.63	40	53	52	48.3	Prevailing winds from some point between—		Days.			Days.	
Min.	29.44	29.38	29.43	—6	9	2½	1.8	N. & E.		3	Clear		8	
Mean	30.08	30.02	30.07					E. & S.		0	Variable }		13	
Range	1.21	1.25	1.20	46	44	49½	46.5	S. & W.		11	Cloudy }			
Mean of month	30.057			...	...	...	26.4	W. & N.		17	Rain or snow fell on		10	
Extreme range	1.27			...	...	...	59.0							

Remarks.

1st. Snow in the morning; about five inches added to the previous quantity, making, probably, two feet on the level. Evening clear.
2d. Very pleasant in the morning. Flurry of snow at 5 P. M. Evening clear, with aurora of considerable brightness, but without streamers.
3d Very pleasant.
4th. Remarkably mild for the season.
5th. Very mild.
6th. Pleasant in the morning; wind at S. W. Evening blustering, with wind at N. W.
7th. Very fine. 8th. Overcast.
9th. Cold, but fine.
10th. Mild; wind light S. W'ly.
11th. Pleasant. Indications of a storm in the afternoon.
12th. Thick fog and mist in the morning. Rain in the afternoon. Clouds broken at 10 P. M.
13th. Very mild. The great snow of the 29th of December is nearly all gone.
14th. Very blustering.
15th. Very fine in the morning. Air raw in the afternoon; wind N. W'ly. Thick haze overhead at 10 P. M., with appearances of storm.
16th. Ground dusted over with fresh snow this morning. Sprinkling of rain in the afternoon.
17th. Snowed moderately from 8 to 9 A. M., the snow melting as it fell.
18th. Began to snow moderately from 11 A. M. to noon, and continued through day and evening.
19th. About an inch of fresh snow on the ground this morning.
20th. Light rain this morning, about two inches of snow having fallen during the night. Mist through the day.
21st. Very mild in the morning; wind S. W'ly, and cloudy. From 3 to 5 P. M., the wind came to N. W., and the thermometer fell rapidly. Evening clear, blustering, and cold.
22d. Cold, but clear and fine. Evening very [illegible]
23d. Very cold and blustering, with occasional flurries of snow.
24th. Pleasant.
25th. Very cold; wind brisk at N. W.
26th. Snowing at sunrise, which ceased from 8 to 9 A. M. About three inches of damp snow.
27th. Very mild. 28th. Very cold.
29th. Cold extreme: wind light N. W. Ther. at sunrise 6° below zero, being 2° lower than at any time since Jan. 24, 1839, when it stood —8°.
30th. Mild. Began to snow gently at 6 P. M.
31st. From two to three inches of fresh fallen snow on the ground this morning.

February, 1854. New Moon, 26d. 11h. 31m. P. M.

Days.	Barometer, reduced to 32° F. Sunrise.	At 2 P. M.	At 10 P. M.	Thermometer. Sunrise.	At 2 P. M.	At 10 P. M.	Daily mean.	Winds. (Direction and Force.) Sunrise.	At 2 P. M.	At 10 P. M.	Weather. (Tenths Cloudy.) Sunrise.	At 2 P. M.	At 10 P. M.	Rain and Snow in Inches of Water.
1	29.39	29.29	29.34	34	49	40	41.0	S. W. 1	S. W. 1	S. W. 1	1	7	0	
2	29.41	29.38	29.48	37	48	34	39.7	S. W. 1	S'ly 1	N'ly 1	10	5	10	
3	29.64	29.72	29.85	19	14	6	13.0	N. E. 2	N. E. 2	N. W. 2	10	Snow	0	
4	29.98	30.03	30.14	2	14	6	7.3	N. W. 1	N. W. 2	N. W. 1	0	0	0	
S 5	30.15	30.03	29.69	1	21	21	14.3	N. W. 1	S. W. 1	N. E. 2	0	Hazy	Snow	0.30
6	29.84	30.03	30.22	14	16	6	12.0	N'ly 3	N. W. 3	N. W. 1	10	0	0	
7	30.25	30.24	30.19	1	24	20	15.0	S. W. 1	S. E. 1	S. E. 1	0	1	10	
8	30.04	29.74	29.29	25	36	42	34.3	N. E. 1	S. E. 1	S. E. 4	Snow	Rain	Rain	1.50
9	29.18	29.44	29.48	42	40	36	39.3	N. W. 2	N. W. 2	S. W. 2	10	0	0	
10	29.56	29.54	29.85	33	39	21	31.0	N. W. 2	N. W. 3	N. W. 2	5	10	0	
11	30.03	30.07	30.18	13	18	11	14.0	N. W. 2	N. W. 3	N. W. 1	0	0	0	
S 12	30.26	30.19	30.23	8	28	24	20.0	N. W. 2	N. W. 2	N. W. 1	0	2	10	
13	30.20	30.00	29.83	27	33	34	31.3	S. E'ly 2	S. E. 2	S. E. 1	9	Hail	Rain	}
14	29.83	29.81	29.82	34	41	34	36.3	N'ly 1	N. E'ly 1	N. E. 2	10	10	Misty	}
15	29.74	...	29.66	35	36	35	35.3	N. E. 1	N. E. 1	N. E. 1	Misty	Misty	Misty	} 0.60
16	29.73	29.70	29.78	35	33	26	31.3	N. E'ly 1	N. W. 2	N. W. 1	10	Snow	2	}
17	29.99	29.99	30.09	20	31	19	23.3	N. W. 2	N. W. 3	N. W. 2	0	3	0	
18	30.04	29.87	29.73	18	35	35	29.3	S. W. 1	S. W. 2	S. W. 3	2	2	6	
S 19	29.72	29.83	30.03	33	35	16	28.0	S. W. 2	N. W. 2	N. W. 2	8	4	0	
20	30.05	...	29.76	8	...	24	...	N. W. 2	...	N. E. 2	0	...	Snow	
21	29.57	29.57	29.76	17	20	18	18.3	N. E. 4	N'ly 4	N. W. 2	Snow	9	0	0.45
22	29.81	29.65	29.50	17	43	36	32.0	S. W. 1	S. W. 2	S. W. 3	0	3	2	
23	29.43	29.45	29.88	20	17	12	16.3	N. W. 4	N. W. 4	N. W. 3	6	10	0	
24	30.00	29.95	30.01	11	26	26	21.0	W. 2	S. W. 2	S. W. 2	8	10	10	
25	30.32	30.44	30.47	13	17	16	15.3	N'ly 2	N. W. 2	E'ly 2	8	0	10	
S 26	30.19	29.88	29.30	24	40	47	37.0	N. E. 2	N. E. 2	S. W'ly 3	10	Rain	Rain	2.00
27	29.31	29.67	30.15	39	35	22	32.0	S. W. 2	N. W. 1	N. W. 2	5	Snow	0	
28	30.38	30.35	30.18	18	32	31	27.0	N. W. 2	N. W. 1	S. W. 2	10	1	10	
Means	29.86	29.84	29.85	21.4	30.4	24.9	...	1.7	1.8	1.9	5.8	5.8	5.0	4.85
									1.8			5.5		
REDUCED TO SEA LEVEL.														
Max.	30.56	30.62	30.65	42	49	47	39.7	Prevailing winds from some point between—		Days.			Days.	
Min.	29.36	29.47	29.47	1	14	6	7.3	N. & E.		6	Clear		6	
Mean	30.04	30.02	30.03					E. & S.		3	Variable		} 11	
Range	1.20	1.15	1.18	41	35	41	32.4	S. & W.		6	Cloudy		}	
Mean of month	30.030			...	...	...	25.6	W. & N.		13	Rain or snow fell on		11	
Extreme range	1.29			...	...	...	48.0							

REMARKS.

1st and 2d. Pleasant.
3d. Began to snow moderately from 7 to 8 A. M. Clouds broken in the afternoon. Evening very clear and cold. Snow one or two inches deep.
4th. Clear and cold.
5th. Began to snow from 6 to 7 P. M.
6th. Very cold, with piercing wind. Snow 6 or 7 inches deep, and much drifted.
7th. Pleasant.
8th. Morning cold, and snowing. Snow turned to rain in afternoon. Amount of snow and rain large.
9th. Ground nearly bare of snow this morning.
10th. Very fine.
11th. Cold, but very fine.
12th. Pleasant. Appearances of storm in the evening.
13th. Began to hail moderately from noon to 1 P. M., which soon turned to rain.
14th. Mild and cloudy. Mist in the evening.
15th. Mist, with occasional sprinkling of rain.
16th. Began to snow from 8 to 9 A. M., and continued till 3 P. M.; quantity small.
17th. Very blustering at mid-day. Clear and fine in the evening.
18th. Pleasant. At 10 P. M., haze, with stars visible.
19th. Mild in the morning; overcast, and wind S'ly. In the afternoon, wind N. W., and cold. Evening very clear.
20th. Mostly clear in morning. Clouds gathering in the afternoon. Began to snow from 9 to 10 P. M.
21st. Snowing at sunrise, and heavy wind at N. E. Snow ceased and clouds broken at 10 A. M. Snow much drifted; five or six inches on a level.
22d. Pleasant.
23d. Very variable; sunshine, clouds, cold, and violent snow-squalls. Evening clear.
24th. Cold and raw in the morning.
25th. Cold and raw. Appearances of storm in the evening.
26th. Began to rain moderately from 9 to 10 A. M.; wind N. E. Wind soon hauled to E., and in the afternoon to S. E., with increased force and heavy rain.
27th. Variable. Flurry of snow from 10 A. M. to noon. Evening clear. Aurora low in the north, but quite bright; no streamers.
28th. Pleasant.

March, 1854. New Moon, 28d. 11h. 43m. A. M.

Days.	Barometer Sunrise.	At 2 P. M.	At 10 P. M.	Thermometer Sunrise.	At 2 P. M.	At 10 P. M.	Daily mean.	Winds Sunrise.	At 2 P. M.	At 10 P. M.	Weather Sunrise.	At 2 P. M.	At 10 P. M.	Rain and Snow
1	30.08	30.02	30.04	28	41	32	33.7	S. W. 2	N. W. 2	N. W. 1	1	2	0	
2	30.09	30.06	30.07	30	47	35	37.3	S. W. 2	S. W. 2	S'ly 1	0	2	10	
3	29.89	29.59	29.73	35	36	33	34.7	S. E. 2	N. E. 2	N'ly 1	Rain	Rain	Misty	0.35
4	29.77	29.65	29.55	33	41	36	36.7	N'ly 1	S. W. 1	S. W. 1	10	10	10	
S 5	29.60	29.65	29.75	35	37	31	34.3	N. W. 1	N. W. 3	N. W. 2	6	2	1	
6	29.92	29.94	30.04	29	37	28	31.3	N. W. 1	N. W. 2	N. W. 1	0	2	0	
7	30.01	29.77	29.67	25	43	37	33.0	S. W. 1	S. W. 2	S. W. 1	3	10	Rain	}
8	29.54	29.35	29.38	35	37	33	35.0	N. E. 1	N. E. 2	N. W. 1	Misty	Rain	8	}
9	29.63	29.71	29.77	34	46	36	38.7	N'ly 1	N. W. 1	S. W. 1	10	10	Rain	} 1.00
10	29.59	29.45	29.33	34	40	35	36.3	N. E. 2	N. E. 2	N'ly 1	Rain	Misty	Misty	}
11	29.52	29.79	30.03	35	45	31	37.0	N. W. 2	N. W. 2	N. W. 1	2	0	0	
S 12	30.12	30.04	29.98	31	49	38	39.3	S. W. 1	S. W'ly 2	S. W'ly 2	0	0	0	
13	29.92	29.80	29.86	38	62	43	47.7	S. W. 2	S. W. 2	S. W. 2	0	4	6	
14	29.87	29.70	29.70	40	50	35	41.7	N. E'ly 2	N. E. 2	N. E. 2	2	6	5	
15	29.75	29.69	29.51	30	55	41	42.0	N. W. 1	W'ly 1	S. W. 1	0	10	10	
16	29.24	29.08	29.18	41	68	52	53.7	S. W'ly 1	S. W. 1	N. W. 2	3	2	2	
17	29.38	29.38	28.88	37	51	43	43.7	N. W. 1	N. W. 2	S. W. 2	0	5	Rain	
18	29.13	29.27	29.66	24	29	21	24.7	N. W. 4	N. W. 5	N. W. 3	0	2	0	
S 19	29.89	29.82	29.79	17	29	24	23.3	N. W. 2	N. W. 3	N. W. 2	0	1	0	
20	29.75	29.84	30.02	24	28	16	22.7	W by N. 2	N'ly 2	N. W. 2	2	10	0	
21	30.08	30.03	30.04	13	29	21	21.0	N. W. 2	N. W. 2	N. W. 1	0	0	0	
22	30.04	29.91	29.71	16	36	31	27.7	S. W. 1	S. W. 2	S'ly 2	0	0	10	
23	29.48	29.27	29.17	32	41	36	36.3	N. E. 1	S. E. 2	W'ly 2	Misty	Rain	10	1.50
24	29.16	29.14	29.26	31	35	22	29.3	N. W. 2	N'ly 3	N. W. 4	1	2	0	
25	29.28	29.22	29.28	19	30	23	24.0	N. W. 3	N. W'ly 3	N. W. 2	3	5	0	
S 26	29.30	29.30	29.43	20	33	25	26.0	N. W. 3	N. W. 3	N. W. 2	0	3	10	
27	29.51	29.54	29.70	23	33	21	25.7	N. W. 2	N. W. 2	N. W. 3	4	1	2	
28	29.77	29.77	29.93	16	27	17	20.0	N. W. 2	N. W. 2	N. W. 2	0	10	1	
29	30.05	30.02	30.13	17	32	24	24.3	N. W. 2	N. W. 2	N. W. 2	0	0	0	
30	30.15	30.10	30.17	17	39	30	28.7	N. 2	S'ly 2	S'ly 1	2	10	10	
31	30.12	30.06	29.89	32	36	34	34.0	E'ly 2	E'ly 2	N. E'ly 1	10	10	Misty	
Means	29.73	29.68	29.70	28.1	40.1	31.1	...	1.8	2.1	1.7	3.2	5.1	5.0	2.85
									1.9			4.4		
REDUCED TO SEA LEVEL.														
Max.	30.33	30.28	30.35	41	68	52	47.7	Prevailing winds from some point between—		Days.			Days.	
Min.	29.31	29.32	29.35	13	27	16	20.0	N. & E.		6	Clear		10	
Mean	29.91	29.86	29.88					E. & S.		0	Variable		} 11	
Range	1.02	0.96	1.00	28	41	36	27.7	S. & W.		8	Cloudy		}	
Mean of month	29.883			...	...	...	33.1	W. & N.		17	Rain or snow fell on		10	
Extreme range	1.04			...	...	...	55.0							

REMARKS.

1st. Very fine.
2d. Very mild and pleasant.
3d. Moderate rain in the morning. Cloudy in the afternoon and evening, with light mist.
4th. Mild; air damp.
5th. Pleasant. 6th. Very fine.
7th. Mild and pleasant in the morning. Cloudy in the afternoon. Light rain in the evening.
8th. Moderate rain and mist. Brief thunder-shower from 7 to 8 P. M.
9th. Mild. Moderate rain in the evening.
10th. Mist, with occasional light rain.
11th. Very fine.
12th. Very fine; evening splendid.
13th. Warmest day since Nov. 30, '53; ther. 62°.
14th. Pleasant in the morning. Air raw at N. E. in the afternoon.
15th. Very mild. Frost out of the ground in open places.
16th. Very fine. At 2½ P. M, ther. nearly 70°, a point above which it has not risen since Sept 20, 1853, when it stood at 77°. Light shower at 5 P. M. At 7 P. M., lightning in the S.W. and N.W. Mostly clear at 10 P. M.
17th. Pleasant through the day. Brisk shower from 10 to 11 P. M., with barometer very low (28.97), and wind very blustering.
18th. Wind heavy during the last night, and extremely violent through the day; a perfect storm of wind.
19th. Wind piercing and cold.
20th. Snow-squalls in the morning. Evening clear and cold.
21st. Pleasant, but cold.
22d. More moderate. Air S'ly in afternoon, and very raw. Evening cloudy; appearances of storm.
23d. One or two inches of snow on the ground this morning; wind N. E., which came to S. E., with rain before noon.
24th. Pleasant in the morning. Evening cold and very blustering.
25th. Very cold and blustering.
26th. Cold, blustering, and most uncomfortable.
27th. Very cold, blustering, and dusty. Aurora in the evening.
28th. Very cold and uncomfortable. Aurora in the evening, with streamers.
29th. Pleasant. At 7½ P. M., a brilliant comet was seen, low down, a little west of northwest.
30th. Pleasant in morning. Mist, with snow-flakes, at 6 P. M. Aurora from 8 to 10 P. M. Comet concealed by the clouds.
31st. Sprinkling of rain and mist in the afternoon and evening.

April, 1854. New Moon, 27d. 1h. 6m. A. M.

DAYS.	Barometer, reduced to 32° F. Sunrise.	At 2 P. M.	At 10 P. M.	Thermometer. Sunrise.	At 2 P. M.	At 10 P. M.	Daily mean.	Winds (Direction and Force.) Sunrise.	At 2 P. M.	At 10 P. M.	Weather (Tenths Cloudy.) Sunrise.	At 2 P. M.	At 10 P. M.	Rain and Snow in Inches of Water
1	29.54	29.45	29.53	39	52	36	42.3	S'ly 1	S. W. 2	N. W'ly 2	Rain	Misty	Rain	1.25
S 2	29.77	29.90	30.17	32	42	28	34.0	N. W. 2	N. W. 2	N. W. 2	0	6	0	
3	30.39	30.38	30.34	22	40	28	30.0	N. W. 1	N. E. 2	S'ly 2	0	0	0	
4	30.28	30.16	30.16	26	46	34	35.3	S. W. 1	S. W. 1	S. W. 1	0	10	3	
5	30.10	30.04	29.92	32	50	37	39.7	S. W. 1	S. W. 2	S. W. 2	0	2	0	
6	29.84	29.64	29.50	38	63	52	51.0	S. W. 1	S'ly 1	S. W. 2	3	8	10	
7	29.54	29.77	30.13	53	59	36	49.3	W. 1	N. W. 2	N. W. 2	1	0	0	
8	30.26	...	29.89	32	...	40	...	N. W. 1	...	S'ly	2	...	6	
S 9	29.78	29.75	29.70	46	56	38	46.7	S. E'ly 1	E'ly 1	N. E. 2	10	10	10	
10	29.57	29.24	29.42	38	46	36	40.0	N. E. 2	N'ly 2	N. E'ly 2	Rain	10	Misty	0.40
11	29.51	29.66	29.87	36	45	32	37.7	N.N.E. 2	N. W. 2	N. E. 1	10	6	0	
12	29.98	29.92	29.97	33	61	37	43.7	N. W'ly 1	S. E'ly 2	S. W. 1	10	5	0	
13	29.91	29.88	30.11	38	65	38	47.0	S. W'ly 2	S. W. 2	N. E. 2	2	9	5	
14	30.28	30.25	30.13	28	43	34	35.0	N. E. 2	N. E. 2	E'ly 2	0	3	10	
15	29.95	29.80	29.72	27	35	32	31.3	N. E. 2	N. E'ly 2	N. E. 2	Snow	10	10	0.60
S 16	29.82	29.87	29.84	32	39	33	34.7	N. E'ly 2	N. E. 3	N. E. 2	10	9	10	
17	29.80	29.52	29.52	31	32	33	32.0	N. E. 2	N. E. 4	N. E. 3	Snow	Snow	Misty	} 0.65
18	29.56	29.62	29.70	32	44	33	36.3	N. E. 2	N. N. E. 2	N. W. 1	Snow	10	0	
19	29.76	29.67	29.63	34	55	43	44.0	N. W. 1	S. W. 2	S. W. 1	3	0	10	
20	29.59	29.51	29.66	40	56	42	46.0	W'ly 1	N. W. 1	N. W. 1	1	2	0	
21	29.76	29.74	29.82	39	61	50	50.0	N. W. 2	N. W. 3	N. W. 1	0	4	0	
22	29.83	29.74	29.55	43	48	42	44.3	W'ly 1	S. W. 1	S. W. 1	3	Rain	10	
S 23	29.49	29.56	29.77	40	49	42	43.7	N. E. 2	N. E. 2	N. E'ly 1	Rain	7	0	1.00
24	29.74	29.79	29.68	38	59	46	47.7	N. W. 2	N. W. 2	S'ly 1	0	0	3	
25	29.64	29.64	29.69	47	68	48	54.3	N. W. 1	N. W. 2	S'ly	0	0	3	
26	29.52	29.42	29.36	49	68	54	57.0	S. W. 1	S. W. 1	S'ly 1	10	8	Rain	
27	29.38	29.41	29.58	60	66	47	57.7	N'ly 2	S. E'ly 2	E'ly 1	5	2	Rain	
28	29.73	29.89	30.03	42	41	38	40.3	N. E. 2	N. E. 2	N. E. 3	Misty	Misty	Rain	} 2.50
29	30.06	30.10	29.95	38	43	47	42.7	N. E. 2	N. E. 2	N. E. 1	Misty	10	10	
S 30	29.86	29.78	29.72	55	57	49	53.7	S. E. 1	S. E. 2	S'ly 2	Rain	Rain	Rain	
Means	29.81	29.76	29.80	38.0	51.3	39.5	...	1.5	1.9	1.6	5.7	6.2	5.7	6.30
									1.7			5.9		
REDUCED TO SEA LEVEL.								Prevailing winds from some point between—		Days.			Days.	
Max.	30.57	30.56	30.52	60	68	54	57.7							
Min.	29.56	29.42	29.54	22	32	28	30.0							
Mean	29.99	29.94	29.98					N. & E.		11	Clear		7	
Range	1.01	1.14	0.98	38	36	26	27.7	E. & S.		4	Variable		} 11	
Mean of month	29.970			...	...	...	42.9	S. & W.		8	Cloudy			
Extreme range	1.15			...	...	...	46.0	W. & N.		7	Rain or snow fell on		12	

REMARKS.

1st. Rain and mist through the day.
2d. Pleasant. The comet very conspicuous this evening, notwithstanding a strong moonlight. Its motion is east and south.
3d. Very fine. Comet again visible.
4th, 5th, and 6th. Very fine.
7th. Very fine, but the air full of dust.
8th. Pleasant.
9th. Cloudy, with appearances of storm.
10th. Light rain and mist.
11th. Cloudy in the morning. Evening still and very clear. Comet not visible in the strong moonlight.
12th. Pleasant. Evening very clear.
13th. Pleasant.
14th. Air very raw and uncomfortable.
15th. The ground this morning covered with three or four inches of snow, and snowing fast. Ceased snowing at about 1 P. M. Snow from five to six inches deep on the level; rather damp and heavy.
16th. Air raw and chilly. Icicles a foot long hung from the eaves of the houses at 5 P. M.
17th. Driving snow and hail nearly all day. Nearly four inches on the level has fallen to-day; very damp and heavy.
18th. Snow again during the night and this morning. Evening clear; wind N. W. The fields heavily covered with snow.
19th. The snow has disappeared rapidly to-day, but the fields are still much covered. For the last five days, they have presented the appearance of midwinter.
20th. Very fine. Snow still lingers in patches.
21st. Very fine. Snow not entirely gone.
22d. Rain began to fall between noon and 1 P. M., and continued till 9 P. M.
23d. Moderate rain in the morning. Clear from 2 to 3 P. M.
24th and 25th. Very fine.
26th. Very mild. Light shower, with lightning, at 9 P. M.
27th. Pleasant. Wind S. E'ly in the afternoon. Began to rain from 9 to 10 P. M.
28th. Mist and rain.
29th. Mist and light rain.
30th. Copious rain throughout the day.

May, 1854. New Moon, 26d. 8h. 40m. P. M.

DAYS.	Barometer At 6 A. M.	At 2 P. M.	At 10 P. M.	Thermometer At 6 A. M.	At 2 P. M.	At 10 P. M.	Daily mean.	Winds At 6 A. M.	At 2 P. M.	At 10 P. M.	Weather At 6 A. M.	At 2 P. M.	At 10 P. M.	Rain
1	29.76	29.73	29.78	47	62	46	51.7	S. W. 2	S. W. 2	S. W. 1	0	2	0	
2	29.76	29.66	29.61	46	74	54	58.0	S. W. 2	S. W. 2	S. W. 1	0	5	10	
3	29.56	29.52	29.47	51	54	47	50.7	S. W. 2	S. E. 2	E'ly 2	10	Rain	Rain	} 1.25
4	29.56	29.58	29.66	46	47	43	45.3	N. E. 2	N. E. 3	N. E. 2	10	Misty	Misty	
5	29.51	29.53	29.40	45	62	52	53.0	N. E. 1	S. E'ly 2	S. W'ly 2	7	8	9	0.20
6	29.50	29.41	29.47	43	49	31	41.0	N. W. 3	N. W. 3	N'ly 2	2	5	0	
S 7	29.46	29.30	29.46	32	57	44	44.3	N. W. 2	N. W. 3	N. W. 2	0	2	0	
8	29.56	29.54	29.65	41	59	48	49.3	N. W. 1	N. W. 2	N. W. 1	1	0	0	
9	29.70	29.68	29.70	48	74	52	58.0	N. W. 1	W'ly 2	S. W. 1	0	2	10	
10	29.68	29.65	29.66	51	64	53	56.0	S. W. 2	S. W. 2	S. E'ly 2	2	10	Rain	
11	29.67	29.74	29.86	54	62	54	56.7	S. W. 2	S. W. 2	S. W. 1	10	9	5	
12	29.94	29.96	30.07	54	69	52	58.3	S. W. 1	S. E'ly 2	S'ly 1	Foggy	5	Hazy	
13	30.16	30.18	30.19	54	73	56	61.0	S. E'ly 1	S. E'ly 2	S. E'ly 1	Foggy	3	3	
S 14	30.18	30.08	29.96	62	66	58	62.0	S'ly 2	S'ly 2	S'ly 2	Sprinl'g	Rain	Rain	1.40
15	29.82	29.73	29.76	60	74	64	66.0	S. 2	S'ly 2	S. W. 1	Rain	2	3	
16	29.81	29.78	29.87	68	78	57	67.7	S. W. 2	E'ly 1	E'ly 1	Foggy	2	0	
17	29.94	29.95	29.86	57	66	58	60.3	S. E'ly 1	S. E. 2	S. E'ly 2	Foggy	10	Foggy	
18	29.79	29.77	29.81	60	74	60	64.7	S. 2	S. W. 3	S. W. 2	Foggy	9	Rain	0.40
19	29.81	29.81	29.85	60	72	55	62.3	S. W. 1	S. W. 2	S. W. 1	10	1	0	
20	29.87	29.83	29.84	57	71	59	62.3	S. W. 1	S. E. 2	E'ly 1	Foggy	5	Foggy	
S 21	29.89	29.88	29.86	60	74	59	64.3	N. W. 2	S'ly 2	S. W'ly 2	5	7	1	
22	29.93	29.93	29.97	60	75	60	65.0	N. W. 2	S. W. 3	N. W. 2	8	3	0	
23	30.05	30.03	30.05	52	61	52	55.0	N. W.	S. E. 2	S. E. 1	0	1	0	
24	30.08	30.01	29.97	52	73	57	60.7	N. W. 1	S. E'ly 2	S'ly 1	0	0	0	
25	29.92	29.79	29.62	53	62	57	57.3	S. W. 2	S. W. 3	S. W. 2	7	Sprin'lg	Rain	} 0.35
26	29.54	29.53	29.60	60	61	58	59.7	N. W. 1	Nl'y 2	N'ly 3	9	Sprinl'g	10	
27	29.71	29.76	29.74	52	63	56	57.0	N. E. 3	N. E. 3	N. E. 1	10	10	0	
S 28	29.75	29.67	29.66	59	80	64	67.7	N'ly 2	W'ly 2	S'ly 1	2	3	2	
29	29.75	29.75	29.75	57	75	56	62.7	N. E. 2	E'ly 2	S'ly 1	10	3	3	
30	29.65	29.56	29.59	55	65	58	59.3	S. E'ly 1	S'ly 2	N. E. 2	10	10	10	
31	29.86	29.89	29.99	48	61	47	52.0	N. E. 3	E'ly 3	N. E. 1	6	4	0	
Means	29.78	29.75	29.77	53.0	66.3	53.8	...	1.7	2.2	1.5	6.4	5.2	5.0	3.60
									1.8			5.5		
REDUCED TO SEA LEVEL.								Prevailing winds from some point between—		Days.			Days.	
Max.	30.36	30.36	30.37	68	80	64	67.7							
Min.	29.64	29.48	29.58	32	47	31	41.0							
Mean	29.96	29.93	29.95					N. & E.		4	Clear		7	
Range	0.72	0.88	0.79	36	33	33	26.7	E. & S.		10	Variable		} 13	
Mean of month	29.947			...	...	...	57.7	S. & W.		10	Cloudy			
Extreme range	0.89			...	...	...	49.0	W. & N.		7	Rain fell on		11	

REMARKS.

1st. Very fine.
2d. Very warm. Appearances of storm in the evening.
3d. Moderate rain through the day and evening.
4th. Rain and mist through the day.
5th. Pleasant in the morning. Shower from 4 to 6 P. M.
6th. Pleasant in the morning. Light flurry of snow at 5 P. M. and blustering.
7th. The ground considerably frozen this morning, and ice formed to the thickness of half an inch in open vessels.
8th. Very fine. Evening splendid.
9th. Pleasant. Sprinkling of rain at 11 P. M.
10th. Shower from 3 to 4 P. M. Sprinkling in the evening.
11th. Cloudy in the morning. Clouds broken in the afternoon.
12th. Pleasant.
13th. Very fine.
14th. Copious shower in the afternoon.
15th. Clouds cleared in the morning. Pleasant in the afternoon, and warm.
16th. Fine. Warmest day since Sept. 7, 1853. Thermometer 78°.
17th. Cloudy; air damp and cool.
18th. Heavy shower at 7½ P. M. and in evening.
19th. Cleared in the morning. Afternoon and evening very fine.
20th. Very fine.
21st. Pleasant. Aurora in evening, not bright.
22d. Very fine.
23d. Fine. Air cool from S. E. in the afternoon and evening.
24th. Very fine.
25th. Cloudy in the morning. Moderate rain in the afternoon.
26th. Dashing showers in the morning. Heavy passing clouds in afternoon, occasionally broken so as to show glimpses of the sun's disk, but not sufficient to afford any accurate observation of the eclipse, which, by computation, began in this place at 4 h. 26 m. 14 s. mean time P. M., and continued 2 h. 20 m. 53 s.
27th. Mist in the morning. Evening clear.
28th. Very pleasant. The warmest day of the season thus far. Thermometer 80°.
29th. Pleasant.
30th. Mist, and occasional sprinkling of rain.
31st. Cold for the season; wind brisk N. W.

June, 1854. New Moon, 25d. 6h. 43m. A. M.

DAYS.	Barometer, reduced to 32° F. At 6 A. M.	At 2 P. M.	At 10 P. M.	Thermometer. At 6 A. M.	At 2 P. M.	At 10 P. M.	Daily mean.	Winds. (Direction and Force.) At 6 A. M.	At 2 P. M.	At 10 P. M.	Weather. (Tenths Cloudy.) At 6 A. M.	At 2 P. M.	At 10 P. M.	Rain and Snow in Inches of Water.
1	30.01	30.00	30.00	46	69	50	55.0	N. E. 1	N. E'ly 2	N'ly 1	10	2	0	
2	30.01	29.94	29.90	51	75	57	61.0	N. W. 2	N. W. 2	N. W. 1	0	0	0	
3	29.88	29.83	29.87	60	82	59	67.0	N. W. 1	S. W'ly 2	W'ly 1	0	4	0	
S 4	29.89	29.82	29.79	57	77	61	65.0	S. E'ly 1	S. W'ly 3	S. W. 2	Foggy	0	0	
5	29.74	29.67	29.70	61	82	62	68.3	S. W. 2	S. W. 2	S. W. 1	0	0	0	
6	29.74	29.75	29.77	64	82	63	69.7	S. W. 2	S. E. 2	S. E'ly 2	Foggy	0	Hazy	
7	29.73	29.67	29.66	59	71	65	65.0	N. E. 2	S. E'ly 2	S. E'ly 1	Rain	10	10	} 1.40
8	29.58	29.37	29.49	65	72	65	67.3	N. E'ly 1	E'ly 2	S. W. 2	Rain	10	8	
9	29.46	29.50	29.58	65	80	62	69.0	N. E. 2	S. W. 3	W. 2	10	4	0	
10	29.60	29.74	29.74	60	69	62	63.7	W. 2	W'ly 3	S. W. 2	0	10	8	
S 11	29.82	29.77	29.79	62	74	64	66.7	S. W. 1	S. W. 2	S. W. 1	9	10	10	
12	29.75	29.68	29.64	62	71	62	65.0	S. W. 1	S. W. 2	S. W. 1	4	Shower	3	
13	29.63	29.61	29.58	62	73	65	66.7	S. W. 1	S. W. 1	S. W. 1	5	10	10	
14	29.57	29.54	29.56	62	79	65	68.7	S. W. 2	S. W. 1	S. W. 2	1	10	10	
15	29.56	29.55	29.56	65	83	67	71.7	S. W. 2	W'ly 2	S'ly 1	5	3	10	
16	29.59	29.71	29.89	65	75	56	65.3	N. W. 2	N. E. 3	N. E. 1	8	3	0	
17	29.98	29.95	29.94	55	72	59	62.0	N. E. 1	N. E. 2	N. E. 1	2	1	2	
S 18	29.91	29.77	29.76	57	80	67	68.0	N. W. 1	S. E. 2	N'ly 2	3	1	0	
19	29.69	29.66	29.68	67	88	67	74.0	W'ly 1	W'ly 2	W'ly 1	2	5, Sh'r	0	1.75
20	29.68	29.67	29.70	68	84	67	73.0	N. W. 1	N. E. 3	N. E. 1	3	5	0	
21	29.76	29.77	29.80	61	67	56	61.3	N. E'ly 2	N. E. 2	N. E. 2	10	10	10	
22	29.86	29.85	29.87	57	63	55	58.3	N. E. 2	N. E. 2	N. E. 2	10	10	10	
23	29.83	29.75	29.73	56	63	60	59.7	N. E. 3	N. E. 2	N. E. 1	Misty	10	10	
24	29.64	29.57	29.58	63	77	63	67.7	S'ly 2	S. W. 2	S. W. 1	10	5	2	
S 25	29.58	29.61	29.72	64	75	59	66.0	N. W. 2	N. W. 2	N. W. 1	0	7	0	
26	29.82	29.78	29.71	55	75	62	64.0	N'ly 2	S. E'ly 2	S'ly 2	9	8	6	
27	29.79	29.74	29.79	64	79	60	67.7	S. W. 2	S'ly 1	Calm	7	7	0	
28	29.74	29.58	29.53	64	74	70	69.3	S'ly 1	S. 3	S.	10	0	0	0.20
29	29.70	29.71	29.74	68	80	62	70.0	N. 2	S'ly 2	S'ly 2	0	6	8	
30	29.68	29.63	29.61	64	63	62	63.0	S. W'ly 2	S. W'ly 1	S. E'ly 1	10	Rain	10	0.35
Means	29.74	29.71	29.72	61.0	75.1	61.5	...	1.7	2.2	1.4	5.9	5.7	4.9	3.60
								1.8			5.5			
REDUCED TO SEA LEVEL.														
Max.	30.19	30.18	30.18	68	88	70	74.0							
Min.	29.64	29.55	29.67	46	63	50	55.0							
Mean	29.92	29.89	29.90											
Range	0.55	0.63	0.51	22	25	20	19.0							
Mean of month	29.903			...	...	...	65.9							
Extreme range	0.64			...	...	...	42.0							

Prevailing winds from some point between— Days.
N. & E. 8
E. & S. 3
S. & W. 15
W. & N. 4

Days.
Clear 4
Variable . . . } 19
Cloudy . . . . }
Rain fell on . . 7

REMARKS.

1st. Cool, but pleasant.
2d. Pleasant.
3d. Warm and very fine.
4th. Very fine.
5th. Very fine; streets dry. Vegetation begins to show want of rain.
6th. Fine, with hot sun.
7th. Fine showers early in the morning. Air damp, and occasional showers through the day.
8th. Copious rain during the night, which continued till 9 A. M.
9th. Rain during the night and up to 8 A. M.; afterwards pleasant. Evening perfectly clear.
10th. Pleasant.
11th. Clouds, but no rain.
12th. Light showers in the afternoon. Mostly clear at 11 P. M.
13th. Alternate clouds and hot sun
14th. Hot sun from 7 to 10 A. M. Cloudy in the afternoon, with thunder, but no rain.
15th. Very damp and sultry. Lightning in the evening and during the night.
16th. Cool in the afternoon and evening.
17th and 18th. Pleasant.
19th. Thermometer 86° at 2 P. M. in the shade, with a current of air. Heavy gust and violent thunderstorm, with heavy rain and hail, from 5 to 6 P. M. The hail-stones were large, some of them being very nearly half an inch in diameter, much flattened, opaque at the centre, and transparent at the surface. The figure of several of the larger ones examined was that of a very flattened ellipsoid.
20th. Pleasant, with hot sun.
21st. Air damp and raw. Cool for the season.
22d. Cloudy, with occasional mist.
23d. Very cool for the season.
24th. Pleasant.
25th. Very fine.
26th. Pleasant.
27th. Cool, but pleasant.
28th. Cool in the morning. Thundershower between 5 and 6 P. M. Evening air close and oppressive.
29th. Air raw in the afternoon, and S'ly in the evening.
30th. Light showers in the morning. Cloudy in the afternoon. Mostly clear at 11 P. M.

July, 1854. New Moon, 24d. 10h. 8m. P. M.

DAYS.	Barometer At 6 A. M.	At 2 P. M.	At 10 P. M.	Thermometer At 6 A. M.	At 2 P. M.	At 10 P. M.	Daily mean.	Winds At 6 A. M.	At 2 P. M.	At 10 P. M.	Weather At 6 A. M.	At 2 P. M.	At 10 P. M.	Rain and Snow
1	29.69	29.83	29.93	63	80	62	68.3	N. W. 2	N. W. 2	N. W. 1	0	2	0	
S 2	29.99	29.95	29.85	63	80	67	66.7	N. W. 1	S'ly 2	S. W. 2	3	2	7	
3	29.76	29.66	29.63	68	88	76	77.3	S. W. 2	S. W. 3	N. W. 1	2	2	0	
4	29.64	29.60	29.60	76	94	81	83.7	N. W. 1	S. W. 2	N. W. 1	1	2	8	
5	29.56	29.59	29.66	81	91	77	83.0	N. W. 2	N. W. 2	N. W. 1	6	2	3	
6	29.82	29.84	29.87	69	85	68	74.0	N. W. 1	N. W. 2	S. W. 2	0	2	2	
7	29.92	29.91	29.93	67	82	70	73.0	S. W. 2	S'ly 2	S'ly 1	3	4	7	
8	29.93	29.90	29.86	68	90	70	76.0	S. W. 1	S. W. 2	S. W. 2	2	5	2	
S 9	29.81	29.73	29.72	74	86	75	78.3	S. W. 2	S'ly 3	S. W'ly 1	10	8	8	
10	29.74	29.78	29.81	72	70	62	68.0	N'ly 2	N. E. 3	N. E. 1	9	10	0	
11	29.82	29.81	29.81	61	76	64	67.0	N. E. 2	N. E. 2	N. E'ly 1	7	8	5	
12	29.83	29.84	29.87	62	70	64	65.3	E'ly 1	S. E. 1	S. E'ly 1	10	10	8	
13	29.99	30.01	30.02	62	78	62	67.3	N. E'ly 1	S. E'ly 2	E'ly 1	7	3	2	
14	29.97	29.92	29.94	57	61	56	58.0	N. E. 1	N. E. 1	N. E. 1	Rain	Rain	Rain	1.65
15	29.92	29.89	29.89	56	67	59	60.7	N. E. 1	N. E'ly 1	N. E'ly 1	10	9	10	
S 16	29.98	29.96	29.96	51	79	66	65.3	N. E. 1	E'ly 1	S. E'ly 1	Foggy	0	Foggy	
17	29.97	29.92	29.85	63	77	69	69.7	S. E'ly 1	S. E'ly 2	S. E'ly 1	Foggy	1	2	
18	29.78	29.73	29.74	68	85	71	74.7	N. E'ly 1	N. E'ly 1	E'ly 1	0	1	2	
19	29.76	29.79	29.72	67	85	72	74.7	N'ly 1	N'ly 1	S. E'ly 1	2	0	0	
20	29.68	29.66	29.71	74	84	71	76.3	S. E'ly 1	S. E'ly 1	E'ly 1	0	1	0	
21	29.73	29.73	29.81	73	86	74	77.7	S'ly 2	S. W. 3	W'ly 1	3	2	7	
22	29.88	29.88	29.90	74	86	77	79.0	S. W. 1	S. W. 2	S. W. 1	5	7	5	
S 23	29.91	29.89	29.89	76	87	74	79.0	S. W. 2	S. W. 3	S. W. 1	10	5	0	
24	29.93	29.92	29.93	77	85	74	78.7	S. W. 3	S. W'ly 3	S. W. 1	6	8	Rain	} 0.80
25	29.84	29.81	29.80	74	79	74	75.7	S. W. 1	S. W. 3	S. W. 2	Rain	10	Misty	
26	29.77	29.71	29.72	74	83	75	77.3	S. W. 2	S. W. 3	S. W. 1	10	5	10	
27	29.80	29.83	29.94	70	79	64	71.0	N. W. 1	N. W. 2	N. W. 1	Sprinl'g	5	0	
28	30.01	29.92	29.93	58	81	66	68.3	N. W. 1	S. W. 1	S. W. 1	0	0	0	
29	29.82	29.73	29.67	70	81	72	74.3	S. W. 2	S. W. 3	S. W. 2	10	8	0	
S 30	29.66	29.66	29.83	72	87	70	76.3	S. W. 2	N. W. 3	N. W. 1	5	0	0	
31	29.86	29.86	29.86	63	82	68	71.0	N. W. 2	N. W. 2	N. W. 1	0	0	0	
Means	29.83	29.81	29.83	67.8	81.4	69.4	...	1.5	2.1	1.1	5.5	4.3	4.1	2.45
								1.6			4.5			
REDUCED TO SEA LEVEL.														
Max.	30.19	30.19	30.20	81	94	81	83.7							
Min.	29.74	29.77	29.78	51	61	56	58.0							
Mean	30.01	29.99	30.01											
Range	0.45	0.42	0.42	30	33	25	25.7							
Mean of month	30.003			...	...	...	72.9							
Extreme range	0.46			...	...	...	43.0							

Prevailing winds from some point between— Days.
N. & E. 9
E. & S. 4
S. & W. 13
W. & N. 5

Days.
Clear 9
Variable . . . } 14
Cloudy . . . . }
Rain fell on . . 8

1st and 2d. Very fine.
3d. Intensely hot. Thermometer in the shade, and in a brisk current of air, stood at 88°; and in the shade, without the current of air, at 93°.
4th. Intensely hot. Ther. in the shade, and in a fresh current of air from S. W., at 1 P. M., stood at 91°—the highest point since June 21, '53, when, under same circumstances, the ther. stood at 95°.
5th. Very hot, but less oppressive than yesterday.
6th. Very fine; warm, but not oppressive.
7th. Very fine.
8th. Hot sun during day. Evening pleasant.
9th. Warm and sultry. Sprinkling of rain from 7 to 8 P. M.
10th. Cloudy in the morning, with damp air at N. E. Sprinkling of rain at 8 A. M.
11th. Pleasant.
12th. Cloudy, with light sprinkling of rain at 8 A. M.
13th. Very fine.
14th. Heavy rain all the morning. Cloudy in afternoon, with mist. Rain again in the evening.
15th. Light clouds in morning. Clouds broken and sun out in the afternoon.
16th. Fog in morning. Very fine during day.
17th. Cloudy and fog in the morning. Cleared at 9 A. M.
18th. Very pleasant, though very warm.
19th. Warm, but not unpleasant.
20th. Very warm.
21st. Very hot at mid-day. Light thunder-showers from 5 to 6 P. M.
22d. Very warm; damp and sultry.
23d. Extremely hot and sultry. At 8 A. M., dew-point 73°.
24th. At 8 A. M., dew-point 71°. Sprinkling of rain from noon to 1 P. M. Fine shower from 10 to 11 P. M.
25th. Heavy showers during the last night and this morning. At 10 A. M., ther. 80°; dew-point 75°. At 5 P. M., dew-point 71°.
26th. At 1 P. M., dew-point 74°. Sun out at mid-day, hot and very sultry.
27th. Sprinkling of rain at 7 A.M.; dew-point 63°. At 5 P. M., dew-point 58°. Evening clear and cool.
28th. Very fine; air dry and bracing. Dew-point fallen to 53°.
29th. Wind S. W'ly. At 6 A. M., dew-point 68°, and at 2 P. M., 69°. Evening fine.
30th. At 6 A. M., dew-point 67°; at 1 P. M., 58°; wind changed from S. W. to N. W. Evening fine.
31st. At 6 A. M., dew-point 56°. Day warm, but fine.

August, 1854. New Moon, 23d. 0h. 52m. P. M.

Days.	Barometer, reduced to 32° F At 6 A. M.	At 2 P. M.	At 10 P. M.	Thermometer. At 6 A. M.	At 2 P. M.	At 10 P. M.	Daily mean.	Winds. (Direction and Force.) At 6 A. M.	At 2 P. M.	At 10 P. M.	Weather. (Tenths Cloudy.) At 6 A. M.	At 2 P. M.	At 10 P. M.	Rain and Snow in Inches of Water.
1	29.84	...	29.66	66	...	73	...	N. W. 2	...	S. W. 3	5	...	8	
2	29.57	29.53	29.64	76	87	79	81.0	S. W. 1	N. W'ly 1	N'ly 1	2	2	1	0.10
3	29.77	29.72	29.68	67	80	66	71.0	S. W'ly 2	W'ly 2	W'ly 1	0	0	2	
4	29.63	29.53	29.53	68	68	65	67.0	S. W. 2	S. W. 2	S. W. 2	Sprin'le	Rain	2	0.10
5	29.68	...	29.61	65	...	65	...	S. W. 1	...	S. W. 1	5	...	Foggy	
S 6	29.61	29.59	29.52	74	84	70	76.0	S. W. 1	S. W. 3	S. W. 3	1	5	9	
7	29.65	29.70	29.78	66	76	64	68.7	N. W. 3	N. W. 2	N. W. 1	1	2	8	
8	29.87	29.88	29.96	58	78	61	65.7	N. W. 1	N. W. 2	N. W. 1	0	2	2	
9	30.02	30.00	29.99	57	77	60	64.7	N. W. 1	N. E. 2	N. E'ly 1	0	2	0	
10	29.99	29.95	29.94	58	75	64	65.7	N. E. 2	N. E. 2	N. E. 2	5	6	10	
11	29.87	29.86	29.88	63	74	62	66.3	N. E. 2	N. E. 2	N. W. 1	10	10	2	
12	29.89	29.87	29.75	66	80	69	71.7	S. W. 2	S. W. 2	S'ly 1	3	2	Misty	
S 13	29.65	29.53	29.53	72	81	76	76.3	S. E'ly 1	S. E'ly 2	S. W'ly 3	Misty	6	3	
14	...	...	...	...	...	...	...	...	...	...	...	...	...	
15	...	...	...	...	...	...	...	...	...	...	...	...	...	
16	...	...	29.75	...	...	64	...	...	...	S. W. 1	...	...	0	
17	29.78	29.76	29.77	62	77	62	67.0	S. W. 1	S. W. 1	S. W. 1	8	10	2	
18	29.90	29.88	29.96	58	76	61	65.0	N. W. 1	S. W. 1	S. W. 1	0	2	0	
19	29.97	...	29.92	60	...	64	...	S. W. 1	...	S. W. 1	5	...	0	
S 20	29.86	29.73	29.74	65	79	62	68.7	S. W. 1	S. W. 3	S. W. 1	5	0	0	
21	29.94	29.92	29.85	63	80	63	68.7	N. W. 1	S. W'ly 2	S. W. 1	3	2	0	
22	29.67	...	...	65	...	...	...	S. W. 2	...	...	2	...	...	
23	...	...	...	...	...	...	...	...	...	...	...	...	...	
24	...	...	...	...	...	...	...	...	...	...	...	...	...	
25	...	29.72	29.83	...	86	71	...	...	N. W. 2	N. W. 1	...	3	10	
26	29.85	29.76	29.70	61	79	63	67.7	N. W. 1	N. W. 1	N'ly 1	3	7	Rain	0.10
S 27	29.81	29.83	29.94	60	67	57	61.3	N. W. 2	N. W. 1	N. W. 1	10	10	7	
28	...	...	30.15	...	...	54	...	...	...	N. W.	...	...	0	
29	30.15	30.09	30.08	50	70	56	58.7	N. W. 1	N. W. 1	N. W. 1	0	0	0	
30	30.06	29.95	29.89	50	70	61	60.8	N'ly 1	S'ly 3	S. W. 1	Foggy	0	0	
31	29.87	29.85	29.94	64	80	65	69.7	S. W. 1	S. W. 1	E'ly 1	5	9	10	
Means	29.83	29.79	29.81	63.1	77.3	65.5	...	1.4	1.8	1.2	4.4	4.3	4.1	0.30
								1.6			4.3			
REDUCED TO SEA LEVEL.														
Max.	30.33	30.27	30.33	74	87	79	81.0							
Min.	29.75	29.71	29.70	50	67	54	58.7							
Mean	30.01	29.97	29.99											
Range	0.58	0.56	0.63	24	20	25	22.3							
Mean of month	29.990			...	...	...	68.6							
Extreme range	0.63			...	...	...	37.0							

Prevailing winds from some point between— Days.
N. & E. 2
E. & S. 1
S. & W. 16
W. & N. 8

Days.
Clear 8
Variable . . . } 14
Cloudy . . . . }
Rain fell on . . 5
(4 days omitted.)

Remarks.

1st. Pleasant in the morning. Cloudy at noon and in the evening.
2d. Light thundershower at 4½ A. M. Day pleasant.
3d. Very fine.
4th. Several light but refreshing showers.
5th. Pleasant.
6th. Pleasant. Sprinkling of rain from 7 to 8 P. M., with thunder.
7th. Very fine. Sprinkling of rain at 7 P. M. Air in the morning very dry. At 2 P. M., dew-point 50°; thermometer 76°.
8th. At 7 A. M., dew-point 51°. Day very fine and dry.
9th. At 7 A. M., dew-point 49°. Day very fine.
10th. At 7 A. M., dew-point 54°. Air damp in the evening, with some appearances of storm.
11th. Cloudy in the morning, with light mist. Evening pleasant, and mostly clear.
12th. Cloudy, with light mist in the afternoon and evening.
13th. Cloudy in the morning. Pleasant in the afternoon and evening.
16th. Very fine.
17th. Overcast with light hazy clouds. Evening mostly clear.
18th. Hazy round the horizon, with light clouds interspersed. Evening clear.
19th. Very pleasant. At 7 A. M., dew-point 52°.
20th. Pleasant. At 7 A. M., dew-point 62°; the ground extremely dry.
21st. Very warm.
25th. Very hot; ground excessively dry, and air full of smoke.
26th. Very warm and sultry in the morning. Light shower at noon, and gentle rain in the evening.
27th. Mostly cloudy.
28th. Pleasant, but cool.
29th. Dew-point 49°. Very dry and very drying.
30th. Morning foggy. Mid-day and afternoon clear and pleasant.
31st. At 7 A. M., dew-point 62°. Warm in the morning. Cool towards evening.

September, 1854. New Moon, 22d. 2h. 55m. A. M.

Days.	Barometer At 6 A. M.	At 2 P. M.	At 10 P. M.	Thermometer At 6 A. M.	At 2 P. M.	At 10 P. M.	Daily mean.	Winds At 6 A. M.	At 2 P. M.	At 10 P. M.	Weather At 6 A. M.	At 2 P. M.	At 10 P. M.	Rain and Snow in Inches of Water.
1	30.03	30.02	30.00	62	63	58	61.0	N. E. 1	N. E. 1	N. E. 1	10	Rain	Rain	
2	29.97	29.94	29.84	59	65	62	62.0	N. E. 2	N. E. 1	E'ly 1	Rain	10	Misty	0.65
S 3	29.70	29.75	29.81	68	78	68	71.3	W'ly 1	S. W. 2	S. W.	10	0	Misty	
4	29.91	29.90	29.89	66	75	65	68.7	N. W. 2	W'ly 1	S. W. 1	0	0	Hazy	
5	29.88	29.78	29.80	65	82	73	73.3	S. W. 1	S. W. 2	S. W. 1	10	5	1	
6	29.80	29.69	29.77	75	88	72	78.3	S. W. 2	S. W. 2	W'ly 1	0	2	Rain	1.10
7	29.73	29.69	29.80	70	83	69	74.0	W'ly 2	W'ly 2	N. W. 1	10	5	0	
8	29.91	29.88	29.78	61	75	66	67.3	N. W. 1	N. W. 2	S. W. 1	0	2	10	
9	29.58	29.49	29.62	76	84	60	73.3	S. W. 3	S. W. 5	N. E. 2	10	10	Rain	} 3.45
S 10	29.71	29.70	29.69	54	52	51	52.3	N. 1	E. 3	N. E. 3	Rain	Rain	10	
11	29.86	29.87	29.89	48	63	51	54.0	N. W. 2	N. W. 2	N. W. 1	0	0	0	
12	29.81	29.75	29.77	58	67	63	62.7	S. W. 2	S. W. 3	N. W. 1	10	10	0	
13	29.96	30.04	30.09	60	65	49	58.0	N'ly 2	N. E. 2	N. E. 1	0	0	1	
14	30.11	30.03	29.85	49	67	61	59.0	N. E. 1	S. E'ly 1	S'ly 1	2	10	Sprin'le	
15	29.66	29.70	29.90	64	74	55	64.3	S'ly 1	N. W. 2	N. W. 2	Rain	5	0	0.45
16	30.03	30.02	30.09	49	63	50	67.3	N. W. 2	N. W. 2	N. W. 2	0	0	0	
S 17	30.11	30.18	30.21	48	63	48	53.0	N. W. 1	N. W. 2	S. W. 1	0	0	0	
18	30.18	30.07	29.98	47	68	57	57.3	S. W. 1	S. W. 2	S. W. 1	0	3	5	
19	29.75	29.64	29.59	65	76	63	68.0	S. W. 2	S. W. 3	S. W. 1	Rain	3	10	} 0.45
20	29.53	29.60	29.88	61	67	48	58.7	N. W. 2	N. W. 3	N. W. 2	6, Sh'r	1	0	
21	30.12	30.10	30.07	38	54	42	44.7	N. W. 1	N. W. 1	S. W. 2	0	5	2	
22	30.29	30.29	30.31	37	59	46	47.3	S. W. 1	S. W. 1	S. W. 1	1	0	0	
23	...	...	...	...	...	...	...	...	...	...	...	...	...	
S 24	29.91	...	29.84	57	...	57	...	W'ly 1	...	S. W'ly 1	0	...	0	
25	29.83	29.80	29.85	56	73	57	62.0	S. W. 1	S. W. 2	S. W. 1	2	3	1	
26	29.85	29.82	29.85	56	76	60	64.0	S. W. 1	S. W. 1	S. W. 1	2	0	0	
27	29.84	29.73	29.72	60	77	65	67.3	S. W. 1	S. W. 2	S. W. 1	6	3	2	
28	29.71	29.71	29.78	67	76	59	67.3	S. W. 1	N. E. 1	E'ly 1	7	7	0	
29	29.96	29.96	30.12	51	61	45	52.3	N'ly 1	N. E. 2	N. E. 1	1	2	0	
30	[illegible]	[illegible]	[illegible]	[illegible]	[illegible]	[illegible]	[illegible]	[illegible]	[illegible]	[illegible]	[illegible]	[illegible]	[illegible]	
Means	29.89	29.87	29.89	57.4	69.4	57.4	...	1.5	1.9	1.3	4.4	3.6	4.0	6.10
								1.6			4.0			
REDUCED TO SEA LEVEL.														
Max.	30.47	30.47	30.49	76	88	73	78.3							
Min.	29.71	29.67	29.77	37	52	42	44.7							
Mean	30.07	30.05	30.07											
Range	0.76	0.80	0.72	39	36	31	33.6							
Mean of month	30.063			...	...	...	61.4							
Extreme range	0.82			...	...	...	51.0							

Prevailing winds from some point between— Days.
N. & E. 6
E. & S. 1
S. & W. 13
W. & N. 10

Days.
Clear 10
Variable . . . } 10
Cloudy . . . . }
Rain fell on . . 9
(1 day omitted.)

Remarks.

1st. Light showers through the day and evening, refreshing to the parched earth.
2d. Appearances of rain during the day. Mist in the evening.
3d. Rain last night. Day pleasant. Thick mist in the evening.
4th. Very fine.
6th. Cloudy in the morning. Clear in the evening. Air warm and sultry.
6th. Very hot during day. Sun partly covered by clouds. Thunder and rain from 8 to 9 P. M., which continued at intervals for several hours.
7th. Cloudy in the morning. Fine in the afternoon and evening.
8th. Very pleasant.
9th. At 6 A. M., temperature 76°; dew-point 72°; wind S. W. Sultry in morning. Wind changed from S. W. to N. E., with showers, in the afternoon. Steady rain after 7 P. M.
10th. Steady rain all day and evening; quantity large.
11th. Very fine.
12th. Cloudy, with occasional mist through the day. Evening mostly clear.
13th. Cool and fine.
14th. Cloudy in the afternoon. Sprinkling of rain in the evening.
15th. Copious shower from 6 to 8 A. M. Afternoon and evening fine.
16th. Cloudless day. Evening cool.
17th and 18th. Very fine.
19th. Pleasant.
20th. Copious shower at 2 A. M., with thunder and a gust of wind
21st. Very cool for the season. White frost in low places; the first in this vicinity.
22d. White frost in low places. Day fine.
23d. Fine.
24th. Very fine.
[illegible]
26th. Very fine. Aurora in the evening, not very bright.
27th. Very fine.
28th. Very pleasant.
29th. Pleasant. Very cool in the afternoon and evening.
30th. Cool, but pleasant.

October, 1854. New Moon, 21d. 4h. 16m. P. M.

DAYS.	Barometer, reduced to 32° F. Sunrise.	At 2 P. M.	At 10 P. M.	Thermometer. Sunrise.	At 2 P. M.	At 10 P. M.	Daily mean.	Winds. (Direction and Force.) Sunrise.	At 2 P. M.	At 10 P. M.	Weather. (Tenths Cloudy.) Sunrise.	At 2 P. M.	At 10 P. M.	Rain and Snow in Inches of Water.
S 1	29.98	29.75	29.49	41	63	60	54.7	S. W'ly 1	S. W. 2	S. W. 1	3	10	Rain	0.10
2	29.44	29.56	29.66	64	64	48	58.7	S. W. 2	N. W. 3	N. W. 1	0	1	0	
3	29.66	29.53	29.35	45	64	63	57.3	N. W. 1	S. E. 3	S. W. 3	3	10	Rain	0.40
4	29.37	29.44	29.66	64	61	50	58.3	S. W. 2	S. W. 2	N. W. 2	10	10	0	
5	29.85	29.98	30.15	45	55	41	47.0	N. W. 2	N. W. 2	N. W. 1	0	5	0	
6	30.27	30.24	30.15	38	64	52	51.3	N. W. 1	S. W. 2	S. W. 1	1	3	0	
7	30.12	29.97	29.95	52	73	59	61.3	S. W. 1	S. W. 2	S. W. 1	1	0	0	
S 8	29.98	29.93	29.94	60	77	61	66.0	N. W. 1	S. W. 1	S. W. 1	5	10	0	
9	29.86	29.67	29.64	60	76	65	67.0	S. W. 1	S. W. 2	S. W. 1	Foggy	5	8	
10	29.91	29.93	30.07	53	60	44	52.3	N. W. 2	N. E. 2	N. E. 2	7	0	0	
11	30.05	29.94	29.88	47	65	60	57.3	N. E. 1	S'ly 3	S'ly 1	9	10	10	
12	29.84	29.74	29.67	60	75	66	67.0	S. W. 2	S'ly 3	S. W. 3	10	5	8	
13	29.75	29.84	29.86	65	58	51	58.0	N'ly 2	N. E. 2	N. E. 2	10	10	8	
14	29.82	...	...	51	65	56	57.3	N. E'ly 1	...	...	10	...	...	
S 15	...	29.23	29.23	49	47	38	44.7	...	N. W. 2	N. E. 2	...	10	Rain	0.90
16	...	29.34	29.54	38	54	47	46.3	...	N. W. 3	S. W. 2	...	0	10	
17	29.57	29.60	29.75	48	54	41	47.7	S. W. 2	S. W. 2	N. E. 2	7	10	Rain	
18	29.88	29.77	29.74	34	53	38	41.7	N. W. 2	N. W. 2	N. W. 2	0	6	0	
19	30.00	30.06	30.20	35	45	36	38.7	N. W. 2	N. E. 2	N'ly 1	0	10	0	
20	30.28	30.29	30.27	33	51	38	40.7	N. W. 1	N. W. 2	N. W. 1	0	2	2	
21	30.26	30.21	30.22	34	54	40	42.7	N. W. 1	N. W. 1	N. W. 1	1	2	0	
S 22	30.18	30.20	30.20	36	55	43	44.7	N. W. 1	N. W. 2	N. W. 1	2	0	0	
23	30.19	30.17	30.18	40	52	43	45.0	N. W. 2	N. E. 3	N. E. 2	0	0	7	
24	30.17	30.12	30.13	43	53	41	45.7	N. E. 3	N. E. 3	N. E. 1	10	8	0	
25	30.15	30.13	30.18	40	63	47	50.0	N'ly 2	N. E. 1	N. E. 1	0	0	0	
26	30.29	30.24	30.24	45	63	47	51.7	N. W. 1	S'ly 1	S'ly 1	0	0	0	
27	30.24	30.14	30.14	44	64	47	51.7	S. W. 1	S. E'ly 2	N'ly 1	6	1	0	
28	30.16	...	30.11	44	...	54	...	N. W. 1	...	S. E. 1	6	...	5	
S 29	...	...	29.96	...	...	61	...	...	...	S. E. 1	Foggy	Misty	Misty	
30	29.91	29.88	29.84	55	69	62	62.0	S'ly 1	S'ly 1	E'ly 1	10	Rain	Rain	} 0.50
31	29.72	29.58	29.57	64	67	62	64.3	S. E'ly 1	S'ly 2	S. W. 2	Rain	10	10	
Means	29.96	29.87	29.90	47.6	60.8	50.4	...	1.5	2.1	1.4	4.8	5.4	4.3	1.90
									1.7			4.8		
REDUCED TO SEA LEVEL.														
Max.	30.47	30.47	30.45	65	77	66	67.3	Prevailing winds from some point between—		Days.			Days.	
Min.	29.55	29.41	29.41	33	45	36	38.7	N. & E.		7	Clear		12	
Mean	30.14	30.05	30.08					E. & S.		5	Variable		} 10	
Range	0.92	1.06	1.04	32	32	30	28.6	S. & W.		10	Cloudy			
Mean of month	30.030			...	...	...	52.9	W. & N.		9	Rain fell on		9	
Extreme range	1.06			...	...	...	44.0							

REMARKS.

1st. Pleasant in the morning. Began to rain from 9 to 10 P. M.
2d. Wind changed from S. W. to N. W. from 6 to 7 A. M., and grew cooler.
3d. Light rain from 3 to 8 P. M.
4th. Pleasant.
5th. Pleasant. Evening cloudless and splendid.
6th and 7th. Very fine.
8th. Pleasant. Evening cloudy.
9th. Pleasant.
10th. Pleasant. Evening splendid.
11th. Pleasant.
12th. Much overcast, with some appearance of storm in the evening.
13th and 14th. Cloudy.
15th Showery through the day. Steady and rather heavy rain in the evening.
16th. Variable. Morning and evening cloudy. Sprinkling of rain at 10 P. M.
17th. Cloudy. Sprinkling of rain in the evening; wind N. E.
18th. Shower from 4 to 5 P. M. Evening clear, with aurora not very bright.
19th. Air raw in the afternoon. Evening clear and cool.
20th. First white frost in the College yard. Day fine.
21st and 22d. Very fine.
23d. Some indications of storm at 11 P. M.
24th. Cloudy in the morning. Evening clear.
25th. Very fine; nearly cloudless.
26th. Very fine and mild.
27th. Fine. Evening splendid.
28th. Very fine through the day. Cloudy in the evening.
29th. Mist, with occasional sprinkling of rain.
30th. Very warm. Sprinkling of rain in the afternoon and evening.
31st. Rain in the morning. Clouds broken in the afternoon and evening.

November, 1854. New Moon, 20d. 4h. 53m. A. M.

DAYS.	Barometer Sunrise.	At 2 P. M.	At 10 P. M.	Thermometer Sunrise.	At 2 P. M.	At 10 P. M.	Daily mean.	Winds Sunrise.	At 2 P. M.	At 10 P. M.	Weather Sunrise.	At 2 P. M.	At 10 P. M.	Rain and Snow
1	29.56	29.51	29.56	54	70	53	59.0	S. W. 2	S. W. 2	N. W. 2	0	3	Shower	0.10
2	29.60	29.69	29.88	44	57	44	48.3	N. W. 2	N. W. 1	N. W. 2	0	...	4	
3	29.85	29.81	29.98	51	62	46	53.0	S. W. 2	S. W. 2	S. W. 1	1	10	Rain	
4	30.05	30.06	30.20	35	43	26	34.7	N. W. 2	N. W. 2	N. W. 2	10	7	0	
S 5	30.33	30.26	30.24	18	31	23	24.0	N. W'ly 2	N. W. 2	N. W. 2	0	0	0	
6	30.13	29.97	29.69	20	42	44	35.3	N. W. 1	S. E. 2	S'ly 2	0	5	9	
7	29.42	29.26	29.30	47	51	37	45.0	S. E'ly 1	S. W'ly 2	N. W. 1	10	Sprin'le	0	
8	29.42	...	29.74	35	...	31	...	N. W. 1	...	N. W. 1	0	...	2	
9	29.90	29.89	30.04	29	44	34	35.7	N. W'ly 2	W'ly 3	W'ly 1	2	0	2	
10	30.09	30.04	30.00	28	54	51	44.3	N. W. 1	S. W.	S. W. 1	0	2	3	
11	29.89	29.77	...	54	56	...	...	S. W. 3	S. E. 3	...	10	Rain	...	} 6.00
S 12	...	...	...	...	...	...	...	S'ly 3	S'ly 2	S'ly 2	Rain	Rain	Rain	
13	...	29.51	29.55	...	64	58	...	...	S'ly 2	S'ly 1	Rain	Rain	Foggy	
14	29.65	29.62	29.59	45	48	35	42.7	N. W. 2	N. W. 2	N. W. 1	5	0	0	
15	29.50	29.44	29.34	33	41	35	36.3	S. W. 1	S. W.	N. E. 1	3	Rain	Rain	} 0.45
16	29.30	29.26	29.31	35	39	37	37.0	N. E. 1	N'ly 2	N. W'ly 1	Rain	10	10	
17	29.33	29.32	29.32	35	44	45	41.3	N. W. 2	N. W. 2	S. W. 2	4	8	10	
18	29.41	29.38	29.48	44	50	44	46.0	S. W. 1	S. W. 1	S. W. 1	10	10	Rain	
S 19	29.44	29.40	29.48	39	44	37	40.0	N. W. 1	N. W. 1	N. W. 1	7	5	0	
20	29.64	29.59	29.71	30	38	27	31.7	N. W. 1	N. W. 2	N. W. 1	0	1	0	
21	29.83	29.80	29.91	27	41	33	33.7	N. W. 1	N. W. 1	N. W. 1	5	1	10	
22	29.80	29.56	29.64	35	43	36	38.0	N. E. 1	N. E. 1	N. E. 2	Rain	Rain	10	0.60
23	29.77	29.69	29.70	31	44	33	36.0	N. W. 1	N. W. 1	N. W. 1	1	0	0	
24	29.62	29.60	29.41	38	66	56	53.3	N. W. 1	S'ly 1	S'ly	Foggy	10	Rain	} 1.10
25	29.05	29.11	...	56	61	...	...	S'ly 2	S. W. 2	...	Rain	5	...	
S 26	...	...	...	...	...	...	...	...	...	...	...	...	...	
27	...	...	29.87	...	...	27	...	...	...	N. W. 1	...	...	0	
28	29.93	29.94	29.93	26	42	28	32.0	N. W. 1	N. W. 1	W'ly 1	0	0	0	
29	29.78	...	...	34	...	...	...	N. E. 1	...	...	Rain	Rain	Rain	1.00
30	...	...	...	...	...	...	...	...	...	...	...	...	...	
Means	29.69	29.64	29.70	36.9	47.0	38.3	...	1.5	1.7	1.3	5.0	5.7	4.4	9.15
									1.5			5.0		
REDUCED TO SEA LEVEL.														
Max.	30.51	30.44	30.42	56	70	56	59.0	Prevailing winds from some point between—		Days.			Days.	
Min.	29.23	29.29	29.48	18	31	23	24.0	N. & E.		3	Clear		8	
Mean	29.87	29.82	29.88					E. & S.		2	Variable		} 6	
Range	1.28	1.15	0.94	38	39	33	35.0	S. & W.		10	Cloudy			
Mean of month	29.859			...	...	...	40.7	W. & N.		13	Rain fell on		14	
Extreme range	1.28			...	...	...	52.0				(2 days omitted.)			

REMARKS.

1st. Pleasant; very mild and warm for the season. Evening showery and cooler.
2d. Pleasant.
3d. Pleasant through the day. Sprinkling of rain in the evening.
4th. Air raw and cold. Evening very cold.
5th. Fresh dahlias and other flowers were gathered in abundance from the garden yesterday, having, to that time, suffered no injury from frost. This morning, the thermometer stood at 18°, with the ground hard frozen.
6th. Ground frozen nearly three inches deep this morning.
7th. Sprinkling of rain in the morning. Evening very clear.
8th. Cool and pleasant.
9th and 10th. Pleasant.
11th. Rain in the afternoon.
12th. Rain all day.
13th. Rain in the morning. Rain and mist in the evening, with fog.
14th. Very fine.
15th. Moderate rain and drizzle, mixed with some snow, began at 11 A. M. and continued.
16th. Light rain and drizzle in the morning. Cloudy in the afternoon and evening.
17th. Variable. Sprinkling of rain in evening.
18th. Sprinkling of rain in morning. Cloudy in the afternoon. Light rain in the evening.
19th. Pleasant.
20th. Very fine.
21st. Very pleasant.
22d. Steady rain in the morning. Rain and mist in the afternoon.
23d. Very fine.
24th. Cloudy. Began to rain at 6 P. M.; heavy rain and violent wind during the evening and night.
25th. Rain in the morning. Pleasant in the afternoon.
26th. Very pleasant.
27th and 28th. Very fine.
29th. Heavy rain.

December, 1854. New Moon, 19d. 4h. 38m. P. M.

DAYS.	Barometer, reduced to 32° F. Sunrise.	At 2 P. M.	At 10 P. M.	Thermometer. Sunrise.	At 2 P. M.	At 10 P. M.	Daily mean.	Winds (Direction and Force.) Sunrise.	At 2 P. M.	At 10 P. M.	Weather (Tenths Cloudy.) Sunrise.	At 2 P. M.	At 10 P. M.	Rain and Snow in Inches of Water.
1	...	29.65	29.62	...	31	26	...	...	N. W. 2	N. W. 1	...	0	10	
2	29.64	29.69	29.89	27	33	20	26.7	N. W. 1	N. W. 2	N. W. 1	10	5	0	
S 3	29.84	29.49	28.93	20	29	36	28.3	N. W. 1	N. E. 2	E'ly 4	9	10	Rain	1.15
4	28.78	28.75	28.86	34	29	17	26.7	S. W. 2	W'ly 2	N. W. 3	3	10	0	
5	28.99	29.11	29.23	13	17	16	15.3	W by N 3	W'ly 3	W'ly 2	2	1	10	
6	29.37	29.32	29.33	20	32	28	26.7	S. W. 2	S. W. 2	S. W. 1	1	5	10	
7	29.27	29.23	29.24	27	34	22	27.7	S. W. 1	S. W. 2	N. W. 2	10	5	3	
8	29.45	...	29.96	16	...	11	...	N. W. 2	...	N. W. 2	1	...	0	
9	30.23	30.29	30.31	10	26	19	18.3	N. W. 2	N. W. 2	N. W. 1	0	0	0	
S 10	30.20	30.09	30.00	27	48	46	40.3	S. W. 2	S. W. 2	S. W. 2	2	10	10	
11	29.74	29.67	29.77	34	38	28	33.3	N. W. 1	W'ly 2	N. W. 2	R'n, sn.	2	0	
12	29.84	29.84	29.90	26	34	17	25.7	N. W. 1	N. W. 2	N. W. 1	5	3	0	
13	29.87	29.66	29.69	18	37	34	29.7	S. W. 2	S. W. 3	S. W. 1	8	0	0	
14	29.73	29.74	29.79	34	47	37	39.3	S. W'ly 1	S. W'ly 2	W'ly 1	8	10	10	
15	29.74	29.68	29.44	31	45	41	39.0	S. W. 1	S. W. 2	N. E'ly 1	0	2	Rain	
16	...	...	29.56	...	...	32	...	...	...	N. W. 1	...	...	2	
S 17	29.83	29.68	29.70	24	29	28	27 0	N. W. 1	N. E'ly 1	N. E'ly 2	7	10	Snow	
18	29.59	29.57	29.70	18	29	10	19.0	W by N 2	N. E'ly 1	N. W. 1	Snow	10	0	
19	29.82	29.78	29.80	3	13	5	7.0	N. W. 1	N. W. 1	N. W. 2	0	3	0	
20	29.78	29.71	29.80	3	16	3	7.3	N. W. 2	N. W. 2	N. W. 1	1	2	0	2.20
21	29.73	29.64	29.80	6	30	23	19.7	S. W. 1	S. W. 2	W'ly 1	5	Snow	5	
22	...	30.21	30.36	9	12	7	9.3	N. E. 1	N. E. 2	N. E. 2	8	6	10	
23	...	...	30.49	...	...	14	...	...	...	N'ly 1	...	...	10	
S 24	30.12	29.94	29.84	32	39	39	36.7	N. E. 1	N. W. 1	N'ly 1	Rain	10	10	
25	29.81	...	29.80	31	...	35	...	S. W. 1	...	W'ly 1	8	...	6	
26	29.82	29.89	29.94	34	44	32	36.7	N. W. 1	N. W. 2	N. W. 1	1	1	2	
27	29.79	29.66	29.78	35	38	35	36.0	E'ly 1	N. E'ly 1	N. E. 2	Rain	Rain	Misty	
28	29.80	...	29.51	35	...	35	...	N. E. 2	...	N. E. 1	Misty	...	Misty	
29	29.41	29.43	29.60	38	34	22	31.3	W'ly 1	N. W. 2	N. W. 2	10	Misty	Snow	
30	29.64	...	...	14	...	...	...	N. W. 3	...	...	10	...	...	
S 31	...	...	...	...	...	...	...	...	...	...	...	...	...	
Means	29.69	29.65	29.71	23.0	31.8	24.8	...	1.5	1.9	1.5	6.5	6.0	5.4	3.35
									1.6			6.0		
REDUCED TO SEA LEVEL.														
Max.	30.41	30.47	30.67	38	48	39	40.3							
Min.	28.96	28.94	29.04	3	12	5	7.0							
Mean	29.87	29.83	29.89											
Range	1.45	1.53	1.63	35	36	34	33.3							
Mean of month	29.863			...	...	...	26.5							
Extreme range	1.73			...	...	...	45.0							

Prevailing winds from some point between— Days.
N. & E. 6
E. & S. 0
S. & W. 9
W. & N. 15

Days.
Clear 6
Variable . . . . } 12
Cloudy . . . . }
Rain or snow fell on 12
(1 day omitted.)

REMARKS.

1st. Cold, but pleasant.
2d. Pleasant. Evening clear and cold.
3d. Began to snow from 1 to 2 P. M. Heavy storm of wind and rain in the evening.
4th. Air very raw. Evening cold.
5th. Wind high and the cold severe. Very thick haze at 10 P. M.
6th. More moderate. Some indications of storm in the evening.
7th. Pleasant in morning. Raw in afternoon. Flurry of snow at 6 P. M. Evening pleasant.
8th. Very cold in the evening.
9th. Clear and cold, but not unpleasant.
10th. Mild, with some appearances of storm.
11th. Rain and snow in the morning. Mostly clear at 2 P. M., and mild.
12th and 13th. Pleasant.
14th. Pleasant in the morning. Sprinkling of rain in the afternoon.
15th. Mild and pleasant in the morning. Began to rain moderately at 6 P. M.
16th. Cloudy; air mild and soft.
17th. Cloudy; air damp and raw. Snow in the evening.
18th. Snow from one to two inches deep this morning. Evening clear and cold.
19th. Very cold, but wind light.
20th. Fine, but very cold.
21st. Flurry of snow in the morning. Evening mostly clear.
22d. Very raw and cold. Flurry of snow in the afternoon.
23d. Cloudy; sharp wind.
24th. Rain in the morning. Afternoon and evening misty.
25th. Pleasant and mild.
26th. Very mild and pleasant.
27th. Moderate rain in the morning. Mist in the afternoon and evening.
28th. Heavy mist through the day.
29th. Fine rain and mist in the morning. Began to snow from 2 to 3 P. M., with wind N. W. Snow continued through the evening.

January, 1855. New Moon, 18d. 3h. 30m. A. M.

DAYS.	Barometer Sunrise.	At 1 P. M.	At 10 P. M.	Thermometer Sunrise.	At 1 P. M.	At 10 P. M.	Daily mean.	Winds Sunrise.	At 1 P. M.	At 10 P. M.	Weather Sunrise.	At 1 P. M.	At 10 P. M.	Rain and Snow
1	...	...	30.40	...	...	19	...	...	...	N. W. 1	...	...	0	
2	30.52	30.58	30.57	17	25	22	21.3	N'ly 1	N. E. 2	N. E. 1	10	10	10	
3	30.56	30.51	30.41	24	38	34	32.0	E'ly 2	S. W. 2	S. W. 2	10	10	10	
4	30.39	30.29	30.23	35	42	39	38.7	S. W'ly 1	S. W. 2	S. W. 1	10	10	10	
5	30.33	30.42	30.64	39	40	30	36.3	N. W'ly 1	N. E. 2	N. E. 1	5	7	4	
6	30.65	30.64	30.56	24	29	28	27.0	N'ly 1	N. E. 2	N. E'ly 1	10	10	10	
S 7	30.35	30.27	30.24	32	54	47	44.3	S'ly 1	S. W. 1	S. W. 3	10	9	Rain	
8	30.54	30.58	30.59	36	39	29	34.7	N. W. 1	N. W. 1	N. W. 1	5	1	4	
9	30.44	30.25	30.08	29	38	33	33.3	N. E. 2	N. E. 2	N. W. 1	10	10	0	
10	30.08	30.16	30.21	30	29	14	24.3	N. W. 1	N. W. 2	N. W. 2	0	0	0	
11	30.13	29.91	29.69	14	31	34	26.3	N. W. 1	S'ly 1	S'ly 1	2	10	10	
12	29.54	29.57	29.59	33	37	34	34.7	S'ly 2	S. W. 2	S. W. 1	4	5	8	
13	...	...	...	...	...	...	...	...	...	...	...	...	...	
S 14	29.77	29.83	29.84	12	16	10	12.7	N. W. 4	N. W. 4	N. W. 3	0	0	7	
15	29.90	29.86	29.84	14	31	31	25.3	S. W. 1	S. W. 1	S. W'ly 1	8	10	10	
16	29.89	29.84	29.92	29	33	24	28.7	S. W. 1	N. E'ly 1	N. E. 2	10	Snow	Snow	
17	29.01	29.93	29.95	20	31	28	26.3	N. W'ly 2	N. E'ly 1	N. E. 1	5	10	10	0.15
18	29.68	29.41	29.30	35	40	33	36 0	N. E. 1	N. E. 1	N. E. 2	Rain	Rain	Rain	} 4.00
19	29.06	29.07	...	32	30	...	...	N. W. 2	N. W. 2	...	Snow	Snow	...	
20	...	...	29.62	...	...	32	...	...	...	N. W. 1	...	...	10	
S 21	29.70	29.77	29.67	26	32	32	30.0	N. W. 1	N. E. 2	N. E. 1	0	10	10	
22	29.20	29.09	29.60	46	46	28	40.0	S. W. 4	S'ly 3	S'ly 2	10	Rain	0	0.60
23	...	...	29.99	...	...	20	...	...	...	N. W. 1	...	...	0	
24	29.97	29.82	29.70	17	31	26	24.7	N. W. 1	E'ly 2	N. E. 2	6	10	Snow	
25	29.69	...	29.71	16	...	19	...	N. W. 2	...	N. W. 1	0	...	0	
26	29.61	29.19	28.82	23	32	33	29.3	E'ly 2	E'ly 4	W'ly 2	10	Snow	Rain	} 0.70
27	28.97	...	29.55	21	...	19	...	W'ly 3	...	W'ly 2	1	...	0	
S 28	29.81	29.77	29.70	21	35	36	30.7	S. W. 2	S. E. 2	S. E'ly 2	7	10	Rain	} 1.00
29	29.40	29.41	29.67	45	45	32	40.7	S'ly 3	S'ly 1	S. W. 2	10	Foggy	0	
30	29.72	...	...	25	...	...	...	S. W'ly 2	...	...	0	...	...	
31	29.73	...	...	22	...	...	...	W.	...	...	2	...	...	
Means	29.88	29.93	29.93	26.5	35.0	28.4	...	1.7	1.9	1.5	6.0	6.4	6.4	6.45
									1.7			6.9		
REDUCED TO SEA LEVEL.														
Max.	30.83	30.82	30.82	46	54	47	44.3							
Min.	29.15	29.25	29.00	12	16	10	12.7							
Mean	30.06	30.10	30.11											
Range	1.68	1.57	1.82	34	38	37	31.6							
Mean of month	30.090			...	...	...	30.0							
Extreme range	1.83			...	...	...	44.0							

Prevailing winds from some point between— Days
N. & E. 10
E. & S. 1
S. & W. 9
W. & N. 10

Days.
Clear 7
Variable . . . . } 12
Cloudy . . . . }
Rain or snow fell on 11
(1 day omitted.)

1st. Very pleasant.
2d. At 10 A. M., barometer 30.67. Appearances of storm in the evening.
3d. Cloudy and air rather raw, with appearances of storm.
4th. Cloudy, and very mild.
5th. Very fine for the season.
6th. Air raw, with appearances of storm.
7th. Very mild. Sprinkling of rain in the morning. Raining at 10 P. M.
8th. Very fine.
9th. Cloudy through the day. Clear at 10 P. M.
10th. Pleasant. Grew cold towards night.
11th. Flurry of snow from 2 to 4 P. M.
12th. Very mild.
14th. Very fine and cold.
15th. Flurry of snow from 11 A. M. to noon; air rather raw.
16th. Began to snow moderately from 11 A. M. to noon.
17th. About two inches of light snow on the ground this morning.
18th. Steady rain all day.
19th. Snow all day from the N. W.; quantity, from three to four inches on the level.
20th. Pleasant.
21st. Sprinkling of rain in the afternoon.
22d. Heavy rain in morning from S'ly. Evening clear, with wind W'ly.
23d. Very fine.
24th. Air raw in the afternoon. Began to snow from 5 to 6 P. M.
25th. Between four and five inches of dry snow on the ground this morning. The day very fine.
26th. Snow from the east all day; snow damp, and wind heavy. At 11 P. M., wind W'ly, and raining lightly.
27th. Very fine. Evening splendid.
28th. Air raw in the afternoon, with wind S'ly. Moderate rain in the morning.
29th. Heavy wind and heavy rain last night. Clouds and fog in the morning. Evening fine.
30th. Fine.
31st. Very fine. Evening splendid.

February, 1855. NEW MOON, 16^d. 1^h. 40^m. P. M.

DAYS	BAROMETER, REDUCED TO 32° F. Sunrise.	At 1 P. M.	At 10 P. M.	THERMOMETER. Sunrise.	At 1 P. M.	At 10 P. M.	Daily mean.	WINDS. (DIRECTION AND FORCE.) Sunrise.	At 1 P. M.	At 10 P. M.	WEATHER. (TENTHS CLOUDY.) Sunrise.	At 1 P. M.	At 10 P. M.	RAIN AND SNOW IN INCHES OF WATER.
1	...	...	...	23	28	20	23.7	N. W. 1	N. W. 1	N'ly	...	...	...	
2	...	...	...	15	30	32	25.7	N. W.	S. W.	S. E.	...	...	...	
3	29.43	...	...	25	30	17	24.0	W'ly 4	W'ly	S. W.	5	...	...	
S 4	29.56	29.51	...	14	19	...	...	W'ly 2	W by N. 3	...	7	10	...	
5	...	29.35	29.48	...	15	7	...	...	N. W. 1	N. W. 1	...	0	0	
6	29.70	29.72	29.93	—3	—7	—14	—8.0	N. W. 2	N. W. 1	N. W. 2	0	0	0	
7	30.00	30.02	29.87	—15	10	7	0.7	N. W. 1	N. E. 1	N. E. 2	0	10	Snow	
8	29.62	29.48	29.41	12	25	18	18.3	N. E'ly 2	N. E. 2	N. E. 2	10	Snow	Snow	1.25
9	29.46	29.54	29.63	16	18	14	16.0	N. E. 3	N. W. 2	N. E'ly 1	Snow	Snow	10	
10	29.74	29.88	29.96	13	22	10	15.0	N. W. 1	N. W. 1	N. W. 1	0	0	0	
S 11	29.91	29.82	29.87	4	29	23	18.7	N. W. 1	N. W. 1	N'ly 1	1	10	0	
12	29.97	30.07	30.15	14	27	18	19.7	N. W. 1	N. W. 1	N. W. 2	0	0	0	
13	30.19	30.18	30.20	16	33	22	23.7	N. W. 1	N. W. 1	N. W. 1	5	2	0	
14	30.08	29.97	29.74	26	38	36	33.3	E'ly 2	E'ly 2	N. E. 2	8	10	Rain	2.80
15	29.61	29.49	29.44	42	42	36	40.0	S. E'ly 2	N. E. 1	N. E. 1	Foggy	Rain	Misty	
16	29.44	29.48	29.56	36	39	36	37.0	N. E. 1	S. W. 1	S. W. 1	Foggy	10	10	
17	29.53	29.48	29.50	35	38	33	35.3	S. W. 1	N. W. 2	N. W. 3	10	10	10	
S 18	29.50	29.49	29.50	31	38	32	33.7	N. W'ly 3	N. W'ly 5	N. W'ly 3	1	1	3	
19	29.52	29.51	29.58	33	38	29	33.3	W by N 3	N. W'ly 3	N. W. 1	8	2	0	
20	29.62	29.56	29.66	31	38	28	32.3	N. W'ly 1	N by W 2	N by W. 3	10	4	10	
21	29.86	29.87	29.90	28	40	28	32.0	N. W. 2	N. W. 3	N. W. 2	3	3	0	
22	29.87	29.75	29.72	25	37	31	31.0	N. W. 1	N. W. 2	N. W. 1	0	0	2	
23	29.66	29.67	29.74	32	26	14	24.0	N. W. 2	N. W'ly 2	N. W. 1	10	10	0	
24	29.82	29.78	29.76	5	17	12	11.3	N. W. 2	N. W. 3	N. W. 2	0	0	0	
S 25	29.67	29.53	29.51	8	18	11	12.3	S. by W. 2	W by N 3	N. W'ly 2	0	2	2	
26	29.42	29.40	29.46	9	23	17	16.3	W. 2	W'ly 3	W'ly 2	0	3	8	
27	29.51	29.56	29.79	14	24	18	18.7	N. W. 2	N. W. 2	N. W. 1	7	0	0	
28	29.96	30.00	30.10	14	29	18	20.3	N. W. 2	N. W. 2	N. W. 1	0	0	0	
Means	29.71	29.68	29.73	18.6	27.3	20.5	...	1.8	1.9	1.6	4.6	4.7	4.0	4.05
									1.8			4.4		
REDUCED TO SEA LEVEL.														
Max.	30.37	30.36	30.38	42	42	36	40.0							
Min.	29.60	29.53	29.59	—15	—7	—14	—8.0							
Mean	29.89	29.86	29.91											
Range	0.77	0.83	0.79	57	49	50	32.0							
Mean of month	29.887			...	...	...	22.1							
Extreme range	0.85			...	...	...	57.0							

Prevailing winds from some point between— Days.
N. & E. 4
E. & S. 0
S. & W. 4
W. & N. 20

Days.
Clear 13
Variable . . . .} 7
Cloudy . . . . .}
Rain or snow fell on 8

REMARKS.

1st and 2d. Fair.
3d. Very fine.
4th. Pleasant.
5th. Snow in the morning. Clear and cold in the evening. Quantity of snow small.
6th. Wind light at about N. W., and cold intense. At 10 P. M., thermometer 14° below zero, which is one degree lower than any record at this station for twenty-four years.
7th. At sunrise, thermometer stood at 15° below zero; wind light at N. W. Began to snow from 5 to 6 P. M., with wind light at N. E.
8th. Cloudy in the morning. Snow in the afternoon and evening. At 4 P. M., thermometer 29°.
9th. Snow from N. E. nearly all day; quantity large, and considerably drifted—from twelve to fourteen inches deep on the level.
10th. Very fine.
11th. Cloudy in afternoon; air raw and chilly.
12th and 13th. Very fine.
14th. Began to rain moderately at 2 P. M.
15th. Rain nearly all day.
16th. Foggy in the morning. Cloudy in the afternoon; very mild.
17th. Cloudy. Showers of rain and snow.
18th. Very fine. Wind brisk at N. W.
19th. Very fine.
20th. Pleasant. Evening cloudy.
21st and 22d. Very fine.
23d. Cloudy in the morning. Flurry of snow from 2 to 4 P. M. Evening cooler, and mostly clear.
24th. Cold, but very fine.
25th. Wind brisk. Air very raw and cold.
26th. Air very raw and uncomfortable.
27th. Very fine.
28th. Very fine; nearly cloudless. Evening very clear.

March, 1855. NEW MOON, 17^d. 11^h. 37^m. P. M.

DAYS	Barometer Sunrise.	At 1 P. M.	At 10 P. M.	Thermometer Sunrise.	At 1 P. M.	At 10 P. M.	Daily mean.	Winds Sunrise.	At 1 P. M.	At 10 P. M.	Weather Sunrise.	At 1 P. M.	At 10 P. M.	Rain and Snow
1	30.18	30.12	30.14	13	32	24	23.0	N. W. 1	N. W. 1	S. W. 1	0	0	0	
2	30.12	30.05	29.99	18	39	24	27.0	N. W. 1	S. W. 1	S. W. 1	0	1	0	
3	29.85	29.69	29.63	22	43	36	33.7	S. W. 1	S. W. 1	S. W'ly 1	0	10	10	
S 4	29.69	29.77	29.99	33	41	31	35.0	W'ly 2	N. W. 2	N. W. 1	8	0	0	
5	29.81	29.61	29.37	33	49	42	41.3	S. W. 2	S. W. 3	S. W. 3	5	3	Rain	0.15
6	29.36	29.34	29.60	42	50	31	41.0	S. W. 2	N. W'ly 3	N. W. 1	5	2	2	
7	29.68	29.60	29.67	21	36	26	27.7	N. W. 2	N. E. 2	N. E. 1	3	9	2	
8	29.74	29.69	29.61	24	35	25	28.0	N'ly 1	N. W'ly 2	N. W. 1	9	2	0	
9	29.52	29.38	29.40	27	37	34	32.7	S. W. 2	S. W. 1	S. W. 1	9	10	Rain	0.10
10	29.45	29.40	29.49	26	31	26	27.7	N'ly 3	N'ly 3	N. W. 3	9	8	5	
S 11	29.64	29.55	29.59	26	38	31	31.7	N. W. 1	N. W. 1	N. W. 1	8	0	0	
12	29.60	29.67	29.90	30	35	28	31.0	N. W'ly 1	N'ly 2	N. E. 1	10	10	0	
13	29.96	29.92	29.66	25	37	32	31.3	N'ly 2	E'ly 2	E'ly 3	5	10	Rain	0.25
14	29.69	29.76	29.94	32	34	26	30.7	N. E. 1	N'ly 2	N'ly 2	Misty	5	10	
15	29.85	29.57	29.56	27	35	34	32.0	N. E. 1	E'ly 2	N. W'ly 1	Snow	Rain	0	
16	29.72	29.79	29.89	34	40	33	35.7	N. W'ly 2	N. W. 1	N. W. 1	8	10	0	
17	29.90	29.75	29.63	34	34	34	34.0	S'ly 1	E'ly 1	E'ly 1	10	Rain	Misty	0.45
S 18	29.72	29.75	29.83	34	43	34	37.0	W'ly 2	W'ly 1	N. W'ly 1	7	10	0	
19	29.85	29.86	29.87	27	42	30	33.0	N. W. 1	N. W'ly 1	S. E'ly 1	0	0	0	
20	29.75	29.70	29.84	33	41	28	34.0	S. W'ly 2	S. W. 4	N. W. 2	10	9	0	
21	29.87	29.91	29.99	22	37	27	28.7	N. W. 2	N. W. 2	N. W. 1	0	0	0	
22	29.99	29.78	29.67	27	37	28	30.7	N. W. 2	N. E. 2	N. W. 1	8	10	5	
23	29.60	29.36	29.21	22	38	35	31.7	N. W. 2	S. W. 3	S. W. 3	0	10	10	
24	29.28	29.08	29.30	34	35	17	28.7	S. W. 2	S. W. 3	N. W. 3	3	10	0	
S 25	29.39	29.38	29.43	18	32	28	26.0	N. W. 2	N. W. 3	N. W. 1	8	2	4	
26	29.53	29.44	29.28	24	44	34	34.0	W'ly 2	S. W. 3	N. E. 1	10	10	Snow	
27	29.27	29.26	29.45	28	38	26	30.7	N. W. 1	W'ly 2	N. W. 2	1	5	1	
28	29.53	29.50	29.52	24	37	26	29.0	N. W. 3	N. W. 3	N. W. 2	5	3	0	
29	29.53	29.48	29.64	26	41	35	34.0	N. W. 2	N. W. 3	N. W. 1	3	2	0	
30	29.65	29.65	29.74	32	57	47	45.3	N. W. 1	W. by S. 2	W'ly 1	5	0	Hazy	
31	29.75	29.66	29.53	35	55	42	44.0	S. W. 2	S'ly 2	S'ly 1	5	2	5	
Means	29.69	29.63	29.66	27.5	39.4	30.8	...	1.7	2.1	1.5	5.6	5.5	3.3	0.85
									1.8			4.8		
REDUCED TO SEA LEVEL.														
Max.	30.36	30.30	30.32	42	57	47	45.3							
Min.	29.46	29.26	29.39	13	31	17	23.0							
Mean	29.87	29.81	29.84											
Range	0.90	1.04	0.93	29	26	30	22.3							
Mean of month	29.840			...	...	...	32.6							
Extreme range	1.10			...	...	...	44.0							

Prevailing winds from some point between— Days.
N. & E. 6
E. & S. 1
S. & W. 8
W. & N. 16

Days.
Clear 7
Variable . . . .} 17
Cloudy . . . . .}
Rain or snow fell on 7

REMARKS.

1st and 2d. Very fine.
3d. Pleasant in the morning. Air raw in the afternoon.
4th. Very fine.
5th. Very blustering and dusty in the morning. Began to rain from 8 to 2 P. M.
6th. Fine.
7th. Air raw and uncomfortable.
8th. Very fine.
9th. Cloudy. Began to rain very gently from 7 to 8 P. M.
10th. Ground covered with snow this morning. Weather very blustering and uncomfortable.
11th. Pleasant. Evening very fine.
12th. Cloudy and raw in the morning. Aurora in the evening, and clear.
13th. Cloudy. Began to snow at 5 P. M., with wind E'ly. Snow turned to rain in the evening.
14th. Air raw and uncomfortable, with occasional rain and hail.
15th. Snowing at sunrise, and ground covered with snow. Rain and drizzle in the afternoon. Evening clear.
16th. Pleasant. Evening very fine.
17th. Began to snow very moderately from 8 to 9 A. M. Snow, rain, and mist in the afternoon.
18th. Pleasant.
19th. Very fine.
20th. Air very raw and uncomfortable.
21st. Cold, but fine.
22d. Pleasant, but cold.
23d. Air very raw and uncomfortable. Appearances of storm in the evening.
24th. Air very raw. Snow in the air in the afternoon. Very cold in the evening.
25th. Wintry cold.
26th. Air raw and uncomfortable. Moderate snow from N. E. in the evening.
27th. Ground covered with snow this morning.
28th. Wind very blustering and cold.
29th. Day blustering. Evening still and splendid.
30th. Very fine. At 1 P. M., thermometer 57°, being the highest point reached since Nov. 26, 1854—a period of 124 days. A bright circle about the moon in the evening.
31st. Very fine. Hazy in the evening. Circle about the moon.

April, 1855. New Moon, 16d. 9h. 57m. P. M.

DAYS.	Barometer, reduced to 32° F. At 6 A. M.	At 2 P. M.	At 10 P. M.	Thermometer. At 6 A. M.	At 2 P. M.	At 10 P. M.	Daily mean.	Winds. (Direction and Force.) At 6 A. M.	At 2 P. M.	At 10 P. M.	Weather. (Tenths Cloudy.) At 6 A. M.	At 2 P. M.	At 10 P. M.	Rain and Snow in Inches of Water
S 1	29.09	28.74	29.05	42	43	24	36.3	N'ly 1	N. W. 3	N. W. 5	Rain	10	0	1.20
2	29.17	29.11	29.39	18	30	27	25.0	N. W. 4	N. W. 4	N. W. 3	0	10	8	
3	29.62	29.67	30.02	24	38	31	31.0	N. W. 2	N. W. 3	N. W. 1	0	0	3	
4	30.14	30.09	30.11	28	51	35	38.0	N. W. 2	S. W. 2	S. W'ly 1	0	2	2	
5	30.00	29.88	29.54	35	51	42	42.7	S. W'ly 1	S. E'ly 2	E'ly 1	5	10	Rain	0.50
6	29.28	29.34	29.44	40	57	46	47.7	N'ly 1	N. W'ly 1	S'ly 1	10	4	10	
7	29.47	29.55	29.69	38	46	34	39.3	N. W. 1	N. W. 2	N. W. 1	10	0	2	
S 8	29.77	29.72	29.82	28	46	34	36.0	N. W. 1	S. W'ly 2	N. W. 1	0	0	0	
9	29.80	29.77	29.82	34	49	38	40.3	N. W. 1	S'ly 2	N. W. 1	3	10	0	
10	29.90	29.84	29.58	34	49	39	40.7	E'ly 1	S. E'ly 2	E'ly 2	2	10	Rain	
11	29.49	29.48	29.47	36	41	36	37.7	N. W'ly	N. W. 3	N. W. 2	10	10	Sprin'le	
12	29.60	29.70	29.85	36	45	38	39.7	N. W. 2	N. W. 4	N. W. 1	10	10	0	
13	29.91	29.89	29.96	36	51	41	42.9	N. W. 1	N. W. 2	N. E. 1	0	3	5	
14	29.89	29.72	29.63	38	47	42	42.3	E'ly 1	S. E'ly 2	W'ly 1	10	Sprin'le	0	
S 15	29.73	29.72	29.78	46	52	42	46.7	S. W'ly 1	S. W. 1	S. W. 1	10	10	0	
16	29.92	29.97	30.04	39	60	47	48.7	S. W. 1	S'ly 2	S'ly 1	0	0	0	
17	30.04	30.01	29.95	44	67	46	52.3	S'ly 1	S. W. 3	S. W. 2	0	8	Rain	
18	29.85	29.77	29.68	49	74	51	58.0	S'ly 2	S. W. 1	W'ly 1	5	9	0	
19	29.54	29.51	29.70	51	76	47	58.0	S. W'ly 1	W'ly 2	N. E. 2	7	10	10	
20	29.67	29.54	29.75	41	39	36	38.7	N. E. 2	N. E. 2	N. E. 2	Misty	Rain	Rain	0.80
21	30.01	29.99	29.99	38	59	45	47.7	S. W. 1	N. W. 1	S'ly 2	0	0	0	
S 22	29.94	29.87	29.86	43	60	50	51.0	S. W. 2	S. W. 2	S. W. 1	3	10	5	
23	30.00	29.91	30.05	45	60	40	48.3	S. W. 1	S. E'ly 2	S'ly 2	0	0	0	
24	29.97	29.86	29.77	41	70	54	55.0	S. W. 1	S. W. 2	S. W. 1	0	3	10	
25	29.72	29.88	30.04	54	65	44	54.3	S. W. 1	N. E. 2	N. E. 2	6	10	8	
26	29.98	29.76	29.60	44	46	49	46.3	N. E. 2	S. E. 2	W'ly 2	10	10	9	
27	29.71	29.79	29.95	42	56	41	46.3	N. W. 2	N. W. 4	N. W. 2	3	3	0	
28	30.01	29.95	30.00	38	54	45	45.7	N. W. 2	N. W. 2	N. W. 1	0	0	Hazy	
S 29	30.10	30.03	30.01	38	43	38	39.7	N. E'ly 1	S. E'ly 2	S. E'ly 1	Snow	Misty	Misty	
30	30.02	29.98	29.81	40	49	48	45.7	E'ly 1	E'ly 2	E'ly 1	Misty	10	10	
Means	29.78	29.73	29.78	38.7	52.5	41.0	...	1.4	2.2	1.5	4.5	6.4	5.1	2.50
								1.7			5.3			
REDUCED TO SEA LEVEL.								Prevailing winds from some point between—		Days.			Days.	
Max.	30.32	30.27	30.29	54	76	54	58.0							
Min.	29.27	28.92	29.23	18	30	24	25.0							
Mean	29.96	29.91	29.96					N. & E.		3	Clear		8	
Range	1.05	1.35	1.06	36	46	30	33.0	E. & S.		5	Variable }		8	
Mean of month	29.943			...	...	...	44.1	S. & W.		9	Cloudy }			
Extreme range	1.40			...	...	...	58.0	W. & N.		13	Rain or snow fell on		14	

REMARKS.

1st. Rain in the morning, with wind light N'ly. Barometer very low; at 1 P. M., it stood at 28.83. At 3 P. M., clouds broken, and wind blustering at N. W. Evening clear and cold, and wind violent.

2d. Very cold for the season, and extremely blustering; few days during the winter more severe and uncomfortable to be out.

3d. More pleasant, but still blustering.

4th. Pleasant.

5th. Pleasant in the morning. Cloudy in the afternoon, with light rain towards night.

6th and 7th. Pleasant.

8th. Very fine. Evening clear.

9th. Sprinkling of rain in the afternoon. Evening clear.

10th. Pleasant in the morning. Began to rain in the evening.

11th. Air raw. Sprinkling of rain in evening.

12th. Cloudy through the day. Evening clear; aurora in the north, accompanied with streamers.

13th. Pleasant.

14th. Sprinkling of rain in the afternoon. Evening mostly clear.

15th. Sprinkling of rain in morning and afternoon. Evening clear.

16th. Very fine.

17th. Pleasant and warm in morning. Cloudy towards night; sprinkling of rain in the evening.

18th. Very warm; prevalence of thin clouds and haze. Sprinkling at 2 P. M. Frequent lightning at the north in the evening. Venus was occulted by the moon, near the western horizon, at 8 h. 46 m. 56 s. P. M., mean time at Providence.

19th. Sprinkling of rain at 2 P. M. Appearances of storm in the evening.

20th. Moderate rain nearly all day.

21st. Very fine.

22d. Broken clouds, with occasional sprinkling of rain.

23d and 24th. Very fine.

25th. Air warm and sultry in the morning; wind S. W. Cooler in the afternoon, with wind N. E.

26th. Cloudy in the morning, with sprinkling of rain. Heavy mist in the afternoon.

27th. Blustering through the day. Evening very fine and clear.

28th. Cool, but pleasant.

29th. Air full of snow from 6 to 8 A. M. Mist in the afternoon and evening.

30th. Cool and misty.

May, 1855. New Moon, 15d. 9h. 5m. P. M.

DAYS.	Barometer At 6 A. M.	At 1 P. M.	At 10 P. M.	Thermometer At 6 A. M.	At 1 P. M.	At 10 P. M.	Daily mean.	Winds At 6 A. M.	At 2 P. M.	At 10 P. M.	Weather At 6 A. M.	At 2 P. M.	At 10 P. M.	Rain
1	29.65	29.68	29.90	45	61	43	49.7	Nl'y 1	N. W. 1	N. E. 3	10	10	10	
2	30.00	29.92	29.94	43	63	44	50.0	N'ly 1	N. W. 1	E'ly 2	10	0	10	
3	29.96	29.85	29.72	40	61	43	48.0	N'ly 2	N'ly 2	N. W. 1	2	4	0	
4	29.64	29.58	29.61	44	60	45	49.7	N'ly 2	N. W. 2	N. E. 2	1	6	Rain	
5	29.59	29.57	29.63	46	63	53	54.0	N'ly 1	N. E. 2	N. W'ly 1	5	10	0	
S 6	29.59	29.46	29.50	54	69	53	58.7	N. W. 2	N. W. 2	N. W. 2	2	5	0	
7	29.66	29.61	29.59	43	60	43	48.7	N. W. 1	N. W. 1	S'ly 2	4	3	2	
8	29.60	29.53	29.42	40	41	40	40.3	N. E. 2	E'ly 4	N. E. 4	9	Rain	Rain	} 1.10
9	29.58	29.66	29.83	41	38	35	38.0	N. E. 4	N. E. 4	N. E. 3	Misty	Rain	Rain	
10	29.81	29.80	29.82	38	53	40	43.7	N'ly 2	N. W. 2	N. W. 1	9	0	0	
11	29.76	29.71	29.75	43	66	46	51.7	N. W. 1	N. W. 2	N. W. 1	5	3	2	
12	29.74	29.74	29.77	47	69	46	54.0	S'ly 1	S'ly 1	S. E'ly 1	5	4	2	
S 13	29.85	29.84	29.87	46	67	51	54.7	S'ly	S. by E. 1	S'ly 1	2	0	0	
14	29.74	29.72	29.77	50	69	61	60.0	S'ly 1	S. W'ly 2	N. W. 1	Foggy	10	10	
15	29.84	29.77	29.68	55	77	64	65.3	N. W. 1	S. W. 2	S. W'ly 1	8	5	2	
16	29.64	29.55	29.58	65	78	62	68.3	S. W. 1	S. W. 3	S. W. 2	Hazy	5	10	
17	29.62	29.70	29.85	53	66	53	57.3	S. W'ly 1	S'ly 2	N. W. 1	Sprin'le	0	0	0.35
18	29.95	29.95	29.94	51	66	52	56.3	N. W. 1	N. W. 2	S. E'ly 2	0	5	2	
19	29.84	29.75	29.70	54	62	48	54.7	S'ly 2	S. E'ly 2	N. E. 2	5	10	Rain	
S 20	29.38	29.38	29.40	51	52	50	51.0	N. E. 3	N. E. 3	N. E. 2	10	Rain	10	0.50
21	29.42	29.46	29.48	47	53	46	48.7	N. W. 2	N. W. 3	N. W. 1	3	8	10	
22	29.56	29.60	29.59	46	47	44	45.7	N. W. 2	N. E. 2	N. E. 2	10	Misty	10	
23	29.70	29.73	29.86	50	65	48	54.3	N. W. 2	N. W. 3	E'ly 1	7	3	0	
24	29.78	29.71	29.73	50	75	61	62.0	S'ly 2	S. E'ly 3	S'ly	8	8	Rain	0.60
25	29.72	29.71	29.75	60	74	59	64.3	N. W. 1	N. W. 2	N. W. 2	10	5	0	
26	29.75	29.72	29.77	52	57	50	53.0	N. W. 2	N. W. 2	N. W. 1	0	0	0	
S 27	29.76	29.62	29.64	48	68	55	57.0	N. W. 2	N. W. 2	N. W. 1	0	0	2	
28	29.80	29.83	29.96	52	67	50	56.3	N. W. 1	S'ly 2	S'ly 2	0	2	2	
29	29.97	30.03	30.05	53	66	52	57.0	S'ly 1	S. E'ly 3	S'ly 2	3	1	1	
30	30.05	30.03	30.05	55	76	61	64.0	S'ly 2	S. W. 3	S. W. 2	2	0	2	
31	30.07	30.01	30.01	62	78	60	66.7	S'ly 2	S. W. 3	S. W. 2	3	2	3	
Means	29.74	29.72	29.75	49.2	63.5	50.3	...	1.6	2.2	1.7	5.9	4.8	4.5	2.55
								1.8			5.1			
REDUCED TO SEA LEVEL.								Prevailing winds from some point between		Days.			Days.	
Max.	30.25	30.21	30.23	65	78	64	68.3							
Min.	29.56	29.56	29.58	38	41	35	38.0							
Mean	29.92	29.90	29.93					N. & E.		4	Clear		11	
Range	0.69	0.65	0.65	27	37	29	30.3	E. & S.		5	Variable }		10	
Mean of month	29.917			...	...	...	54.5	S. & W.		8	Cloudy }			
Extreme range	0.69			...	...	...	43.0	W. & N.		14	Rain fell on		10	

1st. Clouds. Appearances of storm in evening.

2d. Pleasant at mid-day. Air raw in evening.

3d. Pleasant.

4th. Cold and unpleasant. Light rain in the evening.

5th. Clouds, with occasional light sprinklings. Evening clear.

6th. Very fine, but dry, and the air filled with dust.

7th. Pleasant. Windy and cool in afternoon.

8th. Began to rain from 11 A. M. to noon. Storm heavy from N. E. in the afternoon and evening.

9th. Moderate rain, with occasional mixture of snow all day. Wind heavy at N. E.

10th. Very fine.

11th. Pleasant.

12th. Very pleasant. Air cool S. E'ly towards evening.

13th. Pleasant; air hazy.

14th. Mild and pleasant. Sprinkling of rain from 3 to 4 P. M.

15th. Very warm; air thick and hazy near the horizon.

16th. Very warm. Wind blustering in the afternoon, and the air full of dust.

17th. Rain last night. Evening splendid.

18th. Very fine.

19th. Began to rain quite moderately at 6 P. M.

20th. Light rain last night and through the day.

21st. Quite cool for the season.

22d. Very cold for the season. Cloudy, with occasional mist and sprinkling.

23d. Cool. Evening very clear.

24th. Mostly cloudy in the morning. Heavy thunder and rain from 8 to 10 P. M.

25th. Pleasant.

26th. Very fine.

27th. Very fine; nearly cloudless through day.

28th. Very fine.

29th and 30th. Fine.

31st. Fine; sun hot.

June, 1855. New Moon, 14d. 9h. 21m. A. M.

Days	Barometer, reduced to 32° F. At 6 A. M.	At 1 P. M.	At 10 P. M.	Thermometer. At 6 A. M.	At 1 P. M.	At 10 P. M.	Daily mean.	Winds (Direction and Force.) At 6 A. M.	At 1 P. M.	At 10 P. M.	Weather (Tenths Cloudy.) At 6 A. M.	At 1 P. M.	At 10 P. M.	Rain and Snow in Inches of Water.
1	29.91	29.86	29.84	62	77	63	67.3	S. W. 2	S. W. 4	S. W. 3	10	8	10	
2	29.80	29.77	29.79	65	75	62	67.3	S. W. 3	S. W. 3	S. W. 3	Misty	Sprin'l	10	0.60
S 3	29.68	29.68	29.59	64	63	59	62.0	S. E. 4	S. E. 3	S. E. 4	10	Rain	Rain	}
4	29.54	29.52	...	61	69	...	...	S. E. 3	S. E. 2	...	Misty	4	...	
5	29.64	29.63	29.69	50	70	56	58.7	N. W. 2	N. W. 3	N. W. 1	0	3	8	
6	29.75	29.74	29.76	57	74	62	64.3	N. W. 1	W byN. 2	W'ly 1	0	8	10	
7	29.67	29.42	29.25	62	63	63	62.7	S. W'ly 1	S'ly 1	S. W. 4	Sprin'le	10	10	0.15
8	29.25	29.37	29.58	58	73	55	62.0	N. W. 2	W'ly 2	N. W. 1	5	3	0	
9	29.60	29.60	29.62	55	70	59	61.3	N. W. 1	...	N. W. 2	2	2	0	
S 10	29.57	29.47	29.50	63	74	62	66.3	S'ly 2	S. W. 3	S. W'ly 2	10	10	0	
11	29.29	29.37	29.63	63	74	55	64.0	S. W. 1	S. W. 3	N. W. 1	10	0	0	
12	29.67	29.71	29.81	57	68	51	58.7	S. W. 2	S. W. 2	N. W. 1	10, Spr.	7	0	
13	29.83	29.81	29.79	48	68	56	57.3	N. W. 1	N. E. 2	S. W. 1	3	2	0	
14	29.71	29.63	29.72	58	74	54	62.0	N. W. 2	N. W. 2	S'ly 1	2	10	0	
15	29.53	...	29.54	54	72	59	61.7	S. W. 2	S. W. 2	S. W. 1	8	3	10	
16	29.57	29.48	29.61	55	76	62	64.3	N. W. 1	S'ly 1	S. W. 1	0	10	10	
S 17	29.48	29.78	29.84	63	74	58	65.0	N. W. 1	W'ly 2	S. W'ly 1	0	0	0	
18	29.94	29.93	29.96	54	74	55	61.0	N by W 1	N. E. 1	N. E. 1	0	1	0	
19	29.95	29.84	29.75	55	70	56	60.3	N. E. 1	N. E'ly 1	N. E. 1	Hazy	10	Rain	
20	29.70	29.63	29.64	57	74	62	64.3	E'ly 1	S. W'ly 1	N. W. 1	10	8	0	
21	29.62	29.67	29.73	62	78	64	68.0	N. W. 1	N. W. 2	N. W. 1	0	0	0	
22	29.72	29.68	29.58	65	74	66	68.3	S'ly 2	S. W. 3	S'ly 1	3	4	Misty	
23	29.72	29.80	29.85	67	78	68	71.0	N. W. 1	N. E. 2	N. E. 1	2	7	1	
S 24	29.84	29.78	29.71	69	72	64	68.3	S'ly 1	S. E'ly 2	S. E'ly 1	6	10	Rain	0.20
25	29.66	29.67	29.77	64	76	68	69.3	S'ly 1	S. E'ly 1	S. E'ly 1	Foggy	10	10	
26	29.84	...	29.85	68	...	70	...	S'ly 2	...	S. W. 2	10	...	10	
27	29.94	29.94	29.95	71	86	72	76.3	N. W. 1	W'ly 2	S. W. 2	0	0	0	
28	29.86	29.76	29.75	76	80	69	75.0	S. E. 2	S. W. 1	W'ly 1	8	Rain	1	0.30
29	29.73	29.65	28.61	70	90	78	79.3	N. W. 2	W byN 2	W'ly 1	2	2	5	
30	29.62	29.65	28.66	78	95	72	81.7	N. W. 1	W'ly 1	W'ly 1	2	5	2	0.70
Means	29.69	29.67	29.70	61.7	72.0	62.1	...	1.6	2.0	1.5	5.5	5.5	4.6	1.95
									1.7			5.2		
REDUCED TO SEA LEVEL.														
Max.	30.13	30.12	30.14	78	95	78	81.7							
Min.	29.43	29.55	29.43	48	63	51	57.3							
Mean	29.87	29.85	29.88											
Range	0.70	0.57	0.71	30	32	27	24.4							
Mean of month	29.867			...	...	...	65.2							
Extreme range	0.71			...	...	...	47.0							

Prevailing winds from some point between— Days.
N. & E. 4
E. & S. 5
S. & W. 11
W. & N. 10

Days.
Clear 7
Variable . . . } 7
Cloudy . . . . }
Rain fell on . . 16

REMARKS.

1st. Very dusty in the morning. Sprinkling of rain from 6 to 7 P. M.
2d. Cloudy, with occasional showers.
3d. Copious rain through the day.
4th. Pleasant.
5th and 6th. Very fine.
7th. Sprinkling of rain in the morning. Cloudy in the afternoon and evening, with wind strong at S. W. Showers during the night.
8th and 9th. Very fine.
10th. Sprinkling of rain early this morning.
11th. Pleasant.
12th. Sprinkling of rain in the morning. Evening splendid.
13th. Pleasant, but cool for the season.
14th. Pleasant.
15th. Pleasant. Dash of rain from 7 to 8 P. M.
16th. Variable. Sprinkling of rain from 7 to 8 P. M.
17th and 18th. Very fine.
19th. Sprinkling of rain in the afternoon and evening.
20th. Sprinkling and mist in morning. Evening clear.
21st. Very fine.
22d. Fine in the morning. Cloudy in the afternoon. Heavy mist and light rain in the evening.
23d. Very fine.
24th. Cloudy in the morning. Light rain in the afternoon and evening.
25th. Fog and clouds. Brisk shower from 5 to 6 P. M.
26th. Cloudy all day; occasional light showers.
27th. Very fine. Warmest day since Aug. 25, 1854. Thermometer 86° on both days.
28th. Light showers through the day. Thunder from 5 to 6 P. M.
29th. Very hot and uncomfortable.
30th. Excessively hot in the morning. At 1 P. M., 95° in the shade. Heavy shower from 4 to 6 P. M.

July, 1855. New Moon, 13d. 7h. 53m. P. M.

Days	Barometer At 6 A. M.	At 1 P. M.	At 10 P. M.	Thermometer At 6 A. M.	At 1 P. M.	At 10 P. M.	Daily mean.	Winds At 6 A. M.	At 1 P. M.	At 10 P. M.	Weather At 6 A. M.	At 1 P. M.	At 10 P. M.	Rain
S 1	29.68	29.64	29.65	76	93	76	81.7	S. W'ly 1	W'ly 2	Calm	1	0	0	
2	29.66	29.65	29.64	76	90	74	80.0	S. W. 1	S. W. 3	S. W. 1	0	0	0	
3	29.86	29.88	29.91	72	86	66	74.7	N. W. 1	N. W. 2	N. W. 1	5	3	0	
4	29.91	29.86	29.85	68	81	72	73.7	S. E'ly 1	S'ly 2	S. W. 2	0	10	3	
5	29.84	29.83	29.88	70	87	70	75.7	S. W. 1	S. W. 2	S. W. 1	10	8	2	0.25
6	29.90	29.83	29.77	71	78	70	73.0	S. W. 2	S. W. 2	S. W. 1	10	Rain	Rain	1.60
7	29.73	29.62	29.73	70	73	63	68.7	N. E. 2	N. E. 1	N. E. 2	Rain	Rain	Rain	}
S 8	29.76	29.86	29.98	60	73	62	65.0	N'ly 2	N. W. 1	N. W. 1	10	5	0	
9	30.07	30.01	29.99	61	76	61	66.0	N. W. 1	S. W. 1	S. W. 1	0	0	0	
10	29.92	29.86	29.80	63	77	65	68.3	S. W. 1	S. W. 2	S. W. 1	5	4	0	
11	29.75	29.71	29.70	64	74	66	68.0	S. W. 1	S. W. 1	S. W. 1	10	10	0	0.15
12	29.71	29.70	29.72	70	82	68	73.3	S'ly 1	S'ly 2	S. W. 1	5	0	Foggy	
13	29.68	29.62	29.62	70	85	73	76.0	S. W. 1	S. W. 2	S. W. 1	10	4	Sprin'le	
14	29.70	29.75	29.91	70	81	69	73.3	N. W. 1	N. E. 2	N. E. 1	0	3	6	
S 15	30.06	30.05	30.09	71	83	64	72.7	N. E. 1	E'ly 1	S'ly 1	0	2	0	
16	30.09	30.05	30.02	62	80	70	70.7	N. E. 1	S'ly 2	S'ly 2	5	3	10	
17	29.96	29.84	29.80	74	90	76	80.0	S. E'ly 1	S. W'ly 2	Calm	3	1	0	
18	29.82	29.76	29.76	78	90	76	81.3	S'ly 1	S. W. 2	W'ly 1	7	6	0, Sh'r	0.15
19	29.66	29.58	29.61	78	95	81	84.7	S'ly 1	W'ly 2	W'ly 1	2	3	0	
20	29.73	29.78	29.88	75	68	65	68.3	N. E. 2	N. E. 2	N. E. 1	7	10	Rain	0.30
21	29.88	29.88	29.94	61	68	61	63.3	N. E. 2	N. E. 2	N. E. 2	Sprin'le	10	Sprin'le	
S 22	29.98	29.97	29.99	62	74	61	65.7	N. E. 2	N. E. 2	N. E. 1	1	8	3	
23	29.97	...	...	63	...	...	...	N. E. 1	...	...	10	...	...	0.20
24	29.92	29.90	29.84	67	70	68	68.3	S. E. 1	S. E. 1	S. W. 1	10	Misty	Misty	
25	29.78	29.73	29.72	74	87	80	80.3	S. W. 1	W. 1	0	7	5	8	
26	29.74	29.68	29.64	76	86	74	78.7	Calm	S. E. 1	E'ly 1	8	9	Sprin'le	0.65
27	29.57	29.67	29.73	75	78	67	73.3	N. W. 2	N. E'ly 3	N. E. 2	0	8	10	
28	29.78	29.77	29.77	67	76	68	70.3	N. E. 1	N. E. 1	S'ly 1	10	10	7	
S 29	29.77	29.76	29.78	67	73	69	69.7	S. E. 1	N. E. 1	Calm	Rain	10	10	0.15
30	29.78	29.75	29.72	68	80	72	73.3	N. E. 1	N. E. 1	S'ly 1	10	5	8	
31	29.73	29.72	29.80	72	78	72	74.0	S'ly 1	S. W. 2	S. W'ly 1	10	Shower	2	0.10
Means	29.82	29.79	29.81	69.4	80.4	69.0	...	1.2	1.7	1.2	6.0	5.9	5.0	3.25
									1.4			5.6		
REDUCED TO SEA LEVEL.														
Max.	30.27	30.23	30.27	78	95	81	84.7							
Min.	29.75	29.76	29.79	60	68	61	63.3							
Mean	30.00	29.97	29.99											
Range	0.52	0.47	0.48	18	27	20	21.4							
Mean of month	29.987			...	...	...	72.9							
Extreme range	0.52			...	...	...	35.0							

Prevailing winds from some point between— Days.
N. & E. 12
E. & S. 3
S. & W. 14
W. & N. 2

Days.
Clear 8
Variable . . . } 9
Cloudy . . . . }
Rain fell on . . 14

REMARKS.

1st. Very hot. Air fresh at mid-day. Evening perfectly calm and cloudless.
2d. Very warm, with a fresh breeze.
3d. Very fine.
4th. Very fine. Air extremely damp in the evening.
5th. Copious showers from 4 to 5 A. M. Cloudy for the most part during the day; air damp.
6th. Sprinkling of rain in the afternoon. Light shower in the evening.
7th. Heavy showers at intervals during day.
8th. Cloudy in the morning. Pleasant in the afternoon. Evening clear.
9th and 10th. Very fine.
11th. Light showers at intervals during day. Evening clear.
12th. Pleasant. Sprinkling of rain from 5 to 6 P. M.
13th. Sun scorching hot and air damp. Sprinkling of rain from 9 to 10 P. M.
14th. Pleasant.
15th. Very fine. Evening very clear.
16th. Pleasant.
17th. Very hot and sultry. Evening cloudless.
18th. Very hot and sultry. Brisk shower from 2 to 3 P. M.
19th. Intensely hot. From 1 to 2 P. M., thermometer 95° in the shade, exposed to a brisk current of air; at 6 P. M., 89°; at 10 P. M., 81°—being the hottest day since July 13, 1849, when the same thermometer, in the same place, rose to 97°.
20th. Heavy shower from 10 to 11 A. M. Light shower in the afternoon and evening.
21st. Occasional sprinkling of rain. Very cool.
22d. Pleasant.
23d. Pleasant in the morning. Light shower in the afternoon.
24th. Showery in the morning. Drizzling in the afternoon and evening
25th. Sultry and oppressive.
26th. Heat oppressive in the morning. Shower in the afternoon.
27th. Variable; sunshine and clouds.
28th. Cloudy for the most part.
29th. Light rain in the morning. Cloudy and rather sultry in the afternoon and evening.
30th. Cloudy and sultry.
31st. Cloudy in the morning. Light shower from 1 to 2 P. M. Evening pleasant.

August, 1855. New Moon, 12d. 1h. 46m. P. M.

Days.	Barometer, reduced to 32° F. At 6 A. M.	At 1 P. M.	At 10 P. M.	Thermometer. At 6 A. M.	At 1 P. M.	At 10 P. M.	Daily mean.	Winds. (Direction and Force.) At 6 A. M.	At 1 P. M.	At 10 P. M.	Weather. (Tenths Cloudy.) At 6 A. M.	At 1 P. M.	At 10 P. M.	Rain and Snow in Inches of Water.
1	29.85	29.84	29.91	72	84	67	74.3	N. E. 1	N. E. 2	N. E. 1	5	5	2	
2	29.93	29.95	29.98	67	83	66	72.0	N. E. 1	N. E. 2	N. E'ly 1	10	5	0	
3	30.01	29.96	29.97	66	77	66	69.7	S. W. 1	S. W. 2	S. W. 1	0	1	0	
4	29.78	29.64	29.69	64	84	69	72.3	S. W. 1	S. W. 2	S. W. 1	0	2	Rain	0.62
S 5	29.71	29.67	29.65	65	74	66	68.3	N. E. 2	N. E. 2	N. E. 1	3	5	10	
6	29.59	29.58	29.69	62	81	64	69.0	N. W. 1	N. W. 2	N. W. 1	3	5	0	0.20
7	29.81	...	...	62	...	...	...	N. W. 1	...	...	0	...	...	
8	...	...	...	...	...	...	...	...	...	...	...	...	...	} 1.20
9	...	...	29.20	...	...	78	...	...	...	S. W. 3	...	...	3	
10	...	29.38	29.61	...	76	62	...	...	W'ly 2	N. W. 1	...	2	0	
11	29.82	29.88	30.04	57	74	57	62.7	N. W. 2	N. E. 1	N. E. 1	0	3	0	
S 12	29.98	30.08	30.02	56	74	59	63.0	E'ly 1	E'ly 1	E'ly 1	3	2	0	
13	29.80	29.84	29.82	58	78	60	68.3	S. W'ly 1	S. W. 2	W'ly 1	6	10	2	
14	29.85	29.88	29.93	67	80	65	70.7	N. W. 1	N. W. 1	N. W. 1	3	2	0	
15	29.94	29.93	29.81	63	77	67	69.0	N. W. 1	S. W. 2	S. W. 1	1	5	2	
16	29.73	29.63	29.63	71	84	74	76.3	S. W. 2	S. W. 3	S. W. 1	10	4	10	
17	29.53	29.54	29.74	75	91	66	77.3	S. W. 2	S. W. 3	N. W. 2	8	6	0	
18	...	29.94	29.99	...	70	54	...	...	N. W. 2	N. W. 2	...	5	0	
S 19	30.10	30.10	30.15	53	70	55	59.3	N. W. 1	N. W. 2	N. W. 1	0	2	0	
20	30.21	30.14	30.13	57	74	66	65.7	W'ly 1	S. W'ly 2	S. W. 1	0	10	0	
21	30.09	30.02	30.03	60	78	61	66.3	S. W. 2	S. W. 2	S. W. 1	2	0	0	
22	29.98	29.93	29.90	63	83	70	72.0	S. W. 1	S. W. 2	S. W. 1	5	7	Sprin'le	
23	29.74	29.63	29.59	72	83	73	76.0	S. W. 1	S. W. 2	S. W. 1	10	10	10	
24	29.60	29.59	29.73	73	86	70	76.3	N. W. 1	N. W. 2	N. W. 1	0	2	0	
25	29.88	29.93	30.01	68	79	60	69.0	N. W. 1	N. W. 2	N. E'ly 1	0	3	0	
S 26	29.96	29.91	29.80	60	70	68	66.0	N. E. 1	S. E. 1	S'ly 1	7	Rain	10	
27	29.89	29.95	29.97	60	63	51	58.0	N. E. 2	N. E. 3	N. E. 2	10	10	8	
28	29.94	29.78	29.94	48	67	51	55.3	N. E. 1	N. E. 1	N. E. 2	0	0	0	
29	29.87	...	29.71	60	...	59	...	E. N. E. 2	...	S. W. 2	0	...	2	
30	29.73	...	30.00	61	...	51	...	N. W. 2	...	N. W. 2	0	...	0	
31	...	30.12	...	...	68	...	...	...	W'ly 2	...	...	4	...	
Means	29.86	29.84	29.84	63.1	76.9	63.7	...	1.3	1.9	1.3	3.2	4.6	3.0	2.02
								1.5			3.6			
Reduced to sea level.														
Max.	30.39	30.32	30.33	75	91	86	77.3							
Min.	29.71	29.56	29.38	48	63	51	55.3							
Mean	30.04	30.02	30.02											
Range	0.68	0.76	0.95	27	28	35	22.0							
Mean of month	30.027			...	...	...	67.9							
Extreme range	1.01			...	...	...	43.0							

Prevailing winds from some point between— Days.
- N. & E. 7
- E. & S. 2
- S. & W. 11
- W. & N. 10

Days.
- Clear 12
- Variable . . . } 10
- Cloudy . . . . }
- Rain fell on . . 8

(1 day omitted.)

Remarks.

1st. Pleasant.
2d. Pleasant. Evening very clear.
3d. Very fine.
4th. Very hot sun in the morning. Thunder-showers from 6½ to 8 P. M.
5th. Pleasant in the morning. Cool in the afternoon; wind N. E. Evening cloudy.
6th. Shower last night. Pleasant during the day. Evening clear.
8th. Rain in the evening.
9th. Heavy rain in the morning. Evening very warm.
10th. Very fine.
11th. Very fine. Evening splendid.
12th. Very fine. Evening cloudless.
13th. Sprinkling of rain from 3 to 4 P. M. Evening fine.
14th. Very pleasant.
15th. Very fine.
16th. Sultry and warm.
17th. Very warm and sultry at mid-day. Cool and pleasant in the evening.
18th. Very fine.
19th. Very fine. Evening splendid.
20th and 21st. Very fine.
22d. Pleasant. Sprinkling of rain at 6 P. M. and in the evening.
23d. Cloudy; air very damp, with occasional sprinkling of rain.
24th. Very fine. Evening splendid.
25th. Fine day. Evening very fine and cool.
26th. Cloudy; occasional sprinkling of rain.
27th. Very cool for the season.
28th. Very cool; frost in some low places; day splendid.
29th. Fine day.
30th. Very fine.

September, 1855. New Moon, 11d. 5h. 46m. A. M.

Days.	Barometer At 6 A. M.	At 1 P. M.	At 10 P. M.	Thermometer At 6 A. M.	At 1 P. M.	At 10 P. M.	Daily mean.	Winds At 6 A. M.	At 1 P. M.	At 10 P. M.	Weather At 6 A. M.	At 1 P. M.	At 10 P. M.	Rain
1	30.09	...	...	61	...	...	...	S. W'ly 2	...	...	10	...	...	
S 2	29.71	29.68	29.86	78	85	63	75.3	W. 2	W. 3	N. W. 1	7	1	0	
3	29.90	29.88	29.95	57	64	56	59.0	N. W. 1	N. 1	N. E. 1	8	10	3	
4	30.00	30.00	30.13	54	68	50	57.3	N. 2	N. E. 2	N. E. 1	2	5	0	
5	30.16	30.14	30.15	50	70	53	57.7	N. E. 1	N. E. 1	N. E. 1	1	2	0	
6	30.12	30.10	30.13	52	77	57	62.0	N. E. 1	N. E. 1	N. E. 1	0	0	0	
7	30.10	30.01	29.96	56	77	62	65.0	N. E. 1	N. E. 1	S'ly 1	1	5	2	
8	...	...	29.75	63	85	73	73.7	S. W. 1	W'ly 2	N. W'ly 1	1	2	3	
S 9	29.72	29.69	29.68	72	88	71	77.0	W'ly 2	W'ly 2	N. W'ly 1	3	5	0	
10	29.75	29.72	29.78	62	79	61	67.3	N. W. 1	N. W. 2	N. W. 1	0	2	0	
11	29.82	29.80	29.84	58	81	64	67.7	N. W. 1	N. W. 2	N. W. 1	0	0	0	
12	29.82	29.72	29.68	65	90	76	77.0	S. W. 1	W'ly 2	N. W. 2	2	3	0	
13	29.62	29.66	29.89	75	77	58	70.0	S. W. 2	N. W. 3	N. W. 2	5	10	0	
14	30.02	30.02	30.04	52	68	53	57.7	N. W. 1	N. E'ly 2	N. E. 2	0	3	10	
15	30.02	29.95	29.93	52	72	57	60.3	N. E'ly 1	N. E. 1	S'ly 1	10	0	Hazy	
S 16	29.82	29.76	29.78	58	75	62	65.0	E'ly 1	S. W'ly 1	W'ly 1	Foggy	10	0	
17	29.80	29.79	29.75	63	82	66	70.3	S. W. 1	S. W. 2	S. W. 1	5	3	0	
18	29.57	29.42	29.79	70	87	48	68.3	S. W. 2	S. W. 2	N. E. 3	10	10	10	
19	29.90	29.98	30.17	46	56	41	47.7	N. E. 2	N. W. 2	N. W. 1	9	0	0	
20	30.17	30.10	30.03	38	62	47	49.0	N. W. 1	N. W. 2	W'ly	0	0	3	
21	29.90	29.81	29.77	46	70	62	59.3	N. W. 1	N. W. 1	N. W'ly 1	3	10	Rain	
22	29.72	29.74	29.89	56	68	56	60.0	N'ly 1	N. E. 1	N. E. 1	Sprin'le	5	10	
S 23	30.03	30.07	30.16	54	56	51	53.7	N. E. 2	N. E. 2	N. E. 1	Misty	10	5	
24	30.15	30.10	30.09	53	62	48	54.3	N'ly 1	N'ly 2	N'ly 1	2	1	0	
25	29.99	29.88	29.86	47	67	52	55.3	N. W'ly 1	N. W. 1	N. W. 1	8	2	0	
26	29.76	29.64	29.59	53	73	63	63.0	S. W'ly 1	S. W'ly 2	S. W. 3	5	5	7	
27	29.44	29.48	29.68	63	69	54	62.0	S. W. 1	N. W. 1	N. W. 1	Rain	7	0	0.25
28	29.85	29.89	29.91	45	63	47	51.7	N. W. 1	N. W. 2	N. W. 1	0	0	0	
[illegible]	[illegible]	[illegible]	[illegible]	[illegible]	[illegible]	[illegible]	[illegible]	[illegible]	[illegible]	[illegible]	[illegible]	[illegible]	[illegible]	
S 30	30.04	29.96	29.92	48	66	56	56.7	S'ly 1	S. W. 2	S. W. 2	2	10	10	
Means	29.90	29.86	29.90	56.3	72.4	57.1	...	1.3	1.7	1.3	4.5	4.3	2.9	0.25
								1.4			3.9			
Reduced to sea level.														
Max.	30.35	30.32	30.35	78	90	76	77.0							
Min.	29.62	29.60	29.77	38	56	41	47.3							
Mean	30.08	30.04	30.08											
Range	0.73	0.72	0.58	40	34	25	29.7							
Mean of month	30.067			...	...	...	61.9							
Extreme range	0.75			...	...	...	52.0							

Prevailing winds from some point between— Days.
- N. & E. 8
- E. & S. 0
- S. & W. 6
- W. & N. 16

Days.
- Clear 9
- Variable . . . } 16
- Cloudy . . . . }
- Rain fell on . . 5

Remarks.

1st. Cloudy in the morning; brisk wind. Clear in the afternoon.
2d. Clear and pleasant, but windy.
3d. Cloudy and cool.
4th. Cool, but pleasant.
5th and 6th. Very fine.
7th. Very fine. Ground excessively dry.
8th. Very hot sun.
9th. Intensely hot sun.
10th. Very fine.
11th. Very fine. Sun scorching hot at noonday.
12th. Sun extremely hot at mid-day, and vegetation perishing from drought.
13th. Pleasant. Sprinkling of rain about 1 P. M. Evening clear and cool.
14th. Cool and pleasant. Evening cloudy, with some appearances of rain.
15th. Cloudy in the morning. Clear in the afternoon. Drought very severe.
16th. Light sprinkling of rain in the morning, not enough to lay the dust.
17th. Pleasant.
18th. Sun very hot at mid-day. Cloudy at 2 P. M., with the thermometer at 87°. At 4 P. M., wind changed from W'ly to N. E., with a gust and light rain, and a very rapid fall of the temperature. During the eight hours from 2 to 10 P. M., the thermometer fell 39°. The quantity of rain since August 9th, a period of forty days, has been hardly more than enough to lay the dust.
19th. Fine, but cold for the season.
20th. Very cold. Frost this morning in low places.
21st. Pleasant. Began to rain moderately at 10 P. M.
22d. Sprinkling of rain from 7 to 8 A. M.
23d. Mist, and occasional sprinkling of rain.
24th and 25th. Very fine.
26th. Pleasant.
27th. Light rain from 6 to 9 A. M. Evening very clear.
28th. Very fine; nearly cloudless.
29th. Very fine.
30th. Pleasant in the morning. Cloudy in the afternoon, with appearances of rain in the evening.

October, 1855. New Moon, 10d. 10h. 18m. P. M.

Days	Barometer, reduced to 32° F. Sunrise	At 1 P. M.	At 10 P. M.	Thermometer. Sunrise	At 1 P. M.	At 10 P. M.	Daily mean	Winds (Direction and Force.) Sunrise	At 1 P. M.	At 10 P. M.	Weather (Tenths Cloudy.) Sunrise	At 1 P. M.	At 10 P. M.	Rain and Snow in Inches of Water
1	29.75	29.68	29.61	60	66	62	62.7	S. E. 2	S. E. 2	E'ly 3	10	10	Rain	} 1.75
2	29.56	29.52	29.42	64	70	65	66.3	S. E. 2	S. E. 3	S. E'ly 2	Rain	10	Misty	
3	29.46	29.30	29.39	64	70	64	66.0	S'ly 1	S'ly 3	S'ly 1	10	5	8	
4	29.38	29.33	29.37	60	67	53	60.0	N. W. 1	W'ly 2	N. E'ly 1	9	Sprin'le	Rain	0.15
5	29.56	29.64	29.75	52	74	62	62.7	N. W. 1	N. W. 1	N. W. 1	5	0	10	
6	29.68	29.52	29.38	62	74	66	67.3	S. W'ly 1	S'ly 2	S. W'ly 2	7	Rain	Rain	1.25
S 7	29.60	29.64	29.77	48	58	45	50.3	N. W. 2	N. W. 2	N. W. 1	0	0	0	
8	29.81	29.76	29.87	39	58	48	48.3	N. W. 1	N. W. 1	S. W'ly 1	0	3	0	
9	29.88	29.86	29.93	46	60	52	52.7	N. W. 1	S. W. 1	S. W. 1	8	5	0	
10	29.93	29.92	30.02	51	66	48	55.0	S. W. 1	S. W'ly 1	N. E. 1	0	2	0	
11	29.97	29.86	29.77	47	65	52	54.7	N'ly 1	S'ly 1	E'ly 1	5	10	7	
12	29.65	29.58	29.53	52	66	56	58.0	S. E'ly 1	S. E. 3	E'ly 2	5	10	Sprin'le	
13	29.54	29.57	29.70	51	55	47	51.0	S. W. 2	S. W. 2	S. W. 2	10	2	2	
S 14	29.77	29.74	29.62	40	56	47	47.7	E'ly 1	S. E'ly 2	N. E. 2	10	2	Rain	0.15
15	29.76	29.74	29.79	40	54	48	47.3	W'ly 2	N. W'ly 1	S. W'ly 1	0	0	3	
16	29.77	29.76	29.86	48	62	47	52.3	N. W. 1	N. W. 3	N. W. 1	0	2	3	
17	29.91	29.86	29.88	38	52	39	43.0	N. W. 2	N. W. 2	N. W. 1	0	0	0	
18	29.83	29.76	29.83	38	61	45	48.0	N. W. 1	S. W. 1	N. W. 1	2	1	0	
19	29.86	29.85	29.89	41	63	56	53.3	N. W. 1	S'ly 2	S'ly 1	2	3	Foggy	
20	29.93	29.96	29.79	55	64	59	59.3	S'ly 1	S'ly 1	E'ly 1	10	10	Rain	1.00
S 21	29.66	29.57	29.57	56	59	56	57.0	N. E'ly 1	N. E. 1	N. E. 1	10	10	10	
22	29.58	...	29.64	59	...	52	...	S'ly 1	...	S'ly	10	...	10	
23	29.70	29.69	29.75	41	55	46	46.7	N. W. 2	N. W. 1	N'ly 1	3	0	Sprin'le	
24	29.63	29.39	29.38	45	52	54	50.3	N. E. 2	N. E. 2	S. E'ly 1	Misty	Rain	Misty	0.78
25	29.44	29.52	29.77	46	51	37	44.7	S. W. 2	N. W. 2	N. W. 2	10	3	0	
26	29.89	29.88	29.80	35	51	41	42.3	W'ly 2	N by W. 1	S. W. 1	0	3	6	
27	29.64	29.50	29.58	43	53	40	45.3	S. W. 1	S. W. 3	N. W. 1	6	7	0	
S 28	29.17	29.17	29.65	41	48	38	42.3	N. E. 1	N. W. 2	N. W. 1	Rain	Sprin'le	0	0.25
29	29.82	29.85	29.88	33	51	37	40.3	N. W. 1	N. W. 2	S. W. 1	0	0	0	
30	29.74	29.67	29.97	45	59	44	49.3	S. W. 1	S. W. 2	S. W. 1	5	10	0	
31	30.16	30.15	30.11	35	53	41	43.0	N. W. 1	S. W. 1	S. W. 1	0	0	2	
Means	29.71	29.67	29.72	47.6	59.8	49.9	...	1.3	1.8	1.3	5.3	4.9	5.3	5.33
								1.5			5.2			
REDUCED TO SEA LEVEL.														
Max.	30.34	30.33	30.29	64	74	66	67.3							
Min.	29.35	29.35	29.55	33	48	37	40.3							
Mean	29.89	29.85	29.90											
Range	0.99	0.98	0.74	31	26	29	27.0							
Mean of month	29.880			...	...	...	52.4							
Extreme range	0.99			...	...	...	41.0							

Prevailing winds from some point between— Days.
N. & E. 2
E. & S. 5
S. & W. 12
W. & N. 12

Days.
Clear 9
Variable . . . . } 13
Cloudy . . . . }
Rain fell on . . 9

REMARKS.

1st. Wind S. E'ly in morning, with occasional sprinkling of rain. Wind more E'ly in the evening, with sprinkling.
2d. Rain and mist through the day, with heavy rain in the night.
3d. Cloudy for the most part, with occasional mist.
4th. Pleasant in the morning. Sprinkling of rain from 1 to 2 P. M. Moderate rain in evening.
5th. Pleasant.
6th. Cloudy in morning. Began to rain gently from 4 to 5 P. M. Rain in the evening.
7th. Very fine.
8th and 9th. Pleasant.
10th. Pleasant. Evening very clear and cool.
11th. Pleasant.
12th. Cloudy for the most part, with indications of rain.
13th. Pleasant.
14th. Light showers in the morning, and again in the evening.
15th. Pleasant.
16th. Very fine.
17th. Very fine; evening cloudless.
18th. Very fine.
19th. Very mild and pleasant.
20th. Cloudy; air damp. Began to rain at 8 P. M.
21st. Cloudy, with occasional mist. Air mild.
22d. Cloudy, with occasional mist.
23d. Pleasant in the morning. Sprinkling of rain in the evening.
24th. Heavy showers at intervals. I neglected to record the quantity of rain that fell this day, and am indebted to Z. Allen, Esq., for supplying the omission.
25th. Quite cool. Evening splendid.
26th. Pleasant.
27th. Pleasant. Evening fine.
28th. Variable and blustering. Thundershower from 8 to 9 A. M.; then sunshine, followed by clouds and sprinkling of rain. Evening cool and clear. At 10 P. M., barometer stood at 29.20, being the lowest for the month.
29th. Very fine.
30th. Pleasant.
31st. Very fine. Up to the close of this month, there has been no frost on College Hill to injure the most delicate plants.

November, 1855. New Moon, 9d. 2h. 24m. P. M.

Days	Barometer Sunrise	At 1 P. M.	At 10 P. M.	Thermometer Sunrise	At 1 P. M.	At 10 P. M.	Daily mean	Winds Sunrise	At 1 P. M.	At 10 P. M.	Weather Sunrise	At 1 P. M.	At 10 P. M.	Rain and Snow
1	30.01	29.79	29.75	45	61	57	54.3	S'ly 1	S'ly 1	S'ly 1	10	10	Foggy	
2	29.73	29.76	29.92	53	52	47	50.7	N. E. 1	N. E. 2	N. E. 2	Misty	10	10	
3	29.96	29.98	29.97	46	49	45	46.7	N. E. 1	N. E. 1	N. E. 1	10	Sprin'le	Rain	0.75
S 4	29.98	29.99	30.11	44	46	43	44.3	N. E. 2	N. E. 2	N. E. 2	10	10	10	
5	30.16	30.15	30.16	38	47	44	43.0	N. E. 1	N. E. 2	N. E. 2	10	10	10	
6	30.11	30.02	30.01	44	53	46	47.7	N. E. 1	E'ly 2	N. E. 1	10	10	Misty	
7	29.99	29.91	29.88	46	54	49	49.7	N. E. 2	N. E. 1	N. E. 1	Misty	10	10	
8	29.86	29.81	30.00	46	56	47	49.7	N. E. 1	N. E'ly 1	N. W. 1	Misty	Misty	3	
9	30.10	30.09	30.22	40	54	38	44.0	N. W. 1	N. W. 2	N. W. 1	0	1	0	
10	30.24	30.13	30.11	34	51	43	42.7	N. W. 1	N. W. 1	N. W. 1	0	0	2	
S 11	30.07	30.09	30.13	43	54	49	48.7	Calm	Calm	N. E. 1	3	2	10	
12	30.13	30.06	29.92	49	53	49	50.3	N. E. 2	N. E. 2	N. E. 2	10	Rain	Rain	2.15
13	29.86	29.87	29.97	45	56	44	48.3	N. E. 2	N. W. 2	N. W. 1	10	2	0	
14	29.99	29.94	29.95	40	61	45	48.7	N. W. 1	N. W. 1	N. W. 1	2	3	0	
15	29.96	29.92	29.86	42	56	50	49.3	N. W. 1	S'ly 1	S. W'ly 1	2	4	10	
16	29.67	29.44	29.61	52	66	46	54.7	S. W. 2	S. W. 3	N. E. 3	7	9	10	
17	29.92	29.98	29.84	29	36	32	32.3	N. W. 2	N. E. 2	N. E. 2	5	10	Rain	0.60
S 18	29.69	29.75	29.79	35	40	32	35.7	N. E. 1	N. W. 2	N. W. 2	10	4	0	
19	29.83	29.82	29.95	30	39	27	32.0	N. W. 1	N'ly 2	N. W. 1	2	8	1	
20	30.07	30.08	30.11	20	30	25	25.0	N. W. 1	N. W. 2	N. W. 1	0	2	3	
21	29.99	29.66	29.54	28	35	35	32.7	N. E. 1	E'ly 1	N. E'ly 1	Snow	Rain	Misty	0.25
22	29.67	...	30.09	30	28	20	26.0	N. W. 3	N. W. 3	N. W. 1	2	2	0	
23	29.96	29.53	29.37	20	42	43	35.0	S. W. 1	S. W. 2	S. W. 3	7	8	10	
24	29.50	...	29.98	36	...	23	...	N. W. 4	...	N. W. 1	2	...	0	
S 25	30.07	29.86	29.49	23	42	50	38.3	W. 1	S. W. 1	S. W. 2	2	10	Rain	
26	29.39	...	29.39	46	...	38	...	S. W. 2	...	N. W. 2	5	...	0	
27	29.62	29.55	29.40	30	40	37	35.7	N. W. 1	N. W. 1	N. W. 1	0	0	0	
28	29.27	29.16	...	36	47	...	...	N. W. 2	W'ly 2	...	3	5	...	
29	29.24	...	...	32	...	...	...	N'ly 5	...	...	10	...	...	
30	...	29.86	29.91	...	37	29	...	...	N. W. 1	N. W. 1	...	0	1	
Means	29.86	29.85	29.87	38.0	47.6	40.5	...	1.6	1.7	1.4	5.9	6.4	5.4	3.75
								1.6			5.9			
REDUCED TO SEA LEVEL.														
Max.	30.42	30.31	30.40	53	66	57	54.7							
Min.	29.42	29.34	29.55	20	28	20	25.0							
Mean	30.04	30.03	30.05											
Range	1.00	0.97	0.85	33	38	37	29.7							
Mean of month	30.040			...	...	...	42.0							
Extreme range	1.08			...	...	...	46.0							

Prevailing winds from some point between— Days.
N. & E. 11
E. & S. 0
S. & W. 6
W. & N. 13

Days.
Clear 7
Variable . . . . } 15
Cloudy . . . . }
Rain fell on . . 8

REMARKS.

1st. Very mild. Warm fog in the evening.
2d. Cloudy, with some mist.
3d. Cloudy in the morning, with mist. Light rain in the afternoon, increasing in the evening.
4th. Cloudy through the day, with occasional rain.
5th. Cloudy, with some mist.
6th. Mild and cloudy, with occasional mist.
7th. Clouds and mist.
8th. Clouds and mist. Sun appeared for a short time from 10 to 11 A. M. Mostly clear at 10 P. M.
9th, 10th, and 11th. Very fine.
12th. Cloudy in the morning. Began to rain moderately from noon to 1 P. M., and continued through the night.
13th. Very fine. Evening splendid. Looked for meteors—this being the anniversary of the great shower, but none appeared.
14th. Very fine.
15th. Very mild and pleasant.
16th. Pleasant. Appearances of storm in the evening.
17th. Cloudy for the most part. Began to hail and rain from 3 to 4 P. M. Frost this morning, being the first of the season to injure plants on College Hill.
18th. Mild. Cloudy in morning, with sprinkling. Evening clear.
19th. Very fine.
20th. The first cold day of the season.
21st. Light snow in the morning, which melted as it fell. Rain in the afternoon.
22d. Wind cold and searching. Splendid evening.
23d. Cloudy in the afternoon, with appearances of storm.
24th. Very blustering. Cold and splendid evening.
25th. Morning cold. Wind S. W. and fresh in the afternoon. Began to rain moderately from 5 to 6 P. M.
26th. Variable. Pleasant in morning. Sprinkling of rain from 5 to 6 P. M. Evening clear.
27th. Very fine.
28th. Pleasant.
29th. Cloudy in the morning. Clear for the most part in the afternoon.
30th. Very fine.

December, 1855. New Moon, 9d. 5h. 10m. A. M.

DAYS.	BAROMETER, REDUCED TO 32° F. Sunrise.	At 1 P. M.	At 10 P. M.	THERMOMETER. Sunrise.	At 1 P. M.	At 10 P. M.	Daily mean.	WINDS. (DIRECTION AND FORCE.) Sunrise.	At 1 P. M.	At 10 P. M.	WEATHER. (TENTHS CLOUDY.) Sunrise.	At 1 P. M.	At 10 P. M.	RAIN AND SNOW IN INCHES OF WATER
1	29.77	29.68	29.67	31	49	37	39.0	S. W. 1	S. W. 2	S. W. 2	0	1	0	
S 2	29.51	29.30	29.17	38	51	47	45.3	S. W. 1	S. W. 1	W'ly 2	Foggy	10	5	
3	29.37	29.46	29.68	35	46	35	38.7	W'ly 1	N. W. 1	N. W. 1	0	5	0	
4	29.77	29.87	29.96	35	43	34	37.3	N. W. 1	N. W. 2	N. W. 1	0	5	10	
5	29.98	29.90	29.91	32	45	36	37.7	S. W. 1	W'ly 1	S. W. 1	2	0	0	
6	29.89	29.83	29.81	29	44	38	37.0	N. E. 1	N. E. 1	N. E. 1	3	5	10	
7	29.82	29.80	29.91	34	42	31	35.7	N. W. 2	N. W. 2	N. W. 2	8	5	0	
8	29.92	29.88	29.84	26	41	28	31.7	N. W. 1	N. W. 2	N. W. 1	0	0	0	
S 9	29.62	29.18	28.77	32	45	54	43.7	E'ly 1	S. E. 3	S. W. 2	10	Rain	8	1.75
10	28.94	29.10	29.38	37	41	30	36.0	W'ly 3	W'ly 3	N. W. 2	0	0	0	
11	29.51	29.63	29.87	28	25	22	25.0	N. W. 2	N. W. 3	N. W'ly 3	9	4	0	
12	30.20	30.21	30.32	18	29	20	22.3	N. W'ly 2	N. W. 4	N. W. 1	0	0	0	
13	30.30	30.12	30.15	23	30	24	25.7	S. E'ly 1	S'ly 1	S'ly 2	Snow	Snow	2	0.20
14	30.33	30.31	30.32	19	34	26	26.3	N. W. 1	S. W. 1	S. W'ly 1	0	2	5	
15	30.21	30.07	29.97	32	38	35	35.0	E'ly 2	E'ly 1	N. E. 1	Hail	Rain	Misty	
S 16	29.88	29.73	29.59	35	38	50	41.0	S. E'ly 1	N. E. 1	S. W.. 1	Rain	Rain	10	0.85
17	29.64	29.60	29.63	40	47	37	41.3	W'ly 1	N. W. 1	N. W. 1	10	8	0	
18	29.77	29.82	30.04	31	35	26	30.7	N. W. 1	N. W. 3	N. W. 1	0	5	0	
19	30.07	30.00	29.95	24	35	27	28.7	N. W. 2	N. W. 2	N. E. 2	3	3	10	
20	29.99	29.99	30.10	21	30	22	24.3	N. W. 1	N. W. 2	N. W. 1	1	1	0	
21	30.09	29.99	29.79	22	38	41	33.7	N. W. 1	S. W. 1	S. W. 2	9	10	Rain	} 0.70
22	29.76	29.69	29.43	39	41	49	43.0	S. W. 1	S. W. 1	S. W. 3	10	Sprin le	Rain	
S 23	29.46	29.56	29.73	48	53	40	47.0	W S.W. 3	W. 2	W'ly 1	0	0	2	
24	29.95	29.98	30.08	40	42	30	37.3	N. W. 1	N. W. 1	N. E. 3	10	9	10	
25	29.99	29.87	29.45	32	28	29	29.7	N. E. 2	N'ly 2	N'ly 1	10	Rain	Misty	1.10
26	29.14	29.53	29.99	33	22	18	24.3	W'ly 2	N. W. 3	N. W. 2	8	0	0	
27	30.24	30.26	30.28	14	20	16	16.7	N. W. 2	N. W. 2	N. W. 2	0	0	0	
28	30.11	29.95	...	18	29	...	...	S. W. 1	S. W. 2	N. W'ly 1	10	Snow	0	
29	30.07	29.97	29.56	8	18	21	15.7	N'ly 2	N'ly 2	N. E. 2	1	10	Snow	1.50
S 30	29.22	29.41	29.71	32	28	18	26.0	W'ly 2	N. W. 1	N. W. 1	Snow	0	0	
31	29.92	29.93	29.97	10	25	15	16.7	S. W. 1	S. W. 1	S. W. 1	0	2	10	
Means	29.82	29.79	29.80	28.8	36.5	31.2	...	1.5	1.8	1.5	4.9	5.0	4.2	6.10
									1.6			4.7		
REDUCED TO SEA LEVEL.														
Max.	30.51	30.49	30.50	48	53	54	47.0							
Min.	29.12	29.28	28.95	8	18	15	15.7							
Mean	30.00	29.97	29.98											
Range	1.39	1.21	1.55	40	35	39	32.3							
Mean of month	29.983			...	...	...	32.2							
Extreme range	1.56			...	...	...	46.0							

Prevailing winds from some point between— Days.
N. & E. 6
E. & S. 1
S. & W. 8
W. & N. 16

Days.
Clear 10
Variable . . . } 11
Cloudy . . . . }
Rain or snow fell on 10

REMARKS.

1st. Very fine.
2d. Cloudy, with dense fog, in the morning. Stars out at 10 P. M., with wind light at W'ly.
3d, 4th, and 5th. Very fine.
6th. Mild for the season.
7th. Pleasant. Evening cooler, and very clear.
8th. Very fine.
9th. At sunrise, wind very light E'ly; cloudy. Rain began to fall gently about 8 A. M., which gradually increased, and continued through day. Barometer fell rapidly, and wind hauled to S. E. and grew fresh. At 1 P. M., bar. 29.28, wind fresh S.E.; at 6 P. M., 28.98, wind heavy S.E.; at 8 P. M., 28.90, raining moderately, wind high; at 9 P. M., 28.87, wind S. W'ly and abated, with clouds broken and stars out.
10th. Very fine.
11th. Cloudy in the morning. Clear evening, and wind blustering at N. W.
12th. Clear and cold.
13th. Light snow from S. E'ly in the morning.
14th Pleasant. From one to two inches of light snow on the ground.
15th. Wind light E'ly, with moderate rain and mist all day.
16th. Moderate rain nearly all day.
17th. Very mild and pleasant.
18th. Pleasant. Evening very fine; bow around the moon.
19th. Appearances of storm in the evening.
20th. Very fine. Evening cool, but splendid.
21st. Morning cold. Afternoon mild. Sprinkling of rain in the evening.
22d. Light showers through the day. Rain in the evening.
23d. Uncommonly mild and pleasant for the season.
24th. Mild in the morning. Cooler in the afternoon, with the wind hauling N. E, and appearances of storm.
25th. Light rain and mist, which froze as it fell.
26th. Trees covered with ice this morning, and appearing splendidly in the sun. The day cold and blustering
27th. Cold, but fine. The ground and trees still covered with ice.
28th. Snowed moderately from 9 A. M. to 3 P. M. Clear and cold at night.
29th. Cloudy in the afternoon. Began to snow from 5 to 6 P. M.
30th. About nine inches of heavy snow on the ground this morning, and snowing at sunrise. Clear in the afternoon and evening.
31st. Cold, but pleasant.

January, 1856. New Moon, 7d. 6h. 9m. P. M.

DAYS.	Barometer Sunrise.	At 1 P. M.	At 10 P. M.	Thermometer Sunrise.	At 1 P. M.	At 10 P. M.	Daily mean.	Winds Sunrise.	At 1 P. M.	At 10 P. M.	Weather Sunrise.	At 1 P. M.	At 10 P. M.	Rain and Snow
1	29.94	30.02	30.24	15	29	18	20.7	N. W. 1	N. W. 1	N. W. 1	2	3	0	
2	30.31	30.28	30.02	11	24	25	20.0	N. W. 2	N. W. 2	N. E. 1	5	9	Rain	
3	29.72	29.56	29.70	32	32	30	31.3	N. E. 1	N'ly 1	N. W. 2	Rain	Misty	2	1.00
4	30.04	30.21	30.37	16	20	5	13.7	N. W. 2	N. W. 2	N. W. 1	0	0	0	
5	30.34	30.18	29.74	3	11	10	8.0	N. W. 1	N. W. 1	N. E. 3	10	10	Snow	} 2.50
S 6	29.50	29.70	29.91	12	19	13	14.7	N. E. 4	N. W. 2	N. W. 2	Snow	2	0	
7	30.05	30.03	29.79	4	21	21	15.3	N. W. 1	N. W. 1	N'ly 1	1	2	10	
8	29.63	29.50	29.67	27	30	4	20.3	N. W. 1	S. W. 2	N. W. 2	10	2	0	
9	29.80	29.79	29.80	—8	2	—7	—4.3	N. W'ly 1	W. N. W. 2	N. W. 1	0	0	0	
10	29.73	29.74	29.81	—4	10	18	8.0	W. 2	W. S. W. 2	S. W'ly 2	0	0	0	
11	29.94	30.01	30.17	16	27	14	19.0	N. W. 2	N. W. 2	N. W. 1	0	0	0	
12	30.23	30.20	30.07	8	27	21	18.7	N. W. 1	N. W. 1	N. E. 2	0	10	10	
S 13	29.43	29.08	29.13	34	37	31	34.0	N. E. 3	N. E. 2	N. E. 1	Rain	Rain	Misty	
14	29.30	29.36	29.41	24	30	21	25.0	N. E. 1	N'ly 2	N'ly 2	Snow	10	10	1.50
15	29.43	29.41	29.45	16	29	18	21.0	W'ly 1	N. W. 2	N. W. 1	1	4	0	
16	29.51	29.41	29.46	15	31	24	23.3	N. W. 1	N. W. 1	N. W. 1	0	0	3	
17	29.40	29.27	29.43	25	32	30	29.0	W'ly 1	W'ly 1	N. W. 2	Snow	10	10	
18	29.55	29.56	29.60	28	36	23	29.0	W'ly 1	W'ly 1	Calm	8	2	0	
19	29.55	29.53	29.74	18	35	9	20.7	N. W. 1	N. W. 1	N. W. 2	0	10	0	
S 20	29.69	29.53	29.44	6	17	12	11.7	N. W. 2	N'ly 1	N. W. 1	2	10	2	
21	29.49	29.46	29.47	10	20	11	13.7	N. W. 1	N. W. 1	N. W. 1	1	8	2	
22	29.55	29.56	29.66	6	22	14	14.0	N. W. 2	N. W. 2	N. W. 1	0	0	0	
23	29.63	29.64	29.69	15	30	22	22.3	N. W. 2	N. W. 1	N. W. 1	0	2	0	
24	29.77	29.68	29.64	12	31	23	22.0	S. W'ly 1	S. W. 2	S. W. 1	0	0	...	
25	29.88	29.90	30.09	7	6	5	6.0	N. W. 4	N. W. 4	N. W. 2	0	0	0	
26	30.09	29.97	29.95	4	22	14	13.3	N. W. 3	N. W. 2	N. W. 1	0	0	0	
S 27	29.84	29.69	29.54	12	31	22	21.7	N. W. 1	N. W. 1	W'ly 1	3	10	Snow	
28	29.48	29.34	29.61	24	21	16	20.3	N. E. 2	N. E. 2	N. W. 1	Snow	Snow	2	0.25
29	29.70	29.65	29.58	21	31	27	26.3	W'ly 1	S'ly 2	S'ly 1	10	10	10	
30	29.49	29.44	29.54	26	29	16	23.7	S. W'ly 1	W'ly 2	N. W. 1	10	10	0	
31	29.70	29.72	29.73	12	21	14	15.7	N. W. 2	N. W'ly 2	N. W. 1	0	0	0	
Means	29.73	29.69	29.72	14.4	24.6	16.9	...	1.6	1.6	1.4	4.0	5.0	3.3	5.25
									1.5			4.1		
REDUCED TO SEA LEVEL.														
Max.	30.52	30.46	30.55	34	37	31	34.0							
Min.	29.48	29.26	29.31	—8	2	—7	—4.3							
Mean	29.91	29.87	29.90											
Range	1.04	1.20	1.24	42	35	38	38.3							
Mean of month	29.893			...	...	...	18.6							
Extreme range	1.26			...	...	...	45.0							

Prevailing winds from some point between— Days.
N. & E. 5
E. & S. 0
S. & W. 4
W. & N. 22

Days.
Clear 12
Variable . . . } 11
Cloudy . . . . }
Rain or snow fell on 8

1st. Very fine.
2d. Morning cold. Afternoon moderate. Began to mist and rain at 7 to 9 P. M., freezing as it fell.
3d. Mist and light rain in morning. Trees covered with brilliant ice. Mostly clear at 10 P. M.
4th. Fine. Evening still and very cold.
5th. Wind light N. W. in morning. Began to snow from 4 or 5 P. M.; wind N. E. Storm severe.
6th. Violent storm this morning. Snow deep and very badly drifted. Sun appeared at 11 A. M. Quite clear at 2 P. M., with wind changed from N. E. to N. W., and much abated. Snow probably eighteen or twenty inches deep on the level.
7th. Pleasant in the morning. Mild in the afternoon, with some appearances of storm.
8th. Mild. About two inches of light snow fell last night. Grew cold very fast about sunset, with a gust of wind from N. W'ly.
9th. Wind moderate at W. N. W.; cold intense.
10th. More moderate. 11th. Very fine.
12th. Pleasant in the morning. Appearances of storm in the evening.
13th. Heavy wind from N. E., and rain at sunrise, four or five inches of snow having fallen during the night before the rain commenced.
14th. Air full of snow in the morning.
15th. Pleasant. Evening very fine.
16th. Very fine.
17th. Snowing at sunrise this morning; about an inch of fresh snow on the ground.
18th. Very fine. Evening splendid.
19th. Cloudy in the afternoon; wind N. W. At sunset, wind N. E'ly, which again came to N. W., and grew very cold. Very clear at 10 P. M.
20th. Morning cold. 21st. Pleasant.
22d. Very fine. Evening splendid.
23d. Very fine. Evening mild and clear.
24th. Very fine. Evening mild and cloudy.
25th. Very cold; wind high at N. W. As severe a day to be out as any during the winter.
26th. Very fine.
27th. Pleasant. Light snow in the evening.
28th. Moderate snow during the day. Clear in the evening.
29th. Mild and pleasant. From four to five inches of fresh snow on the ground.
30th. Air full of snow in the morning. Evening clear.
31st. Very fine. The great body of snow which fell on the 5th and 6th remains undiminished; the thermometer having risen above the freezing point on but three days during the month; and the whole time of its continuance above that point would, probably, not exceed thirty-six hours.

February, 1856. New Moon, 6d. 5h. 27m. A. M.

Days.	Barometer, reduced to 32° F: Sunrise.	At 1 P. M.	At 10 P. M.	Thermometer: Sunrise.	At 1 P. M.	At 10 P. M.	Daily mean.	Winds (Direction and Force): Sunrise.	At 1 P. M.	At 10 P. M.	Weather (Tenths Cloudy): Sunrise.	At 1 P. M.	At 10 P. M.	Rain and Snow in Inches of Water.
1	29.59	29.51	29.35	15	31	.26	24.0	N. E. 1	N. E. 1	N. E'ly 1	10	Snow	10	
2	29.38	29.29	29.43	21	24	7	17.3	N. W. 1	N. W. 2	N. W. 2	2	0	0	
S 3	29.42	29.36	29.41	0	12	6	6.0	N. W'ly 3	W N W 3	N. W. 2	0	0	0	
4	29.44	29.44	29.52	2	16	7	8.3	N. W. 2	N. W'ly 2	N. W. 1	0	1	0	
5	29.64	29.60	29.93	8	20	11	13.0	N. W'ly 1	N. W. 2	N. W. 2	5	0	0	
6	30.15	...	30.17	8	...	18	...	N. W. 2	...	S. W'ly 1	0	...	10	
7	30.06	29.53	29.53	21	37	34	30.7	S'ly 1	S'ly 2	S. W'ly 1	10	Rain	3	0.50
8	29.64	29.61	29.64	30	34	24	29.3	N. W. 1	N. W. 2	N'ly 1	2	9	10	
9	29.55	29.50	29.72	20	28	14	20.7	N'ly 1	N'ly 1	N. W. 2	Snow	5	0	
S 10	29.92	29.87	29.91	9	25	20	18.0	N. W. 1	N. W. 2	N. W. 1	2	1	10	
11	29.84	29.68	29.31	24	40	36	33.3	S. W'ly 1	S. W'ly 1	S. E'ly 1	8	7	Rain	} 0.25
12	28.94	28.91	29.43	36	36	7	26.3	S. W. 1	S. W. 3	N. W. 3	9	Snow	0	
13	29.74	29.79	29.87	0	8	2	3.3	N. W. 1	N. W. 2	N. W. 1	1	1	2	
14	29.94	29.89	29.85	—3	13	7	5.7	N. W. 1	N. W. 2	N. W. 1	0	1	7	
15	29.72	29.53	29.41	10	25	24	19.7	S. W'ly 1	S. W'ly 1	S. W'ly 1	4	10	Snow	0.05
16	29.14	29.03	29.10	30	40	30	33.3	Calm	S. W. 1	S. W. 1	Foggy	0	5	
S 17	28.90	29.87	29.05	33	20	12	21.7	S'ly 1	N. W. 3	N. W. 4	Foggy	Snow	6	
18	29.14	29.19	29.33	10	18	10	12.7	W. 4	W'ly 4	W'ly 4	0	10	10	
19	29.59	...	29.65	13	...	17	...	N. W'ly 3	....	Nl'y 1	0	...	4	
20	29.57	29.40	29.42	24	32	27	27.7	S. W'ly 1	W'ly 1	S. W. 1	10	10	10	
21	29.40	29.40	29.49	31	38	27	32.0	S. W'ly 2	W'ly 1	N. W. 1	10	5	0	
22	29.51	29.40	29.53	24	41	31	32.0	N. W. 1	N. W. 1	Calm	0	0	Hazy	
23	29.45	29.15	29.25	27	41	34	34.0	S. W'ly 1	S'ly 1	S. W. 2	3	10	10	
S 24	29.33	29.36	29.45	29	32	22	27.7	N. W. 1	N. W. 3	N. W. 2	3	3	0	
25	29.43	29.38	29.40	19	31	24	24.7	N. W. 1	N. W. 2	W'ly 2	0	10	2	
26	29.57	29.52	29.70	19	32	24	25.0	N. W. 1	N. W. 3	N. W. 2	0	0	0	
27	29.73	29.68	29.54	20	39	26	28.3	N. W. 1	N. W. 2	N. W. 1	0	10	0	
28	29.66	29.67	29.73	19	33	25	25.7	N. W. 1	N. W. 2	N. W. 2	0	5	5	
29	29.80	29.80	29.91	20	34	27	27.0	N. W. 2	N. W. 2	N. W. 1	3	2	10	
Means	29.56	29.49	29.55	19.2	28.9	20.0	...	1.4	1.9	1.6	3.9	5.2	5.0	0.80
									1.6			4.7		

REDUCED TO SEA LEVEL.

	Sunrise.	At 1 P. M.	At 10 P. M.	Sunrise.	At 1 P. M.	At 10 P. M.	Daily mean.
Max.	30.33	30.07	30.35	36	41	34	34.0
Min.	29.08	29.09	29.23	—3	8	2	3.3
Mean	29.74	29.67	29.73				
Range	1.25	0.98	1.12	39	33	32	30.7
Mean of month	29.713			...	...	...	22.7
Extreme range	1.27			...	...	...	44.0

Prevailing winds from some point between— Days.
N. & E. 1
E. & S. 0
S. & W. 7
W. & N. 21

Days.
Clear 8
Variable . . . } 13
Cloudy . . . . }
Rain or snow fell on 8

REMARKS.

1st. Cloudy, with a dusting of snow.
2d. Pleasant. Air grew very cold in evening.
3d. Very clear and cold.
4th. Cold, but not severe.
5th. Pleasant.
6th. Fine through the day. Evening cloudy.
7th. Light snow in the morning. Light rain in the afternoon. Clear in the evening.
8th. Pleasant. Some appearances of storm in the evening.
9th. Light snow in the morning—less than one inch deep. Evening clear.
10th. Pleasant.
11th. Pleasant in the morning. Cloudy in the afternoon. Began to rain moderately from 8 to 9 P. M.; wind light S. E'ly.
12th. Warm in the morning. Very heavy and sudden snow-squall at a quarter before 1 P. M., which continued for half an hour, the wind in the mean time changing from S. W. to N. W. The thermometer, which at noon stood at 46°, fell very rapidly after the squall. Evening clear and piercing cold.
13th. Very cold, with light wind.
14th. Cold, but not severe.
15th. Occasional snow-flakes in the air in the morning. Light snow in the evening.
16th. Thick fog in the morning, with a dead calm. Then a brisk shower of fine hail; then sunshine. Evening mild and hazy.
17th. Very mild at sunrise; wind light S'ly, which came to N. W., and grew cooler, before 9 A. M. Severe snow-squall from 1 to 2 P. M. Afternoon and evening very blustering and cold.
18th. Very cold and blustering.
19th. Pleasant.
20th. Cloudy. Weather mild.
21st. Pleasant. Cloudy in the morning. Clear in the evening.
22d. Very fine. Thick haze in the evening, with a fog-bow around the moon.
23d. Pleasant.
24th. Wind brisk and cold.
25th. Pleasant.
26th. Very fine.
27th. Pleasant.
28th. Pleasant. Air chilly towards night.
29th. Pleasant.

March, 1856. New Moon, 6d. 3h. 40m. P. M.

Days.	Barometer: Sunrise.	At 1 P. M.	At 10 P. M.	Thermometer: Sunrise.	At 1 P. M.	At 10 P. M.	Daily mean.	Winds: Sunrise.	At 1 P. M.	At 10 P. M.	Weather: Sunrise.	At 1 P. M.	At 10 P. M.	Rain and Snow in Inches of Water.
1	30.00	29.97	29.82	23	36	28	29.0	N. W. 2	S'l 2	E'l 2	0	0	Snow	} 0.90
S 2	28.98	28.97	29.18	34	41	33	36.0	S'ly 1	N. . 1	N. y 2	10	10	10	
3	29.62	29.67	29.95	22	30	20	24.0	W. 3	W N 4	N. W. 1	0	2	0	
4	30.05	29.85	29.48	16	35	30	27.0	W. 1	S. 3	W' 2	0	5	10	
5	29.69	29.70	29.73	20	32	20	24.0	W. 2	N. 2	N. ly 1	0	8	0	
6	29.50	29.22	29.42	28	42	23	31.0	S. W. 2	S. 2	N. W. 2	10	2	10	0.20
7	29.67	29.72	29.69	17	24	22	21.0	N. W. 2	N. y ly 2	N. W'ly 1	0	0	10	
8	29.58	29.49	29.71	28	40	12	26.7	S. W. 2	S. [illegible] 2	N. W. 4	10	1	0	
S 9	29.80	29.80	29.82	4	13	10	9.0	N. W. 2	W'ly 3	N. W. 2	0	0	10	
10	29.70	29.67	29.72	—2	11	4	4.3	N. W. 1	N. W 3	N. W. 2	0	0	0	
11	29.57	29.42	29.31	6	27	18	17.0	W'ly 2	W.S W 4	W'ly 2	0	10	2	
12	29.33	29.41	29.49	11	23	15	16.3	W'ly 2	N. W'ly 3	N. W. 2	0	0	0	
13	29.57	29.59	29.71	15	31	23	23.0	W'ly 1	N. W. 2	W'ly 1	0	0	0	
14	29.75	29.76	29.80	24	37	27	29.3	N. W. 2	N. W. 2	N. W. 1	7	2	0	
15	29.82	29.73	29.82	29	42	31	34.0	S. W. 2	S. W. 2	N. W. 1	9	5	0	
S 16	29.83	29.76	29.73	25	37	30	30.7	N. W. 2	N. W. 2	W'ly 1	0	7	8	
17	29.81	29.83	29.93	24	38	30	30.7	N. W. 2	N. W. 3	N. W. 1	0	3	0	
18	29.98	29.94	29.97	26	41	29	32.0	N. W. 1	N. W. 2	N. W. 1	0	0	2	
19	29.83	29.58	29.58	28	35	30	31.0	E'ly 1	S. E. 1	S. E. 1	10	Snow	Snow	0.45
20	29.58	29.55	29.60	32	43	31	35.3	Calm	S. W. 1	S. W'ly 1	10	9	8	
21	29.54	29.55	29.59	33	40	34	35.7	S. E'ly 1	N. E. 1	N. E'ly 1	10	10	10	
22	29.58	29.57	29.57	33	42	33	36.0	N. E'ly 1	N. E. 1	N. E. 2	9	2	10	
S 23	29.56	29.54	29.65	28	39	33	33.3	N. E. 2	N. E. 3	N. E'ly 1	5	3	3	
24	29.64	29.53	29.43	28	46	33	35.7	S'ly 1	S. E'ly 2	E'ly 2	2	7	10	
25	29.50	29.50	29.51	32	41	33	35.3	N'ly 2	N'ly 2	N. ly	9	3	0	
26	29.46	29.36	29.38	32	43	32	35.7	N. W. 2	N. W. 3	N. W'	0	2	0	
27	29.35	29.26	29.33	31	41	30	34.0	N. W. 2	N. W. 2	N. W. 2	0	0	0	
28	29.29	29.27	29.34	24	27	20	23.7	N. W. 2	N. W. 4	N. W. 2	2	3	8	
29	29.42	29.39	29.54	21	33	25	26.3	N. W. 2	N. W. 2	N. W. 2	2	2	2	
S 30	29.62	29.60	29.80	24	35	24	27.7	N. W. 2	N. W. 3	N. W. 2	0	0	0	
31	29.89	29.92	30.04	19	31	26	25.3	N. W. 2	N. W. 2	N. W. 1	0	0	0	
Means	29.63	29.59	29.63	23.1	34.7	25.5	...	1.8	2.3	1.6	3.3	3.2	4.3	1.55
									1.9			3.6		

REDUCED TO SEA LEVEL.

	Sunrise.	At 1 P. M.	At 10 P. M.	Sunrise.	At 1 P. M.	At 10 P. M.	Daily mean.
Max.	30.23	30.15	30.22	34	46	34	36.0
Min.	29.16	29.15	29.36	—2	11	4	4.3
Mean	29.81	29.77	29.81				
Range	1.07	1.00	0.86	36	35	30	31.7
Mean of month	29.797			...	...	...	27.8
Extreme range	1.08			...	...	...	48.0

Prevailing winds from some point between— Days.
N. & E. 3
E. & S. 3
S. & W. 6
W. & N. 19

Days.
Clear 11
Variable . . . } 12
Cloudy . . . . }
Rain or snow fell on 7

1st. Mild and pleasant in the morning. Grew chilly and clouded up towards night. Began to snow from 8 to 9 P. M.
2d. About four inches of very wet snow on the ground this morning, being the result of rain and snow during the night. Clouds broken, and sun out at intervals.
3d. Very blustering and cold.
4th. Pleasant in the morning. A sudden and heavy squall of wind from S. W'ly at about 9 P. M., which lasted half an hour, and ended with a blast of snow.
5th. Pleasant.
6th. Mild in the morning. Snowed from 9 A. M. to noon. Clear and pleasant from 2 to 4 P. M. Flurry of snow from 8 to 9 P. M., and colder.
7th. Raw and cold.
8th. Light hurry of snow last night. Very mild in the morning. Grew cold towards night. Evening very cold, and wind blustering at N. W.
9th. Wind piercing, and cold very severe.
10th. Excessively cold. Wind severe and cutting. With the exceptions of January 5th and February 13th, this is the coldest day of the winter, the mean temperature being 4°.3.
11th. More moderate.
12th. Light snow-squall from 9 to 10 A. M. Cold and blustering in the evening.
13th, 14th, and 15th. Very fine.
16th. Pleasant.
17th. Wind rather blustering. Evening splendid.
18th. Very fine.
19th. Snow began to fall gently between 10 and 11 A. M., and continued falling through the day and evening.
20th. From 4 to 5 inches of damp snow on the ground this morning, of which the greater part disappeared during the day.
21st. Mild, with appearances of storm.
22d and 23d. Pleasant.
24th. Pleasant. Appearances of storm in the evening.
25th. Light dusting of snow on the ground this morning. Day pleasant. Evening splendid.
26th and 27th. Very fine.
28th. Very cold and blustering.
29th. The cold continues.
30th. Pleasant.
31st. Cold, but not unpleasant.

April, 1856. New Moon, 4d. 12h. 45m. P. M.

DAYS.	Barometer, reduced to 32° F. At 6 A. M.	At 1 P. M.	At 10 P. M.	Thermometer. At 6 A. M.	At 1 P. M.	At 10 P. M.	Daily mean.	Winds (Direction and Force.) At 6 A. M.	At 1 P. M.	At 10 P. M.	Weather (Tenths Cloudy.) At 6 A. M.	At 1 P. M.	At 10 P. M.	Rain and Snow in Inches of Water.
1	30.20	30.17	30.25	22	42	29	31.0	N. W. 2	N. W. 2	N. W. 2	0	0	0	
2	30.08	30.00	29.87	27	49	37	37.7	S. W.	S. W. 3	S. W. 2	0	0	10	
3	29.68	29.54	29.55	46	48	42	45.3	S'ly 2	S. W. 2	S. W. 1	Rain	10	Foggy	0.70
4	29.56	29.52	29.52	49	50	42	47.0	S. W. 1	S. W. 1	N. W. 1	10	10	10	
5	29.57	29.58	29.52	36	50	38	41.3	N. W. 2	N. W. 2	N. W. 1	0	2	0	
S 6	29.58	29.60	29.67	40	45	40	41.7	N. W. 1	N. E'ly 2	N. E'ly 1	0	10	0	
7	29.71	29.79	29.92	36	56	40	44.0	N'ly 1	S'ly 1	S'ly 1	0	1	0	
8	30.00	30.02	30.06	38	63	48	49.7	N. W. 1	S. W'ly 2	S. W'ly 1	0	0	0	
9	30.09	29.98	29.86	43	69	49	53.7	S'ly 1	S'ly 3	S. W. 3	0	1	3	
10	29.75	29.77	29.92	48	55	38	47.0	W by N 3	N. W. 4	N. W. 1	1	0	0	
11	29.99	29.92	29.62	32	53	38	41.0	N'ly 1	S. W'ly 2	W'ly 1	2	9	3	
12	29.63	29.24	29.37	44	60	43	49.0	S. W. 2	S. W. 3	N. E'ly 4	8	10	Rain	0.25
S 13	29.87	29.88	30.00	27	42	34	34.3	N. W. 2	N. W. 3	N. W. 1	2	0	0	
14	29.99	29.89	29.72	30	52	43	41.7	N. W. 2	S. W. 3	S. W. 2	5	10	10	
15	29.67	29.66	29.78	44	63	44	50.3	N. W'ly 2	S. E'ly 2	N. W'ly 1	9	9	10	
16	29.90	29.95	29.87	43	55	42	46.7	N. E. 1	N. E'ly 1	N. E. 1	10	10	8	
17	29.78	29.56	29.34	43	60	49	50.7	S. W. 1	S'ly 2	N. E. 1	5	6	Rain	0.35
18	29.41	29.46	29.52	48	65	49	54.0	N. W. 1	W'ly 2	W'ly 2	2	5	6	
19	29.76	29.76	29.78	53	69	49	57.0	N. W. 1	S. E'ly 4	S. E'ly 1	0	5	10	
S 20	29.66	29.60	29.64	49	45	38	44.0	N. E. 1	N. E. 3	N. E. 5	Rain	Rain	Rain	} 1.40
21	29.62	29.42	29.41	38	38	39	38.3	N. E. 4	N. E. 5	N. E. 2	Rain	Rain	Misty	
22	29.41	29.46	29.57	42	51	41	44.7	S'ly 1	E'ly 2	S'ly 1	5	10	2	
23	29.71	29.69	29.70	42	68	49	53.0	S. W'ly 2	S. W. 3	S. W. 1	0	10	10	
24	29.66	29.64	29.69	48	56	48	50.7	S. W. 1	N. E. 2	N. E. 2	Misty	10	Rain	0.10
25	29.80	...	30.06	49	...	43	...	N'ly 2	...	N'ly 1	10	...	0	
26	30.18	30.15	30.16	42	58	40	46.7	N. E. 2	N. E. 2	N. E. 2	0	0	0	
S 27	30.06	29.89	29.81	42	67	48	52.3	W'ly 2	S. W. 2	S. W. 3	0	0	0	
28	29.74	29.72	29.76	54	78	44	58.7	S. W. 1	S. W. 1	N. E. 1	1	5	10	
29	29.74	29.68	29.79	43	66	44	51.0	N. E. 1	N. E. 2	N. E. 1	7	0	0	
30	29.87	30.00	30.15	44	67	43	51.3	N. E. 1	S. E'ly 2	N. E. 2	4	3	10	
Means	29.79	29.74	29.76	41.4	56.7	41.7	...	1.5	2.3	1.7	4.0	5.2	5.4	2.80
								1.8			4.9			
REDUCED TO SEA LEVEL.														
Max.	30.38	30.35	30.43	54	78	49	58.7							
Min.	29.59	29.42	29.52	22	38	29	31.0							
Mean	29.97	29.92	29.94											
Range	0.79	0.93	0.91	32	40	20	27.7							
Mean of month	29.943			...	...	...	46.5							
Extreme range	1.01			...	...	...	56.0							

Prevailing winds from some point between— Days.
N. & E. 8
E. & S. 4
S. & W. 13
W. & N. 5

Days.
Clear 9
Variable . . . } 12
Cloudy . . . . }
Rain fell on . . 9

REMARKS.

1st. Very fine.

2d. Thermometer 49° from 1 to 2 P. M. The warmest day since December 23, 1855, being a period of one hundred days.

3d. Rain in the morning. Fog and mist in the afternoon and evening.

4th. Cloudy, with fog and some mist. Very mild.

5th. Pleasant. Afternoon and evening fine.

6th. Clear at sunrise. Cloudy through greater part of day, with signs of rain. Clear at 10 P. M.

7th. Very fine. Warmer at 2 P. M. (ther. 56°) than at any time since Nov. 16, 1855, being 143 days.

8th. Very fine.

9th. Very fine. From 1 to 2 P. M., ther. 69°, being higher than at any time since Oct. 6, 1855, a period of more than six months.

10th. Wind blustering through the day. Evening still and very clear.

11th. Ground crusted with frost this morning.

12th. Cloudy; air damp. Thunder and light rain in evening, with change of wind from S. W. to N. E.

13th. Cool, but very fine.

14th. Air very raw and chilly. Wind S. W.

15th. Cloudy nearly all day. A few drops of rain in the evening.

16th. Mild. A few drops of rain from 11 A. M. to noon.

17th. Warm in morning. Began to rain from 3 to 4 P. M., and continued at intervals during the evening.

18th. Warm and pleasant.

19th. Pleasant.

20th. Rain storm from N. E. Wind very heavy in the evening.

21st. Storm heavy during day. Wind abated in the evening.

22d. Variable; sunshine and sprinkling of rain in turn. Mostly clear at 10 P. M.

23d. Pleasant.

24th. Damp and misty. Began to rain gently from 9 to 10 P. M.; wind N. E.

25th. Pleasant. Evening clear.

26th and 27th. Very fine.

28th. From 10 A. M. to 2 P. M., very hot for the season. From 5 to 6 P. M., wind changed from S. W'ly to N. E., and grew cooler fast.

29th. Pleasant. Evening splendid.

30th. Warm in the morning. Grew cold towards night.

May, 1856. New Moon, 4d. 9h. 35m. A. M.

DAYS.	Barometer At 6 A. M.	At 1 P. M.	At 10 P. M.	Thermometer At 6 A. M.	At 1 P. M.	At 10 P. M.	Daily mean.	Winds At 6 A. M.	At 1 P. M.	At 10 P. M.	Weather At 6 A. M.	At 1 P. M.	At 10 P. M.	Rain and Snow in Inches of Water.
1	30.20	30.08	30.00	41	57	44	47.3	N. E. 2	S. E'ly 2	S'ly 2	8	5	10	
2	29.78	29.66	29.63	41	44	41	42.0	N. E. 1	N. E. 2	N. E. 2	Rain	10	Rain	} 0.75
3	29.61	29.58	29.62	41	44	38	41.0	N. E. 2	N. E. 2	N. E. 1	Rain	Misty	10	
S 4	29.60	29.59	29.73	40	57	36	44.3	N'ly 1	N. W. 2	N. E. 2	1	8	Misty	
5	29.79	29.87	30.02	38	51	42	43.7	N'ly 1	N. E. 2	N. W. 1	7	8	0	
6	30.05	29.92	29.90	42	64	52	52.7	N. W. 1	N. W. 2	S. W'ly 1	0	5	7	
7	29.86	29.69	29.70	43	68	50	53.7	N. W. 1	N. E. 1	S. E'ly 2	2	10	8	
8	29.79	29.74	29.70	47	45	43	45.0	N. E'ly 2	N. E'ly 2	N. E'ly 5	10	Rain	Rain	} 2.40
9	29.49	29.47	29.39	42	39	39	40.0	N. E. 5	N. E. 3	N. E. 5	Rain	Rain	Rain	
10	29.40	29.42	29.48	43	43	40	42.0	N. E. 2	N'ly 3	N. E'ly 3	Misty	Misty	10	
S 11	29.49	29.48	29.53	41	46	46	44.3	N'ly 3	N. E'ly 1	S. E'ly 1	Rain	Rain	8	
12	29.56	29.56	29.67	52	80	70	67.3	S'ly 1	N. W'ly 3	N. W'ly 1	0	4	6	
13	...	30.03	30.15	...	64	48	...	N. E. 1	N. E. 1	S. E'ly 1	3	8	10	
14	30.18	30.15	30.14	48	63	46	52.3	E'ly 2	S. E. 2	S. E. 2	10	5	6	
15	30.09	30.01	29.96	49	61	54	54.7	S'ly 1	S. E. 2	S. E'ly 2	Foggy	10	Foggy	
16	29.89	29.83	29.84	60	70	59	63.0	S. W. 2	S. W. 3	S. W. 2	7	10	Sprin'le	
17	29.86	...	29.84	56	...	55	...	S. W. 1	...	S. W. 1	Rain	...	0	
S 18	29.79	29.72	29.69	53	74	59	62.0	S'ly 1	S. W. 2	S'ly 2	2	2	2	
19	29.63	29.58	29.54	51	72	59	60.7	N. E. 1	S. E. 2	S'ly 1	Foggy	3	7	
20	29.47	29.38	29.54	56	80	60	65.3	S. W. 1	W'ly 2	N. W. 2	7	3	3	0.10
21	29.64	29.63	29.79	52	64	51	55.7	N. W. 2	N. W. 3	N. W. 1	0	0	0	
22	29.85	29.83	29.86	52	70	55	59.0	N. W. 2	N. W. 2	N. W. 1	0	0	0	
23	29.85	29.77	29.73	57	83	64	68.0	N. W. 2	W'ly 2	S. W. 1	0	0	0	
24	29.69	29.62	29.52	66	91	60	72.3	S. W'ly 1	S. W'ly 3	N. W. 2	0	5	Rain	0.10
S 25	29.51	29.45	29.52	52	64	43	53.0	N. W. 2	W'ly 3	N. W. 1	0	2	0	
26	29.44	29.54	29.59	42	53	45	46.7	N'ly 2	N. W. 3	N. E. 1	Rain	10	0	
27	29.64	29.58	29.59	47	74	53	58.0	N. W. 1	S. W'ly 2	S. W. 1	2	2	0	
28	29.36	29.19	29.28	56	63	57	58.7	S. W. 2	S. W. 2	N. W. 2	Rain	10	0	0.75
29	29.31	29.35	29.39	54	66	52	57.3	N. W. 2	S. W. 2	S. W. 1	0	1	Shower	
30	29.41	29.45	29.60	45	60	44	49.7	N. W. 2	S. W. 2	N. W. 2	0	10	0	
31	29.78	29.80	29.94	42	55	45	47.3	N. W. 2	N. W. 3	N. W. 1	2	5	0	
Means	29.70	29.66	29.71	48.8	62.2	50.0	...	1.7	2.2	1.7	5.2	6.2	5.1	4.10
								1.9			5.5			
REDUCED TO SEA LEVEL.														
Max.	30.38	30.33	30.33	66	91	64	72.3							
Min.	29.49	29.37	29.46	38	39	36	40.0							
Mean	29.88	29.84	29.89											
Range	0.89	0.96	0.87	28	52	28	32.3							
Mean of month	29.870			...	...	...	53.5							
Extreme range	1.01			...	...	...	55.0							

Prevailing winds from some point between— Days.
N. & E. 10
E. & S. 4
S. & W. 7
W. & N. 10

Days.
Clear 6
Variable . . . } 11
Cloudy . . . . }
Rain fell on . . 14

1st. Raw and chilly in the afternoon and evening.

2d. Moderate rain in the morning. Mist and rain in the evening.

3d. Rain and mist all day.

4th. Variable. Cloudy in the afternoon. Cold mist from 7 to 9 P. M. Mostly clear at 11 P. M.

5th. Variable and rough. Occasional sprinkling of rain and hail. Evening clear.

6th and 7th. Pleasant.

8th. Moderate rain, increased towards night.

9th. Heavy rain and high wind.

10th. Mist and rain.

11th. Rain all day. Wind changed in the evening.

12th. Pleasant and very warm.

13th. Pleasant. Appearances of rain in the evening.

14th. Pleasant.

15th. Clouds and fog; air chilly.

16th. Rather sultry. Sprinkling of rain in the evening.

17th. Sprinkling of rain in the morning. Evening clear.

18th. Very fine.

19th. Pleasant.

20th. Brisk thundershower at 3 P. M. Mostly clear at 10 P. M.

21st. Very fine; almost cloudless.

22d. Very fine.

23d. Very hot sun at mid-day.

24th. Excessively hot. From 1 to 2 P. M., the thermometer stood at 91° in the shade, exposed to a brisk breeze, being the highest point reached since the 17th of August last, when, under the same circumstances, it stood at the same height. Thunder-gust at 6 P. M. Light showers with thunder in the evening.

25th. Fine, but cool.

26th. Sprinkling, with mist and heavy clouds from N. W.

27th. Very fine.

28th. Rain in the morning. Clear at 6 P. M.

29th. Pleasant. Light showers in the evening.

30th. Pleasant. Very cool in the afternoon and evening.

31st. Cool, but pleasant.

June, 1856. New Moon, 2d. 6h. 32m. P. M.

Days.	Barometer, reduced to 32° F. At 6 A. M.	At 1 P. M.	At 10 P. M.	Thermometer. At 6 A. M.	At 1 P. M.	At 10 P. M.	Daily mean.	Winds. (Direction and Force.) At 6 A. M.	At 1 P. M.	At 10 P. M.	Weather. (Tenths Cloudy.) At 6 A. M.	At 1 P. M.	At 10 P. M.	Rain and Snow in Inches of Water.
S 1	29.97	29.93	29.95	50	74	54	59.3	N. W. 2	N'ly 2	S. W. 1	5	7	0	
2	29.90	29.84	29.79	55	68	59	[illegible]7	S. W. [illegible]	S. W. [illegible]	S. W. [illegible]	0	0	0	
3	29.72	29.66	29.70	64	83	70	3	S. W.	W'ly	S. W.	7	6	0	
4	29.73	29.70	29.71	67	77	67	3	N. E.	S. W.	N'ly	10	6	10	0.25
5	29.83	29.95	30.06	54	62	50	3	N. E.	N. E.	N. E.	10	10	0	
6	30.07	30.00	29.95	52	51	48	3	N. E.	N. E.	N. E.	10	Misty	Rain	
7	29.80	29.77	29.80	50	58	54	0	N. E.	N. E.	N. E.	10	10	10	
S 8	29.76	29.68	29.65	56	64	58	0	S. W.	S. W.	S. W.	10	10	Misty	
9	29.53	29.49	29.60	56	71	60	3	S. E.	S'ly	W'ly	Misty	2	0	0.55
10	29.59	29.62	29.69	60	81	66	0	S. W.	N. W.	S. W'ly	5	3	10	
11	29.70	29.67	29.72	65	80	62	0	N. W.	S. E.	S'ly	1	2	0	
12	29.79	29.76	29.72	61	74	61	3	S'ly	S. E.	S. E.	0	3	10	
13	29.64	29.58	29.62	62	81	67	0	S'ly	S'ly	S'ly	Rain	5	10	
14	29.63	29.61	29.57	66	75	63	0	S'ly	S'ly	W'ly	5	9	Shower	0.35
S 15	29.55	29.55	29.65	62	77	61	7	N. W.	N. W.	N. W.	8	9	0	
16	29.73	29.76	29.83	56	78	60	7	N W.	N. W.	N. W.	0	3	0	
17	29.87	29.85	29.85	59	76	62	7	N W.	S. W.	N. W.	1	4	3	
18	29.83	29.82	29.75	62	67	60	0	S W.	S. W.	S'ly	8	Rain	Rain	} 0.95
19	29.62	29.61	29.69	61	70	61	0	N E.	N. E.	N. E'ly	Rain	10	10	
20	29.75	29.73	29.73	62	79	69	0	N W.	S. E'ly	S'ly	10	2	0	
21	29.78	29.79	29.81	68	92	77	0	N W.	N. W.	N. W.	1	0	0	
S 22	29.77	29.68	29.69	78	94	81	3	N W.	N. W.	W'ly	2	4	5	
23	29.79	29.80	29.85	71	79	61	3	N E.	N. E.	S'ly	5	2	0	
24	29.86	29.83	29.87	60	76	61	7	S ly	S. E.	S. E.	2	0	2	
25	29.82	29.75	29.72	64	72	64	7	S E'ly	S. W.	S. W.	10	10	10	
26	29.69	29.64	29.60	68	86	72	3	S W.	S. W.	S. W.	10	2	7	
27	29.55	29.60	29.73	72	82	64	7	S W.	N.W'ly	N. W.	2	2	0	0.37
28	29.75	29.65	29.60	63	81	71	7	N W.	S. W.	S. W.	3	3	0	
S 29	29.45	29.38	29.41	75	95	81	7	N W'ly	W'ly	W'ly	0	2	0	
30	29.45	29.45	29.47	79	92	81	0	S. W'ly	S. W.	W'ly	8	2	2	
Means	29.73	29.70	29.73	62.6	76.5	64.1	...	1.6	2.3	1.4	5.7	4.3	4.2	2.47
									1.8			4.7		
REDUCED TO SEA LEVEL.														
Max.	30.25	30.18	30.24	79	95	81	84.3							
Min.	29.63	29.56	29.59	50	51	48	50.3							
Mean	29.91	29.88	29.91											
Range	0.62	0.62	0.65	29	44	33	34							
Mean of month	29.900			...	...	...	67							
Extreme range	0.69			...	...	...	47							

Prevailing winds from some point between— Days.
N. & E. 5
E. & S. 6
S. & W. 11
W. & N. 8

Days.
Clear 8
Variable . . . } 13
Cloudy . . . . }
Rain fell on . . 9

Remarks.

1st. Pleasant.
2d. Very fine.
3d. Very fine and very warm.
4th. Cloudy for the most part. Light showers, with thunder, from 7 to 8 P. M. Showers during the night.
5th. Cloudy through the day. Clear at 10 P. M.
6th. Cloudy, with light rain in the evening.
7th. Cloudy, with occasional sprinkling of rain.
8th. Misty through the day and evening.
9th. Heavy thundershower from 3 to 5 A. M. Mostly clear in the evening.
10th. Very warm and damp.
11th. Very fine.
12th. Pleasant. Evening cloudy, with light mist.
13th. Warm and sultry. Slight sprinkling at 2 P. M.
14th. Warm and sultry. Thundershower, with rain and hail at about 9 P. M.
15th. Clouds and sunshine during day. Evening splendid.
16th. Very fine. Evening splendid.
17th. Very fine.
18th. Sprinkling of rain. Evening rainy.
19th. Clouds, with occasional sunshine. Light rain in the morning.
20th. Very fine.
21st. Excessively hot. Wind light N.W'ly, and mostly clear.
22d. Excessively hot. From 1 to 2 P. M., ther. 94° in the shade, exposed to a fresh breeze.
23d. Very fine.
24th. Pleasant.
25th. Variable. Mostly cloudy. Sprinkling of rain from noon to 1 P. M.
26th. Very warm and sultry. Cloudy in the morning. Mostly clear in the afternoon.
27th. Heavy thundershower from 2 to 3 A. M. Evening clear.
28th. Very fine.
29th. At 9 A. M., thermometer 86°; at 11 A. M., 91°; from 1 to 2 P. M., 95° in the shade, exposed to a fresh breeze; at 5 P. M., 92°. The thermometer reached the same point twice last summer, viz: on the 30th of June and on the 19th of July.
30th. Heat intense, though slightly abated.

July, 1856. New Moon, 2d. 4h. 22m. A. M., and 31d. 4h. 0m. P. M.

Days.	Barometer At 6 A. M.	At 1 P. M.	At 10 P. M.	Thermometer At 6 A. M.	At 1 P. M.	At 10 P. M.	Daily mean.	Winds At 6 A. M.	At 1 P. M.	At 10 P. M.	Weather At 6 A. M.	At 1 P. M.	At 10 P. M.	Rain and Snow
1	...	29.77	29.88	65	81	63	69.7	N. W. 3	N. W. 3	N. W. 1	0	0	0	
2	29.95	29.93	29.89	60	76	62	68.0	N. W. 1	S. E. 3	S'ly 1	1	1	5	
3	29.76	29.65	29.60	65	83	67	71.7	S'ly 2	S'ly 3	S. W. 2	1	0	10	
4	29.54	29.47	29.61	68	79	59	68.7	S'ly 2	N. W. 2	N. W. 2	Rain	10	0	0.35
5	29.66	29.68	29.64	58	77	61	62.0	N. W. 1	N. W. 2	S'ly 1	0	2	0	
S 6	29.59	29.53	29.68	65	83	61	69.7	S. W. 3	S. W. 3	W'ly 1	4	1	Rain	0.65
7	29.75	29.81	29.87	57	74	61	64.0	N. E. 2	N. E. 2	N. E. 1	Shower	3	5	
8	29.89	29.94	29.93	60	78	63	67.0	N. E. 2	N. E. 2	E'ly 1	Shower	3	6	0.10
9	29.87	29.81	29.85	58	62	57	59.0	N. E. 2	N. E. 3	N. E. 3	Rain	10	10	1.55
10	29.85	29.82	29.82	60	75	61	65.3	N. E. 2	N. E. 2	N. E. 1	10	9	2	
11	29.80	29.76	29.72	63	76	63	67.3	N. W. 1	S'ly 3	S'ly 1	1	0	5	
12	29.50	29.52	29.59	64	82	70	72.0	S. E'ly 3	S. W'ly 2	W'ly 1	Rain	10	10	1.25
S 13	29.66	29.63	29.71	72	80	75	75.7	S. W. 2	S. W. 2	S. W. 1	5	3	7	
14	29.72	29.75	29.72	75	86	74	78.3	N. W. 2	S. W. 2	S. W. 1	6	0	2	
15	29.63	29.54	29.69	77	88	74	79.7	S. W. 2	S. W. 4	W'ly 2	3	7	5	
16	...	...	...	...	...	...	...	...	...	...	...	...	...	
17	...	...	...	...	...	...	...	...	...	...	...	...	...	
18	...	...	...	...	92	...	...	...	W'ly 3	...	...	...	...	
19	...	...	29.58	...	...	66	...	...	...	N. W. 2	...	...	3	
S 20	29.61	29.64	29.78	63	74	64	67.0	N. W. 2	N. W. 3	N. W. 1	0	4	0	
21	29.89	29.88	29.94	62	81	66	69.7	N. W. 1	N. W. 2	N. W. 1	0	3	0	
22	29.97	29.96	29.98	62	70	66	66.0	N'ly 1	W'ly 1	S. W. 1	2	Shower	0	0.30
23	29.89	29.95	29.87	64	84	72	73.3	S. W. 1	S. W.	S. W. 1	2	1	0	
24	29.99	29.96	29.89	79	88	76	81.0	W'ly	W.	S. W. 1	2	2	0	
25	29.83	29.79	29.74	70	90	78	79.3	W'ly	W.	S. W. 2	3	4	0	
26	29.75	29.74	29.78	73	92	78	81.0	W.	N. W.	W. 1	0	0	0	
S 27	29.75	29.74	29.74	74	91	81	82.0	W'ly	W.	W. 2	0	2	0	
28	29.79	29.80	29.79	72	86	76	78.0	W.	W.	W. 1	2	6	0	
29	29.77	29.74	29.67	72	90	73	78.3	W'ly	S. W.	W'ly 2	2	3	0	
30	29.60	29.60	29.64	72	80	74	75.3	S.	S.	S'ly	10	7	0	
31	29.68	29.75	29.81	70	74	73	72.3	S'ly	W.	S'ly 1	9	10	8	
Means	29.76	29.75	29 76	66.7	81.1	68.4	...	1 8	2.5	1.3	4.2	4.1	3.1	4.20
									1.9			3.8		
REDUCED TO SEA LEVEL.														
Max.	30.17	30.14	30.16	79	92	81	82.0							
Min.	29.68	29.65	29.76	57	62	57	59.0							
Mean	29.94	29.93	29.94											
Range	0.49	0.49	0.40	22	30	24	23.0							
Mean of month	29.937			...	...	...	72.1							
Extreme range	0.52			...	...	...	35.0							

Prevailing winds from some point between— Days.
N. & E. 4
E. & S. 1
S. & W. 13
W. & N. 11

Days.
Clear 10
Variable . . . } 9
Cloudy . . . . }
Rain fell on . . 12
(3 days omitted.)

Remarks.

1st. Very fine.
2d. Very fine; cool and dry.
3d. Pleasant.
4th. Moderate rain in the morning. Evening clear and cool.
5th. Very fine.
6th. Pleasant in the morning. Copious shower, with thunder, from 5 to 6 P. M.
7th. Light shower from 6 to 7 A. M.; air cool.
8th. Shower about 5 A. M. Pleasant in the afternoon.
9th. Heavy rain in the morning. Cloudy in the afternoon and evening.
10th. Cloudy in the morning. Evening mostly clear.
11th. Very fine.
12th. Heavy rain this morning. Pleasant in the afternoon; clouds prevailing.
13th. Very warm and sultry.
14th. Very warm. Fine breeze at mid-day.
15th. Extremely hot and sultry in the morning. Thunder, with a light shower, between 1 and 2 P. M. Cooler in the afternoon.
16th and 17th. Very warm.
18th. Extremely hot.
19th. Cooler and very fine.
20th. Cool and very fine.
21st. Very fine. A few heavy drops of rain from a passing cloud at about 1 P. M.
22d. Fine showers, with thunder, from noon to 2 P. M. Evening clear.
23d. Pleasant.
24th. Hazy at mid-day.
25th. Very warm.
26th. Hazy in the morning. Smoke and haze at mid-day.
27th. Mostly clear. Hazy at mid-day.
28th. Shower at the N. and N. E.
29th. Light shower from 1 to 2 P. M.
30th and 31st. Occasional sprinkling of rain.

August, 1856. New Moon, 30d. 6h. 5m. A. M.

DAYS.	BAROMETER, reduced to 32° F. At 6 A. M.	At 1 P. M.	At 10 P. M.	THERMOMETER. At 6 A. M.	At 1 P. M.	At 10 P. M.	Daily mean.	WINDS. (Direction and Force.) At 6 A. M.	At 1 P. M.	At 10 P. M.	WEATHER. (Tenths Cloudy.) At 6 A. M.	At 1 P. M.	At 10 P. M.	Rain and Snow in Inches of Water.
1	29.86	29.87	29.88	72	80	72	74.7	S.	S.	S.	10	7	0	
2	29.89	29.88	29.83	72	77	71	73.3	S. E. 1	E. 2	E. 1	5	6	10	
S 3	29.77	29.72	29.73	71	87	71	76.3	S. E. 1	E. 1	S. E. 1	10	7	9	
4	29.74	29.75	29.73	70	75	71	72.0	E. N. E. 1	N. E. 1	N. E. 1	10	9	10	
5	29.60	29.57	29.54	71	78	69	72.7	E'ly 1	S. E'ly 1	S. E. 2	10	10	Rain	0.80
6	29.55	29.52	29.54	72	79	69	73.3	S. W. 2	S'ly 3	S'ly 1	10	5	9	
7	29.59	29.63	29.67	66	79	78	74.3	S. W. 1	W'ly 2	S. W'ly 1	0	3	0	
8	29.68	29.67	29.73	70	80	68	72.7	S. W. 2	S. W. 2	S. W. 1	5	Shower	10	1.25
9	29.73	29.70	29.73	68	81	70	73.0	S. W. 1	S. W. 2	S'ly 1	Rain	8	3	0.10
S 10	29.71	29.69	29.71	65	82	66	71.0	N. W. 2	W'ly 2	W'ly 1	0	5	0	
11	29.68	29.60	29.58	66	85	72	74.3	S. W. 1	S. W. 2	S. W. 1	2	7	10	
12	29.55	29.52	29.53	70	85	70	75.0	S. W. 1	S. E'ly 1	S. W. 1	2	9	8	
13	29.54	29.54	29.58	65	83	65	71.0	N. W. 1	S. W'ly 2	Calm	1	7	5	
14	29.58	29.60	29.61	64	83	66	71.0	N. W. 1	S. W'ly 1	S. W. 1	2	2	0	
15	29.63	29.62	29.66	66	82	64	70.7	N'ly 1	N. E. 1	N. E. 1	0	4	5	
16	29.69	29.68	29.75	62	76	65	67.7	N. W. 2	N. W. 2	N. W. 1	0	5	5	
S 17	29.76	...	29.79	64	...	60	...	N. E. 2	N. W. 2	N. W. 1	2	Shower	0	0.50
18	29.81	29.78	29.84	61	72	62	65.0	N'ly 2	N. E. 2	S. E'ly 2	10	5	5	
19	29.77	...	29.63	65	...	65	...	N'ly 2	...	S. E'ly 3	6	...	Rain	
20	29.39	29.27	29.20	65	64	62	63.7	S. E. 3	E. S. E. 3	N. E. 2	Rain	Rain	Rain	} 2.60
21	29.13	29.19	29.36	58	61	58	59.0	N. E. 3	N. N. E.	N. E'ly	Misty	Rain	Misty	
22	29.42	29.51	29.65	58	70	63	63.7	N. W. 2	N. W. 1	N. W. 1	10	2	0	
23	29.76	29.74	29.67	60	78	68	68.7	N. W. 1	S. W. 2	S. W. 1	0	2	8	
S 24	29.57	29.48	29.49	66	78	67	70.3	S. W. 1	W. 2	N. W. 1	9	2	1	
25	29.50	29.50	29.64	58	72	59	63.0	N. W. 1	N. W. 2	N. W. 1	0	5	4	
26	29.81	29.85	29.92	48	66	56	56.7	N. W. 2	N. W. 2	W. 1	0	0	0	
27	30.03	30.02	30.02	49	70	62	60.3	W'ly 1	W. 3	N. W. 1	0	4	0	
28	30.04	29.99	29.92	60	76	67	67.7	S. W. 1	S. 4	S. W. 3	0	2	8	
29	29.78	29.66	29.61	66	68	66	66.7	S. W. 2	S. W. 5	S. W. 2	9	10	10	0.50
30	29.68	29.70	29.77	60	71	60	63.7	N. W. 1	W. 3	N. W. 1	6	3	0	
S 31	29.88	29.92	29.90	54	72	62	62.7	N. W. 1	W. 1	W. 1	0	1	0	
Means	29.68	29.66	29.69	64.0	76.3	69.2	...	1.5	2.0	1.3	4.8	5.7	5.2	5.75
								1.6			5.2			
REDUCED TO SEA LEVEL.														
Max.	30.22	30.20	30.20	72	87	72	76.3							
Min.	29.31	29.37	29.38	48	61	56	56.7							
Mean	29.86	29.84	29.87											
Range	0.91	0.83	0.82	24	26	16	19.6							
Mean of month	29.857			...	...	...	69.8							
Extreme range	0.91			...	...	...	39.0							

Prevailing winds from some point between— Days.
N. & E. 4
E. & S. 5
S. & W. 12
W. & N. 10

Days.
Clear 6
Variable . . . } 13
Cloudy . . . . }
Rain fell on . . 12

REMARKS.

1st. Pleasant.
2d. Overcast in the morning.
3d. Cloudy for the most part. Air sultry and damp.
4th. Mostly cloudy, light rain towards night.
5th. Cloudy, with light showers during the day. Heavy shower in the evening.
6th. Clouds; occasional sunshine and sprinkling of rain.
7th. Fine.
8th. Light showers in the morning. Heavy rain, with thunder, from 4 to 6 P. M. Evening cloudy.
9th. Light showers in the morning. Mostly clear in the evening.
10th, 11th, and 12th. Pleasant.
13th. Pleasant in the morning. Light shower from 4 to 5 P. M.
14th. Fine. Evening splendid.
15th Pleasant. Showers in the afternoon to the north and east of us, but none here.
16th. Very fine; cool and dry.
17th. Pleasant in the morning. Heavy shower from 6 to 7 P. M. Clear at 9 P. M.
18th. Cloudy; air mild.
19th. Cloudy in the afternoon. Rain in the evening.
20th. Steady rain. Wind fresh; changed during the day from S. E'ly to N. E'ly.
21st. Mist, with occasional light rain.
22d and 23d. Pleasant.
24th. Light shower in the morning. Mostly clear at 9 A. M.
25th. Cool and pleasant in the morning. Light shower in the afternoon.
26th. Pleasant, but very cool.
27th. Cool, but pleasant.
28th. Pleasant; air dry.
29th. Shower in the morning. Light shower and brisk wind through the day.
30th. Cloudy in the morning. Evening clear.
31st. Splendid day.

September, 1856. New Moon, 28d. 10h. 40m. P. M.

DAYS.	Barometer Sunrise.	At 1 P. M.	At 10 P. M.	Thermometer Sunrise.	At 1 P. M.	At 10 P. M.	Daily mean.	Winds Sunrise.	At 1 P. M.	At 10 P. M.	Weather Sunrise.	At 1 P. M.	At 10 P. M.	Rain
1	30.14	30.08	30.03	52	68	53	57.7	N. W. 1	N. E'ly 1	N. E'ly 1	4	2	0	
2	29.96	29.96	29.96	49	67	54	56.7	N. N. E. 2	N. E. 3	N. E. 1	7	0	0	
3	30.01	29.99	30.02	53	74	64	63.7	N'ly 1	N'ly 1	N. W'ly 1	2	0	0	
4	30.03	29.98	30.03	58	73	61	64.0	N. W. 1	N. W. 2	N. W. 1	0	0	0	
5	30.04	30.02	30.05	60	82	62	68.0	N. W. 1	N. W. 1	S. W. 1	0	0	0	
6	29.99	29.94	29.95	61	78	62	67.0	S. W. 2	S. W. 2	S. W. 1	3	4	1	
S 7	29.91	29.92	29.99	65	80	62	69.0	S. W. 1	N. E. 2	N. E. 2	3	8	10	
8	29.95	29.87	29.89	60	76	66	67.3	N. E. 1	S. W. 2	S. W. 1	Foggy	10	0	
9	30.01	29.88	29.88	61	80	66	68.7	N. W. 1	N. W. 2	N. W. 1	3	0	0	
10	29.86	29.83	29.80	62	82	68	70.7	N. W. 1	S. W. 3	S. W. 2	0	0	1	
11	29.68	29.54	29.65	70	83	68	73.7	S. W. 2	S. W. 3	N. W'ly 1	10	4	Shower	0.30
12	29.73	29.70	29.68	60	75	60	65.0	N. W. 2	S. W. 2	S. W. 2	5	2	5	
13	29.66	29.66	29.68	58	77	58	64.3	S. W. 1	W'ly 2	N. W. 2	2	3	0	0.10
S 14	29.77	29.78	29.84	56	70	57	61.0	N. W. 2	N. W. 2	N. W. 1	0	0	0	
15	29.84	29.72	29.69	52	76	60	62.7	N. W. 1	S. W. 2	S. W. 2	2	2	5	
16	29.69	29.75	29.85	58	75	53	63.3	N. W. 1	N. W. 2	N. W. 1	0	2	0	
17	29.90	29.79	29.74	49	70	62	60.3	N. W. 1	W'ly 2	S. W. 1	0	5	3	
18	29.75	29.73	29.72	58	76	66	66.7	N. W. 2	N. W. 2	S. W. 1	8	0	0	
19	29.75	29.77	29.86	65	80	61	68.7	S. W. 1	W'ly 2	S. W. 1	3	3	7	
20	29.89	29.83	29.85	59	75	63	65.7	S. W. 1	S. W. 2	W'ly 1	5	10	Rain	2.25
S 21	29.79	29.77	29.72	62	75	61	66.0	N'ly 2	S'ly 2	N. E. 1	9	7	5	
22	29.67	29.64	29.62	60	63	58	60.3	N. E. 1	E'ly 1	N. E. 2	Rain	Rain	Rain	} 1.50
23	29.52	29.47	29.44	58	63	58	59.7	N'ly 1	N'ly 1	N'ly 1	Misty	10	10	
24	29.37	29.44	29.66	53	65	50	56.0	N. W. 1	N. W. 2	N. W. 1	7	5	0	
25	29.74	...	29.78	44	...	48	...	N. W. 1	...	S. W. 1	0	...	0	
26	29.77	29.72	29.76	48	69	54	57.0	S. W. 1	S. W. 3	S. W. 1	0	3	0	
27	29.75	29.73	29.83	53	70	57	60.0	S. W. 1	S. W. 2	N. E. 1	8	5	2	
S 28	29.89	29.87	29.90	48	68	53	56.0	N. by E. 1	N. E'ly 1	S. E'ly 1	0	3	0	
[illegible]	[illegible]	[illegible]	[illegible]	[illegible]	[illegible]	[illegible]	[illegible]	[illegible]	[illegible]	[illegible]	0	0	1	
30	29.72	29.52	29.46	60	70	69	66.3	S. E. 2	S. E. 3	S. E. 5	10	10	Rain	0.95
Means	29.82	29.79	29.80	56.7	73.4	59.6	...	1.3	2.0	1.4	4.3	3.9	3.0	5.10
								1.6			3.7			
REDUCED TO SEA LEVEL.														
Max.	30.32	30.26	30.23	70	83	69	73.7							
Min.	29.55	29.62	29.62	44	63	48	56.0							
Mean	30.00	29.97	29.98											
Range	0.77	0.64	0.61	26	20	21	17.7							
Mean of month	29.983			...	...	...	63.2							
Extreme range	0.77			...	...	...	39.0							

Prevailing winds from some point between— Days.
N. & E. 7
E. & S. 2
S. & W. 10
W. & N. 11

Days.
Clear 11
Variable . . . } 12
Cloudy . . . . }
Rain fell on . . 7

REMARKS.

1st. Thin, hazy clouds in the morning. Cool through the day.
2d. Pleasant, but quite cool for the season.
3d and 4th. Very fine.
5th. Very fine; sun hot at mid-day.
6th. Very fine. Air damp in the afternoon, with prevalence of clouds. Evening clear.
7th. Sultry and very warm in the morning; wind S. W. Cool in the afternoon and evening, with wind N. E.
8th. Mist at sunrise; wind N. E. Light shower at 9 A. M. Wind S. W. in the afternoon. Clear at 10 P. M.
9th. Very fine. Evening splendid.
10th. Very fine.
11th. Very damp and sultry in the morning. Fine shower, with thunder, from 5 to 6 P. M.
12th. Pleasant.
13th. Pleasant in the morning. Brisk shower from 6 to 7 P. M. Clear at 10 P. M.
14th. Very fine. Evening cloudless and splendid.
15th. Pleasant.
16th. Very fine. Evening cool.
17th and 18th. Very fine.
19th. Pleasant.
20th. Sultry and damp in the morning. Began to rain moderately at 2 P. M. Heavy thunder-showers in the afternoon and evening.
21st. Warm; air sultry.
22d. Rain the greater part of the day. Wind light E'ly and N. E.
23d. Light rain at intervals.
24th. Pleasant. Evening quite cool.
25th and 26th. Very fine.
27th. Pleasant.
28th. Pleasant. Heavy clouds at sunset. Clear [illegible]
29th. Pleasant.
30th. Wind heavy at S E all day. Cloudy, with occasional sprinkling of rain. Heavy rain and very high wind late in the evening.

October, 1856. New Moon, 28d. 4h. 46m. P. M.

Days.	Barometer, reduced to 32° F. Sunrise.	At 1 P. M.	At 10 P. M.	Thermometer. Sunrise.	At 1 P. M.	At 10 P. M.	Daily mean.	Winds. (Direction and Force.) Sunrise.	At 1 P. M.	At 10 P. M.	Weather. (Tenths Cloudy.) Sunrise.	At 1 P. M.	At 10 P. M.	Rain and Snow in Inches of Water.
1	29.40	29.42	29.60	59	65	46	56.7	S. W. 1	S. W. 3	W'ly 2	0	1	5	
2	29.76	29.76	29.82	38	58	52	49.3	S. W. 2	W.byS. 2	S. W. 1	0	2	7	
3	29.83	...	29.89	45	...	47	...	S. W'ly 1	...	W'ly 2	0	...	0	
4	30.00	...	30.02	50	...	46	...	N. W'ly 1	...	N. W'ly 1	0	...	0	
S 5	30.09	30.01	29.96	42	62	53	52.3	N'ly 1	N. E'ly 2	S'ly 1	0	0	0	
6	29.88	29.82	29.88	58	72	64	64.3	S. W. 2	S. W. 2	S. W. 1	9	5	10	
7	29.94	29.96	30.10	48	63	46	52.3	N. W. 1	N. W. 2	N. E. 1	2	5	0	
8	30.18	30.12	30.11	41	63	50	51.3	N'ly 1	S'ly 2	S'ly 1	0	0	0	
9	30.07	29.95	29.99	48	73	54	58.3	S'ly 1	S. W. 1	S. W. 1	3	0	0	
10	29.97	29.96	29.92	50	76	56	60.7	S. W. 1	W'ly 1	S. W'ly 1	0	0	0	
11	29.84	...	29.85	50	...	62	...	S. W. 1	...	N'ly 1	0	...	0	
S 12	30.00	29.98	29.94	50	63	50	54.3	N. E'ly 1	E'ly 1	S. W'ly 1	0	0	2	
13	29.77	29.61	29.53	54	70	57	60.3	S. W. 2	S. W. 2	S. W. 1	10	9	Rain	0.35
14	29.77	29.77	30.01	38	44	34	38.7	N'ly 2	N. E'ly 2	N. E. 3	10	10	3	
15	30.10	30.12	30.12	29	44	32	35.0	N. E'ly 2	N. E. 2	N'ly 1	4	0	0	
16	30.04	29.92	29.93	30	54	42	62.0	N'ly 1	S. W. 1	S. W'ly 1	0	0	0	
17	30.00	30.00	29.97	38	57	54	49.7	N. E. 2	N. E. 3	N. E. 3	0	2	7	
18	29.82	29.80	29.87	57	60	51	56.0	S. E. 3	S. W. 2	S. W. 1	Rain	2	8	0.50
S 19	29.92	29.89	29.99	44	63	50	52.3	W byS. 2	W byN 2	N. W'ly 1	0	3	0	
20	30.04	30.03	30.03	46	65	49	53.3	N'ly 1	N. by E. 1	Calm	0	5	0	
21	30.00	29.93	29.85	45	68	53	53.3	W'ly 1	S. E'ly 1	S'ly 1	4	3	0	
22	29.74	29.62	29.61	49	69	56	58.0	S. W. 1	S. W. 1	Calm	Hazy	10	10	
23	29.52	29.50	29.67	52	63	36	50.3	N. W. 1	N. W. 2	N'ly 3	Hazy	3	0	
24	29.83	29.85	29.99	30	41	29	33.3	N. W. 3	N. W. 3	N. W. 1	0	7	0	
25	29.95	29.86	29.88	28	48	39	28.3	N. W. 2	N. W. 2	N. W. 2	0	5	0	
S 26	29.88	29.83	29.86	33	54	40	42.3	N. W. 1	N. W. 1	Calm	5	0	0	
27	29.84	29.80	29.65	37	54	51	47.3	S'ly 1	S'ly 1	S. W. 1	8	10	10	} 0.30
28	29.44	...	29.52	57	56	41	51.3	S. W. 1	N. W. 2	N. W. 1	F'g, sh'r	7	0	
29	29.61	29.66	29.73	39	53	37	43.0	N. W. 1	N. W. 3	Calm	5	7	0	
30	29.66	29.49	29.44	43	62	46	47.0	S. W. 2	S. W. 3	N'ly 2	3	1	5	
31	29.43	29.40	29.63	45	44	32	40.3	W'ly 1	W'ly 3	N. W. 2	6	10	0	
Means	29.85	29.82	29.85	44.3	59.3	46.9	...	1.4	1.9	1.4	3.5	3.8	2.5	1.15
									1.6			3.3		
REDUCED TO SEA LEVEL.														
Max.	30.36	30.30	30.30	59	76	64	64.7							
Min.	29.58	29.58	29.62	28	41	29	28.3							
Mean	30.03	30.00	30.03											
Range	0.78	0.72	0.68	31	35	35	36.4							
Mean of month	30.020			...	...	...	50.2							
Extreme range	0.78			...	...	...	48.0							

Prevailing winds from some point between— Days.
N. & E. 6
E. & S. 1
S. & W. 13
W. & N. 11

Days.
Clear 15
Variable . . . . } 12
Cloudy . . . . }
Rain fell on . . 4

REMARKS.

1st. Very fine.
2d. Very cool in the morning. Day fine.
3d. Fine.
4th and 5th. Very fine.
6th. Variable. Clouds and sunshine; air damp.
7th. Pleasant. Evening cool.
8th and 9th. Very fine.
10th. Fine; air hazy, without clouds. Warm for the season.
11th and 12th. Very fine.
13th. Cloudy and mild. Began to rain moderately at 10 P. M.
14th. Very cold for the season. In the evening, wind fresh from the N. E., while the clouds were moving from W'ly.
15th. Fine, though cold. Black frost this morning. Ice formed in open vessels of water, of the thickness of window glass. This is the first frost on College Hill to injure the most delicate plants.
16th. Very fine. Severe frost this morning.
17th. Pleasant in the morning. Mostly cloudy in the evening.
18th. Rain at 5 A. M. from S. E. During the morning, the wind hauled to S. W., and the clouds became broken.
19th. Very fine.
20th. Pleasant. Warm for the season.
21st. Pleasant and warm.
22d. Warm. Nearly calm all day; air hazy.
23d. Warm in the morning; wind light N. W'ly. Air grew cool in the evening; wind very fresh, and more to the north. Faint aurora in evening.
24th. Cool. Evening very clear.
25th. Pleasant.
26th. Very fine.
27th. Cloudy, with sprinkling of rain in the afternoon.
28th. Shower during the last night. Air warm and damp this morning. Evening clear.
29th. Pleasant. Evening very fine.
30th. Pleasant.
31st. Blustering and cold.

November, 1856. New Moon, 27d. 10h. 53m. A. M.

Days.	Barometer Sunrise.	At 1 P. M.	At 10 P. M.	Thermometer Sunrise.	At 1 P. M.	At 10 P. M.	Daily mean	Winds Sunrise.	At 1 P. M.	At 10 P. M.	Weather Sunrise.	At 1 P. M.	At 10 P. M.	Rain and Snow
1	29.75	29.61	29.60	29	44	52	41.7	N. W. 1	S. W. 3	S. W. 2	0	5	0	
S 2	29.74	29.74	29.86	45	64	54	54.3	S. W. 1	S. W. 1	S. W. 2	0	6	5	
3	29.91	29.85	29.71	47	61	56	54.7	S. W. 1	S'ly 2	S'ly 1	0	10	Rain	0.40
4	29.60	29.50	29.27	61	65	63	63.0	S. W. 2	S. W. 1	S. W. 3	10	10	10	0.10
5	29.47	29.60	29.98	47	40	29	38.7	N. W. 3	N. W. 4	N. W. 1	2	3	0	
6	30.24	30.29	30.40	23	39	29	30.3	N. W. 2	N. W. 1	N. W. 1	0	0	0	
7	30.37	30.31	30.26	38	54	45	45.7	S. W. 2	S. W. 3	S. W. 1	5	10	7	
8	30.15	...	30.01	48	...	46	...	S. W. 1	...	S. W. 2	10	...	Rain	
S 9	29.82	29.81	29.85	41	43	33	39.0	N. W. 2	N'ly 2	N. E. 2	10	10	8	
10	29.92	29.88	29.93	28	36	25	29.7	N. W. 2	N. W. 2	N. W. 1	7	0	0	
11	29.95	29.91	29.98	22	40	31	31.0	N. W. 1	N. W. 1	N. W. 1	0	0	0	
12	29.98	29.95	29.93	27	50	38	38.3	N. W. 1	S. W. 1	W'ly 1	0	10	10	
13	29.93	29.93	29.97	35	49	39	41.0	N. W. 1	N. W. 1	N. W. 1	0	10	10	
14	29.93	29.80	29.71	33	46	37	38.7	N. W. 1	S. W. 1	S. W. 1	5	10	Rain	
15	29.69	29.64	29.67	32	33	27	30.7	N'ly 1	N. W. 2	N. W. 1	Snow	0	0	
S 16	29.64	29.50	29.48	27	46	46	39.7	N. W. 1	S. W. 2	S. W. 2	0	0	3	
17	29.48	29.45	29.60	39	40	30	36.3	S. W. 1	N. W. 2	N. W. 2	10	2	0	
18	29.63	29.66	29.76	27	39	31	32.3	N. W. 1	N. W. 2	N. W. 1	0	10	0	
19	29.79	29.81	30.02	25	40	26	30.3	N. W. 1	N. W. 2	N. W. 2	0	0	0	
20	30.11	30.10	30.17	22	37	27	28.7	N. W. 1	N. W. 1	N. W. 1	0	0	0	
21	30.13	30.06	30.02	23	47	36	35.3	S. W. 1	S. W. 1	S. W. 1	0	5	10	
22	29.75	29.74	29.94	50	58	44	50.7	S. E. 2	S. W. 2	S. W. 1	Rain	2	0	0.45
S 23	30.05	30.02	29.95	34	49	39	40.7	N. W. 1	N. W'ly 1	S. W'ly 1	0	3	10	
24	29.79	29.72	29.89	42	54	45	47.0	S. W. 2	S. W. 3	N. W. 2	Misty	2	3	
25	29.98	29.97	29.80	35	44	40	39.7	N. by E. 1	N. E. 2	N. E. 1	1	10	Rain	
26	29.44	29.40	29.57	44	55	44	47.7	S. E'ly 1	W. 2	N. W. 2	Rain	1	5	0.60
27	29.71	29.68	29.62	35	44	34	37.7	W. 1	W. 2	W. 1	1	9	0	
28	29.71	29.65	29.75	30	42	30	34.0	W. 1	W. 2	N. 2	0	2	2	
29	29.61	29.25	29.24	26	31	25	27.3	N. E. 2	N. E. 3	N. E. 3	Snow	Rain	10	0.50
S 30	29.70	29.74	29.89	22	36	30	29.3	N. W. 3	N. W. 2	N. W. 1	0	0	0	
Means	29.83	29.78	29.83	34.9	45.7	37.7	...	1.4	1.9	1.5	3.7	4.8	4.4	2.00
									1.6			4.3		
REDUCED TO SEA LEVEL.														
Max.	30.55	30.49	30.58	61	65	63	63.0							
Min.	29.62	29.43	29.42	22	31	25	27.3							
Mean	30.01	29.96	30.01											
Range	0.93	1.06	1.16	39	34	38	35.7							
Mean of month	29.993			...	...	...	39.4							
Extreme range	1.16			...	...	...	41.0							

Prevailing winds from some point between— Days.
N. & E. 2
E. & S. 0
S. & W. 12
W. & N. 16

Days.
Clear 9
Variable . . . . } 11
Cloudy . . . . }
Rain or snow fell on 10

REMARKS.

1st. Wind fresh, and dust abundant.
2d. Very fine.
3d. Pleasant in the morning. Cloudy in the afternoon. Began to rain moderately from 8 to 9 P. M.; air warm.
4th. Cloudy, with occasional mist and sprinkling of rain.
5th. Very blustering through the day. Evening clear and cold.
6th. Very fine.
7th. Mild, with some appearances of rain.
8th. Cloudy in the morning. Moderate rain in the evening.
9th. Air raw and misty, with occasional sprinkling of rain
10th. Pleasant. Evening cool and splendid.
11th. Very fine. Evening cloudless and splendid.
12th. Pleasant. Cloudy in the afternoon.
13th. Pleasant.
14th. Cloudy in the afternoon. Light rain in the evening.
15th. Light snow this morning from sunrise to 10 A. M., which melted as it fell.
16th and 17th. Pleasant.
18th. Cool, but pleasant.
19th. Very fine. Evening very clear.
20th. Very fine. Day and evening cloudless.
21st. Pleasant
22d. Brisk rain from the S. E. in the morning. Clear in the afternoon and evening, and very mild, with wind at S. W.
23d. Pleasant.
24th. Mist this morning. Pleasant in the afternoon and evening.
25th. Pleasant in the morning. Cloudy in the afternoon. Began to rain moderately at 5 P. M.
26th. Rain through the night, which continued with mist till 9 A. M.; then clear and pleasant.
27th. Pleasant in the morning. Cloudy at noon. Clear and pleasant in the evening.
28th. Pleasant. Weather hazy at 9 P. M.
29th. Snow from sunrise to 11 A. M., when it turned to rain. Snow from one to two inches deep. Evening cloudy and cold; storm ceased.
30th. Cold, but very fine overhead.

December, 1856. New Moon, 27d. 3h. 37m. A. M.

Days.	Barometer, reduced to 32° F. Sunrise.	At 1 P. M.	At 10 P. M.	Thermometer. Sunrise.	At 1 P. M.	At 10 P. M.	Daily mean.	Winds. (Direction and Force.) Sunrise.	At 1 P. M.	At 10 P. M.	Weather. (Tenths Cloudy.) Sunrise.	At 1 P. M.	At 10 P. M.	Rain and Snow in Inches of Water
1	29.98	29.94	29.91	26	36	30	30.7	N. W. 2	N. W. 1	N. W. 1	8	10	9	
2	29.79	29.69	29.66	22	40	30	30.7	S. W. 1	W'ly 1	W'ly 2	2	0	10	
3	29.38	28.85	29.02	31	39	32	34.0	E'ly 1	E'ly 2	N. W. 3	Misty	Rain	0	0.75
4	29.24	29.41	29.61	29	30	25	28.0	W'ly 3	N. W'ly 4	W'ly 2	2	2	0	
5	29.74	29.79	29.89	24	32	25	27.0	W. N. W. 2	N. W'ly 3	N. W. 2	0	0	0	
6	29.92	29.89	29.91	22	31	23	25.3	N. W. 2	N. W. 2	N. W. 1	0	0	0	
S 7	29.82	29.76	29.78	23	31	20	24.7	W'ly 2	W'ly 2	N. W. 1	3	0	0	
8	29.79	29.79	29.93	11	23	17	17.0	N. W. 1	N. W. 2	N. W. 1	0	2	0	
9	30.03	30.12	30.24	17	25	20	20.7	N. W. 2	N. W. 2	N. W. 1	7	0	0	
10	30.33	30.30	30.31	15	32	23	23.3	N. W. 1	N. W. 1	N. W. 1	0	0	0	
11	30.15	29.89	29.47	27	41	50	39.3	S. W. 1	S. E'ly 2	S'ly 4	10	10	Rain	1.05
12	29.56	29.59	29.75	36	48	35	39.7	S. W. 1	W'ly 2	W'ly 2	2	0	0	
13	29.83	29.91	29.99	30	43	36	36.3	S. W. 1	W by N. 3	S. W. 2	0	1	10	
S 14	29.69	29.25	28.88	36	41	42	39.7	E'ly 3	S. E. 3	W'ly 5	R'n, sn.	Rain	7	2.25
15	29.30	29.67	29.92	31	34	25	30.0	W by S. 4	N. W'ly 2	N. W. 2	2	0	3	
16	29.94	29.87	29.82	20	23	15	19.3	N. W. 2	N. by E. 2	N. by E. 2	7	2	0	
17	29.85	29.95	30.13	18	19	7	14.7	W'ly 2	N. W. 4	N. W. 2	2	0	0	
18	30.33	30.34	30.48	—5	2	—2	—1.7	N. W. 3	N. W. 3	N. W. 2	1	0	1	
19	30.55	30.51	30.42	—2	17	14	9.7	N. W. 1	N. E. 1	N. E. 2	0	7	10	
20	30.19	29.84	29.59	25	38	46	36.3	S. E. 1	S'ly 2	S. W'ly 3	Snow	Rain	Rain	1.15
S 21	29.69	29.80	29.90	31	26	24	27.0	N. W. 2	N. W. 2	N. W. 2	10	10	9	
22	29.82	29.76	29.70	21	24	24	23.0	N. W. 2	N. E'ly 2	N. E'ly 2	10	10	10	
23	29.54	29.52	29.16	27	25	25	25.7	N. E. 2	N. E. 3	N. E'ly 4	Snow	Snow	Snow	0.60
24	29.11	29.04	29.06	22	23	13	19.3	N'ly 3	N. W. 2	N. W. 2	10	10	10	
25	29.12	29.21	29.46	13	20	21	18.0	N. W. 2	N. W. 3	N. W. 1	10	10	0	
26	29.59	29.60	29.62	21	25	14	20.0	N. W. 2	N. W. 3	N. W. 2	9	7	0	
27	29.65	29.66	29.72	10	25	17	17.3	N. W. 1	N. W. 3	N. W. 1	0	0	0	
S 28	29.69	29.59	29.68	16	34	31	27.0	N. W. 1	N. W. 2	N. W'ly 2	0	Misty	10	
29	29.72	29.73	29.80	29	41	28	32.7	S. W. 2	S. W. 1	S. W. 2	7	5	0	
30	29.85	29.87	29.72	28	35	25	29.3	N. W. 2	N. W. 1	N. W. 1	9	5	6	
31	30.00	29.98	30.00	25	28	26	26.3	N. E. 2	N. E. 2	N. E. 2	10	10	10	
Means	29.78	29.75	29.76	21.9	30.0	24.5	...	1.9	2.2	2.0	5.2	4.9	4.4	5.80
								2.1			4.8			
REDUCED TO SEA LEVEL.														
Max.	30.73	30.69	30.64	36	48	50	39.7	Prevailing winds from some point between—		Days.			Days.	
Min.	29.29	29.22	29.06	—5	2	—2	—1.7	N. & E.		6	Clear		11	
Mean	29.96	29.93	29.94					E. & S.		3	Variable		} 12	
Range	1.44	1.47	1.58	41	46	52	41.4	S. & W.		4	Cloudy			
Mean of month	29.943			...	...	...	25.5	W. & N.		18	Rain or snow fell on		8	
Extreme range	1.67			...	...	...	55.0							

Remarks.

1st. Air raw and cold.
2d. Pleasant. Air raw in the afternoon.
3d. Light snow last night. Mist and light rain in morning; bar. falling rapidly. At 1 P. M., bar. 28.95; wind fresh E'ly. At 3 P. M., calm; mist, fog, and light fine rain; bar. 28.80. At 5 P. M., bar. began to rise; wind sprung up at N.W. At 8 P. M., bar. 29.00. Clear at 10 P. M.; wind blustering N.W.
4th. Very blustering.
5th. Cold and blustering. Evening splendid.
6th. Very fine. Evening splendid.
7th. Cold, but fine. Evening again splendid.
8th. Cold, but very fine. Evening perfectly splendid, without a trace of a cloud.
9th. Fine. Evening cloudless; air transparent.
10th. Air mild; very fine. Evening splendid.
11th. Cloudy in morning; air raw; wind S. E'ly. Began to rain from 4 to 5 P. M., and continued during the evening; wind heavy at S. E'ly.
12th. Pleasant. Evening very clear.
13th. Pleasant. Evening cloudy.
14th. Light rain and snow at sunrise; bar. 29.78, falling rapidly. Rain continued A. M.; at 4 P. M., heavy, wind hauling from S. E. to S. W., and bar. 29.05. At 5 P. M., wind light S. W.; light rain. At 6 P. M., bar. 28.97; wind S. W'ly; clouds broken. At 7 P. M., bar. 28.94; at 8 P. M., 28.90, ther. 50°. At 9 P. M., bar. 28.93; at 10 P. M., 28.98, ther. 42°. Wind blustering since 7 P. M. Rain all day.
15th. Blustering.
16th. Air very cold during day and evening.
17th. Wind blustering, and weather severe.
18th. Extremely cold and severe. Ther. this morning, —5°, with cutting wind from N. W.
19th. Pleasant. Barom., reduced to sea level, 30.71, which is higher than at any time since Jan. 6, 1855, when it rose to 30.85.
20th. Light snow at sunrise, which soon turned to mist and rain. Rain continued all day.
21st. Air raw and uncomfortable.
22d. Cold and raw. Air filled with snow.
23d. One or two inches of light snow. Evening very blustering.
24th. Cold and rough. Snow last night, much drifted—about four inches deep on the level.
25th. Blustering snow-gust in morning. Evening clear and pleasant.
26th. Variable and blustering. Evening clear and pleasant.
27th. Very fine.
28th. Clear and pleasant at sunrise. Cloudy, with mist in the afternoon.
29th. Very fine. 30th. Pleasant.
31st. Air rather raw.

January, 1857. New Moon, 25d. 6h. 18m. P. M.

Days.	Barometer Sunrise.	At 1 P. M.	At 10 P. M.	Thermometer Sunrise.	At 1 P. M.	At 10 P. M.	Daily mean.	Winds Sunrise.	At 1 P. M.	At 10 P. M.	Weather Sunrise.	At 1 P. M.	At 10 P. M.	Rain and Snow
1	30.03	30.00	30.08	28	32	24	28.0	N. E. 1	N. E. 2	N. E. 2	Snow	8	10	
2	30.10	30.02	29.98	20	30	24	24.7	N. E. 2	N. E'ly 2	N. E. 2	10	7	10	
3	29.71	29.36	29.21	26	32	24	27.3	N. E. 1	N. E. 2	N. E. 4	Snow	Snow	Snow	1.20
S 4	29.46	29.54	29.78	23	27	19	23.0	N. W. 1	N. W. 3	N. W. 2	2	0	0	
5	29.78	29.75	29.77	17	20	9	15.3	N. W. 2	N. W. 3	N. W. 2	4	5	1	
6	29.77	29.68	29.72	3	13	4	6.7	N. W. 2	N. W. 3	N. W. 3	0	0	0	
7	29.73	29.64	29.60	3	11	6	6.7	N. W. 2	N. W. 3	N. W. 2	2	1	0	
8	29.68	29.69	29.79	0	8	5	4.3	N. W. 3	N. W. 3	N. W. 3	10	2	0	
9	29.82	29.66	29.63	2	20	13	11.7	N. W. 2	W'ly 1	N. W'ly 1	1	3	3	
10	29.63	29.54	29.42	17	27	23	22.3	W'ly 1	S. W. 1	S. W. 1	8	10	Snow	
S 11	29.36	29.39	29.60	21	27	16	21.3	N'ly 2	N. W. 2	N'ly 2	10	Snow	10	
12	29.70	29.78	29.86	4	19	10	11.0	N. W. 1	N. W. 1	N. W. 1	0	0	0	
13	29.84	29.72	29.64	10	30	16	18.7	S. W'ly 1	S. W. 1	S. W. 1	0	9	0	
14	29.62	29.57	29.64	12	28	22	20.7	N. W. 1	N. W. 1	N'ly 2	0	1	Snow	
15	29.67	29.81	30.04	18	20	2	13.3	N. W. 1	N. W. 2	N. W. 3	10	5	0	
16	30.19	30.12	29.95	—3	17	17	10.3	N. W. 2	N. W. 2	S. W'ly 2	0	2	10	
17	29.74	29.67	29.86	19	29	14	20.7	S. W. 1	S. W. 2	N. W'ly 3	3	10	10	
S 18	30.21	30.09	29.89	—9	—4	3	—3.3	N. W. 2	N. W. 2	N. E. 3	10	10	Snow	
19	29.06	28.94	29.17	6	12	8	8.7	N. E. 5	N. E. 4	N. W. 3	Snow	9	2	2.50
20	29.61	29.74	29.85	6	20	16	14.0	N. W. 2	N. W. 3	N. W. 1	0	1	0	
21	29.74	29.69	29.64	21	36	25	27.3	S. E'ly 1	S'ly 1	S'ly 2	Sn., m't	10	7	
22	29.41	29.23	29.47	17	17	—6	9.3	N'ly 2	N'ly 2	N. W. 3	10	10	0	
23	29.79	29.86	30.15	—14	—5	—10	—9.7	W. N. W. 4	W'ly 3	W'ly 1	0	0	0	
24	30.29	30.20	29.97	—14	10	9	1.7	W'ly 1	S. E'ly 2	N. E. 1	2	3	Snow	0.10
S 25	30.05	30.09	30.32	0	15	4	6.3	N. W. 1	N. W. 2	N. W. 1	0	0	0	
26	30.53	30.51	30.36	—2	21	13	10.7	N. W. 2	S'ly 1	S. W'ly 2	0	Hazy	10	
27	30.20	30.07	30.09	32	40	36	36.0	S. W. 2	S. W. 2	S. W. 1	10	Misty	Rain	0.10
28	30.22	30.19	30.14	33	35	30	32.7	N. W. 2	N. E. 2	N. E. 2	7	1	Snow	
29	30.02	29.93	29.93	25	31	29	28.3	N. E. 2	N. E. 1	N'ly 1	[illegible]	[illegible]	[illegible]	0.30
30	[illegible]	[illegible]	[illegible]	[illegible]	[illegible]	[illegible]	[illegible]	[illegible]	[illegible]	[illegible]	[illegible]	[illegible]	[illegible]	
31	30.12	29.85	29.48	26	32	39	32.3	N. E. 3	N. E. 3	E'ly 2	Snow	Hail	Rain	1.40
Means	29.84	29.79	29.81	11.9	22.0	15.0	...	1.8	2.1	2.0	5.1	5.4	5.3	5.50
								2.0			5.3			
REDUCED TO SEA LEVEL.														
Max.	30.71	30.69	30.54	33	40	39	36.0	Prevailing winds from some point between—		Days.			Days.	
Min.	29.21	29.12	29.35	—14	—5	—10	—9.7	N. & E.		7	Clear		9	
Mean	30.02	29.97	29.99					E. & S.		2	Variable		} 7	
Range	1.50	1.57	1.19	47	45	49	45.7	S. & W.		5	Cloudy			
Mean of month	29.993			...	...	...	16.3	W. & N.		17	Rain or snow fell on		15	
Extreme range	1.59			...	...	...	54.0							

Remarks.

1st. Mild. Snow in morning, covering ground.
2d. Appearances of storm.
3d. Began to snow very gently about 6 A. M.; continued to fall fast through the day. At 10 P. M., snowing very fast, with wind heavy at N. E.
4th. Snow about ten inches deep on the level, and somewhat drifted. Day fine.
5th. Pleasant, but cold.
6th and 7th. Very cold.
8th. Excessively cold.
9th. Cold much abated.
10th. Mild and cloudy in morning. Very moderate snow from S. W. in afternoon and evening.
11th. Light snow in morning; quantity small.
12th. Very fine. 13th. Very pleasant.
14th. Pleasant. Light snow in the evening.
15th. Fresh dusting of snow on the ground this morning. Evening very cold.
16th. Pleasant. Evening cloudy, with appearances of storm.
17th. Mild and pleasant. Evening cold.
18th. Ther. this morning —9°, being lower than at any time since Feb. 7, 1855, when it was —16°; wind moderate at N.W. Began to snow at 6 P. M.; wind N. E., pretty brisk; ther. +2°.
19th. Storm of extreme severity last night. Snow this morning very deep, and much drifted; wind heavy at N. E., and cold. Snowed with violence till 11 A. M. Air full of snow P. M. Mostly clear at 10 P. M. About 18 inches of snow on the level.
20th. Very fine.
21st. Pleasant. Air full of snow-mist A. M.
22d. An inch of fresh snow on the ground this morning, and snow still falling, which ceased before noon—amount small. Grew cold very fast towards night. At 10 P. M., thermometer 6° below zero, with a heavy wind.
23d. At sunrise, thermometer 14° below zero, [illegible] This has been the coldest day, and the severest to be out, for a period of twenty-five years; its mean temperature being 9°.7 below zero.
24th. Extremely cold morning. Ther. —14°, but air very calm. Began to snow from 4 to 5 P. M.
25th. Cold, but pleasant. About three inches of extremely light snow fell last night.
26th. Wind S'ly in afternoon, and air very raw. Evening mostly cloudy.
27th. Cloudy, with mist. Light rain in evening.
28th. Mild. Began to snow from 8 to 9 P. M.
29th. Mist and light snow. Stars out at 10 P. M. About an inch of fresh snow fell.
30th. Very fine.
31st. Snow A. M. Heavy rain P. M. and evening.

February, 1857. New Moon, 24d. 4h. 50m. A. M.

DAYS.	BAROMETER, REDUCED TO 32° F. Sunrise.	At 1 P. M.	At 10 P. M.	THERMOMETER. Sunrise.	At 1 P. M.	At 10 P. M.	Daily mean.	WINDS. (DIRECTION AND FORCE.) Sunrise.	At 1 P. M.	At 10 P. M.	WEATHER. (TENTHS CLOUDY.) Sunrise.	At 1 P. M.	At 10 P. M.	RAIN AND SNOW IN INCHES OF WATER.
S 1	29.62	29.60	29.62	32	43	27	34 0	S. W. 1	S. W. 1	S. W. 1	10	10	0	
2	29.65	29.69	29.94	20	21	12	17.7	N. W. 1	N. W. 2	N. W. 1	7	0	0	
3	30.13	30.20	30.29	4	21	14	13.0	N. W. 1	N. W. 1	N. W. 1	0	0	3	
4	30.11	29.96	30.07	26	43	34	34.3	S. W. 1	S. W. 3	S. W. 2	8	10	Rain	
5	30.18	30.20	30.21	35	34	30	33.0	N. E. 1	N. E. 1	N. E. 2	Rain	Foggy	Misty	
6	30.20	30.15	30.53	30	47	38	38.3	N. E. 1	S. W'ly 2	S'ly 2	Foggy	5	7	
7	30.21	30.15	30.07	40	46	41	42.3	S'ly 1	S. S. E. 1	S. E'ly 2	10	Foggy	Foggy	
S 8	29.93	29.85	29.76	45	49	43	45.7	S. W'ly 2	S.S.W. 2	N.W'ly 4	Foggy	Foggy	Rain	1.25
9	30.04	30.17	30.30	28	25	16	23.0	N.W'ly 3	N. W. 4	N.W'ly 3	Snow	0	0	
10	30.19	29.95	30.26	15	30	9	18.0	W'ly 2	S. W'ly 3	N.W'ly 5	0	8	0	
11	30.41	30.39	30.58	2	13	6	7.0	W.N.W. 2	N. W. 2	N. W. 1	0	5	0	
12	30.80	30.77	30.66	—3	14	15	8.7	N. E. 1	N. E. 1	S'ly 2	0	0	10	
13	30.33	30.09	30.08	31	43	34	36.0	S'ly 2	S'ly 3	W'ly 1	10	Rain	0	0.25
14	30.17	30.25	30.25	30	43	30	34.3	S. W'ly 1	S. W'ly 2	S. W. 1	8	2	0	
S 15	30.06	29.98	29.99	40	49	35	41.3	S. W. 2	S. W. 2	S. W. 1	Foggy	3	0	
16	29.99	29.96	29.97	41	55	46	47.3	S. E'ly 2	S. W. 2	S. W. 1	Foggy	Sprin'le	7	
17	29.94	29.87	29.82	41	61	48	50.0	S. E'ly 1	S. W. 2	S'ly 2	Foggy	8	Foggy	
18	29.79	29.76	29.78	45	57	43	48.3	S. W. 1	S. E'ly 1	S'ly 1	Foggy	0	0	
19	29.65	29.77	29.96	35	35	30	33.3	N. E. 1	N. E. 2	N. E. 3	Foggy	10	Snow	
20	30.14	30.09	29.84	28	33	32	31.0	N. E. 2	N. E. 2	N. E. 2	10	10	Rain	0.65
21	29.54	29.55	29.86	33	42	32	35.7	N. E. 1	N.W'ly 2	N. W. 2	10	5	0	
S 22	30.01	29.91	29.86	26	39	28	31.0	N. W. 1	S'ly 2	S'ly 1	0	0	0	
23	29.76	29.67	29.82	27	47	33	35.7	N. W. 1	W'ly 3	W'ly 1	0	10	0	
24	29.89	29.82	29.61	30	48	43	40.3	S. W. 1	S. E. 3	S'ly 1	2	2	1	
25	29.50	29.45	29.57	52	68	45	55.0	S. W. 3	S. W. 3	N. W. 3	9	9	2	
26	29.73	29.83	30.05	31	33	20	28.0	N. W. 2	N. W. 3	N. W. 2	3	2	0	
27	30.12	29.99	29.74	16	29	25	23.3	N. W. 2	N. W. 2	W'ly 1	7	9	10	
28	29.41	29.40	29.43	27	33	28	29.3	W'ly 1	N.W'ly 3	N. W. 1	Snow	0	0	0.20
Means	29.98	29.95	30.00	28.8	39.3	29.9	...	1.5	2.1	1.7	6.9	5.2	4.0	2.36
									1.8			5.4		
REDUCED TO SEA LEVEL.														
Max.	30.98	30.95	30.84	52	68	48	55.0							
Min.	29.59	29.58	29.61	—3	13	6	7.0							
Mean	30.16	30.13	30.18											
Range	1.39	1.37	1.23	55	55	42	48.0							
Mean of month	30.157			...	...	...	32.7							
Extreme range	1.40			...	...	...	71.0							

Prevailing winds from some point between— Days.
N. & E. 4
E. & S. 3
S. & W. 11
W. & N. 10

Days.
Clear 4
Variable . . . . } 14
Cloudy . . . . }
Rain or snow fell on 10

REMARKS.

1st. Very mild. Cloudy in morning. Clouds broken in afternoon. Evening mostly clear. Fog-bow and haze around the moon.
2d. Pleasant. Evening cold.
3d. Pleasant. Fog-bow about moon in evening.
4th. Mild. Light showers in the evening.
5th. Mild. Light rain this morning. Fog and mist through the day.
6th. Mild and pleasant.
7th. Mild. Dense fog all day.
8th. Mild. Fog and mist through day. Heavy showers in the evening.
9th. Grew cold during day. Evening splendid.
10th. Fine. Cold and blustering in evening.
11th. Fine, but cold. Evening very clear.
12th. The barometer at 10 A. M. stood at 30.87, being higher than I have ever before seen it. The wind came round to S'ly early in the afternoon. Evening cloudy, with appearances of storm. Barometer began to fall before noon.
13th. Light rain from S'ly nearly all day. Evening mostly clear.
14th. Very fine.
15th. Very fine. Evening still and clear.
16th. Remarkably mild. Thick fog in the morning. Sprinkling of rain from 1 to 2 P. M.
17th. Very warm for the season. Fog in the morning and evening. Sunshine at mid-day.
18th. Very fine. Snow nearly all gone, and the frost out of the ground in many places.
19th. Light rain at mid-day. Began to snow from 8 to 9 P. M.
20th. About an inch of fresh snow on the ground this morning. Mist through the day. Rain in the evening.
21st. Cloudy in the morning. Ground covered with sleet. Evening clear.
22d. Very fine.
23d. Pleasant in the morning. Cloudy, and air raw.
24th. Very fine.
25th. Pleasant, and very warm for the season. The warmest day since October 22, 1856.
26th. Flurry of snow between 9 and 10 A. M. Evening clear and blustering. Faint aurora low down in the north.
27th. Air raw. Appearances of storm in the evening.
28th. Between two and three inches of fresh snow on the ground this morning. Mostly clear in the afternoon and evening.

March, 1857. New Moon, 25d. 5h. 20m. P. M.

DAYS.	Barometer Sunrise.	At 1 P. M.	At 10 P. M.	Thermometer Sunrise.	At 1 P. M.	At 10 P. M.	Daily mean.	Winds Sunrise.	At 1 P. M.	At 10 P. M.	Weather Sunrise.	At 1 P. M.	At 10 P. M.	Rain and Snow
S 1	29.44	29.40	29.42	20	31	24	25.0	N. W. 2	S'ly 2	N. E. 3	5	10	Snow	
2	29.34	29.22	29.38	24	16	16	18.7	N. E. 4	N. by E. 5	N'ly 4	Snow	Snow	Snow	0.50
3	29.55	29.63	29.79	9	23	17	16.3	N. W. 2	N. W. 2	N. W. 1	3	0	0	
4	29.85	29.85	29.93	19	39	26	28.0	S. W. 1	S. W. 2	S. W. 1	0	3	0	
5	29.99	29.96	29.87	21	39	34	31.3	Calm	S'ly 2	S'ly 2	0	5	10	
6	29.27	29.18	29.54	34	41	24	33.0	E'ly 1	W'ly 2	N. W. 2	Misty	7	0	0.75
7	29.58	29.71	30.02	21	24	15	20.0	N. W. 3	W by N 4	N. W. 2	0	0	0	
S 8	30.22	30.20	30.19	10	27	18	18.3	N. W. 2	N'ly 2	N. W. 1	0	0	0	
9	30.06	29.77	29.33	15	38	32	28.3	E'ly 1	S. E. 3	S'ly 1	1	10	Snow	0.75
10	29.48	29.69	29.93	23	26	14	21.0	W by N 4	W by N 3	N. W. 2	1	0	2	
11	29.98	29.88	29.71	6	34	30	23.3	S. W. 2	S. E'ly 2	S'ly 1	1	10	Snow	
12	29.74	29.85	30.09	26	24	13	21.0	W'ly 2	N. W. 3	N. W. 2	2	0	0	
13	30.30	30.23	30.10	8	27	22	19.0	N. W. 1	S. E. 2	S. E'ly 2	0	0	7	
14	29.84	29.58	29.70	27	43	30	33.3	S'ly 1	S. W'ly 1	N. W. 1	Snow	4	0	0.15
S 15	29.90	29.96	29.99	30	42	28	34.0	W'ly 1	S. E'ly 2	S. E'ly 1	7	0	0	
16	29.90	29.77	29.59	34	46	37	39.0	S'ly 1	S'ly 2	S'ly 1	9	2	Shower	
17	29.65	29.71	29.96	33	48	34	38.3	N. W. 2	N. W. 2	N. W. 1	0	0	0	
18	30.01	29.98	29.86	30	48	40	39.3	S'ly 1	S. E'ly 2	S'ly 2	9	10	2	
19	29.52	29.21	29.10	44	48	36	42.7	S'ly 3	S'ly 2	W'ly 3	10	Shower	10	1.20
20	29.15	29.36	29.69	33	40	30	34.3	W'ly 3	W'ly 3	N. W. 2	3	10	0	
21	29.76	29.73	29.79	29	37	32	32.7	N. E. 1	S'ly 2	S'ly 2	9	10	8	
S 22	29.98	30.08	30.24	30	40	29	33.0	N. W. 3	N'ly 2	N. E. 2	7	10	2	
23	30.26	30.09	29.92	27	37	35	33.0	N. W. 1	S'ly 2	S'ly 2	8	10	10	
24	29.76	29.65	29.58	36	49	41	42.0	S. W'ly 1	S. W'ly 1	S'ly 1	Foggy	10	10	
25	29.41	29.32	29.38	36	50	34	40.0	S. W. 1	N. W. 2	N. W. 3	2	3	0	
26	29.39	29.43	29.57	31	46	35	37.3	N. W. 2	N. W. 2	N. W. 1	0	8	0	
27	29.53	29.47	29.56	31	51	40	40.7	N. W. 1	N. W. 1	N. W. 1	0	3	10	
28	29.56	29.53	29.62	36	48	40	41.3	N'ly 2	N'ly 1	N'ly 1	10	10	10	
S 29	29.63	29.64	29.74	36	52	42	43.3	N.W'ly 1	N. E. 1	N. E. 2	8	10	10	
30	29.81	29.84	29.87	37	52	42	43.7	N'ly 1	N'ly 1	S'ly 1	8	9	10	
31	29.86	29.77	29.69	37	61	40	46.0	N. W. 1	W'ly 1	W'ly 1	2	2	0	
Means	29.73	29.70	29.75	26.9	39.6	30.0	...	1.7	2.1	1.7	4.5	5.6	4.5	3.35
									1.8			4.9		
REDUCED TO SEA LEVEL.														
Max.	30.48	30.41	30.42	44	61	42	46.0							
Min.	29.33	29.36	29.28	6	16	13	16.3							
Mean	29.91	29.88	29.93											
Range	1.15	1.05	1.14	38	45	29	29.7							
Mean of month	29.907			...	...	...	32.2							
Extreme range	1.20			...	...	...	55.0							

Prevailing winds from some point between— Days.
N. & E. 3
E. & S. 6
S. & W. 8
W. & N. 14

Days.
Clear 10
Variable . . . . } 10
Cloudy . . . . }
Rain or snow fell on 11

1st. Air raw. Snow in evening; wind N. E'ly.
2d. Violent snow-storm all day; wind very heavy. Quantity of snow not large, but much drifted.
3d and 4th. Very fine.
5th. Pleasant. Indications of storm in evening.
6th. Rain and snow last night. Foggy this morning and calm, with light mist. Mostly clear in the afternoon and evening.
7th. Very fine overhead, but extremely blustering.
8th. Cool and very clear.
9th. Mostly clear till 8 A. M., and then cloudy. Began to snow from 3 to 4 P. M.
10th. About four inches of snow on the ground this morning. Wind very blustering and cold from about W. by N. Evening clear and cold.
11th. Air very raw in the afternoon. Began to snow very moderately at 7 P. M.
12th. From three to four inches of fresh snow fell last night. Weather cold and very blustering. Evening clear.
13th. Pleasant in the morning. Air S. E'ly and very raw in the afternoon.
14th. Snowing very moderately about sunrise. Mostly clear in the afternoon. Evening very clear. From one to two inches of snow.
15th. Very fine.
16th. Very fine at mid-day. Shower in evening, and thick fog.
17th. Very fine. Evening cloudless, and air very clear.
18th. Pleasant, though cloudy.
19th. Heavy shower in the morning, with some thunder.
20th Snow-squall from 11 A. M. to noon. Evening very clear.
21st. Air raw and unpleasant.
22d. Light flurry of snow last night. Air raw and chilly all day.
23d. Cloudy. Air raw and chilly in morning.
24th. Very mild. Air light at S. W'ly.
25th. Mild and pleasant in the morning. Grew cold in the evening.
26th. Pleasant. Evening clear.
27th Very fine. Evening cloudy.
28th. Cloudy and mild.
29th. Cloudy through the day. Light sprinkling of rain at 5 P. M.
30th. Mild and pleasant, though cloudy.
31st. Very fine.

April, 1857. New Moon, 24d. 2h. 6m. A. M.

DAYS.	BAROMETER, REDUCED TO 32° F.			THERMOMETER.				WINDS. (DIRECTION AND FORCE.)			WEATHER. (TENTHS CLOUDY.)			RELATIVE HUMIDITY.	RAIN AND SNOW IN INCHES OF WATER
	At 6 A. M.	At 1 P. M.	At 10 P. M.	At 6 A. M.	At 1 P. M.	At 10 P. M.	Daily mean.	At 6 A. M.	At 1 P. M.	At 10 P. M.	At 6 A. M.	At 1 P. M.	At 10 P. M.		
1	29.55	29.86	29.21	37	53	43	44.3	W'ly 1	N. W. 3	S'ly 2	7	10	Sprin'le	...	
2	29.63	29.68	30.00	15	22	20	19.0	N. W. 2	N. W. 4	N. W. 2	Snow	2	0	...	
3	30.05	30.10	30.08	18	40	30	29.3	N. W. 1	S. W. 1	S. W'ly 2	0	3	2	...	
4	30.02	29.90	29.99	32	52	36	40.0	S. W. 2	S. W. 2	S. W. 1	8	0	0	...	
S 5	29.96	29.89	29.80	37	59	46	47.0	S'ly 2	S'ly 1	S. W. 2	Foggy	Sprin'le	3	...	
6	29.62	29.43	29.30	48	52	49	49.7	S'ly 3	S. W. 4	S. W. 3	Rain	Rain	Rain	...	1.87
7	29.68	...	30.13	31	...	31	...	N. W. 2	...	S. W'ly 1	2	...	0	...	
8	30.13	30.14	30.08	28	46	35	36.3	W. by S. 1	S'ly 3	S. W. 1	0	1	1	...	
9	30.01	29.89	29.82	34	54	42	43.3	E'ly 1	S'ly 2	S'ly 2	7	10	Rain	...	} 0.50
10	29.75	29.64	29.46	37	43	41	40.3	N. E. 3	N. E. 3	N. E. 2	Rain	10	10	...	
11	29.50	29.54	29.63	43	62	44	49.7	S. W. 1	S. W. 2	S. W. 1	10	5	0	...	
S 12	29.69	29.71	29.73	44	48	44	45.3	S. W. 1	S. W. 1	E'ly 1	10	Rain	Rain	...	0.50
13	29.77	29.77	29.62	39	59	41	46.3	N. W. 1	E'ly 2	N. E. 2	5	10	10	...	
14	29.32	28.97	29.03	41	46	38	41.7	N. E. 4	N. E. 3	N. W. 3	Misty	Rain	0	...	0.62
15	29.16	29.19	29.29	38	54	34	40.7	W'ly 2	S. W. 3	N. W. 3	9	6	0	...	
16	29.47	29.56	29.59	30	51	36	39.0	N. W. 2	S. W. 2	S'ly 2	0	7	10	...	
17	29.48	29.39	29.42	33	43	38	38.0	N. W. 1	N. W. 3	N. W. 4	Snow	10	10	...	
18	29.50	29.66	29.80	37	47	34	39.3	N. W. 2	N. W. 2	N. E. 2	7	10	0	...	
S 19	29.89	29.86	29.79	38	42	38	39.3	N. E. 3	N. E. 3	N. E. 3	Misty	10	10	...	
20	29.55	29.32	29.22	37	40	41	39.3	N. E. 3	N. E. 4	N. E'ly 3	10	Rain	Rain	...	} 2.80
21	29.19	29.30	29.47	34	34	35	34.3	N. E. 4	N. E. 4	N'ly 2	R'n, sn.	Snow	5	...	
22	29.44	29.47	29.50	35	40	37	37.3	N. E'ly 3	N. E. 3	N. E. 2	10	7	10	...	
23	29.48	29.50	29.59	38	50	39	42.3	N. W. 1	N. W. 2	N. W. 1	5	2	0	...	
24	29.59	29.54	29.65	36	58	44	46.0	N. W. 1	N. W. 2	N. W. 1	0	4	0	...	
25	29.64	29.64	29.69	40	55	41	45.3	N. W. 1	N. W. 2	N. W. 1	2	3	0	...	
S 26	29.70	29.68	29.72	39	58	44	47.0	N. W. 1	N. W. 2	N'ly 1	0	3	2	...	
27	29.64	29.46	29.39	42	50	42	44.7	E'ly 1	S. E. 3	N. W. 1	9	Rain	0	...	
28	29.48	29.42	29.84	38	51	43	44.0	N. W. 2	N. W. 3	N. W. 2	0	7	0	...	
29	29.88	29.90	30.01	42	55	40	45.7	N. W. 1	N. W. 1	N. W. 2	2	0	2	...	
30	30.11	30.11	30.22	37	58	38	44.3	N. E. 1	W. by S 2	S'ly 2	1	0	0	...	
Means	29.66	29.62	29.65	35.9	49.0	38.2	...	1.8	2.5	1.9	6.1	6.3	4.2	...	6.29
								2.1			5.5				
REDUCED TO SEA LEVEL.															
Max.	30.31	30.32	30.40	48	62	49	49.7	Prevailing winds from some point between— Days.			Days.				
Min.	29.34	29.15	29.21	15	22	20	19.0	N. & E. 7			Clear 8				
Mean	29.84	29.80	29.83					E. & S. 2			Variable . . . } 10				
Range	0.97	1.17	1.19	33	40	29	30.7	S. & W. 10			Cloudy . . . . }				
Mean of month	29.823			...	...	...	40.1	W. & N. 11			Rain or snow fell on 12				
Extreme range	1.25			...	...	...	47.0								

REMARKS.

1st. Mild. Very dusty A. M.; wind N.W. Sprinkling towards night; wind E'ly.
2d. Flurry of snow last night. Extremely cold this morning; Wind brisk N. W.
3d. Raw and cold for the season. Circle round the moon in the evening.
4th. Very fine. Circle about the moon.
5th. Pleasant. Sprinkling of rain from noon to 1 P. M.
6th. Wind very heavy, with copious rain in the afternoon and evening.
7th. Cool, but fine. Circle about moon.
8th. Very fine.
9th. Very pleasant morning. Cloudy towards night. Began to rain at 6 P. M.
10th. Light rain A. M. Cloudy, mist, and occasional rain in afternoon and evening.
11th. Very fine.
12th. Light rain through day and evening.
13th. Cloudy in the morning. Appearances of storm in the evening.
14th. Morning misty; wind heavy N. E. Wind slightly abated at noon, with copious rain. From 6 to 7 P. M., bar. 29.00; showed indications of rising at 7½ P. M. At 8 P. M., clouds broken. Clear at 10 P. M.
15th. Variable. Snow-gust at 9 to 10 P. M. Clear at 11 P. M.; wind blustering N W.
16th. Ground crusted with frost this morning and in many places, in the shade, white with snow till after 8 A. M.
17th. Half an inch of snow on the ground this morning. Frequent snow-squalls during the day.
18th. Cloudy through the day. Evening very clear; wind N. E.
19th. Air very raw and chilly. Appearances of storm in the evening.
20th. Began to rain from 10 to 11 A. M., and continued through day and evening.
21st Storm very severe. It snowed fast from 6 A. M. till 7 P. M., thawing as it fell in early part of day, but two or three inches accumulated in afternoon. Clouds broken at 9 P. M. Mostly clear at 11 P. M.
22d. Air cold and raw, and the ground in many places covered with snow.
23d. Very pleasant. Snow disappeared.
24th, 25th, and 26th. Very fine.
27th. Moderate rain at intervals. Clear in the evening.
28th and 29th. Very fine.
30th. Very fine. Evening splendid.

May, 1857. New Moon, 23d. 9h. 39m. A. M.

DAYS.	Bar. At 6 A. M.	Bar. At 1 P. M.	Bar. At 10 P. M.	Therm. At 6 A. M.	Therm. At 1 P. M.	Therm. At 10 P. M.	Daily mean.	Winds At 6 A. M.	Winds At 1 P. M.	Winds At 10 P. M.	Weather At 6 A. M.	Weather At 1 P. M.	Weather At 10 P. M.	Relative Humidity	Rain in inches
1	30.24	30.24	30.12	34½	51	40½	42.0	S'ly 1	S'ly 2	S'ly 2	0	4	Hazy	63	
2	30.00	29.86	29.75	44	57	52	51.0	S. E'ly 2	S'ly 2	S'ly 3	10	10	Rain	82	0.65
S 3	29.73	29.72	29.84	55	62	51	56.0	N. W. 1	S'ly 2	S'ly 2	10	5	7	93	
4	29.85	29.83	29.80	51	49	45	48.3	N. E'ly 1	N. E. 1	N. E. 1	Rain	Rain	Misty	100	
5	29.63	29.53	29.58	49	56	50	51.7	N. E. 1	S. W. 2	S. W. 1	Foggy	Misty	8	97	0.73
6	29.59	29.57	29.69	48	62	52	54.0	S. W. 1	S'ly 3	S. W. 1	0	0	0	76	
7	29.75	29.74	29.85	48	65	49	54.0	S. W. 1	S'ly 2	S'ly 1	0	5	0	64	
8	29.87	29.88	30.02	48	66	48	54.0	N. W. 1	N. W. 1	N. W. 1	0	2	0	64	
9	30.03	29.96	29.85	51	71	47	56.3	S. W. 2	S. W. 3	S. W. 1	0	0	0	59	
S 10	29.61	29.44	29.44	53	70	58	60.3	S. W. 3	S. W. 3	N. W. 2	2	0	0	85	
11	29.57	29.68	29.77	43	49	39	43.7	N. W. 2	N. W. 3	N. W. 1	0	2	10	48	
12	29.93	29.89	29.91	37	58	42½	55.7	N. W. 1	N. W. 2	S. W'ly 2	8	0	0	48	
13	29.94	29.85	29.86	37	60	50	49.0	S. W. 1	S'ly 2	S'ly 1	0	0	0	49	
14	29.74	29.60	29.50	45	58	49	50.7	S'ly 1	S'ly 1	S'ly 1	10	10	Rain	78	
15	29.50	29.44	29.41	47	53	44½	48.2	N'ly 1	S'ly 2	...	10	Sprin'le	...	91	
16	29.50	29.64	29.78	43	45	43	43.7	N. E. 2	N. E. 2	N. E. 1	Rain	Rain	10	88	} 1.00
S 17	29.81	29.79	29.89	44	45	44	44.3	N. E. 1	S. E'ly 2	N. W. 2	Rain	Rain	2	80	
18	29.98	29.99	29.96	43	48	40	43.7	N. E. 3	N. E. 2	N'ly 2	10	10	1	78	
19	29.87	29.67	29.57	40	47	45	44.0	N. E. 3	N. E. 4	N. E. 4	10	Rain	Rain	84	0.45
20	29.44	29.38	29.47	43	47½	43	44.4	N. E. 5	N. E. 2	N. E. 2	Misty	Misty	Misty	97	
21	29.49	...	29.59	42½	...	44	...	N. E. 2	...	N'ly 2	Misty	...	5	74	
22	...	...	...	...	...	...	...	...	...	...	...	...	...	...	
23	...	...	29.67	...	...	56	...	...	...	S'ly 1	...	...	0	68	
S 24	29.70	29.72	29.77	57	72	55	61.3	S. W'ly 1	S. W. 1	S. W. 1	1	2	1	77	
25	29.76	29.68	29.72	55	79	60	64.7	S. W. 1	S. W. 2	S'ly 1	1	1	0	57	
26	29.74	29.74	29.87	65	85	48	66.0	S'ly 1	S. W'ly 2	N. E. 2	2	2	2	53	
27	29.92	29.87	29.84	45	64	58	55.7	N. E. 2	N. E. 2	S'ly 2	Foggy	3	2	84	
28	29.70	29.65	29.64	58	63	57	59.3	S. W. 3	S. W. 2	S. W. 1	Rain	10	Misty	83	} 1.15
29	29.46	29.47	29.52	58	63	55	58.7	S'ly 2	S. W. 2	S'ly 1	Rain	5	2	100	
30	[illegible]	[illegible]	29.77	[illegible]	67	[illegible]	[illegible]	N. W. 2	W'ly 3	N. W. 2	2	2	1	68	
S 31	29.83	29.69	29.71	56	59	59	58.0	S. W. 1	S. E. 2	S'ly 1	0	Rain	10	91	[illegible]
Means	29.75	29.72	29.74	46.5	50.7	49.2	...	1.7	2.1	1.6	5.9	5.4	4.5	77	4.33
								1.8			5.3				
REDUCED TO SEA LEVEL.															
Max.	30.42	30.42	30.30	65	85	60	66.0	Prevailing winds from some point between— Days.			Days.				
Min.	29.62	29.56	29.59	34½	45	39	42.0	N. & E. 7			Clear 8				
Mean	29.93	29.90	29.92					E. & S. 3			Variable . . . } 8				
Range	0.80	0.86	0.71	30½	40	21	24.0	S. & W. 16			Cloudy . . . . }				
Mean of month	29.917			...	...	...	52.8	W. & N. 4			Rain fell on . . 14				
Extreme range	0.86			...	...	...	50.5				(1 day omitted.)				

REMARKS.

1st. White frost in abundance this morning. Air cold and raw during the day.
2d. Occasional sprinkling of rain.
3d. Cloudy and mild. Bow round moon.
4th. Moderate rain nearly all day. Fog and mist in the evening.
5th. Light rain at intervals in the morning. Clouds broken in the evening.
6th. Very fine. Evening splendid.
7th and 8th. Very fine.
9th. Very fine. Cherry-trees in bloom.
10th. Pleasant. Sprinkling of rain at 7 P. M., with lightning.
11th. Pleasant. Cool for the season.
12th. Pleasant, but cool.
13th. Clear. Air cold and raw P. M.
14th. Mild. Sprinkling of rain in afternoon. Moderate rain in evening.
15th. Moderate rain P. M. and evening.
16th. Moderate rain till about 3 P. M. Evening cloudy.
17th. Rainy in morning. Brisk shower of rain and hail from 1 to 2 P. M. Mostly clear at 3 P. M.; wind came from S'ly to N. W.
18th. Cloudy all day. Cold for the season. Mostly clear at 10 P. M.
19th Cloudy in morning. Began to rain from 1 to 2 P. M. Rain in the evening.
20th. Mist through day; occasional rain.
21st. Cloudy day; occasional rain.
22d. Pleasant.
23d. Mild and pleasant.
24th. Very fine. 25th. Very warm.
26th. Very hot in morning; wind W'ly. Wind came to N. E. towards night; grew cold fast. Ther. rose to 85° in the shade—higher than at any time since Aug. 12, 1856.
27th. Pleasant. Fog A. M. Clear evening.
28th. Heavy rain this morning. Mist in the afternoon and evening.
[illegible]
30th. Very fine; air remarkably clear.
31st. Brisk rain from 1 to 3 P. M. Evening cloudy.

NOTE.—The column headed "Relative Humidity" is now for the first time introduced into this Record. The number 100 represents the atmosphere saturated with vapor, so that, with the least reduction of temperature, the vapor would be condensed into fog or mist. The results have been deduced from three daily observations with the standard dry and wet-bulb thermometers of the Smithsonian Institution.

June, 1857. New Moon, 21d. 4h. 55m. P. M.

DAYS.	Barometer, reduced to 32° F. At 6 A. M.	At 1 P. M.	At 10 P. M.	Thermometer. At 6 A. M.	At 1 P. M.	At 10 P. M.	Daily mean.	Winds (Direction and Force.) At 6 A. M.	At 1 P. M.	At 10 P. M.	Weather (Tenths Cloudy.) At 6 A. M.	At 1 P. M.	At 10 P. M.	Relative Humidity.	Rain and Snow in Inches of Water.
1	29.65	29.57	29.49	59	68	61	62.7	S'ly 1	S'ly 2	S'ly	Rain	10	Rain	92	0.40
2	29.39	29.36	29.39	61	71	61	64.3	S'ly 1	S. W. 2	S. W. 1	Foggy	7	0	86	
3	29.49	29.45	29.45	58	73	60	63.7	N. W. 1	W'ly 3	S. W. 2	0	0	3	66	
4	29.48	29.53	29.63	60	70	58	62.7	S. W'ly 2	S. W'ly 3	N. W'ly 2	0	1	10	67	
5	29.64	29.58	29.59	53	61	52	55.3	N. W'ly 1	N. W. 2	N. W. 1	10	5	0	70	
6	29.57	29.55	29.54	47	62	52	60.0	N. W. 1	N. W. 3	N. W. 1	0	7	10	65	
S 7	29.46	29.50	29.56	54	63	63	56.3	S'ly 2	S'ly 1	W'ly 1	Rain	10	9	61	
8	29.65	29.71	29.81	51	67	51	56.3	N. E. 1	N. E. 2	S'ly 1	0	3	1	71	
9	29.81	29.81	29.80	52	64	54	56.7	S'ly 1	S'ly 3	S. W. 1	10	8	10	64	
10	29.76	29.71	29.60	56	66	56	59.3	E'ly 1	S'ly 2	S'ly 2	9	9	Rain	85	} 0.45
11	29.40	29.23	29.09	58½	59½	57	58.3	S. E. 2	S. E. 1	S. W. 1	Misty	Rain	2	97	
12	29.16	29.29	29.45	61	73	62½	65.3	W. by S. 3	S. W'ly 3	S. W. 2	0	2	8	59	
13	29.46	29.47	29.48	66	79	67	71.0	S. W. 2	W'ly 2	W'ly 1	2	0	0	62	
S 14	29.59	29.60	29.68	63	76	62	67 0	W'ly 2	N. W. 3	N. W. 1	1	0	0	62	
15	29.75	29.73	29.74	55	75	59	63.0	N. W. 1	N. W. 2	N. W. 1	1	0	1	48	
16	29.76	29.75	29.72	58	61	52	57.0	N. E'ly 1	N. E. 2	S. W'ly 2	10	Rain	Rain	65	
17	29.71	29.71	29.77	54	63	56	57.7	S. W. 2	S'ly 2	S. W. 1	Misty	10	10	81	
18	29.72	29.66	29.69	52	59	53	54.7	N. E'ly 1	N. E. 2	N. E. 1	Rain	Misty	10	98	} 0.75
19	29.71	29.70	29.70	53	57	61	53.7	N. E. 1	N. E. 1	S'ly 1	Rain	Rain	Rain	100	
20	29.70	29.74	29.69	63	68	64	65.0	S. E'ly 1	S'ly 1	S'ly 1	Foggy	10	Foggy	96	
S 21	29.69	29.66	29.67	65	74	63	67.3	S. W. 2	S. W. 2	S. W. 1	10	9	Foggy	90	
22	29.56	29.48	29.37	62	67	58	62.3	S. W. 1	S. W. 2	S. W'ly 2	Foggy	10	1	91	
23	29.37	29.49	29.61	59	67	58	61.3	S. W'ly 3	S. W'ly 3	W'ly 2	1	8	3	60	
24	29.67	29.64	29.65	61	71	61	64.3	N. W'ly 2	N. W. 2	N. W. 1	3	1	0	68	
25	29.62	29.54	29.62	68	82	63	71.0	N. W. 2	W'ly 3	N. W. 1	0	2	2	45	0.30
26	29.57	29.52	29.65	66	80	60	68.7	N. W. 2	N. W. 3	N. W. 1	3	1	0	51	
27	29.66	29.64	29.68	63	79	63	68.3	N. W. 1	N. W. 3	N'ly 1	2	0	0	42	
S 28	29.67	29.65	29.66	65	76	62	67.7	N. E'ly 2	N. E. 2	N. E. 1	2	0	0	52	
29	29.62	29.61	29.62	57	74	58	63.0	S. E'ly 1	S. E'ly 2	S. E'ly 1	5	8	10	72	
30	29.61	29.59	29.60	56	58	55	56.3	S'ly 2	N. E. 2	N. E. 2	10	10	10	87	
Means	29.60	29.58	29.60	58.5	68.8	58.7	...	1.5	2.2	1.2	6.0	5.7	5.3	69.1	1.90
									1.6			5.7			
REDUCED TO SEA LEVEL.															
Max.	29.99	29.99	29.99	68	82	67	71.0								
Min.	29.34	29.41	29.27	47	57	51	53.7								
Mean	29.78	29.76	29.78												
Range	0.65	0.58	0.72	21	23	16	17.3								
Mean of month	29.773			...	...	...	62.0								
Extreme range	0.72			...	...	...	35.0								

Prevailing winds from some point between— Days.
N. & E. 6
E. & S. 4
S. & W. 12
W. & N. 8

Days.
Clear 9
Variable . . . } 11
Cloudy . . . . }
Rain fell on . . 10

REMARKS.

1st. Rain, with heavy thunder at 2 or 3 A. M. Rain again in the evening.
2d. Pleasant. Evening clear.
3d and 4th. Very fine.
5th. Pleasant. Evening cool.
6th. Pleasant. Quite cool for the season.
7th Light rain in the morning Evening pleasant.
8th and 9th. Pleasant.
10th. Pleasant; mostly cloudy. Light sprinkling of rain in the evening.
11th. Light rain and mist all day. Mostly clear at 10 P. M.
12th. Very clear in the morning. Evening mostly cloudy.
13th. Very fine. Sprinkling of rain at 7½ P. M. Evening clear.
14th. Very fine.
15th. Very fine. Evening splendid.
16th Light rain in afternoon and evening. Air cool.
17th. Cool and cloudy.
18th. Occasional light rain and mist. Cold for the season.
19th. Rain and mist. Warmer in the evening, with rain and fog continued.
20th. Warm and foggy, with some mist. The sun out occasionally.
21st. Mild. Sun out occasionally. Fog in the evening.
22d. Brisk shower of hail and rain for a few minutes at 9 A. M. Evening mostly clear, and air dried.
23d. Pleasant and cool.
24th. Fine.
25th. Very fine in the morning. Gust of wind, with thunder and light rain, at 7 P. M. Mostly clear at 10 P. M.
26th. Very fine.
27th. Very fine. Air extremely dry; dew-point below 38° at 1 P. M.
28th. Very fine; air dry. Evening splendid.
29th. Pleasant. Hot sun in the morning. Cloudy for the most part in the afternoon and evening.
30th. Cloudy, with occasional heavy mist. Cold for the season.

July, 1857. New Moon, 20d. 1h. 4m. A. M.

DAYS.	Barometer At 6 A. M.	At 1 P. M.	At 10 P. M.	Thermometer At 6 A. M.	At 1 P. M.	At 10 P. M.	Daily mean.	Winds At 6 A. M.	At 1 P. M.	At 10 P. M.	Weather At 6 A. M.	At 1 P. M.	At 10 P. M.	Relative Humidity.	Rain and Snow in Inches of Water.
1	29.60	29.68	29.78	53	55	53	53.7	N. E. 2	N. E'ly 3	N. E. 2	Misty	10	10	92	
2	29.77	29.82	29.85	49	63	54	55.3	N. E. 1	N. E. 3	N. E. 2	2	10	Rain	72	
3	29.77	29.73	29.71	52	57	56	55.0	N. E. 2	N. E. 2	N. E. 2	Rain	Rain	10	100	0.20
4	29.70	29.73	29.79	56	71	60	62.3	N. E'ly 2	S'ly 1	S'ly 1	10	4	0	85	
S 5	29.87	29.85	29.95	65	78	63	68.7	N. W. 1	N. W. 1	S'ly 1	5	5	0	72	
6	29.91	29.88	29.83	61	72	63	65.3	N. E'ly 1	S. E'ly 2	S. W. 1	Misty	Misty	8	89	
7	29.79	29.76	29.64	65	81	69	71.7	S. W'ly 2	W'ly 3	S. W. 2	5	2	5	72	
8	29.66	29.73	29.86	66	75	61	67.3	N. W. 1	N. W. 3	N. W. 1	0	1	0	64	
9	29.94	29.97	30.04	60	77	66	67.7	N. W. 1	N. W. 2	N. W. 1	0	2	0	58	
10	30.07	30.04	30.05	67	80	64	70.3	N. W. 1	S. W. 2	S. W. 1	0	2	0	68	
11	29.98	29.87	29.85	66	79	71	72.0	S. W'ly 1	S'ly 3	Calm	7	3	0	82	
S 12	29.83	29.76	29.81	70	88	73	77.0	S'ly 1	S. W'ly 1	S'ly 1	3	2	0	68	
13	29.85	29.81	29.82	66	85	69	73.3	E'ly 1	S. E. 2	E'ly 1	7	3	5	75	
14	29.80	29.76	29.77	76	85	71	77.3	S. E. 2	S. E. 3	S. W. 1	5	3	0	88	
15	29.78	29.76	29.80	73	87	69	76.3	S. W. 1	S. W. 3	W'ly 1	7	0	0	70	
16	29.80	29.83	29.84	70	77	68	71.7	S. W. 2	S. W. 3	S. W. 2	3	0	1	84	
17	29.86	29.75	29.77	68	76	71	71.7	S. E. 1	S. E. 1	S'ly 1	Rain	8	10	92	
18	29.77	29.66	29.64	70	79	72	73.7	S. W. 1	S. W'ly 2	S'ly 1	Rain	5	2	84	0.30
S 19	29.60	...	29.57	72	...	74	...	S. W. 2	...	S. W. 2	10	...	3	88	
20	29.55	29.50	29.51	70	84	73	75.7	S. W. 2	S. W. 3	S. W. 1	10	3	10	79	0.70
21	29.47	29.45	29.47	73	79	71	74.3	S. W. 1	S. W. 3	S. W. 1	10	10	10	85	0.10
22	29.55	29.56	29.71	74	82	72	76.0	S. W. 1	S. W'ly 2	S. W. 1	7	5	3	75	
23	29.72	29.70	29.79	66	62	61	63.0	N. E. 3	N. E. 3	N. E. 1	Rain	Misty	Rain	96	1.00
24	29.83	29.85	29.93	62	77	71	70.0	N. E'ly 2	S'ly 2	S'ly 1	Foggy	5	10	92	
25	29.93	29.94	29.98	68	80	71	73.0	S'ly 1	S. W. 2	S. W. 2	Rain	5	0	74	0.60
S 26	29.98	29.96	29.96	72	83	72	75.7	S. W. 1	S. W. 3	S. W. 1	10	5	0	83	
27	29.95	29.86	29.85	73	86	73	77.3	S. W. 2	S. W. 3	S. W. 2	7	1	0	79	
28	29.82	29.74	29.73	74	84	72	76.7	S. W. 4	S. W. 4	S. W. 3	8	2	8	79	
29	29.70	29.77	28.87	70	79	66	71.7	S. W. 2	N. W. 2	N. W. 1	Rain	5	0	82	0.25
30	29.89	29.88	29.79	61	70	62	64.3	N'ly 1	N. E. 2	N.E. 2	9	10	Rain	65	0.30
31	29.73	29.75	29.71	62	67	66	65.0	N. E. 2	N. E. 1	N. E. 2	3	10	10	84	
Means	29.79	29.78	29.80	66.1	76.6	67.0	...	1.5	2.3	1.3	7.0	5.0	4.4	79.9	3.45
									1.7			5.5			
REDUCED TO SEA LEVEL.															
Max.	30.25	30.22	30.23	76	88	74	77.3								
Min.	29.65	29.63	29.65	49	55	53	53.7								
Mean	29.97	29.96	29.98												
Range	0.60	0.59	0.58	27	33	21	23.6								
Mean of month	29.970			...	...	...	69.9								
Extreme range	0.62			...	...	...	35.0								

Prevailing winds from some point between— Days.
N. & E. 6
E. & S. 6
S. & W. 15
W. & N. 4

Days.
Clear 5
Variable . . . } 18
Cloudy . . . . }
Rain fell on . . 8

1st. Cloudy and cold, with occasional heavy mist.
2d. Very cold; thermometer at sunrise 46°. Light rain at 10 P. M.
3d. Cold and unpleasant. Occasional mist and light rain.
4th. Weather warmer. Evening clear.
5th. Pleasant.
6th. Occasional heavy mist in the morning. Air very damp in the evening.
7th. Pleasant; air warm and sultry.
8th. Very fine. Evening nearly cloudless.
9th. Very fine.
10th. Fine.
11th. Warm and sultry. Thunder from 4 to 5 P. M., but no rain. Evening clear.
12th. Very little air stirring, and excessively hot.
13th. Very sultry, with appearances of shower in the afternoon.
14th. Prevalence of clouds through the day. Evening clear.
15th. Fine; sun very hot.
16th. Very fine.
17th. Showery and warm.
18th. Light showers in the morning. Sun out at times, and very hot.
19th. Cloudy in the morning. Very hot sun in the afternoon.
20th. Heavy thundershower about 4 A. M. Day sultry.
21st. Air very damp. Shower from 6 to 7 P. M.
22d. Very fine.
23d. Rainy in the morning. Mist and heavy rain in the evening.
24th. Air very damp. Sun hot at mid-day.
25th. Heavy rain early in the morning. Evening clear.
26th. Very warm and damp. Evening fine.
27th. Pleasant; fresh air, but very damp.
28th. Warm, but pleasant. Air very fresh through the day.
29th. Light rain at 6 A. M.; wind S. W. From 9 to 10 A. M., the wind came to N. W., and the air became cooler and drier. Evening splendid.
30th. Began to rain moderately from 10 to 11 A. M., and continued.
31st. Cloudy, cool, and damp day and evening.

August, 1857. New Moon, 19d. 11h. 18m. A. M.

DAYS.	Barometer, reduced to 32° F — At 6 A. M.	At 1 P. M.	At 10 P. M.	Thermometer — At 6 A. M.	At 1 P. M.	At 10 P. M.	Daily mean.	Winds (Direction and Force.) — At 6 A. M.	At 1 P. M.	At 10 P. M.	Weather (Tenths Cloudy.) — At 6 A. M.	At 1 P. M.	At 10 P. M.	Relative Humidity.	Rain and Snow in Inches of Water.
1	29.65	29.65	...	67	73	...	...	S'ly 1	S. W'ly 2	...	10	9	...	77	
S 2	...	...	...	...	...	...	...	...	...	...	...	...	...	...	
3	...	29.76	29.83	...	77	66	...	...	N. W.	S. W'ly 1	...	7	0	73	
4	29.82	29.80	29.71	71	80	72	74.3	W'ly	S. W. 3	S. W. 2	0	6	10	72	
5	29.54	29.59	29.70	64	69	66	66.3	N'ly 4	W'ly 2	Calm	Rain	10	10	97	1.00
6	29.79	29.86	29.93	68	75	63	68.7	W'ly 1	N. E. 2	N'ly 1	8	6	0	76	
7	30.03	30.02	30.01	68	74	65	69.0	N'ly 1	S. E. 3	S'ly 1	0	4	0	83	
8	29.97	29.88	29.82	65	76	71	70.7	S'ly 1	S. W. 1	S'ly 3	Hazy	8	3	83	
S 9	29.84	29.83	29.85	73	76	64	71.0	N'ly 4	N'ly 1	N. W'ly 1	0	8	0	74	
10	29.80	29.67	29.50	68	74	70	70.7	S'ly 1	S'ly 2	S. E. 3	Foggy	10	Rain	75	0.75
11	29.31	...	...	70	...	...	...	W'ly 3	...	...	5	...	...	87	
12	...	...	...	...	...	...	...	...	...	...	...	...	...	...	
13	...	...	29.62	...	...	75	...	...	...	S. W. 1	...	...	0	66	0.15
14	29.62	29.58	29.55	78	86	73	79.0	S. W. 2	N. W. 2	N. 1	0	2	0	76	0.15
15	29.70	29.61	29.65	76	80	67	74.3	N'ly 3	N'ly 1	N. W'ly 2	8	10	0	72	
S 16	29.83	29.85	29.93	66	73	64	67.7	N. W. 3	N. W. 2	W'ly 1	0	2	10	54	
17	29.93	29.79	29.62	63	69	69	67.0	N'ly 1	S. E. 2	S. W. 1	10	10	Rain	80	0.35
18	29.71	29.77	29.80	60	62	56	59.3	N'ly 2	N'ly 2	N. 1	10	10	0	94	
19	29.82	...	29.88	55	...	59	...	N. W. 1	...	W. 1	0	...	0	95	
20	29.91	29.87	29.89	60	66	60	62.0	S. W. 1	S'ly 2	S'ly 1	Rain	5	0	88	0.05
21	29.95	29.93	29.95	58	73	59	63.3	N. E. 1	S. E'ly 1	N. E. 2	Foggy	8	0	87	
22	29.95	29.83	29.65	59	70	60	63.0	N. E'ly 1	E'ly 1	N. E. 2	8	4	Rain	85	1.15
S 23	29.54	29.48	29.46	64	69	58	63.7	N'ly 1	S. E. 1	N. W. 1	10	Rain	0	90	0.10
24	29.53	29.62	29.83	60	70	58	62.7	W'ly 2	W. 3	N. W. 2	0	4	0	81	
25	29.96	29.97	...	61	70	...	...	N. W. 1	N. W. 1	...	0	2	...	83	
26	...	30.01	30.01	...	74	61	...	...	S'ly 2	N. W. 2	...	4	0	62	
27	30.00	29.94	...	63	71	...	...	S. W. 1	S. W'ly 2	...	0	6	...	81	
28	29.70	29.61	29.51	68	67	69	68.0	S. E. 5	S. E. 4	S'ly 2	Rain	Rain	10	89	1.10
29	29.53	29.53	29.54	69	77	67	71.0	S. W. 2	S. W. 1	W'ly 1	Misty	9	5	86	
S 30	29.61	29.68	29.84	67	77	60	68.0	N. W. 2	N. W. 2	N. W. 2	4	1	0	60	
31	29.86	29.88	29.98	54	77	66	65.7	N. W. 1	N. W. 2	N. W. 1	0	0	0	77	
Means	29.77	29.77	29.76	62.5	73.3	64.7	...	1.8	1.8	1.4	5.1	6.7	3.1	80.1	4.80
								1.6			5.0				

REDUCED TO SEA LEVEL.

	At 6 A. M.	At 1 P. M.	At 10 P. M.	Th. 6 A. M.	1 P. M.	10 P. M.	Daily mean.
Max.	30.21	30.20	30.19	78	86	73	79.0
Min.	29.49	29.66	29.64	54	62	56	59.3
Mean	29.95	29.95	29.94				
Range	0.72	0.54	0.55	24	24	17	19.7
Mean of month	29.947			...	...	...	66.8
Extreme range	0.72			...	...	...	31.0

Prevailing winds from some point between— Days.
N. & E. 3
E. & S. 5
S. & W. 8
W. & N. 12

Days.
Clear 8
Variable . . . } 12
Cloudy . . . . }
Rain fell on . . 9
(2 days omitted.)

REMARKS.

1st. Cool, but pleasant. Cloudy in the morning. Evening fine.
2d. Very fine. Sun very warm at mid-day.
3d. Cool and fine. Evening very calm.
4th. Very fine. Evening very damp.
5th. Heavy rain before 8 A. M. Damp and cloudy during the day and evening.
6th. Cold and very fine. Evening splendid.
7th. Very fine.
8th. Sultry in the morning. Afternoon and evening fine.
9th. Very fine.
10th. Very damp. Appearances of rain during the day. Commenced raining about 8 P. M., with high wind.
11th and 12th. Very fine.
13th. Rain in morning. Sultry through the day. Incessant heat lightning in the N. E. from 8 to 9 P. M.
14th. Very sultry during the day. Thundershower about 8 P. M. Cleared off before 10 P. M.
15th. Very fine. Sun very hot at mid-day. Evening cool.
16th. Very fine.
17th. Cloudy and damp. Began to rain at about 6 P. M.
18th. Cool. Slight sprinkling of rain in the evening.
19th. Very pleasant.
20th. Pleasant.
21st. Very pleasant.
22d. Cloudy and cool. Commenced raining about 8 P. M., and rained heavily.
23d. Shower and sultry in the morning; wind E'ly, which changed to S. W. in the afternoon. Thunder-squall, with rain about 8 P. M. Cleared by 9 P. M.; wind N. W.
24th. Cool, but very fine.
25th and 26th. Very fine.
28th. Pleasant.
28th. Rainy in the morning. Evening cloudy, with mist.
29th. Cloudy, with mist, in the morning. Clouds broken in the evening.
30th. Very fine. Evening without a cloud.
31st. Very fine.

September, 1857. New Moon, 18d. 0h. 25m. A. M.

DAYS.	Barometer — Sunrise.	At 1 P. M.	At 10 P. M.	Thermometer — Sunrise.	At 1 P. M.	At 10 P. M.	Daily mean.	Winds — Sunrise.	At 1 P. M.	At 10 P. M.	Weather — Sunrise.	At 1 P. M.	At 10 P. M.	Relative Humidity.	Rain and Snow in Inches of Water.
1	30.12	30.12	30.15	57	74	60	63.7	N. W. 1	N. W. 2	N. W. 1	2	2	0	60	
2	30.14	30.12	30.13	58	...	62	...	N. W. 1	...	S. W. 1	0	...	0	66	
3	30.15	30.08	30.11	59	77	65	67.0	S. W. 1	S. W. 2	S'ly 1	2	1	1	83	
4	30.10	30.07	30.07	60	77	67	68.0	S. W. 1	S. W. 1	S. W. 1	2	2	3	90	
5	30.01	29.87	29.78	65	81	68	71.3	S. W. 1	S. W. 2	S. W. 1	7	5	2	82	
S 6	29.71	29.78	29.95	70	69	55	64.7	S. W. 2	N. W. 3	N. W. 1	Rain	0	0	64	0.20
7	30.06	30.07	30.19	48	64	50	54.0	N'ly 2	N. E. 2	N. E. 1	0	0	0	50	
8	30.23	30.17	30.10	46	64	53	54.3	Nl'y 1	N'ly 1	S. W. 1	0	0	0	68	
9	30.01	29.93	29.94	54	74	60	62.7	N. W. 1	N. W. 2	S. W. 1	0	0	2	70	
10	29.93	29.88	29.85	60	77	65	67.3	S. W. 1	S. W. 2	S. W. 1	Foggy	0	0	77	
11	29.82	29.76	29.80	66	84	73	74.3	S. W. 1	S. W. 2	S. W. 1	0	0	0	71	
12	29.92	29.94	29.96	62	66	59	62.3	N. E. 2	N. E. 2	N. E. 2	10	10	10	78	
S 13	29.91	29.88	29.86	60	71	68	66.3	N. E. 2	N. E. 1	S'ly 1	10	10	Misty	92	
14	29.78	29.74	29.65	67	75	70	70.6	Calm	S'ly 1	Calm	Foggy	10	Foggy	100	
15	29.59	29.60	29.76	70	74	58	67.3	S. W'ly 1	N. W. 3	N. W. 1	6	0	0	64	
16	29.85	29.85	29.89	55	67	55	59.0	N. W. 2	N'ly 2	N. W. 1	0	4	8	55	
17	29.80	29.59	29.39	57	61	66	61.3	S. W. 1	S. W. 2	S. W. 2	8	10	Rain	89	0.25
18	29.56	29.64	29.87	64	69	48	60.3	N. W. 2	N. W. 3	N. W. 1	5	2	0	63	
19	29.92	29.90	29.88	43	57	46	48.7	N. W. 2	N. E. 2	N. E. 2	2	10	Rain	76	} 1.20
S 20	29.68	29.66	29.76	52	57	54	54.3	N. E. 2	N. E. 2	N. E. 1	Rain	10	10	86	}
21	29.91	29.95	30.02	49	56	46	50.3	N. E. 1	N. E. 2	N'ly 1	10	10	0	58	
22	29.97	29.80	29.66	44	59	52	51.7	N'ly 1	S. E'ly 2	E'ly 1	8	8	10	81	
23	29.42	29.49	29.59	53	59	46	52.7	N. W'ly 1	W'ly 3	N. W. 1	Rain	0	0	70	0.62
24	29.78	29.78	29.89	43	67	53	54.3	N. W. 1	W'ly 2	S. W. 1	0	0	0	74	
25	29.92	29.89	29.87	50	67	55	57.3	S. W. 1	S. W. 1	S. W. 1	2	10	10	67	
26	29.84	29.82	29.90	48	77	59	61.3	N. W. 1	W'ly 2	S. W. 1	1	0	0	69	
S 27	29.96	29.89	29.81	55	70	60	61.7	N. W. 1	S. W'ly 2	S. W'ly 1	1	0	0	77	
28	29.70	29.56	29.66	59	77	54	63.3	S. W. 1	S. W. 3	N. W. 1	0	5	0	70	
29	29.67	29.73	29.87	48	57	41	40.7	N. W. 1	N. W. 2	N. W. 1	0	3	0	66	
30	29.91	29.86	29.92	36	57	39	44.0	N. W. 2	N. W. 2	N. W. 1	0	3	0	48	
Means	29.87	29.85	29.88	55.3	68.6	56.9	...	1.3	2.0	1.1	4.2	3.9	2.9	72.1	2.27
								1.4			3.7				

REDUCED TO SEA LEVEL.

	Sunrise.	At 1 P. M.	At 10 P. M.	Th. Sunrise.	1 P. M.	10 P. M.	Daily mean.
Max.	30.41	30.35	30.37	70	84	73	74.3
Min.	29.60	29.67	29.57	36	56	39	44.0
Mean	30.05	30.03	30.06				
Range	0.81	0.68	0.80	34	28	34	30.3
Mean of month	30.047			...	...	...	68.3
Extreme range	0.84			...	...	...	48.0

Prevailing winds from some point between— Days.
N. & E. 7
E. & S. 0
S. & W. 11
W. & N. 12

Days.
Clear 15
Variable . . . } 9
Cloudy . . . . }
Rain fell on . . 6

REMARKS.

1st and 2d. Very fine.
3d. Very fine. Aurora with streamers in the evening.
4th and 5th. Very fine.
6th. Rain in the morning. From 8 to 9 A. M., wind changed from S. W. to N. W., and the thermometer fell rapidly. Clear in the afternoon and evening.
7th. Cool, but very fine.
8th. Very fine. At 9¼ P. M., a bright meteor passed directly across the bright star Alpha Lyræ, moving towards the S. W. For a moment, the light of the star was lost in that of the meteor.
9th and 10th. Fine.
11th. Fine. Sun very hot at mid-day.
12th. Air cool and dry.
13th. Cloudy, with appearances of rain.
14th. Air warm and very damp. Nearly a dead calm all day.
15th. Very fine. Evening cloudless, and the air very clear.
16th. Pleasant.
17th. Light rain at 11 to 12 A. M. Steady rain in the evening, and warm.
18th. Very fine.
19th. Cloudy in the morning. Rain in the afternoon and evening. Very cold for the season.
20th. Rain in the morning. Cloudy in the afternoon and evening.
21st. Cloudy through the day. Evening clear and very cold.
22d. Cloudy for the most part.
23d. Rain at sunrise. Clear from 9 to 11 A. M. Evening splendid.
24th. Very fine.
25th. Mild and cloudy.
26th and 27th. Very fine.
28th. Pleasant in the morning. Gust of wind at 2 P. M., with sprinkling of rain. Evening clear.
29th. Very fine. Evening splendid and cool for the season.
30th. Pleasant.

October, 1857. New Moon, 17[d.] 4[h.] 30[m.] P. M.

Days.	Barometer, reduced to 32° F. Sunrise.	At 1 P. M.	At 10 P. M.	Thermometer. Sunrise.	At 1 P. M.	At 10 P. M.	Daily mean.	Winds. (Direction and Force.) Sunrise.	At 1 P. M.	At 10 P. M.	Weather. (Tenths Cloudy.) Sunrise.	At 1 P. M.	At 10 P. M.	Relative Humidity.	Rain and Snow in Inches of Water.
1	29.95	29.97	29.96	37	60	55	50.7	N. W. 1	S'ly 2	S'ly 1	0	2	Sprin'le	57	
2	29.94	29.92	29.99	56	68	56	60.0	S. W. 1	S'ly 2	N. E'ly 1	9	5	8	58	
3	30.08	...	30.12	52	...	44	...	N. E. 3	N. E. 2	N'ly 1	10	10	0	58	
S 4	30.08	30.04	30.00	43	57	45	48.3	N'ly 2	N'ly 2	N'ly 1	1	0	0	67	
5	29.97	29.92	29.92	41	59	48	49.3	N'ly 1	N. E'ly 2	N. E'ly 1	0	0	0	64	
6	29.82	29.68	29.69	41	65	55	53.7	N. E'ly 1	N. E'ly 1	N'ly 1	0	3	5	67	
7	29.71	29.72	29.79	50	62	48	53.3	N'ly 2	N. W. 2	N. W. 1	0	0	0	64	
8	29.74	29.74	29.64	43	68	56	55.7	N. W. 1	N. W. 3	N. W. 1	0	0	0	48	
9	29.66	29.70	29.89	53	70	49	57.3	N. W. 1	N. W. 2	N. W. 1	1	0	0	50	
10	29.99	30.04	30.11	41	57	43	47.0	N. W. 2	N. E. 2	N. E. 2	0	5	0	70	
S 11	30.10	30.06	30.06	39	60	48	49.0	N. E'ly 1	S'ly 2	S'ly 1	0	6	0	94	
12	30.01	29.99	30.02	44	67	54	48.3	N. W. 1	S. W'ly 1	S'ly 1	3	1	0	80	
13	29.98	29.94	29.92	48	72	59	59.7	S'ly 1	S. W'ly 2	Calm	8	7	0	86	
14	29.89	29.82	29.76	57	71	59	62.3	Calm	S'ly 1	N. E. 2	Foggy	10	10	93	
15	29.57	29.41	29.23	57	61	60	59.3	N. E. 2	N. E. 2	N. E. 1	Misty	Misty	Rain	98	0.65
16	29.19	29.23	29.16	61	67	59	62.3	S. W. 1	S. W. 2	S. W. 3	8	9	3	89	
17	29.35	...	29.97	46	...	43	...	W. 4	...	N. W. 1	2	...	0	66	
S 18	30.05	30.05	30.16	43	61	43	49.0	W. 1	N. W. 2	N. W. 1	3	0	0	68	
19	30.05	29.85	29.57	43	61	60	54.7	S. W'ly 1	S. W. 2	S. W. 2	4	10	Rain	79	0.25
20	29.52	29.56	29.68	48	47	36	47.0	W. 2	W by N 4	N. W. 2	8	4	0	40	
21	29.82	29.86	30.00	34	43	32	36.3	N. W. 2	N. W. 3	N. W. 1	5	10	0	55	
22	30.09	30.08	30.19	29	48	34	37.0	N. W. 1	N. W. 2	N. W. 1	0	0	0	50	
23	30.20	30.19	30.15	32	52	46	42.7	N. W. 1	S. W'ly 2	W'ly 1	3	10	10	64	
24	30.09	30.02	29.93	47	56	50	51.0	N. W. 1	W'ly 2	S. E'ly 1	10	5	Rain	77	}
S 25	29.69	29.54	29.29	53	55	56	54.3	E. N. E. 3	N. E'ly 3	N. E. 5	10	Rain	Rain	88	} 2.00
26	28.98	28.88	29.05	58	55	54	55.7	N. E. 1	N. E'ly 2	N. E. 1	Misty	Rain	Rain	94	}
27	29.13	29.24	29.47	50	50	41	47.0	N. E. 2	N. E. 4	N'ly 3	10	Misty	Misty	93	
28	29.56	29.57	29.62	36	41	42	39.7	N'ly 3	N'ly 2	N'ly 1	10	10	10	72	
29	29.56	29.49	29.50	42	48	42	44.0	Calm	N. W'ly 1	N. W'ly 1	Rain	6	7	78	
30	29.56	29.60	29.72	40	49	40	43.0	W by N. 2	W. by N. 3	N'ly 1	9	9	5	42	
31	29.78	29.73	29.69	38	49	43	43.3	N. W'ly 1	E'ly 1	E'ly 2	8	10	Rain	56	
Means	29.78	29.75	29.78	45.2	57.9	48.4	...	1.4	2.1	1.4	5.2	5.7	4.4	69.8	2.90
									1.6			5.1			
REDUCED TO SEA LEVEL.															
Max.	30.38	30.37	30.37	61	72	59	62.3								
Min.	29.16	29.06	29.23	29	41	32	36.3								
Mean	29.96	29.93	29.96												
Range	1.22	1.31	1.14	32	31	27	26.0								
Mean of month	29.950			...	...	...	50.5								
Extreme range	1.32			...	...	...	43.0								

Prevailing winds from some point between— Days.
N. & E. 9
E. & S. 2
S. & W. 8
W. & N. 12

Days.
Clear 9
Variable . . . } 13
Cloudy . . . . }
Rain fell on . . 9

Remarks.

1st. Pleasant in the morning. Cloudy towards night. Sprinkling of rain in the evening.
2d. Pleasant.
3d. Cloudy; air raw and cold. Evening very clear.
4th. Very fine. Evening splendid.
5th. Very fine.
6th. Pleasant.
7th, 8th, and 9th. Very fine.
10th. Pleasant. Cool in the afternoon and evening.
11th, 12th, and 13th. Pleasant.
14th. Thick fog in the morning. Began to rain gently from 10 to 11 P. M.; wind N. E.
15th. Mist through the day. Showers in the evening.
16th. Cloudy and mild. Heavy wind during the night.
17th. Very windy during the day. Evening calm and cool.
18th. Very fine.
19th. Cloudy, with appearances of rain.
20th. Very gusty and raw.
21st. Frost this morning, being the first of the season on College Hill. Ice formed in shallow vessels of the thickness of window glass.
22d. Severe black frost this morning. Ice formed three-eighths of an inch thick in open vessels.
23d. Cloudy, and quite cool.
24th. Air mild, with sprinkling of rain in the morning. Rain in the evening.
25th. Began to rain at noon, and rained steadily all the afternoon and evening.
26th. Heavy showers through the day and evening.
27th. Cold rain and mist.
28th. Cloudy, with occasional mist.
29th. Mostly cloudy, with occasional mist and sprinkling.
30th. Cloudy for the most part.
31st. Cloudy. Sprinkling of rain in the evening.

.November, 1857. New Moon, 16[d.] 10[h.] 46[m.] A. M.

Days.	Barometer Sunrise.	At 1 P. M.	At 10 P. M.	Thermometer Sunrise.	At 1 P. M.	At 10 P. M.	Daily mean.	Winds Sunrise.	At 1 P. M.	At 10 P. M.	Weather Sunrise.	At 1 P. M.	At 10 P. M.	Relative Humidity.	Rain and Snow in Inches of Water.
S 1	29.67	29.62	29.66	43	54	43	46.7	N. W. 1	N. W. 1	N. W. 1	5	7	9	59	
2	29.60	29.44	29.50	45	56	41	47.3	S. W. 2	S. W. 3	N. W. 1	10	2	0	57	0.10
3	29.51	29.57	29.76	38	49	39	42.3	N. W. 2	N. W. 3	N. W. 1	0	8	0	58	
4	29.90	29.89	30.02	35	48	35	39.3	N. W. 1	N. W. 2	N. W. 1	0	0	0	60	
5	30.02	29.95	29.73	35	56	56	47.0	N. W. 1	S. W. 2	S. W. 2	5	1	Rain	91	0.40
6	29.50	29.51	29.59	59	66	60	61.7	S. W. 2	S. W. 3	S. W.	Misty	8	10	77	
7	29.63	29.70	29.81	54	64	52	56.7	N. W. 1	N. W. 1	S. W'ly	0	1	1	53	
S 8	29.87	29.88	29.94	50	53	50	51.0	N. E. 1	N. E. 1	N. E'ly 1	Misty	Misty	Misty	100	
9	29.87	29.80	29.81	50	70	62	60.7	N. E. 1	S. W. 3	S'ly 1	Misty	9	3	90	
10	29.76	...	30.01	64	...	41	...	S. W. 3	...	N. W. 1	Shower	...	0	76	0.65
11	30.18	30.15	30.18	33	53	38	41.3	N. W. 1	N. W. 1	N. W. 1	0	0	0	73	
12	30.12	29.96	29.81	32	50	47	43.0	W'ly 1	S. W. 2	S. W. 1	1	10	2	49	
13	29.69	29.56	29.61	48	54	43	48.3	S. W. 1	S. W. 1	S. W. 1	10	9	1	86	
14	29.71	29.77	30.04	35	38	25	32.7	N. W. 1	N. W. 2	N. W. 1	1	5	0	58	
S 15	30.14	30.06	30.09	22	40	25	29.0	N. W. 1	N. W. 2	N. W. 2	0	0	0	55	
16	30.10	29.93	29.65	25	43	46	38.0	N. W. 1	S. E'ly 1	S. E. 2	0	10	Rain	74	0.60
17	29.40	29.26	29.32	45	50	42	45.7	N. W. 1	N. W. 2	N. W. 1	10	8	10	72	
18	29.29	29.25	29.31	35	49	44	42.7	N. W. 1	N. W. 2	W'ly	0	5	10	72	
19	29.25	29.16	29.06	45	55	54	51.3	S'ly 1	S'ly 2	S'ly 3	9	2	10	76	
20	29.17	29.26	29.45	36	36	22	31.3	W. by S. 4	W'ly 3	S. W'ly 3	5	0	0	46	
21	29.54	29.60	29.67	20	34	31	28.3	S. W'ly 3	S. W. 2	S. W. 1	0	0	0	61	
S 22	29.67	29.65	29.83	33	46	35	38.0	S. W. 2	S. W. 3	S'ly 1	0	8	2	63	
23	29.76	29.55	29.20	37	54	49	46.7	S. W. 2	S. 3	S'ly 2	5	5	Rain	80	0.65
24	29.52	29.64	29.73	29	33	31	31.0	N. W. 3	N. W'ly 2	S. W'ly 2	5	2	10	40	
25	29.86	30.14	30.34	23	19	16	19.7	N. W. 3	N. W'ly 4	N. W'ly 1	0	0	0	36	
26	30.43	...	...	17	...	25	...	W'ly 2	...	...	0	...	...	...	
27	30.27	30.15	...	25	42	...	...	S. W'ly 1	W'ly 1	...	0	0	...	35	
28	30.21	30.11	30.14	32	53	43	42.7	N. W'ly 1	N. W'ly 1	S'ly 1	0	7	5	43	
S 29	30.27	30.22	30.32	44	51	41	45.3	N. W'ly 1	S. W'ly 1	E'ly 1	0	8	8	61	
30	...	30.28	30.17	...	47	42	...	...	E'ly 1	N. E'ly 3	...	10	Misty	72	
Means	29.79	29.75	29.78	37.6	48.7	40.6	...	1.6	2.0	1.2	3.8	4.6	4.6	64.6	2.40
									1.6			4.3			
REDUCED TO SEA LEVEL.															
Max.	30.61	30.46	30.52	64	70	62	61.7								
Min.	29.35	29.34	29.24	17.	19	16	19.7								
Mean	29.97	29.93	29.96												
Range	1.26	1.12	1.28	47	51	46	42.0								
Mean of month	29.953			...	...	...	42.3								
Extreme range	1.37			...	...	...	54.0								

Prevailing winds from some point between— Days.
N. & E. 2
E. & S. 1
S. & W. 12
W. & N. 15

Days.
Clear 8
Variable . . . } 15
Cloudy . . . . }
Rain fell on . . 7

Remarks.

1st. Pleasant.
2d. Light shower, with thunder, at 6 P. M.
3d. Pleasant. Evening splendid.
4th. Very fine.
5th. Pleasant through the day. Sprinkling of rain in the evening.
6th. Cloudy for the most part with occasional mist.
7th. Pleasant. Warm for the season.
8th. Mist, with occasional sprinkling during the day.
9th. Very warm and damp for the season.
10th. Showery in the morning. Evening clear.
11th. Very fine.
12th. Pleasant.
13th. Pleasant for the most part. Sprinkling of rain from 11 A. M. to noon. Evening clear. No meteors observed.
14th. Pleasant in the morning. Weather grew cold towards night.
15th. Cold, but fine. Evening splendid.
16th. Pleasant in the morning. Began to rain from 5 to 6 P. M., with wind S. E'ly. Rain continued in the evening.
17th. Cloudy for the most part.
18th. Pleasant.
19th. Cloudy in the evening, with appearances of rain.
20th. Wind blustering and very cold in the afternoon and evening.
21st. Wind chilly and cold all day.
22d. Pleasant.
23d. Mild. Copious rain in the evening, with thunder.
24th. Pleasant.
25th. Cold day; very blustering. Evening clear.
26th. Fine, but cold.
27th. Mild and pleasant.
28th. Pleasant and very mild.
29th. Pleasant.
30th. Cloudy through the day, with mist in the evening.

December, 1857. New Moon, 16d. 5h. 53m. A. M.

Days.	Barometer, reduced to 32° F. Sunrise.	Barometer At 1 P. M.	Barometer At 10 P. M.	Thermometer. Sunrise.	Thermometer At 1 P. M.	Thermometer At 10 P. M.	Thermometer Daily mean.	Winds (Direction and Force.) Sunrise.	Winds At 1 P. M.	Winds At 10 P. M.	Weather (Tenths Cloudy.) Sunrise.	Weather At 1 P. M.	Weather At 10 P. M.	Relative Humidity.	Rain and Snow in Inches of Water
1	29.88	29.77	29.88	49	54	38	47.0	S'ly 3	W'ly 1	N. W. 1	Rain	10	0	90	1.35
2	29.90	29.85	29.78	32	44	37	37.7	N. W. 1	W'ly 1	N. W. 1	0	0	3	53	
3	29.69	29.63	29.76	36	43	33	37.3	N. W. 1	W'ly 3	W'ly 2	0	10	3	59	
4	29.83	29.78	29.97	31	36	27	31.3	N. W. 1	N. W'ly 3	N. W. 1	5	0	0	48	
5	29.93	29.89	30.01	27	28	28	27.7	S. E'ly 1	E'ly 1	E'ly 1	10	Snow	10	83	
S 6	30.07	29.96	29.71	29	36	38	34.3	E'ly 1	E'ly 2	E'ly 3	10	10	Rain	76	0.75
7	29.53	29.79	29.97	38	52	38	42.2	N. W. 2	N. W. 2	N. W. 1	5	0	0	57	
8	29.89	29.75	29.91	35	54	46	45.0	S. W. 1	S. W. 2	S. W. 1	2	10	0	76	
9	29.98	29.79	29.50	42	42	42	42.0	N. E'ly 1	N. E'ly 2	N. E'ly 1	Rain	Rain	10	95	1.00
10	29.39	29.46	29.63	46	45	35	42.0	N. W'ly 1	N. W. 2	N. W. 1	Misty	1	0	67	
11	29.72	29.85	30.16	35	33	20	29.3	N. W'ly 4	N. W. 2	N. W. 1	0	10	0	42	
12	30.28	30.27	30.34	18	34	24	24.0	N. W. 1	N. W. 2	N. W. 1	0	0	0	69	
S 13	30.26	30.13	30.06	25	41	34	33.3	S. W. 1	S. W. 2	S. W. 1	0	1	0	55	
14	29.95	29.85	29.92	35	49	38	40.7	W'ly 1	W'ly 2	W'ly 1	0	0	0	50	
15	30.05	30.16	30.23	36	38	30	31.3	N'ly 1	N. E. 2	N. E. 1	2	10	0	98	
16	30.24	30.09	30.11	31	42	39	37.3	S'ly 1	S. W. 1	S. W. 1	9	10	10	72	
17	30.09	30.00	29.92	36	42	42	40.0	E'ly 1	S'ly 1	S'ly 1	10	10	10	92	
18	29.58	29.33	29.47	45	53	47	48.3	E'ly 1	S. W. 2	W'ly 2	Rain	Misty	0	84	0.40
19	29.74	29.84	30.01	40	43	30	37.7	W by N 2	N. W. 2	N. W. 2	0	0	0	53	
S 20	30.09	30.10	30.24	23	33	25	27.0	N. W. 1	N. W. 2	N. W. 2	0	0	0	50	
21	30.25	30.19	29.9[illegible]	21	34	33	29.3	N. W. 1	S. W'ly 1	E'ly 1	0	3	10	65	
22	29.45	29.16	29.15	43	51	37	43.7	S. E'ly 1	S. W'ly 2	N. W. 2	Rain	8	0	73	0.35
23	29.21	29.22	29.30	33	37	37	35.7	N. W. 1	W by S. 2	S. W. 2	0	8	0	15	
24	29.37	29.55	29.79	32	41	30	34.3	W'ly 3	N. W. 3	N. W. 2	2	0	0	32	
25	29.87	29.73	29.59	16	22	19	19.0	N. E. 1	N. E. 2	N. E. 2	2	10	7	48	
26	29.61	29.57	29.65	21	21	18	20.0	N. N. E. 2	N. E. 2	N. E. 3	10	Snow	Snow	68	0.25
S 27	29.99	30.03	30.12	12	21	9	14.0	N. W. 1	N. W. 1	N. W. 1	0	0	2	64	
28	29.90	29.73	29.84	26	41	34	33.7	S. W. 2	S. W. 3	S. W. 1	10	10	5	73	
29	29.84	29.79	29.84	31	35	31	32.3	N'ly 1	N. E. 1	N. E. 1	10	Snow	Snow	83	
30	29.83	29.75	29.58	28	33	35	32.0	N. E. 1	N. E. 1	N. E. 2	10	Misty	Rain	92	1.10
31	29.01	28.91	29.44	38	43	35	38.7	N. E. 2	W'ly 4	W. by S. 4	Rain	5	0	78	
Means	29.82	29.77	29.83	31.9	39.4	32.5	...	1.4	1.9	1.5	5.1	6.0	3.5	66.4	5.20
								1.6			4.9				
REDUCED TO SEA LEVEL.															
Max.	30.46	30.45	30.52	49	54	47	48.3								
Min.	29.19	29.09	29.33	12	21	9	14.0								
Mean	30.00	29.95	30.01												
Range	1.27	1.36	1.19	37	33	38	34.3								
Mean of month	29.987			...	...	...	34.6								
Extreme range	1.43			...	...	...	45.0								

Prevailing winds from some point between— Days.
N. & E. 7
E. & S. 2
S. & W. 11
W. & N. 11

Days.
Clear 10
Variable . . . } 9
Cloudy . . . . }
Rain or snow fell on 12

REMARKS.

1st. Rain in the morning. Cleared from 5 to 6 P. M. Evening clear.
2d. Very fine.
3d. Air cool, and wind blustering.
4th. Pleasant.
5th. Began to snow from 9 to 10 A. M.; quantity small; ground covered half an inch deep. The first snow of the season.
6th. Snow disappeared during the morning. Began to rain from 3 to 4 P. M.; rain continued through the evening.
7th. Very fine.
8th. Pleasant. Very mild for the season.
9th. Moderate rain through the day.
10th. Mist and light rain in the morning. Evening very clear.
11th. Cloudy at mid-day. Evening very clear and cold.
12th. Cold, but very fine.
13th. Very fine.
14th. Very fine. Evening very clear.
15th. Mild in the morning. Cloudy and air raw in the afternoon. Evening clear.
16th. Mild. Some flakes of snow in the morning.
17th. Mild for the season.
18th. Moderate rain in morning. Clear at 10 P. M.
19th. Very fine; nearly cloudless.
20th. Very fine. Remarkably clear in the evening.
21st. Clear in the morning. Cloudy in the evening, with appearances of storm.
22d. Moderate rain in morning. Sprinkling at 7 P. M. Clear at 10 P. M., with the wind N. W.
23d. Pleasant.
24th. Very blustering.
25th. Cloudy for the most part and air cold.
26th. Began to snow moderately at 7½ A. M.; snowed all day.
27th. Five or six inches of light snow on the ground this morning. Evening cold.
28th. Mild. Ther. rose 30° from 10 last night till 10 A. M. Cloudy; wind brisk S. W.
29th. Began to snow gently from noon to 1 P. M., and continued.
30th. Ground lightly covered with fresh snow this morning. Light rain in evening.
31st. Light rain and mist this morning; wind E'ly. Clouds broken in afternoon; wind S. W. Evening blustering and very clear.

January, 1858. New Moon, 15d. 0h. 24m. A. M.

Days.	Barometer Sunrise.	Barometer At 1 P. M.	Barometer At 10 P. M.	Thermometer Sunrise.	Thermometer At 1 P. M.	Thermometer At 10 P. M.	Thermometer Daily mean.	Winds Sunrise.	Winds At 1 P. M.	Winds At 10 P. M.	Weather Sunrise.	Weather At 1 P. M.	Weather At 10 P. M.	Relative Humidity.	Rain and Snow in Inches of Water
1	29.74	29.60	29.90	32	49	38	39.7	N. W. 1	S. W. 4	W'ly 2	0	1	0	55	
2	30.06	29.92	29.88	38	39	37	38.0	S. W. 1	S. W. 1	S. W. 1	2	10	10	65	
S 3	29.74	29.62	29.51	32	37	39	36.0	N. W. 1	N. W. 1	S. W. 2	0	0	2	35	
4	29.57	29.37	29.40	35	49	43	42.3	S. W. 1	S. W. 3	S. W. 3	5	0	0	43	
5	29.56	29.59	29.71	38	49	35	30.7	S. W. 1	N. W. 1	N. E. 2	5	3	10	40	
6	29.62	29.64	29.81	24	19	18	20.3	N. E. 3	N. E. 3	N. E. 1	Snow	Snow	10	84	0.25
7	29.80	29.88	30.26	20	33	16	23.0	W. by S. 1	N. W. 4	N. W. 2	2	1	0	65	
8	30.45	30.51	30.49	8	18	6	10.7	N. W. 1	N. W. 2	N. W. 1	0	0	1	64	
9	30.33	30.04	29.90	13	36	37	28.7	S. W. 1	S. W. 2	S. W. 2	10	Snow	10	84	
S 10	30.11	30.18	30.28	31	35	27	31.0	N. W. 1	N. W. 1	E'ly 1	0	0	0	52	
11	30.11	29.59	29.41	35	46	55	45.3	S. E. 2	S. E. 3	S. W. 3	10	Rain	Rain	95	1.65
12	29.61	29.82	30.12	42	46	30	39.3	N. W. 1	N. W. 2	N. W. 1	0	0	0	51	
13	30.14	30.04	30.02	25	37	36	32.7	N. E'ly 1	S. E'ly 1	S. W. 1	5	10	10	72	
14	30.07	30.09	30.17	33	40	30	34.3	S. W. 1	S. W. 1	W'ly 1	10	9	0	73	
15	30.24	30.17	29.94	27	42	39	36.0	N. E. 1	E'ly 2	S'ly 3	1	10	Rain	56	} 1.33
16	29.68	29.23	29.33	45	56	43	48.0	S'ly 2	S. W. 3	W'ly 1	Rain	Rain	8	82	
S 17	29.62	29.65	29.77	35	38	27	33.3	N. W. 2	N. W. 2	N. W. 1	1	0	0	58	
18	29.74	29.75	29.86	24	26	24	24.7	N'ly 2	N'ly 1	N. W. 1	10	Snow	0	71	
19	29.87	29.83	29.89	25	36	30	30.3	N. W. 2	N. W. 1	N. W. 1	5	9	2	52	
20	29.94	29.93	30.10	20	34	25	26.3	N. W. 1	N. W. 2	N. W. 1	0	1	1	50	
21	30.10	29.99	29.97	25	42	36	34.3	S'ly 2	S by W. 2	S. W. 2	0	0	0	63	
22	30.15	30.39	30.50	30	25	15	23.3	N'ly 2	N. W. 1	N. W. 1	2	0	0	22	
23	30.56	30.54	30.51	12	31	25	22.0	N'ly 2	N. W. 1	N. W. 1	0	0	0	54	
S 24	30.45	30.34	30.34	33	43	40	38.7	S. W'ly 1	S. W. 2	S. W'ly 2	10	7	9	60	
25	30.25	30.19	30.04	43	53	42	46.0	S. W. 1	S. W. 1	S. W. 1	10	10	0	94	
26	29.99	29.77	29.60	43	57	47	49.0	S'ly 1	S. W. 4	S. W. 1	7	10	0	78	0.10
27	29.59	29.54	29.56	40	50	41	43.7	N. W. 1	N. W. 2	N. W. 2	0	8	10	62	
28	29.56	29.55	29.48	36	35	31	34.0	N. E. 1	N. E. 2	N'ly 2	Misty	Misty	10	85	
29	29.50	29.26	29.37	23	26	27	25.3	N'ly 2	N'ly 2	N'ly 1	10	10	10	71	
30	29.42	29.42	29.40	27	35	26	29.3	N. W'ly 2	N. W. 2	N. W. 1	0	0	1	65	
S 31	29.78	29.81	30.00	17	24	17	19.3	N. W. 1	N. W. 2	N. W. 2	1	2	0	37	
Means	29.91	29.85	29.90	29.4	38.3	31.7	...	1.4	2.0	1.5	4.4	5.2	4.0	62.5	3.33
								1.6			4.5				
REDUCED TO SEA LEVEL.															
Max.	30.74	30.72	30.69	45	57	55	49.0								
Min.	29.60	29.41	29.51	8	18	6	10.7								
Mean	30.00	30.00	30.08												
Range	1.14	1.31	1.18	37	39	49	38.3								
Mean of month	30.067			...	...	...	33.1								
Extreme range	1.33			...	...	...	51.0								

Prevailing winds from some point between— Days.
N. & E. 4
E. & S. 2
S. & W. 10
W. & N. 15

Days.
Clear 14
Variable . . . } 10
Cloudy . . . . }
Rain or snow fell on 7

1st. Very fine.
2d. Mild and pleasant.
3d. Fine for the season.
4th. Very fine.
5th. Very mild for the season. Frost out of the ground in most places.
6th. Snow in the morning, with heavy wind at N. E. Air snowy in the afternoon and evening.
7th. From four to five inches of snow on the ground, considerably drifted. Blustering through the day. Evening clear.
8th. Cold, but fine. Bright aurora in the evening, with streamers during the early part of it; afterwards, strong diffused light, varying in hue from greenish to pink.
9th. Began to snow from 11 A. M. to noon. Sprinkling of rain in the afternoon.
10th. Very fine.
11th. Steady rain in the afternoon and evening.
12th. Very fine. Frost nearly all out of the ground.
13th. Very mild.
14th. Mild and pleasant. Evening very clear.
15th. Began to rain moderately at 10 P. M. Wind fresh E'ly.
16th. Steady rain in the morning; wind from S'ly to S. W. Stars out in the evening. Thermometer 56°, being warmer than at any time since Nov. 10, 1857.
17th. Very fine. Violets in bloom in the garden.
18th. Light dusting of snow from 10 A. M. to 2 P. M.
19th. Pleasant.
20th and 21st. Very fine.
22d. Very fine. Evening splendid.
23d. Very fine.
24th. Very mild for the season.
25th. Mild and pleasant.
26th. Mild. Occasional brisk showers in the afternoon.
27th. Mild and pleasant.
28th. Mist and sleet in the morning. Air chilly, with some snow, in the afternoon.
29th. Cloudy and chilly all day.
30th. Blustering. Evening splendid.
31st. Cold, but pleasant.

February, 1858. New Moon, 13d. 5h. 4m. P. M.

Days	Barometer, reduced to 32° F. Sunrise	At 1 P. M.	At 10 P. M.	Thermometer. Sunrise	At 1 P. M.	At 10 P. M.	Daily mean	Winds (Direction and Force.) Sunrise	At 1 P. M.	At 10 P. M.	Weather (Tenths Cloudy.) Sunrise	At 1 P. M.	At 10 P. M.	Relative Humidity	Rain and Snow in Inches of Water
1	30.17	30.16	29.94	12	27	30	23.0	N. W. 1	E'ly 1	E'ly 3	0	1	Snow	60	} 1.20
2	29.30	29.35	29.39	44	45	37	42.0	S. E'ly 1	S. W'ly 3	W'ly 2	Rain	Misty	5	100	
3	29.63	29.69	29.84	36	42	33	37.0	N. W. 2	N. W. 3	N. W. 1	3	2	0	51	
4	29.88	29.81	29.78	32	39	29	33.3	W'ly 1	W. by N. 2	W'ly 1	9	6	10	48	
5	29.75	29.66	29.71	26	29	23	26.0	N. W. 2	N'ly 2	N'ly 2	9	3	0	43	
6	29.88	29.89	29.95	22	32	22	25.3	N. W. 1	N. W. 2	N. W. 1	3	0	0	51	
S 7	29.86	29.70	29.77	29	39	36	34.7	S. W'ly 1	S. W. 2	S. W. 1	Snow	10	10	76	
8	29.83	29.87	30.00	30	33	23	28.7	N. W. 1	N. W. 3	N. W. 1	5	3	0	49	
9	30.03	29.82	29.34	19	28	43	30.0	N. W. 2	S. W'ly 2	S. E. 3	3	10	Rain	68	0.25
10	29.13	29.17	29.46	42	43	21	35.0	W. by S. 1	W by N 2	N. W. 3	7	3	0	46	
11	29.76	29.79	30.04	10	13	9	10.7	N. W. 2	N. W. 4	N. W. 2	0	2	0	63	
12	30.08	29.99	30.03	7	24	17	16.0	N. W. 1	N. W. 2	N. W. 1	3	2	0	55	
13	30.05	30.04	30.06	8	20	16	14.7	W'ly 1	N'ly 2	N. E'ly 2	3	10	10	77	
S 14	29.82	29.74	29.74	18	22	18	19.3	N. by E. 2	N. E. 2	N. by E. 2	10	Snow	10	75	0.10
15	29.74	29.74	29.85	18	21	15	18.7	N. W. 2	N. W. 3	N. W. 1	1	5	0	55	
16	29.80	29.59	29.65	10	29	11	16.7	N. W. 2	W by N 2	N. W. 4	0	3	0	50	
17	29.69	29.67	29.81	7	20	13	13.3	N. W. 2	N. W. 3	N. W. 2	0	0	0	39	
18	29.83	29.87	29.96	10	20	10	13.3	N. W. 1	N. W. 3	N. W. 1	5	0	1	58	
19	30.04	29.97	29.95	5	23	18	15.3	N. W. 2	N'ly 1	N. E. 1	2	10	Snow	62	} 1.25
20	29.65	29.38	29.36	25	31	22	26.0	N. E. 3	N. E. 3	N. E. 3	Snow	Snow	Snow	78	
S 21	29.55	29.55	29.59	17	34	28	26.3	N. W. 1	N. W. 1	S. W. 1	0	0	10	48	
22	29.75	29.79	29.86	21	26	18	21.7	N. W. 1	N. W. 2	N. E. 1	1	7	10	57	
23	29.91	30.03	30.32	8	18	8	11.3	N. W. 1	N. W. 2	N. W. 1	0	0	0	59	
24	30.17	30.08	29.90	3	28	21	17.3	N. W. 1	N. W. 1	S. W'ly 1	0	0	2	1	
25	29.71	29.52	29.66	28	40	28	32.0	S. W. 1	W'ly 1	N. W. 1	3	0	0	48	
26	29.70	29.70	29.80	25	37	24	28.7	N. W. 1	N. W. 1	N. W. 1	0	7	0	57	
27	29.76	29.72	29.74	17	40	35	30.7	S. W. 1	S. W. 2	S. W. 1	0	5	3	65	
S 28	29.71	29.59	29.51	35	47	39	40.3	S. W. 1	S. W. 2	S. W. 1	1	5	1	73	
Means	29.79	29.75	29.78	20.1	30.3	23.1	...	1.4	2.1	1.6	3.5	4.2	4.3	57	2.80
									1.7			4.0			
Reduced to sea level.															
Max.	30.35	30.34	30.50	44	47	43	42.0								
Min.	29.31	29.35	29.52	3	13	8	10.7								
Mean	29.97	29.93	29.96												
Range	1.04	0.99	0.98	41	34	35	31.3								
Mean of month	29.953			...	...	...	24.5								
Extreme range	1.19			...	...	...	44.0								

Prevailing winds from some point between— Days.
N. & E. 5
E. & S. 0
S. & W. 6
W. & N. 17

Days.
Clear 11
Variable . . . . } 9
Cloudy . . . . }
Rain or snow fell on 8

REMARKS.

1st. Pleasant morning. Cloudy towards night; wind E'ly. Began to snow and hail, with rain, from 9 to 10 P. M.
2d. Rain in morning. Cloudy in afternoon. Mostly clear at 10 P. M., and very mild.
3d. Very fine. Evening very clear. Frost nearly out of the ground.
4th. Pleasant. Appearances of storm in the evening.
5th. Fine.
6th. Very fine. Evening very clear.
7th. Light snow this morning; covering the ground for a short time.
8th. Rather blustering. Air full of dust.
9th. Light snow from 3 to 4 P. M. Moderate rain in the evening.
10th. Very mild morning; wind W. by N. Grew cold towards sunset; wind N. W., and very brisk.
11th. Very cold, and high wind. Extremely severe to be out.
12th. Cold very much abated.
13th. Cloudy in afternoon. Wind N. E'ly in evening, with appearances of storm.
14th. Light snow, about an inch deep.
15th. Fine. Two inches of snow on the ground this morning.
16th. Light flurry of snow at 2 P. M. Afternoon and evening extremely blustering and severe.
17th and 18th. Cold, but fine.
19th. More mild. Cloudy in afternoon. Light snow in the evening.
20th. Driving snow all day. Wind heavy from N. E. in the afternoon.
21st. From seven to nine inches of damp snow on the ground this morning, somewhat drifted.
22d. Pleasant.
23d. Cold, but pleasant.
24th. Ther. 3° this morning—the coldest of the season; more moderate during day.
25th and 26th. Fine. Evening splendid.
27th. Mild and pleasant.
28th. Very mild.

March, 1858. New Moon, 15d. 7h. 4m. A. M.

Days	Barometer Sunrise	At 1 P. M.	At 10 P. M.	Thermometer Sunrise	At 1 P. M.	At 10 P. M.	Daily mean	Winds Sunrise	At 1 P. M.	At 10 P. M.	Weather Sunrise	At 1 P. M.	At 10 P. M.	Relative Humidity	Rain and Snow in Inches of Water
1	29.34	29.41	29.35	40	40	32	37.3	S. W. 1	N. W. 1	N. E'ly 1	10	Sprin'le	Snow	92	0.70
2	29.14	29.19	29.52	29	33	21	27.7	N. E'ly 2	N. W. 2	N. W. 3	Snow	8	10	68	
3	29.75	29.78	29.89	10	21	7	12.7	N. W. 1	N. W. 1	N. W. 1	0	0	0	25	
4	29.95	29.84	29.85	2	22	10	11.3	N. W. 1	N. W. 1	N. W. 2	0	0	0	54	
5	29.77	29.60	29.62	4	17	9	10.0	N. W. 2	N. W. 2	N. W. 2	0	7	10	53	
6	29.63	29.53	29.44	3	20	13	12.0	N. W. 2	N. W. 2	N. W. 2	0	0	0	54	
S 7	29.38	29.37	29.48	12	25	20	19.0	N. W. 1	N. W. 3	N. W. 2	0	1	0	53	
8	29.50	29.41	29.05	13	30	21	21.3	N. W. 2	S'ly 2	N. E. 3	0	10	Snow	41	0.85
9	28.94	28.98	29.21	18	26	20	21.3	N. W. 1	N. W. 3	N. W. 2	9	0	10	67	
10	29.33	29.40	29.60	18	34	26	26.0	W'ly 2	W by N 3	W'ly 1	8	3	0	34	
11	29.54	29.33	29.50	27	47	36	36.7	S'ly 1	S'ly 1	W'ly 4	9	0	0	58	
12	29.82	29.92	29.96	24	36	31	30.3	N. W. 3	N. W. 2	N. W. 1	0	0	0	35	
13	30.13	30.23	30.29	28	33	25	28.7	N. W. 2	N. W. 2	N. W. 1	0	0	0	55	
S 14	30.19	29.92	29.93	25	40	37	34.0	S'ly 1	S. W. 3	S. W'ly 1	8	Sprin'le	10	75	
15	30.03	30.03	30.04	37	49	37	41.0	N. W. 1	S. W. 1	S. W. 1	0	10	10	68	
16	30.02	30.04	29.93	36	40	37	37.7	S'ly 1	S. E'ly 1	S'ly	Misty	10	Foggy	88	
17	29.70	29.53	29.50	38	53	45	45.7	S'ly 1	S'ly 2	S'ly 1	Foggy	9	5	82	
18	29.30	29.36	29.69	49	60	44	51.0	S. W. 3	W. by S. 1	N. W. 2	0	8	0	65	
19	29.87	30.00	30.12	40	45	35	40.0	N. W. 2	N by W 3	N. W. 1	3	6	0	56	
20	30.13	30.04	29.95	29	43	34	35.3	N. W. 2	S. E. 2	S'ly 1	0	0	0	67	
S 21	29.01	29.21	29.23	39	48	44	43.7	S'ly 2	S'ly 1	N. W. 3	Rain	Rain	5	76	0.50
22	29.35	29.46	29.78	38	45	33	38.7	N. W. 3	N. W. 4	N. W. 1	0	6	3	36	
23	29.86	29.78	29.81	28	40	31	33.0	N. W. 2	N. W. 2	N. W. 1	2	5	0	31	
24	29.83	29.75	29.78	26	45	32	34.3	N. W. 1	N. W. 3	N. W. 1	0	2	0	28	
25	29.69	29.49	29.43	29	53	43	41.7	N. W. 1	W by N. 2	W'ly 2	0	0	5	33	
26	29.50	29.48	29.57	33	45	34	37.3	N. W. 2	N. W. 2	N. W. 2	0	0	0	31	
27	29.53	29.52	29.54	11	48	36	38.3	N. W. 2	N. W. 2	N. W. 1	0	0	3	28	
S 28	29.53	29.50	29.58	35	49	37	40.3	S. W'ly 1	S. W. 1	S. W. 1	10	3	0	68	
29	29.62	29.60	29.72	37	56	44	45.7	N. W. 1	N. W. 2	N. E. 1	0	2	9	40	
30	29.83	29.88	29.92	39	52	38	43.0	N. E. 1	N'ly 1	N. W. 2	8	2	2	52	
31	29.91	29.92	29.99	34	54	38	42.0	N'ly 1	N. E. 2	S. E'ly 2	0	2	0	52	
Means	29.65	29.63	29.69	27.5	40.3	30.6	...	1.6	2.0	1.6	3.4	4.0	3.6	53.7	2.05
									1.7			3.7			
Reduced to sea level.															
Max.	30.37	30.41	30.47	49	60	45	51.0								
Min.	29.12	29.16	29.23	2	17	7	10.0								
Mean	29.83	29.81	29.87												
Range	1.25	1.25	1.24	47	43	38	41.0								
Mean of month	29.837			...	...	...	32.8								
Extreme range	1.35			...	...	...	58.0								

Prevailing winds from some point between— Days.
N. & E. 2
E. & S. 2
S. & W. 8
W. & N. 19

Days.
Clear 13
Variable . . . . } 11
Cloudy . . . . }
Rain or snow fell on 6

REMARKS.

1st. Light rain in the morning. Snow in the evening.
2d. From 5 to 6 inches of damp snow on the ground this morning.
3d. Very fine.
4th. Cold, but fine.
5th. Very cold; wind cutting. Flurry of snow at 7 P. M.
6th. Still cold.
7th. Raw and cold.
8th. Began to snow from 5 to 6 P. M.
9th. Seven or eight inches of fresh snow on the ground this morning.
10th. Pleasant. Evening fine.
11th. Mild and pleasant through the day. Very blustering in the evening.
12th. Very fine. Evening splendid.
13th. Very fine. Evening clear. Aurora this evening, somewhat bright, but diffused.
14th. Cloudy. Air raw, with occasional sprinkling of rain.
15th. Very mild for the season. State of the weather favorable for observing the solar eclipse, which began before sunrise and ended at 7 h. 41 m. 29 s. A. M., Providence mean solar time.
16th. Mist and fog.
17th. Very mild.
18th. Very fine. Thermometer 60°; the warmest day since Nov. 10, 1857.
19th. Very fine. Evening splendid.
20th. Very fine. Evening still and very clear.
21st. Moderate rain in the morning; wind S'ly. Clouds broken in the evening, with the wind N. W.
22d. Clear, and very blustering.
23d and 24th. Very fine.
25th. Pleasant in the morning. Sprinkling of rain from 7 to 8 P. M.
26th. Very fine. Frost nearly all out of the ground.
27th and 28th. Very fine.
29th. Fine through the day. Cloudy at 10 P. M.; wind northeast.
30th. Fine.
31st. Very fine.

April, 1858. New Moon, 13d. 6h. 7m. P. M.

Days.	Barometer, reduced to 32° F. At 6 A. M.	At 1 P. M.	At 10 P. M.	Thermometer. At 6 A. M.	At 1 P. M.	At 10 P. M.	Daily mean.	Winds. (Direction and Force.) At 6 A. M.	At 1 P. M.	At 10 P. M.	Weather. (Tenths Cloudy.) At 6 A. M.	At 1 P. M.	At 10 P. M.	Relative Humidity.	Rain and Snow in Inches of Water.
1	30.08	30.01	30.05	35	58	38	43.7	S. W. 1	S. W. 1	S'ly 1	0	0	0	59	
2	30.02	29.95	29.81	33	56	46	45.0	N. E. 1	S. W'ly 2	S'ly 1	5	9	0	70	
3	29.72	29.64	29.71	40	69	55	54.7	N. W. 1	N. W. 1	N. E'ly 1	1	0	0	49	
S 4	29.82	29.83	29.83	45	57	40	47.3	N. E. 1	N. E. 2	N. E. 2	2	0	2	48	
5	29.81	29.70	29.66	35	62	49	48.7	N. E. 1	S. E'ly 2	S'ly 1	0	3	Foggy	71	
6	29.59	29.56	29.71	50	57	39	48.7	S. W. 1	N. W. 2	N. W. 1	10	9	0	68	
7	29.79	29.79	29.93	30	43	33	35.3	N. W. 2	N. W. 3	N. W. 2	0	0	0	0	
8	30.01	29.97	29.97	30	55	45	43.3	N. W. 2	W'ly 2	S. W. 2	0	2	10	36	
9	29.79	29.58	29.51	42	55	48	48.3	S'ly 1	S'ly 1	S'ly 1	Misty	Misty	Foggy	93	0.25
10	29.50	29.59	29.84	46	58	37	47.0	S'ly 1	N. W. 2	N. W. 3	Foggy	7	0	55	
S 11	29.88	29.73	29.77	34	55	45	44.7	N. W. 1	N. W. 2	N. W. 2	0	7	10	30	
12	29.80	29.77	29.73	39	52	38	43.0	N. E. 1	S'ly 1	N. E. 2	10	8	Sprin'le	28	
13	29.56	29.47	29.41	37	43	40	40.0	N. E. 2	N. E. 2	N. E. 2	Misty	Rain	Rain	91	1.10
14	29.25	29.26	29.32	40	57	42	46.3	N. E. 2	N. W. 2	S. W. 1	Rain	7	0	83	
15	29.29	29.30	29.47	43	60	49	50.7	S. W. 2	N. W. 3	S. W. 2	5	5	3	54	
16	29.57	29.53	29.61	47	63	50	53.3	W by N. 2	W. 2	S. W. 2	0	5	5	53	
17	29.71	29.73	29.78	45	60	46	50.3	S. W. 2	W'ly 2	N. W. 2	0	3	0	31	
S 18	29.86	29.89	29.98	38	61	50	49.7	N. W'ly 2	W by N 2	N. W. 1	0	0	3	31	
19	30.10	30.06	30.03	42	60	45	49.0	N'ly 1	S. W'ly 2	S. W'ly 1	5	10	10	31	
20	30.02	29.82	29.49	44	44	40	42.7	N. E. 1	N. E. 1	E'ly 1	10	Rain	Rain	83	1.00
21	29.22	29.32	29.49	39	44	44	42.3	N by W. 2	W'ly 1	N. W'ly 2	10	10	5	74	
22	29.72	29.80	29.82	42	58	45	48.3	N. W. 1	S'ly 2	S'ly 1	0	0	0	67	
23	29.69	29.47	29.53	50	58	46	51.3	S. W. 2	S'ly 2	N. E. 4	10	Rain	Rain	76	0.75
24	29.62	29.63	29.83	40	51	40	43.7	N. W. 3	W'ly 3	N. W. 2	4	7	8	51	
S 25	29.95	29.95	29.96	42	48	34	41.3	N. W. 2	N. W. 1	N. E. 1	0	10	Snow	24	
26	29.86	29.83	29.87	37	50	39	42.0	N. W. 2	N. W. 1	N. E. 1	0	0	10	52	
27	29.87	29.64	29.44	36	33	34	34.3	N'ly 1	N. E. 3	N. E. 3	10	Snow	Snow	34	0.37
28	29.59	29.53	29.65	40	52	44	45.3	W'ly 2	W'ly 2	N. W. 1	8	7	0	35	
29	29.67	29.55	29.57	47	62	47	52.0	N. W. 2	N. W. 1	S. W. 1	0	0	8	41	
30	29.57	29.55	29.58	48	59	53	53.3	S. W. 1	S. W. 1	S'ly 1	Rain	0	0	85	0.16
Means	29.73	29.68	29.71	40.5	54.7	43.4	...	1.5	1.8	1.6	4.7	5.3	5.1	53.4	3.63
									1.6			5.0			
REDUCED TO SEA LEVEL.															
Max.	30.28	30.24	30.23	50	69	55	54.7								
Min.	29.40	29.44	29.50	30	33	33	34.3								
Mean	29.91	29.86	29.89												
Range	0.88	0.80	0.73	20	36	22	20.4								
Mean of month	29.887			...	...	...	46.2								
Extreme range	0.88			...	...	...	39.0								

Prevailing winds from some point between— Days.
N. & E. 5
E. & S. 1
S. & W. 9
W. & N. 15

Days.
Clear 8
Variable . . . . } 12
Cloudy . . . . }
Rain or snow fell on 10

Remarks.

1st. Very fine.
2d. At 6 A. M., surface current of wind from N. E.; upper current from W'ly. A copious white frost this morning.
3d. Very warm for the season.
4th. Very fine.
5th. Pleasant. Dense fog in the evening.
6th. Sprinkling at 6 P. M. Clear at 10 P. M.
7th. Cold, but fine. Wind blustering, and air full of dust.
8th. Pleasant. Cloudy, with appearances of storm in the evening.
9th. Light rain and mist in the morning. Clouds broken in the evening, and foggy. Aurora from 8 to 9 P. M. Streamers shooting up from a cloud at the north; streamers low down, and not well defined.
10th. Pleasant. Aurora in the evening, with faint streamers. At 10 P. M., there was for some time a narrow, white, well-defined auroral bow spanning the heavens from the east to the west, passing a little to the south of the zenith.
11th. Pleasant.
12th. Pleasant in the morning. Air raw in the afternoon. Sprinkling in evening.
13th. Mist and light showers.
14th. Thundershower at 7 A. M; wind N. E.; clouds broken, lower stratum coming from N. E., the upper from S. W.
15th and 16th. Pleasant.
17th. Very fine. Evening splendid.
18th. Very fine.
19th. Cloudy in the afternoon; air raw and chilly.
20th. Began to sprinkle at 10 A. M. Steady but moderate rain in the evening.
21st. Cloudy all day. Clouds broken in the evening.
22d. Very fine. Evening splendid.
23d. Showery in the morning. Fog in the afternoon. Rain after 10 P. M.
24th. Air dry, wind chilly.
25th. Air chilly. Drizzling rain at 5 P. M. Snow at 10 P. M.
26th. Clear during day. Cloudy at night.
27th. Heavy N. E. storm; wind high, air thick with snow, which melted as it fell.
28th. Cool, but very fine.
29th. Very fine.
30th. Showery in the morning. Afternoon and evening fine.

May, 1858. New Moon, 13d. 2h. 40m. A. M.

Days.	Barometer At 6 A. M.	At 1 P. M.	At 10 P. M.	Thermometer At 6 A. M.	At 1 P. M.	At 10 P. M.	Daily mean.	Winds At 6 A. M.	At 1 P. M.	At 10 P. M.	Weather At 6 A. M.	At 1 P. M.	At 10 P. M.	Relative Humidity.	Rain.
1	29.58	29.75	29.94	57	66	52	58.3	N'ly 1	S'ly 1	S. E. 1	0	0	10	63	
S 2	30.10	30.07	30.18	50	58	46	51.3	N. E. 1	E'ly 1	N. W.	Rain	5	0	56	
3	30.29	30.18	30.16	44	58	41	47.7	N. E. 1	N. W. 1	N. W. 1	0	0	0	42	
4	30.10	29.98	29.96	49	57	49	51.7	N'ly 1	S'ly 1	N. W. 2	0	0	0	47	
5	29.90	29.86	29.77	52	60	53	55.0	S. W. 1	S'ly 1	S. E. 1	10	10	6	66	0.20
6	29.58	29.47	29.46	58	60	57	58.3	S. E. 1	S'ly 1	N. E. 1	Rain	10	Misty	79	
7	29.56	29.65	29.79	55	60	53	56.0	N. E. 1	E'ly 2	N. E. 1	10	10	8	75	
8	29.89	29.89	29.88	48	56	46	50.0	N. E. 2	N. E. 2	N. E.	0	5	10	72	
S 9	29.83	29.74	29.72	50	59	49	52.7	N'ly 1	S. E'ly 1	S'ly 1	10	10	9	58	
10	29.66	29.68	29.77	52	69	57	59.3	S'ly 1	N. W. 1	N. E. 1	2	10	10	47	
11	29.82	29.71	29.63	47	59	47	51.0	N. E. 2	N. E. 2	N. E. 3	10	10	Rain	66	1.00
12	29.40	29.39	29.54	56	69	52	59.0	S. W. 1	S. W. 3	N. W. 2	Foggy	5	0	60	
13	29.59	29.70	29.88	50	65	55	56.7	N. W. 3	N. W. 3	N. W. 1	1	3	0	51	
14	29.95	29.87	29.81	48	63	52	54.3	N. W. 1	N. W. 2	N. W. 1	10	2	5	52	
15	29.70	29.64	29.67	54	69	56	59.7	S. W. 1	N. W. 1	N. W. 1	10	2	5	66	
S 16	29.77	29.81	29.92	55	62	51	56.0	N. W. 2	N. W. 2	N. W. 1	10	3	0	29	
17	30.00	29.92	29.79	44	53	45	47.3	S'ly 1	S. W'ly 2	S'ly 2	2	10	Rain	55	
18	29.79	29.79	29.88	43	48	44	45.0	E. 2	E. by N. 1	N. E. 1	Rain	Misty	Misty	86	
19	29.90	29.90	29.84	46	55	45	48.7	N. E. 1	N. E. 2	S. E. 1	10	10	10	66	
20	29.77	29.68	29.63	46	57	47	50.0	N. E. 1	S. W. 1	S. W. 1	Misty	10	Rain	83	1.00
21	29.58	29.61	29.73	47	52	47	48.7	N. 2	N. W. 1	N. W. 1	10	Rain	0	85	
22	29.76	29.89	30.01	45	55	46	48.7	N. W. 1	N. E. 2	S. W. 1	Rain	5	0	60	
S 23	30.02	29.91	29.82	52	70	54	58.7	W. 2	W'ly 1	S. W. 2	0	3	Sprin'le	57	0.15
24	29.42	29.27	29.52	58	75	59	64.0	S. W. 2	S. W. 4	N. W. 2	10	10	0	59	
25	29.59	29.60	29.81	56	62	50	56.0	N. W. 2	N. E. 3	N. E. 2	0	10	10	57	
26	29.82	29.78	29.78	47	57	49	51.0	N. E. 1	N. E. 2	N. E. 2	10	10	Sprin'le	59	
27	29.74	29.80	29.92	47	53	49	49.7	N. E. 2	N. E. 3	N. E. 2	Misty	10	10	66	
28	29.98	30.02	30.09	49	60	43	50.7	N. E. 2	N. E. 4	N. E. 1	0	2	0	52	
29	30.07	30.01	30.01	44	61	44	49.7	N. E. 2	N. E. 3	N. E. 1	0	0	1	55	
S 30	[illegible]	[illegible]	[illegible]	[illegible]	[illegible]	[illegible]	[illegible]	[illegible]	[illegible]	[illegible]	[illegible]	[illegible]	[illegible]	[illegible]	
31	[illegible]	29.88	29.88	47	60	53	53.0	S'ly 1	S'ly 3	S'ly 1	0	0	0	63	
Means	29.81	29.79	29.83	49.6	60.7	49.8	...	1.4	1.9	1.3	6.0	6.0	5.3	61.1	2.35
									1.5			5.8			
REDUCED TO SEA LEVEL.															
Max.	30.47	30.36	30.30	58	75	59	64.0								
Min.	29.58	29.45	29.64	43	48	41	45.0								
Mean	29.99	29.97	30.01												
Range	0.89	0.91	0.72	15	27	18	19.0								
Mean of month	29.990			...	...	...	53.3								
Extreme range	1.02			...	...	...	34.0								

Prevailing winds from some point between— Days.
N. & E. 14
E. & S. 2
S. & W. 7
W. & N. 8

Days.
Clear 7
Variable . . . . } 10
Cloudy . . . . }
Rain fell on . . 14

Remarks.

1st. Very fine.
2d. Showers in the morning. Cleared in the afternoon. Evening fine.
3d and 4th. Very fine.
5th. Showers from 10 A. M. to noon. Afternoon pleasant.
6th. Light showers in the morning.
7th. Clouds and fog.
8th. Rather cool. Cherry-trees in full bloom.
9th. Cloudy. Air raw in the afternoon.
10th. Cloudy, with occasional sprinkling of rain.
11th. Cloudy through the day. Rain in the evening.
12th. Pleasant. Evening clear.
13th. Fine. Evening very clear.
14th. Very fine.
15th. Pleasant. Thundershower at 9 P. M.
16th. Pleasant.
17th. Sprinkling of rain at intervals. In the evening, light showers.
18th. Mist, with occasional light rain.
19th. Cloudy and cool. Clouds broken in the evening.
20th. Mist, sprinkling, and sunshine. In the evening, light rain.
21st. Light showers and sunshine.
22d. Showers in the morning. Evening clear.
23d. Fine in the morning. Sprinkling in the evening.
24th. Cloudy in the morning. Evening clear.
25th. Pleasant.
26th and 27th. Cloudy and cool, with mist and sprinkling.
28th and 29th. Very fine.
30th. [illegible]
31st. Very fine.
Pear-trees in full bloom from 15th to 20th. Apple-trees from 20th to 25th.

June, 1858. New Moon, 11d. 9h. 38m. A. M.

DAYS.	BAROMETER, REDUCED TO 32° F. At 6 A. M.	At 1 P. M.	At 10 P. M.	THERMOMETER. At 6 A. M.	At 1 P. M.	At 10 P. M.	Daily mean.	WINDS. (DIRECTION AND FORCE.) At 6 A. M.	At 1 P. M.	At 10 P. M.	WEATHER. (TENTHS CLOUDY.) At 6 A. M.	At 1 P. M.	At 10 P. M.	RELATIVE HUMIDITY.	RAIN AND SNOW IN INCHES OF WATER.
1	29.86	29.86	29.90	52	66	56	58.0	S'ly 2	S'ly 1	S'ly 1	9	10	10	46.0	
2	29.91	29.88	29.92	52	77	58	62.3	N'ly 1	N. E. 1	S'ly 1	3	1	0	51.0	
3	29.91	29.89	29.93	60	77	62	66.3	N. W. 2	N. E. 2	N. E. 1	0	3	5	42.0	
4	29.92	29.88	29.79	62	72	64	66.0	S'ly 1	S. W. 3	S. W. 3	5	10	10	45.0	
5	29.68	29.69	29.82	64	83	67	71.3	S. W. 2	S. W. 2	S. W. 1	10	7	6	67.0	0.10
S 6	29.82	29.79	29.85	61	76	67	68.0	S'ly 2	S. W. 3	S. W. 4	Rain	5	2	76.0	0.25
7	29.92	29.92	29.90	67	84	64	71.7	S. W. 1	S. W. 2	S. W. 1	3	2	1	71.0	
8	29.85	29.84	29.92	65	80	70	71.7	S. W. 2	S. W. 2	S. W. 1	7	6	0	64.0	
9	29.93	29.86	29.87	65	80	61	68.7	N. E. 1	N. E. 1	N. E. 2	5	3	10	61.0	
10	29.80	29.71	29.59	63	74	68	68.3	E'ly 1	S. E. 3	S. W'ly 3	Foggy	2	0	79.0	
11	29.52	29.54	29.72	73	85	62	73.3	S. W. 3	S. W. 2	N. E. 2	2	Shower	Rain	72.0	} 3.00
12	29.81	29.83	29.72	55	54	50	53.0	N. E. 2	N. E. 2	N. E. 3	Rain	Rain	Rain	86.0	}
S 13	29.60	29.66	29.70	49	56	53	52.7	N. E. 2	N'ly 2	N. E'ly 1	10	10	10	80.0	
14	29.74	29.74	29.82	51	62	53	55.3	N. E'ly 1	N. E. 1	N. E. 1	10	10	10	72.0	
15	29.77	29.76	29.80	49	52	50	50.3	N. E. 1	N. E. 1	N. E. 1	Rain	Rain	Misty	91.0	1.65
16	29.86	29.88	29.94	50	64	56	56.7	N. E. 1	S'ly 2	S'ly 1	10	5	2	76.0	
17	29.97	29.94	29.90	56	64	58	59.3	S'ly 1	S'ly 2	S'ly 1	Foggy	0	5	82.0	
18	29.81	29.68	29.64	59	84	71	71.3	S'ly 1	S'ly 2	S. W'ly 1	2	1	0	67.0	
19	29.73	29.68	29.73	69	79	66	71.3	N. E. 1	S. E'ly 1	S'ly 1	3	2	7	49.0	
S 20	29.74	29.69	29.66	65	81	70	72.0	N. E'ly 2	S. E'ly 1	S'ly 1	0	5	3	63.0	0.05
21	29.65	29.67	29.75	70	81	63	71.7	N. E'ly 1	N. E. 2	N. W. 1	2	2	5	68.0	0.30
22	29.80	29.89	29.99	64	78	60	67.3	N. W. 1	N. E'ly 2	S'ly 1	2	2	4	61.0	
23	30.00	29.97	29.93	62	77	67	68.7	S. W. 2	S. W. 3	S. W. 3	2	3	7	63.0	
24	29.85	29.75	29.76	68	86	74	76.0	S. W. 2	S. W. 2	S. W. 2	8	1	1	42.0	
25	29.72	29.66	29.71	75	91	70	78.7	Calm	W'ly 2	N. E. 2	0	3	7	76.0	
26	29.67	29.71	29.68	67	83	75	75.0	N. E. 1	N. E. 1	N. E. 1	2	5	3	85.0	0.20
S 27	29.73	29.72	29.75	72	86	74	77.3	N. E'ly 1	N. E'ly 1	S'ly 1	5	3	1	76.0	
28	29.69	29.62	29.67	73	88	78	79.7	S. W'ly 1	S. W'ly 1	N. W. 1	6	3	0	68.0	
29	29.69	29.68	29.62	70	85	79	78.0	N. W. 2	N. W. 2	S. W. 1	0	0	0	40.0	
30	29.68	29.64	29.67	68	80	68	72.0	N. W. 2	N. W. 2	N. W. 1	0	0	0	50.0	
Means	29.79	29.77	29.79	62.5	76.2	64.5	...	1.4	1.8	1.5	5.2	4.5	4.6	65.6	5.55
REDUCED TO SEA LEVEL.								1.6			4.8				
Max.	30.18	30.15	30.17	75	91	79	79.7								
Min.	29.70	29.72	29.77	49	52	50	50.3	Prevailing winds from some point between— Days.							
Mean	29.97	29.95	29.97								Days.				
Range	0.48	0.43	0.40	26	39	29	29.4	N. & E. 11			Clear 6				
								E. & S. 3			Variable . . . } 17				
Mean of month	29.963			...	...	...	67.7	S. & W. 13			Cloudy . . . . }				
Extreme range	0.48			...	...	...	42.0	W. & N. 3			Rain fell on . . 8				

REMARKS.

1st. Cloudy and mild.
2d and 3d. Very fine.
4th. Cloudy, with appearances of rain in the afternoon. Shower during the night.
5th. Very warm and damp.
6th. Thundershower from 5 to 6 A. M. Pleasant in the afternoon and evening, with wind strong at S. W.
7th. Pleasant.
8th. Pleasant. Heavy cumulus clouds in the morning.
9th and 10th. Pleasant.
11th. Light shower at 1 P. M. Showery in the afternoon and evening, with thunder. From noon to 2 P. M., air very hot and sultry.
12th. Rain through the day. Rain heavy in the evening, and cold.
13th and 14th. Cloudy.
15th. Heavy rain through the day. Mist in the evening.
16th and 17th. Pleasant.
18th. Very fine.
19th. Pleasant. Sprinkling of rain at 8 P. M.
20th. Thunder and sprinkling of rain in the afternoon and evening.
21st. At 1 P. M., wind N. E., while the clouds came from the N. W. Heavy shower of rain from 4 to 5 P. M.
22d and 23d. Fine.
24th. Extremely warm and sultry.
25th. Excessively hot at mid-day. Evening much cooler, with wind N. E
26th. Warm and sultry. Shower at 3 P. M., with thunder. Thunder and sprinkling at 6 P. M.
27th. Hot and sultry.
28th. Extremely hot.
29th. Hot; air very dry; breeze cool.
30th. Very fine.

July, 1858. New Moon, 10d. 4h. 17m. P. M.

DAYS.	BAROMETER. At 6 A. M.	At 1 P. M.	At 10 P. M.	THERMOMETER. At 6 A. M.	At 1 P. M.	At 10 P. M.	Daily mean.	WINDS. At 6 A. M.	At 1 P. M.	At 10 P. M.	WEATHER. At 6 A. M.	At 1 P. M.	At 10 P. M.	RELATIVE HUMIDITY.	RAIN AND SNOW.
1	29.82	29.74	29.71	60	68	58	62.0	N. W. 2	N. W. 2	N. W. 1	5	9	0	38.7	
2	29.73	29.71	29.75	58	82	63	67.7	N. W. 2	N. W. 2	S. W. 1	1	0	0	51.7	
3	29.73	29.68	29.58	67	68	69	68.0	S. W. 2	S. E. 2	S'ly 1	Rain	Rain	Foggy	89.5	0.50
S 4	29.47	29.51	29.71	70	84	70	74.7	S. W. 1	N. W. 1	N. W. 1	9	8	0	76.9	
5	29.85	29.94	30.07	63	75	61	66.3	N. W. 1	N. E. 2	S'ly 1	2	2	0	67.1	
6	30.08	30.07	30.04	63	82	66	70.3	S. W. 1	S. W'ly 1	S'ly 1	6	2	0	73.8	
7	29.95	29.89	29.79	67	87	71	75.0	S. W. 2	S. W. 2	S. W. 1	0	2	0	57.1	
8	29.86	29.75	29.82	72	88	69	76.7	S. W. 2	S. W. 3	S. W. 1	0	0	0	51.7	
9	29.86	29.88	29.94	71	83	71	75.0	S. W. 2	S. W. 3	S. W. 1	8	8	Foggy	80.0	
10	29.92	29.83	29.83	74	88	76	79.3	S. W. 2	S. W. 3	S. W. 1	10	3	0	73.9	
S 11	29.78	29.74	29.84	78	93	73	81.3	S. W. 1	S. W. 2	S'ly 1	0	1	Shower	63.1	1.35
12	29.86	29.87	29.87	63	64	60	62.3	N. E. 2	N. E. 2	N. E. 2	Misty	10	Misty	89.0	
13	29.81	29.79	29.87	63	82	74	73.0	N. E. 1	S. W. 4	S. W. 2	Misty	8	10	82.3	
14	29.90	29.89	29.96	73	75	70	72.7	S. W'ly 1	S. W. 1	S. W. 2	Shower	Sprin'le	10	85.3	0.15
15	29.93	29.92	29.92	69	76	68	71.0	N. E. 1	S. W. 1	S. W. 1	10	10	10	81.5	
16	29.93	29.92	29.91	65	77	68	70.0	N'ly 1	S. W'ly 1	S. W'ly 1	Foggy	6	1	79.9	
17	29.90	29.85	29.86	67	80	73	73.3	S'ly 1	S. E. 3	S'ly 1	7	0	10	79.5	
S 18	29.84	29.84	29.93	70	75	68	71.0	N. E. 1	N. E. 1	N. E. 1	Rain	10	0	80.2	0.30
19	29.95	29.94	29.94	63	79	65	69.0	N by W. 2	N. W. 3	N. W. 1	0	1	0	54.8	
20	29.87	29.71	29.75	66	82	67	71.7	N. W. 2	W by N 2	S. W. 1	0	5	7	60.4	
21	29.67	29.64	29.61	66	80	70	72.0	S. W. 2	S. W. 3	S. W. 2	3	3	7	71.2	
22	29.53	29.49	29.56	65	75	66	68.7	S. W. 1	S. E'ly 2	S. W. 2	9	10	Shower	77.6	0.35
23	29.60	29.64	29.69	62	75	65	67.3	N. W. 1	N. W. 2	E'ly 1	0	5	2	71.3	
24	29.71	29.73	29.82	62	71	58	63.7	N. E. 2	N. W. 3	N. by E. 2	Sprin'le	8	9	67.3	0.15
S 25	29.89	29.93	30.02	58	65	57	60.0	N. E'ly 2	N. N. E. 2	N. E. 2	10	10	1	70.8	
26	29.99	29.92	29.90	57	73	60	63.3	N. W. 1	S. W. 2	S'ly 1	2	5	0	70.9	
27	29.78	29.66	29.67	65	79	71	71.7	S. W. 2	S. W. 4	S. W. 1	10	8	6	76.0	
28	29.72	29.74	29.80	66	81	66	71.0	N. W. 1	N. W. 2	N. W. 1	9	3	8	48.0	
29	29.81	29.69	29.55	63	75	70	69.3	N. W. 1	S'ly 1	S. W. 1	6	3	10	67.3	} 2.10
30	29.60	29.55	29.58	59	68	59	62.0	N. W. 2	N. E. 1	N'ly 1	10	10	6	82.8	}
31	29.58	29.60	29.67	59	74	65	66.0	N. W. 1	N. W. 1	N. W. 1	4	3	2	67.3	
Means	29.80	29.78	29.81	65.3	77.5	66.7	...	1.5	2.1	1.2	6.2	5.4	5.0	70.5	4.90
REDUCED TO SEA LEVEL.								1.6			5.5				
Max.	30.26	30.25	30.25	78	93	76	81.3								
Min.	29.65	29.67	29.73	57	64	57	60.0	Prevailing winds from some point between— Days.							
Mean	29.98	29.96	29.99								Days.				
Range	0.61	0.58	0.52	21	29	19	21.3	N. & E. 6			Clear 7				
								E. & S. 3			Variable . . . } 17				
Mean of month	29.977			...	...	...	69.8	S. & W. 14			Cloudy . . . . }				
Extreme range	0.61			...	...	...	36.0	W. & N. 8			Rain fell on . . 7				

REMARKS.

1st. Very cool for the season. Air extremely dry.
2d. Very fine.
3d. Rain in the morning. Thick fog in the evening.
4th. Pleasant.
5th and 6th. Very fine.
7th. Sun very hot at mid-day.
8th. Very warm.
9th and 10th. Very warm and sultry.
11th. Hottest day of the season. Heavy shower from 6 to 9 P. M., with some thunder.
12th. Very cool, with mist.
13th. Air very damp morning and evening.
14th. Very damp, with occasional light showers.
15th. Very damp and cloudy. A few stars visible in the evening.
16th. Pleasant.
17th. Warm; air very damp.
18th. Light showers in morning. Evening clear.
19th. Very fine.
20th. Pleasant.
21st. Very fine.
22d. Thundershower from 4 to 5 A. M.
23d. Fine. Shower during the night.
24th. Pleasant. Evening very cool.
25th. Cloudy for the most part, and very cool.
26th. Fine.
27th. Warm and damp.
28th. Pleasant; air very dry.
29th. Cloudy for the most part during the day. Lightning in the evening. Heavy rain during the night.
30th. Cloudy in the morning. Afternoon rainy. Starlight at 11 P. M.
31st. Fine.

August, 1858. New Moon, 8d. 11h. 46m. P. M.

Days.	Barometer, reduced to 32° F. At 6 A. M.	At 1 P. M.	At 10 P. M.	Thermometer. At 6 A. M.	At 1 P. M.	At 10 P. M.	Daily mean.	Winds. (Direction and Force.) At 6 A. M.	At 1 P. M.	At 10 P. M.	Weather. (Tenths Cloudy.) At 6 A. M.	At 1 P. M.	At 10 P. M.	Relative Humidity.	Rain and Snow in Inches of Water.
S 1	29.71	29.71	29.85	63	79	62	68.0	N. W. 1	N. W. 1	N. E. 1	3	2	0	63.7	0.25
2	29.86	29.90	30.00	60	70	61	63.7	N. E. 2	N. E. 2	N. E. 1	10	10	10	74.1	
3	29.98	29.96	29.97	61	67	60	62.7	N. E. 1	N. E. 2	E'ly 1	1	10	Rain	77.3	
4	29.89	29.80	...	60	68	...	...	E.byN. 1	S. E. 2	...	Rain	Rain	...	74.1	2.50
5	...	...	...	...	...	...	...	...	...	...	...	...	...	...	} 0.45
6	...	...	...	...	...	...	...	...	...	...	...	...	...	...	
7	...	...	29.90	...	...	63	...	...	...	N. E. 1	...	...	0	59.5	
S 8	29.89	29.92	29.96	63	75	62	67.7	N. E. 2	N. E. 2	N. E. 1	1	0	0	52.1	
9	29.91	29.88	29.86	59	72	61	64.0	N. E. 1	N. E. 2	N. E. 2	0	1	10	62.5	
10	29.78	29.73	29.73	61	66	65	64.0	N. E. 3	N. E. 3	N. E. 2	10	Misty	Misty	88.2	
11	29.69	29.71	29.78	65	68	65	66.0	N. E. 2	N. E. 2	N. E. 1	Misty	Rain	2	85.0	
12	29.79	29.84	29.98	65	71	65	67.0	N. E. 1	N. E. 2	Calm	Rain	10	1	84.1	1.45
13	30.03	30.12	30.04	63	72	68	66.0	N. E. 1	N. E. 1	N. E. 2	5	8	10	78.6	
14	30.04	30.03	29.89	62	75	64	67.0	N. E. 2	N. E. 2	N. E. 1	5	6	Rain	73.5	0.20
S 15	29.76	29.72	29.74	65	71	69	68.3	N. E. 1	N'ly 1	N'ly 1	10	10	10	84.7	
16	29.78	29.84	29.93	71	78	69	72.7	N'ly	N. W. 1	Calm	10	6	10	76.2	
17	29.95	29.92	29.89	65	79	73	72.3	Calm	S'ly 2	S'ly 1	Misty	5	10	80.2	0.20
18	29.76	29.63	29.59	72	80	78	76.7	S. W. 2	S. W. 2	S. W. 2	10	7	Shower	87.5	0.45
19	29.49	29.61	29.68	71	71	57	66.3	S. W. 1	N. W. 3	N. W. 1	9	3	2	63.8	
20	29.70	29.71	29.78	51	70	60	60.3	N. W. 2	N. W. 2	S. W. 1	0	5	3	60.1	
21	29.74	29.74	29.75	67	77	70	70.3	S. W. 1	S. W. 2	S. W. 1	2	6	3	70.9	
S 22	29.66	29.66	29.70	66	75	64	68.3	S. W. 1	W'ly 2	N. W. 2	8	10	0	62.0	
23	29.76	29.79	29.91	54	67	54	58.3	N. W. 1	N. W. 3	N. W. 1	0	0	0	50.3	
24	29.95	29.88	29.97	49	72	59	60.0	N. W. 1	S. W. 2	S. W. 1	0	0	0	54.6	
25	30.02	30.04	30.15	59	73	60	64.0	N. W. 1	S. W. 1	S. W. 1	0	3	0	62.5	
26	30.12	30.08	30.08	56	72	60	62.7	Calm	S. W. 2	S. E'ly 1	2	0	5	66.7	
27	29.98	...	...	55	...	...	...	S. W. 1	...	...	...	...	...	86.9	} 2.70
28	...	...	29.55	...	...	70	...	...	...	S'ly 1	...	...	Rain	89.8	
S 29	29.50	29.49	29.55	71	80	66	72.3	S'ly 1	S. W. 1	S. W. 1	10	2	0	73.6	
30	29.56	29.61	29.67	62	76	63	67.0	S. W. 1	S. W. 2	S. W.	3	2	0	70.9	
31	29.68	29.70	29.77	63	76	65	64.0	S. W. 1	S. W. 2	S. W. 1	8	3	0	81.3	
Means	29.81	29.81	29.84	62.2	73.1	64.0	...	1.2	1.9	1.1	5.7	5.3	4.7	72.2	8.20
								1.4			5.2				
Reduced to sea level.															
Max.	30.30	30.30	30.33	72	80	78	76.7								
Min.	29.67	29.67	29.73	49	66	54	58.3								
Mean	29.99	29.99	30.02												
Range	0.63	0.63	0.60	23	14	24	18.4								
Mean of month	30.000			...	...	...	66.4								
Extreme range	0.66			...	...	...	31.0								

Prevailing winds from some point between— Days.
N. & E. 12
E. & S. 1
S. & W. 11
W. & N. 5

Days.
Clear 8
Variable . . . } 7
Cloudy . . . . }
Rain fell on . . 13
(3 days omitted.)

REMARKS.

1st. Very fine in morning. Brisk shower from 5 to 8 P. M., with thunder, wind at the same time changing from W'ly to N. E., with a gust.
2d. Cloudy and cool.
3d. Cloudy, began to rain from 10 to 11 P. M.
4th. Rain nearly all day; very heavy from noon to 3 P. M.
5th. Light shower in the afternoon.
6th. Heavy shower in the afternoon.
7th. Cloudy in the morning. Pleasant in the afternoon. Evening clear.
8th. Fine.
9th. Very fine. Air remarkably clear till evening, when it became overcast.
10th. Occasional mist. Sun out for a short time from 3 to 4 P. M.
11th. Mist and occasional light rain during the day. Evening mostly clear.
12th. Heavy rain in the morning. Evening very still and clear.
13th. Pleasant. Overcast at 1 P. M.
14th. Cloudy. Showery in the evening and during the night.
15th. Cloudy. Rain in the night.
16th. Cloudy in the morning. Pleasant in the afternoon. Evening clear.
17th. Brisk shower from 8 to 10 A. M. Thunder at 5 P. M., but no rain.
18th. Clouds and sunshine. Air very damp. Brisk shower, with thunder, from 10 to 11 P. M.
19th. Pleasant.
20th. Pleasant. Air extremely dry in the morning.
21st. Pleasant.
22d. Pleasant. Evening cool and clear.
23d. Very clear and cold for the season.
24th. Very fine. Morning cold for the season.
25th and 26th. Very fine.
27th. Rain in the afternoon and evening.
28th. Heavy rain, with wind S. E. and S'ly.
29th. Cloudy in the morning. Warm and fine in the afternoon.
30th. Pleasant.
31st. Very fine.

September, 1858. New Moon, 7d. 9h. 7m. A. M.

Days.	Barometer At 6 A. M.	At 1 P. M.	At 10 P. M.	Thermometer At 6 A. M.	At 1 P. M.	At 10 P. M.	Daily mean.	Winds At 6 A. M.	At 1 P. M.	At 10 P. M.	Weather At 6 A. M.	At 1 P. M.	At 10 P. M.	Relative Humidity.	Rain and Snow in Inches of Water.
1	29.80	29.81	29.84	63	73	63	66.3	N. W. 1	N. W.	N. W. 1	0	...	0	67.2	
2	29.80	29.77	29.79	64	73	63	66.7	N. W. 1	S. W.	S. W. 1	5	7	0	83.4	
3	29.78	29.75	29.73	65	76	72	71.0	S. W. 1	S. W. 3	S. W. 2	2	3	10	72.4	
4	29.58	29.59	29.61	72	78	69	73.0	S. W. 1	S. W. 2	S. W. 1	10	10	Rain	85.4	0.80
S 5	29.66	29.68	29.74	65	78	68	70.3	W'ly 1	S. W. 2	S. W. 1	1	4	0	74.4	
6	29.80	29.88	29.98	63	75	65	67.7	N. W. 1	N. W.	N. W. 1	0	...	0	52.2	
7	30.01	30.03	30.04	60	77	65	67.3	N. W. 1	S. W. 1	S. W. 1	0	0	0	58.0	
8	30.00	29.93	29.94	62	82	66	70.0	S. W. 1	W by S. 2	N. W. 1	1	0	0	80.8	
9	29.91	29.86	29.89	66	85	68	73.0	S. W'ly 2	S. W'ly 2	S. W'ly 2	0	0	0	71.6	
10	29.86	29.80	29.77	68	83	69	73.3	S. W. 1	S. W. 2	S. W. 1	Foggy	2	0	80.3	
11	29.73	29.65	29.73	72	80	66	72.7	S. W. 2	S. W. 2	S. W'ly 1	10	10	Rain	80.6	0.25
S 12	29.70	29.69	29.84	60	76	59	65.0	W'ly 2	W'ly 2	N. W. 1	0	3	0	70.0	
13	29.92	29.97	30.08	52	69	58	59.9	N'ly 1	N. E. 1	W'ly 1	0	2	0	65.1	
14	30.12	30.11	30.10	51	66	58	58.3	N'ly 1	N. E. 2	N. E. 1	0	2	7	64.5	
15	30.02	29.91	29.78	56	67	63	62.0	N. E'ly 1	S. E'ly 2	E'ly 1	10	10	Rain	59.9	} 1.85
16	29.32	29.10	29.35	66	74	63	67.7	E. S. E. 5	S. E. 4	N. W. 2	Rain	Rain	0	87.3	
17	29.51	29.62	29.89	60	70	55	61.7	N. W. 1	N. W. 3	N. W. 1	5	2	0	55.9	
18	30.04	30.08	30.18	50	65	54	56.3	N. W. 1	N. W. 2	N. W. 1	0	0	4	71.1	
S 19	30.20	30.20	30.25	54	68	54	58.7	N. W. 1	N. E. 1	Calm	8	1	0	64.6	
20	30.20	30.08	29.96	52	76	64	64.0	S. W. 1	S. W. 2	S. W. 1	0	2	0	72.7	
21	29.82	29.73	29.66	62	81	66	69.7	S. W. 1	S. W. 2	N. W. 1	0	2	1	77.8	
22	29.68	29.65	29.83	54	61	45	53.3	N. W. 1	N'ly 3	N. W. 2	0	5	3	51.0	
23	29.94	29.92	29.93	39	55	45	46.6	N. W. 2	N. W. 1	N. W. 1	0	0	1	47.4	
24	29.87	29.78	29.90	46	55	50	50.3	W'ly 1	S. W. 1	N. W. 1	10	Rain	0	77.5	0.15
25	30.04	30.04	30.10	41	58	46	48.3	N. W. 1	N. W. 2	N. W. 1	0	0	0	56.6	
S 26	30.10	30.12	30.19	44	60	48	50.7	N. W. 1	N. E. 1	N. E. 1	0	3	0	60.7	
27	30.18	30.18	30.18	43	60	48	50.3	N. E. 2	N. E. 3	N. E. 2	0	0	0	57.4	
28	30.10	29.95	29.92	45	56	48	49.7	N. E. 2	N. E. 3	N. E. 1	1	0	0	59.0	
29	29.88	29.76	29.73	45	65	56	55.3	N. E. 2	S. W. 2	S. W. 1	0	0	3	56.4	
30	29.65	29.63	29.65	57	76	63	65.3	S. W. 2	S. W. 2	S. W. 1	0	2	10	70.1	
Means	29.87	29.84	29.89	56.6	70.6	59.3	...	1.4	1.8	1.1	2.8	3.2	2.3	67.4	3.05
								1.4			2.4				
Reduced to sea level.															
Max.	30.38	30.38	30.43	72	85	72	73.3								
Min.	29.50	29.29	29.53	39	55	45	48.3								
Mean	30.05	30.02	30.07												
Range	0.88	1.09	0.90	33	30	27	25.0								
Mean of month	30.047			...	...	...	62.2								
Extreme range	1.14			...	...	...	46.0								

Prevailing winds from some point between— Days.
N. & E. 6
E. & S. 2
S. & W. 14
W. & N. 8

Days.
Clear 16
Variable . . . } 9
Cloudy . . . . }
Rain fell on . . 5

REMARKS.

1st. Very fine.
2d. Fine. Evening very clear.
3d. Pleasant.
4th. Shower, with thunder, from 2 to 3 P. M., and again from 10 to 11 P. M.
5th and 6th. Very fine.
7th. Very fine. Aurora this evening.
8th. Very fine.
9th. Very hot sun at mid-day.
10th. Very hot sun at mid-day. Evening splendid.
11th. Began to rain from 2 to 3 P. M. Showers in the afternoon and evening.
12th and 13th. Very fine.
14th. Pleasant.
15th. Cloudy and cool. Began to rain very moderately at 10 P. M.
16th. At sunrise, the wind very heavy at about E. S. E., and raining. The wind was fitful, very heavy at intervals, hauling to S. E. At 5 P. M., barometer had fallen to 28.90, and the wind had lulled. Before 6 P. M., wind came to N. W., with blustering and heavy gusts, and the barometer rose very rapidly.
17th, 18th, and 19th. Very fine.
20th. Fine.
21st. Very warm at mid-day.
22d. Very cool in the evening.
23d. Fine. Evening splendid.
24th. Began to rain moderately at 10 A. M. Evening very clear.
25th. Very fine. Evening clear.
26th. Very fine. White frost in vicinity this morning.
27th, 28th, and 29th. Very fine.
30th. Very fine. Warm for the season.

Note.—The comet (Donati's, or the fifth comet of 1858) became distinctly visible to the naked eye early in the month, and before its close attained a brilliancy surpassing that of any comet for many years, with the exception of the great comet of 1843 for the single day of its passing its perihelion. We have no recollection of so brilliant a comet as that which now lights up the northwestern sky, immediately after the sunlight has disappeared.

October, 1858. New Moon, 6d. 9h. 0m. P. M.

DAYS.	BAROMETER, REDUCED TO 32° F. At 6 A. M.	At 1 P. M.	At 10 P. M.	THERMOMETER. At 6 A. M.	At 1 P. M.	At 10 P. M.	Daily mean.	WINDS. (DIRECTION AND FORCE.) At 6 A. M.	At 1 P. M.	At 10 P. M.	WEATHER. (TENTHS CLOUDY.) At 6 A. M.	At 1 P. M.	At 10 P. M.	RELATIVE HUMIDITY.	RAIN AND SNOW IN INCHES OF WATER.
1	29.53	29.36	29.42	64	68	55	62.3	S. W. 2	S. W. 2	N. W. 3	10	10	2	77.3	0.25
2	29.58	29.62	29.77	48	60	47	51.7	N. W. 2	N. W. 3	N. W. 2	0	0	0	53.2	
S 3	29.70	29.41	29.41	47	71	68	62.0	S. W. 1	S. W. 2	S. W. 3	3	10	10	70.2	
4	29.39	29.39	29.54	68	82	61	70.3	S. W. 2	S. W. 4	N. W. 1	5	1	0	58.8	
5	29.66	29.73	29.91	57	67	53	59.0	N. W. 1	N. W. 2	N. W. 1	9	0	0	60.8	
6	29.92	29.87	29.86	47	63	48	52.7	N. W. 1	N. W. 1	N. W. 1	0	0	0	51.6	
7	29.63	29.37	29.30	41	58	61	53.3	N. W. 1	S. W. 2	S. W. 1	3	Rain	2	86.5	0.15
8	29.41	29.40	29.46	45	54	43	47.3	W'ly	N. W. 3	S. W'ly 1	0	2	5	41.4	
9	29.43	29.42	29.65	41	56	46	47.7	S. W. 2	S. W. 3	N. W. 2	0	5	0	55.0	
S 10	29.77	29.86	30.01	44	60	46	50.0	N'ly 2	N. W. 2	N. W. 1	0	0	0	53.5	
11	29.99	29.99	30.02	44	57	46	49.0	N. W. 1	N. W. 2	N. W. 1	9	8	0	55.3	
12	30.06	30.08	30.10	42	55	47	48.0	N'ly 1	N. E'ly 2	N. E. 2	8	10	0	65.2	
13	30.02	29.87	29.71	56	57	61	58.0	N. E. 1	N. E. 1	E'ly 1	10	Rain	Rain	91.1	1.25
14	29.66	29.65	29.75	56	68	51	58.3	N. W. 1	S. W. 2	S. W. 1	8	0	0	60.8	
15	29.88	29.80	30.11	50	60	46	52.0	N. W. 1	N. W. 3	N. W. 1	Shower	5	0	53.5	
16	30.26	30.27	30.32	42	62	52	52.0	N. W. 1	N. W. 1	N. W. 1	0	2	10	59.8	
S 17	30.40	30.37	30.34	51	63	55	56.3	S. W'ly 1	S. W. 1	S. W. 1	9	5	5	74.8	
18	30.31	30.23	30.20	54	70	55	59.7	S. W. 2	S. W. 2	S. W. 1	3	2	1	70.7	
19	30.11	30.06	30.04	53	76	57	62.0	S. W. 1	S. W. 1	S. W. 1	1	2	0	62.2	
20	29.99	29.94	29.99	51	72	65	59.3	S. W. 1	S. W. 1	S. W. 1	1	0	0	70.5	
21	30.13	30.14	30.16	52	56	50	52.7	N'ly 1	N. E. 3	N. E. 2	1	2	10	70.5	
22	30.08	30.02	30.05	53	62	57	57.3	N. E. 1	E'ly 1	E'ly 1	10	10	10	71.8	
23	29.89	29.74	29.77	56	64	55	58.3	N'ly 1	N. E. 1	N. E. 2	Foggy	9	Foggy	80.5	
S 24	29.72	29.71	29.83	53	53	45	50.3	N. E. 3	N. E. 4	N. E. 3	Rain	10	10	78.7	
25	29.95	29.97	30.04	36	45	39	40.0	N. E. 3	N. E'ly 3	N. E. 2	8	2	0	39.2	
26	30.08	30.04	30.01	33	50	43	42.0	N. E'ly 2	N.N.E. 2	N'ly 2	0	0	0	20.0	
27	29.98	29.97	30.00	41	60	50	50.3	N. W. 2	N. W. 2	N. W. 1	2	3	0	30.8	
28	30.07	30.04	30.20	41	67	44	50.7	N. W. 1	N. W. 1	S. W. 1	0	0	1	40.4	
29	30.25	30.21	30.12	39	55	51	48.3	N. E. 1	S. E. 2	S'ly	2	10	Rain	61.3	
30	29.93	29.81	29.76	56	59	61	58.7	S'ly 2	S. W. 2	S. W. 1	10	Rain	Rain	93.6	1.15
S 31	29.72	29.69	29.91	59	68	52	59.7	Calm	S. W. 2	N. W. 1	Foggy	3	1	71.1	
Means	29.89	29.84	29.90	49.0	61.9	51.6	...	1.3	2.0	1.4	4.9	4.6	3.5	62.9	2.80
									1.6			4.3			
REDUCED TO SEA LEVEL.															
Max.	30.58	30.55	30.52	68	82	68	70.3	Prevailing winds from some point between—		Days.					
Min.	29.57	29.54	29.48	33	45	39	40.0						Days.		
Mean	30.07	30.02	30.08												
Range	1.01	1.01	1.04	35	37	29	30.3	N. & E.		8	Clear		10		
								E. & S.		1	Variable		13 (Variable and Cloudy)		
Mean of month	30.057			...	...	...	54.2	S. & W.		12	Cloudy				
Extreme range	1.10			...	...	...	49.0	W. & N.		10	Rain fell on		8		

REMARKS.

1st. Shower, with thunder, at 5 P. M. Evening clear.
2d. Very fine. Evening clear, and the comet very brilliant.
3d. Warm for the season. Appearances of storm in the evening.
4th. Pleasant. Warm for the season.
5th. Pleasant. Evening very clear. The comet splendid, being about 50′ or 55′ south of Arcturus.
6th. Very fine. Comet again very bright, and about 5° south of Arcturus.
7th. Heavy clouds in the morning. Began to rain moderately at 1 P. M. Mostly clear at 10 P. M.
8th. Very fine.
9th. Fine
10th. Very fine.
11th. Pleasant.
12th. Cloudy through the day. Evening clear.
13th. Began to rain at 10 A. M. Rained heavily at intervals during the day and evening.
14th. Pleasant and warm.
15th. Light shower at 6 A. M. Day blustering. Evening clear.
16th. Pleasant. Sprinkling of rain at 9 P. M.
17th. Pleasant.
18th. Fine.
19th. Fine; very warm for the season.
20th. Very fine.
21st. Cloudy in afternoon and evening.
22d. Mild; cloudy all day.
23d. Mild and cloudy.
24th. Occasional light rain; wind heavy.
25th. Cool, but pleasant.
26th. Light frost this morning—the first of the season on College Hill. Ice formed in shallow vessels of the thickness of window glass.
27th. Brilliant aurora this evening, with streamers which at times were strongly tinged with red and pink light.
28th. Very fine.
29th. Cloudy in the afternoon. Sprinkling of rain in the evening.
30th. Moderate rain.
31st. Pleasant in the afternoon. Aurora in the evening, streamers white, with an occasional greenish hue.

November, 1858. New Moon, 5d. 11h. 41m. A. M.

DAYS.	BAROMETER Sunrise.	At 1 P. M.	At 10 P. M.	THERMOMETER Sunrise.	At 1 P. M.	At 10 P. M.	Daily mean.	WINDS Sunrise.	At 1 P. M.	At 10 P. M.	WEATHER Sunrise.	At 1 P. M.	At 10 P. M.	RELATIVE HUMIDITY.	RAIN AND SNOW IN INCHES OF WATER.
1	29.98	30.01	30.11	48	63	50	53.7	N. W. 2	N. W. 2	N. E. 1	0	0	1	50.8	
2	30.17	30.14	30.16	45	47	44	45.3	N. E. 2	N. E. 2	N. E. 2	10	Misty	10	66.5	
3	30.12	30.11	30.07	47	48	46	47.0	N. E. 2	E'ly 3	N. E. 2	10	10	10	57.5	
4	29.96	29.80	29.77	46	49	50	48.3	N. E. 3	N. E. 3	N. E. 2	Rain	10	Rain	67.2	
5	29.79	29.78	29.81	44	50	48	47.3	N. W. 2	N. W. 1	N. E. 1	10	10	10	77.4	
6	29.67	29.57	29.43	46	49	48	47.7	N. E. 2	N. E. 3	N. E. 2	Rain	Rain	Rain	80.9	1.40
S 7	29.42	29.51	29.60	41	49	45	45.0	N. W. 2	N. W. 3	N. W. 2	Rain	3	0	68.4	
8	29.59	29.54	29.60	42	45	41	42.7	S. W. 2	S. W. 2	W'ly 1	3	2	0	83.2	
9	29.61	29.61	29.61	39	46	38	41.0	S. W'ly 1	N. E. 2	N. E. 2	9	10	2	62.4	
10	29.64	29.73	29.84	35	48	37	40.0	N. W. 1	N. W. 2	N. W. 1	1	2	0	53.3	
11	29.94	29.91	29.92	30	41	28	33.0	N. W. 1	N. W. 2	N. W. 1	1	2	0	40.6	
12	29.86	29.80	29.86	24	32	25	27.0	N. W. 1	N. W. 2	N. W. 1	1	8	0	39.2	
13	29.84	29.63	29.51	25	37	36	82.7	N. W. 1	N. E. 1	N. E. 1	10	10	Rain	66.1	
S 14	29.60	29.73	29.89	28	33	28	29.7	N. W. 3	N. W. 3	N. E. 2	1	0	0	38.5	
15	29.85	29.63	29.61	23	35	28	28.7	N. W. 1	S. W. 2	N. W. 1	3	Snow	0	65.7	
16	29.55	29.46	29.48	21	36	32	29.7	N. W. 2	N. W. 3	N. W. 2	1	7	5	51.8	
17	29.50	29.58	29.66	32	41	34	35.7	N. W. 3	N. W. 4	N. W. 2	0	0	0	43.1	
18	29.69	29.62	29.62	35	45	36	38.7	S. W. 1	W by N. 2	N. W. 1	10	2	0	40.0	
19	29.66	29.58	29.71	38	42	31	37.0	S. W. 2	N. W. 3	N. W. 2	6	3	0	39.0	
20	29.69	29.68	29.72	25	45	34	34.7	S. W. 2	N. W. 2	N. W. 1	0	0	2	53.8	
S 21	29.70	29.59	29.59	31	40	35	35.3	W'ly 1	S. W. 1	S. W. 1	9	10	Snow	67.1	
22	29.76	29.81	29.82	33	43	34	36.7	N. W. 1	N. W. 1	S. W. 1	0	2	3	59.9	
23	29.44	29.22	29.34	39	42	34	38.3	N. E. 3	N. E. 4	N'ly 2	Rain	Rain	Misty	85.0	1.25
24	29.89	29.85	...	34	38	...	...	N. W. 1	N'ly 2	...	10	10	...	61.0	
25	29.44	29.47	29.53	33	32	29	31.3	N. W. 2	N. W. 2	N. W. 2	0	5	0	86.3	
26	29.63	29.63	29.77	33	36	32	33.7	N. W. 2	N'ly 2	N'ly 2	0	10	10	70.9	
27	29.89	29.87	29.85	32	35	31	32.7	N. W. 1	N. W. 1	N. W. 1	10	5	10	33.6	
S 28	29.73	29.59	29.42	31	31	31	31.0	N. E'ly 1	N. E'ly 1	N. E. 2	10	Snow	Snow	75.7	0.75
29	29.46	29.56	29.70	27	30	21	26.0	N'ly 2	N. W. 1	N. W. 1	10	2	2	59.7	
30	29.58	29.52	29.75	23	42	28	31.0	S. W. 1	S. W. 2	W'ly 3	10	2	0	55.1	
Means	29.72	29.68	29.72	34.3	41.7	35.7	...	1.7	2.1	1.5	5.8	5.8	4.2	60.0	2.40
									1.8			5.3			
REDUCED TO SEA LEVEL.															
Max.	30.35	30.32	30.31	48	63	50	53.7	Prevailing winds from some point between—		Days.					
Min.	29.60	29.40	29.52	21	30	21	26.0						Days.		
Mean	29.90	29.86	29.90												
Range	0.75	0.92	0.82	27	33	29	27.7	N. & E.		8	Clear		9		
								E. & S.		0	Variable		10 (Variable and Cloudy)		
Mean of month	29.887			...	...	...	37.2	S. & W.		4	Cloudy				
Extreme range	0.95			...	...	...	42.0	W. & N.		18	Rain or snow fell on		11		

REMARKS.

1st. Very fine.
2d. Cloudy, with mist and occasional fine rain in the morning.
3d. Raw and cold.
4th. Moderate rain at intervals.
5th. Cloudy and mild. Wind light at N. W'ly nearly all day.
6th. Light rain all day; more copious in the evening.
7th. Shower in the morning; pleasant in the afternoon and evening.
8th. Very fine. Evening clear.
9th. Cool, and mostly cloudy.
10th. Very fine.
11th. Air raw and snowy. Heavy black frost this morning; the first of the season to injure dahlias and other hardy plants.
12th. Cold and raw.
13th. Air raw and cold. Began to rain from 8 to 9 P. M.
14th. Ground white with snow this morning: weather wintry.
15th. Fine snow in the air nearly all day. Mostly clear at 10 P. M.
16th. Blustering and cold.
17th. Fine, but cold.
18th. Cloudy in the morning. Fine in the afternoon and evening.
19th. Pleasant. Evening very clear.
20th. Pleasant.
21st. Began to snow very gently from 7 to 8 P. M.
22d. Very fine.
23d. Raw all day, with wind heavy at N. E'ly.
24th. Raw and damp.
25th. Clear and cold.
26th. Cloudy and cold.
27th. Cloudy, with appearances of storm in the evening.
28th. Began to snow very gently from 10 to 11 A. M., and continued through the afternoon and evening
29th. Between five and six inches of damp snow on the ground this morning.
30th. Dusting of snow from 8 to 9 A. M. Pleasant in the afternoon and evening.

December, 1858. New Moon, 5d. 5h. 2m. A. M.

DAYS.	BAROMETER, REDUCED TO 32° F. Sunrise.	At 1 P. M.	At 10 P. M.	THERMOMETER. Sunrise.	At 1 P. M.	At 10 P. M.	Daily mean.	WINDS. (DIRECTION AND FORCE.) Sunrise.	At 1 P. M.	At 10 P. M.	WEATHER. (TENTHS CLOUDY.) Sunrise.	At 1 P. M.	At 10 P. M.	RELATIVE HUMIDITY.	RAIN AND SNOW IN INCHES OF WATER.
1	30.07	30.23	30.31	18	24	18	20.0	N. W. 1	N. W. 2	N. W. 1	0	0	2	30.9	
2	30.22	30.04	29.97	21	34	39	31.3	W'ly 1	S. W. 2	S. W. 1	10	Rain	10	79.0	0.10
3	29.91	29.82	29.84	33	49	38	40.0	S. W. 1	S. W. 1	S. W. 1	2	7	0	62.9	
4	30.06	30.01	29.96	33	30	34	33.3	N. E. 1	N. E. 2	N. E. 2	10	Hail	Rain	79.6	0.30
S 5	29.94	29.76	29.64	31	37	35	34.3	N. E. 2	N. E. 1	N. E. 1	Misty	Rain	Misty	79.3	
6	29.83	29.89	30.09	37	48	33	40.3	S. W. 1	N. W. 1	N. W. 1	0	0	0	46.7	
7	30.12	30.04	29.82	29	40	39	36.0	N. E. 2	N. E. 1	E'ly 1	5	10	Rain	68.9	
8	29.67	29.64	29.78	38	44	33	38.3	N'ly 1	N. W. 2	N. W. 1	Rain	Rain	0	70.5	0.45
9	29.95	30.01	30.19	25	27	21	24.3	N. W. 2	N. W. 4	N. W. 1	0	0	0	74.9	
10	30.25	30.21	30.05	17	29	27	24.3	N. W. 1	N. W. 2	S. W. 2	0	2	3	57.2	
11	29.98	29.93	30.03	27	40	34	33.7	S. W. 1	S. W. 2	W'ly 1	5	10	0	46.2	
S 12	29.95	30.29	30.39	22	31	25	26.0	N. W. 1	N. W. 2	N. E. 2	2	0	10	36.0	
13	30.33	30.03	29.84	31	39	39	36.3	E'ly 1	S. E. 2	S. E'ly 2	10	Misty	Rain	78.0	} 0.35
14	29.80	29.69	29.49	38	47	56	47.0	S'ly 1	S. W'ly 1	S. W. 2	Foggy	10	Foggy	84.7	
15	29.43	29.45	29.59	57	58	50	55.0	S. W. 1	S. W. 3	S. W. 1	Misty	10	10	79.3	
16	29.88	29.90	29.94	35	42	32	36.3	N. W. 1	N. W. 1	N. W. 1	0	0	0	41.4	
17	29.89	29.90	30.04	28	43	28	33.0	N. W. 1	N. W. 1	N. W. 2	0	10	5	51.0	
18	30.08	30.12	30.27	16	19	14	16.3	N. W. 2	N. W. 2	N. W. 2	10	10	5	46.8	
S 19	30.27	30.19	29.97	14	25	29	22.7	N. W. 1	E'ly 2	S. E'ly 1	10	7	8	61.8	
20	29.74	29.76	29.80	37	44	35	38.7	W'ly 2	N. W. 2	N. W. 1	10	0	10	66.3	
21	29.67	29.42	29.03	35	39	41	38.3	E'ly 2	N. E. 2	N. E. 1	Misty	Rain	Rain	84.4	1.00
22	29.04	29.37	29.69	35	39	29	34.3	N. W. 1	N. W. 4	N. W. 3	10	3	0	56.5	
23	29.74	29.68	29.65	28	38	33	33.0	N. W. 1	S. W. 2	S. W. 1	0	10	Snow	60.6	
24	29.77	29.93	30.16	26	28	16	23.3	N. W. 1	N. W. 2	N. W. 1	10	3	0	30.7	
25	30.38	30.40	30.45	12	27	15	18.0	N. W. 1	N. W. 1	N. W. 1	0	0	0	37.1	
S 26	30.32	30.19	30.03	16	35	34	28.3	S. W. 1	S. W. 1	S. W. 1	0	8	10	73.7	
27	29.75	29.63	29.70	37	44	37	39.3	S. W. 1	N. W. 2	N. W. 2	10	2	0	55.0	
28	29.71	29.68	29.80	31	35	25	30.3	N. W. 2	N. W. 3	N. W. 3	0	0	0	33.7	
29	29.85	29.83	29.95	20	33	27	26.7	N. W. 1	N. W. 1	N. E. 1	0	3	10	24.4	
30	30.04	30.16	30.20	20	23	19	20.7	N. E. 2	N. E. 3	N. E. 2	10	Snow	10	60.9	
31	30.09	29.82	29.58	31	37	42	36.7	E'ly 1	S. E. 2	S. E. 1	Snow	Rain	Rain	80.6	1.25
Means	29.93	29.90	29.91	28.3	36.4	31.5	...	1.2	1.9	1.4	5.6	6.0	5.6	59.3	3.45
									1.5			5.7			
REDUCED TO SEA LEVEL.															
Max.	30.56	30.58	30.63	57	58	56	55.0	Prevailing winds from some point between—		Days.			Days.		
Min.	29.22	29.55	29.21	12	19	14	16.3	N. & E.		5	Clear		7		
Mean	30.11	30.08	30.09					E. & S.		3	Variable		} 10		
Range	1.34	1.03	1.42	45	39	42	38.7	S. & W.		7	Cloudy				
Mean of month	30.093			...	...	...	32.1	W. & N.		16	Rain or snow fell on 14				
Extreme range	1.42			...	...	...	46.0								

REMARKS.

1st. Clear and cold.
2d. Began to rain very moderately from 1 to 2 P. M.
3d. Pleasant.
4th. Fine hail began to fall from noon to 1 P. M., which turned to rain before night. light rain in the evening.
5th. Mist and light rain all day.
6th. Very fine.
7th. Cloudy. Sprinkling of rain in the evening.
8th. Light rain in the morning. Evening clear.
9th. Cold and blustering. Evening still and very clear.
10th. Very fine.
11th. Pleasant.
12th. Air raw in the afternoon.
13th. Mist in the morning. Light rain in the evening.
14th. Mist and occasional light rain.
15th. Mist and occasional light rain. In the evening, clouds broken.
16th and 17th. Very fine.
18th. Very cold, with scattering snow-flakes in the air.
19th. Morning cold. Milder in the afternoon; wind light E'ly.
20th. The ground white with snow in the morning; air mild and pleasant.
21st. Light rain in the morning, which increased during the afternoon and evening.
22d. Very blustering.
23d. Pleasant in the morning. Cloudy in the afternoon. Sprinkling of snow in the evening.
24th. Ground covered with snow, nearly two inches deep, this morning. Evening cold.
25th. Fine. Evening very clear.
26th and 27th. Pleasant.
28th. Fine.
29th. Pleasant.
30th. Cold and raw. Air full of snow all day.
31st. Snow in the morning, which soon turned to rain, and continued through the day.

January, 1859. New Moon, 4d. 0h. 18m. A. M.

DAYS.	BAROMETER Sunrise.	At 1 P. M.	At 10 P. M.	THERMOMETER Sunrise.	At 1 P. M.	At 10 P. M.	Daily mean.	WINDS Sunrise.	At 1 P. M.	At 10 P. M.	WEATHER Sunrise.	At 1 P. M.	At 10 P. M.	RELATIVE HUMIDITY.	RAIN AND SNOW.
1	29.59	29.52	29.74	39	41	35	38.3	N. W. 1	N. W. 1	N. W. 2	Rain	7	0	76.2	
S 2	30.12	30.12	30.26	29	35	25	29.7	N. W. 1	N. W. 2	N. E. 1	0	0	0	28.5	
3	30.27	30.18	30.07	22	31	25	26.0	N. E. 1	N. E. 2	N.E. 3	10	10	10	55.3	
4	29.74	29.35	29.59	23	23	29	25.0	N. E. 4	N. E. 4	N. W. 2	Snow	Snow	0	66.1	1.50
5	29.84	29.86	29.95	28	39	33	33.3	N. W. 1	S. W. 2	S. W. 2	0	0	3	54.8	
6	30.03	30.02	29.97	28	41	36	35.0	S. W. 1	S. W. 2	S. W. 1	1	0	10	63.3	
7	29.65	29.40	29.09	41	45	49	45.0	S. W. 1	S. W. 1	S. W. 3	Rain	Rain	10	84.0	0.50
8	29.46	29.68	29.84	24	24	14	20.7	W'ly 3	W.byN 3	N. W. 1	0	0	0	36.1	
S 9	29.94	29.92	30.04	10	19	12	13.7	N. W. 1	N. W. 1	N. W. 1	2	1	0	32.2	
10	30.11	30.21	30.29	—2	—1	—9	—4.0	N. W. 2	N. W. 2	N. W. 2	10	10	0	...	
11	30.34	30.08	29.90	-11	4	—1	—2.7	N. W. 1	N. W. 1	N. E. 1	3	10	5	46.7	
12	29.96	29.94	29.95	—1	13	14	8.7	N. W. 2	N. E'ly 1	N. E. 1	10	Snow	10	65.5	} 0,55
13	29.86	29.79	29.87	15	27	27	23.0	N. W. 1	N. E'ly 1	N. E'ly 1	10	7	6	77.7	
14	29.84	29.73	29.51	30	37	36	34.3	N. E. 1	N. E. 1	N. E. 1	10	Rain	Rain	86.5	
15	29.39	29.25	29.31	35	36	35	35.3	N. E. 1	N. E. 1	W'ly 1	10	Misty	1	83.7	
S 16	29.51	...	29.89	34	37	31	34.0	N. W. 2	N. W. 3	N. W. 1	7	2	0	55.2	
17	29.80	29.78	29.81	35	42	37	38.0	S. W. 1	S. W. 1	S. W. 1	10	10	10	65.5	
18	30.12	30.19	30.15	19	25	24	22.7	N. W. 2	N. W. 2	N. W. 1	5	0	7	39.2	0.10
19	30.12	30.11	30.16	28	36	27	30.3	S. W. 1	S. W.	W'ly 1	8	0	0	53.1	
20	30.16	30.04	29.98	27	47	46	40.0	S'ly 1	S. W. 1	S. W. 2	Foggy	0	2	69.1	
21	29.80	29.67	...	51	54	...	...	S'ly 2	S. W'ly 3	...	Misty	Rain	...	79.6	
22	...	29.79	29.95	...	39	30	...	...	S. W'ly 1	N. W. 2	...	10	5	89.6	
S 23	30.24	30.22	30.36	16	20	16	18.7	N. W. 1	N. W. 2	N'ly 1	0	0	0	42.7	
24	30.51	...	30.43	16	...	23	...	N. W. 1	...	N'ly 1	0	...	0	54.8	
25	30.34	30.25	30.14	30	39	32	33.7	S. W. 1	S'ly 1	S. W'ly 1	0	1	2	55.2	
26	...	30.03	30.20	...	42	32	...	...	N. W. 2	N. W. 1	...	0	0	71.2	
27	30.29	30.21	30.19	24	45	35	34.7	S. W. 1	S. 1	E. 2	1	2	10	52.8	
28	29.95	29.76	29.88	37	38	32	35.7	S. E. 1	N. 3	N. E. 2	Rain	Rain	10	82.9	
29	29.86	29.72	29.78	33	34	34	33.7	N. E. 2	N. E. [illegible]	N. 1	Misty	Misty	Misty	[illegible]	[illegible]
S 30	[illegible]	[illegible]	[illegible]	[illegible]	[illegible]	[illegible]	[illegible]	[illegible]	[illegible]	[illegible] 2	0	2	0	53.2	
31	30.13	30.10	...	22	31	...	...	N. W. 1	N. W. 2	N. W. 2	2	2	1	46.4	
Means	29.90	29.89	29.94	28.0	32.6	27.2	...	1.4	1.7	1.5	5.7	4.9	4.0	59.7	5.75
									1.6			4.9			
REDUCED TO SEA LEVEL.															
Max.	30.69	30.43	30.61	51	54	49	45.0	Prevailing winds from some point between—		Days.			Days.		
Min.	29.57	29.43	29.27	—11	—1	—9	4.0	N. & E.		8	Clear		10		
Mean	30.14	30.07	30.12					E. & S.		0	Variable		} 11		
Range	1.12	1.00	1.34	62	55	58	49.0	S. & W.		10	Cloudy				
Mean of month	30.110			...	...	...	33.1	W. & N.		13	Rain or snow fell on 10				
Extreme range	1.42			...	...	...	65.0								

1st. Clear and cold.
2d. Began to rain gently from 1 to 2 P. M.
3d. Pleasant.
4th. Very severe snow-storm this morning, wind blowing heavily from N. E. The storm continued till about 3 P. M., when the barometer began to rise. Clear at 7 P. M.; wind N. E. Snow from twelve to fifteen inches deep, much drifted.
5th. Very fine.
6th. Mild and pleasant.
7th. Moderate rain and fog all day. At 10 P. M., blustering and warm; rain ceased.
8th. Flurry of snow last night. Air cold
9th. Cold.
10th. Extremely cold. At 10 P. M., 19° colder than any previous night this winter
11th. Excessively cold this morning; 11° below zero by the Smithsonian thermometer, and 14° below by a standard thermometer which I have used for about fifteen years. The coldest morning since Jan. 23 1857, when the standard thermometer, in the same place, stood at the same point— 14° below zero. We have no record in this place of a greater degree of cold than this Snow began to fall at 1 P. M. Mostly clear at 10 P. M.
12th. Two inches of light snow on the ground this morning. Dusting of snow in the afternoon. Weather much moderated
13th. Mild and pleasant.
14th. Began to sprinkle from 12 to 1 P. M rain continued in afternoon and evening.
15th. Fog and mist. Evening mostly clear and mild.
16th. Very fine.
17th. Mild and mostly cloudy.
[illegible] two inches of fresh snow last night.
19th. Fine. Evening splendid.
20th. Very fine.
21st. Cloudy in the morning. Rain in the afternoon and evening.
22d. Cloudy through day. Evening clear
23d and 24th. Clear and cold.
25th and 26th. Pleasant and mild.
27th. Pleasant Cloudy in the evening.
28th. Dusting of snow last night, followed by rain, which continued heavily till 3 P. M.
29th. Misty and drizzling. The ground covered with wet ice, and very slippery.
30th and 31st. Pleasant.

February, 1859. New Moon, 2d. 7h. 56m. P. M.

Days.	Barometer, reduced to 32° F. Sunrise.	At 1 P. M.	At 10 P. M.	Thermometer. Sunrise.	At 1 P. M.	At 10 P. M.	Daily mean.	Winds (Direction and Force.) Sunrise.	At 1 P. M.	At 10 P. M.	Weather (Tenths Cloudy.) Sunrise.	At 1 P. M.	At 10 P. M.	Relative Humidity.	Rain and Snow in Inches of Water.
1	30.04	30.09	...	22	37	...	...	W. 1	N. W. 2	N. W. 2	4	3	...	61.7	
2	29.90	29.81	29.78	28	34	30	30.7	N'ly 1	N. E'ly 2	N. E. 2	6	10	Snow	78.7	
3	29.63	29.50	29.27	34	27	22	27.7	N. E. 3	N. E'ly 3	N. E'ly 2	Misty	Hail	10	76.5	0.15
4	29.50	29.62	29.72	29	38	34	33.7	W'ly 2	W. 3	E'ly 1	0	0	Snow	65.1	
5	30.00	30.06	30.18	29	34	21	28.0	N. W. 1	W'ly 1	N. W. 1	0	0	0	65.5	
S 6	30.16	29.93	29.78	25	38	31	31.3	N. W. 1	E'ly 1	N. E. 1	8	10	Snow	68.8	0.40
7	29.95	30.02	...	29	32	...	...	N. W. 1	N. E. 1	...	6	10	...	78.5	
8	30.20	30.08	30.00	24	34	32	30.0	S. E'ly 1	E'ly 1	S'ly 1	10	10	10	...	
9	29.67	29.40	29.13	36	38	38	37.3	N'ly 1	N. E. 1	N. E. 3	Foggy	Rain	Rain	60.6	
10	29.32	29.61	29.93	34	26	15	25.0	N'ly 3	N'ly 2	N. W. 1	10	0	3	74.6	
11	30.17	30.18	...	15	21	...	...	N. W. 1	W'ly 1	...	6	3	...	27.1	
12	30.02	29.96	29.95	22	24	23	23.0	N. E. 1	N. E. 1	N'ly 1	10	10	10	59.8	
S 13	30.00	29.98	29.95	14	23	16	17.7	N. W. 1	N. W. 1	N. W. 1	0	0	0	34.6	
14	29.86	29.87	29.91	20	33	23	25.3	N. W. 2	W'ly 1	S. W'ly	6	0	6	61.8	
15	29.86	29.74	29.65	33	42	39	38.0	S'ly 1	S. W'ly 2	S'ly 1	10	10	10	71.9	
16	29.60	29.63	29.88	38	45	37	40.0	S. W. 1	S. W'ly 1	W'ly 1	Foggy	6	0	71.8	
17	30.12	30.14	30.23	33	44	36	37.7	N. W. 1	S'ly 1	S'ly 1	0	10	10	45.0	
18	30.04	29.90	29.87	33	34	34	33.7	S'ly 2	S'ly 1	N. W'ly 1	Snow	Rain	10	39.4	0.20
19	29.89	30.00	29.81	34	35	36	35.0	S'ly 1	S. E'ly 1	S'ly 1	Foggy	10	Rain	88.4	0.10
S 20	29.41	29.17	29.18	43	47	44	44.7	W'ly 1	S. W'ly 1	W'ly 1	10	Foggy	2	76.6	0.25
21	29.31	29.36	29.63	33	36	27	32.0	W'ly 4	N. W. 4	N. W. 3	3	3	0	38.1	
22	29.77	29.79	29.85	28	42	36	35.3	W. by N.	N. W. 2	W'ly 1	0	0	10	19.9	
23	29.78	29.69	29.69	36	51	37	41.3	S'ly 1	S. W. 1	S'ly 1	8	2	1	53.0	
24	29.54	29.50	29.91	36	41	27	34.7	N. E'ly 2	N. W. 2	N. W. 3	Foggy	7	0	70.2	0.10
25	30.03	30.04	30.06	20	28	23	23.7	N. W. 2	N. E. 1	N. E. 2	7	10	10	46.1	
26	29.96	29.75	29.71	28	29	18	25.0	N. E. 2	N. E. 3	N. W. 2	10	Snow	0	67.4	0.65
S 27	29.84	29.80	29.68	20	43	40	34.3	S. W'ly 1	S'ly 1	S. W. 2	0	0	2	56.5	
28	29.35	29.54	29.74	40	45	34	39.7	W'ly 2	N. W. 3	N. W. 2	10	0	0	41.5	
Means	29.82	29.79	29.78	29.1	35.7	30.1	...	1.5	1.6	1.5	6.6	5.9	5.8	59.2	1.85
									1.5			6.1			
Reduced to sea level.															
Max.	30.38	30.36	30.41	43	51	44	44.7								
Min.	29.49	29.35	29.31	14	21	15	17.7								
Mean	30.00	29.97	29.96												
Range	0.89	1.01	1.10	29	30	29	27.0								
Mean of month	29.977			...	...	...	24.5								
Extreme range	1.10			...	...	...	37.0								

Prevailing winds from some point between— Days.
N. & E. 9
E. & S. 0
S. & W. 9
W. & N. 10

Days.
Clear 6
Variable . . . .} 12
Cloudy . . . . .}
Rain or snow fell on 10

Remarks.

1st. Pleasant.
2d. Cloudy, with a raw wind.
3d. Rain in the morning. Cloudy in the afternoon.
4th. Clear and pleasant. Cloudy in the evening.
5th. Very pleasant.
6th. Cloudy. Snow in the evening.
7th. Pleasant.
8th. Cloudy and mild.
9th. Fog and moderate rain.
10th. Clear and pleasant.
11th. Pleasant.
12th. Cloudy, with snow at intervals.
13th. Very fine.
14th. Pleasant.
15th. Cloudy. Light rain in afternoon.
16th. Cloudy in the morning. Pleasant in the afternoon.
17th. Mild and pleasant.
18th. Light snow and rain in the morning. Clouds broken in the evening.
19th. Mist in the afternoon. Light rain in the evening.
20th. Clouds and fog in morning. Light rain in afternoon. Evening mostly clear.
21st. Extremely blustering all day.
22d. Very fine. Aurora at 8 P. M. Overcast at 10 P. M.
23d. Pleasant and very mild.
24th. Light rain with snow in the morning. Evening clear and blustering.
25th. Raw and cold.
26th. Snow began to fall from 9 to 10 A. M., and continued till night. Mostly clear at 10 P. M. From four to five inches of snow.
27th. Very fine.
28th. Fine.

March, 1859. New Moon, 4d. 2h. 2m. P. M.

Days.	Barometer Sunrise.	At 1 P. M.	At 10 P. M.	Thermometer Sunrise.	At 1 P. M.	At 10 P. M.	Daily mean.	Winds Sunrise.	At 1 P. M.	At 10 P. M.	Weather Sunrise.	At 1 P. M.	At 10 P. M.	Relative Humidity.	Rain and Snow in Inches of Water.
1	29.84	29.93	30.07	27	25	18	23.3	N. W. 1	N. W. 3	N. W. 2	0	1	0	43.7	
2	30.28	30.24	30.30	13	25	19	19.0	N. W. 2	N. W. 2	N. W. 1	0	0	0	54.1	
3	30.24	30.11	29.80	13	33	30	25.3	N'ly 1	S. W. 2	E'ly 2	2	10	Snow	50.5	
4	29.29	29.15	29.30	39	42	35	38.7	S. E. 2	N. W. 1	N. W. 1	Rain	10	3	77.9	1.20
5	29.25	29.33	29.61	39	46	38	41.0	S. W. 1	N. W. 3	N. W. 1	10	8	3	51.3	
S 6	29.74	29.82	29.98	38	49	37	41.3	N. W. 1	N. W. 2	N. W. 1	0	0	0	52.4	
7	29.98	29.85	29.68	31	47	39	39.0	N. W. 1	S. W. 1	S. W. 1	0	1	Sprin'le	63.6	
8	29.34	29.18	29.24	39	39	30	36.0	E'ly 3	N. E. 3	N. E. 4	Rain	Misty	Misty	83.2	0.10
9	29.45	29.59	29.80	34	41	32	35.7	N. W. 2	N. W. 2	N. W. 2	10	0	0	42.5	
10	29.94	29.98	30.01	32	48	36	38.7	N. W. 2	N. W. 1	N. W. 1	0	0	5	67.0	
11	30.09	30.09	30.06	33	43	41	39.0	W'ly 1	S. E'ly 2	S'ly 2	0	10	7	70.7	
12	29.91	29.78	29.81	44	46	44	44.7	S. W'ly 1	S. E'ly 2	S'ly 1	10	Rain	Foggy	88.5	1.10
S 13	29.95	29.92	30.00	40	60	48	49.3	W'ly 1	S. W'ly 1	S. W. 1	1	2	0	44.3	
14	30.12	30.12	30.08	34	50	41	41.7	N. E. 1	S'ly 2	S'ly 1	0	7	10	57.4	
15	29.65	29.41	29.39	48	51	45	48.0	S. W. 5	S'ly 2	W'ly 3	Rain	Rain	10	82.7	2.50
16	29.61	29.75	30.02	40	45	37	40.7	N. W. 3	N. W. 3	N. W. 1	9	2	.0	42.7	
17	30.08	30.01	29.99	34	59	45	46.0	N. W. 1	S'ly 1	S'ly 1	0	8	10	55.3	
18	29.78	29.48	29.17	44	52	52	49.3	S'ly 2	S. E. 4	S. E. 4	10	Rain	Rain	83.2	1.40
19	28.99	29.01	29.16	46	48	45	46.3	S. W. 4	S. W. 5	S. W. 3	1	5	8	57.4	
S 20	29.40	29.41	29.60	35	44	37	38.7	N. W. 3	N. W. 4	N. W. 3	10	3	7	34.4	
21	29.77	29.79	29.86	32	54	43	43.0	N. W. 1	N. W. 1	W'ly 1	0	0	10	21.0	
22	29.91	29.79	29.67	37	50	42	43.0	N. E. 1	S'ly 1	E'ly 1	9	10	Rain	45.5	0.50
23	29.60	29.69	29.77	39	44	36	39.7	N. E. 2	N'ly 2	N. W. 1	Misty	10	0	72.8	
24	29.81	29.77	29.63	34	50	42	42.0	N. W. 1	S. W. 2	S. E'ly 2	0	10	Rain	55.3	
25	29.46	29.36	29.47	42	41	39	40.7	E'ly 1	N. E. 2	N'ly 2	Rain	Rain	10	86.8	1.00
26	29.40	29.35	29.40	34	46	36	38.7	N'ly 1	N'ly 2	N. W. 1	10	10	5	72.3	
S 27	29.54	29.54	29.60	31	48	43	40.7	N. W. 2	N. W. 2	S'ly 2	0	9	10	56.4	
28	29.65	29.64	29.63	41	60	42	47.7	S'ly 1	S. E'ly 2	N. E. 1	10	2	Foggy	65.1	
29	29.49	29.16	29.08	43	54	53	50.0	N. E. 1	S. E. 3	N'ly 3	Foggy	Rain	0	78.6	0.20
30	29.40	29.39	29.52	42	57	41	46.7	W'ly 2	W'ly 2	N. W. 1	3	0	0	42.9	
31	29.64	29.60	29.67	38	52	39	43.0	N. W. 2	N. W'ly 3	N. W. 5	0	0	0	28.3	
Means	29.70	29.65	29.69	36.1	46.7	38.9	...	1.7	2.2	1.8	5.0	5.7	5.7	59.0	8.00
									1.9			5.5			
Reduced to sea level.															
Max.	30.46	30.42	30.48	48	60	53	50.0								
Min.	29.17	29.19	29.26	13	25	18	19.0								
Mean	29.88	29.83	29.87												
Range	1.29	1.23	1.22	35	35	35	31.0								
Mean of month	29.860			...	...	...	32.8								
Extreme range	1.31			...	...	...	47.0								

Prevailing winds from some point between— Days.
N. & E. 3
E. & S. 6
S. & W. 8
W. & N. 14

Days.
Clear 7
Variable . . . .} 11
Cloudy . . . . .}
Rain or snow fell on 13

Remarks.

1st and 2d. Fine, but cold.
3d. Wind S'ly, cold and raw. Began to snow at 7 P. M.
4th. Rain and mist at sunrise. Cloudy in the morning. Pleasant in the afternoon. From six to seven inches of very damp snow on the ground this morning.
5th. Fine.
6th. Very fine.
7th. Pleasant through the day. Sprinkling of rain at 10 P. M.
8th. Cold and misty, with some rain.
9th. The ground covered with fresh snow this morning, which melted during the day. Evening splendid.
10th. Very fine.
11th. Pleasant.
12th. Began to rain at 10 A. M. Rain continued till 4 P. M. Evening foggy.
13th. Very fine. The warmest day since November 1, 1858.
14th. Pleasant in the morning. Rain towards night.
15th. Steady rain all day. Barometer began to rise at 8 P. M. Evening cloudy, with rain.
16th. Fine. Evening splendid.
17th. Pleasant. Indications of storm in the evening.
18th. Began to rain at 8 A. M.; wind brisk S. E. Rain continued through the day and evening, with wind heavy.
19th. Extremely blustering all day.
20th. Weather continues very blustering and uncomfortable.
21st. Very fine.
22d. Pleasant in the morning. Began to rain at 7 P. M.
23d. Cloudy in the morning. Evening clear.
24th. Pleasant in the morning. Began to rain at 5 P. M.
25th. Rainy day.
26th. Cloudy, with occasional rain.
27th. Pleasant in the morning. Raw in the afternoon. Evening cloudy.
28th. Pleasant. Evening foggy.
29th. Mist and fog in the morning. Rain in the afternoon. Cleared from 9 to 10 P. M.
30th. Pleasant.
31st. Blustering. Heavy squall from 5 to 6 P. M., with dashes of rain. Very high wind in the evening.

April, 1859. New Moon, 3d. 5h. 9m. A. M.

Days.	Barometer, reduced to 32° F. Sunrise.	At 1 P. M.	At 10 P. M.	Thermometer. Sunrise.	At 1 P. M.	At 10 P. M.	Daily mean.	Winds (Direction and Force.) Sunrise.	At 1 P. M.	At 10 P. M.	Weather (Tenths Cloudy.) Sunrise.	At 1 P. M.	At 10 P. M.	Relative Humidity.	Rain and Snow in Inches of Water
1	29.79	29.74	29.84	32	48	38	39.3	N. W. 4	N. W. 5	N. W. 2	0	0	0	41.6	
2	29.85	29.76	29.81	32	54	44	43.3	N. W. 1	N'ly 2	E'ly	0	0	10	39.2	
S 3	29.63	29.45	29.37	43	42	41	42.0	E'ly 1	S. E. 1	S. E. 1	10	Rain	10	71.1	
4	29.31	29.22	29.41	39	47	33	39.7	N. W. 1	N. W. 3	N. W. 4	9	10	0	35.3	
5	29.42	29.34	29.42	30	41	33	34.7	N. W. 2	N. W. 4	N. W. 2	0	3	0	31.2	
6	29.49	29.51	29.60	30	43	38	37.0	N. W. 1	N. W. 4	N. W. 2	0	7	0	31.0	
7	29.64	29.54	29.61	33	52	43	42.7	W by N 1	N. W. 3	N. W. 1	0	1	10	28.3	
8	29.63	29.61	29.70	40	50	40	43.3	N. W. 1	N. W. 2	N. W. 2	0	9	7	36.2	
9	29.90	29.87	30.03	31	42	32	35.0	N. W. 2	N. W. 3	N. W. 1	0	0	0	29.4	
S 10	30.04	29.96	29.94	29	45	37	37.0	N. W. 1	S. W. 2	S. W'ly 1	0	0	0	52.7	
11	29.80	29.63	29.63	40	35	38	37.7	S. E. 1	E'ly 3	S. W'ly 3	10	Rain	Misty	74.5	0.53
12	29.73	29.75	29.81	38	49	43	43.3	N. W. 2	N'ly 1	S. W'ly 1	10	9	5	83.4	
13	29.80	29.77	29.89	45	60	40	48.3	S. E'ly 1	S. W. 2	E'ly 2	10	1	Foggy	70.6	
14	29.92	29.81	29.53	40	40	38	39.3	N. E. 3	S. E'ly 3	N. E. 3	10	Rain	Rain	85.5	0.45
15	29.52	29.49	29.47	37	53	43	44.3	N'ly 2	S'ly 1	S. E'ly	10	1	9	63.1	
16	29.43	29.38	29.60	44	43	39	42.0	S'ly	N'ly 1	N. W. 1	10	10	0	77.0	
S 17	29.63	29.61	29.69	38	55	46	46.3	N. W. 3	S'ly 2	N'ly 1	0	5	10	40.4	
18	29.70	29.70	29.73	38	50	41	43.0	N'ly 1	N. E. 2	N. W. 1	3	10	0	38.0	
19	29.72	29.60	29.60	39	59	46	48.0	N. W. 1	N. W. 2	N. W. 1	0	0	0	29.2	
20	29.59	29.53	29.61	43	59	46	49.3	N. W. 1	N. W. 3	N. W. 1	0	0	5	21.7	
21	29.63	29.57	29.62	42	66	52	53.3	N. W. 1	N. W. 1	S. W. 1	0	0	10	33.1	
22	29.63	29.62	29.46	48	52	42	47.3	N. E. 2	N. E. 2	N. E. 4	10	Rain	Rain	48.7	} 1.05
23	29.22	29.01	28.98	42	55	45	47.3	N. E. 2	S. E. 2	S. W. 4	Rain	10	10	80.1	}
S 24	29.13	29.33	29.64	42	53	46	47.0	W. by S. 1	N. W. 4	N. W. 1	5	2	0	48.3	
25	29.75	29.79	29.80	41	65	49	51.7	N. W. 1	W. by S 2	S. W. 1	0	10	10	61.5	
26	29.72	29.68	29.56	48	59	47	51.3	N'ly 1	N'ly 1	S'ly 2	10	10	Sprin'le	75.2	} 0.25
27	29.58	29.71	29.77	44	56	45	48.3	N. E. 1	S. E'ly 1	N. E. 1	Rain	8	2	63.3	}
28	30.00	29.98	29.99	41	51	39	43.7	N. E. 1	N. E. 2	N. E. 1	9	9	2	36.2	
29	29.94	...	29.75	39	53	42	44.7	N. E. 2	N. E. 2	N. E. 1	1	5	0	39.7	
30	29.69	29.67	29.83	44	69	52	55.0	N. E. 1	N. E. 1	N'ly 1	0	0	0	29.4	
Means	29.66	29.61	29.66	39.1	51.5	41.9	...	1.4	2.2	1.6	4.6	5.3	5.0	49.2	2.28
								1.7			5.0				
REDUCED TO SEA LEVEL.								Prevailing winds from some point between—		Days.			Days.		
Max.	30.22	30.16	30.21	48	69	52	55.0	N. & E.		7	Clear		8		
Min.	29.31	29.19	29.16	29	35	32	34.7	E. & S.		5	Variable		} 14		
Mean	29.84	29.79	29.84					S. & W.		4	Cloudy		}		
Range	0.91	0.97	1.05	19	34	20	20.3	W. & N.		14	Rain fell on		8		
Mean of month	29.823			...	...	...	44.2								
Extreme range	1.06			...	...	...	40.0								

REMARKS.

1st. Cold, and extremely blustering.
2d. Pleasant.
3d. Drizzling rain all day.
4th. Blustering.
5th. Blustering and cold.
6th. Very blustering. Snow-squall between 1 and 2 P. M. Evening clear.
7th. Blustering, but milder.
8th. Pleasant.
9th. Very blustering and cold.
10th. Pleasant.
11th. Cold rain, beginning at 7 A. M., mingled with hail.
12th. Cloudy in the morning. Partially clear in the afternoon.
13th. Pleasant. Towards night, the wind rather fresh from S E'ly, while the upper clouds came from N. W'ly. At 10 P. M., thick fog.
14th. Cold and rainy.
15th. Pleasant. From 3 to 9 P. M., wind rather fresh S. E., while the upper clouds came from W. by N. At 10 P. M., the lower clouds nearly covered the heavens.
16th. Cloudy in the morning. Dashes of rain from noon to 1 P. M., from N. E. Evening clear.
17th. At 1 P. M., wind S'ly, with heavy cumulus clouds from N. W. Evening cloudy.
18th. Cloudy through the day; wind N. E. Evening clear, with wind light at N. W.
19th. Very fine. Evening splendid.
20th. Very fine. Evening hazy.
21st. Pleasant. Air warm and summer-like.
22d. Began to rain moderately between 1 and 2 P. M. Rain heavy in the evening.
23d. Rain in showers through the day.
24th. Blustering.
25th. Warm for the season. Wind S'ly in the afternoon, with clouds from the W.
26th. Cloudy, but mild.
27th. Light rain in the morning. Evening mostly clear.
28th. Very cold for the season.
29th. Pleasant, but cold. Brilliant aurora in the evening. Streamers of great beauty, extending nearly to the zenith. At times, the streamers assumed a pinkish color; and at times the whole northern heavens presented a reddish-pink hue.
30th. Very fine.

May, 1859. New Moon, 2d. 4h. 56m. P. M.

Days.	Barometer Sunrise.	At 1 P. M.	At 10 P. M.	Thermometer Sunrise.	At 1 P. M.	At 10 P. M.	Daily mean.	Winds Sunrise.	At 1 P. M.	At 10 P. M.	Weather Sunrise.	At 1 P. M.	At 10 P. M.	Relative Humidity.	Rain and Snow in Inches of Water
S 1	29.91	29.99	30.00	55	61	46	54.0	N. W. 1	N. W. 1	N. W. 1	0	0	0	65.6	
2	29.95	29.85	30.00	47	69	54	56.7	S. W.	W'ly 1	E'ly 1	0	0	0	69.7	
3	30.04	30.17	30.19	49	62	46	52.3	N. E. 1	E'ly 2	N. W. 1	0	0	0	70.9	
4	30.20	30.15	30.17	51	61	49	53.7	S. W. 1	S'ly 2	S'ly 2	0	0	0	74.6	
5	30.16	...	...	54	...	...	...	S. W. 1	...	...	0	...	...	76.7	
6	...	...	...	...	...	...	...	...	...	...	...	...	...	...	
7	...	...	29.72	...	72	56	...	...	...	S. W. 1	...	...	0	69.0	
S 8	29.66	29.60	29.55	57	68	65	63.3	S. E. 1	S. E. 2	S. E'ly 1	2	2	2	67.4	
9	29.50	29.53	29.68	65	67	47	59.7	S'ly 1	N. E. 3	N. E. 2	10	3	10	75.6	
10	29.70	29.72	29.90	45	47	44	45.3	N. E. 3	N. E. 3	N. E. 2	Rain	Rain	Rain	91.6	} 1.05
11	29.98	30.02	30.04	43	46	44	44.3	N. E. 3	N. E. 4	N. E. 3	Rain	Rain	10	94.1	}
12	30.04	29.94	30.01	44	47	46	45.7	N. E. 4	N. E. 4	N. E. 2	Rain	Misty	10	92.7	}
13	30.00	29.91	29.90	48	72	58	59.3	N. E. 2	N'ly 1	S'ly 1	10	0	Foggy	86.3	
14	29.85	29.94	29.99	57	62	55	58.0	N'ly 1	N. E'ly 3	N. E. 1	3	10	8	86.0	
S 15	30.04	30.08	30.13	52	56	43	50.3	N. E. 2	N. E. 2	N. E. 1	7	10	7	84.0	
16	30.13	30.02	29.97	42	64	44	50.0	N. E. 1	N. E. 2	S. E. 1	0	0	10	77.3	
17	29.86	29.76	29.72	43	59	54	52.0	S. E. 1	S. E. 2	Calm	10	10	Foggy	89.4	
18	29.75	29.76	29.78	55	67	58	60.0	S'ly 1	S'ly 2	S'ly 1	Foggy	10	10	86.5	
19	29.71	29.77	29.82	58	71	59	62.7	S'ly 1	S. E'ly 1	S. E'ly 1	Misty	10	Rain	89.9	} 2.35
20	29.88	29.87	29.97	60	60	53	57.7	N. E. 1	N. E. 2	N. E. 1	Misty	Rain	Misty	92.3	}
21	29.91	29.81	29.78	51	54	52	52.3	N. E. 2	N. E. 2	N. E. 2	Rain	Rain	Rain	94.3	}
S 22	29.60	29.56	29.69	61	60	57	59.3	S'ly 2	S'ly 3	S'ly 1	Rain	Misty	10	91.1	
23	29.87	29.89	29.98	52	69	55	58.7	N. W. 1	N. W. 1	N. W. 1	0	0	0	68.5	
24	30.04	30.06	30.11	53	74	55	60.7	W'ly 1	S. E. 2	S. E. 1	0	0	0	75.9	
25	30.11	30.04	30.02	54	74	56	61.3	S'ly 1	N. W. 1	N. W. 1	10	10	0	74.3	
26	29.96	30.00	29.88	58	80	60	66.0	S. W. 1	S. W. 3	S. W. 1	3	0	2	74.8	
27	29.81	29.72	29.62	57	73	60	63.3	S. W. 1	S. E. 3	S'ly 1	0	0	10	82.6	
28	29.58	29.50	29.75	64	70	57	63.7	S. W. 1	S'ly 3	W'ly 1	10	3	0	75.7	
S 29	29.83	29.77	29.82	52	71	59	60.7	W 1	S. W. [illegible]	S'ly 1	[illegible]	[illegible]	[illegible]	[illegible]	
30	[illegible]	[illegible]	[illegible]	[illegible]	[illegible]	[illegible]	[illegible]	[illegible]	[illegible]	[illegible]	[illegible]	[illegible]	[illegible]	81.1	
31	30.19	30.14	30.14	53	67	53	57.7	E'ly 2	S. W. 3	S. W. 2	0	5	Rain	81.2	
Means	29.90	29.88	29.91	53.1	64.5	53.0	...	1.4	2.3	1.3	5.3	5.0	5.5	80.6	3.40
								1.7			5.3				
REDUCED TO SEA LEVEL.								Prevailing winds from some point between—		Days.			Days.		
Max.	30.38	30.35	30.37	65	80	65	66.0	N. & E.		11	Clear		12		
Min.	29.68	29.68	29.73	42	46	43	44.3	E. & S.		6	Variable		} 9		
Mean	30.08	30.06	30.09					S. & W.		10	Cloudy		}		
Range	0.70	0.67	0.64	23	34	22	21.7	W. & N.		3	Rain fell on		10		
Mean of month	30.077			...	...	...	55.9								
Extreme range	0.70			...	...	...	38.0								

REMARKS.

1st to 4th. Very fine.
5th and 6th. Pleasant.
7th. Very warm.
8th. Warm and hazy.
9th. Cloudy for the most part. Appearance of storm in the evening.
10th. Moderate rain all day.
11th. Cold rain.
12th. Light rain and mist. Cold and raw.
13th. Middle of the day clear and warm.
14th. Cloudy for the most part, but air mild and soft. Sprinkling of rain at 1½ P. M. In the evening, wind light from N. E., while clouds came slowly from W'ly.
15th. In the morning, wind brisk from N. E.; clouds from N. W. Weather pleasant, but cold.
16th. Fine. Evening cloudy.
17th. Light rain in the afternoon. Foggy and calm in the evening.
18th. Mild; air damp. Clouds and sunshine.
19th. Shower from 3 to 4 A. M. Rain in the evening.
20th. Light showers at intervals.
21st. Rainy day.
22d. Light rain in the morning.
23d and 24th. Very fine.
25th. Cloudy, but warm.
26th. Very warm. Evening hazy.
27th. Pleasant.
28th. Showery till noon. Clear at 5 P. M.
29th. Very fine.
30th. Dashes of rain in morning. Pleasant in afternoon. At 2 P. M., wind fresh from S. W., with clouds from N. W.
31st. Pleasant through the day. Began to rain from 9 to 10 P. M.

June, 1859. New Moon, 1d. 2h. 2m. A. M., and 30d. 9h. 33m. A. M.

Days.	Barometer, reduced to 32° F. Sunrise.	Barometer At 1 P. M.	Barometer At 10 P. M.	Thermometer. Sunrise.	Thermometer At 1 P. M.	Thermometer At 10 P. M.	Thermometer Daily mean.	Winds. (Direction and Force.) Sunrise.	Winds At 1 P. M.	Winds At 10 P. M.	Weather. (Tenths Cloudy.) Sunrise.	Weather At 1 P. M.	Weather At 10 P. M.	Relative Humidity.	Rain and Snow in Inches of Water.
1	30.09	30.07	30.03	54	64	62	60.0	S. W. 2	S'ly 2	S'ly 1	10	Rain	10	78.2	0.55
2	29.98	29.89	29.91	65	79	66	70.3	S. W. 3	S. W. 4	S'ly 2	9	5	9	70.4	
3	29.80	29.77	29.75	66	72	66	68.0	S. W. 3	S. W. 2	S. W. 1	10	Rain	Rain	82.7	} 0.62
4	29.72	29.77	29.83	67	57	48	57.3	N. W. 2	N. E. 2	N. E. 2	Rain	Rain	Rain	81.0	
S 5	29.82	29.81	30.00	46	58	47	50.3	N. W. 2	N. W. 2	N. W. 1	8	10	0	57.5	
6	30.03	30.03	30.07	47	68	55	56.7	N. W. 2	S. W. 1	S. W. 2	5	7	0	55.2	
7	30.08	30.02	30.06	56	69	58	61.0	S. W. 2	S. E. 3	S. W. 2	0	5	0	61.8	
8	29.97	29.76	29.60	55	67	62	61.8	S. W. 2	S. W. 4	S. W. 2	2	10	10	79.0	
9	29.62	29.68	29.80	55	67	51	57.7	N. W. 3	N. W. 2	N. W. 1	1	1	0	58.3	
10	29.81	29.69	29.82	53	75	53	60.3	N. W. 1	S. W. 5	S. W. 2	0	1	Rain	58.4	0.25
11	29.92	29.99	30.08	46	60	49	51.7	N. W. 2	N. W. 3	N. W. 1	0	...	0	52.1	
S 12	30.17	30.10	30.14	47	57	54	53.7	N. W. 1	S'ly 3	S. W'ly 2	0	...	0	52.0	
13	30.06	29.98	29.90	55	66	64	61.7	S. W. 2	S. W. 3	S. W. 1	5	10	9	77.1	
14	29.87	29.86	29.87	65	81	65	70.3	S. W. 1	W'ly 2	S'ly 1	10	5	10	77.1	
15	29.69	29.71	29.65	65	85	69	73.0	S. W. 1	S'ly 3	S. W. 3	Foggy	3	1	65.9	
16	29.60	29.59	29.65	70	74	67	70.3	S. W. 3	S. W. 2	S. W. 1	10	Sprin'le	Rain	79.9	} 4.55
17	29.67	29.64	29.41	65	65	60	63.3	N'ly 1	N. E. 2	N. E. 1	9	Rain	Rain	88.7	
18	29.41	29.55	29.74	60	73	59	64.0	N'ly 1	W'ly 2	N. W. 1	1	8	0	74.2	0.10
S 19	29.80	29.80	29.83	57	75	62	64.7	N. W. 1	N. W. 2	S. W. 2	0	3	Hazy	57.9	
20	29.79	29.75	29.69	61	65	60	62.0	S. W. 1	S. W. 3	S. W. 1	10	9	Foggy	75.5	0.05
21	29.58	29.53	29.56	62	68	58	62.7	S. W. 1	S. W. 1	N. E. 1	10	Sprin'le	Misty	84.7	0.05
22	29.57	29.60	29.76	57	70	62	63.0	N. E. 1	S'ly 2	S. W. 1	10	9	Foggy	85.7	
23	29.83	29.87	29.97	63	66	60	63.0	S. E. 2	N. E. 2	N. E. 1	10	Misty	10	84.8	
24	29.92	29.90	29.87	59	64	62	61.7	N. E. 2	N. E. 2	N. E. 2	Misty	Rain	Misty	90.1	0.12
25	29.80	29.69	29.83	63	77	61	67.0	E'ly 1	S. W. 2	N. W. 2	Misty	8	0	74.9	0.15
S 26	29.89	29.89	29.96	62	80	65	69.0	N. W. 1	W'ly 2	N. W. 1	5	3	0	62.0	
27	30.00	29.99	30.00	62	81	66	69.7	N. W. 1	S. W. 3	S. W. 1	1	1	0	58.4	
28	29.99	29.93	29.85	66	76	71	71.0	S. W'ly 2	S. W. 1	S. W.	0	10	8	56.5	
29	29.83	29.70	29.61	74	88	76	79.3	S. W. 1	S'ly 1	S'ly 1	3	1	Rain	67.9	0.62
30	29.54	29.69	29.84	73	73	59	68.3	N. W. 1	N. W. 3	N. W. 1	2	0	0	60 3	
Means	29.83	29.81	29.84	59.9	70.7	60.6	...	1.6	2.4	1.4	5.7	6.5	5.9	70.3	7.06
									1.8			6.0			

REDUCED TO SEA LEVEL.							
Max.	30.35	30.28	30.32	74	88	76	79.3
Min.	29.59	29.71	29.59	46	57	47	50.3
Mean	30.01	29.99	30.02				
Range	0.76	0.57	0.73	28	31	29	29.0
Mean of month	30.007			...	...	...	63.7
Extreme range	0.76			...	...	...	42.0

Prevailing winds from some point between—	Days.
N. & E.	4
E. & S.	0
S. & W.	19
W. & N.	7

	Days.
Clear	6
Variable } Cloudy }	10
Rain fell on	14

REMARKS.

1st. Showery.

2d. Air warm and damp, with very fresh wind.

3d. Showery, with thunder at 9 A. M. Thundershower at 7 P. M.

4th. Light rain through the day.

5th. Variable; cool for the season.

6th. Very fine.

7th. At 2 P. M., wind fresh from S. E., with heavy cumulus clouds moving slowly from N. W'ly. Evening clear.

8th. Dashes of rain in the afternoon, with heavy clouds.

9th. Very fine. Evening splendid.

10th. Pleasant in the morning. At mid-day, wind very strong from S. W. Moderate rain from 6 to 10 P. M.; wind abated.

11th. Very fine; ther. at 5 A. M., 44°. Appearances of frost in low places in vicinity.

12th. At 1 P. M., wind fresh from S'ly, clouds at the same time moving slowly from N. W.; evening clear.

13th. Variable; dashes of rain P. M.

14th. Very warm and sultry.

15th. Very warm.

16th. Cloudy, with showers.

17th. Began to rain at 10 A. M., and continued; from 5 to 10 P. M., incessant and very heavy. The quantity during the day was about four inches, which is more than has fallen in any single day since July 13, 1834. On the night of that day, occurred the most extraordinary rain of which I have any record. It was believed at the time that the quantity was from seven to eight inches. A gauge holding six inches was filled to overflowing.

18th. Pleasant in morning. Light showers at 2 P. M., and from 7 to 8 P. M. Very clear at 10 P. M.

19th. Very fine.

20th. Light rain at intervals through day.

21st. Misty, and occasional sprinkling.

22d and 23d. Cloudy and misty.

24th. Light rain in the afternoon.

25th. Showery. Evening clear.

26th. Fine.

27th. Very warm.

28th. Fine and warm.

29th. Very hot. Heavy squall from W'ly from 7 to 8 P. M., followed by thunder and a little rain.

30th. Very fine.

July, 1859. New Moon, 29d. 4h. 36m. P. M.

Days.	Barometer At 6 A. M.	Barometer At 1 P. M.	Barometer At 10 P. M.	Thermometer At 6 A. M.	Thermometer At 1 P. M.	Thermometer At 10 P. M.	Thermometer Daily mean.	Winds At 6 A. M.	Winds At 1 P. M.	Winds At 10 P. M.	Weather At 6 A. M.	Weather At 1 P. M.	Weather At 10 P. M.	Relative Humidity.	Rain and Snow in Inches of Water.
1	29.87	29.87	29.86	55	75	62	64.0	E'ly 1	S. E'ly 2	S'ly 1	0	0	0	66.3	
2	29.80	29.69	29.62	65	79	73	72.3	S. W'ly 2	S'ly 2	S'ly 3	10	10	8	79.2	
S 3	29.59	29.59	29.69	71	78	62	70.3	S. W. 2	S. W. 2	N. W. 2	10	Shower	10	72.5	0.15
4	29.80	29.99	30.12	54	66	54	58.0	N. W. 2	N'ly 2	N. W. 1	8	3	0	52.9	
5	30.19	30.18	30.18	54	69	54	59.0	N. W. 1	N'ly 3	N. E. 1	0	3	0	53.7	
6	30.11	30.06	30.06	53	72	61	62.0	N. E. 2	N. E. 2	N. E. 1	3	2	0	66.5	
7	30.01	29.98	30.00	60	80	65	68.3	N'ly 2	S. E'ly 1	S. W. 1	2	0	0	69.5	
8	29.97	29.91	29.94	67	84	69	73.3	S. W. 1	S. W. 2	S. W. 1	1	3	5	70.0	
9	29.93	29.95	30.04	68	79	64	70.3	N'ly 1	N. E. 1	N. E. 1	5	2	0	63.4	
S 10	30.03	29.99	30.00	65	83	71	73.0	N. W. 1	W'ly 2	S'ly 1	0	7	0	51.5	
11	29.95	29.86	29.85	67	81	73	73.7	S'ly 1	S. E. 2	S'ly 1	3	0	0	75.5	
12	29.82	29.79	29.78	72	90	71	77.7	S. W. 1	S. W. 1	S'ly	5	6	0	70.4	
13	29.81	29.78	29.83	71	80	72	74.3	S. W. 1	S'ly 1	S'ly 1	10	Rain	6	83.0	0.37
14	29.87	29.91	29.97	68	78	63	69.7	N. W. 2	N. E. 2	N'ly 1	6	4	0	59.1	
15	30.05	29.99	29.96	65	77	65	67.0	N. W. 1	S. W. 2	E'ly 1	0	7	10	59.4	
16	29.88	29.80	29.77	61	72	66	66.3	E'ly 1	S'ly 2	S'ly 1	10	10	10	70.9	
S 17	29.62	29.66	29.70	64	85	70	73.0	N. W. 1	N. W. 2	N. W. 1	2	2	0	64.0	
18	29.70	29.74	29.75	68	81	67	72.0	N'ly 1	N. E'ly 2	E'ly 1	0	6	5	63.5	
19	29.69	29.65	29.57	70	76	68	71.3	S'ly	S'ly	S'ly 1	10	10	10	74.2	
20	29.47	29.38	29.57	68	87	69	74.7	S. W. 1	W'ly 2	N. W. 2	10	2	0	53.9	
21	29.79	29.70	29.72	59	75	63	65.7	N. W. 3	N. W. 3	W'ly 1	0	3	5	46.0	
22	29.65	29.49	29.47	66	80	67	71.0	S. W. 2	S. W. 3	S. W. 1	2	3	Rain	70.8	0.12
23	29.45	...	29.68	63	...	62	...	N. W. 3	...	N. W. 1	0	...	0	66.7	
S 24	29.78	29.76	29.80	61	78	64	67.7	N. W. 2	N. W. 2	N. W. 1	3	2	0	45.9	
25	29.78	29.74	29.75	65	80	66	70.3	S. W'ly 1	S. W. 2	W'ly 1	9	4	0	67.9	0.35
26	29.70	29.62	29.59	69	78	70	72.3	S. W. 2	S. W. 3	W'ly 2	10	10	5	70.0	0.15
27	29.57	29.50	29.56	56	74	62	64.0	N. W. 1	N. W. 3	N. W. 1	0	5	0	59.0	
28	29.59	29.64	29.66	61	77	66	68.0	N. W. 2	N. W. 3	N. W. 1	0	5	0	58.9	
29	29.84	29.85	29.94	60	78	68	68.7	N. W. 1	N. W. 2	S. W. 1	0	5	0	68.1	
30	29.98	29.97	29.97	59	81	66	68.7	N. E. 1	S. E'ly 2	S'ly 1	2	6	2	71.2	
S 31	29.93	29.87	29.86	63	74	66	67.7	S'ly 1	S'ly 1	S'ly 1	8	10	10	64.7	
Means	29.81	29.80	29 81	63.5	78.2	65.8	...	1.4	2.0	1.1	4.2	5.0	3.1	64.8	1.14
									1.5			4.1			

REDUCED TO SEA LEVEL.							
Max.	30.37	30.36	30.36	72	90	73	77.7
Min.	29.63	29.56	29.65	53	66	54	58.0
Mean	29.99	29.98	29.99				
Range	0.74	0.80	0.71	19	24	19	19.7
Mean of month	29.987			...	...	...	69.2
Extreme range	0.81			...	...	...	37.0

Prevailing winds from some point between—	Days.
N. & E.	4
E. & S.	6
S. & W.	11
W. & N.	10

	Days.
Clear	10
Variable } Cloudy }	15
Rain fell on	6

REMARKS.

1st. Very fine.

2d. Cloudy; air very damp.

3d. Cloudy, with light shower.

4th. Very fine.

5th. Fine, but cool. At 6 P. M., wind fresh from N. E., while high clouds were coming from S. W.

6th. Very fine. Evening splendid.

7th and 8th. Very fine.

9th. Pleasant. Sun hot.

10th. Very warm. In the evening, wind light from S'ly, with upper clouds coming from N. E.

11th. Very warm and sultry.

12th. Very hot and damp; no evaporation.

13th Sultry. Light thundershower at 1 P. M.; frequent thunder in the afternoon. Light shower from 7 to 8 P. M.; then moonlight.

14th. Cool, but fine.

15th. Very fine.

16th. Cloudy; air damp.

17th. At 1 P. M., wind from N. W., with high cumulus clouds coming from N. E'ly. Heavy gust of wind from N. E'ly at 7 and 8 P. M. Thunder, with heavy clouds driven in different directions; no rain.

18th. Very pleasant.

19th. Cloudy.

20th. Fine in the afternoon and evening.

21st. Very fine; air extremely dry.

22d. Warm through the day. Shower from 10 to 11 P. M.

23d. Fine. Evening very clear.

24th. Very fine.

25th. Fine in the morning. Shower from 3 to 5 P. M.

26th. Fine shower at 7 P. M.

27th. Fine. Sprinkling of rain at 4 P. M. from a passing cloud.

28th. Very fine.

29th. Pleasant Beginning of solar eclipse lost, by reason of clouds; the end well observed at 6 h. 36 m. 49 s. P. M., Providence mean time.

30th. Pleasant. Sun hot at mid-day.

31st. Cloudy.

August, 1859. New Moon, 27d. 11h. 18m. P. M.

Days.	Barometer, reduced to 32° F. At 6 A. M.	At 2 P. M.	At 10 P. M.	Thermometer. At 6 A. M.	At 2 P. M.	At 10 P. M.	Daily mean.	Winds. (Direction and Force.) At 6 A. M.	At 2 P. M.	At 10 P. M.	Weather. (Tenths Cloudy.) At 6 A. M.	At 2 P. M.	At 10 P. M.	Relative Humidity.	Rain and Snow in Inches of Water.
1	29.83	29.82	29.86	62	79	66	69.0	N. W. 1	S. W. 3	S. W. 1	3	3	1	66.7	
2	29.85	29.85	29.84	67	78	70	71.7	S. W. 1	S. E. 1	S'ly 1	10	8	10	80.4	
3	29.90	29.86	29.87	73	84	71	76.0	S'ly 1	S. W. 1	S. W.	5	3	0	74.1	
4	29.79	29.67	29.64	71	83	75	76.3	S. W. 2	S. W. 2	S. W. 1	10	3	Rain	78.9	
5	29.65	29.64	29.61	76	81	70	75.7	S. W. 1	S. W.	S. W.	10	Rain	10	78.3	0.75
6	29.71	29.75	...	66	79	...	...	N. W. 2	N. W. 2	...	7	0	...	66.9	
S 7	...	...	...	...	...	...	...	...	...	...	...	...	...	...	
8	...	29.80	29.92	...	78	65	...	...	N. W. 1	S. W. 1	...	3	0	62.1	
9	30.01	30.01	30.03	67	81	64	70.7	N. W. 1	S. E. 2	S'ly 1	0	5	0	66.6	
10	30.03	30.04	29.99	68	80	67	71.7	S. W.	S. W. 1	S. W. 1	5	0	3	64.8	
11	29.98	...	29.93	59	...	59	...	N. E. 1	...	S'ly 1	5	...	10	62.9	
12	29.90	...	29.82	66	...	72	...	S'ly 1	...	S. W. 1	10	...	10	86.9	
13	29.74	29.67	29.68	71	74	70	71.7	S. W.	S. W. 1	S. W. 1	Rain	10	5	83.3	0.75
S 14	29.69	29.68	29.69	73	85	73	77.0	N. W.	N. W. 2	S'ly	0	5	10	61.9	
15	29.75	29.81	29.89	72	75	60	69.0	N. W. 2	N. W. 3	N. W. 2	6	4	0	64.0	
16	29.93	29.95	29.97	62	68	65	61.7	N. W. 2	N'ly 3	N. E. 1	10	4	0	44.1	
17	30.00	29.95	29.92	58	73	56	62.3	N. W. 1	N. E. 3	E'ly 1	0	0	0	54.8	
18	29.83	29.72	...	63	80	...	...	N. W. 1	N. W. 1	...	0	0	...	78.1	
19	...	...	...	...	...	...	...	...	...	...	...	...	...	...	0.37
20	29.81	...	29.90	63	75	59	65.7	N'ly 2	N. E. 2	N. E. 1	8	0	0	53.1	
S 21	29.91	29.90	29.93	61	77	61	66.3	N. E. 1	N. E. 2	E'ly 1	0	2	0	55.0	
22	29.94	29.92	29.98	56	75	61	64.0	E'ly 1	E'ly 2	E'ly 1	0	5	0	84.1	
23	30.03	30.02	30.03	60	78	63	67.0	E'ly 1	S'ly 2	S'ly 1	Foggy	2	0	72.5	
24	29.96	29.88	29.80	57	74	69	66.7	N. E'ly 1	S. E. 2	S. E. 1	Foggy	10	Rain	78.9	
25	29.60	29.50	29.73	70	68	66	68.0	S. E. 3	N. E. 3	N. W. 1	Rain	Rain	0	89.5	1.17
26	29.77	29.75	29.76	64	81	68	71.0	N. W. 1	W. 3	W'ly 1	0	2	2	66.3	
27	29.68	29.59	29.59	68	81	64	71.0	N. W. 3	W'ly 2	S. W. 1	10	5	0	86.3	0.20
S 28	29.71	29.67	29.71	56	73	57	62.0	N. W. 1	W'ly 2	N. W. 3	0	2	0	54.3	
29	29.72	29.70	29.74	48	70	57	58.3	N. W. 1	N. W. 2	N. W. 1	0	3	0	44.5	
30	29.80	29.70	29.76	50	72	57	59.7	N. W. 1	N. W. 1	Calm	0	1	1	52.3	
31	29.61	29.58	29.61	57	77	57	63.7	S. W. 1	S. W. 3	S. W. 1	1	5	9	65.3	0.45
Means	29.83	29.79	29.82	66.1	77.0	64.5	...	1.2	1.9	1.0	5.5	3.9	3.4	67.5	3.69
									1.4			4.3			
Reduced to sea level.															
Max.	30.21	30.22	30.21	73	85	75	77.0								
Min.	29.78	29.68	29.77	48	68	56	58.3								
Mean	30.01	29.97	30.00												
Range	0.43	0.54	0.44	25	17	19	18.7								
Mean of month	29.993			...	...	...	69.2								
Extreme range	0.54			...	...	...	37.0								

Prevailing winds from some point between— Days.
N. & E. 5
E. & S. 5
S. & W. 9
W. & N. 10

Days.
Clear 9
Variable . . . } 12
Cloudy . . . . }
Rain fell on . . 8
(2 days omitted.)

REMARKS.

1st. Fine.
2d. Cloudy and sultry. Heavy fog about 8 P. M.
3d. Very damp and sultry. Cloudy in the morning.
4th. Damp and sultry in the afternoon; good deal of wind, and rain after 9 P. M.
5th. Slight showers in the morning, and sultry. Steady rain from 3 to 7 P. M. Evening cloudy.
6th to 9th. Very fine.
10th. Fine.
11th. Fog in the morning. Cloudy in the evening.
12th. Damp. Cloudy most of the day.
13th. Showery. Evening clear.
14th. Pleasant. Quite warm.
15th. Cool, but very fine.
16th. Very fine, though quite cool.
17th. Very cool.
18th. Pleasant.
19th. Showery in the evening.
20th and 21st. Very fine.
22d. Fine. Evening very clear.
23d. Very fine.
24th. Cloudy; air damp. Began to rain at 7 P. M.
25th. Copious rain at intervals till 4 P. M. Evening clear.
26th. Very fine.
27th. Shower, with thunder, from 4 to 5 P. M. Evening clear.
28th. Very fine. Splendid aurora in the evening. Large portions of the heavens often covered with light. approaching to blood red. At 35 or 40 min. past 9 o'clock, rays of red and white light (the red much predominating) met near the zenith, forming a rare and most magnificent display. The central point of light was about 10° south, and a little east of the zenith.
29th. Very fine; sky nearly cloudless. Light show of aurora in the evening.
30th. Very fine.
31st. Thundershowers in the afternoon and evening.

September, 1859. New Moon, 26d. 8h. 48m. A. M.

Days.	Barometer. Sunrise.	At 2 P. M.	At 10 P. M.	Thermometer. Sunrise.	At 2 P. M.	At 10 P. M.	Daily mean.	Winds. Sunrise.	At 2 P. M.	At 10 P. M.	Weather. Sunrise.	At 2 P. M.	At 10 P. M.	Relative Humidity.	Rain and Snow in Inches of Water.
1	29.67	29.63	29.60	53	73	59	61.7	N. W. 1	N. W. 2	N. W. 1	0	2	0	64.1	
2	29.50	29.59	29.77	62	73	54	63.0	S. W. 2	W'ly 2	N. W. 2	5	1	0	56.8	
3	29.79	29.79	29.79	50	71	62	61.0	N. W. 2	N. W. 2	S'ly 1	0	0	5	64.3	
S 4	29.70	29.70	29.89	65	78	60	67.7	S. W. 3	S. W. 2	N. W. 2	Sprin'le	3	1	63.5	
5	29.97	29.97	29.98	52	67	59	59.3	N. W'ly 2	S. W. 1	S. W. 1	5	10	Sprin'le	61.0	
6	30.00	30.00	30.12	54	67	52	57.7	N. W. 2	N. W. 3	N. W. 1	1	2	0	54.3	
7	30.13	30.12	30.11	50	...	52	...	N'ly 1	...	N. W. 1	5	...	0	79.0	
8	30.11	30.08	30.12	50	70	53	57.7	N. W. 1	N. W. 2	N. W. 1	0	3	0	58.1	
9	30.13	30.03	29.97	50	71	55	58.7	N. W. 1	N. W. 1	N. W. 1	0	4	0	61.3	
10	30.12	30.03	29.97	52	74	61	62.3	N. W. 1	S. W. 2	S. W. 1	0	5	Sprin'le	66.5	
S 11	29.77	29.56	29.40	63	74	70	69.0	S. W. 2	S. W. 1	S. W. 1	Sprin'le	10	10	80.9	
12	29.36	29.30	29.33	65	75	65	68.3	N. W'ly 1	S. W. 3	S. W. 1	0	5	0	69.7	
13	29.33	29.24	29.36	59	77	56	64.0	S. W. 1	S. W. 3	N. W. 3	0	10	0	66.0	0.10
14	29.40	29.60	29.93	48	59	46	51.0	N. W. 4	N. W. 5	N. W. 2	0	3	5	48.0	
15	30.08	30.10	30.18	39	57	43	46.3	N. W. 2	N. W. 2	N. W. 1	1	5	0	41.7	
16	30.17	30.11	30.10	39	63	52	51.3	N. W. 1	S. W'ly 1	S. W. 1	8	10	10	41.7	
17	29.96	29.64	29.43	51	54	52	52.3	N. E. 2	N. E'ly 4	N. E. 5	Rain	Rain	Rain	91.0	} 2.40
S 18	29.51	29.59	29.72	52	67	59	59.3	N. E. 4	N.N.E. 3	N. W. 1	Rain	8	0	76.3	}
19	29.75	29.70	29.73	50	72	62	61.3	N. W. 1	S. W. 3	N. W. 1	0	0	1	88.2	
20	29.70	29.72	29.86	65	78	66	69.7	S. W. 2	S. W. 3	S. W. 1	7	10	10	76.9	
21	29.92	29.97	29.93	54	51	53	52.7	N. E. 3	N. E. 4	N. E. 2	10	Rain	Rain	88.3	
22	29.92	29.92	29.92	50	54	52	52.0	N. E'ly 2	N. E. 2	N. E. 2	Misty	Misty	Rain	93.0	
23	29.82	29.78	29.79	52	58	56	55.3	N. E. 1	N. E. 2	N'ly 1	Rain	Misty	10	89.4	1.15
24	29.76	29.70	29.77	56	70	62	62.7	N'ly 2	N. W. 1	N. W. 1	10	5	10	72.8	
S 25	29.77	29.77	29.78	61	65	63	63.0	N. W. 1	N. W. 1	S. W. 1	10	10	Sprin'le	83.1	
26	29.77	29.76	29.80	61	71	62	64.7	S. W. 1	S. W. 1	S. W. 1	Foggy	2	10	75.1	
27	29.82	29.76	29.80	62	78	62	67.3	S. W. 1	S. W. 2	S. W. 1	Foggy	2	0	58.0	
28	29.78	29.76	29.90	64	72	63	66.3	S. W. 1	S. W. 2	N. E. 1	0	0	10	[illegible]	
[illegible]	[illegible]	[illegible]	[illegible]	[illegible]	[illegible]	[illegible]	[illegible]	[illegible]	[illegible]	[illegible] 1	1	1	0	[illegible]	
30	30.22	30.17	30.12	43	63	49	51.7	N. E. 1	S. W. 2	S. W. 1	0	0	0	67.6	
Means	29.83	29.81	29.85	54.3	67.7	56.9	...	1.7	2.2	1.4	5.3	5.3	4.9	69.5	3.65
									1.8			5.2			
Reduced to sea level.															
Max.	30.40	30.35	30.36	65	78	70	69.7								
Min.	29.51	29.44	29.51	39	51	43	46.3								
Mean	30.01	29.99	30.03												
Range	0.89	0.91	0.85	26	27	27	23.4								
Mean of month	30.006			...	...	...	59.6								
Extreme range	0.91			...	...	...	39.0								

Prevailing winds from some point between— Days.
N. & E. 6
E. & S. 0
S. & W. 13
W. & N. 11

Days.
Clear 7
Variable . . . } 11
Cloudy . . . . }
Rain fell on . . 12

REMARKS.

1st. Fine.
2d. Aurora very brilliant from 2 to 4 A. M. Change in weather from 9 to 11 A. M., the wind hauling from S. W. to N'ly, and the air becoming much dryer. Splendid aurora again in the evening; diffused light around the north, with occasional streamers, and broad, brilliant flashes of light running from the horizon to the zenith, and a good deal of red light in the N. W.
3d. Very fine.
4th. Sprinkling of rain at 6 A. M. Pleasant in the afternoon and evening.
5th. Pleasant. Sprinkling at 10 P. M.
6th. Very fine.
7th. Cool and pleasant. Evening clear.
8th and 9th. Fine.
10th. Fine in the morning. Sprinkling of rain from 9 to 10 P. M.
11th. Cloudy, and occasional sprinkling.
12th. Fine.
13th. Cloudy. Heavy dashes of rain from 5 to 6 P. M. Very clear at 10 P. M., and much cooler.
14th. Wind very high, and cold for the season.
15th. Very cool for the season. Evening clear.
16th. Cloudy, with air chilly from S. W. in the afternoon.
17th. Began to rain at sunrise, and rained all day, being very heavy in the afternoon, with high wind.
18th. Light rain and mist in the morning. Cloudy in the afternoon. Evening clear and mild.
19th. Very fine.
[illegible] sultry.
21st. Began to rain moderately at sunrise; rain fine and misty, with strong wind. In evening, wind abated; rain increased.
22d. Mist, and occasional light showers.
23d. Clouds, with occasional rain.
24th. Warm and pleasant.
25th. Cloudy; occasional brief sunshine. Sprinkling of rain in the evening.
26th. Pleasant.
27th. Morning foggy. Evening very clear, warm, and mild.
28th. Brief showers from 5 to 6 P. M., with light thunder.
29th. Cool. Evening very clear.
30th. Fine. Evening very clear.

October, 1859. New Moon, 25d. 7h. 25m. P. M.

DAYS.	BAROMETER, REDUCED TO 32° F. Sunrise.	At 2 P. M.	At 10 P. M.	THERMOMETER. Sunrise.	At 2 P. M.	At 10 P. M.	Daily mean.	WINDS. (DIRECTION AND FORCE.) Sunrise.	At 2 P. M.	At 10 P. M.	WEATHER. (TENTHS CLOUDY.) Sunrise.	At 2 P. M.	At 10 P. M.	RELATIVE HUMIDITY.	RAIN AND SNOW IN INCHES OF WATER.
1	30.06	29.93	29.85	44	68	61	57.7	S. W. 1	S. W. 3	S. W. 1	0	3	2	71.5	
S 2	29.80	29.62	29.73	62	67	58	62.3	S. W. 1	S. W. 2	S. W. 1	Rain	10	2	82.9	0.50
3	29.85	29.85	29.86	48	63	53	54.7	N.W'ly 2	N. W. 3	N. W. 1	0	0	0	59.6	
4	29.80	29.76	29.86	53	78	60	63.7	S. W. 2	S. W. 2	S. W. 1	0	0	0	62.3	
5	29.82	29.75	29.58	54	74	59	62.3	S. W. 1	S. W. 2	N.W'ly 1	Foggy	0	9	68.4	
6	29.40	29.62	29.85	58	62	47	55.7	N. W. 2	N. W. 3	N. W. 1	8	2	0	64.3	
7	29.93	29.82	29.84	42	61	52	51.7	N. W. 1	N. W. 2	S. W. 1	1	2	0	61.5	
8	29.74	29.75	29.79	54	49	48	50.3	S'ly 2	N. E. 2	N. E. 2	Rain	Misty	Rain	91.4	
S 9	29.76	29.77	29.88	42	50	47	46.3	N. E. 3	N. E. 2	N. E. 3	Rain	10	1	71.9	2.00
10	29.89	29.83	29.92	41	45	39	41.7	N. E. 2	N. E. 3	N. E. 1	10	10	0	62.1	
11	29.93	29.90	29.98	38	62	47	49.0	N. W. 1	N. W. 2	N. W. 1	0	0	3	55.4	
12	30.10	30.08	30.11	46	60	47	51.0	N. W. 1	N'ly 1	S'ly 1	0	5	0	54.5	
13	30.04	29.94	29.87	50	66	58	58.0	S. W. 2	S. W. 3	S. W. 2	2	10	5	77.4	
14	29.75	29.55	29.60	60	74	55	63.0	S. W. 2	S. W. 3	S. W. 2	7	3	10	68.5	0.12
15	29.68	29.68	30.00	46	56	38	46.7	N.W'ly 1	N. W. 3	N. W. 1	0	5	0	45.1	
S 16	30.16	30.15	30.22	33	48	38	38.0	N. W. 2	N. W. 2	N. W. 1	0	0	0	53.7	
17	30.16	30.05	29.89	38	60	60	52.7	S. W. 1	S. W. 3	S. W. 3	0	10	Rain	62.2	
18	29.72	29.34	29.51	61	65	47	57.3	S. W. 3	S. W. 3	N. W. 4	Rain	Rain	0	75.3	
19	29.56	29.55	29.53	40	50	40	43.3	N. W. 2	N. W. 3	N. W. 1	0	0	10	49.1	
20	29.45	29.41	29.47	37	45	34	38.7	W'ly 3	N. W. 3	N. W. 1	3	0	0	42.6	
21	29.46	29.47	29.59	33	40	38	35.3	N. W. 2	N. W. 3	N. W. 2	8	3	0	33.8	
22	29.61	29.62	29.72	29	46	42	39.0	S. W. 2	S. W. 2	S. W. 1	0	8	10	49.0	
S 23	29.83	29.83	29.93	39	51	40	43.3	N'ly 1	N. W. 1	N. W. 1	9	0	0	59.0	
24	29.97	29.82	29.78	34	54	47	45.0	N. W. 2	S. W. 2	S. W. 2	0	8	7	48.2	
25	29.61	29.44	29.41	45	58	44	49.0	S. W. 2	N. W. 3	N. W. 1	9	10	10	45.8	
26	29.50	29.44	29.35	29	38	33	33.3	N. W. 3	N. W. 3	N. W. 2	2	0	7	42.0	
27	29.31	29.24	29.38	32	44	35	37.0	N'ly 1	N. W. 2	N. W. 1	10	0	0	35.0	
28	29.43	29.47	29.58	33	48	43	41.3	W'ly 1	W'ly 3	W'ly 1	0	5	0	41.1	
29	29.61	29.66	29.82	33	48	35	38.7	N. W. 1	N. W. 2	N. W. 1	0	0	9	37.5	
S 30	29.91	29.92	29.95	33	44	40	39.0	N. W. 1	N. W. 1	W'ly 1	9	10	10	46.3	
31	29.93	29.90	30.00	37	45	40	40.7	W'ly 1	N. W. 1	N. W. 1	10	10	10	45.9	
Means	29.77	29.71	29.77	42.7	55.5	45.8	...	1.7	2.4	1.4	4.5	4.6	3.7	56.9	2.62
									1.8			4.3			
REDUCED TO SEA LEVEL.															
Max.	30.34	30.33	30.40	62	78	61	63.7								
Min.	29.49	29.42	29.59	29	38	33	33.3	Prevailing winds from some point between—		Days.			Days.		
Mean	29.95	29.89	29.95												
Range	0.85	0.91	0.81	33	40	28	30.4	N. & E.		3	Clear		8		
								E. & S.		0	Variable		} 17		
Mean of month	29.931			...	...	...	48.0	S. & W.		10	Cloudy		} 17		
Extreme range	0.98			...	...	...	49.0	W. & N.		18	Rain fell on		5		

REMARKS.

1st. Fine. Evening hazy, and overcast at times. Aurora visible at 7½ P. M.; delicate streamers at N., shooting up 30° or 40°.

2d. Rain in morning; wind light S. W., and warm. Clouds broken in afternoon. Evening mostly clear. At 7 P. M., faint auroral streamers visible.

3d and 4th. Very fine.

5th. Pleasant. Air warm and damp.

6th. Pleasant. 7th. Very fine.

8th. Light rain in morning; wind S'ly. Between 9 and 10 A. M., wind came to N. E. Rained in heavy showers in afternoon and evening, with thunder.

9th. Cloudy in the morning. Evening mostly clear and cool.

10th. Variable. Evening clear. Slight appearance of white frost on College Hill, being the first of the season.

11th. Fine in the morning. Partly overcast in the afternoon and evening.

12th and 13th. Pleasant.

14th. Pleasant. Shower from 7 to 8 P. M.

15th. Wind high and gusty from 3 to 6 P. M. Evening clear and cold, with wind abated.

16th. Cool, but fine.

17th. Cloudy in the afternoon. Light shower in the evening.

18th. Showery till 5 P. M., when the wind came from S. W. to N. W., with heavy clouds and gust of wind. At 7 P. M., mostly clear, and a very brilliant aurora extening from N. W. to N. E. Brilliant streamers, narrow and well defined, shot from the horizon nearly up to the zenith. It continued till late in the evening, but much less brilliant than at first. On the change of wind, the air, from being very damp, became suddenly extremely dry.

19th. Pleasant. Evening overcast.

20th. Cold and blustering. Aurora in the evening low down in N.; not very bright.

21st. Flurry of snow at 1 A. M. Air cold and blustering. Faint aurora in evening, without streamers.

22d. Cloudy in the afternoon.

23d. Very fine.

24th and 25th. Pleasant.

26th. Air raw and cold.

27th and 28th. Very fine.

29th. Pleasant.

30th. Air raw and wintery.

31st. Cloudy. Air chilly.

November, 1859. New Moon, 24d. 8h. 35m. A. M.

DAYS.	BAROMETER Sunrise.	At 2 P. M.	At 10 P. M.	THERMOMETER Sunrise.	At 2 P. M.	At 10 P. M.	Daily mean.	WINDS Sunrise.	At 2 P. M.	At 10 P. M.	WEATHER Sunrise.	At 2 P. M.	At 10 P. M.	RELATIVE HUMIDITY.	RAIN AND SNOW.
1	30.02	30.00	30.01	36	48	35	39.7	W'ly 1	N. W. 1	N. W. 1	5	7	3	53.6	
2	30.01	29.83	29.92	35	52	37	41.3	N. W. 1	N. W. 2	N. W. 1	10	10	0	42.4	
3	30.10	30.14	30.31	35	48	33	39.0	N. W. 1	N. W. 3	N. W. 1	0	0	0	36.8	
4	30.29	30.05	29.99	35	57	51	47.7	S'ly 1	S. W. 3	S. W. 1	10	2	2	65.1	
5	29.95	29.85	29.93	48	70	57	58.3	S. W. 1	S. W. 1	S. W. 1	1	3	2	52.0	
S 6	30.22	30.25	30.42	44	52	36	44.0	N. W. 1	N. W. 2	N. W. 1	0	2	0	39.0	
7	30.44	30.43	30.41	31	50	36	39.0	N. E. 1	S. E'ly 2	S. E. 1	0	0	0	54.7	
8	30.33	30.24	30.17	31	55	46	44.0	N'ly 1	S. E. 2	S'ly 1	0	0	Foggy	75.6	
9	30.08	29.95	29.90	37	62	49	49.3	S. W. 1	S. E'ly 2	S. W. 1	Foggy	2	0	76.1	
10	29.72	29.49	29.38	52	60	58	56.7	S. W. 1	S. W. 1	S. W. 2	Foggy	Sprin'le	10	84.7	
11	29.40	29.65	29.97	52	46	31	43.0	N'ly 1	N. W. 3	N. W. 2	5	0	0	75.0	
12	30.04	29.99	29.70	31	44	52	42.3	N. E. 1	E'ly 1	S'ly 2	5	Sprin'le	10	68.7	
S 13	29.50	29.27	29.30	60	62	38	53.3	S'ly 4	S. W. 4	N. W. 3	10	Rain	Sprin'le	73.7	0.62
14	29.65	29.81	30.02	32	42	32	35.3	N.W'ly 1	W. 2	W'ly 1	0	5	2	53.7	
15	30.08	30.12	30.27	30	44	35	36.3	N. W. 2	S. E. 1	Calm	0	1	1	50.0	
16	30.33	30.31	30.35	35	45	40	40.0	E'ly 1	E'ly 1	Calm	9	Rain	0	72.2	0.10
17	30.31	30.21	30.20	36	53	40	43.0	S'ly 1	S'ly 1	S'ly 1	Foggy	3	2	80.6	
18	30.21	30.00	29.90	39	65	58	54.0	S. W. 1	S. E. 2	S. W. 2	1	1	Rain	73.8	
19	29.67	29.40	29.38	58	60	55	57.7	S'ly 1	S'ly 3	S'ly 1	Rain	Rain	5	85.0	0.30
S 20	29.56	29.70	30.01	49	44	34	42.3	N. W. 2	N. W. 3	N. W. 2	7	0	0	42.4	
21	30.20	30.24	30.21	33	39	36	36.0	N. W. 2	N. E. 2	E'ly 2	1	10	R'n, h'l	44.0	
22	29.82	29.55	29.63	43	46	40	43.0	N. E. 3	N. W. 2	W'ly 2	Rain	10	10	83.3	0.65
23	29.72	29.81	29.91	40	...	36	...	S. W. 1	...	E'ly 1	5	...	10	75.6	
24	30.09	30.11	30.19	33	35	30	32.7	N. W. 2	N. W. 2	N. W. 3	8	10	8	50.0	
25	30.27	30.18	30.08	29	36	35	33.3	N. W. 2	S. W'ly 1	E'ly 1	9	5	10	51.4	
26	29.52	29.50	29.55	46	53	45	48.0	S'ly 2	N.W'ly 2	Calm	Rain	4	0	63.1	0.60
S 27	29.69	29.65	29.65	37	45	40	40.7	W'ly 2	W.byS. 2	W'ly 1	1	8	10	43.7	
28	29.58	29.53	29.81	37	45	33	38.3	S. W. 1	N. W. 2	N. W. 1	5	2	0	42.9	
29	29.91	29.93	30.00	33	43	34	36.7	W.byN. 1	S'ly 1	S'ly 1	5	2	1	42 5	
30	29.93	29.90	29.95	34	55	46	45.0	S. W. 1	S. W. 2	S. W. 1	0	2	6	66.1	
Means	29.95	29.90	29.95	39.1	50.2	40.7	...	1.4	2.0	1.3	5.3	4.8	4.4	60.6	2.27
									1.6			4.7			
REDUCED TO SEA LEVEL.															
Max.	30.62	30.61	30.60	60	70	58	58.3								
Min.	29.58	29.45	29.48	29	35	30	32.7	Prevailing winds from some point between—		Days.			Days.		
Mean	30.13	30.08	30.13												
Range	1.04	1.16	1.12	31	35	28	25.6	N. & E.		1	Clear		6		
								E. & S.		6	Variable		} 15		
Mean of month	29.936			...	...	...	43.3	S. & W.		13	Cloudy		} 15		
Extreme range	1.17			...	...	...	41.0	W. & N.		10	Rain fell on		9		

REMARKS.

1st. Very fine.

2d. Cloudy, with mist and occasional fine rain in the morning.

3d. Raw and cold.

4th. Moderate rain at intervals.

5th. Cloudy and mild; wind light N. W'ly nearly all day.

6th. Light rain all day; more copious in the evening.

7th. Shower in the morning. Pleasant in the afternoon and evening.

8th. Very fine. Evening clear.

9th. Cool, and mostly cloudy.

10th. Very fine.

11th. Air raw and snowy. Heavy black frost this morning; the first of the season to injure dahlias and other hardy plants.

12th. Cold and raw.

13th. Air raw and cold. Began to rain from 8 to 9 P. M.

14th. Ground white with snow this morning. Weather wintry.

15th. Fine snow in the air nearly all day. Mostly clear at 10 P. M.

16th. Blustering and cold.

17th. Fine, but cold.

18th. Cloudy in the morning. Fine in the afternoon and evening.

19th. Pleasant. Evening very clear.

20th. Pleasant.

21st. Began to snow very gently from 7 to 8 P. M.

22d. Very fine.

23d. Raw all day, with wind heavy at N. E'ly.

24th. Raw and damp.

25th. Clear and cold.

26th. Cloudy and cold.

27th. Cloudy, with appearances of storm in the evening.

28th. Began to snow very gently from 10 to 11 A. M., and continued through afternoon and evening.

29th. Between five and six inches of damp snow on the ground this morning.

30th. Dusting of snow from 8 to 9 A. M. Pleasant in the afternoon and evening.

December, 1859. New Moon, 24d. 0h. 39m. A. M.

Days.	Barometer, reduced to 32° F. Sunrise.	At 2 P. M.	At 10 P. M.	Thermometer. Sunrise.	At 2 P. M.	At 10 P. M.	Daily mean.	Winds. (Direction and Force.) Sunrise.	At 2 P. M.	At 10 P. M.	Weather. (Tenths Cloudy.) Sunrise.	At 2 P. M.	At 10 P. M.	Relative Humidity.	Rain and Snow in Inches of Water.
1	29.88	29.78	29.79	46	61	56	54.3	S. W. 1	S. W. 3	S. W. 1	7	9	6	71.4	
2	29.80	29.76	29.74	55	57	56	56.0	S. W. 2	S. W. 2	S. W. 2	10	10	7	82.8	
3	30.21	30.33	30.46	33	28	26	29.0	N'ly 2	N'ly 3	N. E. 2	10	10	Snow	65.5	
S 4	30.35	30.31	30.18	22	27	27	25.3	N. E. 2	N.N.E. 2	N. E. 2	Snow	Hail	Hail	74.8	0.75
5	30.18	30.21	30.27	28	32	30	30.0	N. E. 2	N.byE. 2	N'ly 1	10	Misty	Foggy	81.6	
6	30.22	30.17	30.03	32	35	38	35.0	N. N. E. 1	N.N.E. 1	N. E'ly 1	Misty	Misty	Misty	82.8	
7	29.82	29.60	29.60	53	61	43	52.3	S. W. 1	S. W. 3	N.W'ly 2	Misty	Rain	Rain	84.4	1.10
8	29.71	29.88	30.06	27	23	14	21.3	N. W. 1	N. W. 3	N. W. 3	10	5	0	67.3	
9	30.13	30.10	29.91	11	25	30	22.0	N. W. 1	N. W. 1	S'ly 1	0	2	10	54.4	
10	29.73	29.78	29.89	25	30	19	24.7	N. W. 2	N. W. 3	N. W. 2	0	3	0	50.1	
S 11	29.87	29.73	29.62	16	28	28	24.0	W'ly 1	W'ly 1	W'ly 1	2	10	10	61.0	
12	29.32	29.50	29.87	39	33	13	28.3	S. W. 3	N. W. 3	N. W. 2	1	3	2	34.5	
13	30.07	30.13	30.24	15	28	20	21.0	W'ly 1	W'ly 1	N. W. 1	0	2	3	33.5	
14	30.11	29.87	29.64	18	21	27	22.0	N.byE. 2	N. E. 4	N. E. 2	10	Snow	Snow	58.4	
15	29.78	29.81	30.01	26	33	30	29.7	N. W. 1	N. W. 2	N. W. 1	9	2	1	60.7	
16	30.04	30.07	30.15	27	30	22	26.3	N. W. 1	N. W. 2	N.W'ly 1	2	0	Hazy	60.1	
17	30.13	30.08	29.88	26	35	37	32.7	N'ly 1	N. E. 2	E'ly 4	10	10	10	55.4	
S 18	29.63	29.52	29.67	41	42	39	40.7	E'ly 4	E.by N. 2	W'ly 2	Rain	Rain	10	84.8	0.80
19	29.71	29.71	29.82	38	46	38	40.7	S. W'ly 1	S. W. 2	W'ly 1	10	2	0	56.4	
20	29.78	29.42	29.17	35	34	37	35.3	S'ly 1	S. E. 1	E'ly 1	10	Snow	Rain	79.8	0.30
21	29.43	29.63	29.75	37	36	28	33.7	S.byW. 2	W'ly 3	N. W. 2	7	5	0	48.1	
22	29.75	29.75	29.73	26	34	26	28.7	N. W. 2	N.W'ly 2	N. W. 1	0	1	2	45.9	
23	29.64	29.59	29.57	23	31	22	25.3	W'ly 1	N. W. 2	N. W. 1	1	0	0	46.8	
24	29.55	29.67	29.86	22	20	12	18.0	N. W. 2	N. W. 4	N. W. 2	7	0	0	34.0	
S 25	29.85	29.79	29.74	16	27	26	23.0	W by S. 2	W.byS. 2	S. W. 2	2	5	10	59.8	
26	29.55	29.47	29.57	29	31	34	31.3	N. W. 1	N'ly 2	N'ly 1	10	10	7	58.6	
27	29.78	29.90	30.14	28	25	8	20.3	N. W. 2	N. W. 2	N. W. 2	1	0	0	37.6	
28	30.19	30.17	30.20	1	9	1	3.7	N. W. 2	N. W. 2	N. W. 3	0	10	0	10.1	
29	30.18	30.10	29.95	—2	15	13	8.7	N. W. 2	N. E'ly 1	N. E. 1	5	7	10	41.4	
30	29.53	29.53	29.79	16	22	18	18.7	N. E. 2	N. E. 2	N. W. 1	Snow	10	0	28.2	0.50
31	29.78	29.83	29.92	19	23	12	18.0	W'ly 1	N. W. 2	N. W. 2	9	2	0	37.1	
Means	29.86	29.84	29.88	26.7	31.7	26.8	...	1.6	2.1	1.7	6.2	6.1	5.4	56.4	3.45

Winds, mean force: 1.8. Weather, mean cloudiness: 5.9.

Reduced to Sea Level.

	Barometer Sunrise.	At 2 P. M.	At 10 P. M.	Thermometer Sunrise.	At 2 P. M.	At 10 P. M.	Daily mean.
Max.	30.53	30.51	30.64	55	61	56	56.0
Min.	29.50	29.60	29.35	—2	9	1	3.7
Mean	30.04	30.02	30.06				
Range	1.03	0.91	1.29	57	52	55	52.3
Mean of month	30.041			...	...	...	28.4
Extreme range	1.29			...	...	...	63.0

Prevailing winds from some point between— Days.
N. & E. 9
E. & S. 1
S. & W. 5
W. & N. 16

Days.
Clear 7
Variable . . . } 14
Cloudy . . . . }
Rain or snow fell on 10

REMARKS.

1st. Rain in the morning. Cleared from 5 to 6 P. M. Evening clear.
2d. Very fine.
3d. Air cool, and wind blustering.
4th. Pleasant.
5th. Began to snow from 9 to 10 A. M.; quantity small; ground covered half an inch deep. The first snow of the season.
6th. Snow disappeared during the morning. Began to rain from 3 to 4 P. M., and continued through the evening.
7th. Very fine.
8th. Pleasant. Very mild for the season.
9th. Moderate rain through the day.
10th. Mist and light rain in the morning. Evening very clear.
11th. Cloudy at mid-day. Evening very clear and cold.
12th. Cold, but very fine.
13th. Very fine.
14th. Very fine. Evening very clear.
15th. Mild in the morning. Cloudy and air raw in the afternoon. Evening clear.
16th. Mild. Some flakes of snow in the morning.
17th. Mild for the season.
18th. Moderate rain in morning. Clear at 10 P. M.
19th. Very fine; nearly cloudless.
20th. Very fine. Remarkably clear in the evening.
21st. Clear in the morning. Cloudy in the evening; appearances of storm.
22d. Moderate rain in morning. Sprinkling at 7 P. M. Clear at 10 P. M., with the wind N. W.
23d. Pleasant.
24th. Very blustering.
25th. Cloudy for most part, and air cold.
26th. Began to snow moderately at 7½ A. M., and continued all day.
27th. Five or six inches of light snow on ground in morning. Evening still and cold.
28th. Mild. The thermometer rose 30° between 10 o'clock last night and 10 this morning. Cloudy; wind brisk at S. W.
29th. Began to snow gently from noon to 1 P. M., and continued.
30th. Ground lightly covered with fresh snow this morning. Light rain in evening.
31st. Light rain and mist this morning; wind E'ly. In the afternoon, wind S. W., and clouds broken. Evening blustering and very clear.

January, 1860. New Moon, 22d. 7h. 8m. P. M.

Days.	Barometer Sunrise.	At 2 P. M.	At 10 P. M.	Thermometer Sunrise.	At 2 P. M.	At 10 P. M.	Daily mean.	Winds Sunrise.	At 2 P. M.	At 10 P. M.	Weather Sunrise.	At 2 P. M.	At 10 P. M.	Relative Humidity.	Rain and Snow in Inches of Water.
S 1	30.02	29.98	30.03	5	17	11	11.0	W'ly 1	N. W. 2	N. W. 1	0	2	3	39.8	
2	30.06	30.01	30.11	6	12	3	7.0	N. W. 1	N. W. 3	N. W. 2	2	0	0	44.3	
3	30.18	30.05	30.04	1	17	23	13.7	N. W. 1	N. W. 2	S. W. 3	0	2	10	38.0	
4	30.01	29.93	29.86	20	30	25	25.0	W'ly 2	S. W. 2	W'ly 2	8	10	3	62.2	
5	30.06	30.18	30.41	11	15	12	12.7	N. W. 2	N. W. 3	N. W. 1	1	0	0	7.6	
6	30.29	30.22	30.18	12	27	26	21.7	W'ly 1	S. W. 2	S. W. 2	0	2	3	52.7	
7	30.06	29.95	29.76	28	38	36	34.0	S. W. 2	S'ly 2	S'ly 2	10	10	Rain	79.2	0.20
S 8	29.68	29.60	29.73	42	44	38	41.3	S'ly 1	S'ly 1	W'ly 1	Foggy	Foggy	0	85.9	
9	29.92	29.95	30.08	36	46	34	38.7	W'ly 1	N. W. 1	N. W. 1	2	1	2	66.1	
10	29.96	29.91	29.92	37	50	37	41.3	S. W. 2	S. W. 2	S. W. 1	10	3	Foggy	71.5	
11	29.72	29.65	29.82	37	46	43	42.0	S. W. 3	S. W. 3	S. W. 2	10	10	Sprin'le	71.9	
12	29.90	29.92	29.99	29	27	18	24.7	N. E. 2	N'ly 2	N. W. 1	Snow	Snow	0	78.3	0.40
13	30.06	30.23	30.26	18	21	13	17.3	N. W. 2	N. W. 2	N'ly 1	1	0	10	46.7	
14	30.04	29.67	29.51	18	27	32	25.7	N. E'ly 1	N. E'ly 1	N. E'ly 1	Snow	Snow	Rain	75.1	0.25
S 15	29.43	29.42	29.53	29	36	34	33.0	N. W. 1	W'ly 2	S. W. 1	2	2	0	80.0	
16	29.58	29.59	29.56	36	48	32	38.7	S. W. 1	S. W. 2	S. W. 1	2	0	0	57.0	
17	29.50	29.39	29.53	33	41	31	35.0	N. W. 1	N. W. 1	N. W. 1	8	10	10	92.8	
18	29.63	29.72	29.65	25	35	32	30.7	S. W. 1	S. W. 2	W'ly 1	6	9	0	71.4	
19	29.56	29.62	29.83	31	38	26	31.7	N'ly 1	N'ly 2	N. W. 1	10	10	0	46.9	
20	29.82	29.73	29.69	29	41	39	36.3	W by S. 2	S. W. 3	S. W. 2	5	8	0	54.0	
21	29.51	29.52	29.71	38	52	41	43.7	S. W. 1	S. W. 2	S. W. 1	0	0	0	49.0	
S 22	29.73	29.66	29.68	38	45	36	39.7	S. W. 1	N. W. 1	N. W. 1	5	2	0	66.9	
23	29.76	29.86	30.03	37	43	33	37.7	N. W. 1	N. W. 2	N. W. 1	0	0	0	42.8	
24	30.05	29.96	29.73	30	48	43	40.3	S. W. 1	S. W. 2	S. W. 3	5	7	10	31.7	
25	29.43	29.43	29.65	45	48	35	42.7	S. W. 3	N. W. 3	N. W. 3	10	3	0	39.9	
26	29.83	29.78	29.74	29	34	26	29.7	W'ly 2	N. W. 2	N'ly 2	1	10	Snow	42.0	0.10
27	29.72	29.63	29.63	18	30	27	25.0	N. W. 2	N'ly 1	N. W. 2	4	3	10	47.3	
28	29.64	29.58	29.69	21	30	23	24.7	N. W. 2	S. W'ly 2	N.W'ly 1	3	10	0	44.7	
S 29	29.99	30.03	29.96	15	30	30	25.0	N. W. 2	N. W. 2	S. W. 2	0	0	0	53.7	0.05
30	29.70	29.62	29.76	39	49	37	41.7	S. W. 2	S. W. 2	S. W. 2	3	1	0	52.1	
31	29.75	29.70	29.88	39	52	12	37.7	S. W. 3	S. W. 3	N. E. 4	1	5	Snow	8.4	
Means	29.89	29.86	29.91	26.8	36.0	28.6	...	1.6	2.0	1.6	4.5	4.9	4.0	54.8	0.80

Winds, mean force: 1.7. Weather, mean cloudiness: 4.5.

Reduced to Sea Level.

	Barometer Sunrise.	At 2 P. M.	At 10 P. M.	Thermometer Sunrise.	At 2 P. M.	At 10 P. M.	Daily mean.
Max.	30.47	30.41	30.59	45	52	43	43.7
Min.	29.61	29.57	29.69	1	12	3	7.0
Mean	30.07	30.04	30.09				
Range	0.86	0.84	0.90	44	40	40	36.7
Mean of month	30.065			...	...	...	30.6
Extreme range	1.02			...	...	...	51.0

Prevailing winds from some point between— Days.
N. & E. 2
E. & S. 0
S. & W. 15
W. & N. 14

Days.
Clear 11
Variable . . . } 12
Cloudy . . . . }
Rain or snow fell on 8

REMARKS.

1st. Pleasant, but cold.
2d. Very cold. Bow round the moon.
3d. Morning intensely cold. Warmer towards night; appearances of storm.
4th. Flurry of snow last night. Dusting of snow from 3 to 9 P. M. Clear at 11 P. M.
5th. Cold, but fine. Evening splendid.
6th. Pleasant. Fog-bow round the moon. At 9 P. M., the moon was surrounded by a brilliant, broad corona of dark orange light; and, outside of that, a well-defined rainbow of about 6° or 7° radius, with bright fog-bow.
7th. Mild. Light rain from 6 to 7 P. M.
8th. Thick fog during the day.
9th. Haze in the evening. Fog-bow round the moon.
10th. Mild and pleasant.
11th. Cloudy. Sprinkling in evening.
12th. About six inches of damp snow fell to-day. Evening clear.
13th. Fine.
14th. Light snow. Rain in the evening.
15th. Fine. Evening very clear.
16th. Very fine.
17th. Pleasant. Overcast in evening.
18th. Pleasant morning. Cloudy afternoon. Light flurry of snow from 7 to 8 P. M. Mostly clear at 10 P. M.
19th. Cloudy day. Evening clear.
20th. Pleasant day. Evening clear.
21st. Very mild and fine.
22d. Pleasant.
23d. Fine; evening very clear.
24th. Pleasant in morning. Air raw in afternoon. Evening cloudy.
25th. Mild and variable day. Evening clear; wind blustering from N. W.
26th. Air raw. Began to snow moderately from 10 to 11 P. M.
27th. Variable. Half inch of light snow on ground this morning.
28th. Morning hazy. About noon, a prismatic bow, distinct but not bright, round the sun, together with another bow of much larger dimensions, sweeping from the sun up to the zenith.
29th. Very fine. Half an inch of snow on the ground this morning.
30th. Very fine.
31st. Morning mild. Wind changeable. From 2 P. M. till the morning of Feb. 1st, the ther. fell 48°. There is but one similar instance in my Record. This was in Jan. 1832, when the fall was 49° in 24 hours.

February, 1860. New Moon, 21d. 2h. 36m. P. M.

Days.	Barometer, reduced to 32° F. Sunrise.	At 2 P. M.	At 10 P. M.	Thermometer. Sunrise.	At 2 P. M.	At 10 P. M.	Daily mean.	Winds. (Direction and Force.) Sunrise.	At 2 P. M.	At 10 P. M.	Weather. (Tenths Cloudy.) Sunrise.	At 2 P. M.	At 10 P. M.	Relative Humidity.	Rain and Snow in Inches of Water.
1	29.97	30.00	30.22	4	6	—1	3.0	N. W. 3	N. W. 3	N. W. 1	Snow	5	0	38.1	0.35
2	30.27	30.30	30.31	—1	15	9	7.7	N. W. 2	N. W. 2	N'ly 3	3	10	10	39.4	
3	30.33	30.29	30.23	12	22	18	17.3	N'ly 3	N'ly 1	N'ly 2	9	8	5	67.4	
4	30.15	30.22	30.33	20	26	23	23.0	N. E'ly 1	N'ly 2	N. E'ly 1	Snow	10	8	76.9	
S 5	30.36	30.30	30.14	25	36	34	31.7	N'ly 1	S'ly 2	S'ly 2	10	10	10	72.7	
6	29.77	29.58	29.50	41	43	44	42.7	S'ly 1	S'ly 1	S. E'ly 1	Foggy	Foggy	Foggy	94.1	0.50
7	29.57	29.67	29.85	44	45	35	41.3	N. W'ly 1	N. W. 2	N. W. 1	5	7	0	65.6	
8	29.89	29.82	29.76	28	41	33	34.0	N. W. 2	S. W'ly 1	S'ly 1	1	3	5	64.6	
9	29.69	29.50	29.27	32	42	38	37.3	W'ly 1	S'ly 2	S'ly 1	0	3	10	48.0	
10	29.24	29.38	29.82	18	19	14	17.0	N. W. 5	N. W. 5	N. W. 4	1	0	0	29.6	0.10
11	29.82	29.81	29.70	11	25	21	19.0	N. W. 3	N. W. 1	S. E'ly 2	6	10	Snow	43.9	
S 12	29.70	29.78	30.02	17	25	18	20.0	N. W. 2	N. W. 3	N. W. 2	1	2	0	51.4	
13	29.98	29.73	29.61	20	44	39	34.3	S. W. 2	S. W. 2	S. W. 1	10	5	10	43.7	
14	29.73	29.86	30.00	31	30	22	27.7	N. E. 2	N. E. 1	N'ly 1	10	10	4	53.5	
15	30.06	29.92	29.77	16	30	27	24.3	N. W. 1	N. E. 2	N. E. 3	8	10	Snow	66.4	} 1.00
16	29.59	29.44	29.53	28	29	23	30.0	N. E. 2	N'ly 2	N'ly 3	Snow	Snow	Snow	31.1	}
17	29.55	29.58	29.67	16	17	9	14.0	N. W. 2	N. W. 3	N. W. 2	2	0	0	40.9	
18	29.61	29.43	28.88	7	16	26	16.3	N. W. 2	N. E. 2	N. W. 2	1	Snow	10	72.5	0.62
S 19	29.00	29.18	29.69	24	23	17	21.3	W'ly 2	N. W'ly 3	N. W. 2	10	5	0	63.0	
20	29.95	29.88	29.90	14	33	29	25.3	N. W. 2	S. W. 2	S'ly 1	3	9	1	43.2	
21	29.99	30.04	30.17	24	44	33	33.7	S. W. 2	S. W. 2	S. W. 1	1	0	0	67.9	
22	30.08	29.85	29.58	32	45	50	42.3	S'ly 1	S'ly 2	S'ly 4	9	10	Rain	83.0	0.87
23	29.50	29.34	29.52	45	54	44	47.7	S'ly 1	S. W. 2	W'ly 1	Foggy	10	0	77.5	
24	29.58	29.58	29.68	35	44	33	37.3	N. W. 2	N. W. 2	N. W. 3	2	5	10	62.2	0.10
25	29.74	...	30.00	28	...	28	...	N. W. 2	...	N. W. 3	1	...	1	43.3	
S 26	30.22	30.20	30.27	22	35	31	29.3	N. W. 2	N. W. 2	N. W. 1	0	0	3	42.2	
27	30.22	30.16	30.17	35	50	43	42.7	S. W. 3	S. W. 4	S. W. 2	4	0	5	50.7	
28	30.21	30.20	30.30	39	55	37	43.7	S. W. 1	E'ly 1	E'ly 1	10	9	Hazy	58.3	
29	30.29	30.26	30.17	36	44	39	39.7	N. E. 1	N. E. 1	N. E. 2	Foggy	10	Foggy	75.7	
Means	29.86	29.83	29.86	24.2	33.9	28.1	...	1.9	2.1	1.9	5.8	6.4	5.7	57.5	3.54
								2.0			6.0				
REDUCED TO SEA LEVEL.								Prevailing winds from some point between—		Days.			Days.		
Max.	30.54	30.48	30.51	45	55	50	47.7	N. & E.		6	Clear		5		
Min.	29.18	29.36	29.06	—1	6	—1	3.0	E. & S.		2	Variable		} 15		
Mean	30.04	30.01	30.04					S. & W.		9	Cloudy		}		
Range	1.36	1.12	1.45	46	49	51	44.7	W. & N.		12	Rain or snow fell on		9		
Mean of month	30.040			...	...	...	28.7								
Extreme range	1.48			...	...	...	56.0								

REMARKS.

1st. Snowing moderately at sunrise, with six or seven inches of snow on the ground, much drifted. Clouds broken in the afternoon; intensely cold. Evening clear.
2d. Blustering, cloudy, and cold.
3d. Cold abated. Light snow in the air.
4th. Air full of snow in the morning; a mere dusting on the ground.
5th. Cloudy; air raw and chilly from S'ly.
6th. Thick fog, with occasional light rain. Clouds prevented the lunar eclipse from being observed this evening.
7th. Pleasant. Sky frequently obscured by clouds through the day. Evening clear.
8th. Pleasant, Fog-bow round the moon in the evening.
9th. Pleasant. Evening overcast.
10th. Heavy gale from N. W. all day, and cold.
11th. Wind abated. Cloudy in afternoon. Began to snow at 7 P. M., with wind S'ly.
12th. Pleasant, and mostly clear.
13th. Pleasant, with appearances of storm in the evening.
14th. Appearances of storm in the morning. Evening bright.
15th. Cloudy. Began to snow from 8 to 9 P. M.
16th. Gentle snow all day—nearly nine inches on the level.
17th. Cold, with cutting wind from N.W. Evening very clear.
18th. Clear and cold at sunrise. Began to snow about noon, and continued. Rain and hail in evening. In the morning, wind N.W.; went round through W., S., E., and N. E., and at 10 P. M. came again to N. W., and grew colder. From 2 to 10 P. M., the barometer fell rapidly to 28.95.
19th. Rough and cold. About four additional inches of snow on the ground.
20th. Pleasant.
21st. Very fine. Diffused aurora in the evening, with faint streamers.
22d. Occasional light rain through day. Steady rain in the evening.
23d. Variable. Warm for season. Shower from 5 to 6 P. M. Evening clear.
24th. Variable; sunshine and clouds.
25th, 26th, and 27th. Pleasant.
28th. Very mild; cloudy for most part.
29th. Cloudy; fog morning and evening.

March, 1860. New Moon, 22d. 8h. 47m. A. M.

Days.	Barometer Sunrise.	At 2 P. M.	At 10 P. M.	Thermometer Sunrise.	At 2 P. M.	At 10 P. M.	Daily mean.	Winds Sunrise.	At 2 P. M.	At 10 P. M.	Weather Sunrise.	At 2 P. M.	At 10 P. M.	Relative Humidity.	Rain and Snow in Inches of Water.
1	29.91	29.68	29.59	38	51	53	47.3	N. E. 1	S. by W. 2	S. W. 1	Misty	Rain	10	90.2	0.65
2	29.84	29.66	29.97	46	53	47	48.7	W'ly 2	W by N 2	W'ly 1	0	0	0	60.8	
3	30.11	29.95	29.62	35	47	48	43.3	N. W. 1	S. W. 3	S. W. 3	2	10	Rain	38.1	0.10
S 4	29.50	29.48	29.73	42	52	35	43.0	W by N 2	N. W. 3	N. W. 2	0	2	0	32.5	
5	29.84	29.65	29.48	28	45	42	38.3	N. W. 2	S. W. 2	S. W. 2	0	3	0	54.0	
6	29.56	29.73	29.93	32	46	32	36.7	N. W. 2	N. E'ly 2	N. E. 1	0	0	2	52.6	
7	29.76	29.67	29.67	32	36	36	34.7	S. E'ly 2	S. E. 2	E'ly 2	Snow	Rain	10	62.5	0.25
8	29.67	29.65	29.54	37	46	43	42.0	S. W. 1	S. W. 2	S. W. 2	Foggy	10	10	82.9	
9	29.26	29.18	29.33	34	41	33	36.0	N. E'ly 3	N'ly 3	N. W. 2	Snow	10	2	77.8	
10	29.36	29.37	29.51	28	35	25	29.3	N. W. 2	N. W. 3	N. W. 1	1	3	0	42.2	
S 11	29.58	29.58	29.79	26	41	32	33.0	S. W. 2	W by N. 3	N. W. 1	3	3	0	41.5	
12	29.68	29.50	29.55	36	43	39	39.3	S'ly 2	S. E. 4	N'ly 1	10	Rain	Foggy	76.8	0.75
13	29.59	29.68	29.63	37	36	38	37.0	N'ly 3	N. E'ly 2	N. E'ly 4	10	Misty	10	73.0	
14	29.51	29.50	29.79	34	37	36	35.7	N. E. 4	N'ly 3	N. W. 2	10	Misty	1	57.1	
15	29.94	30.03	30.19	34	52	36	40.7	N. W. 2	S. by E. 2	S. by E. 2	0	0	0	31.6	
16	30.25	30.20	30.20	36	48	35	39.7	S'ly 1	S. by E. 3	S'ly 1	0	0	0	60.7	
17	30.23	30.17	30.21	32	49	39	40.0	S'ly 1	S. W. 2	W'ly 1	Foggy	8	0	75.8	
S 18	30.22	30.18	30.10	33	59	40	44.0	E'ly 1	S'ly 1	S'ly 1	1	0	0	59.7	
19	30.05	29.91	29.83	36	56	38	43.3	N. by E. 2	S. E. 3	E'ly 2	0	0	9	51.4	
20	29.64	29.42	29.45	38	50	38	42.0	N. by E. 1	S. E. 2	N. W. 1	10	Misty	0	74.4	0.05
21	29.43	29.40	29.42	36	43	28	35.7	N. W. 2	N. W. 3	N. W. 3	0	4	0	68.7	
22	29.36	29.34	29.41	25	28	20	24.3	N. W. 2	N. W. 3	N. W. 2	10	Snow	0	53.7	
23	29.41	29.39	29.37	20	43	33	32.0	N. W. 1	N. W. 2	N. W. 2	7	2	3	56.2	
24	29.23	29.20	29.35	30	43	31	34.7	W by N. 2	N. W. 3	N. W. 2	2	5	5	40.9	
S 25	29.39	29.39	29.60	29	36	31	32.0	W by N. 2	N. W. 3	N. W. 1	10	10	0	33.2	
26	29.65	29.65	29.75	27	46	33	35.3	N. W. 2	S. W. 3	N. W. 2	0	3	0	42.7	
27	29.74	29.73	29.80	30	42	31	34.3	N. W. 2	N. W. 2	N. W. 1	10	5	0	37.6	
28	29.69	29.60	29.55	33	53	40	42.0	S. W. 2	S. W. 4	S. W. 3	0	2	8	34.3	
29	29.54	29.53	29.62	32	47	37	38.7	W. 2	W. by S. 3	S. W. 2	5	7	0	49.3	
30	29.64	29.60	29.61	33	67	52	50.7	S. W. 1	S. W. 3	S. W. 3	2	0	0	33.2	
31	29.55	29.34	29.40	47	71	55	57.7	S. W. 2	S. W. 4	S. W. 2	1	2	3	74.5	
Means	29.68	29.62	29.68	33.4	46.5	37.3	...	1.8	2.7	1.9	4.7	5.1	3.0	55.5	1.80
								2.1			4.2				
REDUCED TO SEA LEVEL.								Prevailing winds from some point between—		Days.			Days.		
Max.	30.43	30.38	30.38	47	71	55	57.7	N. & E.		3	Clear		12		
Min.	29.41	29.38	29.51	20	28	20	24.3	E. & S.		7	Variable		} 10		
Mean	29.86	29.80	29.86					S. & W.		10	Cloudy		}		
Range	1.02	1.00	0.87	27	43	35	33.4	W. & N.		11	Rain or snow fell on		9		
Mean of month	29.840			...	...	...	39.1								
Extreme range	1.05			...	...	...	51.0								

REMARKS.

1st. Fog, with warm, southerly rain.
2d. Fine, evening very clear.
3d. Air raw in afternoon. Began to rain moderately from 8 to 9 P. M.
4th. Clear; blustering. Evening splendid.
5th. Pleasant.
6th. Fine. Air growing hazy at 10 P. M.
7th. Snowing at sunrise; turned to rain.
8th. Cloudy. Light shower in evening.
9th. Snow A. M. Clouds broken P. M. Evening clear. Snow disappeared by night.
10th. Blustering. Evening very clear.
11th. Blustering. Evening still and clear.
12th. Rain began from 8 to 9 A. M.; continued moderately till towards night. Stars appeared dimly through fog in evening.
13th. Misty; occasional fine show in air.
14th. Mist; occasional light rain mixed with snow. Clear at 10 P. M
15th and 16th. Very fine. Sky cloudless.
17th. Much overcast through day. Clear evening; diffused aurora at the north.
18th. Very fine. Light haze in morning.
19th. Very fine day. Evening overcast. Frost out of the ground in most places.
20th. Mist; light drizzling rain. Clouds broken at sunset. Very clear at 10 P. M.
21st. Mostly clear in morning. Cloudy in afternoon. Clear at 10 P. M.; air raw and blustering.
22d. Blustering; snow flurries through the day. Clear at 10 P. M., and cold.
23d. Variable. The ground hard frozen and white with snow this morning.
24th. Blustering; sunshine and clouds. Evening mostly clear.
25th. Cloudy through the day. Air very raw and blustering. Evening clear.
26th. Very fine. Wind changeable all day. Soon after 9 P. M., a bright aurora appeared in the north, with occasional short streamers bristling up from a bank of luminous cloud low down in north. A little past 10, the northern heavens were splendidly lighted up with a reddish-pink light; sky almost cloudless. About 11 P. M., sky wholly overcast; not a star visible.
27th. Variable day. Cloudless evening.
28th. More mild. Mostly clear in the morning. Evening cloudy.
29th. Pleasant. Evening clear.
30th. Very warm and summer-like.
31st. Dry haze and smoke, without clouds, and a red sun. Air very warm and dry.

April, 1860. New Moon, 21d. 0h. 37m. A. M.

Days.	Barometer, reduced to 32° F. Sunrise.	At 2 P. M.	At 10 P. M.	Thermometer. Sunrise.	At 2 P. M.	At 10 P. M.	Daily mean.	Winds (Direction and Force.) Sunrise.	At 2 P. M.	At 10 P. M.	Weather (Tenths Cloudy.) Sunrise.	At 2 P. M.	At 10 P. M.	Relative Humidity.	Rain and Snow in Inches of Water.
S 1	29.34	29.16	29.20	47	68	51	55.3	S. W. 2	S. W. 4	S. W. 2	Hazy	Hazy	Rain	54.5	0.05
2	29.36	29.43	29.60	29	34	24	29.0	N. W. 3	N. W. 4	N. W. 2	10	0	0	52.4	
3	29.72	29.59	29.54	22	45	39	35.3	N. W. 2	S. W. 3	S. W. 1	5	3	5	54.1	
4	29.51	29.36	29.29	43	54	47	48.0	S. W. 1	S. E. 2	S. E. 1	Misty	10	Rain	79.8	0.20
5	29.38	29.37	29.50	47	61	47	51.7	W'ly 2	N. W. 3	S. W. 2	Misty	0	2	42.6	
6	29.57	29.60	29.88	41	52	37	43.3	N. W. 2	N. W. 2	N. E. 2	10	Sprin'le	10	66.3	0.30
7	29.98	29.99	30.01	35	53	37	41.7	N. W. 2	S. W'ly 2	S'ly 2	0	2	7	54.5	
S 8	29.96	29.78	29.70	40	45	52	45.7	S'ly 2	S. E. 3	S. E'ly 2	10	Rain	Misty	81.3	} 0.50
9	29.62	29.62	29.88	48	51	44	47.7	N. E'ly 1	N'ly 2	N'ly 2	Foggy	Misty	10	79.1	
10	29.99	29.91	29.66	41	43	41	41.7	N. E. 3	N. E. 2	E'ly 2	10	Rain	10	54.5	
11	29.51	29.50	29.75	43	47	44	44.7	W'ly 2	N. W. 2	N. W. 2	Sprin'le	10	9	62.7	
12	29.83	29.75	29.71	39	60	46	48.3	N. W. 1	N. W. 2	S. W. 2	0	1	10	41.0	
13	29.57	29.55	29.79	42	52	42	45.3	S. W. 2	N. W. 3	N. W. 2	3	4	0	31.7	
14	29.56	29.51	29.79	42	42	30	38.0	W N W 3	N. W. 2	N. W. 2	2	9	0	45.0	
S 15	29.91	29.89	30.08	26	42	34	34.0	N. W. 2	N. W. 3	N. W. 1	0	0	0	21.4	
16	30.11	30.06	29.85	30	45	42	39.0	N. W. 1	S. W. 3	S. E'ly 2	1	10	Rain	72.6	0.40
17	29.66	29.60	29.83	42	64	51	52.3	S. E'ly 1	S. W. 2	N. W. 1	10	2	0	76.2	0.10
18	30.13	30.19	30.27	39	51	41	43.7	N. W. 3	N. W. 4	N. W. 1	0	0	0	17.3	
19	30.27	30.18	30.01	36	53	47	45.3	N. W. 2	S. E'ly 3	S. W. 1	0	1	1	36.8	
20	29.85	29.62	29.64	47	67	52	55.3	S. W. 1	S. W. 2	S. W. 1	7	10	10	65.2	
21	29.50	29.55	29.71	52	48	40	46.7	N. E. 2	N. E. 3	N. E. 2	9	10	10	47.9	
S 22	29.67	29.62	29.66	40	53	44	45.7	N'ly 1	E'ly 2	S. W'ly 2	10	2	10	54.0	
23	29.61	29.59	29.55	43	60	50	51.0	W'ly 2	S. byE. 3	S. E'ly 1	0	10	7	65.3	
24	29.55	29.59	29.61	45	62	35	47.3	N.byE. 2	N. W. 2	N. W. 3	10	3	0	36.4	
25	29.59	29.52	29.56	33	47	36	38.7	N. W. 2	S. W'ly 3	S. W. 2	0	Sprin'le	10	42.5	
26	29.51	29.56	29.89	32	52	41	41.7	N.byW 2	N. W. 3	N. W. 2	8	10	0	46.4	
27	29.87	29.88	30.01	38	58	45	47.0	N. W. 2	N. W. 3	N. W. 1	0	2	0	34.4	
28	30.07	30.03	30.05	40	59	44	47.7	W byN 1	S. E. 3	S'ly 2	1	2	3	51.1	
S 29	30.03	29.98	29.99	42	60	44	48.7	N. E. 1	S. E. 3	N. W. 2	2	2	3	34.3	
30	29.96	29.96	29.96	40	58	39	45.7	N. E. 2	N. E. 4	N. E. 2	1	1	0	46.7	
Means	29.74	29.67	29.76	39.5	52.8	42.2	...	1.8	2.7	1.7	5.3	5.8	5.2	51.6	1.55
								2.1			5.4				
REDUCED TO SEA LEVEL.															
Max.	30.45	30.37	30.45	52	68	52	55.3								
Min.	29.52	29.34	29.38	22	42	24	29.0								
Mean	29.92	29.85	29.94												
Range	0.93	1.03	1.07	30	26	28	26.3								
Mean of month 29.903				...	...	...	44.8								
Extreme range 1.07				...	...	...	46.0								

Prevailing winds from some point between— Days.
N. & E. 4
E. & S. 7
S. & W. 7
W. & N. 12

Days.
Clear 6
Variable . . . } 11
Cloudy . . . . }
Rain fell on . . 13

REMARKS.

1st. Hazy morning. Cloudy afternoon. Moderate rain began at 9 to 10 P. M.
2d. Cold and blustering. Snow on ground.
3d. Weather more mild.
4th. Mist; sprinkling. Rain in evening.
5th. Pleasant.
6th. Clouds and mist. Heavy shower of rain and hail from 4 to 5 P. M.
7th. Air raw and chilly.
8th. Began to rain at 9 A. M., and continued moderately through the day.
9th. Mist and moderate rain.
10th. Mist; occasional sprinkling of rain.
11th. Mist with occasional sprinkling of rain. Stars out in the evening.
12th. Very fine. Evening cloudy.
13th. Blustering at noon. Evening clear. Aurora from 10 to 11 P. M. From 8 to 9 P. M., a massive bank of white light from N. W. to N. E. About 10, streamers began to shoot up, and soon after Merry Dancers played brilliantly all over the northern heavens. This imposing display lasted till near midnight.
14th. Extremely blustering in morning. Rain from 10 A. M. to noon. Evening very clear, and cold for the season.
15th. Blustering, cold, and wintry. The ground hard frozen this morning. Evening nearly cloudless.
16th. Hazy morning. Rain in afternoon.
17th. Showery from 7 to 10 A. M. Clouds broken at noon. Clear evening.
18th. Very clear. Light clouds in S. W.
19th. Pleasant.
20th. Very mild. Cloudy for most part.
21st. Light rain at intervals in morning.
22d. Cloudy for the most part.
23d. Variable and mild.
24th. Sprinkling in morning; cleared before noon. Evening blustering and very clear. Occultation of Venus by the moon.
25th Variable; mostly cloudy. Thick, heavy shower of snow at 6 P. M. Thermometer 31° at 5 A. M.
26th. Variable; blustering and cold. Air filled with snow several times during morning. Evening very clear.
27th. Fine. Evening cloudless.
28th. Pleasant.
29th. Pleasant. Fog-bow around moon.
30th. Mostly clear, with the air raw and cold for the season.

May, 1860. New Moon, 20d. 1h. 38m. P. M.

Days.	Barometer At 6 A. M.	At 2 P. M.	At 10 P. M.	Thermometer At 6 A. M.	At 2 P. M.	At 10 P. M.	Daily mean.	Winds At 6 A. M.	At 2 P. M.	At 10 P. M.	Weather At 6 A. M.	At 2 P. M.	At 10 P. M.	Relative Humidity.	Rain and Snow in Inches of Water.
1	29.94	29.90	29.93	39	59	44	47.3	N. E. 2	N. E. 3	N. E. 2	10	4	10	70.0	
2	29.87	29.93	...	43	61	...	...	N. E. 3	N. E. 3	...	10	4	0	56.2	
3	...	29.85	29.80	...	63	50	...	...	N'ly 2	N. E. 1	...	10	10	27.2	
4	29.71	29.66	29.70	45	66	52	54.3	N. E. 1	N. E. 3	N. E. 1	5	2	0	59.7	
5	29.70	29.67	29.78	48	76	55	59.7	N. E. 2	N. E. 3	S. E. 1	1	2	1	49.7	
S 6	29.76	29.74	29.76	51	76	54	60.3	N. E. 2	S. E. 2	S'ly 1	Hazy	0	5	48.1	
7	29.62	29.70	29.91	52	65	51	56.0	S. E'ly 1	N. E. 2	N. E. 1	5	5	10	61.0	
8	29.93	29.90	29.96	50	60	53	54.3	N. E. 2	S. E. 2	S. E. 1	10	10	10	54.7	
9	29.91	29.96	30.00	52	58	53	54.3	E'ly 1	S. E. 2	S. E'ly 1	10	10	10	57.4	
10	30.03	30.05	30.12	52	68	52	57.3	E'ly 1	S. by E. 3	S. E. 1	10	9	1	55.5	
11	30.11	30.14	30.16	49	69	53	57.0	E'ly 2	S. by E. 3	S'ly 1	5	0	0	69.2	
12	30.10	30.08	30.04	50	73	58	60.3	S. W. 1	S. W. 3	S. W. 1	0	8	5	65.5	
S 13	30.53	29.79	29.76	58	75	57	63.3	S. W. 2	S'ly 3	S. W. 1	4	1	0	64.3	
14	29.67	29.65	29.76	64	58	47	56.3	N'ly 1	N. E. 4	E'ly 2	5	10	7	74.9	
15	29.71	29.77	29.80	45	63	47	51.7	N. E. 2	N. by E. 3	S. E. 2	3	5	5	69.3	
16	29.79	29.87	30.01	46	62	45	54.3	S. E. 1	S. E. 3	S. E'ly 1	5	3	2	40.3	
17	30.07	30.06	30.08	43	62	48	54.3	N'ly 1	S. E. 3	S. E'ly 2	0	0	0	40.3	
18	29.99	29.00	29.73	47	63	56	55.3	S'ly 1	S. E'ly 3	S'ly 1	10	10	Foggy	74.4	
19	29.52	29.26	29.24	59	66	59	61.3	S. by E. 3	S. by E. 3	S. W. 3	Rain	5	0	79.2	0.22
S 20	29.22	29.42	29.70	58	62	49	56.3	W.byS. 4	N. W. 4	N. W. 1	2	1	0	43.9	
21	29.83	29.81	29.81	43	45	42	43.3	N. W. 1	E. 2	E'ly 1	0	Rain	10	67.2	} 0.33
22	29.69	29.75	29.80	46	53	48	49.0	N. E'ly 2	N. 2	E'ly 1	Rain	10	Foggy	73.6	
23	29.80	29.80	29.86	51	69	51	57.0	N. E. 1	N. by E. 2	S'ly 1	Foggy	1	0	56.7	
24	29.88	29.88	29.90	46	64	51	53.7	N by W. 1	S. by E. 2	S. by E. 2	1	8	0	64.7	
25	29.90	29.74	29.74	49	58	59	55.3	N. W. 1	S. E'ly 3	S'ly 1	0	5, Sh'r	0	92.1	
26	29.70	29.70	29.69	58	64	50	57.3	N.by E. 2	N. E. 3	N. E. 1	2	10	Rain	73.7	0.40
S 27	29.67	29.60	29.69	51	59	51	53.7	N. E. 2	N. E. 2	N. E. 2	10	10	10	69.9	
28	29.65	29.63	29.73	51	62	49	54.0	N. E. 2	N. E. 2	N. E. 1	10	8	0	57.1	
29	29.79	29.82	29.90	49	76	55	60.0	N. N. E. 2	N. E. 2	S'ly 1	[illegible]	0	1	[illegible]	
30	[illegible]	[illegible]	[illegible]	[illegible]	[illegible]	[illegible]	[illegible]	[illegible]	[illegible]	[illegible]	[illegible]	[illegible]	Sprin'le	64.0	
31	29.68	29.60	29.57	56	65	60	60.3	S. 2	S'ly 3	S. W. 1	Rain	Misty	Foggy	85.6	0.70
Means	29.49	29.76	29.82	50.2	62.5	51.6		1.7	2.7	1.3	5.7	5.4	4.8	61.9	1.65
								1.9			5.3				
REDUCED TO SEA LEVEL.															
Max.	30.71	30.26	30.08	64	76	60	63.3								
Min.	29.40	29.44	29.42	39	45	42	43.3								
Mean	29.07	29.94	30.00												
Range	1.31	0.82	0.66	25	31	18	20.0								
Mean of month 29.870				...	...	...	54.8								
Extreme range 1.31				...	...	...	37.0								

Prevailing winds from some point between— Days.
N. & E. 15
E. & S. 12
S. & W. 3
W. & N. 1

Days.
Clear 7
Variable . . . } 16
Cloudy . . . . }
Rain fell on . . 8

REMARKS.

1st. Variable; air raw and damp.
2d. Variable. Evening clear.
3d. Cloudy for the most part.
4th. Variable. Evening clear.
5th. Very warm. Air hazy; no clouds.
6th. Warm. Air hazy, with thin clouds in the afternoon and evening.
7th. Hazy. Overcast in the evening.
8th. Cloudy for the most part. Sun visible at intervals. Occasional sprinkling of rain.
9th. Cloudy; air damp. Appearances of rain.
10th. Cloudy in morning. Clouds broken in afternoon. Evening clear.
11th. Very fine. Ground extremely dry for the season.
12th. Warm. Clear in morning. Haze and clouds in afternoon and evening.
13th. Very warm. Still and cloudless in the evening.
14th. Cloudy through the day. A few drops of rain between noon and 1 P. M. Stars appearing in the evening.
15th. Variable. Air very hazy, giving a red appearance to the sun and moon.
16th. Hazy in morning; sun red. Very raw in the afternoon and evening.
17th. Pleasant. Air hazy; no clouds.
18th. Cloudy, with appearance of rain in the evening.
19th. Moderate rain in morning. Clouds broken at 1 P. M. Evening very clear.
20th. Very blustering. Air extremely dry in the afternoon and evening.
21st. Cold and raw; occasional light rain.
22d. Moderate rain last night. Occasional light rain in the morning.
23d. Very fine after 10 A. M. Evening [illegible]
24th. Heavy clouds at mid-day, with some drops of rain. Cloudless and splendid in the evening.
25th. Very clear in the morning. Heavy clouds in afternoon. Light shower at 5½ P. M. Evening still and cloudless.
26th. Variable. Cloudy in the afternoon. Rain at 8 P. M.
27th. Cloudy.
28th. Cloudy A. M. Evening very clear.
29th. Very fine.
30th. Clear in morning. Cloudy in afternoon, and shower in evening.
31st. Rain in morning, mist and fog in afternoon and evening.

SUMMARIES

OF THE

METEOROLOGICAL REGISTER, PROVIDENCE, R. I.

SUMMARIES.

TABLE I.

MONTHLY AND ANNUAL MEAN HEIGHT OF THE BAROMETER.

Reduced to the Sea Level, and to the Temperature of 32° Fahr.

YEARS.	JANUARY.	FEBRUARY.	MARCH.	APRIL.	MAY.	JUNE.	JULY.	AUGUST.	SEPTEMBER.	OCTOBER.	NOVEMBER.	DECEMBER.	MEAN FOR THE YEAR.
1831	. . .	. . .	. . .	. . .	. . .	. . .	. . .	. . .	. . .	. . .	. . .	29.967	. . .
1832	29.991	30.087	29.943	29.885	29.887	29.847	29.823	29.937	29.933	30.010	29.920	29.890	29.929
1833	29.910	29.913	29.943	29.930	29.993	29.837	29.943	29.967	30.027	29.970	30.020	30.080	29.961
1834	30.150	30.037	30.057	29.980	29.920	29.803	29.943	29.883	30.027	30.043	29.923	30.093	30.072
1835	30.007	30.007	29.963	29.827	29.880	29.890	29.897	29.907	29.987	30.060	29.953	29.947	29.944
1836	29.917	29.990	30.017	30.053	29.990	30.003	29.913	29.983	30.023	29.933	29.933	30.067	29.985
1837	29.673	29.833	30.097	29.753	29.933	29.837	29.847	29.883	30.063	30.033	29.917	29.943	29.901
1838	30.050	29.817	29.957	29.843	29.810	29.850	29.867	29.910	30.003	29.867	30.037	29.903	29.910
1839	29.993	30.043	29.933	29.917	30.070	30.060	30.130	30.133	30.093	30.257	30.127	29.713	30.039
1840	29.940	30.067	29.803	30.033	29.877	29.877	29.933	29.930	30.003	29.967	29.880	29.967	29.940
1841	30.023	29.827	29.937	29.913	29.853	29.857	29.897	30.023	29.920	29.900	29.857	29.923	29.911
1842	29.933	29.933	29.950	29.930	29.870	29.930	29.973	30.040	29.943	29.970	29.980	29.980	29.953
1843	30.037	29.870	29.827	29.907	29.917	29.887	29.897	29.967	29.977	29.850	29.983	29.963	29.924
1844	29.877	30.003	29.960	30.120	29.913	29.930	29.853	29.877	29.980	29.963	29.890	29.837	29.934
1845	29.897	29.883	29.910	29.893	29.880	29.877	29.753	29.947	29.903	30.070	29.793	29.930	29.895
1846	29.837	29.910	29.877	30.020	29.847	. . .	29.957	29.997	30.020	30.110	30.023	29.960	29.960
1847	30.070	29.986	29.983	29.970	29.980	29.920	29.980	30.000	29.953	30.080	30.043	30.063	30.002
1848	30.087	29.850	29.983	30.030	29.853	29.837	29.950	30.040	29.910	29.947	30.040	30.050	29.962
1849	30.080	30.133	30.030	29.937	30.017	29.980	30.053	29.990	30.037	29.963	29.943	29.977	30.012
1850	30.067	29.900	29.863	29.913	29.893	29.967	29.967	29.920	29.983	29.900	29.987	29.963	29.944
1851	29.997	30.153	29.977	29.893	30.003	29.933	29.867	30.003	30.107	29.963	29.933	29.970	29.983
1852	29.867	29.877	29.967	29.693	29.950	29.883	29.957	29.990	30.037	30.000	29.920	29.997	29.928
1853	29.943	29.940	29.830	29.933	29.943	30.027	29.987	29.960	29.990	29.977	30.203	29.873	29.884
1854	30.057	30.030	29.883	29.970	29.947	29.903	30.003	29.990	30.063	30.090	29.859	29.863	29.972
1855	30.090	29.887	29.840	29.943	29.917	29.867	29.987	30.027	30.067	29.880	30.040	29.983	29.961
1856	29.893	29.713	29.797	29.943	29.870	29.900	29.937	29.857	29.983	30.020	29.993	29.943	29.821
1857	29.993	30.157	29.907	29.823	29.917	29.773	29.970	29.947	30.047	29.950	29.953	29.987	29.953
1858	30.067	29.953	29.837	29.887	29.990	29.963	29.977	30.000	30.047	30.057	29.887	30.093	29.980
1859	30.110	29.977	29.860	29.823	30.077	30.007	29.987	29.993	30.006	29.931	29.936	30.041	29.985
1860	30.065	30.040	29.840	29.903	29.870	. . .	. . .	. . .	. . .	. . .	. . .	. . .	. . .
MEANS	29.987	29.959	29.923	29.920	29.902	29.905	29.902	29.968	30.003	29.988	29.963	29.964	29.959

TABLE II.

MONTHLY AND ANNUAL MEAN HEIGHT OF BAROMETER AT SUNRISE, OR 6 A. M.; 1 OR 2 P. M.; AND 10 P. M.

29 inches must be added to each entry to make the full height.

YEARS.	JANUARY.			FEBRUARY.			MARCH.			APRIL.			MAY.			JUNE.			JULY.		
	Sunrise.	1 to 2 P. M.	10 P. M.	Sunrise.	1 to 2 P. M.	10 P. M.	Sunrise.	1 to 2 P. M.	10 P. M.	6 A. M.	1 to 2 P. M.	10 P. M.	6 A. M.	1 to 2 P. M.	10 P. M.	6 A. M.	1 to 2 P. M.	10 P. M.	6 A. M.	1 to 2 P. M.	10 P. M.
1831	. .	. .	. .	. .	. .	. .	. .	. .	. .	. .	. .	. .	. .	. .	. .	. .	. .	. .	. .	. .	. .
1832	0.97	0.99	1.02	1.09	1.09	1.18	0.96	0.93	0.94	0.88	0.88	0.88	0.89	0.86	0.91	0.86	0.82	0.86	0.83	0.81	0.83
1833	0.92	0.90	0.93	0.92	0.89	0.93	0.96	0.92	0.95	0.94	0.91	0.94	1.01	0.97	1.00	0.85	0.81	0.85	0.97	0.91	0.95
1834	1.17	1.12	1.16	1.05	1.02	1.04	1.09	1.03	1.05	1 00	0.97	0.97	0.92	0.90	0.94	0.81	0.78	0.82	0.95	0.94	0.94
1835	1.01	1.00	1.01	1.01	0.99	1.02	0.96	0.95	0.98	0.83	0.81	0.84	0.89	0.86	0.89	0.90	0.87	0.90	0.90	0.89	0.90
1836	0.96	0.92	0.87	1.01	0.98	0.98	1.02	1.01	1.02	1.05	1.05	1.06	0.99	0.98	1.00	1.01	0.99	1.01	0.92	0.91	0.91
1837	0.68	0.65	0.69	0.86	0.78	0.86	1.11	1.09	1.09	0.75	0.72	0.79	0.93	0.92	0.95	0.85	0.82	0.84	0.85	0.84	0.85
1838	1.08	1.02	1.05	0.82	0.80	0.83	0.96	0.95	0.96	0.85	0.83	0.85	0.81	0.80	0.82	0.86	0.84	0.85	0.87	0.86	0.87
1839	1.01	0.98	0.99	1.07	1.03	1.03	0.93	0.92	0.95	0.93	0.90	0.92	1.07	1.07	1.07	1.06	1.04	1.08	1.14	1.12	1.13
1840	0.95	0.92	0.95	1.08	1.06	1.06	0.81	0.81	0.79	1.05	1.02	1.03	0.87	0.88	0.87	0.88	0.87	0.88	0.93	0.94	0.93
1841	1.05	1.02	1.01	0.83	0.79	0.83	0.96	0.90	0.95	0.90	0.92	0.92	0.85	0.83	0.88	0.87	0.84	0.86	0.90	0.90	0.89
1842	0.96	0.91	0.93	0.94	0.93	0.93	0.97	0.92	0.96	0.94	0.93	0.92	0.88	0.85	0.88	0.93	0.93	0.93	0.98	0.97	0.97
1843	1.05	1.04	1.02	0.89	0.84	0.88	0.83	0.80	0.85	0.92	0.89	0.91	0.94	0.89	0.92	0.90	0.87	0.89	0.90	0.89	0.90
1844	0.93	0.80	0.90	1.01	0.98	1.02	0.96	0.95	0.97	1.13	1.11	1.12	0.93	0.90	0.91	0.94	0.92	0.93	0.87	0.84	0.85
1845	0.88	0.89	0.92	0.90	0.87	0.88	0.91	0.88	0.94	0.90	0.88	0.90	0.89	0.87	0.88	0.89	0.86	0.88	0.77	0.74	0.75
1846	0.86	0.81	0.84	0.94	0.88	0.91	0.89	0.85	0.89	1.05	1.00	1.01	0.86	0.83	0.85	. .	. .	. .	0.96	0.95	0.96
1847	1.10	1.06	1.05	1.01	0.98	0.97	0.98	0.98	0.99	0.99	0.94	0.98	0.99	0.96	0.99	0.94	0.89	0.93	0.97	0.98	0.99
1848	1.13	1.04	1.09	0.87	0.82	0.86	1.00	0.96	0.99	1.06	1.01	1.05	0.86	0.83	0.87	0.84	0.83	0.84	0.97	0.93	0.95
1849	1.11	1.05	1.07	1.15	1.11	1.14	1.05	1.01	1.03	0.95	0.92	0.94	1.03	1.00	1.02	1.00	0.96	0.98	1.06	1.03	1.07
1850	1.09	1.05	1.06	0.90	0.88	0.92	0.87	0.84	0.88	0.93	0.88	0.93	0.91	0.87	0.90	0.99	0.94	0.97	0.98	0.95	0.97
1851	1.00	0.98	1.01	1.19	1.12	1.15	0.99	0.96	0.98	0.91	0.88	0.89	1.02	0.98	1.01	0.96	0.90	0.94	0.86	0.86	0.88
1852	0.88	0.85	0.87	0.90	0.85	0.88	1.00	0.95	0.95	0.70	0.68	0.70	0.96	0.94	0.95	0.90	0.86	0.89	0.97	0.94	0.96
1853	0.97	0.93	0.93	0.98	0.91	0.93	0.85	0.80	0.84	0.95	0.91	0.94	0.96	0.93	0.94	1.04	1.01	1.03	1.00	0.97	0.99
1854	1.08	1.02	1.07	1.04	1.02	1.03	0.91	0.86	0.88	0.99	0.94	0.98	0.96	0.93	0.95	0.92	0.89	0.90	1.01	0.99	1.01
1855	1.06	1.10	1.11	0.89	0.86	0.91	0.87	0.81	0.84	0.96	0.91	0.96	0.92	0.90	0.93	0.87	0.85	0.88	1.00	0.97	0.99
1856	0.91	0.87	0.90	0.74	0.67	0.73	0.81	0.77	0.81	0.97	0.92	0.94	0.88	0.84	0.89	0.91	0.88	0.91	0.94	0.93	0.94
1857	1.02	0.97	0.99	1.16	1.13	1.18	0.91	0.88	0.93	0.84	0.80	0.83	0.93	0.90	0.92	0.78	0.76	0.78	0.97	0.96	0.98
1858	1.09	1.03	1.08	0.97	0.93	0.96	0.83	0.81	0.87	0.91	0.86	0.89	0.99	0.97	1.01	0.97	0.95	0.97	0.98	0.96	0.99
1859	1.14	1.07	1.12	1.00	0.97	0.96	0.88	0.83	0.87	0.84	0.79	0.84	1.08	1.06	1.09	1.01	0.99	1.02	0.99	0.98	0.99
1860	1.07	1.04	1.09	1.04	1.01	1.04	0.86	0.80	0.86	0.92	0.85	0.94	0.67	0.94	1.00	. .	. .	. .	. .	. .	. .
MEANS	1.004	0.966	0.991	0.974	0.938	0.963	0.936	0.916	0.931	0.932	0.903	0.926	0.927	0.912	0.939	0.916	0.888	0.912	0.941	0.927	0.941
	0.987			0.958			0.928			0.920			0.926			0.905			0.936		

TABLE II—Concluded.

MONTHLY AND ANNUAL MEAN HEIGHT OF BAROMETER AT SUNRISE, OR 6 A. M.; 1 OR 2 P. M.; AND 10 P. M.

29 inches must be added to each entry to make the full height.

YEARS.	AUGUST.			SEPTEMBER.			OCTOBER.			NOVEMBER.			DECEMBER.			FOR THE YEAR.		
	6 A. M.	1 to 2 P. M.	10 P. M.	6 A. M.	1 to 2 P. M.	10 P. M.	Sun-rise.	1 to 2 P. M.	10 P. M.	Sun-rise.	1 to 2 P. M.	10 P. M.	Sun-rise.	1 to 2 P. M.	10 P. M.	Sun-rise.	1 to 2 P. M.	10 P. M.
1831	. .	. .	. .	. .	. .	. .	. .	. .	. .	. .	. .	. .	0.97	0.92	1.01	. .	. .	. .
1832	0.94	0.93	0.94	0.95	0.92	0.93	1.02	1.00	1.01	0.93	0.91	0.92	0.93	0.92	0.95	0.938	0.922	0.947
1833	0.97	0.96	0.97	1.04	1.00	1.04	0.99	0.94	0.98	1.03	1.02	1.01	1.09	1.06	1.09	0.974	0.941	0.973
1834	0.89	0.87	0.89	1.03	1.01	1.04	1.07	1.02	1.04	0.94	0.91	0.92	1.01	0.96	1.01	0.994	0.961	0.985
1835	0.91	0.90	0.91	0.99	0.97	1.00	1.07	1.04	1.07	0.98	0.93	0.95	0.97	0.93	0.94	0.952	0.920	0.951
1836	0.99	0.98	0.98	1.03	1.01	1.03	0.95	0.90	0.95	0.95	0.92	0.93	1.08	1.04	1.08	0.997	0.974	0.985
1837	0.88	0.88	0.89	1.07	1.06	1.06	1.05	1.00	1.05	0.92	0.92	0.91	0.96	0.91	0.96	0.909	0.883	0.912
1838	0.91	0.90	0.92	1.00	0.99	1.02	0.88	0.84	0.88	1.04	1.01	1.06	0.90	0.88	0.93	0.923	0.893	0.920
1839	1.14	1.13	1.13	1.10	1.08	1.10	1.27	1.25	1.25	1.13	1.11	1.14	0.92	0.86	0.90	1.064	1.041	1.058
1840	0.94	0.93	0.92	1.01	0.98	1.02	0.99	0.96	0.98	0.89	0.87	0.88	0.97	0.96	0.97	0.947	0.933	0.957
1841	1.02	1.01	1.05	0.93	0.91	0.92	0.88	0.89	0.93	0.87	0.84	0.86	0.93	0.93	0.91	0.916	0.898	0.918
1842	1.05	1.05	1.02	0.97	0.91	0.95	0.99	0.94	0.98	1.00	0.96	0.98	0.99	0.96	0.99	0.967	0.938	0.953
1843	0.98	0.95	0.97	0.98	0.96	0.99	0.87	0.81	0.87	1.01	0.96	0.98	0.99	0.94	0.96	0.938	0.962	0.928
1844	0 88	0.86	0.89	1.00	0.96	0.98	0.98	0.94	0.97	0.91	0.88	0.88	0.84	0.84	0.83	0.940	0.915	0.938
1845	0.96	0.92	0.96	0.91	0.92	0.88	1.09	1.05	1.07	0.80	0.75	0.83	0.94	0.91	0.94	0.903	0.878	0.902
1846	1.01	0.99	0.99	1.04	1.00	1.02	1.14	1.08	1.11	1.03	1.00	1.04	0.98	0.94	0.96	0.978	0.939	0.962
1847	1.01	0.99	1.00	0.98	0.91	0.97	1.11	1.04	1.09	1.07	1.01	1.05	1.07	1.05	1.07	1.018	0.983	1.007
1848	1.03	1.01	1.08	0.92	0.89	0.92	0.98	0.92	0.94	1.06	1.00	1.06	1.08	1.03	1.04	0.983	0.939	0.974
1849	1.00	0.98	0.99	1.05	1.02	1.04	0.97	0.93	0.99	0.97	0.92	0.94	1.01	0.96	0.96	1.029	0.991	1.014
1850	0.93	0.91	0.92	1.00	0.94	1.01	0.92	0.87	0.91	1.00	0.97	0.99	0.97	0.93	0.99	0.958	0.919	0.954
1851	1.02	0.99	1.00	1.12	1.08	1.12	0.98	0.94	0.97	0.95	0.91	0.94	0.99	0.95	0.97	0.999	0.963	0.997
1852	1.00	0.97	1.00	1.05	1.02	1.04	1.03	0.98	0.99	0.94	0.89	0.93	0.99	1.00	0.99	0.943	0.903	0.889
1853	0.97	0.95	0.96	1.00	0.98	0.99	1.00	0.95	0.98	1.22	1.18	1.21	0.90	0.84	0.88	0.987	0.947	0.960
1854	1.01	0.97	0.99	1.07	1.05	1.07	1.14	1.05	1.08	0.87	0.82	0.88	0.87	0.83	0.89	0.989	0.948	0.978
1855	1.04	1.02	1.02	1.08	1.04	1.08	0.89	0.85	0.90	1.04	1.03	1.05	1.00	0.97	0.98	0.968	0.943	0.968
1856	0.86	0.84	0.87	1.00	0.97	0.98	1.03	1.00	1.03	1.01	0.96	1.01	0.96	0.93	0.94	0.902	0.882	0.913
1857	0.95	0.95	0.94	1.05	1.03	1.06	0.96	0.93	0.96	0.97	0.93	0.96	1.00	0.95	1.01	0.962	0.933	0.962
1858	0.99	0.99	1.02	1.05	1.02	1.07	1.07	1.02	1.08	0.90	0.86	0.90	1.11	1.08	1.09	0.988	0.957	0.994
1859	1.01	0.97	1.00	1.01	0.99	1.03	0.95	0.89	0.95	1.13	1.08	1.13	1.04	1.02	1.06	1.007	0.970	1.005
1860	. .	. .	. .	. .	. .	. .	. .	. .	. .	. .	. .	. .	. .	. .	. .	. .	. .	. .
MEANS	0.975	0.955	0.972	1.015	0.976	1.013	1.009	0.965	1.000	0.984	0.948	0.994	0.981	0.948	0.976	0.967	0.938	0.962
	0.967			1.001			0.991			0.975			0.968			0.956		

TABLE III.

MONTHLY AND ANNUAL MEAN TEMPERATURES.

YEARS.	JANUARY.	FEBRUARY.	MARCH.	APRIL.	MAY.	JUNE.	JULY.	AUGUST.	SEPTEMBER.	OCTOBER.	NOVEMBER.	DECEMBER.	MEAN FOR THE YEAR.
1831	. .	. .	. .	. .	. .	. .	. .	. .	. .	. .	. .	18.2	. .
1832	28.2	27.6	35.4	40.8	54.2	62.4	64.4	68.4	60.3	51.4	40.8	31.0	47.08
1833	31.8	26.1	31.7	48.3	59.1	62.8	70.1	66.7	61.8	50.7	37.5	30.7	48.11
1834	23.3	33.0	36.1	46.7	52.8	63.6	73.1	69.3	62.8	48.1	37.7	27.5	47.83
1835	25.9	23.5	30.2	41.1	54.9	64.9	71.1	67.9	57.4	54.5	37.7	22.1	45.98
1836	25.4	18.5	30.0	43.1	54.9	59.9	69.5	65.2	60.6	44.6	35.4	28.3	44.62
1837	21.3	24.7	30.3	43.7	54.1	64.2	67.9	65.9	58.1	48.3	39.2	28.2	45.50
1838	32.5	17.9	35.1	40.8	53.5	68.4	75.0	71.0	62.0	47.5	35.3	26.1	47.09
1839	26.3	27.9	34.9	46.7	56.0	62.2	71.7	67.9	62.5	51.5	37.1	30.6	47.94
1840	18.6	32.9	36.0	47.8	57.3	66.6	72.2	71.0	59.4	51.3	39.2	27.7	48.32
1841	30.5	25.1	35.1	42.2	54.1	67.9	70.3	69.2	63.3	45.8	37.5	32.8	47.82
1842	30.9	34.4	39.7	46.3	53.8	64.1	72.9	68.5	60.0	51.0	38.6	29.2	49.12
1843	34.2	22.4	28.7	45.3	54.6	64.5	68.9	69.9	61.3	49.2	37.7	31.1	47.32
1844	20.4	28.2	36.3	50.6	58.5	64.7	68.6	68.1	59.8	50.0	39.3	32.8	48.09
1845	30.7	28.5	36.8	44.6	54.3	64.7	69.1	68.4	57.9	50.8	42.5	24.9	47.77
1846	27.3	21.7	35.6	46.3	53.3	60.6	67.4	71.3	66.2	50.3	44.7	29.8	47.87
1847	29.4	28.8	32.4	43.0	54.3	65.8	72.4	69.2	62.5	50.0	46.1	37.6	49.29
1848	32.3	27.4	34.3	46.8	58.9	66.1	70.2	76.2*	59.7	51.3	37.8	37.3	49.86
1849	24.5	22.4	37.0	43.7	54.2	67.5	71.7	70.6	60.5	50.9	47.5	31.2	48.48
1850	30.5	32.2	34.0	43.1	52.3	67.2	72.4	67.8	60.7	52.9	43.5	29.3	48.99
1851	29.8	32.1	38.5	46.3	56.4	64.2	70.6	67.7	61.0	52.5	36.9	25.5	48.46
1852	23.9	28.6	34.8	41.8	57.1	67.7	72.4	66.6	62.6	52.4	39.6	37.8	48.94
1853	28.3	30.5	36.0	44.4	57.0	66.9	70.6	69.2	62.5	49.4	42.6	28.6	48.83
1854	26.4	25.6	33.1	42.9	57.7	65.9	72.9	68.6	61.4	52.9	40.7	26.5	47.88
1855	30.0	22.1	32.6	44.1	54.5	65.2	72.9	67.9	61.9	52.4	42.0	32.2	48.15
1856	18.6	22.7	27.8	46.5	53.5	67.7	72.1	69.8	63.2	50.2	39.4	25.5	46.83
1857	16.3	32.7	32.2	40.1	52.8	62.0	69.9	66.8	68.3	50.5	42.3	34.6	47.38
1858	33.1	24.5	32.8	46.2	53.3	67.7	69.8	66.4	62.2	54.2	37.2	32.1	48.29
1859	[illegible]	24.5	[illegible]	44.2	55.0	[illegible]	[illegible]	[illegible]	[illegible]	[illegible]	[illegible]	[illegible]	47.66
1860	30.6	28.7	39.1	44.8	54.8	. .	. .	. .	. .	. .	. .	. .	. .
MEANS	27.38	26.78	34.46	44.91	55.17	64.97	70.69	68.74	61.41	50.45	39.98	33.02	48.19

* 13 days omitted.

TABLE IV.

MONTHLY AND ANNUAL MEAN TEMPERATURES AT THE THREE HOURS OF DAILY OBSERVATION, VIZ: SUNRISE, OR 6 A. M.; 1 OR 2 P. M.; AND 10 P. M.

YEARS.	JANUARY.			FEBRUARY.			MARCH.			APRIL.			MAY.			JUNE.			JULY.		
	Sun-rise.	1 to 2 P. M.	10 P. M.	Sun-rise.	1 to 2 P. M.	10 P. M.	Sun-rise.	1 to 2 P. M.	10 P. M.	6 A. M.	1 to 2 P. M.	10 P. M.	6 A. M.	1 to 2 P. M.	10 P. M.	6 A. M.	1 to 2 P. M.	10 P. M.	6 A. M.	1 to 2 P. M.	10 P. M.
1831	. .	. .	. .	. .	. .	. .	. .	. .	. .	. .	. .	. .	. .	. .	. .	. .	. .	. .	. .	. .	. .
1832	23.3	34.8	26.5	23.9	32.4	26.5	29.8	42.6	33.7	35.1	48.0	39.3	47.4	60.5	49.4	55.5	71.8	60.0	59.2	70.1	64.0
1833	29.0	36.7	29.8	19.9	30.4	28.0	26.1	39.3	29.9	40.5	59.5	44.9	53.2	67.9	56.2	57.2	72.1	59.0	64.5	78.6	67.3
1834	19.5	28.0	22.6	28.2	38.7	32.0	30.3	43.5	34.4	40.6	55.2	44.3	46.3	61.6	50.5	57.6	72.1	62.1	67.4	81.2	70.8
1835	22.2	30.6	24.7	19.6	28.4	22.3	25.6	37.8	27.2	36.7	50.4	40.3	47.9	62.9	52.6	59.1	71.2	59.9	65.5	78.7	69.1
1836	22.5	29.7	24.0	13.7	24.5	17.4	24.9	36.6	28.3	36.9	51.3	51.0	48.8	64.7	51.2	54.5	67.8	57.5	64.6	76.3	67.5
1837	16.7	26.7	20.5	21.3	29.7	23.5	25.4	36.4	29.1	37.6	52.0	41.4	47.7	63.4	51.3	58.7	72.4	61.4	62.4	76.1	65.1
1838	28.6	38.0	30.9	12.3	24.4	17.0	30.1	42.4	32.7	34.3	49.2	39.3	47.0	62.5	50.9	63.6	77.2	69.4	69.4	83.7	71.9
1839	22.0	32.5	24.7	23.9	33.0	26.8	29.3	42.6	32.7	40.5	55.6	44.1	50.6	64.5	52.9	56.7	70.3	54.5	67.1	78.5	69.3
1840	14.5	23.9	17.5	28.5	38.1	32.0	30.9	42.7	34.4	41.1	57.2	45.0	53.2	66.2	52.4	61.0	75.0	63.9	67.4	79.8	69.4
1841	27.2	34.4	30.0	20.2	32.2	22.9	29.5	42.3	33.4	37.5	48.7	40.4	48.2	63.2	51.0	61.8	76.1	65.8	64.8	78.2	67.8
1842	26.5	36.2	29.9	30.3	40.1	32.7	34.8	46.3	38.0	41.2	53.5	44.1	47.9	61.7	51.7	58.3	71.8	62.1	68.1	81.1	69.6
1843	30.1	38.7	33.6	18.3	27.5	21.5	24.1	34.4	27.5	41.0	51.5	43.5	49.7	63.1	50.9	58.7	73.7	61.2	62.7	77.5	66.5
1844	16.9	24.5	19.7	22.9	34.6	27.2	32.6	41.6	34.8	43.3	60.1	47.6	52.9	66.9	55.8	59.0	74.2	61.0	63.0	77.4	65.5
1845	28.6	34.7	29.0	23.9	34.3	27.3	32.1	44.0	34.4	39.7	51.6	42.1	48.5	62.6	51.7	58.7	74.2	61.1	63.5	77.8	66.1
1846	23.6	31.9	26.5	17.6	27.2	20.3	30.2	42.6	34.1	39.1	55.8	44.0	48.0	61.0	50.7	55.2	69.6	57.0	62.5	75.6	64.2
1847	25.7	33.9	28.5	23.9	34.7	27.9	27.7	37.8	31.7	36.6	51.6	40.8	48.1	63.3	51.5	60.4	74.1	62.9	66.5	81.3	69.3
1848	28.7	36.9	31.4	22.7	33.2	26.2	29.1	40.6	33.3	40.7	56.3	43.3	53.5	67.0	56.1	59.9	75.1	63.4	64.6	79.0	66.9
1849	20.7	29.0	23.9	17.9	27.8	21.3	32.0	43.1	36.0	39.1	50.4	41.8	48.0	64.5	50.1	60.8	78.0	63.6	65.4	82.3	67.4
1850	26.1	35.5	29.8	27.4	38.2	30.8	29.8	39.6	32.6	38.0	51.6	39.6	47.7	60.0	49.3	60.7	78.3	62.6	66.7	81.6	68.8
1851	26.1	35.6	27.7	27.5	37.6	31.1	33.7	46.3	35.6	40.7	54.4	43.8	50.6	66.4	52.2	58.7	74.3	59.7	66.3	79.2	66.3
1852	20.5	29.0	22.3	24.0	34.6	27.2	29.7	41.3	33.3	37.2	49.0	39.3	51.9	67.0	52.5	63.1	77.5	62.5	67.0	83.7	66.6
1853	24.4	33.6	27.0	26.8	35.4	29.2	32.3	40.5	35.1	39.7	52.0	41.5	51.7	66.7	52.6	60.8	77.6	62.3	65.7	79.3	66.7
1854	23.1	31.2	24.8	21.4	30.4	24.9	28.1	40.1	31.1	38.0	51.3	39.5	53.0	66.3	53.8	61.0	75.1	61.5	67.8	81.4	69.4
1855	26.5	35.0	28.4	18.6	27.3	20.5	27.5	39.4	30.8	38.7	52.5	41.0	49.2	63.5	50.3	61.7	72.0	62.1	69.4	80.4	69.0
1856	14.4	24.6	16.9	19.2	28.9	20.0	23.1	34.7	25.5	41.4	56.7	41.7	48.3	62.2	50.0	62.6	76.5	64.1	66.7	81.1	68.4
1857	11.9	22.0	15.0	28.8	39.3	29.9	26.9	39.6	30.0	35.9	49.0	38.2	46.5	59.7	49.2	58.5	68.8	58.7	66.1	76.6	67.0
1858	29.4	38.3	31.7	20.1	30.3	23.1	27.5	40.3	30.6	40.5	54.7	43.4	49.6	60.7	49.8	62.5	76.2	64.5	65.3	77.5	66.7
1859	28.0	32.6	27.2	29.1	35.7	30.1	36.1	46.7	38.9	39.1	51.5	41.9	53.1	64.5	53.0	59.9	70.7	60.6	63.5	78.2	65.8
1860	26.8	36.0	28.6	24.2	33.9	28.1	33.4	46.5	37.3	39.5	52.8	42.2	50.2	62.5	51.8	. .	. .	. .	. .	. .	. .
MEANS	23.57	32.23	25.97	22.83	32.51	25.78	29.40	41.09	32.98	38.97	52.88	42.05	49.27	63.69	51.77	59.51	73.70	61.58	65.47	81.54	67.59
	27.26			27.04			34.49			44.97			54 91			64.93			71.53		

TABLE IV—Concluded.

MONTHLY AND ANNUAL MEAN TEMPERATURES AT THE THREE HOURS OF DAILY OBSERVATION, VIZ: SUNRISE, OR 6 A. M.; 1 OR 2 P. M.; AND 10 P. M.

YEARS.	AUGUST.			SEPTEMBER.			OCTOBER.			NOVEMBER.			DECEMBER.			FOR THE YEAR.		
	6 A. M.	1 to 2 P. M.	10 P. M.	6 A. M.	1 to 2 P. M.	10 P. M.	Sun-rise.	1 to 2 P. M.	10 P. M.	Sun-rise.	1 to 2 P. M.	10 P. M.	Sun-rise.	1 to 2 P. M.	10 P. M.	Sun-rise.	1 to 2 P. M.	10 P. M.
1831	. .	. .	. .	. .	. .	. .	. .	. .	. .	. .	. .	. .	14.4	22.7	17.5	. .	. .	. .
1832	63.2	76.1	65.9	54.8	68.0	58.0	45.8	58.8	49.6	37.2	46.4	38.8	28.2	34.5	30.2	42.70	53.82	45.16
1833	61.3	74.4	64.4	56.0	70.4	59.0	45.7	57.7	48.8	32.3	43.9	36.2	27.3	34.8	30.1	42.75	55.78	46.13
1834	63.6	77.3	66.9	57.8	70.4	60.1	42.0	55.8	48.1	33.1	43.5	36.4	24.6	32.1	25.9	42.58	54.87	46.26
1835	62.9	75.4	65.4	50.3	67.2	54.7	48.6	62.7	52.3	34.9	45.1	38.3	18.6	26 6	21.1	40.99	53.08	42.33
1836	59.8	73.4	62.7	55.9	67.6	59.0	38.4	53.2	42.0	30.4	41.9	34.1	24.0	34.2	26.6	39.53	51.77	42.61
1837	61.3	73.0	63.4	51.0	67.7	55.7	42.4	56.0	46.5	33.9	46.2	37.5	23.4	34.3	29.9	40.15	52.82	43.77
1838	65.2	79.8	68.1	58.0	68.9	59.0	42.5	55.2	44.9	31.0	41.2	33.5	22.0	31.8	24.4	41.92	54.53	44.07
1839	63.7	74.4	65.5	56.2	70.7	60.7	44.9	60.0	49.8	32.6	42.8	35.9	27.9	34.9	29.1	42.95	54.98	46.22
1840	65.7	78.1	69.1	53.1	68.2	56.9	46.2	58.3	49.4	35.1	44.6	37.8	22.9	33.4	26.9	43.30	55.46	46.45
1841	63.9	75.8	67.8	59.0	69.4	61.4	40.3	53.3	43.8	34.2	42.5	35.7	29.5	38.0	31.0	43.01	54.51	45.92
1842	64.6	74.4	60.6	54.4	68.2	57.5	44.2	60.0	48.8	34.6	44.4	36.7	27.2	32.2	28.1	44.34	55.83	47.15
1843	65.2	76.8	67 6	56.0	68.7	59.2	44.4	55.7	47.6	32.9	43.9	36.4	27.9	35.5	29.8	42.59	53.92	45.44
1844	62.1	76.9	65.2	53.8	68.5	57.0	45.5	56.2	48.4	35.9	43.7	38.3	29.3	37.0	32.0	43.03	55.20	46.04
1845	63.2	77.1	65.1	52.7	64.5	56.5	45.5	58.4	48.4	39.0	48.0	40.6	22.4	29.1	23.2	43.15	54.69	45.46
1846	66.6	79.4	67.9	60.5	74.5	63.5	43.8	58.1	49.0	41.5	49.7	42.9	26.1	33.8	29.5	42.89	54.93	45.80
1847	63.6	77.3	66.8	59.7	68.0	59.8	44.2	58.1	47.7	41.6	52.7	43.9	33.7	43.2	36.0	44.14	56.34	47.23
1848	74.8	82.8	71.0	53.5	68.4	57.1	46.0	58.6	49.2	33.9	44.3	35.3	34.0	41.8	36.0	45.12	57.00	47.43
1849	65.3	78.6	68.0	54.2	70.1	57.1	46.6	57.1	49.1	42.7	53.5	46.2	27.6	35.6	30.4	43.35	55.83	47.16
1850	61.7	76.8	65.0	55.4	69.3	57.5	47.2	61.4	50.0	39.2	50.4	40.9	25.5	34.3	28.2	43.78	56.42	47.93
1851	62.9	76.5	63.8	55.2	70.1	57.6	46.8	60.4	50.3	32.4	43.1	35.1	21.3	30.3	25.0	43.68	56.18	45.68
1852	61.5	75.3	62.9	57.5	70.8	59.5	47.7	59.5	50.1	36.4	44.3	38.1	34.5	42.8	36.1	44.25	56.23	46.70
1853	64.9	76.8	66.8	58.0	70.0	59.4	43.3	58.0	47.0	38.2	49.7	39.8	24.6	34.4	26.8	44.20	56.17	47.85
1854	63.1	77.3	65.5	57.4	69.4	57.4	47.6	60.8	50.4	36.9	47.0	38.3	23.0	31.8	24.8	43.37	55.01	45.12
1855	63.1	76.9	63.7	56.3	72.4	57.1	47.6	59.8	49.9	38.0	47.6	40.5	28.8	36.5	31.2	43.78	55.28	45.46
1856	64.0	76.3	69.2	56.7	73.4	59.6	44.3	59.3	46.9	34.9	45.7	37.7	21.9	30.0	24.5	41.46	54.12	43.71
1857	62.5	73.3	64.7	55.3	68.6	56.9	45.2	57.9	48.4	37.6	48.7	40.6	31.9	39.4	32.5	42.26	53.58	44.18
1858	62.2	73.1	64.0	56.6	70.6	59.3	49.0	61.9	51.6	34.3	41.7	35.7	28.3	36.4	31.5	43.78	55.14	45.99
1859	66.1	77.0	64.5	54.3	67.7	56.9	42.7	55.5	45.8	39.1	50.2	40.7	26.7	31.7	26.8	44.81	55.25	46.02
1860	. .	. .	. .	. .	. .	. .	. .	. .	. .	. .	. .	. .	. .	. .	. .	. .	. .	. .
MEANS	63.86	76.44	65.84	56.70	60.35	58.34	44.94	53.95	48.35	35.85	45.95	38.28	20.12	34.24	28.11	42.998	54.955	45.688
	68.71			61.13			49.08			40.03			20.49			47.880		

TABLE V.

MONTHLY AND ANNUAL MAXIMUM AND MINIMUM TEMPERATURES, AND RANGE.

YEARS.	JANUARY.			FEBRUARY.			MARCH.			APRIL.			MAY.			JUNE.			JULY.		
	Max.	Min.	Range.	Max.	Min.	Range.	Max.	Min.	Range.	Max.	Min.	Range.	Max.	Min.	Range.	Max.	Min.	Range.	Max.	Min.	Range.
1831	. .	. .	. .	. .	. .	. .	. .	. .	. .	. .	. .	. .	. .	. .	. .	. .	. .	. .	. .	. .	. .
1832	54	—7	61	57	—1	58	59	12	47	77	20	57	82	36	46	88	45	43	89	51	38
1833	63	0	63	46	2	44	61	—4	65	82	26	56	87	38	49	83	46	37	91	56	35
1834	51	2	49	54	2	52	66	18	48	75	29	46	78	30	48	85	47	38	93	55	38
1835	53	—9	62	55	0	55	61	—2	63	70	21	49	86	36	50	80	45	35	88	50	38
1836	43	2	41	45	—6	51	49	10	39	68	20	48	81	34	47	84	37	47	89	52	37
1837	44	0	44	41	—4	45	51	4	47	71	27	44	80	28	52	82	45	37	88	57	31
1838	58	3	55	39	1	38	61	15	46	67	23	44	74	36	38	91	50	41	96	58	38
1839	53	—8	61	52	2	50	64	5	59	73	27	46	78	34	44	82	44	38	88	60	28
1840	40	—4	44	61	—5	66	68	8	60	75	28	47	88	36	52	85	45	40	90	58	32
1841	53	0	53	45	2	43	63	11	52	68	24	44	80	34	46	90	42	48	87	54	33
1842	52	3	49	58	9	49	68	15	53	80	23	57	76	36	40	83	43	40	90	58	32
1843	54	8	46	43	2	41	46	12	34	67	25	42	75	42	33	87	41	46	89	54	35
1844	46	—1	47	49	7	42	57	12	45	78	23	55	82	39	43	89	48	41	84	56	28
1845	50	7	43	53	2	51	70	15	55	72	30	42	89	37	52	90	50	40	89	49	40
1846	47	—1	48	44	—2	46	57	8	49	76	28	48	73	37	36	83	45	38	92	50	42
1847	50	7	43	51	6	45	52	17	35	82	15	67	76	35	41	90	49	41	93	52	41
1848	55	—4	59	47	2	45	64	8	56	69	28	41	88	42	46	91	44	47	90	55	35
1849	53	—4	57	45	—1	46	62	17	45	65	24	41	82	39	43	97	47	50	97	51	46
1850	51	9	42	52	0	52	58	11	47	69	25	44	76	39	37	93	45	48	92	54	38
1851	54	1	53	55	0	55	73	17	56	68	30	38	85	35	50	90	46	44	90	52	38
1852	44	—2	46	54	2	52	58	10	48	65	27	38	87	37	50	94½	50	44½	95	56	39
1853	53	6	47	58	7	51	62	10	52	67	32	35	87	38	49	94	46	48	88	58	30
1854	53	—6	59	49	1	48	68	13	55	68	22	46	80	31	49	88	46	42	94	51	43
1855	54	10	44	42	-15	57	57	13	44	76	18	58	78	35	43	95	48	47	95	60	35
1856	37	—8	45	41	—3	44	46	—2	48	78	22	56	91	36	55	95	48	47	92	57	35
1857	40	-14	54	68	—3	71	61	6	55	62	15	47	85	34½	50½	82	47	35	88	49	39
1858	57	6	51	47	3	44	60	2	58	69	30	39	75	41	34	91	49	42	93	57	46
1859	54	-11	65	51	14	37	60	13	47	69	29	40	80	42	38	88	46	42	90	53	37
1860	52	1	51	55	—1	56	71	20	51	68	22	46	76	39	37	. .	. .	. .	. .	. .	. .
Greatest	63	. .	65	68	. .	71	73	. .	65	82	. .	67	91	. .	55	97	. .	50	97	. .	46
Least	. .	—14	41	. .	—15	37	. .	—4	34	. .	15	35	. .	28	33	. .	37	35	. .	49	28
Means	. .	. .	51.1	. .	. .	49.4	. .	. .	50.3	. .	. .	46.9	. .	. .	44.8	. .	. .	42.3	. .	. .	36.7

TABLE V—Concluded.

MONTHLY AND ANNUAL MAXIMUM AND MINIMUM TEMPERATURES, AND RANGE.

YEARS.	AUGUST.			SEPTEMBER.			OCTOBER.			NOVEMBER.			DECEMBER.			FOR THE YEAR.		
	Max.	Min.	Range.	Max.	Min.	Range.	Max.	Min.	Range.	Max.	Min.	Range.	Max.	Min.	Range.	Max.	Min.	Range.
1831	..	..	..	..	..	..	..	..	..	..	..	..	35	—1	36	..	..	..
1832	84	46	38	80	42	38	73	28	45	66	18	48	51	11	40	89	—7	96
1833	86	45	41	86	40	46	73	25	48	66	14	52	43	12	31	91	—4	95
1834	87	54	33	86	33	53	81	26	55	59	20	39	55	—8	63	93	—8	101
1835	86	48	38	84	40	44	74	34	40	67	10	57	43	-12	55	88	—12	100
1836	82	50	32	84	34	50	74	22	52	57	14	43	57	0	57	89	—6	95
1837	86	49	37	82	39	43	74	23	51	69	11	58	50	4	46	88	—4	92
1838	94	49	45	80	44	36	73	28	45	63	4	59	47	8	39	96	1	95
1839	85	50	35	79	40	39	72	26	46	57	16	41	49	4	45	88	—8	96
1840	83	57	26	77	40	37	73	30	43	58	20	38	52	4	48	90	—5	95
1841	87	54	33	81	48	33	68	26	42	68	18	50	54	5	49	90	0	90
1842	82	52	30	83	38	45	72	32	40	60	18	42	46	7	39	90	3	87
1843	82	58	24	83	36	47	72	32	40	65	22	43	44	9	35	89	2	87
1844	84	53	31	80	33	47	68	33	35	61	15	46	56	12	44	89	—1	90
1845	85	47	38	76	39	37	72	26	46	65	15	50	49	7	42	90	2	88
1846	93	55	38	90	45	45	79	28	51	66	22	44	55	10	45	93	—2	95
1847	86	53	33	86	43	43	71	22	49	72	8	64	65	9	56	93	6	87
1848	87	62	25	83	34	49	75	33	42	58	13	45	62	10	52	91	—4	95
1849	84	56	28	83	46	36	67	32	35	67	27	40	55	7	48	97	—4	101
1850	86	49	37	83	39	44	72	29	43	64	24	40	52	7	45	93	0	93
1851	86	53	33	88	35	53	75	30	45	56	19	37	50	—1	51	90	—1	91
1852	86	55	31	83	39	44	73	30	43	63	20	43	63	10	53	95	—2	97
1853	90	52	38	85	35	50	68	32	36	70	15	55	48	4	44	90	4	86
1854	87	50	37	88	37	51	77	33	44	70	18	52	48	3	45	94	—6	100
1855	91	48	43	90	38	52	74	33	41	66	20	46	54	8	46	95	—15	110
1856	87	48	39	83	44	39	76	28	48	65	22	43	50	—5	55	95	—8	103
1857	86	54	32	84	36	48	72	29	43	70	16	54	54	9	45	88	—14	102
1858	80	49	31	85	39	46	82	33	49	63	21	42	58	12	46	93	2	91
1859	85	48	37	78	39	39	78	29	49	70	29	41	61	—2	63	90	—11	101
1860	..	..	..	..	..	..	..	..	..	..	..	..	..	..	..	..	..	..
Greatest	94	..	45	90	..	53	82	..	55	72	..	64	65	..	63	97	..	110
Least	..	45	24	..	33	33	..	22	35	..	4	37	..	—12	31	..	—15	86
Means	..	..	34.4	..	..	44.1	..	..	44.5	..	..	46.9	..	..	47.0	..	..	94.9

TABLE VI.

SHOWING THE NUMBER OF DAYS IN EACH MONTH IN WHICH THE PREVAILING WINDS CAME FROM EACH OF THE FOUR QUARTERS OF THE HORIZON.

The figures 1, 2, 3, and 4, at the head of the monthly columns, indicate the quarters, as follows: 1, from some point between North and East; 2, between East and South; 3, between South and West; 4, between West and North.

YEARS.	JANUARY.				FEBRUARY.				MARCH.				APRIL.				MAY.				JUNE.				JULY.			
	1	2	3	4	1	2	3	4	1	2	3	4	1	2	3	4	1	2	3	4	1	2	3	4	1	2	3	4
1831	..	..	..	..	..	..	..	..	..	..	..	..	..	..	..	..	..	..	..	..	..	..	..	..	..	..	..	..
1832	2	3	9	16*	10	1	6	12	3	1	11	16	14	1	6	9	10	1	10	10	7	3	8	15	5	0	14	12
1833	5	0	13	12*	6	0	7	15	6	0	11	14	6	1	12	11	14	2	9	6	2	1	15	12	1	0	16	14
1834	8	1	8	14	7	1	10	10	4	1	14	12	11	1	14	4	9	3	12	7	5	4	15	6	4	2	19	6
1835	3	1	9	18	7	1	8	12	9	0	10	12	5	1	10	14	10	0	13	8	4	0	15	11	4	0	17	10
1836	11	0	7	13	8	2	4	15	8	0	12	11	7	1	12	10	12	1	11	7	17	5	6	2	9	3	14	5
1837	3	0	6	22	7	1	8	12	8	3	6	14	3	0	11	16	6	3	15	7	7	3	12	8	2	1	13	15
1838	8	0	13	10	4	0	3	21	13	5	5	8	4	6	8	12	6	6	15	4	5	4	15	6	3	4	12	12
1839	7	2	8	14	13	2	6	7	6	2	11	12	12	3	8	7	8	4	14	5	6	1	14	9	2	2	22	5
1840	4	1	9	17	7	1	9	12	5	4	10	12	3	2	15	9*	11	5	11	4	4	4	9	13	4	2	16	6*
1841	11	4	6	10	4	1	8	15	9	2	10	10	9	1	10	10	4	1	17	9	9	1	14	6	4	1	12	11
1842	1	2	18	10	4	3	10	11	7	1	12	11	13	1	6	10	7	5	12	7	3	4	15	8	3	1	21	4
1843	7	1	13	10	6	0	8	14	3	3	5	20	11	5	4	10	11	5	5	10	3	4	13	10	4	5	9	13
1844	1	3	6	21	6	1	9	13	12	2	11	6	13	3	7	7	5	9	10	7	3	3	16	8	9	2	14	4*
1845	6	2	5	18	3	4	8	13	5	5	9	12	9	6	6	9	6	3	15	7	3	1	17	9	4	1	14	12
1846	6	2	10	13	6	0	4	18	5	5	9	12	2	7	11	10	11	8	7	5	10	6	9	5	6	2	10	10*
1847	3	2	12	14	7	5	0	16	3	4	4	20	3	0	14	13	10	7	9	5	5	1	11	13	9	3	13	6
1848	7	1	10	13	3	0	3	23	6	1	9	15	5	1	7	17	8	8	8	5*	7	3	7	13	3	6	12	10
1849	1	0	9	21	14	0	1	13	12	4	5	10	3	6	6	15	11	3	11	6	8	5	8	9	8	3	10	10
1850	7	2	4	18	1	3	8	16	5	1	3	22	3	6	11	10	10	5	6	10	3	5	12	10	9	5	12	5
1851	5	0	13	13	2	3	9	14	5	1	12	13	9	7	5	9	8	2	14	7	8	5	7	10	6	2	14	9
1852	7	0	8	16	2	2	11	14	8	1	8	14	11	1	7	11	7	8	8	8	0	3	15	12	2	6	13	10
1853	7	2	8	14	4	8	3	13	3	2	9	17	5	6	12	7	8	3	14	6	7	5	14	4	2	1	17	11
1854	3	0	11	17	6	3	6	13	6	0	8	17	11	4	8	7	4	10	10	7	8	3	15	4	9	4	13	5
1855	10	1	9	10*	4	0	4	20	6	1	8	16	3	5	9	13	4	5	8	14	4	5	11	10	12	3	14	2
1856	5	0	4	22	1	0	7	21	3	3	6	19	8	4	13	5	10	4	7	10	5	6	11	8	4	1	13	11*
1857	7	2	5	17	4	3	11	10	3	6	8	14	7	2	10	11	7	3	16	4*	6	4	12	8	6	6	15	4
1858	4	2	10	15	5	0	6	17	2	2	8	19	5	1	9	15	14	2	7	8	11	3	13	3	6	3	14	8
1859	8	0	10	13	9	0	9	10	3	6	8	14	7	5	4	14	11	6	10	3*	4	0	19	7	4	6	11	10
1860	2	0	15	14	6	2	9	12	3	7	10	11	4	7	7	12	15	12	3	1	..	..	..	..	..	..	..	..
MEANS	5.5	1.1	9.1	15.0	5.6	1.6	6.7	14.2	5.9	2.5	8.7	13.9	7.4	3.2	9.0	10.6	9.1	4.6	10.8	6.8	5.9	3.3	12.3	8.4	5.2	2.7	14.0	8.6

* Days omitted.

TABLE VI—Concluded.

SHOWING THE NUMBER OF DAYS IN EACH MONTH IN WHICH THE PREVAILING WINDS CAME FROM EACH OF THE FOUR QUARTERS OF THE HORIZON.

The figures 1, 2, 3, and 4, at the head of the monthly columns, indicate the quarters, as follows: 1, from some point between North and East; 2, between East and South; 3, between South and West; 4, between North and West.

YEARS.	AUGUST.				SEPTEMBER.				OCTOBER.				NOVEMBER.				DECEMBER.				FOR THE YEAR.				DAYS OMITTED.
	1	2	3	4	1	2	3	4	1	2	3	4	1	2	3	4	1	2	3	4	1	2	3	4	
1831	..	..	..	..	..	..	..	..	..	..	..	..	..	..	..	..	8	0	3	18*	..	..	..	..	2
1832	3	0	18	10	2	1	18	9	6	1	13	11	3	0	16	11	10	0	7	13*	75	12	138	144	2
1833	4	0	15	12	4	0	14	12	6	2	14	9	3	1	13	13	13	1	8	9	70	8	147	139	1
1834	12	2	9	8	4	5	12	9	3	0	13	15	8	0	12	10	8	0	9	14	83	20	147	115	0
1835	3	2	15	11	4	3	11	12	2	1	21	7	4	0	11	15	5	1	8	17	60	10	148	147	0
1836	4	2	16	9	12	1	11	6	4	2	13	12	6	2	7	15	2	3	9	17	101	21	122	122	0
1837	7	2	12	10	8	2	11	9	7	2	10	11*	4	2	11	13	8	0	14	9	70	19	129	146	1
1838	5	1	14	11	10	0	8	12	3	1	10	17	2	1	10	17	1	1	15	14	64	29	128	144	0
1839	8	3	14	6	1	2	10	17	9	3	13	6	5	3	5	17	15	0	4	12	92	27	129	117	0
1840	2	1	20	8	4	2	10	14	7	3	14	7	13	2	3	12	6	2	8	15	70	29	134	129	4
1841	11	4	12	3*	11	4	13	2	7	1	9	14	10	1	4	15	4	2	8	17	93	23	123	122	4
1842	9	1	9	5	7	0	9	14	2	1	12	16	5	3	3	19	5	0	8	18	66	22	135	133	9
1843	4	8	14	5	12	2	8	8	5	2	8	16	4	2	6	18	7	1	8	15	77	38	101	149	0
1844	3	4	13	7*	11	3	7	8*	7	5	13	6	4	2	11	13	6	1	7	17	81	37	121	120	7
1845	2	3	7	6*	2	4	14	10*	5	4	13	9	2	1	18	9	7	0	4	20	54	34	130	134	13
1846	7	2	12	4*	6	2	14	8	7	4	12	8	16	3	3	8	2	1	9	19	84	42	110	120	9
1847	2	2	9	11*	13	1	6	10	8	1	9	13	3	2	13	12	4	2	11	14	70	30	111	147	7
1848	1	3	9	5*	6	2	6	16	7	2	8	14	3	1	8	18	9	5	5	12	65	39	92	161	9
1849	3	10	10	8	8	3	11	8	11	7	5	8	5	4	8	13	6	2	2	21	90	47	86	142	0
1850	7	4	12	8	6	6	7	11	0	2	16	13	8	4	8	10	8	0	7	16	67	43	106	149	0
1851	1	3	14	13	11	8	6	5	1	9	7	14	4	0	6	20	3	2	8	18	63	42	115	145	0
1852	6	5	11	6*	4	2	10	14	10	3	7	11	7	2	5	16	9	1	9	12	73	34	112	144	3
1853	7	2	17	2*	7	1	11	11	6	0	15	10	5	5	10	10	7	0	5	19	68	35	135	124	3
1854	2	1	16	8*	6	1	13	10*	7	5	10	9	3	2	10	13*	6	0	9	15*	71	33	129	125	7
1855	7	2	11	10*	8	0	6	16	2	5	12	12	11	0	6	13	6	1	8	16	77	28	106	152	2
1856	4	5	12	10	7	2	10	11	6	1	13	11	2	0	12	16	6	3	4	18	61	29	112	162	2
1857	3	5	8	12*	7	0	11	12	9	2	8	12	2	1	12	15	7	2	11	11	68	36	127	130	4
1858	12	1	11	5*	6	2	14	8	8	1	12	10	8	0	4	18	5	3	7	16	86	20	115	142	2
1859	5	5	9	10*	6	0	13	11	3	0	10	18	1	6	13	10	9	1	5	16	70	35	121	136	3
1860	..	..	..	..	..	..	..	..	..	..	..	..	..	..	..	..	..	..	..	..	..	..	..	..	..
MEANS	5.1	2.9	12.1	7.9	6.9	2.0	10.5	10.5	5.4	2.4	11.4	11.0	5.4	1.8	8.9	13.9	6.6	1.2	7.6	15.4	74.0	29.4	121.6	137.2	2.9

* Days omitted.

TABLE VII.

MEAN FORCE OF THE WIND AT THE DIFFERENT HOURS OF OBSERVATION, AND FOR THE MONTH AND YEAR.

YEARS.	JANUARY.				FEBRUARY.				MARCH.				APRIL.				MAY.				JUNE.				JULY.			
	Sunrise.	1 or 2 P. M.	10 P. M.	Mean.	Sunrise.	1 or 2 P. M.	10 P. M.	Mean.	Sunrise.	1 or 2 P. M.	10 P. M.	Mean.	6 A. M.	1 or 2 P. M.	10 P. M.	Mean.	6 A. M.	1 or 2 P. M.	10 P. M.	Mean.	6 A. M.	1 or 2 P. M.	10 P. M.	Mean.	6 A. M.	1 or 2 P. M.	10 P. M.	Mean.
1843	..	..	..	..	1.4	1.7	1.4	1.5	2.2	2.7	2.5	2.5	1.6	1.9	1.6	1.7	1.6	1.7	1.2	1.5	1.7	2.1	1.3	1.7	1.6	2.1	1.2	1.6
1844	1.7	1.9	1.4	1.7	1.3	1.6	1.3	1.4	1.6	1.9	1.7	1.7	1.3	1.9	1.2	1.5	1.7	2.5	1.4	1.9	1.7	2.2	1.4	1.8	1.5	1.8	1.5	1.6
1845	1.5	1.7	1.8	1.7	1.6	1.6	1.4	1.5	1.5	2.3	1.5	1.8	1.7	2.2	1.7	1.9	1.9	2.5	2.0	2.1	1.5	2.2	1.6	1.8	1.5	2.1	1.5	1.7
1846	1.4	1.9	1.7	1.7	1.4	2.1	1.5	1.7	1.5	2.1	1.6	1.7	1.3	1.7	1.4	1.5	1.3	1.7	1.3	1.4	1.3	1.6	1.3	1.4	1.4	1.8	1.3	1.5
1847	1.4	1.6	1.6	1.5	1.3	1.6	1.4	1.4	1.5	1.9	1.5	1.6	1.3	2.1	1.6	1.7	1.4	1.7	1.4	1.5	1.2	1.7	1.2	1.4	1.4	1.9	1.4	1.6
1848	1.2	1.6	1.4	1.4	1.3	1.4	1.2	1.3	1.4	1.5	1.5	1.5	1.1	1.7	1.2	1.3	1.2	1.8	1.2	1.4	1.4	1.8	1.2	1.5	1.1	1.7	1.0	1.3
1849	1.4	1.7	1.5	1.5	1.5	1.6	1.6	1.6	1.5	2.2	1.5	1.7	1.4	1.6	1.3	1.4	1.3	1.6	1.5	1.5	1.3	2.0	1.3	1.5	2.2	2.5	1.4	2.0
1850	1.4	1.6	1.7	1.6	1.4	1.7	1.5	1.5	1.5	2.0	1.6	1.7	1.7	2.3	1.8	1.9	1.7	2.1	1.4	1.7	1.6	2.0	1.2	1.6	1.6	2.1	1.5	1.7
1851	1.6	2.0	1.7	1.8	1.5	2.0	1.7	1.7	1.8	2.1	2.0	2.0	1.9	2.3	1.7	2.0	1.9	2.1	1.7	1.9	1.8	2.4	1.9	2.0	1.8	2.0	1.4	1.7
1852	1.8	2.0	1.7	1.8	1.5	2.1	1.8	1.8	1.9	1.9	1.8	1.9	1.9	2.2	1.8	2.0	1.9	2.2	1.5	1.9	1.5	2.1	1.5	1.7	1.8	2.1	1.4	1.8
1853	1.7	1.9	2.0	1.9	1.7	2.3	1.6	1.9	1.9	2.3	1.7	2.0	1.6	2.0	1.6	1.7	1.8	2.3	1.5	1.9	1.8	2.3	1.5	1.9	1.4	1.8	1.4	1.5
1854	1.5	1.8	1.6	1.6	1.7	1.8	1.9	1.8	1.8	2.1	1.7	1.9	1.5	1.9	1.6	1.7	1.7	2.2	1.5	1.8	1.7	2.2	1.4	1.8	1.5	2.1	1.1	1.6
1855	1.7	1.9	1.5	1.7	1.8	1.9	1.6	1.8	1.7	2.1	1.5	1.8	1.4	2.2	1.5	1.7	1.6	2.2	1.7	1.8	1.6	2.0	1.5	1.7	1.2	1.7	1.2	1.4
1856	1.6	1.6	1.4	1.5	1.4	1.9	1.6	1.6	1.8	2.3	1.6	1.9	1.5	2.3	1.7	1.8	1.7	2.2	1.7	1.9	1.6	2.3	1.4	1.8	1.8	2.5	1.3	1.9
1857	1.8	2.1	2.0	2.0	1.5	2.1	1.7	1.8	1.7	2.1	1.7	1.8	1.8	2.5	1.9	2.1	1.7	2.1	1.6	1.8	1.5	2.2	1.2	1.6	1.5	2.3	1.3	1.7
1858	1.4	2.0	1.5	1.6	1.4	2.1	1.6	1.7	1.6	2.0	1.6	1.7	1.5	1.8	1.6	1.6	1.4	1.9	1.3	1.5	1.4	1.8	1.5	1.6	1.5	2.1	1.2	1.6
1859	1.4	1.7	1.5	1.5	1.5	1.6	1.5	1.5	1.7	2.2	1.8	1.9	1.4	2.2	1.6	1.7	1.4	2.3	1.3	1.7	1.6	2.4	1.4	1.8	1.4	2.0	1.1	1.5
1860	1.6	2.0	1.6	1.7	1.9	2.1	1.9	2.0	1.8	2.7	1.9	2.1	1.8	2.7	1.7	2.1	1.7	2 7	1.3	1.9	..	..	..	..	..	..	..	..
MEANS	1.54	1.82	1.62	1.66	1.51	1.84	1.57	1.64	1.69	2.13	1.71	1.84	1.54	2.08	1.64	1.74	1.61	2.10	1.47	1.73	1.54	2.08	1.40	1.68	1.54	2.04	1.31	1.63

YEARS.	AUGUST.				SEPTEMBER.				OCTOBER.				NOVEMBER.				DECEMBER.				FOR THE YEAR.			
	6 A. M.	1 or 2 P. M.	10 P. M.	Mean.	6 A. M.	1 or 2 P. M.	10 P. M.	Mean.	Sunrise.	1 or 2 P. M.	10 P. M.	Mean.	Sunrise.	1 or 2 P. M.	10 P. M.	Mean.	Sunrise.	1 or 2 P. M.	10 P. M.	Mean.	Sunrise or 6 A. M.	1 or 2 P. M.	10 P. M.	Mean.
1843	1.3	1.8	1.4	1.5	1.4	1.9	1.3	1.5	1.2	2.1	1.3	1.5	1.3	1.5	1.1	1.3	1.4	1.8	1.9	1.7	1.52	1.94	1.47	1.64
1844	1.8	2.1	1.4	1.8	1.7	2.2	1.6	1.8	1.6	2.0	1.3	1.6	1.5	1.7	1.6	1.6	1.5	1.8	1.6	1.6	1.58	1.97	1.45	1.67
1845	1.2	1.6	1.2	1.3	1.4	1.9	1.3	1.5	1.2	1.9	1.3	1.5	1.5	1.7	1.3	1.5	1.5	1.9	1.7	1.7	1.50	1.98	1.53	1.67
1846	1.2	1.5	1.1	1.3	1.2	1.9	1.3	1.5	1.4	1.7	1.5	1.5	1.4	1.9	1.8	1.7	1.3	1.6	1.6	1.5	1.34	1.79	1.45	1.53
1847	1.1	1.4	1.2	1.2	1.4	1.7	1.3	1.5	1.3	1.7	1.2	1.4	1.2	1.4	1.3	1.3	1.4	1.5	1.4	1.4	1.33	1.68	1.38	1.46
1848	1.1	1.6	1.0	1.2	1.1	1.7	1.1	1.3	1.2	1.2	1.0	1.1	1.2	1.3	1.1	1.2	1.1	1.2	1.2	1.2	1.20	1.54	1.18	1.31
1849	1.4	2.4	1.2	1.7	1.3	2.0	1.3	1.5	1.3	2.0	1.5	1.6	1.5	1.5	1.3	1.4	1.5	1.8	1.6	1.6	1.47	1.91	1.42	1.60
1850	1.7	2.3	1.5	1.8	1.1	1.9	1.4	1.5	1.6	1.6	1.3	1.5	1.5	1.7	1.5	1.6	1.6	1.7	1.7	1.7	1.53	1.92	1.51	1.65
1851	1.7	2.0	1.5	1.7	1.4	1.7	1.2	1.4	1.6	2.0	1.5	1.7	1.6	1.8	1.7	1.7	1.7	1.9	1.7	1.8	1.69	2.03	1.64	1.79
1852	1.3	1.9	1.2	1.5	1.5	1.8	1.3	1.5	1.6	2.1	1.6	1.8	1.8	2.0	1.8	1.9	1.8	1.8	1.7	1.8	1.69	2.02	1.59	1.77
1853	1.3	1.6	1.2	1.4	1.5	1.9	1.3	1.6	1.7	2.2	1.4	1.8	1.8	2.0	1.7	1.8	1.8	2.0	1.7	1.8	1.67	2.05	1.55	1.76
1854	1.4	1.8	1.2	1.5	1.5	1.9	1.3	1.6	1.5	2.1	1.4	1.7	1.5	1.7	1.3	1.5	1.5	1.9	1.5	1.6	1.57	1.96	1.46	1.66
1855	1.3	1.9	1.3	1.5	1.3	1.7	1.3	1.4	1.3	1.8	1.3	1.5	1.6	1.7	1.4	1.6	1.5	1.8	1.5	1.6	1.50	1.91	1.44	1.62
1856	1.5	2.0	1.3	1.6	1.3	2.0	1.4	1.6	1.4	1.9	1.4	1.6	1.4	1.9	1.5	1.6	1.9	2.2	2.0	2.0	1.58	2.09	1.53	1.73
1857	1.8	1.8	1.4	1.7	1.3	2.0	1.1	1.5	1.4	2.1	1.4	1.6	1.6	2.0	1.2	1.6	1.4	1.9	1.5	1.6	1.58	2.10	1.50	1.73
1858	1.2	1.9	1.1	1.4	1.4	1.8	1.1	1.4	1.3	2.0	1.4	1.6	1.7	2.1	1.5	1.8	1.2	1.9	1.4	1.5	1.43	1.97	1.41	1.60
1859	1.2	1.9	1.0	1.4	1.7	2.2	1.4	1.8	1.7	2.4	1.4	1.8	1.4	2.0	1.3	1.6	1.6	2.1	1.7	1.8	1.62	2.27	1.48	1.80
1860	..	..	..	..	..	..	..	..	..	..	..	..	..	..	..	..	..	..	..	..	..	..	..	..
MEANS	1.38	1.85	1.25	1.50	1.38	1.89	1.29	1.52	1.43	1.93	1.36	1.58	1.50	1.76	1.44	1.57	1.51	1.81	1.61	1.64	1.52	1.95	1.59	1.64

TABLE VIII.

MEAN CLOUDINESS OF THE SKY AT THE DIFFERENT HOURS OF OBSERVATION, AND THE MEAN FOR THE MONTH AND YEAR.

YEARS.	JANUARY.				FEBRUARY.				MARCH.				APRIL.				MAY.				JUNE.				JULY.			
	Sunrise.	1 or 2 P. M.	10 P. M.	Mean.	Sunrise.	1 or 2 P. M.	10 P. M.	Mean.	Sunrise.	1 or 2 P. M.	10 P. M.	Mean.	6 A. M.	1 or 2 P. M.	10 P. M.	Mean.	6 A. M.	1 or 2 P. M.	10 P. M.	Mean.	6 A. M.	1 or 2 P. M.	10 P. M.	Mean.	6 A. M.	1 or 2 P. M.	10 P. M.	Mean.
1843	..	..	..	..	4.8	4.6	4.0	4.5	3.4	3.4	3.2	3.3	6.5	5.7	5.5	5.9	5.4	4.7	4.2	4.8	3.1	3.8	2.9	3.3	3.7	3.9	3.4	3.7
1844	3.6	2.9	3.4	3.3	3.5	4.3	3.1	3.6	6.1	5.8	6.0	6.0	4.2	4.0	4.3	4.2	4.9	5.0	5.2	5.0	3.6	3 8	3.6	3.7	5.2	5.3	4.8	5.1
1845	6.3	4.8	5.2	5.4	4.5	4.4	4.6	4.5	5.4	5.0	4.3	4.9	6.0	6.0	5.1	5.7	5.0	5.0	5.0	5.0	3.9	2.9	1.9	2.9	3.2	3.6	2.8	3.2
1846	4.8	4.7	5.0	4.8	5.3	4.1	6.0	5.1	4.5	4.5	4.2	4.4	3.5	3.5	3.5	3.5	6.6	6.6	7.1	6.8	5.6	4.8	5.0	5.1	6.4	5.1	4.2	5.2
1847	5.8	4.9	4.1	4.9	6.5	7.1	6.9	6.8	4.7	4.5	3.9	4.4	4.4	5.5	4.8	4.9	4.3	5.3	4.8	4.8	4.8	4.9	4.4	4.7	5.3	4.0	3.8	4.4
1848	5.4	4.9	5.4	5.2	3.8	3.6	2.8	3.4	3.9	4.1	3.5	3.8	4.1	3.6	2.8	3.5	6.4	6.1	5.9	6.1	4.4	5.4	4.0	4 6	4.9	5.5	4.7	5.0
1849	4.2	4.1	4.2	4.2	6.0	5.5	6.2	5.9	5.7	6.2	5.4	5.8	4.2	4.2	5.0	4.5	6.3	6.6	5.5	6.1	4.2	4.1	3.4	3.9	5.0	4.0	3.8	4.3
1850	5 5	5.8	4.6	5.3	3.8	4.0	3.1	3.6	5.0	5.0	3.7	4.6	4.3	5.5	3.9	4.6	5.1	7.6	5.4	6.0	4.7	4.1	3.2	4.0	5.4	5.5	4.9	5.3
1851	4.8	5.0	4.1	4.6	6.1	6.2	4.4	5.6	5.9	6.0	4.6	5.5	4.9	5.7	5.3	5.3	5.3	5.6	4.2	5.0	3.8	4 0	4.4	4.1	5.1	6.1	4.1	5.1
1852	6.4	6.4	4.7	5.8	4.6	4.5	4.4	4.5	5.5	6.1	6.3	6.0	5.4	6.1	6.2	5.9	5.2	4.1	4.1	4.5	4.2	4.5	3.6	4.1	4 3	3.4	3.5	3.7
1853	4.9	5.2	5.2	5.1	5.0	5.5	5.2	5.2	4.4	4.7	4.7	4.6	4.9	5.3	4.4	4.9	5.3	4.5	3.5	4.4	5.1	3.3	4.5	4.3	5.9	5.5	4.1	5.2
1854	5.5	5.7	5.1	5.4	5.8	5.8	5.0	5.5	3.2	5.1	5.0	4.4	5.7	6.2	5.7	5.9	6.4	5.2	5.0	5.5	5.9	5.7	4.9	5.5	5.5	4.3	4.1	4.6
1855	6.0	8.4	6.4	6.9	4.6	4.7	4.0	4.4	5.6	5.5	3.3	4.8	4.5	6.4	5.1	5.3	5.9	4.8	4.5	5.1	5.5	5.5	4.6	5.2	6.0	5.9	5.0	5.6
1856	4.0	5.0	3.3	4.1	3.9	5.2	5.0	4.7	3.3	3.2	4.3	3.6	4.0	5.2	5.4	4.9	5.2	6.2	5.1	5.5	5.7	4 3	4.2	4.7	4.2	4.1	3.1	3.8
1857	5.1	5.4	5.3	5.3	6.9	5.2	4.0	5.4	4.5	5.6	4.5	4.9	6.1	6.3	4.2	5.5	5.9	5.4	4.5	5.3	6.0	5.7	5.3	5.7	7.0	5.0	4.4	5.5
1858	4.4	5.2	4.0	4.5	3.5	4.2	4.3	4.0	3.4	4.0	3.6	3.7	4.7	5.3	5.1	5.0	6.0	6.0	5.3	5.8	5.2	4.5	4.6	4.8	6.2	5.4	5.0	5.5
1859	5.7	4.9	4.0	4.9	6.6	5.9	5.8	6.1	5.0	5.7	5.7	5.5	4.6	5.3	5.0	5.0	5.3	5.0	5.5	5.3	5.7	6.5	5.9	6.0	4.2	5.0	3.1	4.1
1860	4.5	4.9	4.0	4.5	5.8	6.4	5.7	6.0	4.7	5.1	3.0	4.2	5.8	5.8	5.2	5.4	5.7	5.4	4.8	5.3	..	..	..	..	..	..	..	..
MEANS	5.11	5.19	4.59	4.95	5.06	5.07	4.69	4.93	4.68	4.97	4.40	4.69	4.85	5.31	4.81	4.99	5.56	5.51	4.98	5.35	4.79	4.58	4.20	4.51	5.15	4.80	4.04	4.67

YEARS.	AUGUST.				SEPTEMBER.				OCTOBER.				NOVEMBER.				DECEMBER.				FOR THE YEAR.			
	6 A. M.	1 or 2 P. M.	10 P. M.	Mean.	6 A. M.	1 or 2 P. M.	10 P. M.	Mean.	Sunrise.	1 or 2 P. M.	10 P. M.	Mean.	Sunrise.	1 or 2 P. M.	10 P. M.	Mean.	Sunrise.	1 or 2 P. M.	10 P. M.	Mean.	Sunrise or 6 A. M.	1 or 2 P. M.	10 P. M.	Mean.
1843	6.8	5.7	4.1	5.5	4.6	3.1	3.5	3.7	5.1	5.1	3.7	4.6	2.8	4.9	4.6	4.1	5.1	5.0	6.8	5.8	4.66	4.54	4.17	4.46
1844	3.9	4.8	4.1	4.2	4.4	4.0	2.8	3.7	5.1	5.7	4.4	5.1	4.0	5.3	4.7	4.7	5.5	5.5	4.6	5.2	4.50	4.70	4.25	4.48
1845	3.9	3.6	1.7	3.1	3.1	3.7	3.9	3.6	4.5	5.0	3.8	4.4	4.8	5.2	4.8	4.9	4.9	5.7	5.6	5.4	4.63	4.58	4.06	4.42
1846	4.5	4.7	3.4	4.2	3.6	3.4	2.8	3.3	4.0	5.1	5.0	4.7	7.7	6.9	6.4	7.0	4.2	4.2	5.0	4.5	5.06	4.80	4.80	4.89
1847	5.7	3.6	3.2	4.2	6 4	5.9	5.1	5.8	3.7	3.9	3.3	3.6	6.3	5.8	5.7	5.9	6.2	6.3	6.9	6.5	5.34	5.14	4.74	5.07
1848	4.7	4.0	3.3	4.0	4.1	4.8	3.0	4.0	5.2	5.7	4.2	5.0	5.0	4.0	3.0	4.0	6.6	6.8	5.7	6.4	4.87	4.87	4.03	4.59
1849	5.4	4.4	3.7	4.5	3.1	3.5	2.7	3.1	6.2	7.0	5.6	6.2	4.5	5.7	4.9	5.0	5.0	5.2	4.9	5.0	4.98	5.04	4.61	4.88
1850	4.2	4.6	2.5	3.8	5.0	4 2	4.0	4.4	4.7	4.1	2.9	3.9	6.2	5.2	5.0	5.5	5.1	7.8	5.9	6.2	4.92	5.28	4.11	4.77
1851	4.7	5.1	3.5	4.4	4.2	4 0	4.0	4.1	4.7	4.6	3.7	4.3	4.4	5.6	5.0	5.0	4.7	4.7	4.5	4.6	4.88	5.22	4.32	4.81
1852	5.8	6.2	4.3	5.4	4.3	4.8	3.2	4.1	6.4	6.1	5.0	5.8	6.0	6.5	5.2	5.9	6.1	6.8	5.5	6.1	5.35	5.46	4.67	5.16
1853	5.3	5.1	5.3	5.2	5.8	4.9	4.3	5.0	3.5	4.2	3.5	3.7	5.9	5.8	6.1	5.9	5.6	5.6	4.7	5.3	5.13	4.97	4.62	4.91
1854	4.4	4.3	4.1	4.3	4.4	3.6	4.0	4.0	4.8	5.4	4.3	4.8	5.0	5.7	4.4	5.0	6.5	6.0	5.4	6.0	5.26	5.25	4.75	5.09
1855	3.2	4.6	3.0	3.6	4.5	4.3	2.9	3.9	5.3	4.9	5.3	5.2	5.9	6.4	5.4	5.9	4.9	5.0	4.2	4.7	5.16	5.53	4.48	5.06
1856	4.8	5.7	5.2	5.2	4.3	3.9	3.0	3.7	3 5	3.8	2.5	3.3	3.7	4.8	4.4	4.3	5.2	4.9	4.4	4.8	4.32	4.69	4.16	4.39
1857	5.1	6.7	3.1	5.0	4.2	3.9	2.9	3.7	5.2	5.7	4.4	5.1	3.8	4.6	4.6	4.3	5.1	6.0	3.5	4.9	5.41	5.46	4.23	5.03
1858	5.7	5.3	4.7	5.2	2.8	3.2	2.3	2.8	4.9	4.6	3.5	4.3	5.8	5.8	4.2	5.3	5.6	6.0	5.6	5.7	4.85	4.96	4.35	4.72
1859	5.5	3.9	3.4	4.3	5.3	5.3	4 9	5.2	4.5	4.6	3.7	4.3	5.3	4.8	4.4	4.8	6.2	6.1	5.4	5.9	5.33	5.25	4.73	5.12
1860	..	..	..	..	..	..	..	..	..	..	..	..	..	..	..	..	..	..	..	..	..	..	..	..
MEANS	4.92	4.84	3.68	4.48	4.36	4.15	3.49	4.01	4.72	5.03	4.05	4.61	5.12	5.47	4.87	5.15	5.44	5.74	5.21	5.47	4.98	5.04	4.42	4.81

TABLE IX.

MONTHLY AND ANNUAL NUMBER OF DAYS IN WHICH THE WEATHER WAS CLEAR, VARIABLE OR CLOUDY, AND ON WHICH RAIN OR SNOW FELL.

YEARS.	JANUARY.			FEBRUARY.			MARCH.			APRIL.			MAY.			JUNE.			JULY.		
	Clear.	Variable and Cloudy.	Rain or Snow.	Clear.	Variable and Cloudy.	Rain or Snow.	Clear.	Variable and Cloudy.	Rain or Snow.	Clear.	Variable and Cloudy.	Rain.	Clear.	Variable and Cloudy.	Rain.	Clear.	Variable and Cloudy.	Rain.	Clear.	Variable and Cloudy.	Rain.
1831	. .	. .	. .	. .	. .	. .	. .	. .	. .	. .	. .	. .	. .	. .	.	. .	. .	. .	. .	. .	. .
1832	12	11	8	7	11	11	13	12	6	9	14	7	11	10	10	16	11	3	18	7	6
1833	19	7	5	8	7	3*	17	8	6	22	5	3	10	15	6	18	4	8	25	4	2
1834	19	5	7	15	10	3	21	5	5	14	9	7	14	11	6	14	7	9	21	8	2
1835	12	10	9	6	18	4	9	15	7	11	10	9	10	17	4	11	12	7	13	13	5
1836	9	12	10	12	8	9	19	7	5	15	12	3	17	10	4	12	10	8	17	7	7
1837	21	5	5	15	6	7	18	6	7	15	11	4	16	6	9	16	8	6	17	9	5
1838	12	15	4	19	4	5	14	11	6	16	8	6	17	7	7	21	8	1	21	9	1
1839	17	12	2	7	14	7	17	12	2	15	9	6	17	7	7	15	10	5	18	5	8
1840	13	12	6	11	13	5	11	10	10	12	12	6	20	3	8	12	7	11	13	6	9*
1841	10	11	10	16	8	4	17	5	9	7	5	18	10	8	13	15	7	8	16	2	10*
1842	11	12	8	12	5	11	8	15	8	13	8	9	11	7	13	8	13	9	13	9	7*
1843	10	12	9	8	6	14	13	11	7	10	11	9	7	20	4	13	8	9	14	8	9
1844	14	9	8	11	12	6	7	12	12	10	15	5	7	9	15	9	14	7	7	15	7*
1845	7	14	10	11	8	9	7	16	8	6	9	11*	13	12	6	10	11	9	12	13	6
1846	9	13	9	9	11	8	10	13	8	15	9	6	5	15	11	6	13	10*	4	13	11*
1847	9	13	9	4	16	8	12	9	10	7	14	9	12	13	6	8	7	15	10	15	6
1848	7	17	7	15	7	7	11	12	8	15	9	6	5	14	10*	10	14	6	9	17	5
1849	12	12	7	7	11	10	7	15	9	9	14	7	3	22	6	13	9	8	12	12	7
1850	9	10	12	14	7	7	12	9	10	12	9	9	5	8	18	7	14	9	8	10	13
1851	6	19	6	9	9	10	7	15	9	9	8	13	7	10	14	10	11	9	5	10	16
1852	7	11	13	8	11	10	7	11	13	6	11	13	12	11	8	8	12	10	13	12	6
1853	7	15	9	10	8	10	7	14	10	9	8	13	9	14	8	8	13	9	8	13	10
1854	8	13	10	6	11	11	10	11	10	7	11	12	7	13	11	4	19	7	9	14	8
1855	7	12	11*	13	7	8	7	17	7	8	8	14	11	10	10	7	7	16	8	9	14
1856	12	11	8	8	13	8	11	12	7*	9	12	9	6	11	14	8	13	9	10	9	12
1857	9	7	15	4	14	10	10	10	11	8	10	12	8	8	14*	9	11	10	5	18	8
1858	14	10	7	11	9	8	13	11	6*	8	12	10	7	10	14	6	16	8	7	17	7
1859	10	11	10	6	12	10	7	11	13	8	14	8	12	9	10	6	10	14	10	15	6
1860	12	11	8	6	14	9	12	10	9	6	11	13	7	16	8	. . .	. .	. .	. .	. .	. .
MEANS	11.17	11.45	8.34	9.93	10.00	8.00	11.52	11.19	7.07	10.72	9.93	8.86	10.21	11.24	8.45	10.69	10.69	8.59	12.25	11.08	7.90

NOTE.—In this table, those days only are reckoned as "Clear" in which there were but few clouds. In general, if more than one-sixth of the sky, on the average, was covered with clouds, the day is not reckoned as clear.

* Days omitted.

TABLE IX—Concluded.

MONTHLY AND ANNUAL NUMBER OF DAYS IN WHICH THE WEATHER WAS CLEAR, VARIABLE OR CLOUDY, AND ON WHICH RAIN OR SNOW FELL.

YEARS.	AUGUST.			SEPTEMBER.			OCTOBER.			NOVEMBER.			DECEMBER.			FOR THE YEAR.			DAYS OMITTED.
	Clear.	Variable and Cloudy.	Rain.	Clear.	Variable and Cloudy.	Rain.	Clear.	Variable and Cloudy.	Rain.	Clear.	Variable and Cloudy.	Rain or Snow.	Clear.	Variable and Cloudy.	Rain or Snow.	Clear.	Variable and Cloudy.	Rain or Snow.	
1831	. .	. .	. .	. .	. .	. .	. .	. .	. .	. .	. .	. .	13	10	8	. .	. .	. .	. .
1832	16	3	12	21	3	6	16	12	3	18	7	5	11	12	8	168	113	85	0
1833	16	10	5	16	8	6	14	10	7	14	11	5	11	13	7	190	102	63	10
1834	21	7	3	18	6	6	15	11	5	14	11	5	8	15	8	194	105	66	0
1835	17	9	5	13	12	3*	12	16	3	6	19	5	12	16	3	132	167	64	2
1836	20	6	5	14	11	5	18	10	3	12	12	6	17	10	4	182	115	69	0
1837	15	11	5	19	10	1	19	9	2*	21	4	5	16	13	2	208	98	58	1
1838	15	9	7	17	6	7	17	6	8	18	6	6	20	8	3	207	97	61	0
1839	14	13	4	15	13	2	20	7	4	13	12	5	15	10	6	183	124	58	0
1840	10	13	8	17	5	8	13	10	8	9	12	9	19	5	7	160	108	95	3
1841	10	10	10*	10	14	6	13	11	7	11	9	10	10	10	11	145	100	116	4
1842	8	8	8*	10	12	8	20	7	4	14	9	7	7	13	11	135	118	103	9
1843	9	11	11	12	15	3	10	15	6	12	11	7	6	17	8	124	145	96	0
1844	7	13	7*	10	12	7*	8	15	8	10	11	9	9	12	10	109	149	101	7
1845	6	7	5*	12	10	8	10	15	6	7	15	8	11	13	7	112	143	93	17
1846	10	6	9*	11	13	6	8	15	8	4	18	8	10	11	10	101	150	104	10
1847	8	6	10*	9	13	8	13	12	6	6	21	3	5	14	12	103	153	102	7
1848	6	7	5*	9	15	6	10	11	10	12	11	7	7	10	14	116	144	91	15
1849	10	13	8	13	7	10	6	16	9	12	12	6	8	8	15	112	151	102	0
1850	11	8	12	12	10	8	10	15	6	8	18	4	5	12	14	113	130	122	0
1851	12	10	9	12	8	10	11	13	7	8	16	6	11	12	8	107	141	117	0
1852	6	10	12*	13	12	5	10	13	8	8	14	8	4	13	14	102	141	120	3
1853	6	12	12*	11	12	6*	15	9	7	7	17	6	10	13	8	107	148	108	2
1854	8	14	5*	10	10	9*	12	10	9	8	6	14*	6	12	12*	95	144	118	8
1855	12	10	8*	9	16	5	9	13	9	7	15	8	10	11	10	108	135	120	2
1856	6	13	12	11	12	7	15	12	4	9	11	10	11	12	8	116	141	108	1
1857	8	12	9*	15	9	6	9	13	9	8	15	7	10	9	12	103	136	123	3
1858	8	7	13*	16	9	5	10	13	8	9	10	11	7	10	14	116	135	110	4
1859	9	12	8*	9	9	12	10	16	5	5	16	9	5	16	10	97	151	115	2
1860	. .	. .	. .	. .	. .	. .	. .	. .	. .	. .	. .	. .	. .	. .	. .	. .	. .	. .	.
MEANS	11.19	10.00	9.41	13.44	10.82	6.63	13.04	12.39	6.63	10.71	12.91	7.21	10.18	12.10	[illegible]	[illegible]	[illegible]	[illegible]	[illegible]

* Days omitted.

TABLE X.

MONTHLY AND ANNUAL QUANTITY OF RAIN AND SNOW (REDUCED TO WATER) IN INCHES.

YEARS.	JANUARY.	FEBRUARY.	MARCH.	APRIL.	MAY.	JUNE.	JULY.	AUGUST.	SEPTEMBER.	OCTOBER.	NOVEMBER.	DECEMBER.	FOR THE YEAR.
1831	. .	. .	. .	. .	. .	. .	. .	. .	. .	. .	. .	1.95	. .
1832	3.87	4.25	3.20	3.33	4.14	0.33	1.82	3.92	3.50	2.01	3.46	5.63	39.46
1833	1.71	1.55	1.97	3.17	0.99	4.81	1.11	2.15	1.53	5.98	4.50	4.67	34.14
1834	1.57	1.18	1.43	3.13	5.61	5.10	7.58	1.15	3.81	4.64	3.80	2.97	41.92
1835	3.50	1.20	4.60	4.06	1.50	1.95	2.84	2.25	0.83	3.26	1.72	3.25	30.96
1836	5.63	3.45	5.00	2.30	2.51	3.25	1.53	0.72	1.03	2.35	5.25	4.85	37.87
1837	1.40	2.65	3.17	4.65	7.28	2.82	1.38	2.00	0.48	1.29	1.95	2.55	31.62
1838	2.70	2.32	2.70	2.70	3.88	3.30	0.68	3.55	6.76	4.61	3.65	1.08	37.88
1839	0.76	1.50	1.50	3.63	3.79	2.31	5.26	5.00	1.83	3.75	2.80	5.12	36.75
1840	2.80	2.05	3.50	3.45	3.35	2.89	3.38	3.20	2.95	5.17	5.35	3.10	41.19
1841	6.45	1.50	2.86	7.78	2.18	0.98	5.18	5.12	2.85	3.20	4.45	5.86	47.86
1842	1.30	4.05	2.07	2.10	3.40	9.65	1.48	3.35	1.40	1.16	3.82	3.93	37.71
1843	0.60	5.27	5.58	4.84	3.50	2.12	1.83	6.23	2.20	6.45	1.35	3.03	42.50
1844	4.32	1.95	4.75	0.67	1.95	1.15	4.42	1.11	2.83	5.80	3.30	2.75	35.00
1845	3.20	2.70	3.53	2.34	2.75	2.32	3.10	5.63	1.63	3.40	9.08	3.48	43.16
1846	1.82	2.08	2.86	1.75	4.58	1.30	1.44	2.73	2.33	1.85	4.62	3.15	30.51
1847	2.13	2.71	3.17	1.72	2.02	6.98	2.28	5.50	8.35	1.95	5.72	5.97	48.50
1848	4.82	3.80	2.40	0.95	5.00	3.80	1.85	3.73	2.45	4.05	3.80	3.83	40.48
1849	0.80	0.60	5.99	1.62	3.43	1.23	2.00	3.39	3.14	6.55	2.42	3.52	34.79
1850	5.60	3.38	5.19	4.67	5.00	2.60	2.35	7.65	5.00	2.10	2.10	5.85	51.49
1851	1.93	3.87	2.00	7.80	3.58	1.90	5.19	3.77	2.47	3.20	5.05	2.62	43.38
1852	2.70	2.00	3.55	6.65	2.00	1.00	1.68	8.00	1.40	1.30	4.60	3.70	38.58
1853	4.27	5.75	1.35	5.05	4.95	0.90	6.37	8.38	3.80	4.15	4.40	3.90	53.27
1854	1.80	4.85	2.85	6.30	3.60	3.60	2.45	0.30	6.10	1.90	9.15	3.35	37.10
1855	6.45	4.05	0.85	2.50	2.55	1.95	3.25	2.02	0.25	5.33	3.75	6.10	39.05
1856	5.25	0.80	1.55	2.80	4.10	2.47	4.20	5.75	5.10	1.15	2.00	5.80	40.97
1857	5.50	2.36	3.35	6.29	4.33	1.90	3.45	4.80	2.27	2.90	2.40	5.20	44.75
1858	3.33	2.80	2.05	3.63	2.35	5.55	4.90	8.20	3.05	2.80	2.40	3.45	44.51
1859	5.75	1.85	8.00	2.28	3.40	7.06	1.14	3.69	3.65	2.62	2.27	3.45	45.16
1860	0.80	3.54	1.80	1.55	1.65	. .	. .	. .	. .	. .	. .	. .	. .
MEANS	3.19	2.76	3.20	3.56	3.42	3.02	3.01	4.05	3.02	3.38	3.92	3.90	40.38

SMITHSONIAN CONTRIBUTIONS TO KNOWLEDGE.

METEOROLOGICAL OBSERVATIONS

MADE NEAR

WASHINGTON, ARK.,

EXTENDING OVER A PERIOD OF TWENTY YEARS,

FROM 1840 TO 1859, INCLUSIVE.

BY

NATHAN D. SMITH, M.D.

[ACCEPTED FOR PUBLICATION, JANUARY, 1860.]

COLLINS, PRINTER.
PHILADELPHIA.

INTRODUCTION.

THE Meteorological Tables here presented, form one set of a number of daily records, published by the Smithsonian Institution, to exhibit the simultaneous condition of the weather in different parts of the Continent of North America, during a series of years. This set is from the records of Dr. N. D. Smith, of Arkansas, and may be relied on for regularity, and for as much accuracy as the means at the command of the observer would allow him to attain.

The following remarks relative to the instruments and the character of the country, are from the pen of the observer:—

"Agreeable to your request, I herewith transmit to you a copy of my Record of the Weather, for the past twenty years. It has been kept, intermingled with my diary of events and business, for the satisfaction of myself and family, without the expectation of its being appreciated beyond my household circle. But, since you deem it worthy of acceptance, it is freely presented to the Smithsonian Institution.

"My thermometer has hung all the time in the same place, in the open air, in the window-frame, outside of the sash, on the north side of the house, eight feet above the ground, and protected from any injurious reflection. My rain-gauge is a deep tin cup, set on the ground, in an exposed spot in the garden, and the rain measured after every fall, by a rule graduated to tenths of an inch.

"My residence, where the observations were made, is on the summit of the dividing ridge between the waters of the Red River and those of the Washita, fifteen miles northeast of Fulton, and twenty south of the Little Missouri. From this ridge there is no higher level for a long distance; but to the northwest, there is a gradual ascent for about fifty miles to the foot of the mountains.

"It will be seen by the tables that we have sufficient alternations of heat and cold, rain and sunshine, to diversify our weather. A very large proportion of our rains fall in the night-time, and are generally accompanied with thunder. During the summer, we seldom have any but local showers, and these, though sometimes heavy, are of limited extent. Thus, some localities may be deluged with rain, while others, within a few miles, are at the same time parched with drought.

"Hempstead County is bounded on the south by Red River, which winds in a serpentine course through a valley of from eight to twelve miles in width, much the largest portion of which consists of level prairies, slightly elevated above the surrounding timbered land, and was originally clothed with a tall, fine grass. The soil, beneath the dark brown surface mould, is a dark red clay, twenty to thirty feet deep, through which wells have been sunk, into a quicksand filled with water. The surrounding timber is of gigantic size, consisting of black walnut, pecan, mulberry, oak of different species, cottonwood, cedar, osage orange, with many other species, and thickly interspersed with large cane. These prairies are very distinct in their character from those of the uplands, and only resemble them in being destitute of timber. Ascending northwardly from the river valley, we pass over an elevated timber region, generally level, diversified with ridge and valley, finely watered, soil of several varieties, sandy with pine, clay loam with oak, hickory, and dogwood, and occasionally a tract of prairie.

"Washington, the county town, is situated on a sandy pine hill, in about the centre of the county, in latitude 33° 42′, one hundred and fifty miles west of the Mississippi, fourteen miles northeast from Fulton, on Red River, and on an elevation of about six hundred feet above the bed of Red River, immediately south. To the north and west of the town are the upland prairies. These prairies exhibit a very interesting appearance in a geological point of view. Where they join upon the timbered land, the change is abrupt, from tall timber to naked rock. Tall pine, oak, and hickory, with their roots imbedded in a tough ferruginous clay, grow to the very margin, the line of junction resembling the shore of a lake. The naked prairie is the soft limerock that underlies, at various depths, this whole southwestern region. It has been penetrated by the auger, in attempting to procure water by boring Artesian wells, to the depth of four hundred and fifty feet, without any material change in its character, except occasionally a thin stratum of sandstone. The rock is soft enough to be cut with a knife, and yet cisterns excavated in its substance will hold water and preserve it in purity during any length of time. The chemical composition, so far as I have been informed, is 85 per cent. of carbonate of lime, with a small proportion of silica, and intimately combined with alumina, so that, when exposed to the atmosphere, the moisture absorbed causes it to fall to powder. The naked prairie has the appearance of having been denuded of its superstratum of clay and sand, and the surface produces a slight vegetation, which, being loosened by the action of frost, is ever ready to be washed by the rains to lower grounds, forming a soil of increasing depth as it descends, until, in the valleys, it sustains a growth of heavy timber and cane —a deep, black soil, composed essentially of lime and vegetable mould. Many of these valleys, or river and creek bottoms, are of considerable extent, and are continually increasing in width and depth of soil, by accessions of alluvium from higher grounds. This soil has the peculiar property of retaining moisture, and sustaining a drought without material injury, that would be fatal to crops on sandy uplands. The soil is scarcely surpassed in fertility, yielding equally well all the varied products of the North, and the cotton of the South.

"During the heat of summer, continued refreshing breezes pass over the elevated region, which render the climate pleasant and healthful."

The reductions of the observations were made at the Smithsonian Institution.

JOSEPH HENRY,
Secretary S. I.

CONTENTS.

OBSERVATIONS.

SUMMARIES.

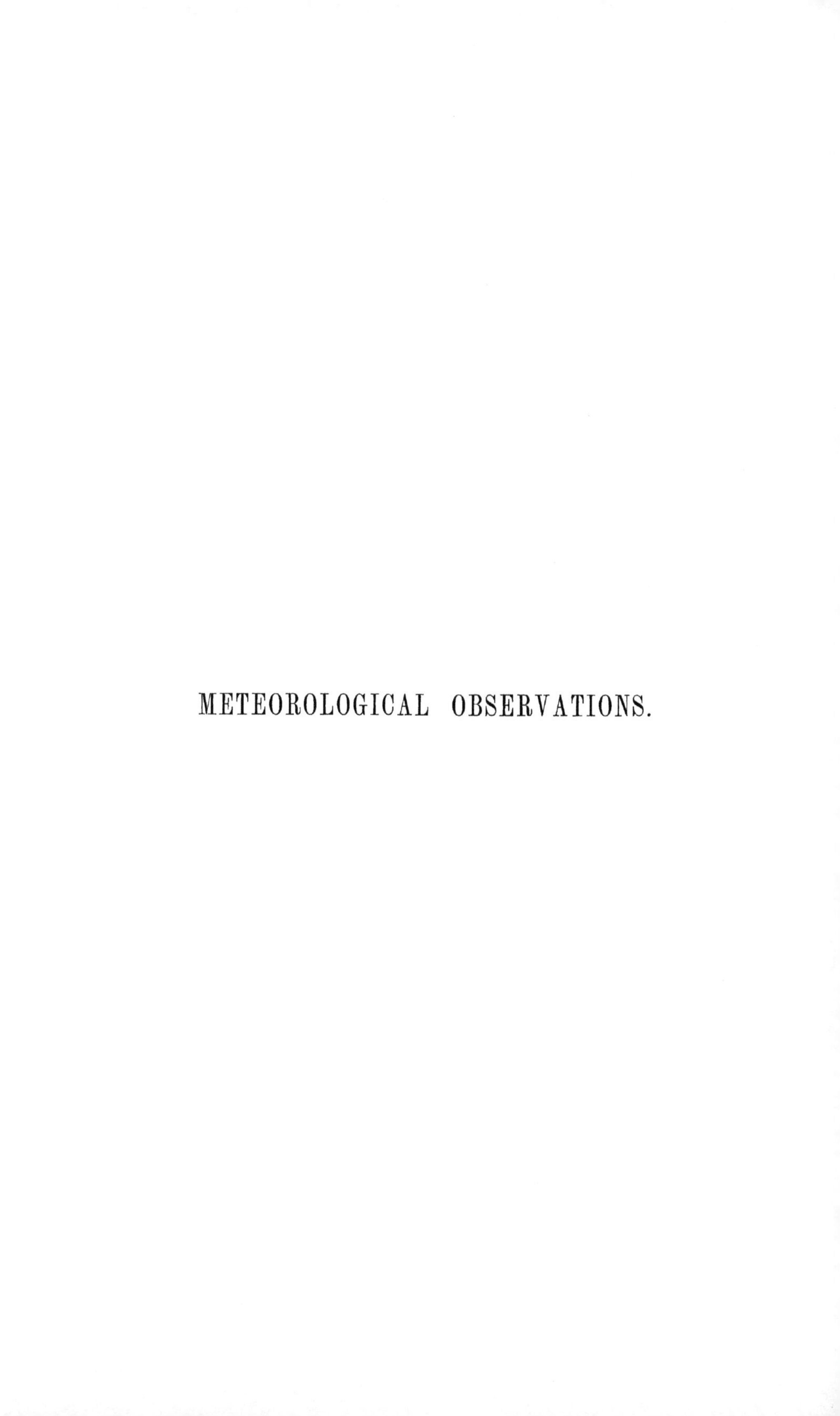

METEOROLOGICAL OBSERVATIONS.

January, 1840.

DAY.	THERMOMETER. Sunrise.	2 P.M.	Mean.	RAIN. Ins.	REMARKS ON THE WEATHER.
1	14	30	22.0	. .	Fair.
2	13	46	29.5	. .	Fair.
3	30	60	45.0	. .	Clouds; fair.
4	28	56	42.0	. .	Fair.
5	40	60	50.0	. .	Cloudy; mist.
6	58	50	54.0	. .	Cloudy.
7	44	50	47.0	. .	Cloudy; mist.
8	44	48	46.0	. .	Cloudy; mist.
9	44	58	51.0	2.0	Cloudy; heavy rain after night.
10	44	58	51.0	. .	Rain; fair at noon.
11	46	50	48.0	. .	Clouds.
12	28	48	38.0	. .	Fair; ice.
13	36	50	43.0	. .	Cloudy.
14	40	48	44.0	1.0	Cloudy; rain.
15	26	40	33.0	. .	Fair.
16	20	40	30.0	. .	Fair.
17	26	50	38.0	. .	Fair.
18	22	40	31.0	. .	Fair.
19	14	44	29.0	. .	Fair.
20	17	56	36.5	1.0	Fair; cloudy; rain after night.
21	46	50	48.0	. .	Rain.
22	46	48	47.0	2.5	Rain; fair at evening.
23	25	60	42.5	. .	Fair.
24	26	60	43.0	. .	Fair.
25	26	60	43.0	. .	Clouds.
26	32	58	45.0	. .	Cloudy. Frogs peeping.
27	50	63	56.5	0.5	Cloudy; rain.
28	60	58	59.0	0.5	Cloudy; rain.
29	55	60	57.5	. .	Cloudy.
30	18	40	29.0	. .	Clouds.
31	24	30	27.0	. .	Cloudy; snow.
Means	33.61	50.61	42.11	7.5	Greatest Rise and Fall of temperature in 24 hours.
Max.	60	63	59.0		
Min.	13	30	22.0		
Range	47	33	37.0		

Extreme range 50

	Sunrise.	2 P.M.
Rise . . .	29	16
Fall . . .	37	20

February, 1840.

DAY.	THERMOMETER. Sunrise.	2 P.M.	Mean.	RAIN. Ins.	REMARKS ON THE WEATHER.
1	20	34	27.0	. .	Cl'dy; ground covered with snow.
2	10	40	25.0	. .	Fair.
3	16	50	33.0	. .	Fair.
4	24	50	37.0	. .	Fair.
5	46	56	51.0	0.5	Clouds; N. wind; rain in night.
6	46	58	52.0	. .	Clouds.
7	36	56	46.0	. .	Fair.
8	40	52	46.0	1.5	Fog; mist; rain at night.
9	50	60	55.0	. .	Cloudy; light showers.
10	35	55	45.0	. .	Fair.
11	27	58	42.5	. .	Fair.
12	48	60	54.0	. .	Cloudy; fair.
13	55	65	60.0	1.5	Cloudy.
14	20	44	32.0	. .	Fair.
15	18	50	34.0	2.5	Fair; cloudy; thunder; rain at
16	36	42	39.0	1.5	Rain. [night.
17	40	50	45.0	. .	Rain.
18	45	60	52.5	. .	Cloudy; mist.
19	60	62	61.0	1.5	Rain.
20	50	60	55.0	. .	Cloudy; fair.
21	38	55	46.5	5.0	Clouds; heavy thunder and rain.
22	54	58	56.0	. .	Rain. Morus mult. buds green.
23	52	62	57.0	. .	Cloudy; fair.
24	38	60	49.0	. .	Fair.
25	35	65	50.0	. .	Fair.
26	50	72	61.0	. .	Clouds.
27	58	75	66.5	. .	Clouds.
28	58	76	67.0	. .	Fair.
29	54	80	67.0	0.5	Fair; thunder; rain at night.
Means	39.97	57.41	48.69	14.5	Greatest Rise and Fall of temperature in 24 hours.
Max.	60	80	67.0		
Min.	10	34	25.0		
Range	50	46	42.0		

Extreme range 70

	Sunrise.	2 P.M.
Rise . . .	22	10
Fall . . .	35	21

March, 1840.

DAY.	THERMOMETER. Sunrise.	2 P.M.	Mean.	RAIN. Ins.	REMARKS ON THE WEATHER.
1	60	70	65.0	0.5	Heavy shower in morning; fair.
2	56	60	58.0	. .	Fair.
3	54	68	61.0	. .	Clouds; fair.
4	47	75	61.0	. .	Fair. Silk-worms hatched.
5	48	72	60.0	. .	Fair.
6	50	74	62.0	. .	Clouds; fair.
7	54	78	66.0	. .	Fair.
8	54	80	67.0	0.1	Fair; wind; thunder; rain at
9	54	80	67.0	0.6	Clouds. [night.
10	48	76	62.0	. .	Fair.
11	42	60	51.0	. .	Fair.
12	42	60	51.0	. .	Fair.
13	33	62	47.5	. .	Fair; frost; smoky; cloudy.
14	59	60	59.5	0.5	Cloudy; rain. Oaks in bloom;
15	46	56	51.0	. .	Cloudy; rain. [vines in leaf.
16	50	58	54.0	1.0	Rain.
17	46	76	61.0	. .	Fair.
18	47	80	63.5	0.3	Fair; thunder and rain at eve.
19	48	80	64.0	. .	Fair.
20	50	42	46.0	. .	Cloudy; rain.
21	38	52	45.0	. .	Cloudy.
22	44	60	52.0	0.5	Cloudy; thunder; rain.
23	52	68	60.0	. .	Cloudy; mist; fair at eve.
24	52	60	56.0	. .	Cloudy.
25	31	60	45.5	. .	Fair; frost.
26	36	70	53.0	. .	Fair; frost.
27	58	74	66.0	. .	Clouds; high wind after night.
28	60	74	67.0	. .	Clouds.
29	48	50	49.0	0.7	Rain.
30	34	48	41.0	. .	Fair; white frost.
31	34	65	49.5	. .	Fair.
Means	47.58	66.06	56.82	4.2	Greatest Rise and Fall of temperature in 24 hours.
Max.	60	80	67.0		
Min.	31	42	41.0		
Range	29	38	26.0		

Extreme range 49

	Sunrise.	2 P.M.
Rise . . .	26	18
Fall . . .	21	38

April, 1840.

DAY.	THERMOMETER. Sunrise.	2 P.M.	Mean.	RAIN. Ins.	REMARKS ON THE WEATHER.
1	50	60	55.0	. .	Cloudy.
2	50	67	58.5	. .	Fair; clouds.
3	50	70	60.0	0.5	Clouds; thunder; rain at night.
4	60	74	67.0	. .	Flying clouds from south.
5	60	70	65.0	. .	Fog; cloudy. [at night.
6	64	74	67.0	1.5	Shower in morning; thunder; rain
7	61	70	65.5	0.3	Cloudy; shower at noon.
8	51	61	56.0	. .	Clouds.
9	46	74	60.0	. .	Fair. [night.
10	60	68	64.0	2.8	Cloudy; thunder; heavy rain at
11	60	72	66.0	1.5	Cloudy; showers; rain. First
12	44	61	52.5	. .	Fair. [swarm of bees.
13	50	58	54.0	. .	Cloudy.
14	58	72	65.0	0.5	Cloudy; thunder; rain at night.
15	60	75	67.5	. .	Fair.
16	56	83	69.5	. .	Fair. [night.
17	66	80	73.0	0.1	Cloudy; fair; thunder; rain at
18	51	50	50.5	0.2	Cloudy; thunder; rain.
19	49	54	51.5	. .	Cloudy; shower.
20	52	70	61.0	0.1	Rain.
21	60	76	68.0	. .	Cloudy. Silk-worms spinning.
22	66	76	71.0	. .	Cloudy.
23	67	80	73.5	0.2	Rain in morning; fair at noon.
24	68	83	75.5	. .	Clouds; fair.
25	68	80	74.0	1.5	Clouds; thunder; rain at night.
26	60	68	64.0	. .	Fair.
27	46	49	47.5	0.8	Thunder; hail and rain.
28	58	62	60.0	0.7	Cloudy; rain.
29	56	76	66.0	1.3	Thunder; rain. [P.M.
30	64	70	67.0	1.6	Cloudy; fair; heavy shower at 4
Means	57.03	69.43	63.23	13.6	Greatest Rise and Fall of temperature in 24 hours.
Max.	68	83	75.5		
Min.	44	49	47.5		
Range	24	34	28.0		

Extreme range 39

	Sunrise.	2 P.M.
Rise . . .	16	16
Fall . . .	16	30

May, 1840.

DAY.	THERMOMETER. Sun-rise.	THERMOMETER. 3 P. M.	THERMOMETER. Mean.	RAIN. Ins.	REMARKS ON THE WEATHER.
1	62	68	65.0	1.5	Cloudy; heavy rain at night.
2	66	77	71.5	. .	Cl'dy; sh'r at 12; thunder, wind,
3	60	78	69.0	. .	Fair; windy. [rain at night.
4	58	78	68.0	. .	Fair.
5	58	80	69.0	. .	Fair. [rain at night.
6	64	72	68.0	2.8	Cloudy; rain; heavy thunder and
7	68	76	72.0	. .	Cloudy; fair. Reeling silk.
8	58	74	66.0	. .	Fair.
9	52	66	59.0	. .	Cloudy; fair.
10	46	66	56.0	. .	Fair.
11	48	73	60.5	. .	Fair.
12	56	70	63.0	. .	Cloudy.
13	58	72	65.0	. .	Cloudy.
14	64	70	67.0	. .	Cloudy.
15	58	76	67.0	. .	Fair.
16	60	82	71.0	. .	Fair.
17	66	78	72.0	. .	Cloudy; fair.
18	66	82	74.0	0.5	Fair; shower after night.
19	70	80	75.0	. .	Fog; fair.
20	56	80	68.0	. .	Fair.
21	54	78	66.0	. .	Fair.
22	60	80	70.0	. .	Fair. [eve.
23	66	82	74.0	0.4	Fair; thunder, rain, and hail at
24	64	68	66.0	0.5	Fair; cloudy; showery.
25	58	72	65.0	. .	Fog; fair.
26	56	74	65.0	. .	Fair; clouds; light sprinkle.
27	60	80	70.0	. .	Fair.
28	68	78	73.0	. .	Cloudy; sprinkle.
29	62	80	71.0	. .	Fair.
30	62	80	71.0	. .	Fair.
31	. .	. .	. .	. .	
Means	60.13	75.67	67.90	5.7	
Max.	70	82	75.0		
Min.	46	66	56.0		
Range	24	16	19.0		
Extreme range 36					

Greatest Rise and Fall of temperature in 24 hours.	Sunrise.	3 P. M.
Rise . . .	8	9
Fall . . .	14	14

June, 1840.

DAY.	THERMOMETER. Sun-rise.	THERMOMETER. 3 P. M.	THERMOMETER. Mean.	RAIN. Ins.	REMARKS ON THE WEATHER.
1	64	85	74.5	. .	Fair. Second crop of silk-worms
2	76	86	81.0	. .	Fair. [hatched.
3	68	88	78.0	. .	Fair.
4	60	84	72.0	. .	Fair.
5	74	82	78.0	0.3	Fair; thunder, wind, and rain at
6	. .	. .	. .	. .	[night.
7	66	77	71.5	. .	Fair.
8	56	76	66.0	. .	Fair.
9	57	82	69.5	. .	Fair.
10	64	82	73.0	. .	Fair.
11	66	82	74.0	. .	Fair.
12	64	85	74.5	. .	Fair.
13	64	84	74.0	. .	Fair.
14	66	88	77.0	. .	Fair.
15	70	87	78.5	. .	Fair.
16	66	82	74.0	. .	Fair.
17	70	80	75.0	. .	Fair.
18	68	84	76.0	. .	Fair.
19	70	85	77.5	. .	Fog; fair.
20	68	82	75.0	. .	Fog; clouds.
21	70	83	76.5	. .	Clouds.
22	70	78	74.0	. .	Cloudy; mist in the morning.
23	72	78	75.0	0.4	Cloudy; rain.
24	74	84	79.0	0.2	Cloudy and showers. Silk-worms
25	74	84	79.0	. .	Clouds. [spinning.
26	74	87	80.5	. .	Fair.
27	74	84	79.0	. .	Clouds.
28	74	86	80.0	. .	Fair.
29	74	88	81.0	. .	Fair.
30	74	92	83.0	. .	Fair.
Means	68.52	83.62	76.07	0.9	
Max.	76	92	83.0		
Min.	56	76	66.0		
Range	20	16	17.0		
Extreme range 36					

Greatest Rise and Fall of temperature in 24 hours.	Sunrise.	3 P. M.
Rise . . .	14	6
Fall . . .	10	5

July, 1840.

DAY.	THERMOMETER. Sun-rise.	THERMOMETER. 3 P. M.	THERMOMETER. Mean.	RAIN. Ins.	REMARKS ON THE WEATHER.
1	70	84	77.0	. .	Cloudy.
2	68	82	75.0	. .	Fair.
3	59	70	64.5	. .	Fair; clouds.
4	64	70	67.0	0.2	Cloudy; rain at noon.
5	68	78	73.0	. .	Fair.
6	66	74	70.0	. .	Fair.
7	72	78	75.0	1.4	Cloudy; thunder: rain at 2 P. M.
8	70	80	75.0	0.5	Cloudy; thunder; rain at 4 P. M.
9	72	84	78.0	. .	Clouds.
10	74	87	85.5	. .	Cloudy; fair.
11	74	86	75.0	. .	Clouds.
12	74	84	79.0	. .	Clouds.
13	72	88	80.0	. .	Fair.
14	74	99	81.0	. .	Fog; fair.
15	70	88	79.0	. .	Fair.
16	74	88	81.0	. .	Clouds; fair.
17	74	88	81.0	. .	Clouds.
18	72	85	78.5	. .	Clouds; sprinkle at 3 P. M.
19	74	84	79.0	. .	Clouds; sprinkle at 4 P. M.
20	72	88	80.0	. .	Clouds.
21	70	86	78.0	. .	Clouds.
22	74	86	80.0	0.2	Clouds; rain at night. 3d crop of
23	70	88	79.0	. .	Fair. [silk-worms hatched.
24	68	86	77.0	. .	Fair.
25	67	88	77.5	. .	Fair.
26	70	88	79.0	. .	Fair.
27	70	90	80.0	. .	Fair.
28	74	90	82.0	. .	Fair.
29	70	90	80.0	. .	Fair.
30	70	84	77.0	0.2	Fair; rain at 3 P. M.
31	74	87	80.5	. .	Fog; fair.
Means	70.64	84.42	77.53	2.5	
Max.	74	90	85.5		
Min.	59	70	64.5		
Range	15	20	21.0		
Extreme range 31					

Greatest Rise and Fall of temperature in 24 hours.	Sunrise.	3 P. M.
Rise . . .	6	8
Fall . . .	9	12

August, 1840.

DAY.	THERMOMETER. Sun-rise.	THERMOMETER. 3 P. M.	THERMOMETER. Mean.	RAIN Ins.	REMARKS ON THE WEATHER.
1	70	88	79.0	. .	Fair.
2	70	92	81.0	. .	Fair; clouds.
3	70	90	80.0	. .	Clouds.
4	74	91	82.5	. .	Cloudy.
5	70	90	80.0	. .	Fair.
6	74	90	82.0	. .	Cloudy.
7	74	92	83.0	0.2	Fair; shower at night.
8	62	80	71.0	. .	Cloudy.
9	54	82	68.0	. .	Fair.
10	54	87	70.5	. .	Fair.
11	54	86	70.0	. .	Fair.
12	56	88	72.0	. .	Fair.
13	64	85	79.5	. .	Fair.
14	60	88	74.0	. .	Fair.
15	54	87	70.5	. .	Sprinkle at night.
16	60	84	72.0	. .	Slight sprinkle at noon.
17	60	88	74.0	. .	
18	64	90	77.0	0.2	Clouds; shower at 3 P. M.
19	60	88	74.0	0.2	Clouds; shower at 2 P. M.
20	64	92	78.0	0.4	Clouds; shower at 5 P. M.
21	70	90	80.0	. .	
22	70	92	81.0	. .	
23	70	92	81.0	0.3	Shower at 3 P. M.
24	66	90	78.0	. .	
25	68	89	78.5	. .	
26	66	93	74.5	. .	
27	70	94	82.0	. .	
28	70	93	81.5	. .	
29	70	92	81.0	. .	
30	72	90	81.0	. .	
31	72	86	79.0	. .	
Means	65.55	89.00	77.27	1.3	
Max.	74	94	83.0		
Min.	54	80	68.0		
Range	20	14	15.0		
Extreme range 40					

Greatest Rise and Fall of temperature in 24 hours.	Sunrise.	3 P. M.
Rise . . .	8	5
Fall . . .	12	12

September, 1840.

DAY.	THERMOMETER. Sunrise.	3 P. M.	Mean.	RAIN. Ins.	REMARKS ON THE WEATHER.
1	60	84	72.0	. .	Fair.
2	58	82	70.0	. .	Fair; clouds; sprinkle in night.
3	66	78	72.0	. .	Cloudy; fair.
4	54	76	65.0	. .	Fair.
5	48	76	62.0	. .	Fair.
6	50	84	67.0	. .	Fair.
7	60	88	74.0	. .	Smoky; fire in the woods.
8	60	91	75.5	. .	Smoky; rain after night.
9	70	80	75.0	0.8	Thunder; rain.
10	60	82	71.0	. .	Fair.
11	56	75	65.5	. .	Fair.
12	50	76	63.0	. .	Fair.
13	50	78	64.0	. .	Fair; clouds.
14	54	78	66.0	. .	Fair.
15	52	82	67.0	. .	Fair.
16	54	86	70.0	. .	Fair.
17	68	80	74.0	0.1	Cloudy; rain at night.
18	56	76	66.0	. .	Cloudy; wind from S. W.
19	43	70	56.5	. .	Fair.
20	48	77	62.5	. .	Fair.
21	54	76	65.0	. .	Fair.
22	50	74	62.0	. .	Fair.
23	54	72	63.0	. .	Cloudy; fair.
24	66	73	69.5	. .	Cloudy; mist.
25	66	82	74.0	. .	Cloudy; fair.
26	60	84	72.0	0.7	Fair; shower at 3 P. M.
27	66	70	68.0	0.3	Fair; shower at noon.
28	66	70	68.0	0.4	Rain; thunder.
29	68	68	68.0	0.5	Rain; thunder.
30	64	78	71.0	. .	Fog; fair.
Means	57.70	78.20	67.95	2.8	
Max.	70	91	75.5		
Min.	43	68	56.5		
Range	27	23	19.0		
Extreme range 48					

Greatest Rise and Fall of temperature in 24 hours.

	Sunrise.	3 P. M.
Rise	10	9
Fall	13	11

November, 1840.

DAY.	THERMOMETER. Sunrise.	3 P. M.	Mean.	RAIN. Ins.	REMARKS ON THE WEATHER.
1	34	60	47.0	. .	Fair.
2	40	62	51.0	. .	Fair; cloudy.
3	48	64	56.0	. .	Cloudy.
4	40	68	54.0	. .	Fair.
5	52	72	62.0	. .	Fair.
6	56	60	58.0	0.2	Rain.
7	56	70	63.0	. .	Fair.
8	36	62	49.0	. .	Fair.
9	34	64	49.0	. .	Fair.
10	48	60	54.0	1.6	Cloudy; thunder and rain at night.
11	48	60	54.0	. .	Fair.
12	34	64	49.0	. .	Fair.
13	33	66	49.5	. .	Fair.
14	44	66	55.0	. .	Fair.
15	36	40	38.0	. .	Fair.
16	40	54	47.0	. .	Fair.
17	40	36	38.0	. .	Cloudy; fair.
18	26	46	36.0	. .	Fair; ice.
19	24	48	36.0	. .	Fair; ice.
20	45	65	55.0	1.7	Cloudy; thunder and rain at night.
21	56	58	57.0	. .	Rain; fair at 1 P. M.
22	32	36	34.0	. .	Cloudy.
23	27	34	30.5	0.3	Cloudy; rain at night.
24	33	34	33.5	. .	Snow.
25	23	30	26.5	. .	Cloudy; snow; fair at noon.
26	18	48	33.0	. .	Fair.
27	26	56	41.0	. .	Fair.
28	30	40	35.0	. .	Fair.
29	46	68	57.0	. .	Fair.
30	46	60	53.0	. .	Clouds.
Means	38.37	55.03	46.70	3.8	
Max.	56	72	63.0		
Min.	18	30	26.5		
Range	38	42	36.5		
Extreme range 54					

Greatest Rise and Fall of temperature in 24 hours.

	Sunrise.	3 P. M.
Rise	21	28
Fall	24	26

October, 1840.

DAY.	THERMOMETER. Sunrise.	3 P. M.	Mean.	RAIN. Ins.	REMARKS ON THE WEATHER.
1	64	81	72.5	. .	Fair.
2	74	60	67.0	0.2	Rain; fair.
3	35	60	47.5	. .	Fair; white frost.
4	37	70	53.5	. .	Fair; white frost.
5	40	70	55.0	. .	Fair; white frost.
6	. .	. .	. .	. .	
7	50	80	65.0	. .	Fair.
8	68	80	74.0	0.2	Cloudy; rain in the night.
9	70	80	75.0	. .	Cloudy.
10	70	83	76.5	. .	Cloudy; fair.
11	69	76	72.5	. .	Clouds; thunder.
12	62	74	68.0	2.7	Fog; rain; heavy rain in night.
13	66	76	71.0	1.8	Rain; thunder showers.
14	68	70	69.0	. .	Cloudy.
15	70	72	71.0	1.0	Rain; thunder.
16	63	72	67.5	1.0	Thunder; rain; fair at 2 P. M.
17	70	70	70.0	. .	Clouds.
18	70	74	72.0	0.2	Cloudy; shower at 1 P. M. and at
19	60	70	65.0	. .	Fair. [night.
20	54	72	63.0	0.2	Clouds; thunder and hail in the
21	58	66	62.0	. .	Fair. [night.
22	40	64	52.0	. .	Frost; fair.
23	40	66	53.0	. .	Frost; fair.
24	44	56	50.0	. .	Clouds; fair.
25	30	56	43.0	. .	Fair; white frost.
26	36	55	45.5	. .	Fair; white frost.
27	40	60	50.0	0.7	Cloudy; rain at night.
28	56	56	56.0	. .	Rain.
29	36	56	46.0	. .	Fair; white frost.
30	40	56	48.0	. .	Fair.
31	32	60	46.0	. .	Fair; white frost.
Means	53.73	68.03	60.88	8.0	
Max.	74	83	76.5		
Min.	30	55	43.0		
Range	44	28	33.5		
Extreme range 53					

Greatest Rise and Fall of temperature in 24 hours.

	Sunrise.	3 P. M.
Rise	18	10
Fall	20	21

December, 1840.

DAY.	THERMOMETER. Sunrise.	3 P. M.	Mean.	RAIN. Ins.	REMARKS ON THE WEATHER.
1	42	40	41.0	. .	Cloudy.
2	40	40	40.0	. .	Cloudy.
3	42	44	43.0	0.7	Rain.
4	34	34	34.0	. .	Snow.
5	28	44	36.0	. .	Fair.
6	27	46	36.5	. .	Fair.
7	42	60	51.0	. .	Cloudy.
8	50	62	56.0	. .	Clouds.
9	58	66	62.0	. .	Clouds; fair. [night.
10	57	66	61.5	0.3	Fog; fair; thunder and rain at
11	60	66	63.0	0.2	Cloudy; shower at 2 P. M.
12	40	44	42.0	. .	Fair.
13	33	40	36.5	. .	Fair.
14	40	66	53.0	. .	Cloudy; fair.
15	40	72	56.0	. .	Fair.
16	48	56	52.0	. .	Fair.
17	28	50	39.0	. .	Fair.
18	32	40	36.0	. .	Cloudy; fair at noon.
19	36	40	38.0	0.5	Cloudy; rain at night.
20	36	44	40.0	. .	Cloudy.
21	40	52	46.0	. .	Fair; cloudy.
22	44	54	49.0	. .	Cloudy.
23	40	48	44.0	. .	Cloudy; fair.
24	24	30	27.0	. .	Cloudy; fair.
25	28	50	39.0	. .	Fair.
26	36	58	47.0	. .	Fair.
27	32	40	36.0	. .	Fair.
28	24	30	27.0	. .	Fair.
29	34	44	39.0	1.0	Fair; rain at night.
30	34	36	35.0	. .	Cloudy.
31	27	29	28.0	. .	Cloudy; snow.
Means	37.94	48.10	43.02	2.7	
Max.	60	72	63		
Min.	24	29	27		
Range	36	43	36		
Extreme range 48					

Greatest Rise and Fall of temperature in 24 hours.

	Sunrise.	3 P. M.
Rise	15	26
Fall	20	22

January, 1841.

DAY.	THERMOMETER. Sunrise.	THERMOMETER. 2 P. M.	THERMOMETER. Mean.	RAIN. Ins.	REMARKS ON THE WEATHER.
1	16	36	26.0	. .	Fair.
2	26	36	31.0	. .	Fair.
3	14	48	31.0	. .	Fair.
4	25	46	35.5	. .	Cloudy.
5	42	64	53.0	1.0	Fog; mist; fair; thunder and rain
6	58	48	53.0	. .	Rain; thunder. [at night.
7	33	36	34.5	. .	Cloudy.
8	33	34	33.5	. .	Cloudy.
9	36	40	38.0	0.2	Cloudy; rain.
10	40	42	41.0	0.2	Rain.
11	42	47	44.5	. .	Fair.
12	38	42	40.0	. .	Cloudy.
13	36	38	37.0	0.2	Rain.
14	28	45	36.5	. .	Mist; fair.
15	30	45	37.5	2.0	Cloudy; heavy rain at night.
16	50	40	45.0	. .	Mist; snow and sleet at night.
17	3	12	7.5	. .	Fair; ground white with snow.
18	4	21	12.5	. .	Fair; cloudy; snow at night.
19	19	24	21.5	. .	Cloudy; mist.
20	26	34	30.0	. .	Cloudy; mist.
21	30	37	33.5	. .	Cloudy; fair.
22	24	42	33.0	. .	Fair; trees loaded with icicles.
23	30	40	35.0	. .	Fair; trees loaded with icicles.
24	40	59	49.5	. .	Fair.
25	34	60	47.0	. .	Fair.
26	50	62	56.0	. .	Cloudy; mist; fair.
27	50	65	57.5	. .	Fair.
28	50	52	51.0	0.2	Cloudy; rain.
29	42	50	46.0	. .	Fair.
30	42	48	45.0	0.7	Cloudy; rain.
31	40	44	42.0	0.5	Cloudy; rain.
Means	33.26	43.13	38.19	5.0	
Max.	58	65	57.5		
Min.	3	12	7.5		
Range	55	53	50.0		
Extreme range 62					

Greatest Rise and Fall of temperature in 24 hours.

	Sunrise.	2 P. M.
Rise . . .	20	19
Fall . . .	47	28

March, 1841.

DAY.	THERMOMETER. Sunrise.	THERMOMETER. 2 P. M.	THERMOMETER. Mean.	RAIN. Ins.	REMARKS ON THE WEATHER.
1	48	50	49.0	. .	Smoky.
2	52	60	56.0	0.7	Thunder and rain in morning.
3	38	44	41.0	. .	Fair.
4	50	64	57.0	0.2	Cloudy; thunder and rain at night.
5	52	54	53.0	0.1	Cloudy; thunder and rain at night.
6	42	48	45.0	. .	Fair.
7	36	50	43.0	. .	Fair. Morus buds green.
8	28	50	39.0	1.2	Fair; thunder and rain at night.
9	40	45	42.5	. .	Rain; thunder.
10	36	37	36.5	0.7	Snow and rain.
11	32	36	34.0	. .	Snow.
12	30	46	38.0	. .	Fair.
13	28	32	30.0	. .	Fair.
14	40	68	54.0	. .	Fair.
15	50	68	59.0	. .	Fair.
16	48	62	55.0	. .	Fair.
17	35	62	48.5	. .	Fair.
18	36	70	53.0	. .	Fair.
19	45	75	60.0	. .	Clouds. Oaks in bloom.
20	52	60	56.0	. .	Fair.
21	56	64	60.0	. .	Cloudy; thunder; rain at night.
22	60	58	59.0	0.7	Cloudy; rain.
23	32	60	46.0	. .	Fair; white frost. Vegetation
24	40	70	55.0	. .	Fair. [killed.
25	56	75	65.5	. .	Clouds. Silk-worms hatched.
26	66	70	68.0	2.4	Cloudy; thunder; rain.
27	60	70	65.0	2.6	Cloudy; thunder; rain and hail
28	60	62	61.0	. .	Fair. [at night.
29	40	50	45.0	. .	Fair.
30	40	59	49.5	. .	Fair.
31	48	72	60.0	. .	Cloudy; fair at eve.
Means	44.39	57.77	51.08	8.6	
Max.	66	75	68.0		
Min.	28	32	30.0		
Range	38	43	38.0		
Extreme range 47					

Greatest Rise and Fall of temperature in 24 hours.

	Sunrise.	2 P. M.
Rise . . .	16	36
Fall . . .	28	16

February, 1841.

DAY.	THERMOMETER. Sunrise.	THERMOMETER. 2 P. M.	THERMOMETER. Mean.	RAIN. Ins.	REMARKS ON THE WEATHER.
1	40	48	44.0	. .	Cloudy.
2	32	52	42.0	. .	Fair.
3	40	50	45.0	. .	Fair.
4	32	52	42.0	. .	Fair.
5	44	50	47.0	0.2	Cloudy; rain at night.
6	38	40	39.0	. .	Cloudy; rain.
7	34	42	38.0	. .	Cloudy; fair.
8	34	40	37.0	. .	Cloudy.
9	36	46	41.0	. .	Cloudy; fair.
10	28	30	29.0	. .	Cloudy.
11	18	33	25.5	. .	Fair.
12	18	42	30.0	. .	Fair.
13	26	35	30.5	. .	Fair.
14	26	35	30.5	. .	Fair.
15	24	42	33.0	. .	Fair.
16	,26	58	42.0	. .	Fair.
17	32	65	48.5	. .	Fair.
18	30	65	47.5	. .	Fair; smoky; fire in the woods.
19	40	62	51.0	. .	Smoky; clouds.
20	36	40	38.0	. .	Smoky.
21	42	60	51.0	. .	Smoky.
22	40	66	53.0	. .	Smoky.
23	40	76	58.0	. .	Smoky.
24	43	50	46.5	. .	Smoky.
25	38	52	45.0	. .	Smoky.
26	40	60	50.0	0.2	Smoky; rain at night.
27	44	52	48.0	. .	Fair.
28	32	60	46.0	. .	Fair.
Means	34.04	50.11	42.07	0.4	
Max.	44	76	58.0		
Min.	18	30	25.5		
Range	26	46	32.5		
Extreme range 58					

Greatest Rise and Fall of temperature in 24 hours.

	Sunrise.	2 P. M.
Rise . . .	12	20
Fall . . .	10	26

April, 1841.

DAY.	THERMOMETER. Sunrise.	THERMOMETER. 2 P. M.	THERMOMETER. Mean.	RAIN. Ins.	REMARKS ON THE WEATHER.
1	54	72	63.0	. .	Clouds. [rain at night.
2	58	64	61.0	0.4	Cl'dy; sh'r in morning; thunder;
3	50	56	53.0	1.2	Cloudy; showers; rain and hail.
4	50	60	55.0	. .	Cloudy; fair.
5	44	70	57.0	. .	Fair.
6	48	74	61.0	. .	Fair.
7	54	76	65.0	. .	Cloudy; fair.
8	56	80	68.0	. .	Fair.
9	64	82	73.0	. .	Clouds; fair.
10	66	76	71.0	. .	Cloudy.
11	54	60	57.0	. .	Cloudy.
12	47	50	48.5	. .	Fair.
13	48	76	62.0	. .	Fair; thunder at night; sprinkle.
14	54	70	62.0	. .	Fair.
15	52	64	58.0	0.2	Fair; clouds; shower at 3 P. M.
16	54	76	65.0	. .	Fair; showers. [after night.
17	66	80	73.0	1.0	Cloudy; thunder, rain, and hail
18	54	68	61.0	. .	Fair.*
19	44	70	57.0	0.2	Fair; thunder; rain at night.
20	61	70	65.5	. .	Fair.
21	46	76	61.0	. .	Fair.
22	54	78	66.0	. .	Fair.
23	58	76	67.0	. .	Fair.
24	58	80	69.0	. .	Fair.
25	58	82	70.0	. .	Fair.
26	68	70	69.0	0.5	Cloudy; rain.
27	52	54	53.0	1.7	Rain.
28	56	72	64.0	0.2	Rain; high wind at night.
29	45	62	53.5	. .	Fair; windy. Silk-worms spin-
30	42	70	56.0	. .	Fair. [ning.
Means	53.83	70.47	62.15	5.4	
Max.	68	82	73.0		
Min.	42	50	48.5		
Range	20	32	24.5		
Extreme range 40					

Greatest Rise and Fall of temperature in 24 hours.

	Sunrise.	2 P. M.
Rise . . .	17	26
Fall . . .	16	16

* April 18. Meteor at 3 P. M., N. W.; explosion like the sharp rattle of a wagon over rough ground, 45° above the horizon, leaving fragments of clouds on the clear sky.

May, 1841.

DAY.	THERMOMETER. Sunrise.	THERMOMETER. 3 P. M.	THERMOMETER. Mean.	RAIN. Ins.	REMARKS ON THE WEATHER.
1	44	78	61.0	. .	Fair.
2	52	78	65.0	. .	Fair.
3	60	76	68.0	. .	Cloudy.
4	66	76	71.0	1.2	Cloudy; thunder; rain at night.
5	60	76	68.0	. .	Fair.
6	58	76	67.0	2.0	Thundershower A. M.; fair; thun-
7	58	70	64.0	. .	Fair. [der; rain at night.
8	54	60	57.0	2.5	Cloudy; thunder, rain, and hail.
9	58	60	59.0	. .	Cloudy; rain.
10	54	82	68.0	. .	Fair.
11	54	80	67.0	. .	Fair.
12	60	85	72.5	. .	Fair.
13	64	78	71.0	. .	Cloudy; fair.
14	54	62	58.0	. .	Fair.
15	44	69	56.5	. .	Fair.
16	50	70	60.0	. .	Fair.
17	46	77	61.5	. .	Fair.
18	50	80	65.0	. .	Fair.
19	50	80	65.0	. .	Cloudy.
20	50	84	67.0	. .	Fair.
21	60	80	70.0	. .	Cloudy; sprinkle.
22	65	83	74.0	. .	Fair.
23	65	82	73.5	0.5	Cloudy; thunder; rain at 4 P. M.
24	65	78	71.5	. .	Cloudy; sprinkle at night.
25	66	72	69.0	. .	Cloudy.
26	62	80	71.0	. .	Fair.
27	58	82	70.0	. .	Fair.
28	58	84	71.0	. .	Fair.
29	66	87	76.5	. .	Fair; shower at 3 P. M. [2 P. M.
30	62	70	66.0	0.7	Fair; cl'dy; thunder; rain; hail at
31	60	86	73.0	0.3	Fair; cl'dy; thunder; rain 4 P. M.
Means	57.19	76.81	67.0	7.2	
Max.	66	87	76.5		
Min.	44	60	56.5		
Range	22	27	20.0		

Extreme range 43

Greatest Rise and Fall of temperature in 24 hours.

	Sunrise.	3 P. M.
Rise . . .	10	22
Fall . . .	10	16

June, 1841.

DAY.	THERMOMETER. Sunrise.	THERMOMETER. 3 P. M.	THERMOMETER. Mean.	RAIN. Ins.	REMARKS ON THE WEATHER.
1	60	84	72.0	. .	Fair.
2	60	88	74.0	. .	Fair.
3	62	88	75.0	. .	Fair.
4	64	90	77.0	. .	Fair.
5	66	91	78.5	. .	Fair.
6	64	88	76.0	. .	Fair.
7	64	89	76.5	. .	Fair.
8	66	92	79.0	. .	Fair.
9	66	92	79.0	. .	Fair.
10	70	88	79.0	. .	Fair.
11	70	87	78.5	. .	Cloudy; rain.
12	64	80	72.0	. .	Fair. [after night.
13	66	78	72.0	1.0	Fair; thunder; rain at 3 P. M. and
14	68	76	72.0	0.3	Fair; shower at 3 P. M.
15	70	68	69.0	0.7	Cloudy; rain at 3 P. M.
16	68	85	76.5	. .	Cloudy.
17	70	80	75.0	. .	Clouds.
18	70	80	75.0	. .	Clouds.
19	70	85	77.5	. .	Fair.
20	70	85	77.5	. .	Clouds; sprinkle at noon.
21	76	64	70.0	1.5	Cloudy; heavy rain at 9 A. M.
22	66	83	74.5	1.5	Rain; fair.
23	66	76	71.0	. .	Fair.
24	56	76	66.0	. .	Fair.
25	54	76	65.0	. .	Fair.
26	52	80	66.0	. .	Fair.
27	56	85	70.5	. .	Fair.
28	60	86	73.0	. .	Fair.
29	60	88	74.0	. .	Fair.
30	70	84	77.0	. .	Cloudy; fair.
Means	64.80	83.07	73.93	5.0	
Max.	76	92	79.0		
Min.	52	64	65.0		
Range	24	28	14.0		

Extreme range 40

Greatest Rise and Fall of temperature in 24 hours.

	Sunrise.	3 P. M.
Rise . . .	10	19
Fall . . .	10	21

July, 1841.

DAY.	THERMOMETER. Sunrise.	THERMOMETER. 3 P. M.	THERMOMETER. Mean.	RAIN. Ins.	REMARKS ON THE WEATHER.
1	70	88	79.0	. .	Cloudy; fair.
2	72	90	81.0	. .	Fair.
3	70	88	79.0	. .	Fair.
4	70	92	81.0	. .	Fair.
5	72	92	82.0	. .	
6	72	93	82.5	. .	
7	74	86	80.0	. .	
8	70	90	80.0	. .	
9	68	90	79.0	. .	
10	68	94	81.0	. .	
11	68	92	80.0	. .	
12	70	90	80.0	. .	
13	70	92	81.0	. .	
14	75	91	83.0	. .	
15	72	95	83.5	. .	
16	70	96	83.0	. .	
17	70	96	83.0	. .	
18	72	88	80.0	0.2	Cloudy; thunder and rain.
19	66	88	77.0	. .	Fair.
20	66	91	78.5	. .	Fair.
21	66	90	78.0	. .	Fair.
22	70	90	80.0	. .	Fair.
23	70	91	80.5	. .	Fair.
24	70	94	82.0	. .	Fair.
25	70	93	81.5	. .	Fair; thunder and wind at 3 P.M.;
26	66	92	79.0	. .	Fair. [sprinkle at night.
27	66	95	80.5	. .	Fair.
28	70	95	82.5	. .	
29	72	96	84.0	. .	
30	74	80	77.0	1.2	Cloudy; thunder; rain and hail at
31	64	85	74.5	. .	[2 P. M.
Means	69.77	91.07	80.42	1.4	
Max.	75	96	84.0		
Min.	64	80	74.5		
Range	11	16	9.5		

Extreme range 32

Greatest Rise and Fall of temperature in 24 hours.

	Sunrise.	3 P. M.
Rise . . .	5	5
Fall . . .	10	16

August, 1841.

DAY.	THERMOMETER. Sunrise.	THERMOMETER. 3 P. M.	THERMOMETER. Mean.	RAIN. Ins.	REMARKS ON THE WEATHER.
1	64	84	74.0	. .	Fair.
2	58	84	71.0	. .	Fair.
3	60	86	73.0	. .	Cloudy.
4	66	88	77.0	. .	Fair.
5	66	88	77.0	. .	Fair.
6	66	92	79.0	. .	Fair.
7	70	94	82.0	. .	Fair.
8	74	86	80.0	. .	Showery; fair at 2 P. M.
9	74	87	80.5	0.4	Rain.
10	72	76	74.0	0.5	Fog; rain.
11	70	86	78.0	. .	Fair; clouds.
12	66	85	75.5	. .	Fair.
13	64	84	74.0	. .	Fair.
14	64	88	76.0	. .	Fair.
15	64	88	76.0	. .	Fair.
16	64	90	77.0	. .	Fair.
17	68	90	79.0	. .	Fair.
18	70	92	81.0	. .	Fair.
19	70	93	81.5	0.4	Cloudy; rain at 4 P. M.
20	70	83	76.5	. .	Clouds; sprinkle.
21	70	82	76.0	. .	Cloudy; thunder.
22	70	85	77.5	. .	Fair.
23	70	74	72.0	. .	Cloudy; sprinkle.
24	70	74	72.0	. .	Cloudy.
25	66	84	75.0	. .	Fair.
26	66	87	76.5	. .	Fair.
27	66	89	77.5	0.3	Clouds; fair.
28	70	86	78.0	. .	Fair.
29	70	86	78.0	1.4	Fair; rain and thunder at night.
30	68	80	74.0	. .	Cloudy; fair.
31	65	86	75.5	. .	Fair.
Means	67.45	85.71	76.58	3.0	
Max.	74	94	82.0		
Min.	58	74	71.0		
Range	16	20	11.0		

Extreme range 36

Greatest Rise and Fall of temperature in 24 hours.

	Sunrise.	3 P. M.
Rise . . .	6	10
Fall . . .	6	11

September, 1841.

DAY.	THERMOMETER. Sunrise.	THERMOMETER. 3 P. M.	THERMOMETER. Mean.	RAIN. Ins.	REMARKS ON THE WEATHER.
1	68	80	74.0	0.4	Fair; cloudy; rain at 3 P. M.
2	66	88	77.0	. .	Fair.
3	68	88	78.0	. .	Fair.
4	70	86	78.0	. .	Fair; shower at noon.
5	68	74	71.0	2.2	Rain; thunder.
6	68	83	75.5	. .	Cloudy; fair.
7	72	86	79.0	. .	Cloudy; fair.
8	72	86	79.0	. .	Fair; slight shower at noon.
9	72	86	79.0	. .	Fair.
10	70	75	72.5	. .	Fair.
11	62	72	67.0	. .	Clouds.
12	60	78	69.0	. .	Fair.
13	55	66	60.5	. .	Fair.
14	54	77	65.5	. .	Fair; clouds.
15	60	80	70.0	. .	Fair.
16	62	78	70.0	. .	Fair.
17	56	78	67.0	. .	Fair.
18	56	78	67.0	. .	Fair.
19	59	80	69.5	. .	Fair.
20	66	83	74.5	1.0	Cloudy; rain; fair; thunder; rain
21	62	58	60.0	. .	Cloudy. [at night.
22	52	67	59.5	. .	Fair.
23	52	69	60.5	. .	Fair.
24	44	66	55.0	. .	Fair.
25	46	80	63.0	. .	Fair.
26	60	80	70.0	1.0	Fair; thunder; rain at night.
27	60	80	70.0	. .	Fair.
28	56	76	66.0	. .	Cloudy.
29	56	70	63.0	. .	Fair.
30	50	67	58.5	. .	Fair.
Means	60.73	77.17	68.95	4.6	
Max.	72	88	79.0		
Min.	44	58	55.0		
Range	28	30	24.0		

Extreme range 44

Greatest Rise and Fall of temperature in 24 hours.

	Sunrise.	3 P. M.
Rise . . .	14	14
Fall . . .	10	25

October, 1841.

DAY.	THERMOMETER. Sunrise.	THERMOMETER. 3 P. M.	THERMOMETER. Mean.	RAIN. Ins.	REMARKS ON THE WEATHER.
1	46	68	57.0	. .	Fair.
2	48	62	55.0	. .	Fair.
3	40	62	51.0	. .	Fair.
4	42	63	52.5	. .	Fair.
5	40	68	54.0	. .	Fair.
6	44	72	58.0	. .	Fair.
7	50	75	62.5	. .	Fair.
8	70	70	70.0	. .	Cloudy.
9	70	76	73.0	1.0	Rain; thunder.
10	67	80	73.5	0.5	Cloudy; rain.
11	70	74	72.0	0.4	Cloudy; rain.
12	62	72	67.0	. .	Cloudy; fair.
13	60	66	63.0	. .	Fair.
14	44	63	53.5	. .	Fair.
15	42	66	54.0	. .	Clouds.
16	52	70	61.0	. .	Fair.
17	50	64	57.0	. .	Fair.
18	43	71	57.0	. .	Fair.
19	58	70	64.0	. .	Fair.
20	44	60	52.0	. .	Fair.
21	44	60	52.0	. .	
22	36	50	43.0	. .	Fair; first sign of frost.
23	30	50	40.0	. .	Fair; killing frost.
24	33	50	41.5	. .	Fair.
25	24	50	37.0	. .	Fair.
26	28	62	45.0	. .	Fair.
27	58	57	57.5	0.2	Cloudy; thunder; rain.
28	56	60	58.0	3.2	Thunder; rain.
29	66	70	68.0	2.2	Fair; thunder; rain at night.
30	62	72	67.0	0.8	Rain.
31	59	60	59.5	. .	Rain.
Means	49.61	64.93	57.27	[illegible]	
Max.	70	80	73.5		
Min.	24	50	37.0		
Range	46	30	36.5		

Extreme range 56

Greatest Rise and Fall of [illegible]

	Sunrise.	3 P. M.
Rise . . .	30	12
Fall . . .	16	12

November, 1841.

DAY.	THERMOMETER. Sunrise.	THERMOMETER. 2 P. M.	THERMOMETER. Mean.	RAIN. Ins.	REMARKS ON THE WEATHER.
1	46	60	53.0	. .	Fair.
2	36	46	41.0	. .	Fair.
3	42	64	53.0	. .	Fair.
4	35	60	47.5	. .	Fair.
5	35	50	42.5	. .	Fair.
6	30	45	37.5	. .	Fair.
7	36	64	50.0	. .	Fair.
8	51	60	55.5	. .	Cloudy.
9	64	70	67.0	0.2	Rain.
10	59	72	65.5	0.8	Cloudy; rain at night.
11	64	66	65.0	0.5	Rain.
12	55	66	60.5	. .	Fair.
13	44	60	52.0	. .	Fair.
14	46	50	48.0	. .	Fair.
15	34	58	46.0	. .	Fair.
16	34	67	50.5	. .	Fair.
17	50	70	60.0	. .	Fair.
18	64	70	67.0	. .	Cloudy.
19	58	66	62.0	. .	Fair.
20	52	76	64.0	. .	Fair.
21	69	64	66.5	0.4	Thunder shower in morning; fair.
22	36	60	48.0	. .	Fair.
23	42	60	51.0	. .	Fair. [night.
24	54	66	60.0	0.7	Fair; smoky; thunder; rain at
25	48	40	44.0	. .	Cloudy; cold north wind.
26	30	34	32.0	. .	Cloudy; cold north wind.
27	27	28	27.5	. .	Cloudy; snow.
28	23	38	30.5	. .	Fair.
29	15	38	26.5	. .	Fair.
30	18	46	32.0	. .	Fair.
Means	43.23	57.13	50.18	2.6	
Max.	69	76	67.0		
Min.	15	28	26.5		
Range	54	48	40.5		

Extreme range 61

Greatest Rise and Fall of temperature in 24 hours.

	Sunrise.	2 P. M.
Rise . . .	17	19
Fall . . .	33	26

December, 1841.

DAY.	THERMOMETER. Sunrise.	THERMOMETER. 2 P. M.	THERMOMETER. Mean.	RAIN. Ins.	REMARKS ON THE WEATHER.
1	28	40	34.0	0.5	Fair; cloudy; rain at night.
2	39	47	43.0	. .	Rain.
3	46	54	50.0	. .	Cloudy; fair.
4	36	40	38.0	. .	Fair.
5	30	52	41.0	. .	Fair.
6	28	57	42.5	. .	Fair.
7	35	55	45.0	. .	Cloudy.
8	55	60	57.5	. .	Cloudy.
9	60	64	62.0	0.3	Rain.
10	57	67	62.0	. .	Fair.
11	31	56	43.5	. .	Fair.
12	46	50	48.0	0.3	Cloudy; thunder; rain.
13	48	55	51.5	. .	Fair.
14	39	62	50.5	. .	Fair.
15	49	60	54.5	. .	Clouds and wind at night.
16	33	50	41.5	. .	Fair.
17	23	45	34.0	. .	Fair.
18	22	45	33.5	. .	Fair.
19	45	58	51.5	. .	Cloudy.
20	56	57	56.5	1.2	Cloudy; sprinkle; rain.
21	41	42	41.5	0.5	Cloudy; thunder; rain.
22	58	50	54.0	. .	Cloudy.
23	22	40	31.0	. .	Fair.
24	21	33	27.0	. .	Fair.
25	24	37	30.5	. .	Fair.
26	24	33	28.5	. .	Cloudy; snow flakes.
27	28	30	29.0	. .	Cloudy; sleet.
28	32	37	34.5	. .	Cloudy; fair at noon.
29	34	34	34.0	0.2	Snow in large flakes; rain.
30	26	45	35.5	. .	Fair.
31	23	50	36.5	. .	Fair.
Means	36.74	48.55	42.64	[illegible]	
Max.	60	67	62.0		
Min.	21	30	27.0		
Range	39	37	.35.0		

Extreme range 46

Greatest Rise and Fall of [illegible]

	Sunrise.	2 P. M.
Rise . . .	23	13
Fall . . .	35	15

January, 1842.

DAY.	THERMOMETER. Sun-rise.	2 P. M.	Mean.	RAIN. Ins.	REMARKS ON THE WEATHER.
1	28	50	39.0	. .	Fair.
2	40	50	45.0	. .	Cloudy.
3	25	52	38.5	. .	Fair.
4	28	52	40.0	. .	Fair.
5	46	65	55.5	. .	Cloudy. Frogs.
6	64	69	66.5	1.0	Rain.
7	57	64	60.5	. .	Fair.
8	49	64	56.5	0.5	Fair; cloudy; rain at night.
9	44	47	45.5	0.5	Cloudy; rain.
10	42	48	45.0	. .	Cloudy.
11	32	50	41.0	. .	Fair.
12	30	50	40.0	. .	Fair.
13	30	55	42.5	. .	Fair.
14	38	62	50.0	. .	Fair.
15	28	56	42.0	. .	Fair.
16	28	56	42.0	. .	Fair.
17	34	61	47.5	. .	Fair.
18	42	61	51.5	. .	Fair.
19	50	42	46.0	0.1	Cloudy; rain.
20	28	40	34.0	. .	Fair.
21	28	52	40.0	. .	Fair.
22	24	48	36.0	. .	Fair.
23	28	48	38.0	. .	Cloudy.
24	38	42	40.0	1.3	Cloudy; rain.
25	38	44	41.0	. .	Rain.
26	36	50	43.0	. .	Fair.
27	30	56	43.0	. .	Fair. [bees at work.
28	44	62	53.0	. .	Clouds; fair. Elms in bloom;
29	53	65	59.0	. .	Clouds; fair.
30	40	66	53.0	. .	Clouds; fair.
31	60	59	59.5	. .	Clouds; fair.
Means	38.13	54.39	46.26	3.4	
Max.	64	69	66.5		
Min.	24	40	34.0		
Range	40	29	32.5		
Extreme range 45					

Greatest Rise and Fall of temperature in 24 hours.

	Sunrise.	2 P. M.
Rise . . .	20	13
Fall . . .	22	19

February, 1842.

DAY.	THERMOMETER. Sun-rise.	2 P. M.	Mean.	RAIN. Ins.	REMARKS ON THE WEATHER.
1	34	54	44.0	. .	Fair.
2	56	54	55.0	1.8	Thunder; rain.
3	54	66	60.0	. .	Cloudy; fair.
4	43	52	47.5	. .	Fair; windy; clouds. Morus buds
5	30	50	40.0	. .	Fair. [green.
6	48	59	53.5	. .	Cloudy.
7	28	50	39.0	. .	Fair.
8	20	36	28.0	. .	Fair.
9	24	47	35.5	. .	Fair.
10	46	58	52.0	. .	Cloudy.
11	54	58	56.0	0.1	Rain.
12	38	50	44.0	1.0	Cloudy; rain.
13	28	56	42.0	. .	Fair; icicles glittering from the
14	34	49	41.5	. .	Fair. [trees.
15	36	59	47.5	. .	Fair.
16	30	50	40.0	. .	Fair.
17	31	50	40.5	. .	Fair.
18	54	64	59.0	. .	Cloudy.
19	25	45	35.0	. .	Fair.
20	27	44	35.5	. .	Fair.
21	22	45	33.5	. .	Fair.
22	25	58	41.5	. .	Fair. Peach blooms.
23	40	65	52.5	0.8	Smoky; thunder; rain at night.
24	50	55	52.5	. .	Fair.
25	48	55	51.5	. .	Fair.
26	32	64	48.0	. .	Fair.
27	52	67	59.5	. .	Smoky; sprinkle.
28	63	72	67.5	. .	Cloudy; fair.
Means	38.29	54.71	46.50	3.7	
Max.	63	72	67.5		
Min.	20	36	28.0		
Range	43	36	39.5		
Extreme range 52					

Greatest Rise and Fall of temperature in 24 hours.

	Sunrise.	2 P. M.
Rise . . .	23	14
Fall . . .	29	19

March, 1842.

DAY.	THERMOMETER. Sun-rise.	2 P. M.	Mean.	RAIN. Ins.	REMARKS ON THE WEATHER.
1	67	70	68.5	0.8	Cloudy; thunder; rain.
2	54	70	62.0	0.8	Cloudy; thunder; rain.
3	54	78	66.0	1.7	Cloudy; thunder; rain.
4	56	70	63.0	. .	Cloudy; fair.
5	50	70	60.0	. .	Fair.
6	64	70	67.0	. .	Cloudy.
7	46	59	52.5	. .	Fair.
8	46	64	55.0	. .	Fair.
9	64	76	70.0	. .	Cloudy.
10	69	82	75.5	. .	Fair. Cattle flies troublesome.
11	50	84	67.0	0.7	Cloudy; thunder; rain.
12	34	40	37.0	. .	Fair; rain at night.
13	40	44	42.0	0.2	Cloudy; rain.
14	38	64	51.0	. .	Fair.
15	32	64	48.0	. .	Fair; white frost.
16	40	60	50.0	. .	Fair.
17	56	66	61.0	. .	Clouds; sprinkle.
18	53	70	61.5	. .	Fair. Grape-vine leaves.
19	54	70	62.0	. .	Fair.
20	60	76	68.0	. .	Fair. Apple blooms.
21	62	72	67.0	. .	Cloudy. Silk-worms hatched.
22	58	80	69.0	. .	Fair.
23	60	82	71.0	. .	Fair.
24	66	80	73.0	. .	Cloudy; sprinkle in the night.
25	58	76	67.0	. .	Fair.
26	50	74	62.0	. .	Fair; smoky.
27	55	74	64.5	. .	Fair; smoky.
28	51	75	63.0	. .	Fair; smoky.
29	54	76	65.0	. .	Fair; smoky.
30	64	70	67.0	0.4	Cloudy; rain.
31	57	67	62.0	. .	
Means	53.61	70.10	61.85	4.6	
Max.	69	84	75.5		
Min.	32	40	37.0		
Range	37	44	38.5		
Extreme range 52					

Greatest Rise and Fall of temperature in 24 hours.

	Sunrise.	2 P. M.
Rise . . .	18	20
Fall . . .	19	44

April, 1842.

DAY.	THERMOMETER. Sun-rise.	2 P. M.	Mean.	RAIN. Ins.	REMARKS ON THE WEATHER.
1	40	73	56.5	. .	Fair. Ripe strawberries.
2	58	72	65.0	0.1	Fair; cloudy; light showers; fair.
3	67	75	71.0	. .	Cloudy. Seringa in bloom.
4	66	78	72.0	1.2	Cloudy; fair; shower at night.
5	59	70	64.5	1.7	Cloudy, thunder; rain.
6	62	70	66.0	. .	Fair.
7	60	70	65.0	. .	Fair.
8	48	70	59.0	. .	Fair.
9	46	76	61.0	. .	Fair.
10	59	79	69.0	. .	Fair. Ripe mulberries.
11	64	80	72.0	. .	Fair.
12	65	78	71.5	0.5	Cloudy; wind and rain at night.
13	60	70	65.0	. .	Fair.
14	42	64	53.0	. .	Fair.
15	45	73	59.0	. .	Fair.
16	54	59	56.5	0.5	Rain.
17	50	50	50.0	. .	Cloudy; rain.
18	49	68	58.5	. .	Fair.
19	44	70	57.0	. .	Fair.
20	45	75	60.0	. .	Fair.
21	50	79	64.5	. .	Fair.
22	53	80	66.5	. .	Fair. Silk-worms spinning.
23	56	80	68.0	. .	Fair.
24	56	76	66.0	. .	Clouds.
25	42	56	49.0	. .	Fair.
26	. .	. .	. .	. .	
27	39	70	54.5	. .	Fair.
28	47	74	60.5	. .	Fair.
29	50	60	55.0	. .	Fair.
30	61	79	70.0	. .	Clouds.
Means	53.00	71.52	62.26	4.0	
Max.	67	80	72.0		
Min.	39	50	49.0		
Range	28	30	23.0		
Extreme range 41					

Greatest Rise and Fall of temperature in 24 hours.

	Sunrise.	2 P. M.
Rise . . .	18	19
Fall . . .	18	20

May, 1842.

DAY.	THERMOMETER. Sun-rise.	THERMOMETER. 3 P. M.	THERMOMETER. Mean.	RAIN. Ins.	REMARKS ON THE WEATHER.
1	69	80	74.5	. .	Clouds; fair. } First appearance of locusts, which appeared also at this season in 1829.
2	66	80	73.0	. .	Fair.
3	48	68	58.0	. .	Fair; cloudy.
4	42	66	54.0	. .	Fair.
5	40	67	53.5	. .	Fair.
6	40	72	56.0	. .	Fair.
7	45	78	61.5	. .	Fair.
8	60	80	70.0	. .	Clouds; fair.
9	54	80	67.0	. .	Fair.
10	62	81	71.5	. .	Fair.
11	62	81	71.5	. .	Fair.
12	64	80	72.0	0.1	Clouds; thunder; showers.
13	65	73	69.0	. .	Clouds; thunder; showers.
14	60	64	62.0	. .	Clouds; thunder; sprinkle.
15	54	75	64.5	. .	Fair.
16	56	60	58.0	. .	Rain; thunder.
17	58	74	66.0	0.5	Rain; thunder.
18	54	80	67.0	. .	Rain.
19	66	82	74.0	. .	Fair.
20	66	84	75.0	. .	Fair.
21	64	63	63.5	. .	Fair.
22	65	78	71.5	0.5	Rain; fair.
23	64	83	73.5	. .	Fair; showers.
24	65	74	69.5	0.3	Rain.
25	60	78	69.0	. .	Fair; clouds.
26	62	75	68.5	. .	Clouds.
27	66	72	69.0	0.4	Clouds; rain.
28	65	80	72.5	. .	Clouds.
29	68	82	75.0	0.3	Rain.
30	66	88	77.0	. .	Fair.
31	70	86	78.0	. .	Fair.
Means	59.55	76.26	67.91	2.1	Greatest Rise and Fall of temperature in 24 hours.
Max.	70	88	78.0		
Min.	40	60	53 5		
Range	30	28	24.5		
Extreme range 48					

	Sunrise.	3 P. M.
Rise . . .	15	15
Fall . . .	18	21

June, 1842.

DAY.	THERMOMETER. Sun-rise.	THERMOMETER. 3 P. M.	THERMOMETER. Mean.	RAIN. Ins.	REMARKS ON THE WEATHER.
1	70	88	79.0	. .	Fair.
2	74	86	80.0	. .	Clouds; fair.
3	70	90	80.0	. .	Fair.
4	70	87	78.5	. .	Fair.
5	70	85	77.5	. .	Fair; clouds.
6	70	82	76.0	0.8	Cloudy; thunder; rain.
7	68	82	75.0	. .	Cloudy; thunder; rain.
8	70	87	78.5	0.2	Fair.
9	70	76	73.0	. .	Cloudy; shower.
10	65	82	73.5	. .	Fair.
11	58	80	69.0	. .	Fair.
12	60	72	66.0	. .	Cloudy; rain.
13	60	80	70.0	. .	Fair.
14	54	78	66.0	. .	Fair; clouds.
15	60	78	69.0	. .	Clouds.
16	60	77	68.5	. .	Clouds.
17	69	70	69.5	1.2	Fair; thunder; rain.
18	68	84	76.0	0.3	Cloudy; thunder; rain.
19	68	72	70.0	. .	Cloudy; mist.
20	66	80	73.0	. .	Cloudy.
21	70	85	77.5	. .	Fair.
22	72	72	72.0	1.0	Rain.
23	68	76	72.0	0.4	Rain; mist; showers.
24	68	80	74.0	0.2	Showers.
25	70	85	77.5	. .	Fair.
26	70	85	77.5	. .	Fair.
27	70	86	78.0	0.3	Shower.
28	66	86	76.0	0.1	Fair; shower at night.
29	67	89	75.0	. .	Fair.
30	72	88	80.0	1.0	Fair; rain at night.
Means	66.90	81.60	74.25	5.5	Greatest Rise and Fall of temperature in 24 hours.
Max.	74	90	80.0		
Min.	54	70	66.0		
Range	20	20	14.0		
Extreme range 36					

	Sunrise.	3 P. M.
Rise . . .	9	14
Fall . . .	7	13

July, 1842.

DAY.	THERMOMETER. Sun-rise.	THERMOMETER. 3 P. M.	THERMOMETER. Mean.	RAIN. Ins.	REMARKS ON THE WEATHER.
1	64	68	66.0	0.2	Rain.
2	56	79	67.5	. .	Fair. Ripe peaches.
3	54	86	70.0	. .	Fair.
4	60	81	70.5	. .	Cloudy.
5	60	78	69.0	. .	Cloudy; smoky.
6	66	86	76.0	. .	Cloudy.
7	70	89	79.5	. .	Fog; fair.
8	70	91	80.5	. .	Fog; fair.
9	70	90	80.0	. .	Fair.
10	76	88	82.0	. .	Fair.
11	70	89	79.5	. .	Fair.
12	68	90	79.0	. .	Fair.
13	68	91	79.5	. .	Fair.
14	70	86	78.0	. .	Fair.
15	70	86	78.0	. .	Fair.
16	66	86	76.0	. .	Fair.
17	66	89	77.5	. .	Fair.
18	68	89	78.5	. .	Fair.
19	70	91	80.5	. .	Fair.
20	72	92	82.0	. .	Fair.
21	68	80	74.0	0.2	Fair; shower.
22	70	88	79.0	. .	Fair.
23	68	86	77.0	. .	Fair.
24	70	85	77.5	. .	Fair,
25	71	87	79.0	0.8	Cloudy; thunder; rain.
26	72	85	78.5	0.6	Cloudy; thunder; rain.
27	73	86	79.5	. .	Fair.
28	75	87	81.0	. .	Fair.
29	70	91	80.5	. .	Fair.
30	70	93	81.5	. .	Fair.
31	70	86	78.0	. .	Fair.
Means	68.09	86.42	77.26	1.8	Greatest Rise and Fall of temperature in 24 hours.
Max.	76	93	82.0		
Min.	54	68	66.0		
Range	22	25	16.0		
Extreme range 39					

	Sunrise.	3 P. M.
Rise . . .	6	11
Fall . . .	8	20

August, 1842.

DAY.	THERMOMETER. Sun-rise.	THERMOMETER. 3 P. M.	THERMOMETER. Mean.	RAIN. Ins.	REMARKS ON THE WEATHER.
1	62	77	69.5	. .	Fair.
2	54	78	66.0	. .	Fair.
3	53	76	64.5	. .	Fair.
4	53	79	66.0	. .	Fair.
5	54	81	67.5	. .	Fair.
6	59	86	72.5	. .	Fair.
7	63	88	75.5	. .	Fair.
8	68	82	75.0	. .	Fair.
9	66	86	76.0	0.5	Cloudy; thunder; rain.
10	66	85	75.5	. .	Fair; clouds.
11	70	84	77.0	0.8	Cloudy; thunder; rain.
12	72	78	75.0	1.2	Rain; fair; shower.
13	72	81	76.5	0.6	Rain; fair; shower.
14	72	80	76.0	. .	Fog; fair.
15	68	80	74.0	. .	Fair.
16	64	82	73.0	. .	Fair.
17	64	85	74.5	. .	Fair.
18	60	86	73.0	. .	Fair.
19	60	88	74.0	. .	Fair.
20	64	80	72.0	1.0	Cloudy; thunder; rain.
21	66	78	72.0	. .	Rain.
22	68	80	74.0	. .	Cloudy; fair.
23	64	82	73.0	. .	Fair.
24	66	83	74.5	. .	Cloudy; fair.
25	62	83	72.5	. .	Fair.
26	64	86	75.0	. .	Fair.
27	66	86	76.0	. .	Fair.
28	64	86	75.0	. .	Fair.
29	66	88	77.0	. .	Fair.
30	66	89	77.5	. .	Fair.
31	66	88	77.0	. .	Fair.
Means	63.93	82.93	73.43	4.1	Greatest Rise and Fall of temperature in 24 hours.
Max.	72	89	77.5		
Min.	53	76	64.5		
Range	10	13	13.0		
Extreme range 36					

	Sunrise.	3 P. M.
Rise . . .	5	5
Fall . . .	8	9

September, 1842.

DAY.	THERMOMETER. Sun-rise.	3 P. M.	Mean.	RAIN. Ins.	REMARKS ON THE WEATHER.
1	66	88	77.0	..	Fair. [P. M.
2	64	86	75.0	0.2	Fog; fair; shower from E. at 3
3	66	84	75.0	..	Fog; fair; shower from E. from 3
4	66	84	75.0	..	Fog; fair. [to 5 P. M.
5	66	90	78.0	..	Fair.
6	67	87	77.0	..	Fair.
7	72	90	81.0	..	Fair.
8	70	89	79.5	..	Fair.
9	68	90	79.0	..	Fair.
10	70	92	81.0	..	Fair.
11	68	88	78.0	0.2	Fair; shower at 5 P. M.
12	72	85	78.5	1.3	Cloudy; thunder; rain at night.
13	70	74	72.0	..	Cloudy; rain.
14	64	72	68.0	..	Cloudy.
15	57	72	64.5	..	Fair.
16	50	72	61.0	..	Fair.
17	50	72	61.0	..	Fair.
18	50	72	61.0	..	Fair.
19	54	74	64.0	..	Clouds; sprinkle from W.
20	64	81	72.5	..	Cloudy.
21	68	76	72.0	..	Cloudy.
22	62	74	68.0	..	Cloudy; sprinkle.
23	58	71	64.5	..	Cloudy.
24	64	68	66.0	..	Cloudy.
25	56	81	68.5	..	Fair.
26	56	78	67.0	..	Fair.
27	60	76	68.0	..	Fog; fair.
28	56	78	67.0	..	Fair.
29	62	78	70.0	..	Fair.
30	48	71	59.5	..	
Means	62.13	79.77	70.95	1.7	
Max.	72	92	81.0		
Min.	48	68	59.5		
Range	24	24	21.5		

Extreme range 44

Greatest Rise and Fall of temperature in 24 hours.

	Sunrise.	3 P. M.
Rise . . .	10	13
Fall . . .	14	11

October, 1842.

DAY.	THERMOMETER. Sun-rise.	3 P. M.	Mean.	RAIN. Ins.	REMARKS ON THE WEATHER.
1	46	78	62.0	..	Fair.
2	43	78	60.5	..	Fair.
3	44	80	62.0	..	Fair.
4	50	80	65.0	..	Fair.
5	53	80	66.5	..	Fair.
6	56	82	69.0	..	Fair.
7	58	82	70.0	1.8	Fair; cloudy; thunder; rain at
8	65	63	64.0	0.2	Rain. [night.
9	48	51	49 5	..	Rain.
10	40	62	51.0	..	Fair.
11	43	70	56.5	..	Fair.
12	48	74	61.0	..	Fair.
13	48	74	61.0	..	Fair.
14	48	70	59.0	..	Fair.
15	41	65	53.0	..	Fair.
16	42	72	57.0	..	Fair.
17	46	74	60.0	..	Fair.
18	54	70	62.0	..	Fair; smoky; fire in the woods.
19	48	57	52.5	..	Cloudy; smoky; wind N.W.
20	46	60	53.0	..	Cloudy; fair; wind N.W.
21	50	56	53.0	0.3	Cloudy; rain.
22	56	64	60.0	0.2	Cloudy; rain.
23	64	68	66.0	0.2	Cloudy; rain.
24	62	65	63.5	..	Cloudy; rain from W.
25	36	62	49.0	..	Fair; frost.
26	32	61	46.5	..	Fair; killing frost.
27	32	61	46 5	..	Fair.
28	34	64	49.0	..	Fair.
29	34	65	49.5	..	Fair.
30	34	67	50.5	..	Fair.
31	36	69	52.5	..	Fair.
Means	46.35	68.52	57.44	2.7	
Max.	64	82	70.0		
Min.	32	51	46.5		
Range	32	31	23.5		

Extreme range 50

Greatest Rise and Fall of temperature in 24 hours.

	Sunrise.	3 P. M.
Rise . . .	8	11
Fall . . .	26	10

November, 1842.

DAY.	THERMOMETER. Sun-rise.	2 P. M.	Mean.	RAIN. Ins.	REMARKS ON THE WEATHER.
1	41	72	56.5	..	Fair.
2	47	74	60.5	..	Fair.
3	54	74	64.0	..	Fair.
4	54	74	64.0	..	Fair.
5	54	74	64.0	0.2	Fair; rain.
6	50	60	55.0	..	Fair; clouds.
7	41	61	51.0	..	Fair.
8	50	56	53.0	..	Cl'dy; fair; high wind from N.W.
9	34	56	45.0	..	Fair.
10	30	50	40.0	..	Fair.
11	42	50	46.0	1.2	Rain.
12	28	46	37.0	..	Fair.
13	31	50	40.5	..	Fair.
14	46	58	52.0	..	Fair.
15	40	49	44.5	1.0	Cloudy; rain.
16	50	50	50.0	0.3	Fog; rain.
17	28	31	29.5	..	Cloudy; fair.
18	16	34	25.0	..	Fair.
19	16	32	24.0	..	Fair.
20	16	42	29.0	..	Fair.
21	28	44	36.0	..	Cloudy.
22	23	46	34.5	..	Fair.
23	30	42	36.0	..	Fair; high N.W. wind.
24	15	40	27.5	..	Fair.
25	32	51	41.5	..	Fair.
26	42	60	51.0	..	Fair.
27	36	43	39.5	..	Cloudy.
28	29	34	31.5	..	Rain; freezing.
29	34	42	38.0	..	Fair; cloudy.
30	32	52	42.0	..	Fair.
Means	35.63	51.57	43.60	2.7	
Max.	54	74	64.0		
Min.	15	31	24 0		
Range	39	43	40.0		

Extreme range 59

Greatest Rise and Fall of temperature in 24 hours.

	Sunrise	2 P. M.
Rise . . .	15	11
Fall . . .	22	19

December, 1842.

DAY.	THERMOMETER. Sun-rise	2 P. M.	Mean.	RAIN. Ins.	REMARKS ON THE WEATHER.
1	27	53	40.0	..	Fair.
2	40	64	52.0	..	Fair.
3	50	66	58.0	..	Fair.
4	53	68	60.5	..	Fair.
5	64	70	67.0	..	Clouds.
6	42	46	44.0	1.8	Cloudy; rain.
7	44	54	49.0	2.6	Cloudy; thunder; rain.
8	35	41	38.0	0.2	Fair; cloudy.
9	27	45	36.0	..	Fair.
10	26	45	35.5	..	Fair.
11	27	40	33.5	..	Fair.
12	25	37	31.0	..	Fair.
13	31	35	33.0	..	Fair.
14	24	35	29.5	..	Fair.
15	24	44	34.0	..	Fair.
16	32	54	43.0	..	Fair.
17	28	46	37.0	..	Fair.
18	40	49	44.5	..	Cloudy; sprinkle.
19	44	49	46.5	..	Cloudy.
20	42	46	44.0	..	Cloudy; fair.
21	32	50	41.0	..	Fair.
22	34	39	36.5	..	Fair.
23	15	36	25.5	..	Fair.
24	35	40	37.5	..	Fair.
25	31	40	35.5	0.3	Rain.
26	40	54	47.0	..	Cloudy.
27	46	56	51.0	0.4	Rain.
28	52	54	53.0	..	Cloudy; fair.
29	30	46	38.0	..	Fair.
30	28	34	31.0	..	Fair.
31	20	50	35.0	..	
Means	35.10	47.94	41.52	5.3	
Max.	64	70	67.0		
Min.	15	34	25.5		
Range	49	36	41.5		

Extreme range 55

Greatest Rise and Fall of temperature in 24 hours.

	Sunrise.	2 P. M.
Rise . . .	20	16
Fall . . .	22	24

January, 1843.

DAY.	THERMOMETER. Sun-rise.	THERMOMETER. 2 P. M.	THERMOMETER. Mean.	RAIN. Ins.	REMARKS ON THE WEATHER.
1	28	56	42.0	..	Fair.
2	34	54	44.0	..	Fair.
3	28	38	33.0	..	Fair.
4	21	58	39.5	..	Fair.
5	38	62	50.0	..	Fog; clouds.
6	58	68	63.0	0.2	Fair; thunder; rain from S.W. at
7	36	42	39.0	..	Clouds; fair. [4 P. M.
8	18	40	29.0	..	Fair; cloudy; rain and sleet at
9	33	38	35.5	0.5	Rain. [night.
10	27	47	37.0	..	Fair.
11	28	42	35.0	..	Cloudy.
12	17	34	25.5	..	Fair.
13	15	40	27.5	..	Fair.
14	22	57	39.5	..	Fair.
15	28	60	44.0	..	
16	42	62	52.0	..	
17	38	64	51.0	..	Cloudy.
18	52	64	58.0	..	Cloudy.
19	58	64	61.0	..	Cloudy.
20	59	62	60.5	0.7	Cloudy; rain; fair.
21	59	68	63.5	0.3	Rain; fair.
22	58	65	61.5	..	Fog; clouds.
23	54	69	61.5	..	Fair.
24	53	65	59.0	..	Clouds; fair.
25	42	65	53.5	..	Clouds; fair.
26	58	66	62.0	0.2	Clouds; thunder; rain at night.
27	36	56	46.0	..	Fair.
28	25	52	38.5	..	Fair.
29	39	37	38.0	..	Cloudy; rain.
30	32	41	36.5	0.1	Snow.
31	32	30	31.0	..	Fair; cold N. wind.
Means	37.68	53.74	45.71	2.9	
Max.	59	69	63.5		
Min.	15	30	25.5		
Range	44	39	38.0		

Extreme range 54

Greatest Rise and Fall of temperature in 24 hours.

	Sunrise.	2 P. M.
Rise . . .	20	20
Fall . . .	22	26

February, 1843.

DAY.	THERMOMETER. Sun-rise.	THERMOMETER. 2 P. M.	THERMOMETER. Mean.	RAIN. Ins.	REMARKS ON THE WEATHER.
1	23	38	30.5	..	Fair.
2	24	54	39.0	..	Fair.
3	34	60	47.0	..	Cloudy.
4	54	68	61.0	0.2	Cloudy; thunder and rain at night.
5	32	44	38.0	..	Fair; white frost.
6	20	40	30.0	..	Fair.
7	26	35	30.5	..	Cloudy; sleet at night.
8	25	34	29.5	..	Cloudy.
9	34	48	41.0	..	Cloudy.
10	50	52	51.0	..	Fair.
11	26	54	40.0	..	Fair.
12	42	60	51.0	..	Fair.
13	58	58	58.0	0.6	Cloudy; thunder; rain at night.
14	22	24	23.0	..	Ground covered with snow.
15	8	34	21.0	..	Fair.
16	28	45	36.5	..	Clouds.
17	24	58	41.0	..	Fair.
18	35	58	46.5	0.3	Cloudy; thunder; rain at night
19	42	58	50.0	..	Clouds; fair. [from S.W.
20	32	58	45.0	..	Fair.
21	30	60	45.0	..	Fair.
22	56	66	61.0	..	Fair.
23	36	40	38.0	..	Cloudy.
24	35	49	42.0	..	Fair.
25	21	56	38.5	..	Fair.
26	32	66	49.0	..	Fair.
27	32	47	39.5	0.5	Smoky; cloudy; thunder; rain at
28	30	32	31.0	..	Sleet. [night.
Means	29.39	45.03	37.21	1.6	
Max.	58	68	61.0		
Min.	8	24	21.0		
Range	50	44	40.0		

Extreme range 60

Greatest Rise and Fall of [illegible]

	Sunrise.	2 P. M.
Rise . . .	26	16
Fall . .	36	34

March, 1843.

DAY.	THERMOMETER. Sun-rise.	THERMOMETER. 2 P. M.	THERMOMETER. Mean.	RAIN. Ins.	REMARKS ON THE WEATHER.
1	18	33	25.5	..	Fair; cloudy.
2	16	33	24.5	..	Fair.
3	22	40	31.0	0.5	Cloudy; rain at night.
4	30	32	31.0	0.5	Rain; freezing; trees covered with
5	28	34	31.0	..	Cloudy; rain. [ice.
6	30	34	32.0	1.3	Cloudy.
7	36	46	41.0	..	Rain.
8	40	46	43.0	..	Cloudy; thunder; rain.
9	44	62	53.0	0.3	Cloudy; mist; thunder; rain at
10	37	44	40.5	..	Cloudy; fair. [night.
11	24	44	34.0	..	Fair; cloudy; comet.
12	24	40	32.0	..	Fair.
13	14	41	27.5	..	Fair.
14	20	60	40.0	..	Fair; thunder; rain at night
15	30	24	27.0	1.5	Rain and hail; snow 4 ins. deep.
16	6	30	18.0	..	Fair.
17	22	29	25.5	..	Fair.
18	22	50	36.0	..	Cloudy; fair.
19	32	38	35.0	..	Fair.
20	22	36	29.0	..	Cloudy.
21	29	48	38.5	..	Cloudy; sleet; fair.
22	28	40	34.0	..	Cloudy.
23	16	36	26.0	..	Fair.
24	29	39	34.0	..	Snow 4 inches deep.
25	12	46	29.0	..	Fair.
26	..	..	..	..	
27	46	38	42.0	1.5	Thunder; rain in the morning.
28	22	45	33.5	..	Fair.
29	32	66	49.0	..	Fair.
30	54	70	62.0	..	Cloudy.
31	48	60	54.0	0.2	Cloudy; rain at night.
Means	27.77	42.80	35.28	5.8	
Max.	54	70	62.0		
Min.	6	24	18.0		
Range	48	46	44.0		

Extreme range 64

Greatest Rise and Fall of temperature in 24 hours.

	Sunrise.	2 P. M.
Rise . . .	34	21
Fall . . .	24	36

April, 1843.

DAY.	THERMOMETER. Sun-rise.	THERMOMETER. 2 P. M.	THERMOMETER. Mean.	RAIN. Ins.	REMARKS ON THE WEATHER.
1	30	60	45.0	..	Fair.
2	42	64	53.0	..	Cloudy.
3	50	60	55.0	..	Cloudy.
4	42	62	52.0	..	Fair.
5	38	70	54.0	..	Fair.
6	42	66	54.0	..	Fair; smoky; fire in the woods.
7	39	78	58.5	..	Smoky.
8	54	84	69.0	..	Smoky.
9	54	76	65.0	..	Smoky.
10	48	76	62.0	..	Smoky.
11	60	82	71.0	..	Smoky.
12	54	75	64.5	..	Smoky.
13	50	70	60.0	..	Smoky.
14	50	82	66.0	0.7	Smoky; thunder, rain at night.
15	64	70	67.0	1.2	Rain; heavy thunder at night.
16	60	70	65.0	0.1	Rain.
17	54	64	59.0	..	Fair.
18	42	63	52.5	..	Fair.
19	48	68	58.0	..	Cloudy; thunder; rain.
20	58	65	61.5	1.0	Cloudy; thunder; rain.
21	51	70	60.5	2.2	Cloudy; thunder; rain.
22	60	76	68.0	..	Fair.
23	54	85	69.5	3.0	Cloudy; thunder and rain at 4
24	70	81	75.5	..	Cloudy. [P. M., one hour.
25	66	86	76.0	..	Cloudy.
26	66	76	71.0	0.2	Cloudy; showers.
27	60	64	62.0	..	Fair.
28	46	60	53.0	0.8	Rain; thunder.
29	55	66	60.5	..	
30	50	60	55.0	..	
Means	51.90	70.97	61.43	[illegible]	
Max.	70	86	76.0		
Min.	30	60	45.0		
Range	40	26	31.0		

Extreme range 56

Greatest Rise and Fall of [illegible]

	Sunrise.	2 P. M.
Rise . . .	16	12
Fall . . .	18	12

May, 1843.

DAY.	THERMOMETER. Sun-rise.	THERMOMETER. 3 P. M.	THERMOMETER. Mean.	RAIN. Ins.	REMARKS ON THE WEATHER.
1	47	72	59.5	0.2	Fair; rain at night.
2	54	72	63.0	. .	Cloudy; fair.
3	50	76	63.0	. .	Fair.
4	54	77	65.5	. .	Fair.
5	64	74	69.0	1.5	Fair; thunder; rain at night.
6	60	76	68.0	0.7	Cloudy; thunder; rain at night.
7	58	57	57.5	0.8	Rain.
8	50	57	53.5	0.2	Rain.
9	58	68	63.0	. .	Rain in the morning; fair at eve.
10	55	70	62.5	. .	Cloudy; fair.
11	56	80	68.0	. .	Fair.
12	66	82	74.0	. .	Fair.
13	60	82	71.0	1.0	Fair; thunder; rain at night.
14	68	74	71.0	. .	Rain.
15	66	84	75.0	. .	Fair.
16	64	76	70.0	. .	Fair; rain at night.
17	64	60	62.0	0.5	Rain.
18	55	66	60.5	0.2	Rain.
19	60	72	66.0	. .	Cloudy; fair.
20	50	75	62.5	. .	Fair.
21	63	68	65.5	0.2	Rain; showers.
22	50	78	64.0	. .	Fair.
23	58	82	70.0	. .	Fair.
24	56	82	69.0	. .	Fair.
25	70	84	77.0	0.4	Rain in the morning; fair at eve.
26	67	84	75.5	. .	Cloudy; fair.
27	72	85	78.5	. .	Clouds; shower.
28	70	80	75.0	. .	Fair.
29	54	68	61.0	. .	Fair.
30	46	76	61.0	. .	Fair.
31	50	80	65.0	. .	Fair.
Means	58.55	74.74	66.64	5.7	
Max.	72	85	78.5		
Min.	46	57	53.5		
Range	26	28	25.0		
Extreme range 39					

Greatest Rise and Fall of temperature in 24 hours.

	Sunrise.	3 P. M.
Rise . . .	14	12
Fall . . .	16	19

June, 1843.

DAY.	THERMOMETER. Sun-rise.	THERMOMETER. 3 P. M.	THERMOMETER. Mean.	RAIN. Ins.	REMARKS ON THE WEATHER.
1	52	80	66.0	. .	Fair.
2	58	80	69.0	. .	Fair.
3	64	85	74.5	. .	Fair.
4	64	84	74.0	. .	Fair.
5	72	80	76.0	1.0	Cloudy; thunder; rain.
6	56	76	66.0	. .	Fair.
7	59	86	72.5	. .	Fair.
8	66	87	76.5	. .	Fair.
9	74	82	78.0	1.5	Clouds; showers; thunder; rain
10	59	60	59.5	. .	Rain; fair. [at night.
11	50	72	61.0	. .	Fair.
12	54	74	64.0	. .	Fair.
13	64	82	73.0	. .	Fog; fair.
14	60	86	73.0	. .	Fair.
15	68	87	77.5	. .	Fair.
16	68	87	77.5	. .	Cloudy; shower at 10 A. M.; fair.
17	74	90	82.0	0.6	Fog; fair; thunder; rain at night
18	67	72	69.5	. .	Rain from S. W. [S. W.
19	66	88	77.0	. .	Fog; fair; shower at 3 P. M.
20	70	84	77.0	. .	Fair.
21	66	84	75.0	. .	Fair.
22	70	86	78.0	. .	Fair.
23	70	83	76.5	0.3	Cloudy; showers; thunder; rain
24	68	72	70.0	. .	Fog; fair. [at night.
25	62	84	73.0	. .	Fog; fair.
26	66	73	69.5	0.2	Cloudy; showers.
27	66	84	75.0	. .	Fog; fair.
28	70	88	79.0	. .	Fair.
29	70	90	80.0	. .	Fair.
30	70	90	80.0	. .	Fair.
Means	64.77	81.87	73.32	3.6	
Max.	74	90	82.0		
Min.	50	60	59.5		
Range	24	30	22.5		
Extreme range 40					

Greatest Rise and Fall of temperature in 24 hours.

	Sunrise.	3 P. M.
Rise . . .	10	16
Fall . . .	16	22

July, 1843.

DAY.	THERMOMETER. Sun-rise.	THERMOMETER. 3 P. M.	THERMOMETER. Mean.	RAIN. Ins.	REMARKS ON THE WEATHER.
1	74	80	77.0	. .	Cloudy.
2	68	80	74.0	. .	Fair; cloudy; sprinkle.
3	64	80	72.0	. .	Fair.
4	56	80	68.0	. .	Fair.
5	56	89	72.5	. .	Fair.
6	70	90	80.0	. .	Fair.
7	68	90	79.0	. .	Fair.
8	72	90	81.0	. .	Fair.
9	74	84	79.0	1.5	Fog; showers.
10	70	82	76.0	. .	Rain.
11	72	80	76.0	. .	Showery.
12	68	80	74.0	. .	Showery.
13	66	87	76.5	. .	Fog; fair.
14	66	89	77.5	. .	Fair.
15	70	90	80.0	. .	Fair.
16	70	91	80.5	. .	Fair.
17	72	92	82.0	. .	Fair.
18	72	86	79.0	. .	Fair.
19	72	90	81.0	. .	Fair.
20	68	88	78.0	. .	Fair; clouds; shower at 2 P. M.
21	66	85	75.5	0.2	Clouds; shower at 3 P. M. and at
22	64	85	74.5	. .	Clouds; fair. [night.
23	64	87	75.5	. .	Clouds; fair.
24	66	88	77.0	. .	Fair.
25	68	89	78.5	. .	Fair.
26	68	89	78.5	. .	Fair.
27	70	92	81.0	. .	Fair.
28	70	90	80.0	. .	Fair; clouds.
29	70	90	80.0	. .	Fair; clouds; shower at noon and
30	70	74	72.0	1.0	Rain; thunder. [at night.
31	62	79	70.5	. .	Fair.
Means	67.94	86.00	76.97	2.7	
Max.	74	92	82.0		
Min.	56	74	68.0		
Range	18	18	14.0		
Extreme range 36					

Greatest Rise and Fall of temperature in 24 hours.

	Sunrise.	3 P. M.
Rise . . .	14	9
Fall . . .	8	16

August, 1843.

DAY.	THERMOMETER. Sun-rise.	THERMOMETER. 3 P. M.	THERMOMETER. Mean.	RAIN. Ins.	REMARKS ON THE WEATHER.
1	56	78	67.0	. .	Fair.
2	56	80	68.0	. .	Fair.
3	54	78	66.0	. .	Fair.
4	54	82	68.0	. .	Fair.
5	60	85	72.5	. .	Fair.
6	60	85	72.5	. .	Fair; clouds.
7	64	85	74.5	. .	Fair; shower at 2 P. M.
8	66	80	73.0	. .	Fog; fair; clouds.
9	66	86	76.0	. .	Fog.
10	60	87	73.5	1.2	Fog; thunder; rain at night.
11	70	87	78.5	0.5	Clouds; rain at night.
12	66	80	73.0	. .	Fog; rain.
13	70	84	77.0	. .	Clouds.
14	62	84	73.0	. .	Clouds.
15	70	80	75.0	. .	Clouds.
16	52	84	68.0	. .	Fair.
17	68	86	77.0	. .	Fair.
18	68	80	74.0	. .	Fair; clouds.
19	60	83	71.5	. .	Fair; clouds.
20	62	80	71.0	. .	Cloudy; smoky.
21	60	78	69.0	. .	Cloudy; smoky.
22	58	76	67.0	. .	Fair.
23	56	79	67.5	. .	Fair.
24	54	80	67.0	. .	Fair.
25	56	84	70.0	1.0	Cloudy; rain at night.
26	60	74	67.0	0.4	Cloudy; rain.
27	60	70	65.0	. .	Fair.
28	60	80	70.0	. .	Fair.
29	58	78	68.0	. .	Fair.
30	62	78	70.0	. .	Fair.
31	60	84	72.0	. .	Fair.
Means	60.90	81.13	71.02	3.1	
Max	70	87	78.5		
Min.	52	70	65.0		
Range	18	17	13.5		
Extreme range 35					

Greatest Rise and Fall of temperature in 24 hours.

	Sunrise.	3 P. M.
Rise . . .	16	10
Fall . . .	18	10

September, 1843.

DAY.	THERMOMETER. Sunrise.	THERMOMETER. 3 P. M.	THERMOMETER. Mean.	RAIN. Ins.	REMARKS ON THE WEATHER.
1	66	88	77.0	..	Fair; shower.
2	70	84	77.0	..	Fair; clouds.
3	66	85	75.5	..	Fog; clouds.
4	66	84	75.0	..	Fair; clouds.
5	68	85	76.5	..	Fair; shower.
6	68	84	76.0	..	Fog; fair; cloudy.
7	64	84	74.0	..	Fog; fair. [thunder.
8	67	87	77.0	0.4	Fair; clouds; shower at 2 P. M.;
9	70	80	75.0	0.4	Fair; clouds; thunder; rain at 3
10	68	80	74.0	..	Fair; clouds. [P. M.
11	72	80	76.0	0.4	Fog; rain; fair.
12	64	76	70.0	..	Mist.
13	70	84	77.0	2.0	Cloudy; thunder; rain at night.
14	68	80	74.0	..	Cloudy; fair.
15	58	76	67.0	..	Cloudy.
16	66	86	76.0	..	Clouds.
17	72	84	78.0	..	Clouds.
18	70	85	77.5	..	Fair.
19	70	84	77.0	0.2	Fair; shower at 3 P. M.
20	68	84	76.0	..	Fair.
21	68	86	77.0	..	Fair.
22	66	85	75.5	..	Fair; shower at 4 P. M.
23	68	84	76.0	0.2	Clouds; shower at 4 P. M.
24	72	80	76.0	1.2	Cloudy; thunder; rain at 3 P. M.
25	66	76	71.0	..	Fog; rain at 3 P. M.
26	66	72	69.0	..	Clouds; fair.
27	52	65	58.5	0.4	Cloudy; rain at night.
28	58	60	59.0	0.9	Cloudy; rain.
29	66	72	69.0	1.0	Rain.
30	68	70	69.0	..	Rain; fair.
Means	66.70	80.33	73.52	7.1	Greatest Rise and Fall of temperature in 24 hours.
Max.	72	88	78.0		
Min.	52	60	58.5		
Range	20	28	19.5		
Extreme range 36					

	Sunrise.	3 P. M.
Rise . . .	8	12
Fall . . .	14	7

November, 1843.

DAY.	THERMOMETER. Sunrise.	THERMOMETER. 2 P. M.	THERMOMETER. Mean.	RAIN. Ins.	REMARKS ON THE WEATHER.
1	50	56	53.0	..	Fair.
2	30	54	42.0	..	Fair; killing frost.
3	36	59	47.5	..	Fair.
4	54	62	58.0	..	Cloudy; rain.
5	53	48	50.5	2.3	Rain.
6	46	50	48.0	..	Rain.
7	44	53	48.5	..	Cloudy; fair.
8	32	52	42.0	..	Fair; cloudy; sprinkle at night.
9	55	67	61.0	..	Cloudy; fair.
10	46	70	58.0	..	Fair.
11	38	50	44.0	..	Fair.
12	36	40	38.0	..	Fair.
13	28	51	39.5	0.2	Cloudy; rain at night.
14	44	50	47.0	0.4	Cloudy; rain.
15	52	60	56.0	..	Cloudy; fair.
16	54	66	60.0	1.0	Cloudy; thunder; rain at night.
17	52	62	57.0	..	Fair.
18	36	57	46.5	..	Fair; cloudy.
19	50	55	52.5	0.4	Cloudy; rain.
20	48	60	54.0	..	Cloudy.
21	48	64	56.0	..	Fog; fair.
22	38	67	52.5	1.2	Fair; rain at night.
23	58	66	62.0	0.3	Rain; fair.
24	36	50	43.0	..	Fair.
25	43	50	46.5	1.8	Cloudy; rain.
26	48	53	50.5	0.4	Rain.
27	52	53	52.5	1.3	Rain.
28	55	58	56.5	1.5	Thunder; rain.
29	43	45	44.0	0.5	Rain; sleet.
30	33	36	34.5	..	Rain; sleet.
Means	44.60	55.47	50.03	11.3	Greatest Rise and Fall of temperature in 24 hours.
Max.	58	70	62.0		
Min.	28	36	34.5		
Range	30	34	27.5		
Extreme range 42					

	Sunrise.	2 P. M.
Rise . . .	23	15
Fall . . .	22	20

October, 1843.

DAY.	THERMOMETER. Sunrise.	THERMOMETER. 3 P. M.	THERMOMETER. Mean.	RAIN. Ins.	REMARKS ON THE WEATHER.
1	52	69	60.5	..	Fair.
2	51	75	63.0	..	Fair.
3	55	70	62.5	..	Fair.
4	54	63	58.5	1.2	Cloudy; rain.
5	57	67	62.0	..	Cloudy; rain.
6	67	68	67.5	0.8	Cloudy; rain.
7	64	64	64.0	0.5	Rain.
8	46	68	57.0	..	Fair.
9	54	68	61.0	..	Fair.
10	45	70	57.5	..	Fair.
11	58	76	67.0	..	Clouds; sprinkle.
12	54	60	57.0	..	Fair.
13	39	60	49.5	..	Fair.
14	37	59	48.0	..	Fair.
15	40	60	50.0	..	Fair.
16	44	58	51.0	..	Fair.
17	40	60	50.0	..	Fair.
18	52	72	62.0	..	Clouds; fair.
19	46	66	56.0	..	Fair.
20	56	74	65.0	..	Fair.
21	61	77	69.0	..	Cloudy; thunder; rain at night.
22	49	60	54.5	0.3	Rain at night.
23	49	60	54.5	2.0	Rain; thunder.
24	58	72	65.0	0.5	Rain.
25	49	46	47.5	0.4	Rain.
26	39	38	38.5	..	Fair.
27	36	39	37.5	..	Fair.
28	36	54	45.0	..	Clouds.
29	46	46	46.0	0.4	Cloudy; rain.
30	36	55	45.5	..	Fog; fair.
31	32	60	46.0	0.7	Fair; white frost; rain at night.
Means	48.45	62.39	55.42	6.8	Greatest Rise and Fall of temperature in 24 hours.
Max.	67	77	69.0		
Min.	32	38	37.5		
Range	35	39	31.5		
Extreme range 45					

	Sunrise.	3 P. M.
Rise . . .	13	15
Fall . . .	18	26

December, 1843.

DAY.	THERMOMETER. Sunrise.	THERMOMETER. 2 P. M.	THERMOMETER. Mean.	RAIN. Ins.	REMARKS ON THE WEATHER.
1	32	43	37.5	..	Fair.
2	27	50	38.5	..	Fair.
3	26	52	39.0	..	Fair.
4	44	54	49.0	..	Fair.
5	32	42	37.0	0.8	Cloudy; rain at night.
6	34	40	37.0	..	Rain.
7	32	46	39.0	..	Fair.
8	33	48	40.5	..	Cloudy.
9	38	50	44.0	..	Fair.
10	38	57	47.5	0.8	Cloudy; rain at night.
11	50	56	53.0	..	Cloudy; fair.
12	32	44	38.0	..	Fair.
13	26	45	35.5	..	Fair.
14	42	50	46.0	1.3	Cloudy; rain at night.
15	54	62	58.0	0.2	Rain.
16	54	54	54.0	..	Fog; cloudy.
17	32	52	42.0	..	Fair.
18	30	52	41.0	..	Fair.
19	36	54	45.0	..	Fair.
20	36	54	45.0	..	Fair.
21	46	54	50.0	..	Cloudy.
22	34	56	45.0	..	Fair.
23	36	60	48.0	..	Fair.
24	40	60	50.0	..	Fair.
25	40	60	50.0	..	Fair.
26	40	52	46.0	..	Fair.
27	30	50	40.0	..	Fair.
28	30	50	40.0	..	Fair.
29	29	52	40.5	..	Fair.
30	46	60	53.0	0.5	Rain.
31	50	55	52.5	..	Rain.
Means	37.06	52.06	44.56	3.6	Greatest Rise and Fall of temperature in 24 hours.
Max.	54	62	58.0		
Min.	26	40	35.5		
Range	28	22	22.5		
Extreme range 36					

	Sunrise	2 P. M.
Rise . . .	18	12
Fall . . .	22	12

January, 1844.

DAY.	THERMOMETER. Sunrise.	THERMOMETER. 2 P. M.	THERMOMETER. Mean.	RAIN. Ins.	REMARKS ON THE WEATHER.
1	50	48	49.0	..	Fair.
2	33	40	36.5	..	Fair.
3	28	42	35.0	..	Fair.
4	26	42	34.0	..	Fair.
5	26	42	34.0	..	Fair.
6	40	44	42.0	0.2	Rain.
7	44	46	45.0	..	Cloudy.
8	36	42	39.0	..	Cloudy; rain.
9	42	44	43.0	..	Cloudy; rain.
10	44	44	44.0	0.5	Cloudy; rain.
11	40	44	42.0	0.7	Cloudy; rain.
12	57	58	57.5	0.3	Cloudy: rain; fair at 2 P. M.
13	32	45	38.5	0.4	Fair; cloudy; sleet at night.
14	40	45	42.5	0.3	Cloudy; rain.
15	45	54	49.5	..	Fair.
16	37	37	37.0	..	Cloudy; snow; fair at noon.
17	26	38	32.0	..	Fair.
18	28	53	40.5	..	Fair; rain at night.
19	42	55	48.5	0.3	Cloudy; rain at night.
20	55	64	59.5	..	Fog; fair.
21	42	66	54.0	..	Fog; fair.
22	65	70	67.5	..	Cloudy; sprinkle.
23	50	63	56.5	..	Fog; fair.
24	32	59	45.5	..	Fair.
25	32	60	46.0	..	Fair.
26	33	42	37.5	..	Cloudy; fair.
27	27	52	39.5	..	Cloudy.
28	26	54	40.0	..	Fair.
29	26	33	29.5	..	Cloudy; rain; icicles.
30	34	50	42.0	0.3	Cloudy; rain.
31	44	48	46.0	..	Cloudy; rain.
Means	39.40	50.80	45.10	3.0	Greatest Rise and Fall of temperature in 24 hours.
Max.	65	70	67.5		
Min.	26	33	29.5		
Range	39	37	38.0		
Extreme range 44					

	Sunrise.	2 P. M.
Rise . . .	23	17
Fall . . .	25	21

February, 1844.

DAY.	THERMOMETER. Sunrise.	THERMOMETER. 2 P. M.	THERMOMETER. Mean.	RAIN. Ins.	REMARKS ON THE WEATHER.
1	60	70	65.0	..	Cloudy; rain at night.
2	46	44	45.0	1.3	Rain.
3	44	45	44.5	1.5	Cloudy; thunder; rain.
4	45	49	47.0	..	Fair; cloudy.
5	32	48	40.0	..	Fair.
6	28	48	38.0	0.2	Fair; rain and sleet at night.
7	36	40	38.0	..	Fair.
8	25	40	32.5	..	Cloudy.
9	25	45	35.0	..	Fair.
10	24	46	35.0	..	Fair.
11	30	49	39.5	..	Fair; cloudy; sprinkle at night.
12	30	58	44.0	..	Fair; cloudy.
13	48	62	55.0	..	Fair; smoky.
14	34	67	50.5	..	Fair.
15	40	66	53.0	..	Fair.
16	32	70	51.0	..	Fair.
17	32	66	49.0	..	
18	40	59	49.5	..	Cloudy; fair.
19	42	66	54.0	..	Smoky.
20	42	66	54.0	..	Smoky.
21	36	62	49.0	..	Smoky.
22	36	64	50.0	..	Smoky.
23	36	72	54.0	..	Smoky.
24	36	72	54.0	..	
25	36	69	52.5	..	Fair. Morus leaves.
26	50	72	61.0	..	Fair.
27	56	78	67.0	..	Fair.
28	55	72	63.5	..	
29	58	71	64.5	..	Cloudy; rain at night.
Means	39.10	59.86	49.48	3.0	Greatest Rise and Fall of temperature in 24 hours.
Max.	60	78	67.0		
Min.	24	40	32.5		
Range	36	38	24.5		
Extreme range 54					

	Sunrise.	2 P. M.
Rise . . .	18	22
Fall . . .	14	26

March, 1844.

DAY.	THERMOMETER. Sunrise.	THERMOMETER. 2 P. M.	THERMOMETER. Mean.	RAIN. Ins.	REMARKS ON THE WEATHER.
1	56	55	55.5	1.0	Cloudy; rain.
2	38	50	44.0	..	Clouds.
3	38	50	44.0	..	Fair.
4	29	50	39.5	..	Fair. Morus buds killed.
5	30	50	40.0	..	Fair.
6	..	..	..	..	
7	40	60	50.0	..	Cloudy.
8	50	70	60.0	..	Fog; fair.
9	44	60	52.0	..	Cloudy; fair.
10	44	56	50.0	..	Cloudy; rain.
11	50	60	55.0	1.8	Cloudy; thunder; rain.
12	54	70	62.0	..	Fair.
13	50	60	55.0	0.2	Cloudy; rain.
14	54	64	59.0	..	Fair.
15	46	54	50.0	..	Cloudy.
16	42	50	46.0	..	Cloudy; fair.
17	40	56	48.0	..	Fair.
18	38	65	51.5	..	Fair.
19	40	74	57.0	..	Fair.
20	50	60	55.0	..	Fair.
21	34	58	46.0	..	Fair.
22	44	50	47.0	..	Fair.
23	30	54	42.0	..	Fair. Morus leaves killed.
24	36	66	51.0	..	Smoky.
25	50	71	60.5	..	Cloudy; fair.
26	56	64	60.0	1.3	Cloudy; thunder; rain at 4 P. M.
27	55	70	62.5	1.0	Thunder; rain and hail at eve.
28	50	74	62.0	1.3	Fair; cloudy; rain at night.
29	54	38	46.0	0.2	Rain; snow—roofs covered.
30	32	50	41.0	..	Cloudy; fair. Ripe strawberries.
31	30	54	42.0	..	Fair.
Means	43.47	58.77	51.12	6.8	Greatest Rise and Fall of temperature in 24 hours.
Max.	56	74	62.5		
Min.	29	38	39.5		
Range	27	36	23.0		
Extreme range 45					

	Sunrise.	2 P. M.
Rise . . .	14	12
Fall . . .	22	36

April, 1844.

DAY.	THERMOMETER. Sunrise.	THERMOMETER. 2 P. M.	THERMOMETER. Mean.	RAIN. Ins.	REMARKS ON THE WEATHER.
1	38	64	51.0	..	Fair.
2	44	68	56.0	..	Fair.
3	52	74	63.0	..	Fair.
4	60	74	67.0	..	Cloudy.
5	60	72	66.0	..	Cloudy.
6	62	76	69.0	..	Cloudy.
7	64	76	70.0	..	Cloudy.
8	66	66	66.0	0.5	Cloudy; rain at 2 P. M. Silk-
9	56	77	66.5	..	Fair. [worms hatched.
10	56	78	67.0	..	Fair.
11	58	76	67.0	0.5	Fair; cloudy; rain at night.
12	62	74	68.0	0.5	Fair; cloudy; rain at 4 P. M.
13	66	64	65.0	0.7	Cloudy; rain.
14	62	60	61.0	1.8	Cloudy; rain.
15	62	72	67.0	0.3	Rain.
16	64	66	65.0	0.5	Rain.
17	57	54	55.5	0.7	Rain.
18	54	66	60.0	0.4	Rain.
19	55	66	60.5	..	Cloudy; fair.
20	52	75	63.5	..	Cloudy; fair.
21	60	78	69.0	..	Cloudy; fair.
22	68	74	71.0	1.0	Cloudy; thunder; rain at night.
23	..	..	..	..	
24	66	81	73.5	..	Fair; clouds; sprinkle.
25	65	80	72.5	..	Fair.
26	66	78	72.0	..	Cloudy; sprinkle at night.
27	66	75	70.5	0.5	Cloudy; rain; thunder at night.
28	60	68	64.0	0.3	Rain.
29	58	66	62.0	..	Rain.
30	62	68	65.0	..	Cloudy; fair.
Means	59.34	71.24	65.29	7.7	Greatest Rise and Fall of temperature in 24 hours.
Max.	68	81	73.5		
Min.	38	54	51.0		
Range	30	27	22.5		
Extreme range 43					

	Sunrise.	2 P. M.
Rise . . .	8	12
Fall . . .	10	12

May, 1844.

DAY.	THERMOMETER. Sun-rise.	2 P. M.	Mean.	RAIN. Ins.	REMARKS ON THE WEATHER.
1	64	72	68.0	0.2	Fair; cloudy; rain at night.
2	68	78	73.0	..	Clouds.
3	66	76	71.0	..	Fair.
4	52	76	64.0	..	Fair; sprinkle at night. Cocoons.
5	52	76	64.0	0.2	Cloudy; showers.
6	58	78	68.0	..	Fair.
7	54	82	68.0	..	Fair; clouds.
8	60	82	71.0	..	Fair.
9	60	82	71.0	..	Fair.
10	66	82	74.0	..	Fair.
11	66	82	74.0	..	Fair.
12	66	82	74.0	..	Fair.
13	66	82	74.0	..	Fair.
14	66	84	75.0	..	Fair.
15	67	84	75.5	..	Fair.
16	68	82	75.0	..	Fair; clouds; rain at night.
17	68	82	75.0	0.8	Cloudy; thunder; rain.
18	68	80	74.0	..	Cloudy.
19	68	82	75.0	..	Cloudy; sprinkle.
20	70	64	67.0	0.4	Rain.
21	57	62	59.5	0.5	Rain; fair.
22	50	77	63.5	..	Fair.
23	60	82	71.0	..	Fair.
24	72	84	78.0	..	Cloudy; fair.
25	72	70	71.0	0.5	Cloudy; rain.
26	64	78	71.0	..	Cloudy; fair.
27	60	80	70.0	..	Fair.
28	68	80	74.0	1.5	Cloudy; thunder; rain at noon.
29	62	68	65.0	..	Fair.
30	50	68	59.0	..	Fair.
31	54	76	65.0	..	Fair.
Means	62.64	77.84	70.24	4.1	
Max.	72	84	78.0		
Min.	50	62	59.0		
Range	22	22	19.0		
Extreme range 34					

Greatest Rise and Fall of temperature in 24 hours.

	Sunrise.	2 P. M.
Rise . . .	12	15
Fall . . .	14	18

June, 1844.

DAY.	THERMOMETER. Sun-rise.	2 P. M.	Mean.	RAIN. Ins.	REMARKS ON THE WEATHER.
1	60	76	68.0	..	Fair.
2	60	84	72.0	..	Fair.
3	62	86	74.0	..	Fair.
4	64	87	75.5	..	Fair; thunder; rain at 2 P. M.
5	66	86	76.0	..	Fair.
6	68	88	78.0	..	Fair.
7	68	88	78.0	..	Fair; thunder; clouds.
8	66	86	76.0	..	Fair.
9	68	88	78.0	0.2	Clouds; thunder; rain at noon.
10	68	82	75.0	0.4	Clouds; thunder; rain 4 P. M. and
11	72	82	77.0	0.5	Clouds; thunder; rain. [night.
12	72	78	75.0	0.3	Clouds; thunder; rain.
13	68	80	74.0	0.2	Clouds; thunder; rain at night.
14	68	84	76.0	..	Clouds.
15	68	85	76.5	..	Clouds.
16	74	86	80.0	..	Fair.
17	72	82	77.0	0.4	Cloudy; thunder; showers.
18	74	86	80.0	..	Clouds; fair.
19	74	88	81.0	..	Clouds; fair.
20	75	88	81.5	0.2	Clouds; shower at 3 P. M.
21	66	84	75.0	..	Fair.
22	64	82	73.0	..	Fair.
23	60	82	71.0	..	Fair.
24	64	87	75.5	0.4	Fair; cl'ds; sh'rs; thunder from S.
25	70	82	76.0	0.4	Clouds; showers; thunder from S.
26	72	84	78.0	0.2	Clouds; showers 10 A. M., 5 P. M.
27	74	86	80.0	0.3	Fog; clouds; sh'rs at noon; fair.
28	73	86	79.5	0.5	Fog; fair; showers at 4 P. M.
29	72	86	79.0	0.2	
30	74	86	80.0	1.2	Cloudy; thunder; rain at 1 and 5 [P. M.
Means	68.53	84.50	76.52	[illegible]	
Max.	75	88	81.5		
Min.	60	76	68.0		
Range	15	12	13.5		
Extreme range 28					

Greatest Rise and Fall of temperature in 24 hours.

	Sunrise.	2 P. M.
Rise . . .	6	8
Fall . . .	9	6

July, 1844.

DAY.	THERMOMETER. Sun-rise.	3 P. M.	Mean.	RAIN. Ins.	REMARKS ON THE WEATHER.
1	70	90	80.0	0.3	Fair; thunder; rain at 4 P. M.
2	70	86	78.0	..	Fair.
3	72	88	80.0	..	Cloudy.
4	74	91	82.5	..	Fair; clouds.
5	70	90	80.0	..	Fair.
6	70	90	80.0	..	Fair.
7	70	90	80.0	..	Fair.
8	72	91	81.5	..	Fair.
9	74	91	82.5	..	Fair.
10	74	92	83.0	..	Fair; shower at night.
11	76	86	81.0	..	Cloudy; fair.
12	76	90	83.0	..	Fair.
13	76	90	83.0	..	Fair.
14	66	90	78.0	..	Fair.
15	74	90	82.0	..	Clouds.
16	76	92	84.0	..	Fair.
17	72	92	82.0	..	Fair.
18	70	92	81.0	..	Fair.
19	70	92	81.0	0.2	Clouds; rain at 6 P. M.
20	72	80	76.0	..	Cloudy.
21	72	80	76.0	0.7	Cloudy; rain at 4 P. M.
22	72	86	79.0	..	Cloudy.
23	70	88	79.0	..	Fair.
24	70	90	80.0	..	Clouds.
25	70	88	79.0	..	Clouds; sprinkle.
26	70	90	80.0	..	Fair.
27	72	92	82.0	..	Fair.
28	74	94	84.0	..	Fair.
29	72	94	83.0	..	Fair.
30	72	92	82.0	..	Fair.
31	74	94	84.0	..	Fair.
Means	72.00	89.71	80.85	1.2	
Max.	76	94	84.0		
Min.	66	80	76.0		
Range	10	14	8.0		
Extreme range 28					

Greatest Rise and Fall of temperature in 24 hours.

	Sunrise.	3 P. M.
Rise . . .	8	6
Fall . . .	10	12

August, 1844.

DAY.	THERMOMETER. Sun-rise.	3 P. M.	Mean.	RAIN. Ins.	REMARKS ON THE WEATHER.
1	75	94	84.5	..	Fair.
2	70	94	82.0	..	Fair.
3	70	94	82.0	..	Fair.
4	76	96	86.0	0.2	Fair; thunder shower at 5 P. M.
5	70	90	80.0	0.3	Cloudy; thunder shower at 2 P.M.
6	70	89	79.5	..	Cloudy; fair. [and at night.
7	68	90	79.0	..	Cloudy.
8	72	94	83.0	..	Cloudy.
9	72	94	83.0	..	Cloudy.
10	74	90	82.0	..	Cloudy.
11	74	88	81.0	..	Cloudy.
12	68	76	72.0	0.2	Cloudy; rain at 9 A. M.
13	64	75	69.5	0.3	Cloudy; thunder; rain.
14	66	82	74.0	..	Fog; fair.
15	64	87	75.5	..	Fair.
16	64	90	77.0	..	Fair.
17	68	90	79.0	..	Fair; clouds.
18	70	91	80.5	..	Fair; clouds.
19	72	92	82.0	..	Fair; clouds.
20	72	92	82.0	..	Fair; clouds.
21	74	94	84.0	..	Fair; clouds.
22	74	94	84.0	..	Fair; clouds.
23	74	80	77.0	0.3	Cloudy; thunder; rain at 9 A. M.
24	72	88	80.0	..	Fog; fair.
25	74	76	75.0	..	Fair; cloudy.
26	66	85	75.5	..	Cloudy; fair.
27	60	86	73.0	..	Fair.
28	64	80	72.0	..	Fair.
29	62	82	72.0	..	Cloudy; fair.
30	66	90	78.0	..	Clouds; smoky.
31	70	86	78.0	..	Fair.
Means	[illegible]	[illegible]	78.77	[illegible]	
Max.	76	96	86.0		
Min.	60	75	69.5		
Range	16	21	16.5		
Extreme range 36					

Greatest Rise and Fall of temperature in 24 hours.

	Sunrise.	3 P. M.
Rise . . .	6	9
Fall . . .	8	14

September, 1844.

DAY.	THERMOMETER. Sun-rise.	THERMOMETER. 3 P. M.	THERMOMETER. Mean.	RAIN. Ins.	REMARKS ON THE WEATHER.
1	70	90	80.0	..	Fair.
2	66	90	78.0	..	Fair.
3	66	93	79.5	0.2	Clouds; shower.
4	70	90	80.0	..	Clouds; thunder.
5	70	88	79.0	..	Cloudy.
6	66	92	79.0	..	Fog; fair.
7	66	86	76.0	0.4	Cloudy; rain at night.
8	70	80	75.0	..	Cloudy; rain.
9	64	83	73.5	..	Fair.
10	63	88	75.5	..	Fair.
11	64	88	76.0	..	Fair; cloudy.
12	70	76	73.0	1.7	Cloudy; thunder; rain.
13	64	74	69.0	0.3	Cloudy; thunder; rain.
14	60	84	72.0	..	Fair.
15	62	82	72.0	..	Fair.
16	62	86	74.0	..	Fair.
17	66	85	75.5	..	Clouds.
18	64	87	75.5	..	Fair.
19	64	85	74.5	..	Fair.
20	61	85	73.0	..	Fair.
21	61	68	64.5	..	Clouds.
22	44	68	56.0	..	Fair.
23	43	74	58.5	..	Fair.
24	45	80	62.5	..	
25	60	64	62.0	0.4	Cloudy; rain from N. W.
26	55	60	57.5	1.6	Cloudy; rain.
27	50	52	51.0	..	Cloudy; rain.
28	50	60	55.0	..	Fair.
29	37	60	48.5	..	Fair; frost in the low ground.
30	36	64	50.0	..	
Means	59.63	78.73	69.18	4.6	
Max.	70	93	80.0		
Min.	36	52	48.5		
Range	34	41	31.5		

Extreme range 57

Greatest Rise and Fall of temperature in 24 hours.

	Sunrise.	3 P. M.
Rise . . .	15	10
Fall . . .	17	17

October, 1844.

DAY.	THERMOMETER. Sun-rise.	THERMOMETER. 3 P. M.	THERMOMETER. Mean.	RAIN. Ins.	REMARKS ON THE WEATHER.
1	46	70	58.0	..	Fair.
2	50	76	63.0	..	Fair; cloudy.
3	50	70	60.0	..	Fair.
4	48	74	61.0	..	Smoky; fair.
5	50	74	62.0	..	Smoky.
6	52	74	63.0	..	Smoky.
7	48	72	60.0	..	Fair.
8	42	70	56.0	..	Fair.
9	42	72	57.0	..	Fair.
10	50	76	63.0	..	Cloudy.
11	..	..	..	..	
12	38	76	57.0	..	Fair.
13	50	70	60.0	0.9	Cloudy; rain at night; thunder.
14	60	68	64.0	..	Cloudy.
15	48	66	57.0	0.1	Fog; fair; thunder; rain at night.
16	60	70	65.0	0.4	Cloudy; thunder; rain at 5 P. M.
17	56	51	53.5	1.0	Mist; rain.
18	46	46	46.0	..	Rain; fair.
19	30	54	42.0	..	Fair; killing frost.
20	40	57	48.5	..	Fair.
21	48	70	59.0	..	Cloudy; fair.
22	54	70	62.0	..	Fog; fair.
23	64	76	70.0	0.3	Cloudy; rain.
24	70	80	75.0	..	Cloudy; fair.
25	70	70	70.0	0.4	Cloudy; rain.
26	62	74	68.0	1.1	Fog; cloudy; rain.
27	56	56	56.0	..	Rain.
28	46	56	51.0	..	Cloudy.
29	32	50	41.0	..	Fair.
30	32	56	44.0	..	Fair.
31	36	76	56.0	..	Clouds; sprinkle at night.
Means	49.20	67.33	58.27	4.2	
Max.	70	80	75.0		
Min.	30	50	41.0		
Range	40	30	34.0		

Extreme range 50

Greatest Rise and Fall of temperature in 24 hours.

	Sunrise.	3 P. M.
Rise . . .	12	20
Fall . . .	16	19

November, 1844.

DAY.	THERMOMETER. Sun-rise.	THERMOMETER. 2 P. M.	THERMOMETER. Mean.	RAIN. Ins.	REMARKS ON THE WEATHER.
1	60	70	65.0	..	Cloudy.
2	62	76	69.0	0.1	Fog; fair; shower at night.
3	64	66	65.0	..	Fair; clouds; showery.
4	44	56	50.0	..	Fair.
5	50	60	55.0	..	Cloudy.
6	48	60	54.0	..	Cloudy.
7	46	65	55.5	..	Cloudy; fair.
8	48	70	59.0	..	Fair.
9	58	74	66.0	..	Cloudy; fair.
10	62	66	64.0	0.7	Cloudy; thunder; rain.
11	60	70	65.0	0.3	Cloudy; thunder; rain.
12	40	40	40.0	0.5	Cloudy; thunder; rain.
13	26	40	33.0	..	Fair.
14	24	46	35.0	..	Fair.
15	24	54	39.0	..	Fair.
16	48	64	56.0	..	Fair; rain at night.
17	52	48	50.0	1.0	Rain.
18	40	50	45.0	..	Cloudy; fair.
19	34	50	42.0	..	Fair.
20	29	60	44.5	..	Fair.
21	44	51	47.5	..	Fog; cloudy.
22	30	52	41.0	..	Fair.
23	30	62	46.0	..	Fair.
24	34	50	42.0	..	Fair.
25	38	45	41.5	..	Cloudy.
26	40	64	52.0	..	Cloudy.
27	54	64	59.0	..	Fog; clouds.
28	56	68	62.0	..	Fog; clouds.
29	58	73	65.5	..	Fog; fair.
30	64	74	69.0	..	Fair.
Means	45.57	59.60	52.58	2.6	
Max.	64	76	69.0		
Min.	24	40	33.0		
Range	40	36	36.0		

Extreme range 52

Greatest Rise and Fall of temperature in 24 hours.

	Sunrise.	2 P. M.
Rise . . .	24	19
Fall . . .	20	30

December, 1844.

DAY.	THERMOMETER. Sun-rise.	THERMOMETER. 2 P. M.	THERMOMETER. Mean.	RAIN. Ins.	REMARKS ON THE WEATHER.
1	44	44	44.0	..	Clouds.
2	44	50	47.0	..	Cloudy; fair.
3	43	50	46.5	..	Cloudy; mist.
4	54	68	61.0	..	Cloudy.
5	36	42	39.0	1.5	Fair; cloudy; thunder; rain at 2 P. M.
6	36	31	33.5	..	Rain; snow.
7	24	38	31.0	..	Fair.
8	22	42	32.0	..	
9	28	40	34.0	..	Clouds; fair.
10	16	40	28.0	..	Fair.
11	21	41	31.0	..	Fair.
12	31	54	42.5	..	Fair.
13	31	52	41.5	..	Fair.
14	26	54	40.0	..	Fair.
15	30	59	44.5	..	Fair.
16	24	36	30.0	..	Fair.
17	24	36	30.0	..	Fair.
18	17	41	29.0	..	Fair.
19	18	54	36.0	..	Fair.
20	42	56	49.0	..	Fair.
21	40	62	51.0	..	Fair.
22	40	48	44.0	..	Fair.
23	26	60	43.0	..	Fair.
24	44	64	54.0	..	Fair; smoky.
25	63	70	66.5	0.1	Fair; shower at night.
26	45	50	47.5	..	Fair.
27	25	50	37.5	..	Fair.
28	30	60	45.0	..	Fair.
29	32	62	47.0	..	Fair; smoky.
30	48	65	56.5	..	Fair; smoky.
31	56	56	56.0	..	Clouds.
Means	34.19	50.81	42.50	1.6	
Max.	63	70	66.5		
Min.	16	31	28.0		
Range	47	39	38.5		

Extreme range 54

Greatest Rise and Fall of temperature in 24 hours.

	Sunrise.	2 P. M.
Rise . . .	24	18
Fall . . .	20	30

January, 1845.

DAY.	THERMOMETER. Sunrise.	2 P. M.	Mean.	RAIN. Ins.	REMARKS ON THE WEATHER.
1	46	60	53 0	..	Fair.
2	58	66	62.0	..	Cloudy.
3	62	66	64.0	..	Fair.
4	32	60	46.0	..	Fair.
5	60	49	54.5	3.0	Cloudy; thunder; rain.
6	44	46	45.0	..	Fair.
7	38	42	40.0	..	Clouds.
8	26	54	40.0	..	Fair.
9	36	50	43.0	0.3	Mist; cloudy; rain at night.
10	40	46	43.0	..	Cloudy; fair.
11	26	56	41.0	..	Fair.
12	28	60	44.0	..	Fair.
13	46	70	58.0	..	Clouds; fair.
14	42	62	52.0	..	Fog; clouds.
15	66	66	66.0	1.0	Cloudy; thunder; rain.
16	62	72	67.0	..	Cloudy.
17	36	36	36.0	..	Cloudy.
18	27	34	30.5	..	Cloudy; snow.
19	34	36	35.0	..	Cloudy; snow 2 inches deep.
20	34	44	39.0	..	Fair.
21	26	54	40.0	..	Fair.
22	32	50	41.0	0.5	Cloudy; thunder; rain.
23	32	50	41.0	..	Fair.
24	32	50	41.0	..	Fair.
25	26	52	39.0	..	Fair.
26	36	58	47 0	..	Clouds.
27	60	60	60.0	2.2	Cloudy; thunder; rain.
28	40	50	45.0	0.2	Rain; fair.
29	30	60	45.0	..	Fair.
30	26	60	43.0	..	Fair.
31	26	60	43.0	..	
Means	39.00	54.16	46.58	7.2	
Max.	66	72	67.0		
Min.	26	34	30.5		
Range	40	38	36.5		

Extreme range 46

Greatest Rise and Fall of temperature in 24 hours.

	Sunrise.	2 P. M.
Rise . . .	28	10
Fall . . .	30	36

February, 1845.

DAY.	THERMOMETER. Sunrise.	2 P. M.	Mean.	RAIN. Ins.	REMARKS ON THE WEATHER.
1	50	62	56.0	..	Clouds; fair.
2	36	52	44.0	..	Fair; cloudy.
3	46	52	49.0	1.0	Cloudy; rain.
4	28	43	35.5	..	Fair.
5	28	48	38.0	..	Fair.
6	24	48	36.0	..	Cloudy.
7	46	60	53.0	..	Cloudy; fair.
8	30	60	45.0	..	Fair.
9	30	64	47.0	..	Fair.
10	34	68	51.0	..	Fair.
11	58	74	66.0	..	Cloudy; fair.
12	62	76	69.0	..	Cloudy; fair.
13	66	76	71.0	..	Cloudy.
14	52	62	57.0	..	Rain; fair.
15	30	54	42.0	..	Fair.
16	34	48	41.0	..	Fair.
17	36	68	52.0	..	Fair.
18	40	70	55.0	..	Fair.
19	64	74	69.0	0.5	Cl'dy; thunder; hail; rain at night.
20	48	68	58.0	0.8	Fair; cl'dy; thunder; hail; rain at night.
21	48	62	55.0	0.5	Thunder; rain.
22	42	50	46.0	..	Fair.
23	30	58	44.0	..	Fair.
24	32	60	46.0	..	Fair.
25	40	68	54.0	..	Fair.
26	36	70	53.0	..	Fair.
27	40	60	50.0	..	Fair.
28	28	62	45.0	..	Fair.
Means	40.64	61.32	50.98	[illegible]	
Max.	66	76	71.0		
Min.	24	43	35.5		
Range	42	33	35.5		

Extreme range 52

[illegible] temperature in 24 hours.

	Sunrise.	2 P. M.
Rise . . .	24	20
Fall . . .	22	14

March, 1845.

DAY.	THERMOMETER. Sunrise.	2 P. M.	Mean.	RAIN. Ins.	REMARKS ON THE WEATHER.
1	52	62	57.0	1.0	Showers; mist.
2	64	69	66.5	0.4	Rain; fair.
3	44	49	46.5	1.5	Cloudy; rain.
4	46	46	46.0	0.2	Cloudy; rain.
5	32	60	46.0	..	Fair.
6	42	72	57.0	..	Fair.
7	62	72	67.0	0.8	Cloudy; mist; thunder; rain.
8	56	66	61.0	0.7	Rain.
9	48	45	46.5	0.6	Rain.
10	40	47	43.5	..	Fair.
11	28	53	40.5	..	Fair.
12	32	58	45.0	..	Fair.
13	36	66	51.0	..	Fair.
14	40	58	49.0	..	Fair.
15	28	57	42.5	..	Fair.
16	40	72	56.0	..	Fair.
17	48	80	64.0	..	Cloudy; smoky.
18	44	48	46.0	..	Cloudy; smoky.
19	34	44	39.0	..	Smoky.
20	25	49	37.0	..	Fair.
21	40	56	48.0	..	Fair; smoky.
22	44	50	47.0	1.0	Smoky; rain.
23	46	50	48.0	1.0	Rain.
24	46	60	53.0	..	Fair.
25	32	60	46.0	..	Fair.
26	32	70	51.0	..	Fair.
27	54	74	64.0	..	Fair.
28	50	76	63.0	..	Fair.
29	60	80	70.0	..	Clouds; fair.
30	66	76	71.0	..	Cloudy; shower.
31	60	60	60.0	0.2	Shower at sunrise.
Means	44.23	60.81	52.52	7.4	
Max.	66	80	71.0		
Min.	25	44	37.0		
Range	41	36	34.0		

Extreme range 55

Greatest Rise and Fall of temperature in 24 hours.

	Sunrise.	2 P. M.
Rise . . .	24	15
Fall . . .	20	32

April, 1845.

DAY.	THERMOMETER. Sunrise.	2 P. M.	Mean.	RAIN. Ins.	REMARKS ON THE WEATHER.
1	32	70	51.0	..	Fair.
2	36	78	57.0	..	Fair.
3	40	80	60.0	..	Fair.
4	62	80	71.0	..	Clouds; fair.
5	62	70	66.0	0.5	Fair; thunder; rain at 2 P. M.
6	50	56	53.0	..	Cloudy.
7	32	66	49.0	..	Fair.
8	40	66	53.0	..	Fair.
9	40	66	53.0	..	Fair.
10	56	80	68.0	..	Fair.
11	56	82	69.0	..	Fair; clouds.
12	56	82	69.0	..	Clouds.
13	56	80	68.0	..	Clouds; rain at 3 P. M.
14	64	81	72.5	0.2	Rain.
15	64	78	71.0	..	Clouds; showery.
16	68	80	74.0	0.2	Clouds; rain at night.
17	60	80	70.0	..	Clouds; showery.
18	70	83	76.5	0.4	Clouds; thunder; rain at night.
19	62	80	71.0	..	Fair.
20	66	80	73.0	..	Cloudy; sprinkle.
21	66	80	73.0	0.3	Rain.
22	70	82	76.0	2.0	Cloudy; thunder; hail; rain.
23	60	80	70.0	..	Cloudy.
24	70	80	75.0	0.7	Cloudy; rain at 3 P. M.
25	46	71	58.5	..	Fair.
26	50	80	65.0	..	Clouds; fair.
27	64	82	73.0	..	Clouds.
28	64	82	73.0	..	Fair.
29	64	84	74.0	..	Fair.
30	68	82	75.0	1.2	Cloudy; thunder; rain at night.
Means	[illegible]	[illegible]	[illegible]	5.5	
Max.	70	84	76.5		
Min.	32	56	49.0		
Range	38	28	27.5		

Extreme range 52

[illegible] temperature in 24 hours.

	Sunrise.	2 P. M.
Rise . . .	22	14
Fall . . .	28	14

May, 1845.

DAY.	THERMOMETER. Sunrise.	THERMOMETER. 3 P. M.	THERMOMETER. Mean.	RAIN. Ins.	REMARKS ON THE WEATHER.
1	60	66	63.0	0.8	Cloudy; rain; thunder from N.W.
2	50	52	51.0	0.6	Rain; thunder from N.W.
3	52	66	59.0	1.0	Cloudy; rain; thunder from N.W.
4	62	68	65.0	1.5	Rain from N.W.
5	62	56	59.0	0.2	Rain.
6	50	64	57.0	. .	Rain; cloudy.
7	48	74	61.0	. .	Fair.
8	48	75	61.5	. .	Fair; cloudy.
9	50	77	63.5	. .	Fair.
10	52	80	66.0	. .	Fair.
11	52	80	66.0	. .	Fair.
12	58	82	70.0	. .	Fair.
13	62	84	73.0	. .	Fair; thunder; sprinkle at night.
14	60	72	66.0	. .	Cloudy; fair.
15	50	74	62.0	. .	Fair.
16	48	74	61.0	. .	Fair.
17	46	76	61.0	. .	Fair.
18	50	80	65.0	. .	Fair.
19	54	84	69.0	0.2	Fair; clouds; rain at night.
20	64	84	74.0	. .	Clouds.
21	64	84	74.0	. .	Fair.
22	64	88	76.0	. .	Fair.
23	64	84	74.0	. .	Fair.
24	70	80	75.0	0.3	Cloudy; rain.
25	60	76	68.0	0.2	Cloudy; rain.
26	60	76	68.0	. .	Cloudy; fair.
27	60	84	72.0	. .	Fair.
28	64	85	74.5	0.3	Clouds; fair; rain at 5 P. M.
29	62	86	74.0	. .	Fog; fair.
30	60	80	70.0	. .	Fair.
31	54	84	69.0	. .	Fair.
Means	56.76	76.01	66.69	5.1	
Max.	70	88	76.0		
Min.	46	52	51.0		
Range	24	36	25.0		
Extreme range 42					

Greatest Rise and Fall of temperature in 24 hours.

	Sunrise.	3 P. M.
Rise . . .	10	14
Fall . . .	12	16

June, 1845.

DAY.	THERMOMETER. Sunrise.	THERMOMETER. 3 P. M.	THERMOMETER. Mean.	RAIN. Ins.	REMARKS ON THE WEATHER.
1	60	84	72.0	. .	Fair.
2	74	78	76.0	2.0	Cloudy; thunder; rain.
3	66	76	71.0	1.2	Cloudy; thunder; rain.
4	66	84	75.0	2.0	Cloudy; thunder; rain.
5	60	84	72.0	. .	Fair.
6	64	86	75.0	. .	Fair.
7	66	86	76.0	. .	Fair.
8	66	86	76.0	0.2	Fair; cloudy; rain at night.
9	70	85	77.5	. .	Rain; fair.
10	70	87	78.5	. .	Fair; clouds.
11	70	87	78.5	. .	Clouds.
12	70	88	79.0	. .	Clouds; fair.
13	70	88	79.0	0.5	Clouds; rain at night.
14	64	86	75.0	. .	Clouds; fair.
15	66	85	75.5	. .	Fair.
16	66	86	76.0	. .	Fair.
17	70	80	75.0	. .	Cloudy; fair.
18	70	86	78.0	. .	Cloudy.
19	71	86	78.5	. .	Fair.
20	70	89	79.5	. .	Clouds; fair
21	70	88	79.0	. .	Fair.
22	70	88	79.0	. .	Fair.
23	70	88	79.0	. .	Fair.
24	70	88	79.0	. .	Fair.
25	70	86	78.0	. .	Clouds, sprinkle.
26	66	80	73.0	0.4	Fair; thunder, rain at 3 P. M.
27	68	88	78.0	. .	Fair.
28	70	88	79.0	. .	Fair.
29	70	82	76.0	0.2	Clouds; shower 10 A. M.
30	66	82	74.0	0.3	Fog; shower at 4 P. M.
Means	67.97	85.17	76.57	6.8	
Max.	74	89	79.5		
Min.	60	76	71.0		
Range	14	13	8.5		
Extreme range 29					

Greatest Rise and Fall of temperature in 24 hours.

	Sunrise.	3 P. M.
Rise . . .	14	8
Fall . . .	8	6

July, 1845.

DAY.	THERMOMETER. Sunrise.	THERMOMETER. 3 P. M.	THERMOMETER. Mean.	RAIN. Ins.	REMARKS ON THE WEATHER.
1	70	86	78.0	. .	Fog; clouds.
2	70	83	76.5	0.8	Clouds; sh'r at 3 P. M.; thunder.
3	70	80	75.0	1.5	Cloudy; thunder; rain.
4	70	86	78.0	. .	Fair; clouds.
5	70	84	77.0	. .	Clouds.
6	70	88	79.0	. .	Clouds; showers.
7	72	85	78.5	. .	Clouds; fair.
8	72	90	81.0	. .	Fair; clouds.
9	72	90	81.0	. .	Fair.
10	72	92	82.0	0.3	Fair; rain at night.
11	72	84	78.0	. .	Fair.
12	72	90	81.0	. .	Fair.
13	70	92	81.0	. .	Fair.
14	72	92	82.0	. .	Fair.
15	74	90	82.0	. .	Fair.
16	74	90	82.0	. .	Fair.
17	72	90	81.0	. .	Fair.
18	74	90	82.0	. .	Fair.
19	72	90	81.0	. .	Fair.
20	70	94	82.0	. .	Fair.
21	72	94	83.0	. .	Fair.
22	72	92	82.0	. .	Fair.
23	72	92	82.0	. .	Fair.
24	70	89	79.5	. .	
25	70	90	80.0	. .	
26	72	93	82.5	0.1	Clouds; thunder; rain at night.
27	72	90	81.0	. .	Fair.
28	72	89	80.5	. .	Fair.
29	74	88	81.0	. .	Cloudy; thunder; sprinkle.
30	70	84	77.0	. .	
31	64	80	72.0	. .	
Means	71.29	88.61	79.95	2.7	
Max.	74	94	83.0		
Min.	64	80	72.0		
Range	10	14	11.0		
Extreme range 30					

Greatest Rise and Fall of temperature in 24 hours.

	Sunrise.	3 P. M.
Rise . . .	4	6
Fall . . .	6	8

August, 1845.

DAY.	THERMOMETER. Sunrise.	THERMOMETER. 3 P. M.	THERMOMETER. Mean.	RAIN Ins.	REMARKS ON THE WEATHER.
1	64	79	71.5	. .	Clouds.
2	64	84	74.0	. .	Clouds; fair.
3	64	82	73.0	. .	Fair.
4	64	84	74.0	. .	Fair.
5	64	86	75.0	. .	Fair.
6	64	86	75.0	. .	Fair; smoky.
7	70	84	77.0	. .	Cloudy.
8	66	80	73.0	0.2	Cloudy; rain.
9	70	78	74.0	0.1	Cloudy; rain.
10	70	74	72.0	. .	Cloudy; rain.
11	68	84	76.0	. .	Fair; clouds.
12	70	85	77.5	. .	Fair; clouds.
13	76	80	78.0	0.1	Cloudy; rain.
14	76	80	78.0	. .	Cloudy.
15	72	85	78.5	. .	Cloudy.
16	72	90	81.0	. .	Cloudy; fair.
17	66	92	79.0	. .	Fair.
18	70	92	81.0	. .	Fair.
19	72	92	82.0	. .	Fair.
20	72	93	82.5	. .	Fair.
21	74	93	83.5	. .	Fair.
22	72	94	83.0	. .	Fair; clouds; thunder.
23	72	92	82.0	0.1	Clouds; thunder; rain.
24	74	88	81.0	. .	Fair.
25	74	89	81.5	. .	Fair.
26	76	88	82.0	. .	Fair.
27	72	89	80.5	. .	Fair; clouds; thunder.
28	74	86	80.0	0.2	Fair, clouds; thunder; rain at 12.
29	74	79	76.5	. .	Fair.
30	74	80	77.0	. .	Fog; fair.
31	73	81	77.0	. .	
Means	70.42	85.45	77.94	0.7	
Max	76	94	83.5		
Min.	64	74	71.5		
Range	12	20	12.0		
Extreme range 30					

Greatest Rise and Fall of temperature in 24 hours.

	Sunrise.	3 P. M.
Rise . . .	6	10
Fall . . .	6	7

September, 1845.

DAY.	THERMOMETER. Sunrise.	THERMOMETER. 3 P. M.	THERMOMETER. Mean.	RAIN. Ins.	REMARKS ON THE WEATHER.
1	73	82	77.5	. .	Fair.
2	74	88	81.0	. .	Fair.
3	78	89	83.5	. .	Fair.
4	74	88	81.0	. .	Fair.
5	76	86	81.0	. .	Fair.
6	74	86	80.0	. .	Fair.
7	73	86	79 5	. .	Fair.
8	74	86	80.0	. .	Fair.
9	72	84	78.0	0.5	Cloudy; rain.
10	70	77	73.5	. .	Fair.
11	68	76	72.0	. .	Fair.
12	70	84	77.0	. .	Fair.
13	73	83	78.0	. .	Fair.
14	68	00	75.5	. .	Fair.
15	62	74	68.0	. .	Fair.
16	61	74	67.5	. .	Fair.
17	65	75	70.0	. .	Fair.
18	67	76	71.5	. .	Fair.
19	62	82	72.0	. .	Fair.
20	70	72	71.0	0.4	Cloudy; rain.
21	62	72	67.0	. .	Fair.
22	54	70	62.0	. .	Fair.
23	58	76	67.0	. .	Fair.
24	62	74	68.0	. .	Fair.
25	58	76	67.0	. .	Fair.
26	58	80	69.0	. .	Fair.
27	60	80	70.0	1.0	Cloudy; rain.
28	70	76	73.0	0.2	Cloudy; rain.
29	74	74	74.0	. .	
30	. .	. .	. .	. .	
Means	67.50	79.62	73.60	2.1	
Max.	78	89	83.5		
Min.	54	70	62.0		
Range	24	19	21.5		

Extreme range 35

Greatest Rise and Fall of temperature in 24 hours.

	Sunrise.	3 P. M.
Rise . . .	10	8
Fall . . .	8	10

October, 1845.

DAY.	THERMOMETER. Sunrise.	THERMOMETER. 3 P. M.	THERMOMETER. Mean.	RAIN. Ins.	REMARKS ON THE WEATHER.
1	48	78	63.0	. .	Fair.
2	50	78	64.0	. .	Fair.
3	50	78	64.0	. .	Fair.
4	56	78	67.0	. .	Fair; clouds.
5	42	61	51.5	. .	Fair.
6	44	56	50.0	. .	Clouds; sprinkle.
7	54	58	56.0	0.1	Cloudy; rain.
8	56	60	58.0	. .	Cloudy.
9	42	64	53.0	. .	Mist; fair.
10	52	60	56.0	. .	Fair.
11	40	54	47.0	. .	Fair; clouds.
12	30	60	45.0	. .	Fair; killing frost.
13	34	65	49.5	. .	Fair.
14	40	74	57.0	. .	Fair.
15	46	57	51.5	. .	Clouds; fair.
16	30	60	45.0	. .	Fair.
17	30	70	50.0	. .	Fair.
18	34	76	55.0	. .	Fair.
19	54	74	64.0	. .	Cloudy.
20	64	70	67.0	. .	Cloudy; sprinkle.
21	46	60	53.0	. .	Fair.
22	34	60	47.0	. .	Fair.
23	36	60	48.0	. .	Fair.
24	50	70	60.0	. .	Cloudy.
25	48	70	59.0	. .	Smoky; fire in the woods.
26	42	74	58.0	. .	Smoky.
27	48	74	61.0	. .	Smoky.
28	46	76	61.0	. .	Smoky.
29	58	70	64.0	. .	Clouds.
30	65	74	69.5	0.5	Clouds; rain.
31	66	76	71.0	0.2	Clouds; rain.
Means	46.29	67.58	56.93	[illegible]	
Max.	66	78	71.0		
Min.	30	54	45.0		
Range	36	24	26.0		

Extreme range 48

Greatest Rise and Fall of temperature in 24 hours.

	Sunrise.	3 P. M.
Rise . . .	20	10
Fall . . .	26	17

November, 1845.

DAY.	THERMOMETER. Sunrise.	THERMOMETER. 2 P. M.	THERMOMETER. Mean.	RAIN. Ins.	REMARKS ON THE WEATHER.
1	62	80	71.0	. .	Fog; fair.
2	48	70	59.0	. .	Fair.
3	38	66	52.0	. .	Fair.
4	36	70	53.0	. .	Smoky; rain.
5	58	76	67.0	. .	Cloudy.
6	56	66	61.0	0.5	Smoky; rain.
7	52	52	52.0	. .	Rain.
8	46	54	50.0	. .	Cloudy; fair.
9	28	48	38.0	. .	Fair.
10	28	50	39.0	. .	Clouds; fair.
11	32	58	45.0	. .	Fair.
12	32	60	46.0	. .	Fair.
13	30	60	45.0	. .	Fair.
14	50	62	56.0	. .	Cloudy; sprinkle.
15	46	70	58.0	. .	Cloudy; fair.
16	50	68	59.0	0.3	Cloudy; rain.
17	60	76	68.0	. .	Cloudy; fair.
18	50	62	56.0	. .	Fair.
19	32	64	48.0	. .	Smoky.
20	40	64	52.0	. .	Smoky.
21	50	70	60.0	. .	Smoky.
22	30	46	38.0	. .	Smoky.
23	25	50	37.5	. .	Smoky; rain at night.
24	26	64	45.0	0.3	Smoky; rain at night.
25	26	64	45.0	. .	Smoky.
26	42	36	39.0	0.1	Rain.
27	24	36	30.0	. .	Fair.
28	18	30	24.0	. .	Fair; cloudy.
29	20	30	25.0	. .	Cloudy; snow at night.
30	19	22	20.5	. .	Cloudy; snow fell all day; 3 inches deep.
Means	38.47	57.47	47.97	1.2	
Max.	62	76	71.0		
Min.	18	22	20.5		
Range	44	54	50.5		

Extreme range 58

Greatest Rise and Fall of temperature in 24 hours.

	Sunrise.	2 P. M.
Rise . . .	22	14
Fall . . .	20	28

December, 1845.

DAY.	THERMOMETER. Sunrise.	THERMOMETER. 2 P. M.	THERMOMETER. Mean.	RAIN. Ins.	REMARKS ON THE WEATHER.
1	—6	26	10.0	. .	Fair; snow 4½ inches deep.
2	10	26	18.0	. .	Cloudy; snow.
3	12	30	21.0	. .	Fair.
4	12	34	23.0	. .	Fair.
5	18	42	30.0	. .	Fair; cloudy; rain at night.
6	30	36	33.0	1.5	Rain; snow melting.
7	36	39	37.5	0.2	Rain.
8	42	46	44.0	. .	Rain.
9	38	42	40.0	. .	Fair.
10	28	44	36.0	. .	Fair.
11	34	38	36 0	1.2	Cloudy; snow; sleet.
12	30	40	35.0	. .	Fair.
13	42	45	43.5	0.3	Rain.
14	42	46	44.0	. .	Cloudy.
15	32	52	42.0	. .	Fair.
16	26	48	37.0	0.2	Fair; cloudy; rain at night.
17	44	54	49.0	. .	Rain; fair.
18	28	48	38.0	. .	Fair.
19	20	32	26.0	. .	Fair; clouds.
20	8	29	18.5	. .	Fair.
21	12	45	28.5	. .	Fair.
22	28	58	43.0	. .	Fair; clouds.
23	46	50	48.0	0.3	Cloudy; rain.
24	40	50	45.0	. .	Cloudy.
25	38	37	37.5	. .	Cloudy.
26	16	32	24.0	. .	Fair.
27	16	40	28.0	. .	Fair.
28	18	52	35.0	. .	Fair.
29	42	54	48.0	. .	Cloudy; sprinkle.
30	38	60	49.0	. .	Fog; fair.
31	50	58	54.0	0.7	Heavy rain at night.
Means	[illegible]	[illegible]	[illegible]	4.4	
Max.	50	60	54.0		
Min	—6	26	10.0		
Range	56	34	44.0		

Extreme range 66

Greatest Rise and Fall of temperature in 24 hours.

	Sunrise.	2 P. M.
Rise . . .	24	16
Fall . . .	25	16

January, 1846.

DAY.	THERMOMETER. Sunrise.	2 P. M.	Mean.	RAIN. Ins.	REMARKS ON THE WEATHER.
1	58	56	57.0	..	Cloudy.
2	36	56	46.0	..	Fair.
3	44	56	50.0	..	Fair.
4	28	54	41.0	..	Fair.
5	30	58	44.0	0.3	Fair; cloudy; rain at night.
6	42	52	47.0	..	Rain; fair.
7	27	55	41.0	..	Fog; fair.
8	30	58	44.0	..	Fog; fair.
9	24	42	33.0	..	Fair.
10	18	40	29.0	..	Fair.
11	25	48	36.5	..	Fair.
12	22	51	36.5	..	Fair.
13	30	54	42.0	..	Fair.
14	36	56	46.0	0.3	Cloudy; rain at night.
15	44	50	47.0	..	Cloudy.
16	46	54	50.0	0.2	Rain.
17	26	56	41.0	..	Fair.
18	28	50	39.0	..	Fair.
19	38	42	40.0	1.5	Rain.
20	38	42	40.0	..	Rain.
21	38	48	43.0	..	Clouds; fair.
22	26	59	42.5	..	Fair.
23	24	50	37.0	..	Fair.
24	28	54	41.0	..	Fair; cloudy.
25	40	58	49.0	..	Cloudy; fair.
26	42	60	51.0	..	Fair.
27	38	66	52.0	..	Fair.
28	40	64	52.0	..	Fair.
29	58	64	61.0	0.4	Rain.
30	46	52	49.0	..	Fair.
31	34	41	37.5	..	Cloudy.
Means	34.97	53.10	44.03	2.7	
Max.	58	66	61.0		
Min.	18	40	29.0		
Range	40	26	32.0		
Extreme range 48					

Greatest Rise and Fall of temperature in 24 hours.

	Sunrise.	2 P. M.
Rise . . .	18	11
Fall . . .	22	16

February, 1846.

DAY.	THERMOMETER. Sunrise.	2 P. M.	Mean.	RAIN. Ins.	REMARKS ON THE WEATHER.
1	25	50	37.5	..	Fair.
2	32	60	46.0	...	Fair.
3	32	64	48.0	..	Fair.
4	34	58	46.0	..	Fair; cloudy.
5	42	44	43.0	0.8	Cloudy; rain.
6	42	46	44.0	0.2	Cloudy; rain.
7	36	60	48.0	0.3	Fog; thunder; rain and hail at night.
8	36	40	38.0	..	Cloudy.
9	23	49	36.0	..	Fair; cloudy.
10	34	50	42.0	..	Cloudy.
11	44	60	52.0	..	Fog; fair.
12	44	54	49.0	0.3	Cloudy; rain at night.
13	38	40	39.0	1.0	Cloudy; rain.
14	36	40	38.0	..	Cloudy; rain; snow.
15	26	52	39.0	..	Fair.
16	30	60	45.0	..	Fair.
17	44	66	55.0	0.4	Fair; cloudy; rain at night.
18	36	32	34.0	0.7	Cloudy; rain; sleet; snow at night.
19	28	38	33.0	..	Cloudy; fair at eve.
20	26	44	35.0	..	Fair; snow at night.
21	34	42	38.0	..	Cloudy; fair.
22	36	58	47.0	..	Cloudy; fair.
23	34	56	45.0	..	Fair; cloudy.
24	46	56	51.0	0.3	Cloudy; rain.
25	31	34	32.5	..	Cloudy.
26	24	31	27.5	..	Cloudy.
27	28	38	33.0	..	Cloudy; mist.
28	50	70	60.0	0.2	Rain.
Means	34.68	49.71	42.20	4.2	
Max.	50	70	60.0		
Min.	23	31	27.5		
Range	27	39	32.5		
Extreme range 47					

Greatest Rise and Fall of temperature in 24 hours.

	Sunrise.	2 P. M.
Rise . . .	22	32
Fall . . .	15	34

March, 1846.

DAY.	THERMOMETER. Sunrise.	2 P. M.	Mean.	RAIN. Ins.	REMARKS ON THE WEATHER.
1	45	50	47.5	..	Cloudy.
2	27	56	41.5	..	Fair.
3	32	62	47.0	..	Fair.
4	42	68	55.0	..	Clouds; fair.
5	42	72	57.0	..	Smoky. Peach blooms.
6	56	72	64.0	..	Smoky; sprinkle at night.
7	50	72	61.0	..	Fog; fair.
8	46	73	59.5	..	Fair; clouds.
9	46	76	61.0	0.4	Cloudy; thunder; rain.
10	52	64	58.0	0.3	Cloudy; thunder; rain.
11	40	60	50.0	..	Fair.
12	48	50	49.0	..	Cloudy.
13	38	60	49.0	..	Fair.
14	38	72	55.0	..	Fair.
15	44	70	57.0	..	Smoky.
16	38	65	51.5	..	Smoky.
17	48	65	56.5	..	Smoky; sprinkle.
18	60	72	66.0	1.0	Smoky; heavy rain at night.
19	60	64	62.0	0.7	Rain.
20	48	54	51.0	..	Fair.
21	42	64	53.0	0.4	Cloudy; rain at night.
22	48	50	49.0	0.3	Rain.
23	50	72	61.0	..	Fog; fair.
24	35	52	43.5	..	Fair.
25	30	56	43.0	..	Fair.
26	39	66	52.5	..	Fair.
27	42	72	57.0	0.5	Fair; rain at night.
28	42	48	45.0	..	Rain.
29	34	60	47.0	..	Fair.
30	40	60	50.0	..	Cloudy.
31	46	56	51.0	..	Fair; cloudy.
Means	43.48	63.00	53.24	3.6	
Max.	60	76	66.0		
Min.	27	48	41.5		
Range	33	28	24.5		
Extreme range 49					

Greatest Rise and Fall of temperature in 24 hours.

	Sunrise.	2 P. M.
Rise . . .	14	22
Fall . . .	18	24

April, 1846.

DAY.	THERMOMETER. Sunrise.	2 P. M.	Mean.	RAIN. Ins.	REMARKS ON THE WEATHER.
1	50	56	53.0	0.3	Rain.
2	50	72	61.0	...	Mist; fair.
3	60	66	63.0	1.0	Cloudy; rain at night.
4	60	70	65.0	..	Mist; cloudy.
5	56	71	63.5	2.2	Cloudy; thunder; rain.
6	60	66	63.0	..	Rain.
7	58	60	59.0	..	Fair.
8	38	60	49.0	..	Fair.
9	48	70	59.0	..	Cloudy.
10	62	64	63.0	0.7	Cloudy; rain.
11	48	47	47.5	..	Rain.
12	38	50	44.0	..	Fair.
13	30	65	47.5	..	Fair.
14	36	70	53.0	..	Fair.
15	42	78	60.0	..	Fair.
16	46	80	63.0	..	Fair.
17	50	81	65.5	..	Fair.
18	50	84	67.0	..	Fair.
19	56	81	68.5	..	Fair; shower at 3 P. M.
20	56	80	68.0	0.1	Cloudy; fair; shower at 3 P. M.
21	66	78	72.0	..	Cloudy; fair.
22	58	78	68.0	..	Fog; fair.
23	64	80	72.0	..	Cloudy; fair.
24	70	71	70.5	0.3	Rain.
25	60	76	68.0	2.1	Cloudy; thunder; rain at night.
26	58	73	65.5	0.2	Fair; rain at night.
27	50	64	57.0	..	Fair; showers.
28	52	72	62.0	..	Fair.
29	54	66	60.0	..	Cloudy.
30	54	66	60.0	..	Fair.
Means	52.67	69.83	61.25	6.9	
Max.	70	84	72.0		
Min.	30	47	44.0		
Range	40	37	28.0		
Extreme range 54					

Greatest Rise and Fall of temperature in 24 hours.

	Sunrise.	2 P. M.
Rise . . .	14	16
Fall . . .	20	17

May, 1846.

DAY.	THERMOMETER. Sunrise.	THERMOMETER. 3 P. M.	THERMOMETER. Mean.	RAIN. Ins.	REMARKS ON THE WEATHER.
1	60	72	66.0	. .	Fair.
2	44	74	59.0	. .	Fair.
3	46	80	63.0	. .	Fair.
4	62	70	66.0	. .	Cloudy; showers.
5	62	56	59.0	. .	Cloudy.
6	64	82	73.0	. .	Cloudy.
7	60	76	68.0	. .	Fair.
8	50	76	63.0	. .	Fair.
9	56	80	68.0	. .	Fair.
10	54	80	67.0	. .	Fair.
11	50	80	65.0	. .	Cloudy.
12	60	85	72.5	. .	Cloudy; fair.
13	64	72	68.0	0.7	Cloudy; rain; fair.
14	62	70	66.0	0.3	Cloudy; rain; fair.
15	50	78	64.0	. .	Fair.
16	48	81	64.5	. .	Fair.
17	48	82	65.0	. .	Fair.
18	50	86	68.0	. .	Fair.
19	60	85	72.5	. .	Fair.
20	60	84	72.0	. .	Fair.
21	60	84	72.0	. .	Fair.
22	64	84	74.0	. .	Fair.
23	64	82	73.0	. .	Clouds; fair.
24	64	78	71.0	. .	Clouds; shower; fair.
25	70	82	76.0	. .	Fair.
26	70	86	78.0	. .	Fair.
27	73	87	80.0	2.0	Cloudy; rain; thunder at night.
28	70	80	75.0	. .	Cloudy.
29	64	82	73.0	0.1	Rain; fair.
30	64	78	71.0	0.4	Rain; fair.
31	64	82	73.0	. .	Fair; shower.
Means	59.26	79.16	69.21	3.5	
Max.	73	87	80.0		
Min.	44	56	59.0		
Range	29	31	21.0		
Extreme range 43					

Greatest Rise and Fall of temperature in 24 hours.

	Sunrise.	3 P. M.
Rise . . .	16	26
Fall . . .	16	14

June, 1846.

DAY.	THERMOMETER. Sunrise.	THERMOMETER. 3 P. M.	THERMOMETER. Mean.	RAIN. Ins.	REMARKS ON THE WEATHER.
1	70	76	73.0	. .	Cloudy; fair.
2	48	79	63.5	. .	Fair.
3	68	86	77.0	. .	Rain; fair.
4	64	86	75.0	0.8	Cloudy; thunder; rain.
5	60	70	65.0	0.2	Rain.
6	60	76	68.0	. .	Fog: fair.
7	60	80	70.0	. .	Fog; fair.
8	60	80	70.0	. .	Clouds; fair.
9	58	78	68.0	. .	Fair.
10	56	80	68.0	. .	Fair.
11	64	76	70.0	. .	Cloudy; shower.
12	60	78	69.0	. .	Cloudy.
13	60	83	71.5	. .	Fair.
14	60	84	72.0	. .	Fair.
15	58	82	70.0	. .	Fair.
16	60	84	72.0	. .	Fair.
17	62	86	74.0	. .	Fair.
18	70	84	77.0	. .	Clouds; shower at 2 P. M.
19	70	82	76.0	0.3	Cloudy; shower at 2 P. M.
20	72	82	77.0	0.5	Cloudy; rain.
21	72	74	73.0	1.7	Cloudy; thunder; rain.
22	70	80	75.0	. .	Cloudy; fair.
23	66	80	73.0	. .	Cloudy.
24	68	86	77.0	0.2	Cloudy; rain at 3 P. M.
25	70	80	75.0	. .	Fair.
26	70	86	78.0	. .	Fair.
27	66	86	76.0	. .	Fair.
28	70	86	78.0	. .	Fair.
29	68	87	77.5	. .	Fair.
30	70	92	81.0	0.5	Cloudy; thunder; rain at night.
Means	64.33	81.63	72.98	4.2	
Max.	72	92	81.0		
Min.	48	70	63.5		
Range	24	22	17.5		
Extreme range 44					

Greatest Rise and Fall of temperature in 24 hours.

	Sunrise.	3 P. M.
Rise . . .	20	7
Fall . . .	22	16

July, 1846.

DAY.	THERMOMETER. Sunrise.	THERMOMETER. 3 P. M.	THERMOMETER. Mean.	RAIN. Ins.	REMARKS ON THE WEATHER.
1	70	86	78.0	. .	Fair.
2	68	88	78.0	. .	Fair.
3	70	90	80.0	. .	Fair.
4	70	90	80.0	. .	Fair.
5	70	90	80.0	. .	Fair.
6	70	90	80.0	. .	Fair; rain at eve.
7	70	88	79.0	1.5	Clouds; rain at 4 P. M.
8	72	87	79.5	. .	Fog; clouds.
9	74	82	78.0	0.2	Clouds; rain at 1 P. M.
10	72	88	80.0	. .	Fair; clouds; thunder.
11	74	82	78.0	. .	Clouds.
12	70	90	80.0	0.5	Clouds; thunder; rain at night.
13	70	90	00.0	0.2	Fair; clouds; rain at night.
14	70	88	79.0	. .	Fair; clouds; rain at night.
15	72	80	76.0	0.4	Cloudy; rain at 2 P. M.
16	68	78	73.0	. .	Rain.
17	60	76	68.0	. .	Fair.
18	60	76	68.0	. .	Fair.
19	58	80	69.0	. .	Fair.
20	60	82	71.0	. .	Fair.
21	60	86	73.0	. .	Fair.
22	74	84	79.0	0.2	Cloudy; showers at 1 and 3 P. M.
23	76	80	78.0	. .	Cloudy; shower at 2 P. M.
24	72	86	79.0	. .	Fair.
25	70	89	79.5	. .	Fair.
26	72	90	81.0	. .	
27	74	92	83.0	. .	Clouds; thunder.
28	70	90	80.0	. .	Clouds; thunder.
29	70	90	80.0	. .	Fair.
30	76	78	77.0	0.5	Rain.
31	70	88	79.0	. .	Cloudy; fair.
Means	69.42	85.61	77.52	3.5	
Max.	76	92	83.0		
Min.	58	76	68.0		
Range	18	16	15.0		
Extreme range 34					

Greatest Rise and Fall of temperature in 24 hours.

	Sunrise.	3 P. M.
Rise . . .	14	10
Fall . . .	8	12

August, 1846.

DAY.	THERMOMETER. Sunrise.	THERMOMETER. 3 P. M.	THERMOMETER. Mean.	RAIN. Ins.	REMARKS ON THE WEATHER.
1	70	89	79.5	. .	Fair.
2	70	88	79.0	. .	Fair.
3	70	88	79.0	. .	Clouds; fair.
4	70	78	74.0	. .	Clouds; fair; shower at noon.
5	68	76	72.0	0.1	Cloudy; shower at 1 P. M.
6	70	78	74.0	. .	Fog; shower.
7	70	82	76.0	. .	Cloudy.
8	72	82	77.0	0.1	Cloudy; shower at 3 P. M.
9	72	78	75.0	0.1	Cloudy; shower at 3 P. M.
10	72	78	75.0	0.1	Cloudy; shower at 1 P. M.
11	66	66	66.0	. .	Fair; shower at 4 P. M.
12	68	86	77.0	. .	Fair; cloudy.
13	74	86	80.0	. .	Fog; fair; cloudy; shower at 12.
14	72	82	77.0	. .	Cloudy; shower at 10 A. M.
15	72	86	79.0	0.2	Fair; shower at night.
16	78	88	83.0	. .	Cloudy; fair.
17	74	90	82.0	. .	Fair; shower at 3 P. M.
18	74	90	82.0	. .	Fair.
19	74	90	82.0	0.2	Fair; shower at 5 P. M.
20	74	82	78.0	0.2	Fair; shower at 3 A. M.
21	74	82	78.0	. .	Cloudy.
22	74	76	75.0	. .	Cloudy; shower at noon.
23	60	79	69.5	. .	Fair.
24	58	76	67.0	. .	Fair.
25	60	81	70.5	. .	Fair.
26	60	82	71.0	. .	Fair.
27	58	84	71.0	. .	Fair.
28	64	86	75.0	. .	Fair.
29	62	87	74.5	. .	Fair.
30	68	86	77.0	. .	Fair.
31	66	86	76.0	. .	Fair.
Means	68.84	82.84	75.84	1.0	
Max.	78	90	83.0		
Min.	58	66	66.0		
Range	20	24	17.0		
Extreme range 32					

Greatest Rise and Fall of temperature in 24 hours.

	Sunrise.	3 P. M.
Rise . . .	6	20
Fall . . .	14	12

September, 1846.

DAY.	THERMOMETER. Sunrise.	THERMOMETER. 3 P. M.	THERMOMETER. Mean.	RAIN. Ins.	REMARKS ON THE WEATHER.
1	68	84	76.0	. .	Clouds; fair.
2	70	76	73.0	. .	Clouds; shower at 3 P. M.
3	72	76	74.0	. .	Fair.
4	72	86	79.0	. .	Fair.
5	72	86	79.0	. .	Fair; shower at 3 P. M.
6	71	82	76.5	0.2	Fog; shower at 3 P. M.
7	74	80	77.0	0.1	Cloudy; showers; rain at night.
8	72	80	76.0	0.5	Cloudy; shower.
9	71	80	75.5	. .	Fair.
10	70	86	78.0	. .	Fair.
11	68	89	78.5	. .	Fair.
12	74	84	79.0	. .	Fair.
13	70	89	79.5	. .	Fair.
14	72	90	81.0	. .	Fair.
15	70	92	81.0	. .	Fair.
16	70	92	81.0	. .	Fair.
17	70	92	81.0	. .	Fair.
18	62	82	72.0	. .	Fair.
19	56	78	67.0	. .	Fair.
20	56	76	66.0	. .	Fair.
21	56	84	70.0	. .	Fair.
22	60	85	72.5	. .	Fair.
23	64	84	74.0	. .	Fair.
24	56	84	70.0	. .	Fair.
25	64	68	66.0	1.0	Cloudy; rain.
26	64	65	64.5	. .	Cloudy; rain.
27	52	70	61.0	. .	Fair.
28	48	72	60.0	. .	Fair.
29	46	72	59.0	. .	
30	46	72	59.0	. .	
Means	64.53	81.20	72.87	1.8	Greatest Rise and Fall of temperature in 24 hours.
Max.	74	92	81.0		
Min.	46	65	59.0		
Range	28	27	22.0		
Extreme range 46					

	Sunrise.	3 P. M.
Rise . . .	8	10
Fall . . .	12	16

October, 1846.

DAY.	THERMOMETER. Sunrise.	THERMOMETER. 3 P. M.	THERMOMETER. Mean.	RAIN. Ins.	REMARKS ON THE WEATHER.
1	52	80	66.0	. .	Fair.
2	50	76	63.0	. .	Fair; smoky.
3	52	78	65.0	. .	Fair.
4	60	78	69.0	. .	Fair.
5	66	80	73.0	. .	Cloudy.
6	66	80	73.0	. .	Fair.
7	56	82	69.0	. .	Fair.
8	66	80	73.0	. .	Fair.
9	60	80	70.0	. .	Fair.
10	54	76	65.0	. .	Fair.
11	60	80	70.0	. .	Cloudy; fair.
12	64	70	67.0	. .	Cloudy; fair.
13	40	66	53.0	. .	Fair.
14	46	70	58.0	. .	Fair.
15	48	70	59.0	. .	Fair.
16	56	70	63.0	. .	Fair.
17	48	50	49.0	. .	Cloudy.
18	32	56	44.0	. .	Fair; white frost.
19	28	60	44.0	. .	Fair; killing frost.
20	34	64	49.0	. .	Clouds.
21	38	60	49.0	. .	Smoky; fire in the woods.
22	38	70	54.0	. .	Smoky.
23	48	70	59.0	. .	Smoky.
24	52	76	64.0	. .	Smoky.
25	48	76	62.0	. .	Smoky.
26	60	74	67.0	0.8	Cloudy; thunder; rain at night.
27	58	70	64.0	. .	Fog.
28	46	62	54.0	. .	Fair.
29	44	60	52.0	1.2	Cloudy; rain.
30	48	54	51.0	. .	Cloudy.
31	52	52	52.0	0.8	Cloudy; rain.
Means	50.64	70.00	60.32	2.8	Greatest Rise and Fall of temperature in 24 hours.
Max.	66	82	73.0		
Min.	28	50	44.0		
Range	38	32	29.0		
Extreme range 54					

	Sunrise.	3 P. M.
Rise . . .	12	10
Fall . . .	24	20

November, 1846.

DAY.	THERMOMETER. Sunrise.	THERMOMETER. 2 P. M.	THERMOMETER. Mean.	RAIN. Ins.	REMARKS ON THE WEATHER.
1	50	56	53.0	0.1	Rain.
2	50	60	55.0	. .	Cloudy; fair.
3	42	64	53.0	. .	Fog; fair.
4	54	66	60.0	. .	Clouds; fair.
5	42	63	52.5	. .	Fair.
6	36	54	45.0	. .	Fair.
7	38	66	52.0	. .	Fair.
8	40	68	54.0	. .	Fair.
9	58	72	65.0	0.1	Cloudy; showers.
10	45	70	57.5	. .	Fair.
11	42	70	56.0	. .	Fair.
12	50	70	60.0	. .	Fair.
13	54	64	59.0	0.5	Cloudy; thunder; rain.
14	32	60	46.0	. .	Fair.
15	54	70	62.0	. .	Cloudy.
16	64	65	64.5	1.0	Cloudy; rain.
17	42	60	51.0	. .	Fair.
18	46	50	48.0	0.1	Rain.
19	30	50	40.0	. .	Fair.
20	28	50	39.0	. .	Fair.
21	38	62	50.0	. .	Fair.
22	40	50	45.0	. .	Fair.
23	28	58	43.0	0.2	Fair; cloudy; shower at night.
24	54	42	48.0	. .	Rain.
25	28	42	35.0	. .	Fair.
26	20	46	33.0	. .	Fair.
27	46	70	58.0	. .	Cloudy; fair.
28	52	73	62.5	. .	Fog; fair.
29	50	62	56.0	0.3	Cloudy; mist; shower at night.
30	56	64	60.0	. .	Rain; cloudy.
Means	43.63	60.57	52.10	2.3	Greatest Rise and Fall of temperature in 24 hours.
Max.	64	73	65.0		
Min.	20	42	33.0		
Range	44	31	32.0		
Extreme range 53					

	Sunrise.	2 P. M.
Rise . . .	26	24
Fall . . .	26	16

December, 1846.

DAY.	THERMOMETER. Sunrise.	THERMOMETER. 2 P. M.	THERMOMETER. Mean.	RAIN. Ins.	REMARKS ON THE WEATHER.
1	64	70	67.0	0.3	Cloudy; thunder; rain at night.
2	66	60	63.0	. .	Fair.
3	30	56	43.0	. .	Fair.
4	30	56	43.0	. .	Fair.
5	46	50	48.0	1.0	Rain.
6	55	70	62.5	0.3	Rain.
7	64	72	68.0	1.0	Thunder; rain.
8	36	38	37.0	. .	Snow.
9	28	42	35.0	. .	Fair; cloudy.
10	32	46	39.0	. .	Fair.
11	24	46	35.0	. .	Fair.
12	26	48	37.0	. .	Fair.
13	44	48	46.0	1.0	Rain.
14	52	60	56.0	. .	Rain.
15	50	60	55.0	0.5	Fair; cloudy; rain at night.
16	52	60	56.0	. .	Fair.
17	32	46	39.0	. .	Fair.
18	32	44	38.0	. .	Fair.
19	30	44	37.0	. .	Fair.
20	26	42	34.0	. .	Cloudy.
21	37	44	40.5	. .	Cloudy.
22	46	54	50.0	. .	Cloudy.
23	38	56	47.0	. .	
24	56	64	60.0	. .	Cloudy.
25	52	65	58.5	. .	Fog; fair.
26	52	68	60.0	. .	Cloudy; fair.
27	60	72	66.0	. .	Cloudy.
28	60	70	65.0	. .	Cloudy.
29	52	66	59.0	. .	Fair.
30	30	56	43.0	. .	Fair.
31	64	56	60.0	0.8	Cloudy; thunder; rain at night.
Means	44.06	55.79	49.92	4.9	Greatest Rise and Fall of temperature in 24 hours.
Max.	66	72	68.0		
Min.	24	38	34.0		
Range	42	34	34.0		
Extreme range 48					

	Sunrise.	2 P. M.
Rise . . .	34	20
Fall . . .	36	34

January, 1847.

Day.	Thermometer. Sunrise.	Thermometer. 2 P. M.	Thermometer. Mean.	Rain. Ins.	Remarks on the Weather.
1	36	44	40.0	. .	Clouds; fair.
2	24	44	34.0	. .	Fair.
3	24	50	37.0	0.4	Fair; cloudy; thunder; rain at night.
4	42	46	44.0	. .	Fair.
5	28	54	41.0	. .	Fair.
6	46	30	38.0	. .	Cloudy; high north wind.
7	10	27	18.5	. .	Fair.
8	16	44	30.0	. .	Fair; cloudy.
9	32	32	32.0	0.5	Rain; sleet.
10	23	24	23.5	. .	Snow covering the ground.
11	10	34	22.0	. .	Fair; icicles glittering on trees.
12	16	42	29.0	. .	Fair.
13	44	58	51.0	. .	Cloudy.
14	60	70	65.0	. .	Fair.
15	64	72	68.0	. .	Clouds.
16	34	38	36.0	. .	Clouds.
17	22	45	33.5	. .	Fair.
18	50	30	40.0	. .	Mist; cloudy.
19	18	18	18.0	. .	Cloudy; sleet.
20	18	30	24.0	. .	Snow.
21	13	32	22.5	. .	Fair.
22	16	38	27.0	. .	Fair.
23	40	45	42.5	0.1	Rain.
24	50	60	55.0	. .	Fog; fair.
25	54	74	64.0	0.7	Cloudy; thunder; rain; hail at night.
26	32	46	39.0	. .	Fair.
27	24	36	30.0	. .	Cloudy.
28	32	34	33.0	1.0	Cloudy; rain.
29	36	44	40.0	. .	Cloudy.
30	22	50	36.0	. .	Fair.
31	30	60	45.0	. .	Fair.
Means	31.16	43.58	37.37	2.7	Greatest Rise and Fall of temperature in 24 hours.
Max.	64	74	68.0		
Min.	10	18	18.0		
Range	54	56	50.0		
Extreme range 64					

	Sunrise.	2 P. M.
Rise . . .	28	17
Fall . . .	36	34

February, 1847.

Day.	Thermometer. Sunrise.	Thermometer. 2 P. M.	Thermometer. Mean.	Rain. Ins.	Remarks on the Weather.
1	30	60	45.0	0.4	Fair; cloudy; rain at night.
2	52	34	43.0	. .	Cloudy.
3	16	34	25.0	. .	Fair.
4	23	52	37.5	. .	Fair.
5	48	60	54.0	. .	Cloudy.
6	56	64	60.0	. .	Cloudy; fair.
7	42	60	51.0	. .	Fair.
8	40	68	54.0	. .	Fair.
9	50	60	55.0	. .	Cloudy; north wind.
10	30	34	32.0	. .	Fair.
11	22	36	29.0	. .	Fair.
12	24	52	38.0	. .	Fair.
13	32	60	46.0	. .	Fair; smoky.
14	32	70	51.0	0.8	Smoky; rain.
15	55	58	56.5	0.7	Cloudy; rain at night.
16	64	69	66.5	0.8	Cloudy; rain.
17	46	44	45.0	0.8	Cloudy; rain.
18	46	59	52.5	. .	Cloudy; rain.
19	40	62	51.0	. .	Fog; fair.
20	62	56	59.0	2.2	Cloudy; rain.
21	30	44	37.0	. .	Fair.
22	28	48	38.0	. .	Fair.
23	28	54	41.0	. .	Fair.
24	48	54	51.0	. .	Fair.
25	30	56	43.0	1.0	Fair; cloudy; rain at night.
26	40	46	43.0	. .	Cloudy.
27	30	40	35.0	. .	Cloudy; fair.
28	28	52	40.0	. .	Cloudy.
Means	38.29	53.07	45.60	6.7	Greatest Rise and Fall of temperature in 24 hours.
Max.	64	70	66.5		
Min.	16	34	25.0		
Range	48	36	41.5		
Extreme range 54					

	Sunrise.	2 P. M.
Rise . . .	25	18
Fall . . .	36	26

March, 1847.

Day.	Thermometer. Sunrise.	Thermometer. 2 P. M.	Thermometer. Mean.	Rain. Ins.	Remarks on the Weather.
1	32	48	40.0	0.4	Cloudy; rain at night.
2	40	43	41.5	1.4	Cloudy; thunder; rain.
3	40	46	43.0	. .	Rain.
4	40	46	43.0	. .	Cloudy; fair.
5	30	54	42.0	. .	Fog; cloudy.
6	48	59	53.5	. .	Cloudy.
7	59	43	51.0	1.5	Cloudy; thunder; rain.
8	40	40	40.0	1.0	Cloudy; thunder; rain.
9	42	42	42.0	0.7	Rain.
10	36	32	34.0	1.8	Cloudy; thunder; rain.
11	32	34	33.0	0.8	Rain.
12	35	40	37.5	. .	Cloudy; rain; snow at night.
13	32	37	34.5	. .	Cloudy.
14	24	44	34.0	. .	Fair.
15	24	44	34.0	. .	Fair.
16	26	61	43.5	. .	Fair.
17	42	65	53.5	. .	Fair.
18	56	73	64.5	. .	Clouds; fair.
19	52	69	60.5	2.0	Fair; cloudy; thunder; rain at night.
20	52	42	47.0	. .	Cloudy.
21	34	56	45.0	. .	Fair.
22	46	62	54.0	. .	Cloudy; fair.
23	40	62	51.0	. .	Fair.
24	44	62	53.0	. .	Fair.
25	45	38	41.5	. .	Smoky; cloudy; rain.
26	26	56	41.0	. .	Fair; ground frozen.
27	28	68	48.0	. .	Fair.
28	44	72	58.0	. .	Fair.
29	50	74	62.0	. .	Fair.
30	60	66	63.0	. .	Cloudy.
31	56	75	65.5	. .	Smoky.
Means	40.48	53.32	46.90	9.6	Greatest Rise and Fall of temperature in 24 hours.
Max.	60	75	65.5		
Min.	24	32	33.0		
Range	36	43	32.5		
Extreme range 51					

	Sunrise.	2 P. M.
Rise . . .	18	18
Fall . . .	19	27

April, 1847.

Day.	Thermometer. Sunrise.	Thermometer. 2 P. M.	Thermometer. Mean.	Rain. Ins.	Remarks on the Weather.
1	58	78	68.0	. .	Smoky.
2	68	78	73.0	. .	Clouds.
3	64	85	74.5	. .	Fair.
4	64	80	72.0	. .	Cloudy; fair.
5	70	81	75.5	. .	Cloudy.
6	56	80	68.0	. .	Smoky.
7	60	80	70.0	. .	Smoky.
8	60	62	61.0	0.4	Thunder; rain.
9	56	72	64.0	2.5	Thunder; rain.
10	64	72	68.0	0.4	Thunder; rain at night.
11	52	60	56.0	. .	Fair; showers.
12	46	76	61.0	. .	Fair.
13	50	76	63.0	. .	Fair.
14	54	80	67.0	0.4	Cloudy; thunder; rain at night.
15	46	63	54.5	. .	Rain; fair.
16	40	68	54.0	. .	Fair.
17	44	74	59.0	. .	Fair.
18	46	75	60.5	. .	Fair.
19	50	78	64.0	. .	Smoky.
20	57	76	66.5	. .	Smoky.
21	62	76	69.0	. .	Smoky.
22	68	76	72.0	1.4	Cloudy; thunder; rain at night.
23	62	72	67.0	. .	Cloudy; fair.
24	50	58	54.0	. .	Cloudy.
25	44	70	57.0	. .	Fair.
26	42	74	58.0	. .	Fair.
27	46	78	62.0	. .	Fair.
28	56	80	68.0	0.3	Clouds; thunder; rain at night.
29	60	66	63.0	. .	Rain.
30	62	80	71.0	0.6	Cloudy; rain at night.
Means	55.23	74.13	64.68	6.0	Greatest Rise and Fall of temperature in 24 hours.
Max.	70	85	75.5		
Min.	40	58	54.0		
Range	30	27	21.5		
Extreme range 45					

	Sunrise.	2 P. M.
Rise . . .	10	16
Fall . . .	14	19

May, 1847.

DAY.	THERMOMETER. Sun-rise.	THERMOMETER. 3 P. M.	THERMOMETER. Mean.	RAIN. Ins.	REMARKS ON THE WEATHER.
1	60	68	64.0	. .	Clouds.
2	48	64	56.0	. .	Fair.
3	44	64	54.0	. .	Fair.
4	52	60	56.0	0.2	Cloudy; rain.
5	42	72	57.0	. .	Fair.
6	56	74	65.0	. .	Cloudy; shower.
7	64	80	72.0	0.7	Cloudy; thunder; rain at night.
8	58	74	66.0	. .	Fair.
9	48	75	61.5	. .	Fair.
10	58	80	69.0	. .	Cloudy.
11	64	82	73.0	. .	Cloudy; thunder; sprinkle.
12	50	78	64.0	. .	Fair.
13	48	80	64.0	. .	Fair.
14	50	80	67.0	. .	Fair.
15	58	72	65.0	0.1	Cloudy; rain.
16	60	82	71.0	. .	Cloudy.
17	52	74	63.0	. .	Fair.
18	52	80	66.0	. .	Fair.
19	58	78	68.0	0.3	Cloudy; rain at night.
20	62	78	70.0	0.2	Cloudy; thunder; rain at night.
21	68	74	71.0	. .	Cloudy.
22	52	75	63.5	. .	Fair.
23	50	78	64.0	1.4	Fair; cloudy; thunder; rain at night.
24	62	76	69.0	. .	Cloudy.
25	58	62	60.0	. .	Cloudy.
26	54	74	64.0	. .	Cloudy.
27	50	82	66.0	. .	Fair.
28	60	85	72.5	. .	Fair.
29	64	84	74.0	. .	Fair.
30	68	85	76.5	0.2	Cloudy; rain at night.
31	72	84	78.0	0.8	Cloudy; rain at night.
Means	56.32	75.93	66.13	3.9	
Max.	72	85	78.0		
Min.	42	60	54.0		
Range	30	25	24.0		
Extreme range 43					

Greatest Rise and Fall of temperature in 24 hours.

	Sunrise.	3 P. M.
Rise . . .	14	12
Fall . . .	16	14

June, 1847.

DAY.	THERMOMETER. Sun-rise.	THERMOMETER. 3 P. M.	THERMOMETER. Mean.	RAIN. Ins.	REMARKS ON THE WEATHER.
1	68	84	76.0	. .	Cloudy.
2	72	86	79.0	. .	Cloudy.
3	72	82	77.0	. .	Cloudy.
4	66	78	72.0	. .	Cloudy.
5	66	82	74.0	. .	Cloudy.
6	62	85	73.5	. .	Fair.
7	64	85	74.5	0.2	Cloudy; thunder; rain.
8	70	85	77.5	0.2	Cloudy; thunder; rain at night.
9	74	86	80.0	0.8	Cloudy; thunder; rain at 6 P. M.
10	66	80	73.0	. .	Cloudy; fair.
11	58	80	69.0	. .	Fair.
12	70	88	79.0	. .	Fair.
13	72	87	79.5	. .	Cloudy; fair.
14	74	86	80.0	. .	Cloudy; fair.
15	66	80	73.0	. .	Cloudy.
16	70	86	78.0	. .	Fair.
17	70	84	77.0	. .	Fair.
18	72	84	78.0	. .	Clouds.
19	74	76	75.0	0.2	Cloudy; rain.
20	66	80	73.0	. .	Fair.
21	56	80	68.0	. .	Fair.
22	56	82	69.0	. .	Fair.
23	58	82	70.0	. .	Fair.
24	60	84	72.0	. .	Fair.
25	60	80	70.0	0.4	Fair; cloudy; rain at 2 P. M.; thunder.
26	66	88	77.0	0.3	Cloudy; rain at 4 P. M.; thunder.
27	68	82	75.0	. .	Cloudy.
28	70	82	76.0	1.9	Cloudy; thunder; rain at night.
29	66	81	73.5	. .	Rain.
30	68	76	72.0	. .	
Means	66.67	82.70	74.68	4.0	
Max.	74	88	80.0		
Min.	56	76	68.0		
Range	18	12	12.0		
Extreme range 32					

Greatest Rise and Fall of temperature in 24 hours.

	Sunrise.	3 P. M.
Rise . . .	12	8
Fall . . .	10	8

July, 1847.

DAY.	THERMOMETER. Sun-rise.	THERMOMETER. 3 P. M.	THERMOMETER. Mean.	RAIN. Ins.	REMARKS ON THE WEATHER.
1	66	72	69.0	. .	Fair.
2	60	82	71.0	. .	Fair.
3	64	86	75.0	. .	Fair.
4	64	86	75.0	. .	Fair.
5	68	80	74.0	0.2	Clouds; showers.
6	74	84	79.0	0.6	Hazy; cloudy; rain at 7 P. M.
7	72	86	79.0	. .	Fair.
8	74	84	79.0	. .	Cloudy.
9	70	86	78.0	. .	Fog; clouds.
10	70	80	75.0	1.0	Cloudy; rain.
11	72	85	78.5	. .	Cloudy; fair.
12	70	88	79.0	. .	Fair.
13	70	86	78.0	. .	Fair.
14	70	86	78.0	. .	Fair.
15	70	90	80.0	. .	Fair.
16	70	92	81.0	. .	Fair.
17	70	91	80.5	. .	Fair.
18	70	76	73.0	0.3	Fair; cloudy; rain at 3 P. M.
19	66	88	77.0	. .	Fog; clouds.
20	68	89	78.5	0.2	Clouds; shower.
21	70	84	77.0	. .	Clouds.
22	72	86	79.0	0.7	Cloudy; rain.
23	68	86	77.0	0.8	Cloudy.
24	70	89	79.5	. .	Fair.
25	70	91	80.5	. .	Fair.
26	70	90	80.0	. .	Cloudy.
27	72	88	80.0	1.4	Cloudy; rain.
28	74	82	78.0	. .	
29	72	84	78.0	0.3	Cloudy; rain.
30	68	80	74.0	. .	Fair.
31	. .	. .	. .	. .	
Means	69.47	85.23	77.35	5.5	
Max.	74	92	81.0		
Min.	60	72	69.0		
Range	14	20	12.0		
Extreme range 32					

Greatest Rise and Fall of temperature in 24 hours.

	Sunrise.	3 P. M.
Rise . . .	6	12
Fall . . .	6	15

August, 1847.

DAY.	THERMOMETER. Sun-rise.	THERMOMETER. 3 P. M.	THERMOMETER. Mean.	RAIN. Ins.	REMARKS ON THE WEATHER.
1	56	82	69.0	. .	Fair.
2	56	84	70.0	. .	Fair.
3	65	90	77.5	. .	Fair.
4	70	89	79.5	. .	Fair; cloudy.
5	70	92	81.0	. .	Cloudy.
6	68	82	75.0	. .	Fair.
7	60	82	71.0	. .	Fair.
8	60	82	71.0	. .	Fair.
9	60	84	72.0	. .	Fair.
10	60	85	72.5	. .	Fair.
11	60	88	74.0	. .	Fair.
12	66	89	77.5	. .	Fair.
13	66	92	79.0	. .	Fair.
14	68	92	80.0	. .	Fair.
15	68	86	77.0	. .	Fair.
16	70	88	79.0	. .	Fog; clouds.
17	66	92	79.0	. .	Fair.
18	72	90	81.0	. .	Fair.
19	70	92	81.0	. .	Fog; fair.
20	70	80	75.0	. .	Cloudy; rain.
21	64	76	70.0	0.8	Rain.
22	66	82	74.0	1.0	Rain.
23	70	78	74.0	1.8	Rain.
24	60	78	69.0	1.1	Rain.
25	70	82	76.0	. .	Fog; clouds.
26	64	84	74.0	. .	Fair.
27	70	78	74.0	1.5	Cloudy; rain.
28	68	80	74.0	1.2	Cloudy; rain.
29	58	78	68.0	. .	Fair.
30	60	82	71.0	. .	Fair.
31	58	82	70.0	. .	Fair.
Means	64.81	84.55	74.68	7·4	
Max.	72	92	81.0		
Min.	56	76	68.0		
Range	16	16	13.0		
Extreme range 36					

Greatest Rise and Fall of temperature in 24 hours.

	Sunrise.	3 P. M.
Rise . . .	10	6
Fall . . .	12	12

September, 1847.

DAY.	THERMOMETER. Sunrise.	3 P. M.	Mean.	RAIN. Ins.	REMARKS ON THE WEATHER.
1	66	86	76.0	..	Fair.
2	66	85	75.5	..	Fair.
3	68	86	77.0	..	Fair.
4	66	86	76.0	..	Fair.
5	66	88	77.0	..	Fair.
6	70	88	79.0	..	Fog; fair; sprinkle at night.
7	74	86	80.0	1.5	Cloudy; rain at night.
8	66	70	68.0	..	Rain; fair.
9	53	73	63.0	..	Fair.
10	46	72	59.0	..	Fair.
11	46	75	60.5	..	Fair.
12	56	75	65.5	..	Fair.
13	56	75	65.5	..	Fair.
14	51	75	63.0	..	Fair.
15	54	80	67.0	..	Fair.
16	54	80	67.0	..	Fair.
17	60	82	71.0	..	Fair.
18	60	82	71.0	..	Fair.
19	54	75	64.5	..	Fair.
20	48	75	61.5	..	Fair.
21	48	75	61.5	..	Fair.
22	52	74	63.0	..	
23	60	76	68.0	..	Cloudy; fair.
24	56	82	69.0	..	Fair.
25	60	82	71.0	..	Fair.
26	66	88	77.0	..	Fair.
27	68	88	78.0	..	Fair.
28	70	76	73.0	..	Fair.
29	50	76	63.0	..	Fair.
30	60	78	69.0	..	Cloudy.
Means	59.00	79.63	69.32	1.5	Greatest Rise and Fall of temperature in 24 hours.
Max.	74	88	80.0		
Min.	46	70	59.0		
Range	28	18	21.0		
Extreme range 42					

	Sunrise.	3 P. M.
Rise . . .	10	6
Fall . . .	20	16

October, 1847.

DAY.	THERMOMETER. Sunrise.	3 P. M.	Mean.	RAIN. Ins.	REMARKS ON THE WEATHER.
1	68	78	73.0	..	Fog; clouds; shower.
2	60	86	73.0	..	Fog; clouds; shower.
3	56	82	69.0	..	Fog; fair.
4	58	83	70.5	..	Clouds.
5	58	82	70.0	..	Fair.
6	..	..	..	..	
7	56	78	67.0	..	Fair.
8	50	76	63.0	..	Clouds; fair.
9	52	80	66.0	..	Fair.
10	52	80	66.0	..	Fair.
11	50	80	65.0	..	Fair.
12	58	84	71.0	..	Fair.
13	38	70	54.0	..	Fair.
14	38	66	52.0	..	Fair.
15	36	66	51.0	..	Fair.
16	44	76	60.0	..	Fair.
17	46	78	62.0	..	Fair.
18	52	80	66.0	..	Fair.
19	56	62	59.0	..	Cloudy; sprinkle.
20	52	70	61.0	..	Cloudy; fair.
21	60	80	70.0	..	Cloudy; showers at night.
22	70	50	60.0	0.5	Cloudy; rain.
23	48	48	48.0	0.4	Cloudy; rain.
24	45	60	52.5	..	Cloudy; fair.
25	32	66	49.0	..	Fair; killing frost.
26	34	56	45.0	..	Fair.
27	30	54	42.0	..	Fair.
28	32	56	44.0	..	Fair.
29	32	64	48.0	..	
30	36	70	53.0	..	
31	56	76	66.0	0.2	Clouds; shower at night.
Means	48.50	71.23	59.87	1.1	Greatest Rise and Fall of temperature in 24 hours.
Max.	70	86	73.0		
Min.	30	48	42.0		
Range	40	38	31.0		
Extreme range 56					

	Sunrise.	3 P. M.
Rise . . .	20	12
Fall . . .	22	30

November, 1847.

DAY.	THERMOMETER. Sunrise.	2 P. M.	Mean.	RAIN. Ins.	REMARKS ON THE WEATHER.
1	64	76	70.0	..	Clouds; fair.
2	60	76	68.0	..	Clouds.
3	64	74	69.0	..	Clouds.
4	58	78	68.0	..	Fog; cloudy.
5	56	66	61.0	..	Fog; cloudy.
6	68	70	69.0	0.2	Cloudy; shower at 9 A. M.; fair at eve.
7	58	78	68.0	..	Fair.
8	70	70	70.0	0.8	Cloudy; thunder; rain and hail.
9	34	56	45.0	0.2	Fair; cloudy; rain at night.
10	42	52	47.0	0.2	Cloudy; rain at night.
11	40	44	42.0	..	Cloudy.
12	42	49	45.5	0.3	Cloudy; rain.
13	66	60	63.0	..	Cloudy; fair.
14	32	58	45.0	..	Fair.
15	32	65	48.5	..	Fair.
16	32	70	51.0	..	Fair.
17	54	72	63.0	..	Cloudy.
18	48	50	49.0	1.3	Rain.
19	26	50	38.0	..	Fair.
20	25	52	38.5	0.5	Fair; cloudy; rain at night.
21	46	58	52.0	0.2	Cloudy; rain at night.
22	52	60	56.0	1.5	Rain.
23	42	56	49.0	..	Fair.
24	38	45	41.5	..	Cloudy.
25	38	38	38.0	..	Fair.
26	16	34	25.0	..	Fair.
27	20	46	33.0	..	Fair.
28	24	54	39.0	..	Fair.
29	30	47	38.5	..	Fair.
30	28	56	42.0	0.4	Fair; cloudy; rain at night.
Means	43.50	58.67	51.08	5.6	Greatest Rise and Fall of temperature in 24 hours.
Max.	70	78	70.0		
Min.	16	34	25.0		
Range	54	44	45.0		
Extreme range 62					

	Sunrise.	2 P. M.
Rise . . .	24	12
Fall . . .	36	22

December, 1847.

DAY.	THERMOMETER. Sunrise.	2 P. M.	Mean.	RAIN. Ins.	REMARKS ON THE WEATHER.
1	42	47	44.5	..	Rain.
2	36	40	38.0	..	Cloudy.
3	24	44	34.0	..	Fair.
4	24	54	39.0	..	Fair.
5	26	58	42.0	..	Fair.
6	30	60	45.0	..	Fair.
7	52	62	57.0	0.5	Cloudy; showers.
8	42	52	47.0	0.4	Fair; cloudy; thunder; rain at night.
9	60	62	61.0	..	Cloudy; fair.
10	30	56	43.0	..	Fair.
11	26	60	43.0	..	Fair.
12	40	42	41.0	0.5	Rain.
13	32	40	36.0	..	Cloudy; fair.
14	26	40	33.0	..	Fair.
15	24	40	32.0	..	Fair.
16	25	40	32.5	..	Fair.
17	20	40	30.0	..	Fair.
18	18	50	34.0	..	Fair.
19	28	56	42.0	..	Fair.
20	36	40	38.0	..	Fair.
21	12	36	24.0	..	Fair.
22	24	50	37.0	..	Fair.
23	28	60	44.0	..	Fair.
24	32	54	43.0	..	Fair.
25	33	46	39.5	..	Clouds.
26	24	42	33.0	..	Fair.
27	30	50	40.0	0.2	Cloudy; showers.
28	50	65	57.5	0.2	Cloudy; smoky; showers.
29	56	60	58.0	..	Cloudy; showers.
30	60	72	66.0	..	Cloudy; fair.
31	..	..	..	2.5	Cloudy; rain.
Means	33.00	50.60	41.80	4.3	Greatest Rise and Fall of temperature in 24 hours.
Max.	60	72	66.0		
Min.	12	36	24.0		
Range	48	36	42.0		
Extreme range 60					

	Sunrise.	2 P. M.
Rise . . .	22	15
Fall . . .	30	18

January, 1848.

DAY.	THERMOMETER. Sunrise.	THERMOMETER. 2 P. M.	THERMOMETER. Mean.	RAIN. Ins.	REMARKS ON THE WEATHER.
1	36	48	42.0	. .	Fair.
2	24	50	37.0	. .	Fair.
3	38	62	50.0	. .	Clouds; fair.
4	33	60	46.5	. .	Fog; fair.
5	52	68	60.0	. .	Fog; fair.
6	34	45	39.5	. .	Fair.
7	30	60	45.0	. .	Fair.
8	52	72	62.0	. .	Fair.
9	18	29	23.5	. .	Fair.
10	12	40	26.0	. .	Fair.
11	32	52	42.0	. .	Fair.
12	50	58	54.0	. .	Fair.
13	55	73	64.0	. .	Cloudy.
14	62	74	68.0	. .	Cloudy; fair.
15	64	66	65.0	1.8	Cloudy; rain at night.
16	50	62	56.0	0.2	Cloudy; rain.
17	46	56	51.0	. .	Fair.
18	32	60	46.0	. .	Fair.
19	32	58	45.0	. .	Fair.
20	30	60	45.0	. .	Fair.
21	32	64	48.0	. .	Fair.
22	32	64	48.0	. .	Fair.
23	34	64	49.0	0.2	Cloudy; rain at night.
24	46	64	55.0	. .	Cloudy; rain.
25	54	64	59.0	0.4	Rain.
26	53	64	58.5	. .	Fair.
27	42	60	51.0	. .	Fair.
28	34	60	47.0	. .	Cloudy.
29	48	52	50.0	0.5	Cloudy; rain.
30	50	68	59.0	. .	Fair.
31	30	50	40.0	. .	Fair.
Means	39.90	58.94	49.42	3.1	Greatest Rise and Fall of temperature in 24 hours.
Max.	64	74	68.0		
Min.	12	29	23.5		
Range	52	45	44.5		
Extreme range 62					

	Sunrise.	2 P. M.
Rise . . .	22	16
Fall . . .	34	43

February, 1848.

DAY.	THERMOMETER. Sunrise.	THERMOMETER. 2 P. M.	THERMOMETER. Mean.	RAIN. Ins.	REMARKS ON THE WEATHER.
1	26	50	38.0	. .	Fair; cloudy.
2	32	58	45.0	. .	Cloudy; fair.
3	44	58	51.0	. .	Fog; mist.
4	32	58	45.0	. .	Fair.
5	26	58	42.0	. .	Fair.
6	28	48	38.0	. .	Fair.
7	24	58	41.0	. .	Fair.
8	34	60	47.0	. .	Fair.
9	46	66	56.0	0.2	Smoky; cloudy; rain.
10	56	70	63.0	. .	Clouds; fair.
11	48	70	59.0	. .	Fog; fair.
12	40	66	53.0	. .	Smoky.
13	36	63	49.5	. .	Cloudy.
14	59	70	64.5	. .	Smoky.
15	62	66	64.0	. .	Cloudy.
16	63	68	65.5	0.7	Cloudy; rain.
17	56	62	59.0	0.5	Cloudy.
18	64	72	68.0	. .	Rain; fair.
19	66	75	70.5	0.5	Cloudy; thunder; rain at night.
20	60	70	65.0	. .	Cloudy; fair.
21	50	54	52.0	0.5	Cloudy, rain.
22	46	50	48.0	. .	Cloudy; rain.
23	42	42	42.0	. .	Cloudy; snow and sleet at night.
24	30	34	32.0	0.3	Clouds; roofs and fences covered
25	28	50	39.0	. .	Fair. [with snow.
26	34	54	44.0	. .	Clouds; fair.
27	32	56	44.0	. .	Fair.
28	34	70	52.0	. .	Fair.
29	40	62	51.0	. .	Smoky.
Means	42.69	59.93	51.31	2.7	Greatest Rise and Fall of temperature in 24 hours.
Max.	66	75	70.5		
Min.	24	34	32.0		
Range	42	41	38.5		
Extreme range 51					

	Sunrise.	2 P. M.
Rise . . .	23	14
Fall . . .	12	18

March, 1848.

DAY.	THERMOMETER. Sunrise.	THERMOMETER. 2 P. M.	THERMOMETER. Mean.	RAIN. Ins.	REMARKS ON THE WEATHER.
1	38	37	37.5	1.2	Rain; cold N. W. wind.
2	36	47	41.5	. .	Cloudy.
3	28	36	32.0	. .	Fair.
4	22	44	33.0	. .	Fair.
5	32	46	39.0	. .	Fair.
6	24	42	33.0	. .	Fair.
7	32	68	50.0	. .	Fair.
8	56	46	51.0	0.4	Rain.
9	33	46	39.5	. .	Fair.
10	32	60	46.0	. .	Fair.
11	36	72	54.0	. .	Fair.
12	56	74	65.0	. .	Cloudy; fair.
13	36	58	47.0	. .	Fair; smoky.
14	30	68	49.0	. .	Smoky.
15	48	70	59.0	. .	Smoky.
16	42	76	59.0	. .	Smoky.
17	56	76	66.0	. .	Smoky.
18	64	66	65.0	0.2	Cloudy; shower at 3 P. M.
19	64	76	70.0	0.8	Cloudy; hail and rain at night;
20	63	77	70.0	0.2	Fair; shower at night. [thunder.
21	60	79	69.5	. .	Fair.
22	50	70	60.0	. .	Fair.
23	40	66	53.0	. .	Fair.
24	44	74	59.0	. .	Fair.
25	64	83	73.5	. .	Cloudy.
26	66	48	57.0	1.7	Rain.
27	44	56	50.0	. .	Rain.
28	36	62	49.0	. .	Fair.
29	40	70	55.0	. .	Fair.
30	60	76	68.0	. .	Cloudy.
31	66	56	61.0	0.2	Cloudy; rain.
Means	45.10	62.10	53.60	4.7	Greatest Rise and Fall of temperature in 24 hours.
Max.	66	83	73.5		
Min.	22	36	32.0		
Range	44	47	41.5		
Extreme range 61					

	Sunrise.	2 P. M.
Rise . . .	24	26
Fall . . .	23	35

April, 1848.

DAY.	THERMOMETER. Sunrise.	THERMOMETER. 2 P. M.	THERMOMETER. Mean.	RAIN. Ins.	REMARKS ON THE WEATHER.
1	32	62	47.0	. .	Fair.
2	40	60	50.0	. .	Fair.
3	58	74	66.0	1.2	Cloudy; thunder; rain at night.
4	58	57	57.5	0.7	Rain.
5	46	54	50.0	0.3	Rain.
6	48	52	50.0	0.2	Rain.
7	52	56	54.0	. .	Cloudy.
8	44	73	58.5	. .	Fog; fair; clouds.
9	52	74	63.0	. .	Fair.
10	56	80	68.0	. .	Fair.
11	62	78	70.0	. .	Cloudy.
12	62	80	71.0	0.2	Cloudy; rain at night.
13	60	70	65.0	0.2	Cloudy; showers.
14	44	70	57.0	. .	Fair.
15	42	66	54.0	. .	Fair.
16	40	68	54.0	. .	Fair.
17	46	70	58.0	. .	Cloudy.
18	54	70	62.0	. .	Fair; cloudy.
19	40	62	51.0	. .	Fair; cloudy.
20	44	68	56.0	. .	Cloudy.
21	42	70	56.0	. .	Fair; cloudy.
22	54	80	67.0	. .	Cloudy; fair.
23	50	82	66.0	. .	Fair.
24	52	82	67.0	1.0	Fair; thunder; rain at night.
25	46	48	47.0	1.5	Rain.
26	46	52	49.0	. .	Rain.
27	44	70	57.0	. .	Fair.
28	50	80	65.0	. .	Fair.
29	60	54	57.0	0.5	Rain.
30	52	70	61.0	. .	Cloudy.
Means	49.20	67.73	58.47	5.8	Greatest Rise and Fall of temperature in 24 hours.
Max.	62	82	71.0		
Min.	32	48	47.0		
Range	30	34	24.0		
Extreme range 50					

	Sunrise.	2 P. M.
Rise . . .	18	18
Fall . . .	34	34

May, 1848.

DAY.	THERMOMETER. Sunrise.	THERMOMETER. 3 P. M.	THERMOMETER. Mean.	RAIN. Ins.	REMARKS ON THE WEATHER.
1	60	76	68.0	..	Cloudy; fair.
2	66	84	75.0	..	Cloudy; fair.
3	72	82	77.0	..	Cloudy; thermometer broken.
4	..	..	..	0.3	Cloudy; showers; fair at eve.
5	..	..	..	..	Cloudy; warm; fair.
6	..	..	..	..	Cloudy; warm; flying clouds.
7	..	..	..	0.3	Fair; breezes; clouds; hail; rain.
8	..	..	..	0.2	Fair; breezes; clouds; showers.
9	..	..	..	0.7	Clouds; showery; rain at night.
10	..	..	..	..	Fair; cool and breezy.
11	..	..	..	..	Fair.
12	..	..	..	..	Fair.
13		..	..	..	Clouds.
14		..	..	..	Clouds.
15		..	..	..	Fair; warm; shower at night.
16		..	..	0.2	Clouds; breezes; shower at night.
17	Thermometer broken	..	..	..	Clouds; showery.
18		..	..	..	Fair.
19		..	..	0.8	Clouds; breezes; thunder; hail;
20		..	..	..	Cloudy. [rain at night.
21		..	..	0.4	Shower in the morning; fair.
22		..	..	0.3	Cloudy; shower at night.
23	..	..	..	1.5	Cl'dy; thunder; heavy rain A. M.
24	..	..	..	0.5	Cloudy; rain at night.
25	..	..	..	..	Fog; mist; fair; clouds; warm.
26	..	..	..	..	Clouds; warm; fair.
27	..	..	..	0.2	Fair; wind and rain at night.
28	..	..	..	..	Clouds; breezes.
29	..	..	..	..	Fair; cool; pleasant.
30	..	..	..	..	Fair.
31	..	..	..	..	Fair.
Means	..	..	..	5.4	Greatest Rise and Fall of temperature in 24 hours.
Max.	..	..	..		
Min.	..	..	..		
Range	..	..	..		
Extreme range ..					

	Sunrise.	3 P. M.
Rise . . .	..	..
Fall . . .	..	..

July, 1848.

DAY.	THERMOMETER. Sunrise.	THERMOMETER. 3 P. M.	THERMOMETER. Mean.	RAIN. Ins.	REMARKS ON THE WEATHER.
1	74	86	80.0	0.8	Cloudy; thunder; rain at 3 P. M.
2	73	78	75.5	0.3	Rain.
3	70	83	76.5	..	Fog; fair.
4	72	84	78.0	0.3	Cloudy; thunder; rain at 12 M.
5	74	86	80.0	..	Fair.
6	74	90	82.0	0.8	Fair; thunder; rain at night.
7	75	88	81.5	..	Cloudy; fair.
8	66	84	75.0	0.2	Fair; rain at night.
9	72	84	78.0	..	Cloudy; fair.
10	66	86	76.0	..	Fair.
11	70	88	79.0	..	Fair.
12	70	88	79.0	..	Fair.
13	70	90	80.0	..	Fair.
14	72	91	81.5	..	Fair.
15	78	89	83.5	..	Cloudy; shower at 4 P. M.
16	74	83	78.5	..	Fair.
17	66	84	75.0	..	Fair.
18	66	82	74.0	..	Fair.
19	66	86	76.0	..	Fair.
20	76	77	76.5	1.7	Cloudy; thunder; rain.
21	74	82	78.0	0.3	Fog; cloudy; rain.
22	68	84	76.0	..	Fair.
23	70	84	77.0	..	Fair.
24	74	82	78.0	0.2	Cloudy; rain at 2 P. M.
25	70	84	77.0	..	Fog; fair; rain at 2 P. M.
26	74	86	80.0	..	Fair; showers.
27	74	84	79.0	..	Fog; fair; clouds.
28	76	86	81.0	0.2	Cloudy; rain.
29	76	76	76.0	0.2	Cloudy; rain.
30	74	80	77.0	1.4	Cloudy; thunder; rain.
31	74	78	76.0	0.3	Cloudy.
Means	71.87	84.29	78.08	6.7	Greatest Rise and Fall of temperature in 24 hours.
Max.	78	91	83.5		
Min.	66	76	74.0		
Range	12	15	9.5		
Extreme range 25					

	Sunrise.	3 P. M.
Rise . . .	10	6
Fall . . .	9	10

June, 1848.

DAY.	THERMOMETER. Sunrise.	THERMOMETER. 3 P. M.	THERMOMETER. Mean.	RAIN. Ins.	REMARKS ON THE WEATHER.
1	..	..	..	..	Fair; pleasant.
2	..	..	..	..	Fair.
3	..	..	..	..	Fair.
4	..	..	..	0.2	Rain; fair at 9 A. M.
5	..	..	..	0.4	Rain at 10.30 A. M.
6	..	..	..	..	Cloudy; sprinkle.
7		..	..	0.4	Cloudy; rain.
8		..	..	2.5	Cold; heavy rain.
9		..	..	0.3	Fog; cloudy; rain.
10		..	..	0.3	Fair; pleasant; sh'r after night.
11	Thermometer broken	..	..	..	Clouds; fair; shower at 1 P. M.
12		..	..	0.2	Fair; clouds; shower at 1 P. M.
13		..	..	..	Fair and pleasant.
14		..	..	..	Fair and pleasant.
15		..	..	..	Light showers.
16		..	..	..	Cloudy; mist; showers.
17	..	..	..	0.5	Fog; clouds; rain.
18	..	..	..	..	Mist; fair.
19	..	.	..	..	Fair; clouds; breezes; shower at 5
20	..	..	..	..	Fair. [P. M.
21	..	..	..	..	Fair.
22	..	89	..	..	Fair.
23	74	91	82.5	..	Fair; clouds.
24	72	78	75.0	2.1	Heavy rain in morning; thunder.
25	75	85	80.0	..	Cloudy; sprinkle at 2 P. M.; fair.
26	73	86	79.5	..	Fair.
27	73	86	79.5	..	Fair.
28	74	82	78.0	2.0	Heavy rain in morning; thunder.
29	74	84	79.0	..	Fog; fair.
30	72	80	76.0	..	Fog; fair.
Means	..	..	..	8.9	Greatest Rise and Fall of temperature in 24 hours.
Max.	..	..	..		
Min.	..	..	..		
Range	..	..	..		
Extreme range ..					

	Sunrise.	3 P. M.
Rise . . .	..	..
Fall . . .	..	..

August, 1848.

DAY.	THERMOMETER. Sunrise.	THERMOMETER. 3 P. M.	THERMOMETER. Mean.	RAIN. Ins.	REMARKS ON THE WEATHER.
1	68	80	74.0	..	Fog; clouds.
2	72	86	79.0	0.1	Cloudy; shower.
3	78	86	82.0	..	Cloudy; fair.
4	76	86	81.0	0.4	Cloudy; rain; thunder.
5	70	80	75.0	..	Fog; fair.
6	66	82	74.0	..	Fair.
7	68	82	75.0	..	Fair.
8	64	82	73.0	..	Fair.
9	64	84	74.0	..	Fair.
10	66	84	75.0	..	Fair.
11	68	85	76.5	..	Fair.
12	68	87	77.5	..	Fair.
13	70	89	79.5	..	Fair.
14	70	90	80.0	..	Fair.
15	70	84	77.0	..	Fair; clouds.
16	70	86	78.0	..	Fair; clouds.
17	74	82	78.0	1.2	Cloudy; thunder; rain.
18	74	80	77.0	..	Cloudy; showers.
19	70	82	76.0	..	Fair; clouds.
20	70	88	79.0	..	Fair; clouds.
21	72	80	76.0	..	Clouds.
22	70	80	75.0	..	Fair.
23	72	76	74.0	..	Fair.
24	74	85	79.5	..	Fair.
25	75	86	80.5	..	Fair.
26	75	86	80.5	..	Fair.
27	70	88	79.0	..	Fair.
28	70	88	79.0	..	Fair.
29	72	90	81.0	..	Fair.
30	74	90	82.0	..	Fair.
31	72	90	81.0	0.5	Cloudy; rain at 4 P. M.
Means	70.71	84.65	77.68	2.2	Greatest Rise and Fall of temperature in 24 hours.
Max.	78	90	82.0		
Min.	64	76	73.0		
Range	14	14	9.0		
Extreme range 26					

	Sunrise.	3 P. M.
Rise . . .	6	9
Fall . . .	6	8

September, 1848.

DAY.	THERMOMETER. Sunrise.	3 P. M.	Mean.	RAIN. Ins.	REMARKS ON THE WEATHER.
1	72	84	78.0	. .	Clouds.
2	72	88	80.0	. .	Clouds; thunder.
3	74	88	81.0	. .	Clouds.
4	74	88	81.0	0.5	Clouds; rain at 4 P. M.
5	74	76	75.0	. .	Fair.
6	60	76	68.0	. .	Fair.
7	60	76	68.0	. .	Fair.
8	58	76	67.0	. .	Fair.
9	60	78	69.0	. .	Fair; clouds.
10	64	78	71.0	. .	Fair.
11	70	78	74.0	0.5	Cloudy; rain at night.
12	72	80	76.0	. .	Cloudy; rain.
13	74	84	79.0	. .	Cloudy.
14	76	88	82.0	. .	Cloudy.
15	74	78	76.0	. .	Fair.
16	58	72	65.0	. .	Fair.
17	58	76	67.0	. .	Fair.
18	56	78	67.0	. .	Fair.
19	60	76	68.0	. .	Fair.
20	62	70	66.0	. .	Fair.
21	52	72	62.0	. .	Fair.
22	52	71	61.5	. .	Fair.
23	54	68	61.0	. .	Fair.
24	52	72	62.0	. .	Fair.
25	52	74	63.0	. .	Fair; clouds.
26	52	74	63.0	. .	Fair.
27	58	75	66.5	. .	Fair; clouds.
28	58	75	66.5	. .	Fair; clouds.
29	58	76	67.0	. .	Fair; clouds.
30	58	68	63.0	. .	
Means	62.47	77.10	69.78	1.0	Greatest Rise and Fall of temperature in 24 hours.
Max.	76	88	82.0		
Min.	52	68	61.0		
Range	24	20	21.0		
Extreme range 36					

	Sunrise.	3 P. M.
Rise . . .	6	4
Fall . . .	16	12

October, 1848.

DAY.	THERMOMETER. Sunrise.	3 P. M.	Mean.	RAIN. Ins.	REMARKS ON THE WEATHER.
1	42	62	52.0	. .	Fair.
2	37	68	52.5	. .	Fair.
3	48	80	64.0	. .	Smoky.
4	58	82	70.0	. .	Smoky.
5	56	81	68.5	. .	Fair.
6	56	81	68.5	. .	Fog; fair.
7	56	80	68.0	. .	Fair.
8	52	80	66.0	. .	Fair.
9	48	78	63.0	. .	Fair.
10	50	80	65.0	. .	Fair.
11	52	78	65.0	. .	Fair.
12	52	80	66.0	. .	Fair.
13	54	78	66.0	. .	Clouds.
14	60	80	70.0	1.0	Cloudy; thunder; rain at night.
15	64	76	70.0	0.3	Cloudy; thunder; rain at night.
16	65	76	70.5	. .	Fair.
17	48	66	57.0	. .	Fair.
18	50	56	53.0	0.3	Cloudy; rain.
19	44	62	53.0	. .	Fair.
20	34	64	49.0	. .	Fair.
21	40	70	55.0	. .	Fair.
22	60	65	62.5	. .	Cloudy; rain.
23	68	74	71.0	1.0	Cloudy; rain; fair at eve.
24	64	68	66.0	. .	Cloudy.
25	64	76	70.0	. .	Cloudy; fair.
26	56	78	67.0	. .	Fog; fair.
27	64	80	72.0	. .	Fair.
28	56	74	65.0	. .	Fair.
29	42	66	54.0	0.2	Fair; cloudy; rain at night.
30	54	60	57.0	. .	Cloudy; fair.
31	34	64	49.0	. .	Fair.
Means	52.52	73.00	62.76	2.8	Greatest Rise and Fall of temperature in 24 hours.
Max.	68	82	72.0		
Min.	34	56	49.0		
Range	34	26	23.0		
Extreme range 48					

	Sunrise.	3 P. M.
Rise . . .	20	12
Fall . . .	20	10

November, 1848.

DAY.	THERMOMETER. Sunrise.	2 P. M.	Mean.	RAIN. Ins.	REMARKS ON THE WEATHER.
1	32	58	45.0	. .	Fair; frost.
2	32	60	46.0	. .	Fair; killing frost; sh'rs at night.
3	60	65	62.5	0.7	Cloudy; rain; snow at night.
4	32	48	40.0	. .	Cloudy; fair.
5	24	58	41.0	. .	Fair.
6	32	62	47.0	. .	Fair.
7	28	56	42.0	. .	Fair.
8	38	60	49.0	. .	Clouds.
9	52	54	53.0	. .	Cloudy.
10	38	58	48.0	2.1	Cloudy; thunder; rain at night.
11	52	56	54.0	. .	Rain.
12	54	56	55.0	. .	Cloudy.
13	50	50	50.0	0.4	Cloudy; rain at night.
14	48	60	54.0	. .	Cloudy.
15	46	53	49.5	1.7	Fair; cloudy; rain at night.
16	46	48	47.0	1.1	Rain.
17	42	50	46.0	. .	Cloudy; fair.
18	24	50	37.0	. .	Fair.
19	20	49	34.5	. .	Fair.
20	38	42	40.0	. .	Sleet in the morning; fair.
21	32	53	42.5	. .	Fair; cloudy.
22	34	63	48.5	. .	Fair.
23	32	53	42.5	. .	Fair.
24	34	63	48.5	. .	Fair.
25	62	64	63.0	. .	Cloudy; fair.
26	42	58	50.0	. .	Fair.
27	38	56	47.0	. .	Fair.
28	20	52	36.0	. .	Fair; clouds.
29	34	58	46.0	0.4	Fair; rain; fair.
30	40	44	42.0	0.5	Cloudy; rain; sleet.
Means	38.53	55.23	46.88	6.9	Greatest Rise and Fall of temperature in 24 hours.
Max.	62	65	63.0		
Min.	20	42	34.5		
Range	42	23	28.5		
Extreme range 45					

	Sunrise.	2 P. M.
Rise . . .	28	10
Fall . . .	28	17

December, 1848.

DAY.	THERMOMETER. Sunrise.	2 P. M.	Mean.	RAIN. Ins.	REMARKS ON THE WEATHER.
1	37	44	40.5	0.1	Rain.
2	32	52	42.0	. .	Fair.
3	52	70	61.0	. .	Clouds.
4	62	73	67.5	. .	Clouds.
5	68	60	64.0	3.0	Cloudy; thunder; rain.
6	40	40	40.0	2.0	Rain.
7	38	42	40.0	0.5	Rain.
8	30	39	34.5	0.9	Cloudy; fair; thunder; rain at night.
9	38	44	41.0	0.8	Rain.
10	32	40	36.0	. .	Cloudy; fair.
11	24	32	28.0	. .	Fair.
12	24	48	36.0	. .	Fair.
13	26	62	44.0	. .	Fair; showers at night.
14	56	46	51.0	0.2	Showers; fair.
15	20	46	33.0	. .	Fair.
16	28	50	39.0	. .	Fair.
17	28	68	48.0	. .	Fair.
18	62	72	67.0	. .	Cloudy.
19	68	74	71.0	0.5	Cloudy; rain.
20	56	50	53.0	. .	Cloudy; rain.
21	50	50	50.0	. .	Rain.
22	26	24	25.0	. .	Sleet; ground covered with ice.
23	26	31	28.5	. .	Cloudy; mist.
24	34	38	36.0	0.5	Mist; freezing; trees coated with ice.
25	32	46	39.0	. .	Fair; icicles sparkling in the sunshine.
26	28	38	33.0	0.5	Cloudy; rain; sleet.
27	30	44	37.0	. .	Fair; clouds.
28	36	40	38.0	0.8	Cloudy; rain; sleet.
29	38	42	40.0	. .	Cloudy.
30	24	50	37.0	. .	Fair.
31	24	53	38.5	. .	Fair; cloudy.
Means	37.71	48.65	43.18	9.8	Greatest Rise and Fall of temperature in 24 hours.
Max.	68	74	71.0		
Min.	20	24	25.0		
Range	48	50	46.0		
Extreme range 54					

	Sunrise.	2 P. M.
Rise . . .	34	18
Fall . . .	36	24

January, 1849.

DAY.	THERMOMETER. Sunrise.	THERMOMETER. 2 P. M.	THERMOMETER. Mean.	RAIN. Ins.	REMARKS ON THE WEATHER.
1	30	60	45.0	..	Fair.
2	36	56	43.0	..	Fair; cloudy.
3	46	46	46.0	0.1	Rain.
4	36	42	39.0	..	Cloudy; snow-flakes.
5	35	40	37.5	..	Cloudy.
6	34	40	37.0	0.8	Cloudy; rain at night.
7	38	46	42.0	..	Cloudy.
8	36	40	38.0	..	Cloudy.
9	23	36	29.5	..	Cloudy; fair at eve.
10	18	40	29.0	..	Fair.
11	28	50	39.0	0.5	Cloudy; rain at night.
12	48	52	50.0	3.0	Cloudy; thunder; rain at night.
13	62	40	51.0	1.5	Rain.
14	30	38	34.0	0.3	Sleet.
15	36	50	43.0	..	Cloudy.
16	36	40	38.0	0.2	Cloudy; rain.
17	42	46	44.0	0.8	Rain; sleet.
18	34	34	34.0	0.2	Rain; sleet; snow.
19	30	40	35.0	..	Cloudy.
20	36	40	38.0	..	Mist.
21	50	50	50.0	..	Mist.
22	37	40	38.5	..	Fair.
23	28	40	34.0	..	Fair.
24	52	70	61.0	..	Cloudy; mist.
25	66	60	63.0	1.2	Rain; fair.
26	32	52	42.0	..	Fair.
27	30	40	35.0	..	Fair.
28	46	66	56.0	..	Cloudy.
29	62	76	69.0	..	Cloudy.
30	66	72	69.0	..	Cloudy.
31	58	72	65.0	0.3	Cloudy; rain at night.
Means	40.03	48.65	44.34	2.7	Greatest Rise and Fall of temperature in 24 hours.
Max.	66	76	69.0		
Min.	18	34	29.0		
Range	48	42	40.0		
Extreme range 58					

	Sunrise.	2 P. M.
Rise . . .	24	30
Fall . . .	34	12

February, 1849.

DAY.	THERMOMETER. Sunrise.	THERMOMETER. 2 P. M.	THERMOMETER. Mean.	RAIN. Ins.	REMARKS ON THE WEATHER.
1	52	60	56.0	1.5	Cloudy; thunder; rain.
2	50	60	55.0	0.8	Rain.
3	32	40	36.0	1.5	Fair; rain at night.
4	38	40	39.0	0.3	Rain.
5	28	44	36.0	..	Fair.
6	30	60	45.0	..	Fair.
7	32	54	43.0	..	Cloudy.
8	48	50	49.0	0.7	Rain.
9	32	48	40.0	..	Fair; clouds.
10	26	50	38.0	..	Fair.
11	42	50	46.0	1.0	Rain.
12	30	48	39.0	..	Fair.
13	32	59	45.5	..	Clouds; fair.
14	34	44	39.0	..	Cloudy.
15	25	32	28.5	..	Cloudy; snow.
16	20	40	30.0	..	Clouds; fair.
17	26	34	30.0	..	Fair; windy.
18	6	26	16.0	..	Fair.
19	20	43	31.5	..	Cloudy.
20	46	60	53.0	..	Cloudy.
21	62	66	64.0	..	Cloudy; mist.
22	58	72	65.0	..	Fair.
23	50	76	63.0	..	Clouds.
24	56	78	67.0	..	Clouds.
25	52	70	61.0	..	Fair.
26	52	76	64.0	..	Fair.
27	50	76	63.0	..	Fair.
28	50	78	64.0	..	Smoky.
Means	38.54	54.79	46.66	[illegible]	[illegible]
Max.	62	78	67.0		
Min.	6	26	16.0		
Range	56	52	51.0		
Extreme range 72					

	Sunrise.	2 P. M.
Rise . . .	26	17
Fall . . .	20	20

March, 1849.

DAY.	THERMOMETER. Sunrise.	THERMOMETER. 2 P. M.	THERMOMETER. Mean.	RAIN. Ins.	REMARKS ON THE WEATHER.
1	48	78	63.0	..	Fair; smoky.
2	52	70	61.0	..	Smoky; cloudy.
3	48	54	51.0	0.5	Rain.
4	48	70	59.0	0.2	Rain.
5	62	74	68.0	0.5	Fair; clouds; showers at night.
6	66	66	66.0	..	Cloudy.
7	60	70	65.0	..	Fair.
8	48	72	60.0	..	Cloudy.
9	66	80	73.0	..	Cloudy.
10	64	80	72.0	..	Fair.
11	65	82	73.5	0.3	Cloudy; shower at night.
12	60	68	64.0	1.8	Rain.
13	60	72	66.0	0.4	Rain.
14	60	76	68.0	0.4	Cloudy; shower at 4 P. M.
15	56	72	64.0	..	Fair; clouds.
16	52	74	63.0	0.2	Fair; shower at night.
17	58	78	68.0	1.0	Cloudy; thunder; rain and hail at night.
18	60	70	65.0	..	Cloudy; fair.
19	50	80	65.0	0.2	Cloudy; wind and shower at night.
20	70	80	75.0	0.2	Shower at night.
21	54	70	62.0	..	Fair.
22	38	70	54.0	..	Fair.
23	48	78	59.0	..	Fair.
24	50	80	65.0	..	Fair.
25	52	64	58.0	..	Fair.
26	36	63	49.5	..	Fair.
27	34	60	47.0	..	Fair.
28	50	60	55.0	..	Fair; shower at night.
29	52	66	59.0	..	Cloudy.
30	52	70	61.0	..	Smoky.
31	50	78	64.0	..	Smoky.
Means	53.58	71.77	62.68	5.7	Greatest Rise and Fall of temperature in 24 hours.
Max.	70	82	75.0		
Min.	34	54	47.0		
Range	36	28	28.0		
Extreme range 48					

	Sunrise.	2 P. M.
Rise . . .	20	16
Fall . . .	16	16

April, 1849.

DAY.	THERMOMETER. Sunrise.	THERMOMETER. 2 P. M.	THERMOMETER. Mean.	RAIN. Ins.	REMARKS ON THE WEATHER.
1	50	76	63.0	..	Fair.
2	54	70	62.0	..	Cloudy.
3	60	68	64.0	0.8	Rain.
4	50	70	60.0	..	Fair.
5	48	80	64.0	..	Fair.
6	66	84	75.0	..	Fair.
7	70	84	77.0	0.3	Cloudy; showers.
8	64	76	70.0	0.3	Rain; showers.
9	65	74	69.5	..	Cloudy; showers.
10	54	74	64.0	..	Fair.
11	56	80	68.0	..	Fair.
12	58	66	62.0	..	Cloudy; rain.
13	60	70	65.0	0.7	Cloudy; rain.
14	50	60	55.0	0.3	Cloudy; rain at night.
15	38	52	45.0	..	Cloudy.
16	32	66	49.0	..	Fair; frost. Vegetation killed.
17	36	66	51.0	..	Fair.
18	36	60	48.0	..	Fair.
19	38	70	54.0	..	Fair.
20	38	70	54.0	..	Fair.
21	44	78	61.0	..	Fair; clouds.
22	60	78	69.0	0.2	Cloudy; showers.
23	64	72	68.0	..	Fair; cloudy; showers.
24	64	64	64.0	..	Fog; cloudy; showers.
25	56	70	63.0	0.1	Cloudy; showers.
26	56	76	66.0	..	
27	56	78	67.0	..	Fog; fair.
28	50	85	67.5	..	Fair.
29	60	86	73.0	..	Fair.
30	60	86	73.0	..	Fair.
Means	52.10	72.07	62.02	[illegible]	[illegible]
Max.	70	86	77.0		
Min.	32	52	45.0		
Range	38	34	32.0		
Extreme range 54					

	Sunrise.	2 P. M.
Rise . . .	18	14
Fall . . .	12	14

May, 1849.

DAY.	THERMOMETER. Sunrise.	THERMOMETER. 3 P. M.	THERMOMETER. Mean.	RAIN. Ins.	REMARKS ON THE WEATHER.
1	68	85	76.5	..	Clouds; fair.
2	64	87	75.5	..	Fair.
3	66	84	75.0	..	Fair.
4	70	80	75.0	..	Cloudy; sprinkle.
5	70	76	73.0	..	Cloudy.
6	70	78	74.0	0.8	Fog; cl'dy; thunder; rain at night.
7	62	74	68.0	0.4	Cloudy; rain.
8	64	74	69.0	0.3	Cloudy; rain.
9	60	66	63.0	..	Cloudy; rain.
10	52	76	64.0	..	Fair.
11	60	80	70.0	..	Fair.
12	64	80	72.0	..	Clouds; fair.
13	64	85	74.5	..	Clouds.
14	56	85	70.5	..	Clouds.
15	64	72	68.0	0.3	Clouds; rain.
16	64	72	68.0	..	Fog; fair.
17	66	80	73.0	..	Cloudy; fair.
18	60	79	69.5	..	Fair; clouds.
19	62	80	71.0	..	Clouds.
20	62	82	72.0	..	Fair; clouds.
21	70	76	73.0	0.4	Cloudy; rain.
22	70	85	77.5	0.2	Rain; fair.
23	60	76	68.0	0.2	Fair; shower at night.
24	62	86	74.0	..	Clouds; fair.
25	74	78	76.0	0.7	Rain; cloudy.
26	64	82	73.0	..	Fair.
27	64	76	70.0	..	Fair.
28	54	82	68.0	..	Fair.
29	54	80	67.0	..	Fair; cloudy.
30	70	82	76.0	..	Cloudy; fair.
31	66	83	74.5	0.2	Rain; fair.
Means	63.74	79.39	71.56	3.5	
Max.	74	87	77.5		
Min.	54	66	63.0		
Range	20	21	14.5		

Extreme range 33

Greatest Rise and Fall of temperature in 24 hours.

	Sunrise.	3 P. M.
Rise . . .	16	10
Fall . . .	10	13

June, 1849.

DAY.	THERMOMETER. Sunrise.	THERMOMETER. 3 P. M.	THERMOMETER. Mean.	RAIN. Ins.	REMARKS ON THE WEATHER.
1	60	82	71.0	..	Fair.
2	64	82	73.0	..	Clouds.
3	64	86	75.0	..	Clouds.
4	70	82	76.0	0.2	Clouds; rain A. M.; fair at eve.
5	70	76	73.0	0.2	Cloudy; rain; showers.
6	70	85	77.5	0.2	Cloudy; rain; showers.
7	70	90	80.0	0.3	Cloudy; rain; showers.
8	76	90	83.0	..	Cloudy; fair.
9	66	84	75.0	0.2	Cloudy; fair; showers.
10	70	85	77.5	..	Cloudy; fair.
11	72	90	81.0	..	Fair.
12	70	88	79.0	0.2	Cloudy; showers; fair.
13	70	88	79.0	..	Cloudy; fair.
14	70	90	80.0	..	Cloudy; fair.
15	70	90	80.0	..	Cloudy; fair.
16	68	88	78.0	..	Fair.
17	68	88	78.0	..	Fair.
18	70	88	79.0	0.2	Cloudy; shower.
19	68	86	77.0	0.1	Fog; shower.
20	66	88	77.0	..	Fair.
21	66	88	77.0	..	Fair.
22	70	91	80.5	..	Fair; cloudy.
23	70	86	78.0	..	Fair; cloudy.
24	74	80	77.0	0.8	Cloudy; rain; thunder.
25	72	78	75.0	0.2	Cloudy; rain.
26	72	82	77.0	0.1	Cloudy; rain.
27	72	86	79.0	..	Cloudy; fair.
28	74	88	81.0	..	Cloudy; fair.
29	76	84	80.0	0.3	Cloudy; rain.
30	72	86	79.0	0.2	Fog; rain.
Means	69.67	85.83	77.75	3.2	
Max.	76	91	83.0		
Min.	60	76	71.0		
Range	16	15	12.0		

Extreme range 31

Greatest Rise and Fall of temperature in 24 hours.

	Sunrise.	3 P. M.
Rise . . .	6	9
Fall . . .	10	6

July, 1849.

DAY.	THERMOMETER. Sunrise.	THERMOMETER. 3 P. M.	THERMOMETER. Mean.	RAIN. Ins.	REMARKS ON THE WEATHER.
1	76	88	82.0	1.0	Thunder; heavy rain A. M.; fair
2	76	84	80.0	1.3	Thunder; rain. [at eve.
3	76	88	82.0	0.3	Clouds; showers. [night.
4	76	84	80.0	3.5	Thunder; sh'rs heavy and in the
5	74	76	75.0	3.1	Thunder; rain—6 ins. in 24 h'rs.
6	74	84	79.0	0.3	Fog; rain.
7	76	84	80.0	..	Cloudy.
8	76	90	83.0	..	Cloudy; fair.
9	74	91	82.5	..	Fair.
10	73	90	81.5	..	Fair; clouds.
11	74	88	81.0	0.3	Fog; clouds; rain at night.
12	74	88	81.0	0.2	Fog; clouds; rain at night.
13	74	84	79.0	..	Rain.
14	74	84	79.0	..	Cloudy.
15	74	84	79.0	..	Fog; clouds.
16	74	86	80.0	..	Clouds.
17	70	90	80.0	..	Fair.
18	74	78	76 0	1.2	Rain; thunder.
19	74	76	75.0	1.8	Rain; thunder.
20	72	78	75.0	2.5	Rain; thunder.
21	74	90	82.0	..	Cloudy; fair.
22	70	90	80.0	..	Fair.
23	76	82	79.0	2.0	Cloudy; thunder; rain.
24	74	86	80.0	0.4	Cloudy; thunder; rain.
25	75	84	79.5	1.0	Fair; thunder; rain.
26	72	84	78.0	..	Fog; cloudy; rain at night.
27	74	84	79.0	0.2	Cloudy; rain.
28	..	..	..	..	
29	74	89	81.5	..	Fair.
30	74	86	80.0	0.2	Cloudy; rain.
31	70	80	75.0	0.2	Rain.
Means	73.93	85.00	79.47	19.5	
Max.	76	91	83.0		
Min.	70	76	75.0		
Range	6	15	8.0		

Extreme range 21

Greatest Rise and Fall of temperature in 24 hours.

	Sunrise.	3 P. M.
Rise . . .	6	12
Fall . . .	4	12

August, 1849.

DAY.	THERMOMETER. Sunrise.	THERMOMETER. 3 P. M.	THERMOMETER. Mean.	RAIN. Ins.	REMARKS ON THE WEATHER.
1	72	83	77.5	..	Cloudy.
2	72	84	78.0	..	Cloudy; showers.
3	72	87	79.5	..	Cloudy; showers.
4	74	82	78.0	0.1	Cloudy; showers.
5	72	86	79.0	..	Cloudy; showers.
6	74	85	79.5	0.1	Cloudy; showers.
7	72	88	80.0	0.1	Cloudy; showers.
8	72	86	79.0	..	Cloudy; fair.
9	74	90	82.0	0.5	Fair; shower at night.
10	72	84	78.0	..	Clouds; shower at night.
11	71	90	80.5	..	Fog; fair.
12	74	92	83.0	..	Fair.
13	74	93	83.5	..	Fair.
14	76	92	84.0	..	Fair; clouds; thunder.
15	74	92	83.0	..	Fair.
16	74	92	83.0	..	Fog; fair.
17	76	92	84.0	..	Fair.
18	76	90	83.0	..	Fair.
19	75	90	82.5	..	Fair.
20	72	92	82.0	..	Fair.
21	72	93	82.5	..	Fair.
22	72	92	82.0	..	Fair.
23	74	94	84.0	..	Fair.
24	76	94	85.0	..	Fair.
25	74	94	84.0	1.0	Cloudy; thunder; rain at night.
26	72	80	76.0	..	Cloudy.
27	74	80	77.0	..	Cloudy.
28	68	81	74.5	..	Cloudy.
29	70	88	79.0	..	Cloudy.
30	76	78	77.0	0.2	Rain.
31	68	76	72.0	2.1	Thunder; rain.
Means	73.03	87.74	80.39	4.1	
Max.	76	94	85.0		
Min.	68	76	72.0		
Range	8	18	13.0		

Extreme range 26

Greatest Rise and Fall of temperature in 24 hours.

	Sunrise.	3 P. M.
Rise . . .	3	6
Fall . . .	8	14

September, 1849.

DAY.	THERMOMETER. Sunrise.	THERMOMETER. 3 P. M.	THERMOMETER. Mean.	RAIN. Ins.	REMARKS ON THE WEATHER.
1	65	78	71.5	..	Fair.
2	58	78	68.0	..	Fair.
3	62	80	71.0	..	Fair.
4	64	86	75.0	..	Fair.
5	68	88	78.0	1.0	Cloudy; thunder; rain at night.
6	70	80	75.0	..	Cloudy.
7	62	80	71.0	..	Fair.
8	58	76	67.0	..	Fair.
9	58	80	69.0	..	Fair.
10	58	84	71.0	..	Fair.
11	60	80	70.0	..	Fair.
12	60	81	70.5	..	Fair.
13	58	84	71.0	..	Fair.
14	76	84	80.0	..	Fair; clouds.
15	70	87	78.5	..	Fog; clouds.
16	72	80	76.0	..	Fog; fair.
17	74	87	80.5	..	Fog; fair.
18	74	89	81.5	..	Fog.
19	77	90	83.5	..	Fair.
20	72	90	81.0	0.2	Fair; shower at night.
21	70	80	75.0	0.3	Fog; cloudy; shower at 3 P. M.
22	70	84	77.0	..	Cloudy.
23	64	76	70.0	..	Fair.
24	55	78	66.5	..	Fair; clouds.
25	56	78	67.0	..	Fair.
26	66	82	74.0	..	Cloudy; fair.
27	56	76	66.0	..	Fair.
28	56	81	68.5	..	Cloudy.
29	72	84	78.0	0.1	Rain; fair.
30	74	89	81.5	..	Cloudy.
Means	65.17	82.33	73.75	1.6	
Max.	77	90	83.5		
Min.	55	76	66.0		
Range	22	14	17.5		
Extreme range 35					

Greatest Rise and Fall of temperature in 24 hours.

	Sunrise.	3 P. M.
Rise . . .	18	7
Fall . . .	9	8

October, 1849.

DAY.	THERMOMETER. Sunrise.	THERMOMETER. 3 P. M.	THERMOMETER. Mean.	RAIN. Ins.	REMARKS ON THE WEATHER.
1	74	84	79.0	..	Clouds.
2	50	76	63.0	..	Fair; sprinkle at night.
3	54	78	66.0	..	Fair.
4	56	84	70.0	..	Fair; clouds.
5	73	70	71.5	..	Cloudy.
6	46	66	56.0	..	Fair.
7	46	66	56.0	..	Fair.
8	40	64	52.0	..	Fair.
9	42	72	57.0	..	Fair.
10	58	70	64.0	..	Fair.
11	51	76	63.5	..	Fair.
12	60	88	64.0	..	Fair.
13	46	64	55.0	..	Fair; cloudy.
14	58	72	65.0	2.8	Cloudy; thunder; rain at night.
15	64	67	65.5	..	Cloudy; rain.
16	48	64	56.0	..	Fair.
17	40	60	50.0	..	Fair.
18	38	50	44.0	..	Fair.
19	39	50	44.5	..	Fair.
20	50	67	58.5	0.2	Cloudy; shower at night.
21	50	70	60.0	..	Fair.
22	44	78	61.0	..	Fair.
23	45	75	60.0	..	Fair.
24	46	77	61.5	..	Fair.
25	44	70	57.0	..	Fair.
26	46	66	56.0	..	Fair.
27	52	72	62.0	..	Fair.
28	50	76	63.0	..	Fair; clouds.
29	54	76	65.0	0.3	Cloudy; thunder; rain at night.
30	50	65	57.5	..	Fair.
31	50	70	60.0	..	Fair.
Means	50.45	69.77	60.11	3.3	
Max.	74	84	79.0		
Min.	38	50	44.0		
Range	36	34	35.0		
Extreme range 46					

Greatest Rise and Fall of temperature in 24 hours.

	Sunrise.	3 P. M.
Rise . . .	17	17
Fall . . .	27	14

November, 1849.

DAY.	THERMOMETER. Sunrise.	THERMOMETER. 2 P. M.	THERMOMETER. Mean.	RAIN. Ins.	REMARKS ON THE WEATHER.
1	48	70	59.0	..	Fair.
2	58	75	66.5	..	Fair.
3	60	76	68.0	..	Fair; clouds.
4	70	80	75.0	0.2	Cloudy; thunder; rain.
5	70	76	73.0	1.7	Cloudy; thunder; rain.
6	62	70	66.0	..	Fair.
7	46	70	58.0	..	Fair.
8	38	62	50.0	..	Fair.
9	38	70	54.0	..	Fair.
10	52	60	56.0	0.7	Cloudy; rain.
11	54	64	59.0	..	Rain.
12	50	68	59.0	..	Rain.
13	42	68	55.0	..	Fair.
14	46	74	60.0	..	Fair.
15	50	75	62.5	..	Fair; clouds.
16	62	75	68.5	0.4	Cloudy; thunder; rain at night.
17	56	70	63.0	..	Cloudy; fair.
18	34	62	48.0	..	Cloudy; thunder; rain at night.
19	50	50	50.0	0.2	Rain.
20	46	50	48.0	..	Cloudy.
21	52	70	61.0	0.3	Cloudy; rain at night.
22	60	70	65.0	..	Fair.
23	66	76	71.0	..	Cloudy; thunder; rain at night.
24	58	56	57.0	1.4	Rain.
25	38	54	46.0	..	Fair.
26	34	54	44.0	..	Fair.
27	30	56	43.0	..	Fair; killing frost.
28	40	62	51.0	..	Fair.
29	46	64	55.0	..	Fair.
30	34	62	48.0	1.5	Cloudy; rain at night.
Means	49.67	66.30	57.98	6.4	
Max.	70	80	75.0		
Min.	30	50	43.0		
Range	40	30	32.0		
Extreme range 50					

Greatest Rise and Fall of temperature in 24 hours.

	Sunrise.	2 P. M.
Rise . . .	16	20
Fall . . .	22	20

December, 1849.

DAY.	THERMOMETER. Sunrise.	THERMOMETER. 2 P. M.	THERMOMETER. Mean.	RAIN. Ins.	REMARKS ON THE WEATHER.
1	50	44	47.0	0.8	Rain; snow at night.
2	34	44	39.0	..	Cloudy; snow.
3	28	54	41.0	..	Fair.
4	32	68	50.0	..	Fair.
5	50	62	56.0	..	Cloudy.
6	42	42	42.0	0.5	Rain.
7	38	46	42.0	1.7	Rain.
8	46	56	51.0	0.2	Rain.
9	35	30	32.5	..	Cloudy; snow.
10	24	30	27.0	..	Snow.
11	10	32	21.0	..	Fair; snow 8 inches deep.
12	24	32	28.0	..	Cloudy; rain at night; icy.
13	30	40	35.0	..	Cloudy; icy.
14	36	40	38.0	..	Cloudy; snow melting.
15	42	56	49.0	1.0	Rain.
16	62	46	54.0	..	Fair; cloudy.
17	24	40	32.0	..	Fair.
18	30	50	40.0	0.4	Cloudy; thunder; rain at night.
19	58	68	63.0	0.2	Rain.
20	64	60	62.0	..	Cloudy; fair.
21	36	60	48.0	..	Fair.
22	38	54	46.0	..	Fair.
23	40	63	51.5	..	Hazy; fair.
24	40	64	52.0	..	Fair.
25	36	50	43.0	..	Fair.
26	50	62	56.0	..	Cloudy; mist.
27	60	60	60.0	0.2	Rain.
28	54	70	62.0	0.5	Fog; mist; thunder; rain at night.
29	52	42	47.0	..	Cloudy; wind; snow and sleet.
30	27	30	28.5	0.2	Snow covering the ground 2 ins. deep.
31	18	32	25.0	..	Fair.
Means	39.03	49.26	44.15	5.7	
Max.	64	70	63.0		
Min.	10	30	21.0		
Range	54	40	42.0		
Extreme range 60					

Greatest Rise and Fall of temperature in 24 hours.

	Sunrise.	2 P. M.
Rise . . .	28	18
Fall . . .	38	28

January, 1850.

DAY.	THERMOMETER. Sun-rise.	THERMOMETER. 2 P. M.	THERMOMETER. Mean.	RAIN. Ins.	REMARKS ON THE WEATHER.
1	30	40	35.0	..	Cloudy.
2	36	44	40.0	0.8	Mist; rain.
3	45	50	47.5	..	Cloudy.
4	30	46	38.0	..	Fair.
5	36	40	38.0	1.0	Cloudy; sleet; rain.
6	40	44	42.0	0.7	Cloudy; thunder; rain at night.
7	46	50	48.0	..	Rain.
8	32	52	42.0	..	Fair.
9	30	54	42.0	..	Fair.
10	30	60	45.0	..	Fair.
11	46	62	54.0	..	Fair.
12	44	56	50.0	..	Cloudy.
13	38	50	44.0	..	Fair.
14	30	50	40.0	..	Fair.
15	46	52	49.0	0.8	Cloudy; rain.
16	50	60	55.0	1.8	Mist; thunder; rain at night.
17	54	56	55.0	..	Thunder; rain.
18	46	52	49.0	..	Fog; fair.
19	42	42	42.0	3.0	Thunder; rain.
20	56	60	58.0	..	Rain.
21	38	44	41.0	..	Fair.
22	28	52	40.0	..	Cloudy.
23	46	52	49.0	1.5	Thunder; hail; rain.
24	62	62	62.0	0.9	Cloudy; rain.
25	50	54	52.0	0.4	Fog; rain.
26	54	62	58.0	..	Fog; fair.
27	54	66	60.0	..	Fog; fair.
28	48	56	52.0	..	Fair.
29	28	52	40.0	..	Fair.
30	28	58	43.0	..	Fair.
31	40	64	52.0	..	Fair.
Means	41.39	52.97	47.18	10.9	
Max.	62	64	62.0		
Min.	28	40	35.0		
Range	34	24	27.0		

Extreme range 36

Greatest Rise and Fall of temperature in 24 hours.	Sunrise.	2 P. M.
Rise . . .	18	18
Fall . . .	20	16

February, 1850.

DAY.	THERMOMETER. Sun-rise.	THERMOMETER. 2 P. M.	THERMOMETER. Mean.	RAIN. Ins.	REMARKS ON THE WEATHER.
1	50	60	55.0	1.0	Cloudy; rain.
2	54	42	48.0	..	Cloudy.
3	28	32	30.0	..	Fair.
4	14	30	22.0	..	Fair.
5	22	46	34 0	..	Fair; cloudy.
6	42	60	51.0	..	Cloudy.
7	56	60	58 0	0.2	Rain.
8	56	60	58.0	1.3	Rain.
9	36	56	46.0	..	Fair.
10	30	50	40.0	..	Fair.
11	36	62	49.0	0.9	Cloudy; thunder; rain at night.
12	44	44	44.0	..	Cloudy; rain; snow at night.
13	34	34	34.0	..	Snow fell all day—3 inches deep.
14	32	44	38.0	..	Fair.
15	30	42	36.0	..	Fair; cloudy.
16	26	46	36.0	..	Fair.
17	28	60	44.0	..	Fair.
18	36	60	48.0	..	Fair.
19	56	66	61.0	..	Cloudy; fair.
20	66	66	66.0	..	Cloudy.
21	64	46	55.0	1.8	Thunder; rain.
22	40	54	47.0	..	Fair.
23	32	50	41.0	..	Fair.
24	54	64	59.0	..	Fair.
25	58	72	65.0	..	Cloudy; mist.
26	62	76	69.0	..	Fog; fair.
27	54	70	62.0	..	Fair.
28	70	78	74.0	..	Cloudy.
Means	43.21	54.64	48.93	5.2	
Max.	70	78	74.0		
Min.	14	30	22.0		
Range	56	48	52.0		

Extreme range 64

Greatest Rise and Fall of temperature in 24 hours.	Sunrise.	2 P. M.
Rise . . .	20	16
Fall . . .	24	20

March, 1850.

DAY.	THERMOMETER. Sun-rise.	THERMOMETER. 2 P. M.	THERMOMETER. Mean.	RAIN. Ins.	REMARKS ON THE WEATHER.
1	50	70	60.0	..	Fair.
2	52	70	61.0	..	Cloudy.
3	44	50	47.0	..	Fair.
4	32	56	44.0	..	Fair; cloudy.
5	48	65	56.5	1.2	Cloudy; thunder; rain at night.
6	54	64	59.0	..	Cloudy; fair.
7	38	68	53.0	..	Fair.
8	44	74	59.0	..	Fair.
9	62	66	64.0	..	Cloudy.
10	44	56	50.0	..	Cloudy; rain at night.
11	38	64	51 0	..	Fair.
12	36	64	50.0	0.2	Cloudy; rain at night.
13	64	78	71.0	..	Cloudy.
14	68	76	72.0	0.4	Cloudy; thunder; rain at night.
15	60	80	70.0	0.2	Fog; thunder; hail at night.
16	70	80	75.0	..	Fair.
17	70	80	75.0	..	Fair.
18	46	60	53.0	..	Fair.
19	50	48	49.0	0.5	Thunder; rain; hail.
20	46	56	51.0	..	Cloudy; rain.
21	56	64	60.0	1.0	Cloudy; rain.
22	50	50	50.0	..	Cloudy.
23	32	50	41.0	..	Fair.
24	32	64	48.0	..	Fair.
25	48	70	59.0	..	Clouds.
26	52	52	52.0	..	Clouds.
27	35	46	40.5	..	Clouds; fair.
28	28	56	42.0	..	Fair.
29	32	64	48.0	..	Fair.
30	38	68	53.0	..	Fair.
31	..	..	..	..	
Means	47.30	63.63	55.47	3.5	
Max.	70	80	75.0		
Min.	28	46	40.5		
Range	42	34	34.5		

Extreme range 52

Greatest Rise and Fall of temperature in 24 hours.	Sunrise.	2 P. M.
Rise . . .	28	14
Fall . . .	24	20

April, 1850.

DAY.	THERMOMETER. Sun-rise.	THERMOMETER. 2 P. M.	THERMOMETER. Mean.	RAIN. Ins.	REMARKS ON THE WEATHER.
1	50	74	62.0	2.3	Cloudy; rain at night.
2	58	70	64.0	0.5	Cloudy; shower at 5 P. M.
3	52	72	62.0	..	Fair.
4	46	68	57.0	..	Fair; clouds.
5	48	56	52.0	..	Fair.
6	44	62	53.0	..	Fair.
7	36	70	53.0	..	Fair.
8	48	70	59.0	..	Clouds.
9	62	70	66.0	0.2	Clouds; rain.
10	48	54	51.0	..	Clouds; rain.
11	40	60	50.0	..	Cloudy; sleet.
12	40	64	52.0	..	Fair.
13	38	70	54.0	..	Fair.
14	42	82	62.0	..	Fair.
15	58	76	67.0	..	Cloudy.
16	66	76	71.0	0.5	Cloudy; thunder; rain.
17	56	86	71.0	..	Fair.
18	58	80	69.0	..	Fair.
19	70	78	74.0	0.2	Cloudy; rain.
20	70	70	70.0	1.0	Cloudy; thunder; rain.
21	70	80	75.0	..	Cloudy; thunder.
22	68	64	66.0	3.8	Cloudy; thunder; rain.
23	50	48	49.0	..	Cloudy; rain.
24	44	52	48.0	0.5	Cloudy; rain.
25	50	62	56.0	0.4	Cloudy; rain.
26	60	76	68.0	..	Fog; fair.
27	66	82	74.0	0.3	Cloudy; thunder; rain.
28	48	64	56.0	..	Fair.
29	44	72	58.0	..	Fair.
30	54	80	67.0	..	Fair; clouds.
Means	52.80	69.60	61.20	9.7	
Max.	70	86	75.0		
Min.	36	48	48.0		
Range	34	38	27.0		

Extreme range 50

Greatest Rise and Fall of temperature in 24 hours.	Sunrise.	2 P. M.
Rise . . .	16	14
Fall . . .	18	16

May, 1850.

DAY.	THERMOMETER. Sunrise.	THERMOMETER. 3 P. M.	THERMOMETER. Mean.	RAIN. Ins.	REMARKS ON THE WEATHER.
1	60	63	61.5	..	Clouds.
2	56	64	60.0	0.2	Clouds; rain.
3	60	70	65.0	..	Fog; rain; fair.
4	58	60	59.0	0.8	Cloudy; rain.
5	50	62	56.0	..	Cloudy; rain.
6	44	70	57.0	..	Fair.
7	54	66	60.0	0.2	Cloudy; rain.
8	58	74	66.0	..	Cloudy; fair.
9	58	76	67.0	..	Fair.
10	60	75	67.5	1.0	Cloudy; thunder; rain at night.
11	52	60	56.0	..	Cloudy.
12	46	68	57.0	..	Fair.
13	58	56	57.0	0.4	Cloudy; thunder; rain.
14	56	62	59.0	..	Rain.
15	52	76	64.0	..	Fair.
16	56	76	66.0	..	Fair.
17	61	82	71.5	..	Fair.
18	58	75	66.5	..	Fair.
19	56	76	66.0	..	Fair.
20	60	80	70.0	..	Cloudy.
21	60	82	71.0	..	Fair.
22	70	84	77.0	..	Fair.
23	64	84	74.0	..	Fair.
24	66	87	76.5	..	
25	66	87	76.5	..	Clouds; fair.
26	68	87	77.5	..	Fair.
27	64	88	76.0	..	Fair.
28	68	90	79 0	..	Fair.
29	66	68	67.0	1.0	Cloudy; thunder; rain.
30	66	64	65.0	0.4	Cloudy; thunder; rain.
31	56	80	68.0	..	Fair.
Means	58.94	73.94	66.44	4.0	
Max.	70	90	79.0		
Min.	44	56	56.0		
Range	26	34	23.0		

Extreme range 46

Greatest Rise and Fall of temperature in 24 hours.

	Sunrise.	3 P. M.
Rise . . .	12	16
Fall . . .	10	17

July, 1850.

DAY.	THERMOMETER. Sunrise.	THERMOMETER. 3 P. M.	THERMOMETER. Mean.	RAIN. Ins.	REMARKS ON THE WEATHER.
1	56	80	68.0	0.7	Thunder; rain; fair.
2	68	86	77.0	..	Fog; fair; shower.
3	76	90	83.0	..	Cloudy; fair.
4	74	90	82.0	..	Fair.
5	70	90	80.0	..	Fair.
6	72	91	81.5	0.1	Fair; cloudy; showers.
7	72	92	82.0	..	Fair.
8	72	90	81.0	..	Fair.
9	74	80	77.0	..	Fog; fair; clouds; showers.
10	70	90	80.0	..	Fair; clouds.
11	72	94	83.0	..	Fair.
12	74	94	84.0	..	Fair.
13	74	80	77.0	1.0	Cloudy; thunder; rain.
14	74	86	80.0	1.0	Cloudy; thunder; rain.
15	70	87	78.5	..	Fair.
16	74	86	80.0	..	Cloudy; fair.
17	74	90	82.0	..	Cloudy; fair.
18	70	86	78 0	0.4	Fair; thunder; rain at eve.
19	68	86	77.0	..	Fair.
20	64	86	75.0	..	Fair.
21	66	92	79.0	..	Fair.
22	70	92	81.0	..	Fair; clouds; showers.
23	76	90	83.0	..	Cloudy; fair.
24	70	90	80.0	0.8	Fair; clouds; thunder; rain.
25	70	86	78.0	..	Clouds.
26	74	80	77.0	0.4	Fair; clouds; shower at 3 P. M.
27	70	80	75.0	0.3	Cloudy; shower at 12 M.
28	74	87	80.5	..	Cloudy.
29	74	88	81.0	..	Cloudy; fair.
30	74	88	81.0	..	Cloudy; sprinkle.
31	72	90	81.0	..	Fair.
Means	71.23	87.65	79.44	4.7	
Max.	76	94	84.0		
Min.	56	80	68.0		
Range	20	14	16.0		

Extreme range 38

Greatest Rise and Fall of temperature in 24 hours.

	Sunrise.	3 P. M.
Rise . . .	12	10
Fall . . .	20	14

June, 1850.

DAY.	THERMOMETER. Sunrise.	THERMOMETER. 3 P. M.	THERMOMETER. Mean.	RAIN. Ins.	REMARKS ON THE WEATHER.
1	56	80	68.0	..	Fair.
2	60	86	73.0	..	Fair.
3	60	82	71.0	..	Fair.
4	66	84	75.0	..	Fair.
5	74	88	81.0	0.2	Cloudy; rain.
6	70	84	77.0	..	Clouds.
7	72	85	78.5	0.1	Clouds; rain.
8	72	82	77.0	0.1	Clouds; thunder; rain.
9	72	82	77.0	1.3	Clouds; thunder; rain at night.
10	68	74	71.0	..	Clouds; rain.
11	64	78	71.0	..	Clouds.
12	64	82	73.0	0.4	Clouds; rain at night.
13	72	76	74.0	0.4	Clouds; rain.
14	74	78	76.0	0.5	Clouds; thunder; rain.
15	72	82	77.0	..	Clouds; rain.
16	72	84	78.0	..	Clouds; fair.
17	74	86	80.0	..	Fair; showers.
18	72	85	78.5	..	Fair; showers.
19	74	87	80.5	..	Fair; showers.
20	72	90	81.0	..	Fair.
21	70	86	78.0	..	Fog; fair.
22	72	86	79.0	..	Fair.
23	72	80	76.0	..	Fair; clouds; thunder.
24	70	88	79.0	..	Fair; clouds; thunder.
25	72	92	82.0	..	Fair; clouds; thunder.
26	72	90	81.0	1.0	Fair; clouds; thunder; rain.
27	70	85	77.5	..	Clouds; fair.
28	70	86	78.0	..	Fair.
29	70	88	79.0	..	Fair.
30	76	90	83.0	..	
Means	69.80	84.20	77.00	[illegible]	
Max.	76	92	83.0		
Min.	56	74	68.0		
Range	20	18	15.0		

Extreme range 36

Greatest Rise and Fall of temperature in 24 hours.

	Sunrise.	3 P. M.
Rise . . .	8	8
Fall . . .	4	8

August, 1850.

DAY.	THERMOMETER. Sunrise.	THERMOMETER. 3 P. M.	THERMOMETER. Mean.	RAIN. Ins.	REMARKS ON THE WEATHER.
1	74	90	82.0	..	Fair.
2	72	91	81.5	..	Fair.
3	74	92	83.0	..	Fair.
4	74	92	83.0	..	Fair.
5	74	96	85.0	..	Fair; clouds.
6	74	97	85.5	..	Fair; clouds.
7	74	96	85.0	..	Fair; clouds.
8	75	96	85.5	..	Fair; clouds; thunder.
9	75	98	86.5	0.1	Fair; clouds; thunder; shower.
10	75	96	85.5	..	Fair.
11	76	98	87.0	..	Fair.
12	80	100	90.0	..	Fair; clouds; thunder.
13	76	101	88.5	..	Fair; clouds; thunder.
14	78	100	89.0	..	Fair; clouds; thunder.
15	76	96	86.0	..	Fair; clouds; thunder; sprinkle.
16	72	92	82.0	..	Fair; clouds; thunder.
17	74	96	85.0	..	Fair; clouds; thunder.
18	74	94	84.0	..	Fair; clouds.
19	76	94	85.0	..	Fair; clouds.
20	76	95	85.5	..	Fair; clouds.
21	76	96	86.0	..	Fair; clouds.
22	74	96	85.0	..	Cloudy; thunder; sprinkle.
23	72	94	83.0	..	Fair.
24	74	98	86.0	..	Fair.
25	72	95	83.5	1.5	Fair; thunder; rain at night.
26	70	86	78.0	1.8	Cloudy; thunder; rain at night.
27	72	76	74.0	2.3	Cloudy; thunder; rain at night.
28	70	76	73.0	0.8	Cloudy; thunder; rain at night.
29	76	83	79.5	0.6	Rain.
30	70	78	74.0	0.2	Cloudy; showers.
31	..	..	..	..	
Means	74.17	92.93	83.55	[illegible]	
Max	80	101	90.0		
Min.	70	76	73.0		
Range	10	25	17.0		

Extreme range 31

Greatest Rise and Fall of temperature in 24 hours.

	Sunrise.	3 P. M.
Rise . . .	4	7
Fall . . .	6	10

September, 1850.

DAY.	THERMOMETER. Sun-rise.	3 P. M.	Mean.	RAIN. Ins.	REMARKS ON THE WEATHER.
1	56	74	65.0	..	Fair.
2	54	76	65.0	..	Fair.
3	56	76	66.0	..	Fair.
4	60	86	73.0	..	Fair; clouds.
5	68	86	77.0	..	Fair; clouds; thunder.
6	62	68	65.0	0.8	Thunder; rain.
7	64	76	70.0	0.2	Cloudy; fair.
8	62	78	70.0	..	Fog; fair.
9	62	80	71.0	..	Fair; clouds.
10	64	80	72.0	..	Fair.
11	62	84	73.0	..	Fair.
12	66	86	76.0	..	Fair.
13	68	87	77.5	..	Fog; fair.
14	70	88	79.0	..	Fog; fair.
15	72	88	80.0	..	Fog.
16	66	78	72.0	..	Fog.
17	62	84	73.0	..	Fog; fair.
18	62	86	74.0	..	Fair.
19	68	84	76.0	..	Fair.
20	56	80	68.0	..	Fair.
21	58	80	69.0	0.2	Cloudy; thunder; rain.
22	66	86	76.0	..	Fog; fair.
23	70	86	78.0	..	Fog; fair.
24	72	86	79.0	..	Fair.
25	68	86	77.0	..	Fair.
26	70	86	78.0	..	Fair.
27	66	88	77.0	..	Fair.
28	70	86	78.0	..	Fair.
29	62	80	71.0	..	Fair.
30	52	76	64.0	..	Fair.
Means	63.80	82.17	72.98	1.2	Greatest Rise and Fall of temperature in 24 hours.
Max.	72	88	80.0		
Min.	52	68	64.0		
Range	20	20	16.0		
Extreme range 36					

	Sunrise.	3 P. M.
Rise . . .	8	10
Fall . . .	14	18

October, 1850.

DAY.	THERMOMETER. Sun-rise.	3 P. M.	Mean.	RAIN. Ins.	REMARKS ON THE WEATHER.
1	54	80	67.0	..	Fair.
2	58	82	70.0	..	Fair.
3	56	80	68.0	..	Fair.
4	48	80	64.0	..	Fair.
5	52	78	65.0	..	Fog; fair.
6	46	66	56.0	..	Fair; clouds.
7	47	71	59.0	..	Smoky; clouds.
8	56	70	63.0	..	Smoky; clouds; sprinkle.
9	60	76	68.0	1.5	Cloudy; rain at night.
10	73	82	77.5	..	Cloudy; rain.
11	76	82	79.0	0.5	Cloudy; rain; fair.
12	64	80	72.0	..	Fair.
13	62	66	64.0	0.3	Cloudy; thunder; rain at night.
14	62	66	64.0	2.0	Cloudy; thunder; rain.
15	64	80	72.0	..	Rain; fair.
16	70	82	76.0	..	Fair.
17	66	80	73.0	0.4	Fair; thunder; rain at night.
18	62	62	62.0	..	Cloudy; fair.
19	42	63	52.5	..	Fair.
20	40	64	52.0	..	Fair.
21	54	74	64.0	..	Fair.
22	54	74	64.0	..	Fair.
23	54	76	65.0	..	Fair.
24	56	72	64.0	..	Fog; clouds; wind.
25	36	50	43.0	..	Fair.
26	32	56	44.0	..	Fair; killing frost.
27	32	60	46.0	..	Fair; killing frost.
28	34	66	50.0	..	Fair.
29	46	70	58.0	..	Fair.
30	46	70	58.0	..	Fair.
31	46	70	58.0	..	
Means	53.16	71.87	62.52	4.7	Greatest Rise and Fall of temperature in 24 hours.
Max.	76	82	79.0		
Min.	32	50	43.0		
Range	44	32	36.0		
Extreme range 50					

	Sunrise.	3 P. M.
Rise . . .	14	10
Fall . . .	20	22

November, 1850.

DAY.	THERMOMETER. Sun-rise.	2 P. M.	Mean.	RAIN. Ins.	REMARKS ON THE WEATHER.
1	40	70	55.0	..	Fair.
2	60	78	69.0	..	Fair; clouds.
3	56	78	67.0	..	Fair; clouds.
4	56	76	66.0	..	Fair.
5	64	78	71.0	1.4	Cloudy; thunder; rain at night.
6	50	48	49.0	0.2	Rain.
7	38	50	44.0	..	Fair.
8	42	54	48.0	..	Rainbow in the morning; cloudy; sprinkle.
9	46	52	49.0	0.1	Cloudy; rain.
10	46	54	50.0	..	Cloudy; fair.
11	36	52	44.0	..	Fair.
12	36	52	44.0	..	Fair.
13	36	60	48.0	..	Fair.
14	36	66	51.0	..	Fair.
15	46	54	50.0	..	Cloudy; sprinkle.
16	30	44	37.0	..	Fair.
17	22	50	36.0	..	Fair.
18	36	54	45.0	..	Cloudy; rain.
19	48	52	50.0	1.8	Rain.
20	46	56	51.0	..	Cloudy.
21	38	56	47.0	..	Fog; fair.
22	44	60	52.0	..	Fog; fair.
23	34	68	51.0	..	Fair.
24	34	68	51.0	..	Fair.
25	60	64	62.0	1.0	Cloudy; rain.
26	66	66	66.0	0.4	Cloudy; thunder; rain.
27	72	58	65.0	0.3	Cloudy; rain.
28	34	46	40.0	..	Fair.
29	30	58	44.0	..	Fair.
30	36	60	48.0	..	Fair; clouds.
Means	43.93	59.40	51.67	5.2	Greatest Rise and Fall of temperature in 24 hours.
Max.	72	78	71.0		
Min.	30	44	36.0		
Range	42	34	35.0		
Extreme range 48					

	Sunrise.	2 P. M.
Rise . . .	26	12
Fall . . .	38	30

December, 1850.

DAY.	THERMOMETER. Sun-rise.	2 P. M.	Mean.	RAIN. Ins.	REMARKS ON THE WEATHER.
1	56	70	63.0	..	Clouds; fair.
2	66	74	70.0	0.2	Clouds; rain at night.
3	38	46	42.0	0.1	Cloudy; rain at night.
4	38	36	37.0	0.1	Cloudy; rain.
5	24	32	28.0	..	Cloudy; sleet.
6	24	26	25.0	..	Cloudy; sleet; snow.
7	12	28	20.0	..	Fair; snow 2 inches deep.
8	12	37	24.5	..	Fair.
9	24	48	36.0	..	Fair.
10	26	56	41.0	..	Fair.
11	40	60	50.0	..	Fair.
12	54	56	55.0	..	Fair.
13	44	50	47.0	..	Cloudy; fair.
14	42	48	45.0	..	Cloudy.
15	46	58	52.0	1.0	Cloudy; rain.
16	54	56	55.0	..	Cloudy; fair.
17	44	48	46.0	..	Cloudy.
18	42	56	49.0	0.4	Cloudy; rain at night.
19	48	52	50.0	..	Cloudy; rain.
20	42	42	42.0	..	Cloudy.
21	42	44	43.0	2.0	Rain.
22	44	48	46.0	..	Rain.
23	36	56	46.0	..	Fair.
24	32	50	41.0	..	Fair; cloudy.
25	40	44	42.0	0.5	Rain.
26	44	42	43.0	..	Rain.
27	38	40	39.0	..	Rain.
28	40	36	38.0	1.0	Rain.
29	32	36	34.0	..	Cloudy.
30	32	36	34.0	..	Cloudy; fair.
31	24	32	28.0	..	Fair.
Means	38.07	46.55	42.31	5.3	Greatest Rise and Fall of temperature in 24 hours.
Max.	66	74	70.0		
Min.	12	26	20.0		
Range	54	48	50.0		
Extreme range 62					

	Sunrise.	2 P. M.
Rise . . .	20	11
Fall . . .	28	28

January, 1851.

DAY.	THERMOMETER. Sunrise.	THERMOMETER. 2 P. M.	THERMOMETER. Mean.	RAIN. Ins.	REMARKS ON THE WEATHER.
1	24	50	37.0	. .	Fair.
2	26	50	38.0	. .	Fair.
3	30	50	40.0	. .	Fair.
4	30	62	46.0	. .	Fair.
5	36	60	48.0	. .	Cloudy.
6	52	60	56.0	. .	Fair.
7	40	70	55.0	. .	Fair.
8	56	66	61.0	0.5	Fair; cloudy; rain.
9	40	56	48.0	. .	Fair.
10	34	56	45.0	. .	Fair.
11	34	56	45.0	. .	Fair.
12	30	66	48.0	. .	Fair.
13	34	64	49.0	. .	Fair.
14	42	66	54.0	. .	Fair.
15	58	70	64.0	. .	Clouds; fair.
16	56	56	56.0	. .	Fair; smoky.
17	26	36	31.0	. .	Cloudy; windy.
18	20	36	28.0	. .	Fair.
19	18	46	32.0	. .	Fair.
20	26	49	37.5	. .	Smoky.
21	36	64	50.0	0.7	Smoky; rain at night.
22	56	56	56.0	. .	Cloudy.
23	34	60	47.0	. .	Fair.
24	28	60	44.0	. .	Fair.
25	30	62	46.0	. .	Fair.
26	44	66	55.0	. .	Smoky.
27	52	64	58.0	0.1	Cloudy; rain.
28	62	68	65.0	. .	Cloudy; fair.
29	24	38	31.0	. .	Fair.
30	24	38	31.0	. .	Fair.
31	24	38	31.0	. .	Fair.
Means	36.32	56.10	46.21	1.3	Greatest Rise and Fall of temperature in 24 hours.
Max.	62	70	65.0		
Min.	18	36	28.0		
Range	44	34	37.0		
Extreme range 52					

	Sunrise.	2 P. M.
Rise . . .	20	18
Fall . . .	38	30

February, 1851.

DAY.	THERMOMETER. Sunrise.	THERMOMETER. 2 P. M.	THERMOMETER. Mean.	RAIN. Ins.	REMARKS ON THE WEATHER.
1	36	36	36.0	1.2	Rain.
2	38	40	39.0	. .	Rain.
3	37	46	41.5	. .	Cloudy; fair.
4	37	50	43.5	. .	Fog; fair.
5	34	60	47.0	. .	Fair.
6	36	60	48.0	. .	Fair.
7	36	64	50.0	0.1	Cloudy; rain at night.
8	60	70	65.0	0.2	Cloudy; thunder; rain at night.
9	58	66	62.0	2.7	Cloudy; rain.
10	40	50	45.0	. .	Fair.
11	30	46	38.0	. .	Fair.
12	32	50	41.0	0.2	Cloudy; rain at night.
13	44	50	47.0	0.5	Rain.
14	52	68	60.0	1.8	Rain; thunder.
15	28	40	34.0	. .	Fair.
16	20	42	31.0	. .	Fair.
17	22	50	36.0	. .	Fair.
18	36	58	47.0	. .	Cloudy.
19	48	56	52.0	4.0	Thunder; rain.
20	56	50	53.0	. .	Rain; fair at eve.
21	32	60	46.0	. .	Fair.
22	46	58	52.0	0.2	Cloudy; rain.
23	64	76	70.0	. .	Fair; clouds.
24	44	60	52.0	. .	Fair.
25	44	70	57.0	. .	Fair.
26	66	74	70.0	1.0	Cloudy; thunder; rain at night.
27	52	40	46.0	0.8	Rain.
28	. .	. .	. .	. .	
Means	41.78	55.18	48.48	12.7	Greatest Rise and Fall of temperature in 24 hours.
Max.	66	76	70.0		
Min.	20	36	31.0		
Range	46	40	39.0		
Extreme range 56					

	Sunrise.	2 P. M.
Rise . . .	24	18
Fall . . .	24	34

March, 1851.

DAY.	THERMOMETER. Sunrise.	THERMOMETER. 2 P. M.	THERMOMETER. Mean.	RAIN. Ins.	REMARKS ON THE WEATHER.
1	28	48	38.0	. .	Fair.
2	28	58	43.0	. .	Fair.
3	28	56	42.0	. .	Fair.
4	36	64	50.0	. .	Fair.
5	58	64	61.0	2.0	Cloudy; thunder; rain at night.
6	36	38	37.0	0.3	Rain.
7	34	56	45.0	. .	Snow in the morning; fair.
8	32	60	46.0	. .	Fair.
9	34	62	48.0	. .	Fair.
10	36	64	50.0	. .	Fair.
11	42	72	57.0	. .	Fair.
12	50	74	62.0	. .	Fair.
13	52	70	61.0	0.5	Smoky; rain.
14	53	70	61.5	. .	Fair.
15	56	70	63.0	. .	Fair.
16	52	70	61.0	. .	Fair.
17	42	72	57.0	. .	Smoky.
18	46	74	60.0	. .	Smoky.
19	38	70	54.0	. .	Smoky.
20	46	72	59.0	. .	Smoky.
21	60	74	67.0	0.3	Smoky; thunder; rain at night.
22	50	70	60.0	. .	Fair.
23	48	60	54.0	. .	Cloudy; fair.
24	38	67	52.5	. .	Smoky.
25	44	75	59.5	. .	Smoky.
26	55	74	64.5	. .	Smoky.
27	60	76	68.0	. .	Cloudy.
28	60	80	70.0	. .	Cloudy; thunder.
29	64	78	71.0	. .	Cloudy; fair.
30	60	76	68.0	1.0	Cloudy; thunder; rain.
31	62	68	65.0	0.4	Cloudy; rain.
Means	46.06	67.16	56.61	4.5	Greatest Rise and Fall of temperature in 24 hours.
Max.	64	80	71.0		
Min.	28	38	37.0		
Range	36	42	34.0		
Extreme range 52					

	Sunrise.	2 P. M.
Rise . . .	22	18
Fall . . .	24	26

April, 1851.

DAY.	THERMOMETER. Sunrise.	THERMOMETER. 2 P. M.	THERMOMETER. Mean.	RAIN. Ins.	REMARKS ON THE WEATHER.
1	64	76	70.0	0.1	Rain; fair.
2	60	76	68.0	. .	Cloudy; fair.
3	66	68	67.0	. .	Rain; fair.
4	60	70	65.0	0.2	Cloudy; rain.
5	50	60	55.0	. .	Fair.
6	40	66	53.0	1.2	Fair; thunder; rain at night.
7	54	60	57.0	. .	Rain.
8	36	60	48.0	. .	Fair.
9	38	68	53.0	. .	Fair.
10	42	78	60.0	. .	Fair; clouds.
11	68	70	69.0	0.7	Cloudy; rain at night.
12	60	70	65.0	. .	Rain.
13	54	74	64.0	. .	Fair.
14	48	62	55.0	. .	Fair.
15	43	69	56.0	. .	Fair.
16	44	74	59.0	. .	Fair.
17	44	72	58.0	. .	Fair.
18	54	82	68.0	. .	Cloudy; fair.
19	66	80	73.0	0.1	Fog; cl'dy; thunder; rain at night.
20	50	58	54.0	0.1	Fair; cloudy; thunder; showers.
21	46	66	56.0	. .	Fair.
22	46	58	52.0	0.2	Cloudy; rain at night.
23	52	62	57.0	. .	Cloudy.
24	42	68	55.0	. .	Fog; fair.
25	50	76	63.0	. .	Fair.
26	48	84	66.0	. .	Fair.
27	54	76	65.0	. .	Clouds.
28	56	76	66.0	. .	Fair.
29	56	80	68.0	. .	Fair.
30	48	80	64.0	. .	Fair.
Means	51.30	70.63	60.97	2.6	Greatest Rise and Fall of temperature in 24 hours.
Max.	68	84	73.0		
Min.	36	58	52.0		
Range	32	26	21.0		
Extreme range 46					

	Sunrise.	2 P. M.
Rise . . .	26	10
Fall . . .	18	22

May, 1851.

DAY.	THERMOMETER. Sunrise.	THERMOMETER. 3 P. M.	THERMOMETER. Mean.	RAIN. Ins.	REMARKS ON THE WEATHER.
1	38	70	54.0	..	Fair; frost in the low grounds.
2	44	74	59.0	..	Fair; clouds.
3	58	68	63.0	1.7	Cloudy; thunder; rain.
4	58	68	63.0	0.3	Rain; fair.
5	46	70	58.0	..	Fair.
6	46	72	59.0	..	Fair.
7	54	66	60.0	0.5	Cloudy; rain.
8	60	78	69.0	..	Rain; fair.
9	62	82	72.0	0.3	Cloudy; thunder; hail at noon.
10	72	84	78.0	..	Cloudy; fair.
11	74	84	79.0	..	Cloudy; fair.
12	70	85	77.5	..	Fair.
13	70	84	77.0	0.1	Rain; fair.
14	62	84	73.0	..	Fair.
15	64	86	75.0	..	Fair.
16	68	85	76.5	..	Fair; clouds.
17	65	85	75.0	..	Fair; clouds.
18	68	85	76.5	..	Cloudy; fair.
19	70	86	78.0	..	Cloudy.
20	76	86	81.0	..	Clouds.
21	74	86	80.0	..	Clouds.
22	72	84	78.0	..	Clouds; thunder; rain at night.
23	70	74	72.0	1.0	Rain.
24	62	76	69.0	..	Rain.
25	70	84	77.0	..	Fog; fair.
26	66	86	76.0	..	Clouds; fair.
27	70	86	78.0	..	Clouds; fair.
28	72	86	79.0	..	Clouds; fair.
29	70	86	78.0	..	Clouds; fair.
30	70	86	78.0	..	Fair.
31	70	88	79.0	..	Fair.
Means	64.22	80.77	72.50	3.9	Greatest Rise and Fall of temperature in 24 hours.
Max.	76	88	81.0		
Min.	38	66	54.0		
Range	38	22	27.0		

Extreme range 50

	Sunrise.	3 P. M.
Rise . . .	14	12
Fall . . .	10	10

June, 1851.

DAY.	THERMOMETER. Sunrise.	THERMOMETER. 3 P. M.	THERMOMETER. Mean.	RAIN. Ins.	REMARKS ON THE WEATHER.
1	68	88	78.0	..	Fair.
2	70	88	79.0	..	Fair.
3	72	87	79.5	..	Fair.
4	70	88	79.0	..	Fair.
5	72	89	80.5	..	Fair.
6	74	70	72.0	0.7	Cloudy; rain.
7	70	86	78.0	0.3	Fog; rain.
8	72	88	80.0	0.1	Fair; thunder; high wind at night; rain.
9	68	86	77.0	..	Cloudy; fair.
10	62	86	74.0	..	Cloudy; fair.
11	70	86	78.0	..	Hazy.
12	70	89	79.5	..	Fair.
13	72	88	80.0	..	Cloudy; fair.
14	70	92	81.0	..	Fair.
15	72	92	82.0	..	Fair.
16	72	92	82.0	..	Fair.
17	72	94	83.0	1.3	Fair; cloudy; thunder; rain at 4 P. M.
18	72	82	77.0	..	Cloudy; fair.
19	66	84	75.0	..	Fog; fair.
20	66	85	75.5	..	Fair.
21	64	86	75.0	0.2	Fair; cloudy; rain at night.
22	70	90	80.0	..	Cloudy.
23	70	90	80.0	..	Clouds.
24	68	90	79.0	..	Fair.
25	68	92	80.0	..	Fair.
26	72	91	81.5	..	Clouds.
27	72	89	80.5	..	Clouds.
28	72	90	81.0	..	Clouds.
29	74	84	79.0	0.2	Clouds; rain at night.
30	64	86	75.0	..	Fair.
Means	69.80	87.60	78.70	2.8	Greatest Rise and Fall of temperature in 24 hours.
Max.	74	94	83.0		
Min.	62	70	72.0		
Range	12	24	11.0		

Extreme range 32

	Sunrise.	3 P. M.
Rise . . .	8	16
Fall . . .	10	19

July, 1851.

DAY.	THERMOMETER. Sunrise.	THERMOMETER. 3 P. M.	THERMOMETER. Mean.	RAIN. Ins.	REMARKS ON THE WEATHER.
1	62	88	75.0	..	Fair; clouds.
2	62	90	76.0	..	Clouds.
3	64	92	78.0	..	Clouds.
4	70	93	81.5	..	
5	72	94	83.0	0.1	Smoky; showers.
6	72	94	83.0	..	Fair.
7	74	92	83.0	..	Clouds.
8	72	86	79.0	..	Fair; cloudy.
9	74	94	84.0	..	Clouds; fair.
10	76	92	84.0	0.8	Cloudy; thunder; rain at 2 P. M.
11	70	90	80.0	..	Fog; clouds.
12	72	94	83.0	..	Fair; clouds.
13	72	94	83.0	..	Fair; clouds.
14	74	94	84.0	..	Fair; clouds.
15	74	98	86.0	..	Fair; clouds.
16	74	97	85.5	..	Fair.
17	76	96	86.0	..	Clouds; fair.
18	74	94	84.0	..	Fair; clouds; thunder.
19	76	84	80.0	0.4	Cloudy; thunder; rain.
20	64	88	76.0	..	Fair.
21	62	90	76.0	..	Fair.
22	64	94	79.0	..	Fair; smoky.
23	70	86	78.0	..	Fair; smoky; sprinkle.
24	73	98	85.5	..	Smoky; clouds; thunder.
25	70	97	83.5	..	Smoky.
26	74	94	84.0	..	Fair; clouds.
27	70	92	81.0	..	Fair; clouds.
28	73	92	82.5	..	Fog; eclipse of the sun; clouds; fair.
29	74	96	85.0	..	Fair; smoky.
30	74	100	87.0	..	Smoky; cloudy.
31	72	90	81.0	0.7	Smoky; cloudy; rain at night.
Means	70.97	92.68	81.82	2.0	Greatest Rise and Fall of temperature in 24 hours.
Max.	76	100	87.0		
Min.	62	84	75.0		
Range	14	16	12.0		

Extreme range 38

	Sunrise.	3 P. M.
Rise . . .	6	12
Fall . . .	12	10

August, 1851.

DAY.	THERMOMETER. Sunrise.	THERMOMETER. 3 P. M.	THERMOMETER. Mean.	RAIN. Ins.	REMARKS ON THE WEATHER.
1	74	84	79.0	..	Cloudy; rain.
2	74	87	80.5	0.8	Mist; rain.
3	74	84	79.0	0.1	Fog; thunder; rain.
4	66	86	76.0	..	Fair.
5	64	88	76.0	..	Fair.
6	66	92	79.0	..	Fair.
7	70	94	82.0	..	Fair.
8	74	96	85.0	..	Fair.
9	74	97	85.5	..	Fair.
10	74	96	85.0	..	Fair.
11	76	94	85.0	..	Fair.
12	76	97	86.5	..	Fair.
13	76	100	88.0	..	Fair.
14	76	102	89.0	..	Fair.
15	78	101	89.5	..	Fair.
16	78	100	89.0	..	Fair.
17	78	100	89.0	..	Fair.
18	76	98	87.0	0.1	Clouds; rain at night.
19	76	95	85.5	..	Fog; clouds; thunder.
20	74	95	84.5	..	Cloudy.
21	72	94	83.0	0.7	Cloudy; thunder; rain at 4 P. M.
22	68	90	79.0	..	Fair.
23	68	92	80.0	..	Fair.
24	70	95	82.5	..	Fair.
25	76	95	85.5	..	Fair.
26	76	96	86.0	1.0	Cloudy; thunder; rain at 2 P. M.
27	72	86	79.0	..	Cloudy; fair.
28	72	86	79.0	..	Cloudy.
29	70	90	80.0	..	Fog; fair.
30	70	90	80.0	..	Fair.
31	70	90	80.0	..	Fair.
Means	72.84	93.21	83.03	2.7	Greatest Rise and Fall of temperature in 24 hours.
Max.	78	102	89.5		
Min.	64	84	76.0		
Range	14	18	13.5		

Extreme range 38

	Sunrise.	3 P. M.
Rise . . .	4	4
Fall . . .	8	10

September, 1851.

DAY.	THERMOMETER. Sunrise.	THERMOMETER. 3 P. M.	THERMOMETER. Mean.	RAIN. Ins.	REMARKS ON THE WEATHER.
1	70	92	81.0	..	Fair.
2	66	90	78.0	..	Fair; clouds.
3	68	92	80.0	..	Fair.
4	70	94	82.0	..	Fair.
5	70	95	82.5	..	Fair.
6	68	94	81.0	..	Fair.
7	68	98	83.0	..	Fair; smoky.
8	72	98	85.0	..	Smoky.
9	70	86	78.0	..	Cloudy; thunder.
10	60	80	70.0	0.6	Fair; clouds; shower from south.
11	72	84	78.0	..	Cloudy; fair.
12	66	92	79.0	..	Fair.
13	70	92	81.0	..	Fair.
14	68	94	81.0	..	Fair.
15	74	92	83.0	..	Fair.
16	74	92	83.0	..	Clouds.
17	70	86	78.0	..	Fair.
18	72	82	77.0	..	Cloudy; sprinkle.
19	68	80	74.0	..	Cloudy.
20	62	88	75.0	..	Fair.
21	62	88	75.0	..	Fair.
22	60	86	73.0	..	Fair.
23	58	90	74.0	..	Fair.
24	68	88	78.0	..	Cloudy.
25	65	84	74.5	..	Cloudy.
26	56	88	72.0	..	Cloudy.
27	58	74	66.0	..	Fair.
28	43	72	57.5	..	Fair.
29	44	76	60.0	..	Smoky.
30	44	80	62.0	..	Smoky.
Means	64.53	87.57	76.05	0.6	Greatest Rise and Fall of temperature in 24 hours.
Max.	74	98	85.0		
Min.	43	72	57.5		
Range	31	26	27.5		
Extreme range 55					

	Sunrise.	3 P. M.
Rise . . .	12	8
Fall . . .	15	14

October, 1851.

DAY.	THERMOMETER. Sunrise.	THERMOMETER. 3 P. M.	THERMOMETER. Mean.	RAIN. Ins.	REMARKS ON THE WEATHER.
1	46	80	63.0	..	Smoky.
2	48	84	66.0	..	Smoky.
3	54	86	70.0	..	Smoky.
4	56	86	71.0	..	Smoky.
5	58	86	72.0	..	Smoky.
6	60	82	71.0	..	Smoky.
7	62	80	71.0	..	Smoky; cloudy; sprinkle.
8	62	82	72.0	..	Smoky; cloudy; fair.
9	70	86	78 0	..	Clouds.
10	72	78	75.0	0.5	Rain at 10 A. M.
11	66	62	64.0	0.5	Cloudy; rain.
12	47	66	56.5	..	Fair.
13	40	70	55.0	..	Fair.
14	44	78	61.0	..	Fair.
15	40	70	55.0	..	Fair; cloudy.
16	42	74	58.0	..	Fair.
17	42	75	58.5	..	Fair.
18	46	74	60.0	..	Fair.
19	42	78	60.0	..	Fair.
20	50	78	64.0	..	Cloudy.
21	52	66	59.0	..	Cloudy.
22	40	62	51.0	..	Fair.
23	33	64	48.5	..	Fair.
24	38	72	55.0	..	Smoky.
25	52	70	61.0	..	Smoky.
26	40	64	52.0	..	Fair.
27	36	72	54 0	..	Smoky.
28	62	70	66.0	0.2	Fair; cloudy; rain.
29	60	74	67.0	..	Fair.
30	60	76	68.0	..	Fair.
31	42	78	60.0	..	Fair.
Means	50.39	74.94	62.66	1.2	Greatest Rise and Fall of temperature in 24 hours.
Max.	72	86	78.0		
Min.	33	62	48.5		
Range	30	24	29.5		
Extreme range 53					

	Sunrise.	3 P. M.
Rise . . .	26	8
Fall . . .	19	16

November, 1851.

DAY.	THERMOMETER. Sunrise.	THERMOMETER. 2 P. M.	THERMOMETER. Mean.	RAIN. Ins.	REMARKS ON THE WEATHER.
1	68	80	74.0	..	Cloudy.
2	40	72	56.0	..	Smoky; fair.
3	42	72	57.0	..	Smoky; fair.
4	38	74	56.0	..	Smoky; fair.
5	52	54	53.0	..	Smoky; windy.
6	28	52	40.0	..	Fair; killing frost.
7	24	52	38.0	..	Smoky.
8	30	68	49.0	..	Smoky.
9	60	62	61.0	0.1	Cloudy; rain.
10	57	60	58.5	1.4	Cloudy; rain.
11	50	60	55.0	1.3	Rain.
12	60	62	61.0	0.2	Rain.
13	46	50	48.0	..	Cloudy; fair at eve.
14	38	54	46.0	..	Cloudy.
15	32	50	41.0	..	Fair.
16	42	62	52.0	..	Fair.
17	40	64	52.0	..	Fair.
18	48	60	54.0	..	Cloudy.
19	50	70	60 0	..	Fair.
20	46	48	47.0	..	Cloudy.
21	30	60	45.0	..	Fair.
22	36	60	48.0	..	Clouds.
23	36	50	43.0	..	Fair.
24	28	40	34.0	..	Fair.
25	18	48	33.0	..	Fair.
26	32	64	48.0	..	Fair.
27	50	54	52.0	0.1	Cloudy; rain; fair.
28	28	48	38.0	..	Fair.
29	38	44	41.0	0.3	Rain.
30	38	46	42.0	..	Cloudy; fair.
Means	40.83	58.00	49.42	3.4	Greatest Rise and Fall of temperature in 24 hours.
Max.	68	80	74.0		
Min.	18	40	33.0		
Range	50	40	41.0		
Extreme range 62					

	Sunrise.	2 P. M.
Rise . . .	30	16
Fall . . .	28	22

December, 1851.

DAY.	THERMOMETER. Sunrise	THERMOMETER. 2 P. M.	THERMOMETER. Mean.	RAIN. Ins.	REMARKS ON THE WEATHER.
1	42	52	47.0	..	Cloudy.
2	32	54	43.0	..	Fair.
3	24	48	36.0	..	Fair.
4	22	48	35.0	..	Fair.
5	26	58	42.0	..	Fair.
6	34	64	49.0	..	Clouds.
7	50	72	61.0	..	Fair.
8	60	73	66.5	..	Cloudy.
9	56	74	65.0	0.5	Cloudy; rain at night.
10	50	70	60.0	..	Rain; fair at eve.
11	36	52	44.0	..	Fair.
12	42	56	49.0	..	Cloudy.
13	32	60	46.0	..	Fair.
14	32	50	41.0	.	Fair; cloudy; rain.
15	26	30	28.0	0.2	Cloudy; snow.
16	22	32	27.0	..	Cloudy.
17	22	30	26.0	..	Fair.
18	12	34	23.0	..	Fair.
19	20	48	34.0	..	Fair.
20	26	48	37.0	..	Fair.
21	36	37	36.5	..	Fair.
22	32	38	35.0	0.1	Cloudy; rain.
23	24	44	34.0	..	Fair.
24	38	52	45.0	..	Cloudy.
25	62	70	66.0	0.3	Cloudy; rain.
26	46	48	47.0	0.7	Cloudy; thunder; rain.
27	48	58	53.0	0.6	Cloudy; thunder; rain.
28	46	70	58.0	..	Fair.
29	66	74	70.0	1.4	Cloudy; rain at night.
30	..	..	..	..	
31	..	..	..	..	
Means	36.60	53.21	44.06	3.8	Greatest Rise and Fall of temperature in 24 hours.
Max.	66	74	70.0		
Min.	12	30	23.0		
Range	54	44	47.0		
Extreme range 62					

	Sunrise.	2 P. M.
Rise . . .	24	18
Fall . . .	16	22

January, 1852.

DAY.	THERMOMETER. Sun-rise.	2 P. M.	Mean.	RAIN. Ins.	REMARKS ON THE WEATHER.
1	30	36	33.0	..	Cloudy; mist; trees covered with ice; fair at eve.
2	30	50	40.0	..	Fair.
3	28	60	44.0	..	Fair.
4	48	60	54 0	..	Fair.
5	38	45	41.5	..	Fair.
6	24	40	32.0	..	Fair.
7	24	46	35.0	..	Fair.
8	44	60	52.0	..	Cloudy.
9	40	60	50.0	..	Cloudy.
10	40	48	44.0	..	Fair.
11	24	40	32.0	..	Cloudy.
12	27	34	30.5	..	Cloudy.
13	9	28	18.5	..	Fair.
14	19	40	29.5	..	Fair.
15	24	46	35.0	..	Fair.
16	34	56	45.0	..	Fair.
17	48	60	54.0	0.8	Fair; cloudy; rain at night.
18	26	24	25.0	..	Snow; fair.
19	4	21	12.5	..	Fair.
20	10	31	20.5	..	Fair.
21	21	40	30.5	..	Fair.
22	16	36	26.0	..	Fair.
23	18	48	33.0	..	Fair.
24	32	50	41.0	1.5	Cloudy; rain at night.
25	38	46	42.0	..	Rain.
26	32	54	43.0	..	Fair.
27	36	62	49.0	..	Fair.
28	32	66	49.0	0.5	Cloudy; rain.
29	52	66	59.0	..	Cloudy.
30	66	60	63.0	..	Fair.
31	40	50	45.0	..	Fair.
Means	30.77	47.19	38.98	2.8	Greatest Rise and Fall of temperature in 24 hours.
Max.	66	66	63.0		
Min.	4	21	12.5		
Range	62	45	50.5		
Extreme range 62					

	Sunrise.	2 P. M.
Rise . . .	20	14
Fall . . .	36	38

February, 1852.

DAY.	THERMOMETER. Sun-rise.	2 P. M.	Mean.	RAIN. Ins.	REMARKS ON THE WEATHER.
1	32	58	45.0	..	Fair.
2	30	62	46.0	..	Fair.
3	34	68	51.0	..	Fair.
4	62	69	65.5	..	Cloudy.
5	64	68	66.0	0.2	Cloudy; rain.
6	60	76	68.0	..	Fair.
7	53	60	56.5	0.3	Cloudy; rain at night.
8	44	46	45.0	..	Rain.
9	44	46	45.0	1.5	Cloudy; rain.
10	47	50	48.5	..	Cloudy; fair at eve.
11	36	50	43.0	..	Fair.
12	28	62	45 0	..	Fair.
13	52	64	58.0	..	Cloudy; fair.
14	30	56	43.0	..	Fair.
15	44	66	55.0	..	Fair.
16	32	64	48.0	..	Fair.
17	48	62	55.0	0.5	Smoky; rain at night.
18	40	39	39.5	..	Rain.
19	38	49	43.5	..	Cloudy.
20	48	60	54.0	1.3	Rain.
21	53	65	59.0	0.7	Rain.
22	52	72	62.0	0.5	Fog; fair; thunder; rain at night.
23	56	66	61.0	..	Rain; fair.
24	56	78	67.0	..	Fair; windy.
25	50	64	57.0	..	Fair.
26	..	..	..	..	
27	46	52	49.0	2.5	Rain.
28	54	60	57.0	0.5	Rain; fair.
29	30	63	46.5	..	Fair.
Means	45.11	60.54	52.82	8.0	Greatest Rise and Fall of temperature in 24 hours.
Max.	64	78	68.0		
Min.	28	39	39.5		
Range	38	39	28.5		
Extreme range 50					

	Sunrise.	2 P. M.
Rise . . .	28	12
Fall . . .	24	23

March, 1852.

DAY.	THERMOMETER. Sun-rise.	2 P. M.	Mean.	RAIN. Ins.	REMARKS ON THE WEATHER.
1	53	72	62.5	..	Fair.
2	48	56	52.0	..	Cloudy; windy.
3	49	68	58.5	..	Cloudy.
4	50	77	63.5	0.1	Cloudy; showers.
5	66	72	69.0	0.2	Cloudy; showers.
6	64	60	62.0	..	Fog; mist; cloudy.
7	54	70	62.0	..	Cloudy; fair.
8	56	78	67.0	..	Fair; clouds.
9	69	68	68.5	..	Cloudy.
10	53	70	61.5	0.4	Cloudy; rain at night.
11	60	72	66.0	0.3	Cloudy; rain at 3 P. M.
12	66	66	67.0	2.6	Cloudy; rain; thunder.
13	60	72	66.0	..	Fair.
14	54	71	62.5	..	Fair.
15	42	74	58.0	..	Fair.
16	54	78	66.0	..	Fair.
17	32	32	32.0	..	Cloudy; snow.
18	30	50	40.0	..	Fair. Vegetation killed.
19	28	58	43.0	..	Fair.
20	30	60	45.0	0.2	Cloudy; rain at night.
21	50	65	57.5	..	Cloudy; fair.
22	36	74	55.0	..	Fair.
23	42	74	58.0	..	Fair.
24	50	76	63.0	..	Fair.
25	54	90	72.0	..	Fair.
26	60	85	72.5	..	Fair.
27	60	76	68.0	..	Smoky.
28	56	86	71.0	..	Smoky.
29	70	85	77.5	1.0	Cloudy; thunder; rain at night.
30	62	68	65.0	..	Fair.
31	..	..	..	..	
Means	51.93	70.17	61.05	4.8	Greatest Rise and Fall of temperature in 24 hours.
Max.	70	90	77.5		
Min.	28	32	32.0		
Range	42	58	45.5		
Extreme range 62					

	Sunrise.	2 P. M.
Rise . . .	23	18
Fall . . .	22	46

April, 1852.

DAY.	THERMOMETER. Sun-rise.	2 P. M.	Mean.	RAIN. Ins.	REMARKS ON THE WEATHER.
1	42	72	57.0	..	Fair.
2	48	70	59.0	..	Fair.
3	60	72	66.0	0.5	Cloudy; showers.
4	70	78	74.0	..	Cloudy; showers.
5	50	52	51.0	..	Cloudy.
6	36	36	36.0	..	Fair.
7	44	70	57.0	..	Fair.
8	42	72	57.0	..	Fair.
9	42	76	59.0	..	Fair.
10	64	68	66.0	1.5	Cloudy; thunder; rain.
11	58	74	66.0	0.3	Fair; clouds; rain at night.
12	58	76	67.0	0.5	Fog; fair.
13	52	72	62.0	0.4	Cloudy; rain at night.
14	62	74	68.0	..	Cloudy; showers.
15	50	73	61.5	..	Fair.
16	60	76	68.0	..	Clouds; fair.
17	52	70	61.0	..	Clouds.
18	42	74	58.0	..	Fair.
19	52	58	55.0	0.1	Cloudy; rain.
20	43	62	52.5	..	Fair.
21	38	66	52.0	..	Fair.
22	40	78	59.0	..	Fair.
23	52	80	66.0	0.5	Cloudy; thunder; rain.
24	62	76	69.0	..	Rain; fair.
25	63	84	73.5	..	Cloudy; fair.
26	54	84	69.0	..	Fair.
27	42	80	61.0	..	
28	44	70	57.0	..	
29	60	80	70.0	..	Clouds.
30	74	90	82.0	..	Fair.
Means	51.87	72.10	61.98	3.8	Greatest Rise and Fall of temperature in 24 hours.
Max.	74	90	82.0		
Min.	36	36	36.0		
Range	38	54	46.0		
Extreme range 54					

	Sunrise.	2 P. M.
Rise . . .	22	34
Fall . . .	20	26

May, 1852.

DAY.	THERMOMETER. Sunrise.	THERMOMETER. 3 P. M.	THERMOMETER. Mean.	RAIN. Ins.	REMARKS ON THE WEATHER.
1	62	90	76.0	..	Fair.
2	74	88	81.0	..	Cloudy; fair.
3	70	84	77.0	..	Clouds; thunder.
4	70	84	77.0	..	Clouds; fair.
5	70	86	78.0	0.3	Clouds; thunder; rain at night.
6	68	67	67.5	0.4	Clouds; thunder; rain at night.
7	66	76	71.0	0.2	Clouds; rain.
8	68	78	73.0	..	Fair.
9	68	80	74.0	0.2	Cloudy; showers.
10	67	76	71.5	0.4	Cloudy; thunder; rain at night.
11	68	76	72.0	..	Cloudy.
12	68	76	72.0	..	Cloudy.
13	68	74	71.0	..	Cloudy.
14	70	86	78.0	..	Fog; fair.
15	66	84	75.0	..	Fair.
16	68	80	74.0	1.0	Cloudy; thunder; rain at night.
17	60	74	67.0	..	Fog; fair.
18	54	74	64.0	..	Fair.
19	57	70	63.5	..	Fair.
20	62	74	68.0	..	Cloudy; fair.
21	62	84	73.0	..	Cloudy; fair.
22	70	82	76.0	..	Cloudy; fair.
23	66	84	75.0	..	Fair; clouds; thunder.
24	66	84	75.0	0.3	Fog; clouds; shower at 2 P. M.
25	70	74	72.0	..	Cloudy; rain.
26	67	74	70.5	0.2	Cloudy; shower at 3 P. M.
27	68	82	75.0	..	Cloudy; fair.
28	66	84	75.0	..	Fair.
29	70	87	78.5	0.3	Fair; shower at 11 A. M.
30	74	85	79.5	..	Cloudy; fair.
31	70	86	78.0	..	Fair.
Means	66.87	80.10	73.48	3.3	
Max.	74	90	81.0		
Min.	54	67	63.5		
Range	20	23	17.5		
Extreme range 36					

Greatest Rise and Fall of temperature in 24 hours.

	Sunrise.	3 P. M.
Rise . . .	12	12
Fall . . .	12	19

June, 1852.

DAY.	THERMOMETER. Sunrise.	THERMOMETER. 3 P. M.	THERMOMETER. Mean.	RAIN. Ins.	REMARKS ON THE WEATHER.
1	66	88	77.0	..	Fair.
2	66	90	78.0	..	Fair.
3	66	90	78.0	..	Fair.
4	70	80	75.0	..	Cloudy; fair.
5	56	78	67.0	..	Fair.
6	56	78	67.0	..	Fair; clouds.
7	62	78	70.0	..	Fair.
8	56	78	67.0	..	Fair.
9	54	82	68.0	..	Fair.
10	60	82	71.0	..	Fair.
11	56	82	69.0	..	Fair.
12	62	86	74.0	..	Fair.
13	62	87	74.5	..	
14	70	83	76.5	..	Cloudy.
15	62	87	74.5	0.3	Cloudy; shower at night.
16	70	86	78.0	..	Cloudy.
17	74	86	80.0	..	Cloudy.
18	68	86	77.0	..	Fair.
19	74	86	80.0	..	Clouds.
20	72	80	76.0	1.0	Rain.
21	74	87	80.5	..	Fog; fair.
22	72	88	80.0	..	Cloudy.
23	78	86	82.0	1.2	Cloudy; thunder; rain at night.
24	76	74	75.0	..	Rain.
25	56	78	67.0	..	Fair.
26	56	79	67.5	..	Fair.
27	60	83	71.5	0.4	Fair; rain at night.
28	70	80	75.0	..	Rain; fair.
29	66	86	76.0	..	Fog.
30	70	91	80.5	..	Fair; cloudy.
Means	65.33	83.50	74.42	2.9	
Max.	78	91	82.0		
Min.	54	74	67.0		
Range	24	17	15.0		
Extreme range 37					

Greatest Rise and Fall of temperature in 24 hours.

	Sunrise.	3 P. M.
Rise . . .	10	7
Fall . . .	20	12

July, 1852.

DAY.	THERMOMETER. Sunrise.	THERMOMETER. 3 P. M.	THERMOMETER. Mean.	RAIN. Ins.	REMARKS ON THE WEATHER.
1	76	90	83.0	3.6	Cloudy; thunder; rain at 4 P. M.
2	72	80	76.0	4.0	Cloudy; thunder; rain.
3	66	76	71.0	5.0	Cloudy; rain.
4	70	86	78.0	0.4	Cloudy; rain.
5	70	88	79.0	..	Fair.
6	70	87	78.5	..	Fair.
7	76	88	82.0	..	Fair.
8	76	88	82.0	..	Fair.
9	75	82	78.5	0.8	Cloudy; rain at noon.
10	72	88	80.0	0.5	Cloudy; rain at 5 P. M.
11	70	90	80.0	..	Fair.
12	70	88	79.0	..	Fair.
13	72	90	81.0	0.1	Clouds; shower at 4 P. M.
14	72	81	76.5	..	Clouds.
15	72	86	79.0	..	Fog; clouds.
16	70	84	77.0	..	Clouds; thunder.
17	68	85	76.5	..	Fair.
18	65	85	75.0	..	Fair.
19	66	86	76.0	..	Fair.
20	66	82	74.0	..	Fair; clouds.
21	66	85	75.5	..	Fair; clouds.
22	70	86	78.0	..	Fair.
23	70	91	80.5	..	Fair.
24	70	88	79.0	..	Clouds; thunder.
25	70	82	76.0	0.7	Clouds; rain at 10 A. M.
26	72	88	80.0	..	Clouds; thunder.
27	70	91	80.5	..	Fair.
28	72	91	81.5	..	Fair.
29	72	92	82.0	..	Fair.
30	72	92	82.0	..	Fair.
31	72	88	80.0	..	Fair.
Means	70.65	86.58	78.61	15.1	
Max.	76	92	83.0		
Min.	65	76	71.0		
Range	11	16	12.0		
Extreme range 27					

Greatest Rise and Fall of temperature in 24 hours.

	Sunrise.	3 P. M.
Rise . . .	6	10
Fall . . .	6	10

August, 1852.

DAY.	THERMOMETER. Sunrise.	THERMOMETER. 3 P. M.	THERMOMETER. Mean.	RAIN. Ins.	REMARKS ON THE WEATHER.
1	70	86	78.0	..	Fair.
2	68	92	80.0	..	Clouds.
3	68	92	80.0	1.7	Clouds; rain at night.
4	72	87	79.5	..	Clouds; fair.
5	72	88	80.0	..	Fair.
6	68	88	78.0	..	Fair.
7	70	88	79.0	..	Fair.
8	70	88	79.0	..	Fair.
9	72	82	77.0	..	Cloudy; showers.
10	74	74	74.0	4.0	Thunder; rain.
11	68	83	75.5	..	Fair.
12	66	82	74.0	..	Fair.
13	60	84	72.0	..	Fair.
14	66	86	76.0	..	Fair.
15	70	86	78.0	..	Cloudy.
16	70	85	77.5	..	Cloudy; fair.
17	70	82	76.0	2.0	Cloudy; thunder; rain at night.
18	72	78	75.0	..	Cloudy; rain.
19	72	72	72.0	0.3	Cloudy; rain.
20	72	83	77.5	2.2	Cloudy; rain.
21	74	86	80.0	..	Cloudy; fair.
22	72	86	79.0	0.2	Cloudy; shower.
23	70	92	81.0	..	Fair; thunder.
24	72	90	81.0	1.3	Cloudy; thunder; rain.
25	72	86	79.0	..	Fog; fair.
26	72	88	80.0	0.1	Fair; shower at 1 P. M.
27	72	88	80.0	..	Fair.
28	66	84	75.0	..	Fair.
29	60	84	72.0	..	Fair.
30	68	88	78.0	..	Fair.
31	72	86	79.0	..	Cloudy.
Means	69.68	85.90	77.48	11.8	
Max.	74	92	81.0		
Min.	60	72	72.0		
Range	14	20	9.0		
Extreme range 32					

Greatest Rise and Fall of temperature in 24 hours.

	Sunrise.	3 P. M.
Rise . . .	8	11
Fall . . .	6	8

September, 1852.

DAY.	THERMOMETER. Sunrise.	THERMOMETER. 3 P. M.	THERMOMETER. Mean.	RAIN. Ins.	REMARKS ON THE WEATHER.
1	72	88	80.0	..	Fair.
2	74	80	77.0	0.5	Cloudy; rain.
3	68	82	75.0	..	Fair.
4	62	82	72.0	..	Fair.
5	62	80	71.0	..	Fair.
6	64	84	74.0	..	Fair.
7	66	84	75.0	0.2	Fair.
8	68	83	75.5	..	Fair.
9	65	85	75.0	..	Fair.
10	66	85	75.5	..	Fair.
11	70	86	78.0	..	Fair.
12	58	78	68.0	..	Fair.
13	56	80	68.0	..	Fair.
14	60	78	69.0	..	Clouds.
15	62	82	72.0	..	Fog; fair.
16	62	84	73.0	..	Fair.
17	66	84	75.0	..	Fair; clouds; rain at night.
18	72	78	75.0	2.5	Rain.
19	70	78	74.0	..	Rain.
20	70	74	72.0	..	Rain; fair.
21	52	74	63.0	..	Fair.
22	54	78	66.0	..	Fair.
23	64	84	74.0	..	Clouds.
24	74	84	79.0	0.2	Clouds; rain.
25	74	76	75.0	0.5	Clouds; rain.
26	58	74	66.0	..	Fair.
27	54	74	64.0	..	Fair.
28	66	79	72.5	..	Fair.
29	58	80	69.0	..	Fair.
30	62	78	70.0	..	Fair.
Means	64.30	80.53	72.42	3.9	
Max.	74	88	80.0		
Min.	52	74	63.0		
Range	22	14	17.0		

Extreme range 36

Greatest Rise and Fall of temperature in 24 hours.

	Sunrise.	3 P. M.
Rise . . .	12	6
Fall . . .	18	8

October, 1852.

DAY.	THERMOMETER. Sunrise.	THERMOMETER. 3 P. M.	THERMOMETER. Mean.	RAIN. Ins.	REMARKS ON THE WEATHER.
1	66	82	74.0	..	Fair; clouds.
2	78	80	79.0	..	Cloudy; mist.
3	74	82	78.0	..	Cloudy.
4	70	80	75.0	..	Cloudy.
5	70	81	75.5	..	Cloudy.
6	68	82	75.0	..	Cloudy.
7	70	84	77.0	0.2	Fair; clouds; shower at night.
8	72	74	73.0	0.6	Cloudy; rain.
9	62	66	64.0	..	Cloudy; fair.
10	50	72	61.0	..	Fair.
11	50	74	62.0	..	Fair.
12	60	60	60.0	..	Cloudy.
13	52	66	59.0	0.2	Rain.
14	49	74	61.5	..	Fair.
15	50	76	63.0	..	Fair.
16	54	78	66.0	..	Fair.
17	56	80	68.0	..	Fair.
18	56	80	68.0	..	Fair.
19	54	78	66.0	..	Fair.
20	54	78	66.0	..	Fair.
21	60	76	68.0	..	Clouds.
22	60	78	69.0	..	Fair; clouds.
23	62	78	70.0	..	Fog; fair.
24	56	74	65.0	..	Fog; fair.
25	60	70	65.0	0.1	Cloudy; rain.
26	66	76	71.0	..	Cloudy; fair.
27	64	65	64.5	..	Cloudy; rain.
28	60	66	63.0	1.3	Rain.
29	54	54	54.0	..	Cloudy.
30	50	62	56.0	..	Cloudy.
31	44	63	53.5	..	
Means	59.71	73.84	66.78	2.4	
Max.	78	84	79.0		
Min.	44	54	53.5		
Range	34	30	25.5		

Extreme range 40

Greatest Rise and Fall of temperature in 24 hours.

	Sunrise.	3 P. M.
Rise . . .	12	8
Fall . . .	12	14

November, 1852.

DAY.	THERMOMETER. Sunrise.	THERMOMETER. 2 P. M.	THERMOMETER. Mean.	RAIN. Ins.	REMARKS ON THE WEATHER.
1	56	68	62.0	..	Fair.
2	48	70	59.0	..	Cloudy.
3	60	72	66 0	..	Cloudy.
4	72	72	72.0	1.0	Cloudy; rain.
5	74	72	73.0	2.0	Rain.
6	54	56	55.0	..	Fair.
7	40	59	49.5	..	Fair.
8	40	66	53.0	..	Fair.
9	39	60	49.5	..	Fair.
10	38	64	51.0	..	Fair.
11	61	64	62.5	0.2	Rain; fair.
12	30	52	41.0	..	Fair; killing frost.
13	35	58	46.5	..	Fair.
14	36	58	47.0	..	Fair; cloudy.
15	30	58	44.0	..	Fair; cloudy.
16	46	56	51.0	1.3	Cloudy; rain.
17	48	52	50.0	0.2	Rain.
18	36	47	41.5	..	Cloudy.
19	30	52	41.0	..	Fair.
20	42	56	49.0	..	Cloudy.
21	44	48	46.0	1.6	Rain.
22	42	50	46.0	..	Cloudy; fair.
23	30	56	43.0	1.0	Fair; cl'dy; thunder; r'n at night.
24	50	61	55.5	..	Cloudy; fair.
25	44	52	48.0	0.4	Rain.
26	34	48	41.0	..	Fair.
27	28	57	42.5	..	Fair.
28	40	65	52.5	..	Fair.
29	54	68	61.0	..	Cloudy.
30	56	68	62.0	..	Cloudy; sprinkle.
Means	44.57	59.50	52.03	7.7	
Max.	74	72	73.0		
Min.	28	47	41.0		
Range	46	25	32.0		

Extreme range 44

Greatest Rise and Fall of temperature in 24 hours.

	Sunrise.	2 P. M.
Rise . . .	23	8
Fall . . .	31	16

December, 1852.

DAY.	THERMOMETER. Sunrise.	THERMOMETER. 2 P. M.	THERMOMETER. Mean.	RAIN. Ins.	REMARKS ON THE WEATHER.
1	50	66	58.0	..	Fair.
2	56	60	58.0	0.2	Rain.
3	48	58	53.0	..	Fair; clouds.
4	38	64	51.0	..	Fair.
5	44	70	57.0	..	Fair; cloudy.
6	67	74	70.5	0.1	Cloudy; thunder; hail from north
7	40	50	45.0	..	Fair. [breaking windows.
8	36	56	46.0	..	Fair.
9	32	54	43.0	..	Fair; cloudy.
10	28	54	41.0	..	Fair.
11	32	54	43.0	..	Fair; cloudy.
12	51	50	50.5	0.1	Cloudy; rain.
13	28	46	37.0	..	Fair.
14	38	46	42.0	..	Cloudy.
15	42	46	44.0	0.8	Cloudy; mist; thunder; rain at
16	64	56	55.0	..	Fair. [night.
17	26	50	38.0	..	Fair.
18	36	62	49.0	..	Fair.
19	58	73	65.5	..	Cloudy; fair.
20	68	78	73.0	..	Cloudy; fair.
21	32	36	34.0	..	Cloudy.
22	32	37	34.5	..	Cloudy; rain.
23	56	72	64.0	0.7	Fog; rain.
24	54	52	53.0	0.6	Cloudy; thunder; rain.
25	48	52	50.0	0.3	Cloudy; rain.
26	37	54	45.5	..	Cloudy; fair.
27	64	70	67.0	..	Cloudy; rain; fair.
28	25	42	33.5	..	Fair.
29	28	50	39.0	..	Fair.
30	44	58	51.0	0.2	Cloudy; rain.
31	64	51	57.5	..	Cloudy; fair.
Means	43.74	56.16	49.95	3.0	
Max.	68	78	73.0		
Min.	25	36	33.5		
Range	43	42	39.5		

Extreme range 53

Greatest Rise and Fall of temperature in 24 hours.

	Sunrise.	2 P. M.
Rise . . .	27	35
Fall . . .	39	42

January, 1853.

DAY.	THERMOMETER. Sun-rise.	THERMOMETER. 2 P. M.	THERMOMETER. Mean.	RAIN. Ins.	REMARKS ON THE WEATHER.
1	25	50	37.5	..	Fair.
2	32	56	44.0	..	Fair.
3	17	32	24.5	..	Fair.
4	19	42	30.5	..	Fair.
5	24	52	38.0	..	Fair.
6	26	60	43.0	..	Fair.
7	42	66	54.0	..	Fair.
8	56	60	58.0	0.1	Cloudy; sprinkle; rain.
9	50	68	59.0	..	Fog; fair.
10	54	60	57.0	..	Cloudy; fair.
11	52	54	53.0	..	Cloudy.
12	44	48	46.0	..	Cloudy; mist.
13	44	50	47.0	..	Cloudy; fair.
14	36	46	41.0	..	Fair.
15	38	50	44.0	..	Fair.
16	38	50	44.0	..	Fair.
17	27	52	39.5	..	Fair; clouds.
18	28	50	39.0	..	Fair.
19	40	50	45.0	..	Cloudy.
20	34	54	44.0	..	Cloudy.
21	35	42	38.5	1.0	Cloudy; sleet; rain.
22	40	42	41.0	..	Cloudy.
23	32	58	45.0	..	Fair.
24	40	56	48.0	..	Fair.
25	36	56	46.0	..	Fair.
26	36	46	41.0	..	Fair.
27	25	50	37.5	..	Fair.
28	30	58	44.0	..	Fair.
29	34	66	50.0	..	Fair.
30	38	66	52.0	..	Cloudy.
31	40	66	53.0	..	Cloudy; fair.
Means	35.87	53.42	44.65	1.1	Greatest Rise and Fall of temperature in 24 hours.
Max.	56	68	59.0		Sunrise. / 2 P. M.
Min.	17	32	24.5		Rise . . . 16 / 16
Range	39	36	34.5		Fall . . . 39 / 24
Extreme range 51					

February, 1853.

DAY.	THERMOMETER. Sun-rise.	THERMOMETER. 2 P. M.	THERMOMETER. Mean.	RAIN. Ins.	REMARKS ON THE WEATHER.
1	52	70	61.0	0.1	Cloudy; rain.
2	46	60	53.0	..	Fair.
3	46	63	54.5	..	Cloudy.
4	50	44	47.0	0.5	Cloudy; rain; snow. [snow.
5	30	28	29 0	..	Cl'dy; ground covered with frozen
6	19	32	25.5	..	Fair; icicles glittering from trees.
7	24	44	34.0	..	Fair; icicles glittering from trees.
8	30	44	37.0	..	Cloudy; fair.
9	32	46	39.0	..	Cloudy.
10	27	60	43.5	..	Fair.
11	36	65	50.5	..	Fair.
12	46	68	57.0	..	Cloudy; fair.
13	42	62	52.0	..	Fair.
14	46	48	47.0	..	Cloudy.
15	48	49	48.5	1.0	Cloudy; rain.
16	46	56	51.0	..	Fair.
17	32	62	47.0	..	Fair.
18	45	58	51.5	..	Cloudy; rain.
19	36	50	43.0	0.6	Cloudy; snow; fair.
20	32	50	41.0	..	Fair; clouds.
21	50	70	60.0	..	Fair.
22	56	38	47.0	1.2	Cloudy; rain; snow.
23	30	42	36.0	2.2	Fair; ground covered with snow,
24	30	53	41.5	..	Fair; sleighs running. [frozen.
25	30	66	48.0	..	Fair.
26	44	66	55.0	..	Cloudy.
27	60	76	68.0	..	Fair.
28	60	66	63.0	..	Fair; clouds.
Means	40.18	54.86	47.52	5.6	Greatest Rise and Fall of temperature in 24 hours.
Max.	60	76	68.0		Sunrise. / 2 P. M.
Min.	19	28	25.5		Rise . . . 18 / 20
Range	41	48	42.5		Fall . . . 26 / 32
Extreme range 57					

March, 1853.

DAY.	THERMOMETER. Sun-rise.	THERMOMETER. 2 P. M.	THERMOMETER. Mean.	RAIN. Ins.	REMARKS ON THE WEATHER.
1	32	66	49.0	..	Fair.
2	38	66	52.0	..	Fair.
3	42	50	46.0	..	Cloudy.
4	32	60	46.0	..	Fair.
5	48	61	54.5	..	Fair.
6	32	64	48.0	..	Fair.
7	48	76	62.0	0.5	Smoky; thunder; rain at night.
8	60	74	67.0	..	Rain; fair.
9	34	48	41.0	..	Cloudy.
10	42	44	43.0	0.6	Cloudy; rain.
11	44	60	52 0	..	Cloudy.
12	50	52	51.0	0.4	Cloudy; mist; rain.
13	44	41	42.5	1.2	Cloudy; rain.
14	38	48	43.0	..	Cloudy; fair.
15	30	54	42.0	..	Fair.
16	36	62	49.0	..	Cloudy.
17	55	68	61.5	0.4	Cloudy; rain.
18	42	66	54.0	..	Fair.
19	36	60	48.0	2.6	Fair; cl'dy; thunder; r'n at night.
20	52	62	57.0	0.3	Cloudy; thunder; rain.
21	56	64	60.0	2.4	Rain.
22	56	74	65.0	..	Cloudy; fair.
23	50	72	61.0	..	Fair.
24	48	74	61.0	..	Fair.
25	56	74	65.0	0.7	Cloudy; thunder; rain at night.
26	50	60	55.0	..	Cloudy; fair.
27	36	62	49.0	..	Fair.
28	36	68	52.0	..	Fair.
29	40	76	58.0	..	Fair.
30	50	78	64.0	..	Fair.
31	58	80	69.0	..	Fair; clouds.
Means	44.23	63.35	53.79	9.1	Greatest Rise and Fall of temperature in 24 hours.
Max.	60	80	69.0		Sunrise. / 2 P. M.
Min.	30	41	41.0		Rise . . . 19 / 16
Range	30	39	28.0		Fall . . . 28 / 26
Extreme range 50					

April, 1853.

DAY.	THERMOMETER. Sun-rise.	THERMOMETER. 2 P. M.	THERMOMETER. Mean.	RAIN. Ins.	REMARKS ON THE WEATHER.
1	60	82	71.0	..	Fair.
2	64	84	74.0	..	Smoky.
3	68	70	69.0	..	Smoky; sprinkle.
4	44	62	53.0	..	Fair.
5	40	76	58.0	..	Fair.
6	52	84	68.0	..	Fair.
7	54	80	67.0	..	Smoky; fair.
8	56	83	69.5	0.1	Fair; cl'dy; thunder; r'n at night.
9	60	62	61.0	0.4	Cloudy; thunder; rain.
10	50	54	52.0	0.6	Cloudy; rain.
11	50	76	63.0	..	Cloudy; fair.
12	56	80	68.0	..	Fair; clouds.
13	70	72	71.0	0.4	Cloudy; rain.
14	50	72	61.0	..	Fair.
15	50	56	53.0	0.6	Cloudy; rain.
16	56	66	61.0	0.7	Cloudy; rain.
17	48	64	56.0	..	Fair.
18	50	78	64.0	..	Fair.
19	58	75	66.5	..	Fair; cloudy.
20	65	84	74.5	..	Cloudy.
21	68	84	76.0	..	Cloudy; showers.
22	68	84	76.0	..	Fair; cloudy; showers.
23	70	80	75.0	0.7	Cloudy; sh'r; fair; thunder; rain
24	70	80	75.0	..	Cloudy. [at night.
25	45	70	57.5	..	Fair.
26	45	72	58.5	..	Fair; cloudy.
27	56	76	66.0	..	Clouds.
28	60	80	70.0	0.5	Clouds; shower at night.
29	66	80	73.0	..	Clouds.
30	66	80	73.0	..	Fog; fair.
Means	57.17	74.87	66.02	4.0	Greatest Rise and Fall of temperature in 24 hours.
Max.	70	84	76.0		Sunrise. / 2 P. M.
Min.	40	54	52.0		Rise . . . 14 / 22
Range	30	30	24.0		Fall . . . 25 / 21
Extreme range 44					

May, 1853.

DAY.	THERMOMETER. Sun-rise.	3 P. M.	Mean.	RAIN. Ins.	REMARKS ON THE WEATHER.
1	68	70	69.0	0.4	Cloudy; showers.
2	64	72	68.0	2.4	Cloudy; thunder; rain.
3	66	72	69.0	0.3	Cloudy; rain.
4	58	78	68.0	0.2	Cloudy; rain; fair.
5	62	83	72.5	. .	Cloudy; fair.
6	64	78	71.0	. .	Fair; clouds.
7	64	72	68.0	. .	Clouds.
8	66	74	70.0	. .	Fair.
9	52	82	67.0	. .	Fair.
10	52	63	57.5	. .	Cloudy; sprinkle.
11	52	80	66.0	. .	Cloudy; fair.
12	64	63	63.5	1.7	Cloudy; thunder; rain.
13	62	76	69.0	. .	Fog; cloudy.
14	68	84	76.0	. .	Cloudy.
15	66	84	75.0	. .	Fair.
16	68	83	75.5	. .	Fair.
17	68	85	76.5	. .	Fair.
18	70	84	77.0	. .	Fair.
19	62	72	67.0	. .	Cloudy; fair.
20	58	73	65.5	. .	Fair.
21	54	84	69.0	. .	Fair.
22	60	86	73.0	2.0	Fair; cl'dy; thunder; r'n at night.
23	64	74	69.0	. .	Cloudy.
24	54	76	65.0	. .	Fair.
25	60	68	64.0	. .	Cloudy; rain at night.
26	58	70	64.0	2.0	Cloudy; rain at night.
27	58	72	65.0	. .	Cloudy.
28	64	80	72.0	0.7	Cloudy; rain at night.
29	70	84	77.0	. .	Fair.
30	68	84	76.0	. .	Fog; fair.
31	66	84	75.0	. .	Fair.
Means	62.26	77.10	69.68	9.7	Greatest Rise and Fall of temperature in 24 hours.
Max.	70	86	77.0		
Min.	52	63	57.5		
Range	18	23	19.5		
Extreme range 84					

	Sunrise.	3 P. M.
Rise . . .	12	17
Fall . . .	14	19

June, 1853.

DAY.	THERMOMETER. Sun-rise.	3 P. M.	Mean.	RAIN. Ins.	REMARKS ON THE WEATHER.
1	68	89	78.5	. .	Fair; clouds.
2	72	88	80.0	. .	Cloudy.
3	70	90	80.0	. .	Fair.
4	74	86	80.0	. .	Fair; clouds.
5	70	88	79.0	. .	Fog; fair.
6	74	78	76.0	0.8	Cloudy; rain.
7	66	83	74.5	. .	Fair.
8	66	80	73.0	. .	Fair.
9	60	86	73.0	. .	Fair.
10	60	90	75.0	. .	Fair.
11	66	90	78.0	. .	Fair.
12	66	88	77.0	. .	Fair.
13	67	87	77.0	0.2	Fair; cloudy; rain at eve.
14	66	88	77.0	. .	Fair.
15	70	86	78.0	. .	Clouds; fair.
16	66	88	77.0	. .	Fair; clouds.
17	68	91	79.5	. .	Fair.
18	68	91	79.5	. .	Fair.
19	68	92	80.0	. .	Fair.
20	66	90	78.0	. .	Fair.
21	70	92	81.0	. .	Cloudy; shower.
22	78	88	83.0	. .	Cloudy.
23	78	80	79.0	0.6	Cloudy; rain.
24	64	76	70.0	. .	Fair; clouds.
25	58	82	70.0	. .	Fair.
26	60	80	70.0	. .	Fair.
27	68	90	79.0	. .	Fair.
28	70	94	82.0	. .	Fair.
29	72	92	82.0	. .	Fair.
30	74	92	83.0	. .	Fair.
Means	68.10	87.17	77.63	1.6	Greatest Rise and Fall of temperature in 24 hours.
Max.	78	94	83.0		
Min.	58	76	70.0		
Range	20	18	13.0		
Extreme range 36					

	Sunrise.	3 P. M.
Rise . . .	8	10
Fall . . .	14	10

July, 1853.

DAY.	THERMOMETER. Sun-rise.	3 P. M.	Mean.	RAIN. Ins.	REMARKS ON THE WEATHER.
1	74	92	83.0	. .	Fair.
2	74	82	78.0	0.1	Cloudy; rain.
3	74	84	79.0	. .	Cloudy; rain.
4	72	88	80.0	. .	Cloudy; fair.
5	72	80	76.0	0.5	Cloudy; rain.
6	72	82	77.0	0.3	Cloudy; rain.
7	70	88	79.0	. .	Fog; fair.
8	74	88	81.0	. .	Fog; fair.
9	74	84	79.0	2.7	Cloudy; thunder; rain.
10	74	80	77.0	. .	Cloudy.
11	76	88	82.0	1.4	Cloudy; thunder; rain.
12	72	90	81.0	. .	Fog; fair.
13	74	90	82.0	. .	Fog; fair; clouds.
14	74	90	82.0	. .	Fair.
15	74	93	83.5	. .	Cloudy.
16	76	86	81.0	0.6	Cloudy; thunder; rain.
17	72	90	81.0	. .	Fog; fair.
18	74	90	82.0	. .	Cloudy.
19	76	92	84.0	. .	Cloudy.
20	72	90	81.0	. .	Cloudy.
21	76	90	83.0	0.6	Cloudy; rain.
22	74	84	79.0	. .	Cloudy.
23	70	90	80.0	. .	Cloudy.
24	74	86	80.0	. .	Cloudy.
25	74	92	83.0	. .	Fair.
26	68	80	74.0	. .	Fair.
27	62	80	71.0	. .	Fair.
28	62	81	71.5	. .	Fair.
29	62	76	69.0	. .	Cloudy.
30	66	84	75.0	. .	Cloudy.
31	72	86	79.0	1.3	Cloudy; rain.
Means	71.94	86.32	79.13	7.5	Greatest Rise and Fall of temperature in 24 hours.
Max.	76	93	84.0		
Min.	62	76	69.0		
Range	14	17	15.0		
Extreme range 31					

	Sunrise.	3 P. M.
Rise . . .	6	8
Fall . . .	6	10

August, 1853.

DAY.	THERMOMETER. Sun-rise.	3 P. M.	Mean.	RAIN. Ins.	REMARKS ON THE WEATHER.
1	74	85	79.5	0.2	Cloudy; rain at 5 P. M.
2	74	84	79.0	. .	Cloudy; rain.
3	74	90	82.0	. .	Fair.
4	74	90	82.0	. .	Fair.
5	74	92	83.0	. .	Fair; clouds; rain at night.
6	74	88	81.0	0.5	Cloudy; rain.
7	76	88	82.0	. .	Cloudy.
8	72	88	80.0	. .	Cloudy.
9	73	90	81.5	. .	Fog; mist.
10	74	90	82.0	. .	Fair.
11	70	90	80.0	. .	Fair.
12	74	88	81.0	. .	Fair.
13	70	92	81.0	. .	Fair.
14	70	92	81.0	. .	Fair; clouds.
15	70	92	81.0	0.1	Fair; clouds; rain at night.
16	70	91	80.5	0.2	Cloudy; rain at 2 P. M.
17	70	91	80.5	. .	Fair.
18	71	91	81.0	. .	Fair.
19	74	94	84.0	. .	Fair.
20	74	94	84.0	. .	Fair.
21	74	94	84.0	. .	Fair.
22	74	96	85.0	. .	Fair.
23	74	95	84.5	. .	Fair.
24	76	90	83.0	. .	Clouds.
25	74	96	85.0	. .	Clouds.
26	70	90	80.0	. .	Clouds.
27	72	80	76.0	0.1	Clouds; rain.
28	64	82	73.0	. .	Fair.
29	68	90	79.0	. .	Fair.
30	70	92	81.0	. .	Fair; clouds; sprinkle.
31	70	93	81.5	. .	Clouds.
Means	72.19	90.26	81.23	1.1	Greatest Rise and Fall of temperature in 24 hours.
Max.	76	96	85.0		
Min.	64	80	73.0		
Range	12	16	12.0		
Extreme range 32					

	Sunrise.	3 P. M.
Rise . . .	4	8
Fall . . .	8	10

September, 1853.

DAY.	THERMOMETER. Sun-rise.	3 P. M.	Mean.	RAIN. Ins.	REMARKS ON THE WEATHER.
1	70	94	82.0	. .	Fair.
2	72	94	83.0	. .	Fair.
3	70	94	82.0	. .	Fair.
4	72	94	83.0	. .	Fair.
5	72	88	80.0	. .	Clouds.
6	70	89	79.5	. .	Fog; clouds.
7	70	80	75.0	. .	Clouds.
8	68	74	71.0	3.0	Cloudy; thunder; rain at night.
9	69	80	74.5	. .	Rain.
10	64	80	72.0	. .	Fair.
11	62	84	73.0	. .	Fair.
12	64	86	75.0	. .	Fair; clouds.
13	74	76	75.0	1.5	Cloudy; rain.
14	74	72	73.0	2.7	Rain.
15	68	86	77.0	. .	Cloudy.
16	72	86	79.0	. .	Fair; clouds.
17	74	84	79.0	. .	Clouds.
18	76	80	78.0	0.7	Cloudy; rain.
19	79	80	79.5	. .	Cloudy; fair.
20	62	80	71.0	. .	Fair.
21	56	72	64.0	. .	Fair.
22	50	72	61.0	. .	Fair.
23	50	72	61.0	. .	Fair.
24	51	77	64.0	. .	Fair.
25	50	78	64.0	. .	Fair.
26	55	80	67.5	. .	Fair.
27	58	80	69.0	. .	Fair.
28	58	80	69.0	. .	Fair.
29	58	82	70.0	. .	Fair.
30	68	79	73.5	0.1	Cloudy; rain at night.
Means	65.20	81.77	73.48	8.0	Greatest Rise and Fall of temperature in 24 hours.
Max.	79	94	83.0		
Min.	50	72	61.0		
Range	29	22	22.0		
Extreme range 44					

	Sunrise.	3 P. M.
Rise . . .	10	14
Fall . . .	17	10

October, 1853.

DAY.	THERMOMETER. Sun-rise.	3 P. M.	Mean.	RAIN. Ins.	REMARKS ON THE WEATHER.
1	68	76	72.0	0.1	Cloudy; rain; fair.
2	52	70	61.0	. .	Fair.
3	48	72	60.0	. .	Fair.
4	48	74	61.0	. .	Fair.
5	50	80	65.0	. .	Fair.
6	56	80	68.0	. .	Fair.
7	60	80	70.0	. .	Fair.
8	50	81	65.5	. .	Fair.
9	54	82	68 0	. .	Fair.
10	60	82	71.0	. .	Fair.
11	60	75	67.5	. .	Cloudy.
12	64	80	72.0	. .	Fog; fair.
13	64	76	70.0	. .	Cloudy.
14	66	70	68.0	0.7	Cloudy; rain.
15	53	67	60.0	. .	Cloudy; rain.
16	60	66	63.0	0.5	Cloudy; rain.
17	60	72	66.0	. .	Fair.
18	56	74	65.0	. .	Fair.
19	58	72	65.0	. .	Fair.
20	52	74	63.0	. .	Fair.
21	54	78	66.0	1.0	Fair; cl'dy; thunder; r'n at night.
22	48	62	55.0	. .	Fair.
23	48	53	50.5	. .	Cloudy.
24	35	56	45.5	. .	Cloudy.
25	36	62	49.0	. .	Fair.
26	60	66	63.0	0.5	Cloudy; rain.
27	43	50	46.5	. .	Cloudy.
28	34	62	48.0	. .	Fair; frost.
29	37	62	49.5	. .	Fair.
30	37	66	51.5	. .	Fair.
31	44	72	58.0	. .	Fair.
Means	52.10	70.71	61.40	2.8	Greatest Rise and Fall of temperature in 24 hours.
Max.	68	82	72.0		
Min.	34	50	45.5		
Range	34	32	26.5		
Extreme range 48					

	Sunrise.	3 P. M.
Rise . . .	24	12
Fall . . .	17	16

November, 1853.

DAY.	THERMOMETER. Sun-rise.	2 P. M.	Mean.	RAIN. Ins.	REMARKS ON THE WEATHER.
1	48	70	59.0	. .	Fair; clouds.
2	60	66	63.0	. .	Cloudy.
3	46	60	53.0	. .	Fair.
4	36	64	50.0	. .	Fair.
5	36	68	52.0	. .	Fair.
6	44	68	56.0	. .	Fair.
7	42	70	56.0	. .	Fair.
8	58	70	64.0	0.5	Cloudy; rain.
9	38	57	47.5	. .	Fair.
10	30	59	44.5	. .	Fair.
11	46	72	59.0	. .	Cloudy.
12	54	72	63.0	. .	Fair.
13	36	66	51.0	. .	Fair.
14	32	68	50 0	. .	Fair; killing frost.
15	56	74	65.0	. .	Cloudy.
16	67	76	71.5	. .	Cloudy; mist.
17	66	78	72.0	. .	Cloudy.
18	58	74	66.0	. .	Fair; clouds; sprinkle.
19	60	76	68 0	1.5	Cloudy; rain at night.
20	66	68	67.0	. .	Rain.
21	58	70	64.0	. .	Fair.
22	44	68	56.0	. .	Fair.
23	46	70	58.0	. .	Fair.
24	40	56	48.0	. .	Fair; cloudy.
25	48	52	50.0	. .	Cloudy.
26	46	54	50.0	. .	Cloudy.
27	52	72	62.0	. .	Fair; clouds.
28	61	70	65.5	0.5	Cloudy; rain.
29	54	64	59.0	. .	Fair.
30	40	60	50.0	. .	Fair.
Means	48.93	67.07	58.00	2.5	Greatest Rise and Fall of temperature in 24 hours.
Max.	67	78	72.0		
Min.	30	52	44.5		
Range	37	26	27.5		
Extreme range 48					

	Sunrise.	2 P. M.
Rise . . .	24	18
Fall . . .	20	14

December, 1853.

DAY.	THERMOMETER. Sun-rise	2 P. M.	Mean.	RAIN. Ins.	REMARKS ON THE WEATHER.
1	32	68	50.0	. .	Fair.
2	39	68	53.5	. .	Fair.
3	40	56	48.0	. .	Fair.
4	35	70	52.5	. .	Fair.
5	54	72	63.0	. .	Fair.
6	50	72	61.0	. .	Fair.
7	52	42	47.0	0.7	Cloudy; thunder; rain.
8	34	42	38.0	. .	Fair.
9	26	54	40.0	. .	Fair.
10	32	54	43.0	. .	Fair.
11	44	54	49.0	. .	Fair; cloudy.
12	34	62	48.0	. .	Fair.
13	34	54	44.0	0.4	Fair; cloudy; rain at night.
14	44	56	50.0	. .	Cloudy.
15	46	60	53.0	. .	Cloudy.
16	50	54	52.0	0.1	Cloudy; rain.
17	40	50	45.0	. .	Cloudy; windy.
18	29	54	41.5	. .	Fair.
19	28	40	34.0	. .	Fair.
20	22	40	31.0	. .	Cloudy; sleet.
21	32	40	36.0	. .	Cloudy; ground covered with ice.
22	40	48	44.0	0.4	Mist; fog; rain at night.
23	40	39	39.5	. .	Cloudy; rain and sleet at night.
24	28	37	32.5	. .	Snow—2.5 inches.
25	32	40	36.0	0.6	Cloudy; snow.
26	34	50	42.0	. .	Fair.
27	40	57	48.5	. .	Cloudy.
28	38	54	46.0	. .	Fair.
29	29	57	43.0	. .	Fair.
30	42	54	48.0	. .	Fair.
31	. .	. .	. .	. .	
Means	37.33	53.27	45.30	2.2	Greatest Rise and Fall of temperature in 24 hours.
Max.	54	72	63.0		
Min.	22	37	31.0		
Range	32	35	32.0		
Extreme range 50					

	Sunrise.	2 P. M.
Rise . . .	19	14
Fall . . .	18	30

January, 1854.

DAY.	THERMOMETER. Sunrise.	THERMOMETER. 2 P. M.	THERMOMETER. Mean.	RAIN. Ins.	REMARKS ON THE WEATHER.
1	32	56	44.0	..	Fair.
2	32	66	49.0	..	Fair.
3	46	67	56.5	..	Fair.
4	34	70	52.0	..	Fair.
5	62	68	65.0	..	Clouds.
6	23	30	26.5	..	Fair.
7	24	30	27.0	..	Cloudy.
8	28	38	33.0	0.1	Cloudy; snow; sleet; ground co-
9	29	44	36.5	..	Cloudy; fair. [vered.
10	36	39	37.5	2.0	Cloudy; rain at night; thunder.
11	40	41	40.5	..	Cloudy.
12	26	48	37.0	..	Fair.
13	28	50	39.0	..	Fair.
14	26	44	35.0	..	Fair.
15	38	70	54.0	..	Cloudy; fair.
16	64	50	57.0	0.6	Cloudy; rain.
17	32	40	36.0	..	Cloudy.
18	39	45	42.0	..	Cloudy; rain at night.
19	40	64	52.0	0.5	Rain.
20	68	67	67.5	0.1	Fair; clouds; rain.
21	11	25	18.0	..	Fair.
22	10	38	24.0	..	Fair.
23	24	36	30.0	..	Fair; cloudy.
24	24	36	30.0	..	Cloudy; sleet.
25	36	46	41.0	0.3	Rain; sleet.
26	59	70	64.5	..	Fog; cloudy.
27	40	50	45.0	..	Cloudy.
28	22	46	34.0	..	Fair.
29	26	57	41.5	..	Clouds; fair.
30	30	60	45.0	..	Fair.
31	36	66	51.0	..	
Means	34.36	50.23	42.29	3.6	Greatest Rise and Fall of temperature in 24 hours.
Max.	68	70	67.5		
Min.	10	25	18.0		
Range	58	45	49.5		
Extreme range 60					

	Sunrise.	2 P. M.
Rise . . .	28	26
Fall . . .	57	42

February, 1854.

DAY.	THERMOMETER. Sunrise.	THERMOMETER. 2 P. M.	THERMOMETER. Mean.	RAIN. Ins.	REMARKS ON THE WEATHER.
1	42	70	56.0	..	Fair.
2	54	55	54.5	..	Cloudy.
3	25	44	34.5	..	Fair.
4	22	56	39.0	..	Fair.
5	37	60	48.5	..	Smoky.
6	49	66	57.5	..	Cloudy.
7	56	68	62.0	0.5	Cloudy; thunder; rain at night.
8	52	60	56.0	..	Cloudy.
9	30	50	40.0	..	Fair.
10	36	68	52.0	..	Fair.
11	36	65	50.5	..	Fair.
12	58	69	63.5	..	Cloudy.
13	64	74	69.0	..	Cloudy.
14	40	60	50.0	..	Cloudy.
15	40	44	42.0	..	Cloudy.
16	21	50	35.5	..	Fair.
17	22	56	39.0	..	Fair.
18	32	56	44.0	..	Smoky.
19	45	54	49.5	1.0	Cloudy; rain.
20	48	54	51.0	..	Cloudy.
21	32	60	46.0	..	Fair.
22	36	60	48.0	..	Fair.
23	36	58	47.0	..	Fair.
24	36	60	48.0	..	Smoky.
25	50	49	49.5	1.2	Cloudy; rain.
26	46	58	52.0	..	Cloudy; fair.
27	30	66	48.0	..	Fair.
28	46	72	59.0	..	Fair.
Means	40.04	59.36	49.70	2.7	Greatest Rise and Fall of temperature in 24 hours.
Max.	64	74	69.0		
Min.	21	44	34.5		
Range	43	30	34.5		
Extreme range 53					

	Sunrise.	2 P. M.
Rise . . .	22	18
Fall . . .	29	16

March, 1854.

DAY.	THERMOMETER. Sunrise.	THERMOMETER. 2 P. M.	THERMOMETER. Mean.	RAIN. Ins.	REMARKS ON THE WEATHER.
1	62	74	68.0	0.3	Cloudy; rain.
2	66	68	67.0	..	Cloudy; fair.
3	36	60	48.0	..	Fair; cloudy.
4	46	68	57.0	..	Fog; cloudy; fair.
5	36	72	54.0	..	Fair.
6	58	68	63.0	..	Cloudy; rain.
7	64	68	66.0	0.7	Cloudy; rain.
8	64	71	67.5	2.0	Cloudy; rain.
9	63	60	61.5	0.8	Cloudy; rain.
10	46	56	51.0	..	Cloudy; fair.
11	32	62	47.0	..	Fair.
12	36	68	52.0	..	Fair.
13	56	72	64.0	..	Cloudy.
14	64	75	69.5	..	Fog; cloudy.
15	66	78	72.0	..	Cloudy.
16	66	86	76.0	..	Fair.
17	66	87	76.5	..	Fair.
18	62	68	65.0	..	Fair; smoky.
19	50	46	48.0	..	Cloudy.
20	46	60	53.0	..	Cloudy.
21	52	66	59.0	0.1	Cloudy; rain.
22	58	80	69.0	..	Fog; fair.
23	54	74	64.0	..	Cloudy.
24	50	80	65.0	..	Fair.
25	50	58	54.0	..	Fair.
26	38	58	48.0	..	Fair.
27	34	68	51.0	..	Smoky. [windows broken.
28	42	78	60.0	..	Cloudy; thunder; rain; and hail;
29	58	84	71.0	2.0	Fog; cloudy; thunder.
30	60	84	72.0	..	
31	..	..	..	..	
Means	52.70	69.90	61.30	5.9	Greatest Rise and Fall of temperature in 24 hours.
Max.	66	87	76.5		
Min.	32	46	47.0		
Range	34	41	29.5		
Extreme range 55					

	Sunrise.	2 P. M.
Rise . . .	22	14
Fall . . .	30	22

April, 1854.

DAY.	THERMOMETER. Sunrise.	THERMOMETER. 2 P. M.	THERMOMETER. Mean.	RAIN. Ins.	REMARKS ON THE WEATHER.
1	34	60	47.0	..	Fair.
2	34	60	47.0	..	Fair.
3	44	72	58.0	..	Fair.
4	58	72	65.0	1.0	Cloudy; rain at night.
5	62	72	67.0	..	Cloudy; fair.
6	54	74	64.0	..	Fog; fair.
7	54	82	68.0	..	Fair.
8	61	80	70.5	0.3	Cloudy; rain at night.
9	54	68	61.0	..	Fair.
10	44	65	54.5	..	Fair; cloudy.
11	50	72	61.0	1.3	Cloudy; thunder; rain at night.
12	54	78	66.0	..	Rain; fair.
13	66	76	71.0	..	Cloudy; fair.
14	65	76	70.5	..	Cloudy; fair.
15	52	60	56.0	..	Cloudy.
16	42	64	53.0	..	Fair.
17	36	68	52.0	..	Fair.
18	44	70	57.0	..	Clouds.
19	52	80	66.0	..	Cloudy; fair.
20	60	82	71.0	..	Fair.
21	66	81	73.5	..	Cloudy.
22	62	84	73.0	..	Cloudy; fair.
23	66	82	74.0	..	Cloudy; fair.
24	64	78	71.0	..	Cloudy; showers at night.
25	70	88	79.0	..	Cloudy; fair.
26	72	86	79.0	0.5	Cl'ds; fair; thunder; rain at night.
27	66	72	69.0	..	Fair.
28	44	64	54.0	..	Fair.
29	38	64	51.0	..	Fair.
30	44	74	59.0	..	Fair.
Means	53.73	73.47	63.60	3.1	Greatest Rise and Fall of temperature in 24 hours.
Max.	72	88	79.0		
Min.	34	60	47.0		
Range	38	28	32.0		
Extreme range 54					

	Sunrise.	2 P. M.
Rise . . .	14	12
Fall . . .	22	16

May, 1854.

DAY.	THERMOMETER. Sun-rise.	3 P. M.	Mean.	RAIN. Ins.	REMARKS ON THE WEATHER.
1	46	76	61.0	..	Fair.
2	54	78	66.0	..	Fair.
3	56	76	66.0	..	Cloudy.
4	58	76	67.0	0.1	Cloudy; rain.
5	60	76	68.0	..	Cloudy; rain.
6	61	76	68.5	1.0	Cloudy; rain; fair.
7	58	81	69.5	..	Fog; fair.
8	60	80	70.0	..	Fair.
9	70	80	75.0	3.1	Cloudy; thunder; rain at night.
10	66	76	71.0	..	Cloudy.
11	58	78	68.0	..	Fair.
12	68	74	71.0	2.0	Cloudy; rain.
13	68	80	74.0	..	Cloudy; rain.
14	64	80	72.0	..	Fair
15	60	84	72.0	..	Fair.
16	74	80	77.0	0.5	Cloudy; showers.
17	64	78	71.0	..	Fair.
18	54	80	67.0	..	Fair.
19	54	85	69.5	..	Fair.
20	62	84	73.0	..	Fair; cl'dy; r'n at night; thunder.
21	66	80	73.0	1.5	Fog; cloudy; rain at night.
22	64	70	67.0	3.5	Cloudy; rain.
23	67	76	71.5	0.6	Cloudy; rain.
24	66	82	74.0	0.6	Cloudy; rain.
25	66	74	70.0	0.7	Cloudy; rain. [at night.
26	66	76	71.0	0.5	Fog; fair; eclipse of the sun; rain
27	70	80	75.0	0.4	Fog; cloudy; rain at 10 A. M.
28	70	82	76.0	0.1	Cloudy; thunder; rain.
29	66	86	76.0	..	Cloudy; fair.
30	76	80	78.0	1.4	Cloudy; thunder; rain at night.
31	68	84	76.0	..	Cloudy; fair.
Means	63.23	78.97	71.10	16.0	Greatest Rise and Fall of temperature in 24 hours.
Max.	76	86	78.0		
Min.	46	70	61.0		
Range	30	16	17.0		
Extreme range 40					

	Sunrise.	3 P. M.
Rise . . .	14	6
Fall . . .	10	10

June, 1854.

DAY.	THERMOMETER. Sun-rise.	3 P. M.	Mean.	RAIN. Ins.	REMARKS ON THE WEATHER.
1	70	84	77.0	..	Fog; fair.
2	64	75	69.5	..	Fair; clouds.
3	62	78	70.0	..	Fog; fair.
4	62	70	66.0	..	Clouds.
5	68	82	75.0	..	Clouds; fair.
6	66	86	76.0	..	Fair; clouds; thunder.
7	70	86	78.0	..	Fair.
8	62	80	71.0	0.2	Cloudy; rain; fair.
9	62	76	69.0	1.5	Cloudy; rain at night.
10	64	80	72.0	..	Cloudy.
11	66	80	73.0	..	Fog; fair.
12	70	78	74.0	0.4	Cloudy; showers.
13	72	82	77.0	..	Cloudy; fair.
14	70	84	77.0	..	Fog; fair.
15	74	76	75.0	0.8	Cloudy; rain.
16	74	88	81.0	..	Cloudy; rain.
17	76	90	83.0	..	Cloudy; fair.
18	74	90	82.0	..	Fair.
19	74	90	82.0	..	Fair.
20	76	90	83.0	0.2	Fair; shower at night.
21	70	88	79.0	..	Fog; fair.
22	69	86	77.5	..	Fair.
23	64	86	75.0	..	Fair.
24	70	92	81.0	..	Fair.
25	72	94	83.0	..	Fair.
26	76	92	84.0	..	Fair.
27	74	94	84.0	..	Fair.
28	74	94	84.0	..	Fair.
29	74	93	83.5	..	Fair.
30	70	94	82.0	..	Fair.
Means	69.63	85.27	77.45	3.1	Greatest Rise and Fall of temperature in 24 hours.
Max.	76	94	84.0		
Min.	62	70	66.0		
Range	14	24	18.0		
Extreme range 32					

	Sunrise.	3 P. M.
Rise . . .	6	12
Fall . . .	8	8

July, 1854.

DAY.	THERMOMETER. Sun-rise.	3 P. M.	Mean.	RAIN. Ins.	REMARKS ON THE WEATHER.
1	73	93	83.0	..	Fair; showers.
2	73	94	83.5	..	Fair.
3	76	94	85.0	0.1	Fair; shower at eve.
4	74	92	83.0	..	Fair.
5	74	94	84.0	..	Fog; fair.
6	74	92	83.0	..	Fair.
7	74	93	83.5	..	Fair.
8	74	94	84.0	..	Fair.
9	74	76	75.0	1.0	Cloudy; thunder; rain.
10	72	81	76.5	..	Cloudy.
11	68	84	76.0	..	Fair.
12	62	88	75.0	..	Fair.
13	64	88	76.0	..	Fair. [P. M.
14	72	78	75.0	0.4	Fair; cloudy; shower from S. at 2
15	74	86	80.0	0.3	Cloudy; fair; shower from S. at 2
16	74	86	80.0	..	Fog; fair. [P. M.
17	74	90	82.0	..	Fair.
18	76	94	85.0	0.5	Fair; shower from S. at 4 P. M.
19	74	92	83.0	..	Fog; fair.
20	74	92	83.0	..	Fair; shower from S. E. at 2 P. M.
21	74	92	83.0	..	Fair.
22	72	94	83.0	..	Fair.
23	72	94	83.0	..	Fair.
24	74	96	85.0	..	Fair.
25	76	97	86.5	..	Fair.
26	76	88	82.0	..	Fair.
27	72	92	82.0	..	Fair.
28	72	93	82.5	..	Fair.
29	76	95	85.5	..	Fair.
30	74	95	84.5	..	Fair.
31	76	92	84.0	..	Fair.
Means	73.03	90.61	81.82	2.3	Greatest Rise and Fall of temperature in 24 hours.
Max.	76	97	86.5		
Min.	62	76	75.0		
Range	14	21.	11.5		
Extreme range 35					

	Sunrise.	3 P. M.
Rise . . .	8	8
Fall . . .	6	18

August, 1854.

DAY.	THERMOMETER. Sun-rise.	3 P. M.	Mean.	RAIN. Ins.	REMARKS ON THE WEATHER.
1	74	95	84.5	..	Fair.
2	74	96	85.0	..	Fair.
3	74	96	85.0	..	Fair.
4	74	96	85.0	..	Fair; smoky; thunder.
5	74	96	85.0	0.1	Clouds; shower at 4 P. M.
6	72	95	83.5	..	Clouds; thunder.
7	74	84	79.0	..	Clouds; shower.
8	74	92	83.0	..	Fog; fair.
9	78	94	86.0	..	Clouds; fair.
10	78	94	86.0	..	Hazy; smoky.
11	78	93	85.5	..	Fair.
12	78	92	85.0	..	Fair.
13	78	94	86.0	..	Fair.
14	78	92	85.0	..	Fair.
15	80	92	86.0	..	Fair.
16	78	84	81.0	..	Fair; cloudy.
17	78	80	79.0	0.5	Cloudy; rain.
18	74	76	75.0	2.1	Cloudy; rain.
19	74	83	78.5	..	Cloudy.
20	72	85	78.5	..	Fog; fair; clouds.
21	72	86	79.0	..	Fair.
22	72	86	79 0	..	Fair.
23	72	86	79.0	..	Cloudy; fair.
24	72	86	79.0	0.5	Fair; clouds; rain.
25	76	82	79.0	..	Cloudy; rain.
26	72	86	79.0	..	Fair.
27	72	88	80.0	..	Fair.
28	74	89	81.5	..	Fair.
29	70	90	80.0	..	Fair.
30	78	90	84.0	..	Fair.
31	76	88	82.0	0.2	Fair; shower at 2 P. M.
Means	74.84	89.22	82.03	3.4	Greatest Rise and Fall of temperature in 24 hours.
Max.	80	96	86.0		
Min.	70	76	75.0		
Range	10	20	11.0		
Extreme range 26					

	Sunrise.	3 P. M.
Rise . . .	8	8
Fall . . .	4	11

September, 1854.

DAY.	THERMOMETER. Sunrise.	THERMOMETER. 3 P. M.	THERMOMETER. Mean.	RAIN. Ins.	REMARKS ON THE WEATHER.
1	78	85	81.5	..	Fair.
2	74	88	81.0	..	Fair.
3	72	84	78.0	..	Fair; clouds.
4	72	88	80.0	..	Fair.
5	72	86	79.0	..	Fair; clouds.
6	72	87	79.5	..	Fair; clouds.
7	74	90	82.0	..	Fair.
8	72	90	81.0	..	Fair.
9	74	93	83.5	..	Fair.
10	74	92	83.0	..	Fair.
11	74	92	83.0	..	Fair.
12	74	90	82.0	..	Fair; clouds; sprinkle.
13	74	90	82.0	..	Fair.
14	72	86	79.0	..	Fair; clouds; sprinkle.
15	72	84	78.0	..	Fair.
16	62	86	74.0	..	Fair.
17	66	86	76.0	..	Fair.
18	72	74	73.0	2.5	Cloudy; rain.
19	72	70	71.0	..	Cloudy; rain.
20	70	68	69.0	..	Cloudy.
21	60	76	68.0	..	Fair.
22	64	76	70.0	..	Cloudy.
23	70	79	74.5	..	Cloudy; rain.
24	74	82	78.0	0.8	Cloudy; rain.
25	72	75	73.5	0.1	Cloudy; rain.
26	70	76	73.0	..	Fog; rain.
27	69	80	74.5	3.4	Rain.
28	72	84	78.0	1.5	Rain.
29	70	84	77.0	..	Fair; clouds.
30	71	82	76.5	..	Fair; clouds.
Means	71.13	83.43	77.28	8.3	
Max.	78	93	83.5		
Min.	60	68	68.0		
Range	18	25	15.5		
Extreme range 33					

Greatest Rise and Fall of temperature in 24 hours.

	Sunrise.	3 P. M.
Rise . . .	6	8
Fall . . .	10	12

October, 1854.

DAY.	THERMOMETER. Sunrise.	THERMOMETER. 3 P. M.	THERMOMETER. Mean.	RAIN. Ins.	REMARKS ON THE WEATHER.
1	72	84	78.0	0.2	Clouds; shower at noon.
2	72	84	78.0	..	Fair.
3	72	87	79.5	..	Fair; clouds.
4	54	72	63.0	..	Fair.
5	48	74	61.0	..	Fair.
6	50	76	63.0	..	Fair.
7	52	76	64.0	..	Fair.
8	52	76	64.0	..	Fair.
9	52	76	64.0	..	Fair; clouds.
10	60	79	69.5	..	Fair.
11	64	84	74.0	0.1	Fair; clouds; sh'r at 2 P. M. and at night.
12	74	81	77.5	..	Cloudy.
13	74	82	78.0	..	Cloudy; rain.
14	74	84	79.0	..	Cloudy.
15	66	60	63.0	2.0	Cloudy; rain.
16	62	72	67.0	..	Cloudy; fair.
17	50	68	59.0	..	Fair.
18	56	71	63.5	..	Fair.
19	56	72	64.0	..	Fair.
20	60	74	67.0	..	Cloudy.
21	56	78	67.0	..	Fair.
22	62	72	67.0	..	Cloudy.
23	56	66	61.0	..	Fog; cloudy.
24	48	63	55.5	..	Cloudy.
25	57	66	61.5	..	Fog; cloudy.
26	50	72	61.0	..	Fair.
27	50	75	62.5	..	Fair.
28	62	68	65.0	..	Cloudy; fair.
29	56	64	60.0	1.6	Fair; cloudy; rain.
30	58	70	64.0	0.1	Fog; cloudy; rain.
31	52	76	64.0	..	Fair.
Means	58.94	74.26	66.60	4.0	
Max.	74	87	79.5		
Min.	48	60	55.5		
Range	26	27	24.0		
Extreme range 39					

Greatest Rise and Fall of temperature in 24 hours.

	Sunrise.	3 P. M.
Rise . . .	12	12
Fall . . .	18	24

November, 1854.

DAY.	THERMOMETER. Sunrise.	THERMOMETER. 2 P. M.	THERMOMETER. Mean.	RAIN. Ins.	REMARKS ON THE WEATHER.
1	50	70	63.0	..	Fair.
2	52	69	60.5	..	Fair.
3	56	64	60.0	..	Cloudy; rain.
4	60	57	58.5	0.2	Cloudy; rain.
5	37	50	43.5	..	Fair.
6	42	50	46.0	..	Fair.
7	46	74	60.0	..	Fair.
8	48	76	62.0	..	Fair.
9	52	66	59.0	..	Fair.
10	60	64	62.0	0.2	Fair; cloudy; rain at night.
11	44	64	54.0	..	Fair; cloudy.
12	34	56	45.0	..	Clouds; north wind.
13	26	54	40.0	..	Fair; killing frost.
14	30	64	47.0	..	Fair.
15	46	74	60.0	..	Fair.
16	36	64	50.0	..	Fair.
17	38	70	54.0	..	Fair.
18	40	52	46.0	..	Fair; north wind.
19	25	52	38.5	..	Fair.
20	32	71	51.5	..	Fair.
21	66	66	66.0	..	Cloudy.
22	50	66	58.0	0.2	Cloudy; fair; cloudy; r'n at night.
23	62	66	64.0	0.8	Cloudy; rain.
24	48	56	52.0	..	Fair.
25	44	44	44.0	..	Cloudy.
26	38	46	42.0	..	Fair.
27	27	52	39.5	..	Fair.
28	28	60	44.0	..	Fair.
29	32	70	51.0	..	Fair.
30	50	68	59.0	0.3	Cloudy; rain at night.
Means	43.50	61.85	52.67	1.7	
Max.	66	76	66.0		
Min.	25	44	38.5		
Range	41	32	27.5		
Extreme range 51					

Greatest Rise and Fall of temperature in 24 hours.

	Sunrise.	2 P. M.
Rise . . .	34	24
Fall . . .	23	18

December, 1854.

DAY.	THERMOMETER. Sunrise.	THERMOMETER. 2 P. M.	THERMOMETER. Mean.	RAIN. Ins.	REMARKS ON THE WEATHER.
1	62	60	61.0	..	Cloudy.
2	52	66	59.0	..	Cloudy.
3	42	58	50.0	..	Fair; windy.
4	36	44	40.0	..	Cloudy; snow at night.
5	24	38	31.0	..	Fair; ground covered with snow.
6	24	48	36.0	..	Fair.
7	30	56	43.0	..	Fair.
8	34	56	45.0	..	Fair.
9	38	64	51.0	1.0	Cloudy; rain at night.
10	54	54	54.0	0.1	Rain.
11	32	52	42.0	..	Fair.
12	28	54	41.0	..	Fair.
13	..	..	..	..	
14	34	56	45.0	..	Fair.
15	44	62	53.0	..	Fair.
16	36	62	49.0	..	Fair.
17	40	56	48.0	..	Fair.
18	26	44	35.0	..	Cloudy.
19	28	42	35.0	..	Fair.
20	20	45	32.5	..	Fair.
21	30	57	43.5	..	Fair.
22	38	61	49.5	..	Cloudy.
23	56	56	56.0	2.7	Cloudy; rain.
24	55	62	58.5	..	Cloudy; rain.
25	57	58	57.5	1.3	Cloudy; rain.
26	48	60	54.0	..	Cloudy; rain; fog; fair.
27	38	68	53.0	..	Fair.
28	58	53	55.5	..	Fair; windy.
29	32	58	45.0	..	Fair.
30	34	60	47.0	..	Fair.
31	40	68	54.0	..	Fair.
Means	39.00	55.93	47.47	5.1	
Max.	62	68	61.0		
Min.	20	38	31.0		
Range	42	30	30.0		
Extreme range 48					

Greatest Rise and Fall of temperature in 24 hours.

	Sunrise.	2 P. M.
Rise . . .	18	12
Fall . . .	26	14

January, 1855.

DAY.	THERMOMETER. Sun-rise.	2 P. M.	Mean.	RAIN. Ins.	REMARKS ON THE WEATHER.
1	56	58	57.0	..	Clouds.
2	62	72	67.0	..	Clouds; fair.
3	62	60	61.0	0.8	Clouds; rain.
4	30	56	43.0	..	Clouds; rain.
5	42	52	47.0	..	Clouds; rain.
6	64	57	60.5	2.8	Clouds; rain.
7	34	42	38.0	..	Clouds.
8	34	39	36.5	..	Clouds.
9	41	48	44.5	0.8	Mist; rain.
10	48	58	53.0	..	Mist; rain.
11	58	68	63.0	..	Mist; rain.
12	58	74	66.0	..	Cloudy; fair.
13	48	52	50.0	..	Fair; windy.
14	28	50	39.0	..	Fair.
15	29	58	43.5	..	Fair.
16	32	62	47.0	..	Fair.
17	32	66	49.0	..	Fair.
18	34	66	50.0	..	Fair.
19	52	68	60.0	..	Fair; clouds.
20	52	70	61.0	..	Cloudy; fair.
21	28	32	30.0	..	Fair; snow.
22	20	44	32.0	..	Fair.
23	38	56	47.0	..	Clouds.
24	36	64	50.0	..	Smoky.
25	46	66	56.0	..	Smoky.
26	28	43	35.5	..	Fair; wind; clouds; snow-flakes.
27	35	58	46.5	..	Fair.
28	28	42	35.0	..	Fair.
29	19	34	26.5	..	Fair.
30	12	33	22.5	..	Fair.
31	14	43	28.5	..	Fair.
Means	38.71	54.55	46.63	4.4	Greatest Rise and Fall of temperature in 24 hours.
Max.	64	74	67.0		
Min.	12	32	22.5		
Range	52	42	44.5		

Extreme range 62

	Sunrise.	2 P. M.
Rise . . .	22	15
Fall . . .	32	38

February, 1855.

DAY.	THERMOMETER. Sun-rise.	2 P. M.	Mean.	RAIN. Ins.	REMARKS ON THE WEATHER.
1	20	53	36.5	..	Fair.
2	26	56	41.0	..	Fair.
3	30	40	35.0	..	Smoky.
4	24	64	44.0	..	Smoky.
5	48	72	60.0	..	Smoky.
6	42	77	59.5	..	Smoky; shower at night.
7	58	72	65.0	..	Smoky.
8	50	66	58.0	..	Smoky.
9	34	53	43.5	..	Fair.
10	32	58	45.0	..	Smoky.
11	30	65	47.5	..	Smoky.
12	58	64	61.0	0.8	Cloudy; thunder; rain and hail at noon.
13	38	60	49.0	..	Fair.
14	31	60	45.5	..	Fair; clouds.
15	34	50	42.0	..	Fair; smoky.
16	26	56	41.0	..	Smoky.
17	28	60	44.0	..	Smoky.
18	42	52	47.0	..	Cloudy.
19	39	53	46.0	0.1	Cloudy; rain; fair.
20	27	58	42.5	..	Fair.
21	32	62	47.0	..	Smoky.
22	48	65	56.5	1.0	Cloudy; thunder; rain at night.
23	40	38	39.0	0.4	Rain.
24	30	38	34.0	..	Snow.
25	30	34	32.0	..	Cloudy.
26	19	34	26.5	..	Fair.
27	24	32	28.0	..	Cloudy; snow-flakes.
28	16	44	30.0	..	Fair.
Means	34.14	54.86	44.50	[illegible]	Greatest Rise and Fall of [illegible]
Max.	58	77	65.0		
Min.	16	32	26.5		
Range	42	45	38.5		

Extreme range 61

	Sunrise.	2 P. M.
Rise . . .	28	24
Fall . . .	20	27

March, 1855.

DAY.	THERMOMETER. Sun-rise.	2 P. M.	Mean.	RAIN. Ins.	REMARKS ON THE WEATHER.
1	20	54	37.0	..	Fair; cloudy.
2	40	56	48.0	..	Cloudy.
3	56	64	60.0	..	Cloudy; fair.
4	40	68	54.0	..	Fair.
5	52	70	61.0	..	Cloudy.
6	62	78	70.0	..	Cloudy.
7	52	80	66.0	..	Fair.
8	60	82	71.0	..	Smoky.
9	56	74	65.0	..	Smoky.
10	50	68	59.0	0.1	Smoky; thunder; rain at night.
11	60	70	65.0	0.1	Clouds; rain at night.
12	62	64	63.0	0.8	Clouds; thunder; rain.
13	47	68	57.5	..	Fair.
14	58	83	70.5	..	Cloudy; fair; wind.
15	46	54	50.0	..	Cloudy.
16	44	53	48.5	..	Cloudy.
17	38	43	40.5	..	Cloudy; snow-flakes.
18	30	58	44.0	..	Fair; ice.
19	30	68	49.0	..	Fair.
20	30	46	38.0	..	Smoky.
21	36	56	46.0	..	Smoky.
22	30	54	42.0	..	Smoky.
23	30	64	47.0	..	Smoky.
24	42	72	57.0	..	Smoky.
25	36	64	50.0	..	Smoky.
26	50	60	55.0	..	Smoky; wind.
27	30	52	41.0	..	Fair.
28	32	50	41.0	..	Smoky; wind.
29	32	55	43.5	..	Smoky.
30	44	43	43.5	1.0	Cloudy; rain.
31	32	56	44.0	..	Fog; fair; white frost.
Means	42.81	62.16	52.48	2.0	Greatest Rise and Fall of temperature in 24 hours.
Max.	62	83	71.0		
Min.	20	43	37.0		
Range	42	40	34.0		

Extreme range 63

	Sunrise	2 P. M.
Rise . . .	20	15
Fall . . .	15	29

April, 1855.

DAY.	THERMOMETER. Sun-rise.	2 P. M.	Mean.	RAIN. Ins.	REMARKS ON THE WEATHER.
1	48	62	55.0	..	Cloudy; thunder at night.
2	48	58	53 0	0.5	Cloudy; rain.
3	50	60	55.0	2.5	Cloudy; thunder; rain at night.
4	60	62	61.0	..	Cloudy; rain.
5	58	62	60.0	0.5	Cloudy; rain at night.
6	52	64	58 0	..	Cloudy; rain.
7	42	62	52.0	..	Fair.
8	52	83	67.5	..	Fair.
9	58	78	68.0	..	Fair; cloudy.
10	62	74	68.0	..	Cloudy.
11	58	64	61 0	..	Cloudy.
12	50	82	66.0	..	Cloudy.
13	64	85	74.5	..	Cloudy; thunder.
14	68	85	76.5	..	Cloudy.
15	64	82	73.0	..	Cloudy; fair.
16	62	87	74.5	..	Fair.
17	66	87	76.5	..	Fair.
18	68	88	78.0	..	Fair.
19	68	82	75.0	0.1	Fair; cloudy; thunder; rain.
20	60	70	65.0	..	Cloudy.
21	52	82	67.0	..	Fair.
22	60	87	73.5	..	Clouds.
23	58	88	73.0	..	Fair.
24	62	92	77.0	..	
25	60	86	73.0	..	Fair; hazy.
26	62	86	74.0	..	Fog; hazy.
27	64	80	72.0	..	Cloudy.
28	64	82	73.0	..	Cloudy.
29	64	83	73.5	..	Hazy.
30	68	84	76.0	..	Fair; clouds.
Means	59.07	77.57	68.32	[illegible]	Greatest Rise and Fall of temperature in 24 hours.
Max.	68	92	78.0		
Min.	42	58	52.0		
Range	26	34	26.0		

Extreme range 50

	Sunrise.	2 P. M.
Rise . . .	16	21
Fall . . .	10	12

May, 1855.

DAY.	THERMOMETER. Sunrise.	THERMOMETER. 3 P. M.	THERMOMETER. Mean.	RAIN. Ins.	REMARKS ON THE WEATHER.
1	73	84	78.5	..	Cloudy; thunder; sprinkle.
2	68	80	74.0	..	Fair; clouds. First appearance of
3	60	78	69.0	..	Fair; clouds. [locusts.
4	60	74	67.0	..	Fair; clouds.
5	56	74	65.0	..	Fair; clouds.
6	61	80	70.5	..	Fair; clouds.
7	64	86	75.0	..	Fair; clouds.
8	62	80	71.0	..	Fair; clouds.
9	56	66	61.0	0.1	Cloudy; rain.
10	56	74	65.0	..	Fair.
11	54	76	65.0	0.2	Fair; cloudy; rain at night.
12	54	80	67.0	0.5	Cloudy; thunder; rain.
13	64	74	69.0	..	Cloudy.
14	64	80	72.0	..	Fog; cloudy.
15	64	82	73.0	..	Fair; clouds.
16	64	86	75.0	..	Fair.
17	74	87	80.5	..	Fair.
18	74	86	80.0	0.1	Clouds; rain.
19	74	86	80.0	..	Clouds.
20	68	90	79.0	..	Fair.
21	72	91	81.5	..	Fair.
22	74	90	82.0	..	Cloudy; fair.
23	72	92	82.0	..	Fair.
24	74	90	82.0	..	Cloudy; fair.
25	72	92	82.0	..	Fair.
26	72	90	81.0	..	Fair; clouds.
27	72	90	81.0	..	Fair; clouds.
28	72	85	78.5	..	Fair; clouds; thunder.
29	69	86	77.5	..	Fair; cloudy.
30	74	82	78.0	..	R'n; thun'r; N. wind; r'n at night.
31	66	80	73.0	1.8	Fair. [Timber & crops damaged.
Means	66.42	82.94	74.68	2.7	Greatest Rise and Fall of temperature in 24 hours.
Max.	74	92	82.0		
Min.	54	66	61.0		
Range	20	26	21.0		

Extreme range 38

	Sunrise.	3 P. M.
Rise . . .	10	8
Fall . . .	8	14

June, 1855.

DAY.	THERMOMETER. Sunrise.	THERMOMETER. 3 P. M.	THERMOMETER. Mean.	RAIN. Ins.	REMARKS ON THE WEATHER.
1	68	78	73.0	..	Fair.
2	54	76	65.0	..	Fair.
3	56	70	63.0	0.1	Fair; cloudy; rain.
4	60	86	73.0	..	Cloudy; fair.
5	70	86	78.0	..	Cloudy; fair.
6	74	84	79.0	0.7	Cloudy; thunder; rain at night.
7	66	76	71.0	..	Rain; fair.
8	60	80	70.0	..	Fair.
9	60	84	72.0	..	Fair.
10	64	85	74.5	..	Fair.
11	57	80	68.5	..	Fair.
12	60	86	73.0	..	Fair.
13	70	82	76.0	..	Fair.
14	62	84	73.0	..	Fair.
15	66	88	77.0	..	Fair.
16	70	89	79.5	..	Fair.
17	74	88	81.0	..	Cloudy; fair.
18	74	87	80.5	..	Cloudy; thunder.
19	76	86	81.0	0.3	Cloudy; thunder; rain at 1 P. M.
20	70	82	76.0	0.1	Cloudy; thunder; rain at 1 P. M.
21	71	78	74.5	..	Cloudy.
22	74	86	80.0	0.3	Cloudy; thunder; rain at night.
23	74	76	75.0	0.3	Cloudy; rain.
24	70	80	75.0	..	Cloudy.
25	66	82	74.0	1.8	Cloudy; thunder; rain.
26	70	91	80.5	..	Fair.
27	76	90	83.0	..	Fair.
28	74	88	81.0	..	Fair; clouds.
29	74	88	81.0	..	Clouds.
30	74	84	79.0	..	
Means	67.80	83.33	75.57	3.6	Greatest Rise and Fall of temperature in 24 hours.
Max.	76	91	83.0		
Min.	54	70	63.0		
Range	22	21	20.0		

Extreme range 37

	Sunrise.	3 P. M.
Rise	10	16
Fall . . .	14	10

July, 1855.

DAY.	THERMOMETER. Sunrise.	THERMOMETER. 3 P. M.	THERMOMETER. Mean.	RAIN. Ins.	REMARKS ON THE WEATHER.
1	65	86	75.5	..	Fair.
2	66	90	78.0	..	Fair.
3	66	90	78.0	..	Fair.
4	66	96	81.0	..	Fair.
5	66	94	80.0	..	Fair.
6	76	93	84.5	..	Clouds; fair.
7	76	94	85.0	..	Clouds; fair.
8	76	96	86.0	..	Fair; clouds.
9	76	93	84.5	..	Fair.
10	76	92	84.0	..	Fair.
11	72	93	82 5	..	Fair.
12	72	94	83.0	..	Fair.
13	76	94	85.0	..	Fair.
14	70	94	82.0	..	Fair.
15	70	94	82.0	..	Fair.
16	78	94	86.0	0.4	Fair; cloudy; thunder; rain at 4
17	74	90	82.0	..	Fog; fair. [P. M.
18	76	94	85.0	..	Clouds.
19	76	92	84.0	0.2	Clouds; shower at 5 P. M.
20	76	86	81.0	..	Clouds.
21	74	90	82.0	0.1	Clouds; shower in the night.
22	76	78	77.0	1.0	Clouds; rain at noon.
23	76	84	80.0	..	Clouds.
24	76	83	79.5	0.4	Clouds; rain at night.
25	74	78	76.0	..	Rain.
26	74	82	78.0	..	Cloudy; rain at night.
27	74	76	75.0	2.5	Rain.
28	74	86	80.0	..	Clouds.
29	76	83	79.5	..	Fair; shower at 3 P. M.
30	74	86	80.0	..	Clouds.
31	75	88	81.5	..	Clouds; thunder.
Means	73.29	89.13	81.21	4.6	Greatest Rise and Fall of temperature in 24 hours.
Max.	78	96	86.0		
Min.	65	76	75.0		
Range	13	20	11.0		

Extreme range 31

	Sunrise.	3 P. M.
Rise . . .	10	10
Fall . . .	9	12

August, 1855.

DAY.	THERMOMETER. Sunrise.	THERMOMETER. 3 P. M.	THERMOMETER. Mean.	RAIN. Ins.	REMARKS ON THE WEATHER.
1	74	88	81.0	..	Fog; fair.
2	74	90	82.0	..	Fair; clouds.
3	74	90	82.0	..	Fair.
4	74	91	82.5	..	Fair.
5	74	91	82 5	..	Fair.
6	76	90	83.0	..	Fair.
7	74	90	82 0	..	Fair.
8	78	90	84.0	..	Cloudy.
9	78	90	84.0	0.4	Cloudy; rain at 5 P. M.
10	78	90	84.0	..	Cloudy.
11	78	92	85.0	..	Fair.
12	74	90	82.0	..	Fair; clouds.
13	70	90	80.0	..	Fair; clouds.
14	70	94	82.0	..	Fair; clouds.
15	74	96	85.0	..	Fair; clouds.
16	76	95	85.5	..	Fair.
17	78	74	76.0	..	Cloudy.
18	66	80	73.0	..	Fair.
19	60	84	72.0	..	Fair.
20	66	84	75.0	..	Fair.
21	70	90	80.0	..	Fair.
22	72	84	78.0	..	Cloudy; rain at night.
23	74	75	74.5	0.5	Rain.
24	72	78	75.0	..	Cloudy; rain.
25	72	78	75.0	0.4	Rain.
26	74	76	75.0	..	Rain.
27	73	80	76.5	1.3	Rain.
28	70	78	74.0	1.5	Rain.
29	70	86	78.0	..	
30	72	88	80.0	..	Fair.
31	70	90	80.0	..	Fair.
Means	72.74	86.52	79.63	4.1	Greatest Rise and Fall of temperature in 24 hours.
Max.	78	96	85.5		
Min.	60	74	72.0		
Range	18	22	13.5		

Extreme range 36

	Sunrise.	3 P. M.
Rise . . .	6	6
Fall . . .	12	21

September, 1855.

DAY.	THERMOMETER. Sunrise.	THERMOMETER. 3 P. M.	THERMOMETER. Mean.	RAIN. Ins.	REMARKS ON THE WEATHER.
1	76	76	76.0	2.3	Cloudy; heavy rain.
2	76	64	70.0	..	Cloudy; thunder.
3	76	80	78.0	0.5	Cloudy; thunder; rain.
4	72	86	79.0	..	Fog; fair; rain at night.
5	74	88	81.0	..	Fog; fair.
6	72	88	81.0	..	Fog; fair.
7	72	84	78.0	..	Fog; thunder.
8	72	84	78.0	0.3	Fog; thunder; shower at 3 P. M.
9	71	82	76.5	..	Fog; clouds.
10	74	78	76.0	0.4	Cloudy; rain.
11	74	84	79.0	0.2	Cloudy; rain.
12	74	88	81.0	..	Cloudy.
13	73	86	79.5	..	Cloudy.
14	73	86	79.5	..	Fog; cloudy.
15	72	88	80.0	..	Fair; cloudy.
16	72	90	81.0	..	Fair.
17	74	90	82.0	..	Fair.
18	74	88	81.0	..	Fair.
19	72	89	80.5	..	Fair.
20	72	89	80.5	..	Fair.
21	70	88	79.0	..	Fair.
22	70	90	80.0	..	Fog; fair.
23	68	88	78.0	..	Fog; fair.
24	70	89	79.5	..	Fair.
25	70	86	78.0	0.7	Clouds; thunder; rain at night.
26	70	78	74.0	..	Cloudy; fair.
27	54	72	63.0	..	Fair.
28	54	72	63.0	..	Fair; cloudy; rain at night.
29	65	69	67.0	1.8	Rain.
30	53	72	62.5	..	Fair.

	Sunrise.	3 P. M.	Mean.	Rain. Ins.
Means	70.37	83.07	76.72	6.2
Max.	76	90	82.0	
Min.	53	64	62.5	
Range	23	26	19.5	

Extreme range 37

Greatest Rise and Fall of temperature in 24 hours.

	Sunrise.	3 P. M.
Rise . . .	11	16
Fall . . .	16	14

November, 1855.

DAY.	THERMOMETER. Sunrise.	THERMOMETER. 2 P. M.	THERMOMETER. Mean.	RAIN. Ins.	REMARKS ON THE WEATHER.
1	64	74	69.0	..	Cloudy.
2	68	72	70.0	3.7	Rain; thunder; heavy at night.
3	64	68	66 0	1.0	Rain; thunder.
4	68	80	74.0	1.4	Rain; thunder.
5	56	66	61.0	..	Cloudy; fair.
6	46	60	53.0	..	Cloudy.
7	37	68	52.5	..	Fair.
8	42	74	58.0	..	Fair.
9	42	72	57.0	..	
10	48	64	56.0	..	Cloudy.
11	66	66	66.0	0.1	Mist; rain; fair.
12	54	66	60.0	..	Cloudy; fair.
13	48	72	60.0	..	Cloudy; fair.
14	61	70	65.5	..	Cloudy.
15	68	80	74.0	..	Cloudy.
16	70	66	68.0	0.6	Cloudy; shower at 1 P. M.
17	42	54	48.0	..	Fair.
18	33	58	45.5	..	Fair; white frost.
19	32	58	45.0	..	Fair.
20	46	64	55.0	..	Fair.
21	46	54	50.0	0.1	Cloudy; rain.
22	38	58	48.0	..	Cloudy.
23	46	57	51.5	0.8	Cloudy; mist; rain at night.
24	52	53	52.5	1.0	Rain.
25	54	65	59.5	..	Rain; cloudy.
26	42	60	51.0	..	Fair.
27	39	58	48.5	..	Fair.
28	38	64	51.0	..	Fair.
29	32	58	45.0	..	Fair.
30	39	60	49.5	..	Fair.

	Sunrise.	2 P. M.	Mean.	Rain. Ins.
Means	49.37	64.83	57.10	8.7
Max.	70	80	74.0	
Min.	32	53	45.0	
Range	38	27	29.0	

Extreme range 48

Greatest Rise and Fall of temperature in 24 hours.

	Sunrise.	2 P. M.
Rise . . .	18	12
Fall . . .	28	14

October, 1855.

DAY.	THERMOMETER. Sunrise.	THERMOMETER. 3 P. M.	THERMOMETER. Mean.	RAIN. Ins.	REMARKS ON THE WEATHER.
1	57	73	65.0	..	Cloudy; fair.
2	52	74	63.0	..	Fair.
3	52	74	63.0	..	Fair.
4	64	72	68.0	1.5	Cloudy; thunder; rain.
5	60	56	58.0	..	Rain.
6	40	60	50.0	..	Fair.
7	39	68	53.5	..	Fair.
8	50	60	55.0	..	Fair.
9	53	77	65.0	..	Fair.
10	52	76	64.0	..	Fair.
11	54	78	66.0	..	Fair.
12	42	68	55.0	..	Fair.
13	42	68	55.0	..	Fair.
14	50	70	60.0	..	Fair.
15	58	70	64.0	..	Cloudy.
16	58	66	62.0	..	Cloudy.
17	54	72	63.0	..	Cloudy; fair.
18	48	74	61.0	..	Smoky.
19	54	78	66.0	..	Fair.
20	54	74	64.0	..	Cloudy.
21	66	67	66.5	0.3	Cloudy; thunder; rain at night.
22	48	50	49.0	..	
23	48	50	49.0	..	Fair.
24	34	48	41.0	..	Fair; white frost.
25	28	50	39.0	..	Fair; killing frost.
26	35	70	52.5	..	Fair.
27	50	77	63.5	..	Fog; fair.
28	56	79	67.5	..	Fog; fair.
29	56	74	65.0	..	Cloudy; fair.
30	55	70	62.5	..	Fair.
31	58	76	67.0	..	Fair.

	Sunrise.	3 P. M.	Mean.	Rain. Ins.
Means	50.55	68.35	59.45	[illegible]
Max.	66	79	68.0	
Min.	28	48	39.0	
Range	38	31	29.0	

Extreme range 51

Greatest Rise and Fall of [illegible]

	Sunrise.	3 P. M.
Rise . . .	15	20
Fall . . .	20	17

December, 1855.

DAY.	THERMOMETER. Sunrise.	THERMOMETER. 2 P. M.	THERMOMETER. Mean.	RAIN. Ins.	REMARKS ON THE WEATHER.
1	40	60	50.0	..	Fair.
2	44	58	51.0	..	Fair.
3	30	50	40.0	..	Fair.
4	33	54	43.5	..	Fair.
5	34	56	45.0	..	Fair.
6	32	62	47.0	..	Fair.
7	47	64	55.5	..	Fair; cloudy.
8	60	64	62.0	1.0	Cloudy; rain.
9	42	52	47.0	..	Fair.
10	32	62	47.0	..	Fair.
11	32	60	46.0	..	Fair.
12	54	67	60.5	..	Cloudy; fair.
13	60	67	63.5	2.3	Cloudy; rain.
14	50	50	50.0	..	Rain; fair.
15	36	52	44.0	0.3	Fair; cloudy; rain.
16	45	56	50.5	..	Fog; fair.
17	34	52	43.0	..	Fair.
18	30	40	35 0	..	Fair.
19	34	54	44.0	..	Fair.
20	34	62	48.0	..	Fair.
21	64	70	67.0	..	Fair.
22	42	56	49.0	..	Fair.
23	32	35	33.5	..	Fair.
24	24	22	23.0	..	Fair.
25	20	20	20.0	..	Fair.
26	10	30	20.0	..	Fair.
27	19	46	32.5	..	Fair.
28	36	42	39.0	..	Cloudy; mist.
29	40	32	36.0	..	Mist; fair.
30	10	26	18.0	..	Fair.
31	18	35	26.5	..	Fair.

	Sunrise.	2 P. M.	Mean.	Rain. Ins.
Means	36.06	50.19	43.13	[illegible]
Max.	64	70	67.0	
Min.	10	20	18.0	
Range	54	50	40.0	

Extreme range 60

Greatest Rise and Fall of [illegible]

	Sunrise.	2 P. M.
Rise . . .	30	16
Fall . . .	30	21

January, 1856.

DAY.	THERMOMETER. Sunrise.	2 P. M.	Mean.	RAIN. Ins.	REMARKS ON THE WEATHER.
1	14	40	27.0	..	Fair.
2	32	44	38.0	..	Cloudy.
3	24	41	32.5	..	Fair.
4	20	58	39.0	..	Fair.
5	20	49	34.5	..	Fair.
6	30	53	41.5	..	Fair; clouds.
7	48	50	49.0	..	Cloudy; fair.
8	28	28	28.0	..	Cloudy.
9	23	26	24.5	..	Cloudy.
10	16	28	22.0	..	Fair; cloudy; sleet at night.
11	26	40	33.0	1.0	Cl'y; gr'nd covered with ice, sleet,
12	30	40	35.0	..	Cl'y; snow 8 in. deep. [and snow.
13	27	53	40.0	..	Fair.
14	32	36	34.0	..	Cloudy; fair.
15	24	32	28.0	..	Cloudy.
16	18	42	30.0	..	Fair.
17	24	54	39.0	..	Fair.
18	27	54	40.5	..	Fair.
19	42	42	42.0	..	Cloudy.
20	26	36	31.0	..	Fair. } Ground slippery, and
21	10	30	20.0	..	Fair. } dangerous travelling;
22	20	36	28.0	..	Fair. } many injuries and
23	24	36	30.0	..	Cloudy. } some deaths from fall-
24	36	40	38.0	..	Cloudy. } ing on the ice.
25	40	38	39.0	3.7	Cloudy; rain heavy all day.
26	36	42	39.0	1.4	Cloudy; snow; old ice yet; rain.
27	26	28	27.0	..	Cloudy; snow; wind.
28	20	38	29.0	..	Fair.
29	26	44	35.0	..	Fair.
30	21	42	31.5	..	Fair.
31	42	54	48.0	..	Cloudy; old ice yet.
Means	26.84	41.10	33.97	6.1	Greatest Rise and Fall of temperature in 24 hours.
Max.	48	58	49.0		
Min.	10	26	20.0		
Range	38	32	29.0		
Extreme range 48					

	Sunrise.	2 P. M.
Rise . . .	21	17
Fall . . .	20	22

February, 1856.

DAY.	THERMOMETER. Sunrise.	2 P. M.	Mean.	RAIN. Ins.	REMARKS ON THE WEATHER.
1	30	62	46.0	..	Fair.
2	34	40	37.0	..	Cloudy; snow at night.
3	8	24	16.0	..	Fair; ground covered with snow.
4	8	30	19.0	..	Fair.
5	16	32	24.0	1.5	Cloudy; sleet; rain at night.
6	34	36	35.0	..	Rain; ground covered with ice;
7	28	40	34.0	..	Cloudy; fair. [snow.
8	29	43	36.0	..	Cloudy; fair; snow at night.
9	24	52	38.0	..	Fair.
10	36	62	49.0	..	Cl'dy; fair; thunder; rain at night.
11	34	51	42.5	..	Fair.
12	33	62	47.5	..	Fair.
13	38	62	50.0	..	Fair.
14	30	66	48.0	..	Fair.
15	48	68	58.0	..	Fair.
16	47	74	60.5	..	Fair.
17	30	52	41.0	..	Fair.
18	30	62	46.0	..	Hazy; rain at night..
19	44	47	45.5	..	Rain.
20	44	48	46.0	1.8	Rain.
21	44	55	49.5	..	Cloudy.
22	49	62	55.5	..	Fog; rain; fair.
23	42	56	49.0	..	Fair.
24	36	52	44.0	..	Fair; cloudy.
25	39	62	50.5	..	Fair.
26	48	51	49.5	1.6	Rain.
27	47	63	55.0	..	Fair.
28	43	68	55.5	..	Fair.
29	44	60	52.0	0.6	Cloudy; rain at night.
Means	35.07	53.17	44.12	5.5	Greatest Rise and Fall of temperature in 24 hours.
Max.	49	74	60.5		
Min.	8	24	16.0		
Range	41	50	44.5		
Extreme range 66					

	Sunrise.	2 P. M.
Rise . . .	18	12
Fall . . .	26	22

March, 1856.

DAY.	THERMOMETER. Sunrise.	2 P. M.	Mean.	RAIN. Ins.	REMARKS ON THE WEATHER.
1	40	44	42.0	0.1	Rain.
2	26	50	38.0	..	Fair; ground frozen.
3	30	60	45.0	..	Fair.
4	42	64	53.0	..	Cloudy.
5	41	60	50.5	..	Cloudy.
6	46	66	56.0	..	Cloudy; fair.
7	39	54	46.5	..	Fair; cloudy; rain.
8	44	66	55.0	..	Fair.
9	40	60	50.0	0.1	Fair; cloudy; rain.
10	36	48	42.0	..	Fair; cloudy; rain at night.
11	42	50	46.0	0.5	Rain.
12	42	43	42.5	0.4	Cloudy; rain at night; snow.
13	36	46	41.0	..	Rain; snow.
14	32	50	41.0	..	Fair; cloudy; rain.
15	40	58	49.0	..	Cloudy; rain at night.
16	46	48	47.0	..	Rain.
17	40	46	43.0	0.8	Rain.
18	44	58	51.0	..	Cloudy; fair at eve.
19	36	62	49.0	..	Fair.
20	42	76	59.0	..	Fair.
21	44	68	56.0	..	Fair.
22	42	64	53.0	..	Fair.
23	48	78	63.0	..	Fair.
24	58	84	71.0	..	Smoky; fair.
25	58	80	69.0	..	Smoky; fair.
26	58	76	67.0	..	Smoky; fair.
27	44	59	51.5	..	Fair.
28	41	62	51.5	0.1	Smoky; cloudy; rain at night.
29	54	60	57.0	0.1	Thunder; rain.
30	50	82	66.0	..	Smoky; fair.
31	43	58	50.5	..	Cloudy; fair.
Means	42.71	60.65	51.68	2.1	Greatest Rise and Fall of temperature in 24 hours.
Max.	58	84	71.0		
Min.	26	43	38.0		
Range	32	41	33.0		
Extreme range 58					

	Sunrise.	2 P. M.
Rise . . .	13	22
Fall . . .	14	24

April, 1856.

DAY.	THERMOMETER. Sunrise.	2 P. M.	Mean.	RAIN. Ins.	REMARKS ON THE WEATHER.
1	48	64	56.0	0.4	Cloudy; smoky; thunder; rain at
2	64	80	72.0	..	Fair. [night.
3	49	82	65.5	..	Fair.
4	58	76	67.0	..	Fair.
5	42	72	57.0	..	Fair.
6	46	80	63.0	..	Fair; smoky; windy.
7	44	76	60.0	..	Smoky.
8	46	84	65.0	..	Smoky.
9	60	86	73.0	..	Smoky.
10	60	87	73.5	..	Smoky.
11	60	80	70.0	..	Smoky.
12	66	80	73.0	..	Smoky.
13	66	86	76.0	..	Smoky.
14	63	80	71.5	..	Smoky; cloudy; sprinkle.
15	78	88	83.0	..	Cloudy; fair.
16	70	85	77.5	1.0	Fair; cl'dy; thunder; r'n at night.
17	62	78	70.0	..	Cloudy; fair.
18	50	82	66.0	..	Fair.
19	58	68	63.0	..	Fair.
20	42	75	58.5	..	Eclipse; fair.
21	47	74	60.5	..	Fair; clouds; thunder.
22	62	78	70.0	..	Smoky; rain; cloudy; thunder.
23	59	82	70.5	..	Fog; fair.
24	58	88	73.0	0.1	Fog; fair; thunder; rain at night.
25	70	84	77.0	..	Fair; cloudy; thunder; rain.
26	70	84	77.0	0.5	Fair; cloudy; thunder; rain.
27	64	76	70.0	..	Fog; cloudy.
28	62	72	67.0	..	Cloudy; shower at noon.
29	66	78	72.0	1.2	Cl'y; thunder; r'n at night; wind.
30	60	80	70.0	..	Cloudy; thunder; rain at 3 P. M.
Means	58.33	79.50	68.92	3.2	Greatest Rise and Fall of temperature in 24 hours.
Max.	78	88	77.5		
Min.	42	64	56.0		
Range	36	24	21.5		
Extreme range 46					

	Sunrise.	2 P. M.
Rise . . .	16	16
Fall . . .	16	14

May, 1856.

DAY.	THERMOMETER.			RAIN.	REMARKS ON THE WEATHER.
	Sunrise.	3 P. M.	Mean.	Ins.	
1	58	79	68.5	..	Fair.
2	58	85	71.5	..	Fair.
3	60	82	71.0	..	Fog; fair; clouds.
4	72	86	79.0	..	Cloudy; fair.
5	74	80	77.0	0.1	Cloudy; thunder; rain.
6	58	82	70.0	..	Fair.
7	58.	80	69.0	..	Fair.
8	52	70	61.0	..	Fair; cloudy.
9	49	73	61.0	..	Cloudy.
10	58	72	65.0	..	Fair; cloudy.
11	50	78	64.0	..	Clouds; fair.
12	50	80	65.0	..	Fair; clouds.
13	60	78	69.0	0.6	Cloudy; thunder; rain.
14	60	82	71.0	..	Fair; clouds; thunder.
15	66	83	74.5	..	Fog; clouds.
16	68	84	76.0	0.3	Cloudy; thunder; wind and rain [at 3 P. M.
17	60	76	68.0	..	Fair; clouds.
18	50	76	63.0	..	Fair.
19	52	82	67.0	..	Fair.
20	56	90	73.0	..	Fair.
21	70	90	80.0	..	Fair.
22	58	91	74.5	..	Fair.
23	64	91	77.5	..	Fair.
24	64	88	76.0	..	Fair.
25	62	90	76.0	..	Fair.
26	66	92	79.0	..	Fair.
27	66	94	80.0	..	Clouds; thunder.
28	63	80	71.5	..	Fair; breezes; dry; dusty.
29	60	85	72.5	..	Fair.
30	64	80	72.0	..	Fair; clouds.
31	58	82	70.0	..	Fair.
Means	60.13	82.61	71.37	1.0	
Max.	74	94	80.0		
Min.	49	70	61.0		
Range	25	24	19.0		

Extreme range 45

Greatest Rise and Fall of temperature in 24 hours.	Sunrise.	3 P. M.
Rise . . .	14	8
Fall . . .	16	14

June, 1856.

DAY.	THERMOMETER.			RAIN.	REMARKS ON THE WEATHER.
	Sunrise.	3 P. M.	Mean.	Ins.	
1	60	88	74.0	..	Fair.
2	64	90	77.0	..	Fair.
3	70	90	80.0	..	Fair.
4	72	91	81.5	..	Fair.
5	72	92	82.0	..	Fair.
6	72	93	82.5	..	Fair; clouds.
7	72	95	83.5	..	Fair.
8	70	95	82.5	..	Fair.
9	78	82	80.0	0.6	Cloudy; thunder; rain at 2 P. M.
10	68	86	78.0	..	Fair.
11	68	88	77.0	..	Fair.
12	71	92	81.5	..	
13	73	92	82.5	..	Cloudy; thunder.
14	68	90	79.0	..	Fair.
15	58	84	71.0	..	Fair.
16	68	90	79.0	..	Cloudy.
17	78	90	84.0	..	Cloudy.
18	76	90	83.0	0.8	Cloudy; thunder; rain at 4 P. M.
19	70	78	74.0	1.5	Cloudy; thunder; rain.
20	72	82	77.0	..	Cloudy; thunder.
21	72	88	80.0	0.1	Cloudy; thunder; rain.
22	72	88	80.0	..	Fog; fair; thunder.
23	72	88	80.0	..	Fair; clouds; thunder.
24	70	90	80.0	..	Fair.
25	70	90	80.0	..	Fair; clouds.
26	74	92	83.0	..	Fair.
27	72	90	81.0	..	Fair.
28	72	88	80.0	..	Fair.
29	74	92	83.0	..	Fair.
30	74	92	83.0	..	
Means	70.73	89.20	79.97	[illegible]	
Max.	78	95	84.0		
Min.	58	78	74.0		
Range	20	17	10.0		

Extreme range 37

Greatest Rise and Fall of temperature in 24 hours.	Sunrise.	3 P. M.
Rise . . .	10	6
Fall . . .	10	13

July, 1856.

DAY.	THERMOMETER.			RAIN.	REMARKS ON THE WEATHER.
	Sunrise.	3 P. M.	Mean.	Ins.	
1	74	92	83.0	..	Clouds; fair.
2	76	96	86.0	..	Fair.
3	76	95	85.5	..	Fair.
4	76	99	87.5	..	Fair.
5	80	102	91.0	1.0	Cloudy; thunder; rain at 4 P. M.
6	76	75	75.5	0.3	Cloudy; thunder; rain.
7	72	80	76.0	0.2	Cloudy; thunder; rain.
8	74	86	80.0	0.6	Cloudy; thunder; rain at night.
9	74	90	82.0	..	Cloudy.
10	74	94	84.0	0.7	Fair; thunder; rain at night.
11	74	87	80.5	..	Fair.
12	66	86	76.0	..	Fair.
13	68	92	80.0	..	Fair.
14	74	92	83.0	..	Fair.
15	75	92	83.5	..	Fair.
16	73	94	83.5	..	Fair.
17	74	94	84.0	..	Fair.
18	73	94	83.5	..	Cloudy; fair.
19	76	86	81.0	0.1	Cloudy; thunder; rain.
20	70	92	81.0	..	Fair.
21	66	90	78.0	..	Fair.
22	70	86	78.0	..	Fair; cloudy.
23	64	90	77.0	..	Fair.
24	66	92	79.0	..	Fair.
25	68	93	80.5	..	Fair.
26	68	92	80.0	..	Fair.
27	74	84	79.0	0.3	Cloudy; thunder; rain at 1 P. M.
28	72	92	82.0	..	Fair.
29	74	90	82.0	..	Fair.
30	72	96	84.0	0.4	Clouds; thunder; rain at night.
31	72	84	78.0	1.0	Cloudy; thunder; rain.
Means	72.29	90.55	81.42	4.6	
Max.	80	102	91.0		
Min.	64	75	75.5		
Range	16	27	15.5		

Extreme range 38

Greatest Rise and Fall of temperature in 24 hours.	Sunrise.	3 P. M.
Rise . . .	6	8
Fall . . .	8	27

August, 1856.

DAY.	THERMOMETER.			RAIN.	REMARKS ON THE WEATHER.
	Sunrise.	3 P. M.	Mean.	Ins.	
1	72	86	79.0	2.0	Cloudy; thunder; rain.
2	72	86	79.0	..	Clouds.
3	72	68	70.0	0.1	Fair; cloudy; thunder; rain.
4	72	90	81.0	..	Fog; fair.
5	72	84	78.0	..	Fair; clouds; thunder.
6	68	90	79.0	..	Fair.
7	70	94	82.0	..	Fair.
8	76	92	84.0	..	Cloudy.
9	74	92	83.0	..	Cloudy; fair.
10	70	94	82.0	..	Fair.
11	68	94	81.0	..	Fair.
12	74	88	81.0	..	Fair; cloudy.
13	70	92	81.0	..	Fair.
14	70	92	81.0	..	Fair.
15	72	82	77.0	..	Cloudy; thunder; sprinkle.
16	72	82	77.0	..	Cloudy.
17	72	96	84.0	..	Cloudy; fair.
18	76	99	87.5	..	Fair; thunder.
19	76	98	87.0	..	Fair.
20	72	93	82.5	..	Fair.
21	72	96	84.0	..	Smoky.
22	78	98	88.0	..	Cloudy; fair.
23	76	96	86.0	..	Fair.
24	76	90	83.0	..	Cloudy.
25	72	90	81.0	..	Fair; cloudy.
26	67	86	76.5	..	Smoky.
27	70	90	80.0	..	Cloudy; fair.
28	68	86	77.0	..	Smoky.
29	68	92	80.0	..	Fair.
30	70	88	79.0	..	Fair.
31	64	86	75.0	..	Fair.
Means	71.65	90.00	80.82	[illegible]	
Max.	78	99	88.0		
Min.	64	68	70.0		
Range	14	31	18.0		

Extreme range 35

Greatest Rise and Fall of temperature in 24 hours.	Sunrise.	3 P. M.
Rise . . .	6	22
Fall . . .	6	18

September, 1856.

DAY.	THERMOMETER. Sunrise.	THERMOMETER. 2 P. M.	THERMOMETER. Mean.	RAIN. Ins.	REMARKS ON THE WEATHER.
1	56	86	71.0	. .	Smoky; dusty; sprinkle.
2	62	80	71.0	. .	Smoky.
3	70	80	75.0	. .	Cloudy.
4	70	84	77.0	0.7	Smoky; thunder; rain at noon.
5	72	84	78.0	0.8	Cloudy; mist; thunder; rain.
6	74	84	79.0	. .	Cloudy; fair.
7	72	86	79.0	. .	Cloudy; fair.
8	74	90	82.0	. .	Fair.
9	72	88	80.0	. .	Fair; clouds.
10	72	90	81.0	. .	Fair; clouds.
11	72	92	82.0	. .	Fair.
12	73	90	81.5	. .	Clouds; thunder.
13	68	88	78.0	. .	Fair.
14	68	88	78.0	. .	Fair.
15	63	88	75.5	. .	Fair.
16	64	90	77.0	. .	Fair.
17	66	90	78.0	. .	Fair; clouds.
18	70	82	76.0	. .	Fair; breezes.
19	62	78	70.0	. .	Fair; clouds.
20	58	72	65.0	. .	Cloudy; rain at night.
21	56	58	57.0	2.0	Rain.
22	58	70	64.0	. .	Fair.
23	48	64	56.0	. .	Fair.
24	42	69	55.5	. .	Fair.
25	44	74	59.0	. .	Fair.
26	50	76	63.0	. .	Fair.
27	50	80	65.0	. .	Fair.
28	56	72	64.0	0.3	Cloudy; rain.
29	48	66	57.0	. .	Fair.
30	42	62	52.0	. .	Fair.
Means	61.73	80.03	70.88	3.8	
Max.	74	92	82.0		
Min.	42	58	52.0		
Range	32	34	30.0		
Extreme range 50					

Greatest Rise and Fall of temperature in 24 hours.

	Sunrise.	2 P. M.
Rise . . .	8	12
Fall . . .	10	14

November, 1856.

DAY.	THERMOMETER. Sunrise.	THERMOMETER. 2 P. M.	THERMOMETER. Mean.	RAIN. Ins.	REMARKS ON THE WEATHER.
1	51	72	61.5	. .	Fair.
2	63	72	67.5	0.3	Cloudy; thunder; rain at night.
3	70	68	69.0	. .	Cloudy; windy.
4	36	60	48.0	. .	Fair.
5	32	58	45.0	. .	Fair; killing frost.
6	40	64	52.0	. .	Cloudy; windy.
7	62	66	64.0	1.0	Cloudy; rain.
8	24	42	33.0	. .	Fair; ground frozen.
9	24	46	35.0	. .	Fair.
10	22	56	39.0	. .	Fair.
11	32	60	46.0	. .	Fair.
12	30	64	47.0	. .	Fair.
13	30	62	46.0	. .	Fair.
14	36	66	51.0	. .	Fair.
15	40	70	55.0	. .	Fair.
16	44	70	57.0	. .	Fair; clouds.
17	36	50	43.0	. .	Fair; windy.
18	24	52	38.0	. .	Fair.
19	30	54	42.0	0.1	Cloudy; rain at night.
20	44	54	49.0	1.0	Cloudy; rain.
21	46	54	50.0	. .	Cloudy; fair.
22	34	50	42.0	. .	Fair.
23	52	66	59.0	. .	Fair.
24	40	70	55.0	. .	Fair; clouds.
25	60	70	65.0	. .	Fair.
26	44	70	57.0	2.0	Fair; cl'dy; thunder; r'n at night.
27	46	50	48.0	. .	Cloudy; rain.
28	48	52	50.0	2.3	Cloudy; thunder; rain.
29	48	56	52.0	. .	Cloudy; fair.
30	39	62	50.5	. .	Cloudy; fair.
Means	40.90	60.20	50.55	6.7	
Max.	70	72	69.0		
Min.	22	42	33.0		
Range	48	30	36.0		
Extreme range 50					

Greatest Rise and Fall of temperature in 24 hours.

	Sunrise.	2 P. M.
Rise . . .	22	16
Fall . . .	38	24

October, 1856.

DAY.	THERMOMETER. Sunrise.	THERMOMETER. 2 P. M.	THERMOMETER. Mean.	RAIN. Ins.	REMARKS ON THE WEATHER.
1	38	73	55.5	. .	Fair.
2	50	82	66.0	. .	Fair.
3	64	80	72.0	. .	Fair.
4	64	84	74.0	. .	Fair.
5	64	82	73.0	. .	Fair.
6	64	82	73.0	. .	Fair.
7	62	84	73.0	. .	Fair.
8	59	83	71.0	. .	Fair.
9	68	70	69.0	. .	Cloudy; thunder; rain.
10	70	74	72.0	2.2	Cloudy; thunder; rain.
11	70	78	74.0	0.3	Fog; rain.
12	70	80	75.0	0.1	Fog; thunder; rain at night.
13	70	76	73.0	. .	Cloudy; rain.
14	58	60	59.0	. .	Cloudy.
15	39	57	48.0	. .	Cloudy; fair.
16	34	60	47.0	. .	Fair; white frost.
17	34	64	49.0	. .	Fair.
18	38	64	51.0	. .	Fair.
19	54	76	65.0	. .	Clouds; fair.
20	64	70	67.0	0.2	Clouds; rain.
21	64	80	72.0	. .	Fair.
22	70	76	73.0	0.5	Fog; mist; thunder; rain.
23	70	80	75.0	. .	Rain.
24	72	75	73.5	0.5	Rain; fair.
25	46	70	58.0	. .	Fair.
26	52	64	58.0	0.5	Fair; cloudy; showers.
27	52	64	58.0	. .	Fair.
28	40	68	54.0	. .	Fair.
29	40	70	55.0	. .	Fair.
30	48	60	54.0	. .	Fair; windy.
31	37	68	52.5	. .	Fair.
Means	55.64	72.71	64.18	4.3	
Max.	72	84	75.0		
Min.	34	57	47.0		
Range	38	27	28.0		
Extreme range 50					

Greatest Rise and Fall of temperature in 24 hours.

	Sunrise.	2 P. M.
Rise . . .	16	12
Fall . . .	26	16

December, 1856.

DAY.	THERMOMETER. Sunrise.	THERMOMETER. 2 P. M.	THERMOMETER. Mean.	RAIN. Ins.	REMARKS ON THE WEATHER.
1	58	60	59.0	0.4	Cloudy; rain.
2	46	43	44.5	. .	Cloudy; rain; fair.
3	24	40	32.0	. .	Fair; ground frozen.
4	22	42	32.0	. .	Fair; ground frozen.
5	30	44	37.0	. .	Cloudy.
6	22	44	33.0	. .	Fair.
7	22	50	36.0	. .	Fair.
8	20	52	36.0	. .	Fair.
9	40	50	45.0	1.4	Cloudy; thunder; rain.
10	52	60	56.0	. .	Cloudy; rain; wind; sleet.
11	30	58	44.0	. .	Fair.
12	32	60	46.0	. .	Fair; clouds; rain at night.
13	54	60	57.0	1.0	Cloudy; thunder; rain.
14	24	42	33.0	. .	Fair.
15	32	48	40.0	. .	Fair.
16	26	50	38.0	. .	Fair.
17	30	52	41.0	. .	Fair.
18	48	58	53.0	. .	Fair.
19	60	56	58.0	0.4	Cloudy; rain.
20	24	38	31.0	. .	Fair.
21	21	42	31.5	. .	Fair.
22	25	42	33.5	. .	Fair.
23	24	40	32.0	. .	Fair.
24	24	56	40.0	. .	Fair.
25	36	65	50.5	. .	Fog; cloudy.
26	60	70	65.0	. .	Cloudy.
27	64	64	64.0	0.2	Cloudy; thunder; rain; fair.
28	30	54	42.0	. .	Fair.
29	38	60	49.0	. .	Fair.
30	34	48	41.0	0.4	Fair; thunder; rain at night.
31	34	43	38.5	. .	Rain.
Means	35.03	51.32	43.18	3.8	
Max.	64	70	65.0		
Min.	20	38	31.0		
Range	44	32	34.0		
Extreme range 50					

Greatest Rise and Fall of temperature in 24 hours.

	Sunrise.	2 P. M.
Rise . . .	24	10
Fall . . .	36	18

January, 1857.

DAY.	THERMOMETER. Sun-rise.	THERMOMETER. 2 P. M.	THERMOMETER. Mean.	RAIN. Ins.	REMARKS ON THE WEATHER.
1	38	44	41.0	..	Cloudy; fair.
2	40	48	44.0	..	Cloudy; mist.
3	19	36	27.5	..	Fair.
4	22	44	33.0	..	Fair; cloudy.
5	42	40	41.0	..	Cloudy; mist.
6	38	44	41.0	..	Cloudy.
7	28	30	29.0	..	Snow; sleet; ground covered.
8	24	28	26.0	..	Sleet. [snow.
9	26	34	30.0	..	Cloudy; trees loaded with ice and
10	18	32	25.0	..	Fair; icicles glittering.
11	18	36	27.0	..	Fair; ice 1.5 inch thick.
12	15	36	25.5	..	Fair; ice 1.5 inch thick.
13	24	40	32.0	..	Fair; ice 1.5 inch thick.
14	24	50	37.0	..	Fair.
15	26	50	38.0	..	Fair.
16	34	50	42.0	1.4	Cloudy; snow melting.
17	38	35	36.5	..	Cloudy; mist; rain.
18	4	23	13.5	..	Fair.
19	12	38	25.0	..	Fair.
20	36	43	39.5	..	Cloudy; mist; fair.
21	30	44	37.0	..	Fair.
22	25	42	33.5	..	Fair.
23	30	34	32.0	..	Cloudy.
24	20	50	35.0	..	Fair.
25	36	44	40.0	..	Fog; mist.
26	46	66	56.0	..	Fog; rain; snow disappearing.
27	60	66	63.0	..	Cloudy; thunder; snow all gone.
28	42	50	46.0	0.3	Cloudy; rain at night.
29	38	50	44.0	..	Cloudy; fair.
30	42	56	49.0	..	Cloudy; fair.
31	36	52	44.0	..	Fair; cloudy.
Means	30.03	43.07	36.55	1.7	
Max.	60	66	63.0		
Min.	4	23	13.5		
Range	56	43	49.5		
Extreme range 62					

Greatest Rise and Fall of temperature in 24 hours.

	Sunrise.	2 P. M.
Rise . . .	24	22
Fall . . .	34	16

February, 1857.

DAY.	THERMOMETER. Sun-rise.	THERMOMETER. 2 P. M.	THERMOMETER. Mean.	RAIN. Ins.	REMARKS ON THE WEATHER.
1	38	60	49.0	..	Cloudy; fair.
2	36	70	53.0	..	Fair.
3	58	74	66.0	..	Cloudy; fair.
4	62	74	68.0	..	Cloudy; fair.
5	62	72	67.0	..	Fair.
6	66	72	69.0	1.0	Cloudy; thunder; rain at night.
7	56	44	50.0	..	Rain; fair.
8	24	42	33.0	..	Fair.
9	20	48	34.0	..	Fair.
10	24	50	37.0	..	Fair.
11	26	57	41.5	..	Fair.
12	50	64	57.0	..	Fair.
13	56	66	61.0	0.2	Smoky; thunder; rain.
14	62	72	67.0	1.0	Cloudy; mist; thunder; rain at
15	58	69	63.5	..	Cloudy. [night.
16	62	74	68.0	..	Mist; fair.
17	64	76	70.0	..	Cloudy; fair.
18	66	75	70.5	1.3	Cloudy; thunder; rain at night.
19	64	65	64.5	2.5	Cloudy; thunder; rain.
20	44	50	47.0	..	Cloudy.
21	40	56	48.0	..	Fair.
22	42	62	52.0	..	Fair.
23	42	68	55.0	0.4	Cloudy; rain at night.
24	62	72	67.0	..	Rain; fair.
25	48	76	62.0	..	Fair.
26	48	78	63.0	..	Fair.
27	58	78	68.0	0.4	Fair; cl'ds; thunder; r'n at night.
28	60	58	59.0	0.2	Fog; mist; rain.
Means	49.93	65.07	57.50	7.0	
Max.	66	78	70.5		
Min.	20	42	33.0		
Range	46	36	37.5		
Extreme range 58					

Greatest Rise and Fall of temperature in 24 hours.

	Sunrise.	2 P. M.
Rise . . .	22	10
Fall . . .	32	28

March, 1857.

DAY.	THERMOMETER. Sun-rise.	THERMOMETER. 2 P. M.	THERMOMETER. Mean.	RAIN. Ins.	REMARKS ON THE WEATHER.
1	50	64	57.0	..	Fair.
2	34	52	43.0	..	Fair.
3	40	64	52.0	..	Fair.
4	48	66	57.0	..	Cloudy.
5	46	56	51.0	..	Cloudy; fair.
6	26	53	39.5	..	Fair; ice.
7	28	48	38.0	..	Fair.
8	36	52	44.0	..	Cloudy; rain.
9	40	48	44.0	..	Cloudy; fair.
10	35	58	46.5	..	Cloudy.
11	42	46	44.0	..	Fair; windy.
12	24	46	35.0	..	Fair.
13	22	55	38.5	..	Smoky.
14	32	62	47.0	..	Smoky.
15	37	58	47.5	..	Smoky.
16	34	72	53.0	..	Smoky.
17	48	66	57.0	..	Smoky; cloudy.
18	47	62	54.5	..	Smoky. Martins.
19	36	73	54.5	..	Smoky.
20	54	82	68.0	..	Fair.
21	54	72	63.0	..	Smoky.
22	60	80	70.0	..	Smoky; cloudy; windy.
23	58	82	70.0	..	Fair.
24	60	82	71.0	..	Fair.
25	56	78	67.0	..	Eclipse of sun; only half observed
26	54	84	69.0	..	Sm'ky. [before obscur'd by sm'ke.
27	58	87	72.5	..	Smoky; thunder at night.
28	60	82	71.0	..	Smoky.
29	58	80	69.0	..	Smoky.
30	56	78	67.0	..	Smoky.
31	56	78	67.0	1.4	Cloudy; thunder; rain at night.
Means	44.81	66.65	55.73	1.4	
Max.	60	87	72.5		
Min.	22	46	35.0		
Range	38	41	37.5		
Extreme range 65					

Greatest Rise and Fall of temperature in 24 hours.

	Sunrise.	2 P. M.
Rise . . .	18	14
Fall . . .	20	12

April, 1857.

DAY.	THERMOMETER. Sun-rise.	THERMOMETER. 2 P. M.	THERMOMETER. Mean.	RAIN. Ins.	REMARKS ON THE WEATHER.
1	58	37	57.5	..	Fog; cloudy.
2	46	50	48 0	..	Fair.
3	38	64	51.0	..	Fair.
4	56	70	63.0	..	Cloudy. [at night.
5	64	39	51.5	0.2	Cl'dy; thunder; rain; hail; freeze
6	24	50	37 0	..	Fair. Vegetation killed.*
7	40	70	55.0	..	Fair.
8	59	56	57.5	..	Cloudy; sprinkle.
9	34	66	50.0	..	Fair; white frost.
10	44	76	60.0	..	Fair; cloudy.
11	44	41	42 5	0.4	Cloudy; rain.
12	32	57	44.5	..	Fair; white frost; ice.
13	40	58	49.0	..	Fair; white frost.
14	32	63	47.5	..	Fair; white frost; ice.
15	36	70	53.0	..	Smoky.
16	40	68	54.0	..	Fair.
17	60	76	68.0	0.2	Cloudy; thunder; rain at night.
18	46	59	52 5	..	Cloudy.
19	34	64	49 0	..	Fair; white frost.
20	38	78	58.0	..	Fair.
21	56	70	63.0	..	Fair; windy.
22	42	60	51.0	..	Fair; windy.
23	36	70	53.0	..	Fair.
24	38	75	56.5	..	Fair; smoky.
25	56	88	62.0	..	Smoky.
26	66	64	65.0	..	Cloudy; rain.
27	42	70	56.0	..	Cloudy.
28	47	80	63.5	..	Fair. [night—ground covered.
29	56	82	69.0	0.3	Cl'dy; thunder; hail and r'n after
30	62	60	61.0	2.3	Cloudy; rain.
Means	45.53	64.37	54.95	3.4	
Max.	66	88	69.0		
Min.	24	39	37.0		
Range	42	49	32.0		
Extreme range 64					

Greatest Rise and Fall of temperature in 24 hours.

	Sunrise.	2 P. M.
Rise . . .	20	20
Fall . . .	40	31

* April 6. Vegetation was, at this time, far advanced; peaches and apples large as bird eggs; corn up, and flowers out; leaves in the forest fully grown. All were killed, and the tree-tops bore the appearance of fire having run over them. Wheat in the ear killed to the ground. Grass that had become sufficient for pasturage destroyed, and starvation produced among the cattle.

A similar freeze took place on the 6th of April, 1827, just thirty years before, producing precisely similar effects.

May, 1857.

DAY.	THERMOMETER. Sunrise.	THERMOMETER. 3 P. M.	THERMOMETER. Mean.	RAIN. Ins.	REMARKS ON THE WEATHER.
1	55	70	62.5	. .	Fog; cloudy.
2	48	74	61.0	. .	Fair.
3	55	68	61.5	. .	Cloudy; fair.
4	42	76	59.0	. .	Fair.
5	60	82	71.0	. .	Fair.
6	58	83	70.5	. .	Fair.
7	56	83	69.5	. .	Fair.
8	64	84	74.0	. .	Fair; cloudy.
9	66	86	76.0	. .	Clouds; fair.
10	70	88	79.0	. .	Cloudy; fair.
11	70	84	77.0	. .	Cloudy.
12	65	84	74.5	. .	Cloudy.
13	74	78	76.0	0.1	Cloudy; thunder; rain at night.
14	68	85	76.5	0.2	Cloudy; thunder; rain.
15	58	86	72.0	1.3	Fair; thunder; rain and hail at night.
16	62	62	62.0	0.8	Cloudy; thunder; rain.
17	62	67	64.5	. .	Cloudy; rain.
18	48	70	59.0	. .	Fair.
19	50	76	63.0	. .	Fair.
20	54	69	61.5	. .	Cloudy.
21	46	78	62.0	. .	Fair.
22	48	82	65.0	. .	Fair.
23	50	82	66.0	. .	Fair.
24	56	83	69.5	. .	Fair.
25	68	72	70.0	0.1	Cloudy; rain.
26	64	76	70.0	. .	Cloudy; fair.
27	57	88	72.5	0.8	Cloudy; thunder; rain at night.
28	62	78	70.0	. .	Cloudy; fair.
29	58	81	69.5	0.3	Cloudy; thunder; rain.
30	68	83	75.5	. .	Cloudy.
31	60	76	68.0	. .	Cloudy.
Means	58.77	78.52	68.65	3.6	Greatest Rise and Fall of temperature in 24 hours.
Max.	74	88	79.0		
Min.	42	62	59.0		
Range	32	26	20.0		
Extreme range 46					

	Sunrise.	3 P. M.
Rise . . .	18	10
Fall . . .	14	24

June, 1857.

DAY.	THERMOMETER. Sunrise.	THERMOMETER. 3 P. M.	THERMOMETER. Mean.	RAIN. Ins.	REMARKS ON THE WEATHER.
1	56	77	66.5	. .	Fog; clouds.
2	56	80	68.0	. .	Fair.
3	54	84	69.0	. .	Fair.
4	62	88	75.0	. .	Fair.
5	64	88	76.0	. .	Fair.
6	68	90	79.0	. .	Fair.
7	70	88	79.0	. .	Clouds.
8	74	92	83.0	0.7	Cloudy; thunder; rain at night.
9	74	92	83.0	. .	Cloudy; thunder.
10	70	90	80.0	. .	Fog; fair.
11	70	90	80.0	. .	Fair.
12	70	88	79.0	. .	Fair.
13	72	88	80.0	. .	Fair; cloudy.
14	74	88	81.0	0.2	Cloudy; thunder; rain at night.
15	76	76	76.0	0.3	Cloudy; thunder; rain.
16	74	76	75.0	0.3	Cloudy; rain; showery all day.
17	68	80	74.0	. .	Fair.
18	65	76	70.5	. .	Fair; breezes.
19	60	80	70.0	. .	Fair.
20	67	80	73.5	. .	Fair.
21	67	81	74.0	. .	Fair.
22	61	81	71.0	. .	Fair.
23	63	81	72.0	. .	Fair.
24	62	80	71.0	. .	Fair.
25	70	84	77.0	. .	Fair; clouds; thunder.
26	74	80	77.0	0.4	Cloudy; rain.
27	74	86	80.0	. .	Cloudy.
28	74	90	82.0	. .	Cloudy.
29	70	87	78.5	. .	Fair.
30	74	86	80.0	. .	Fair.
Means	67.77	84.23	76.00	1.9	Greatest Rise and Fall of temperature in 24 hours.
Max.	76	92	83.0		
Min.	54	76	66.5		
Range	22	16	16.5		
Extreme range 38					

	Sunrise.	3 P. M.
Rise . . .	8	6
Fall . . .	6	12

July, 1857.

DAY.	THERMOMETER. Sunrise.	THERMOMETER. 3 P. M.	THERMOMETER. Mean.	RAIN. Ins.	REMARKS ON THE WEATHER.
1	74	74	74.0	0.6	Cloudy; thunder; rain.
2	72	80	76.0	. .	Cloudy.
3	64	76	70.0	. .	Fair; clouds.
4	64	76	70.0	. .	Fair.
5	64	79	71.5	. .	Cloudy.
6	64	82	73.0	. .	Fair; clouds.
7	66	84	75.0	. .	Fair.
8	66	86	76.0	. .	Fair.
9	70	86	78.0	. .	Fair.
10	70	86	78.0	0.1	Fair; thunder; rain.
11	74	86	75.0	. .	Fair.
12	74	85	79.5	0.1	Cloudy; rain.
13	74	88	81.0	. .	Fair.
14	74	92	83.0	. .	Fair.
15	76	94	85.0	. .	Fair.
16	76	96	86.0	. .	Fair.
17	76	98	87.0	. .	Fair; thunder.
18	76	94	85.0	. .	Fair.
19	76	96	86.0	. .	Fair.
20	76	94	85.0	. .	Fair; clouds.
21	76	94	85.0	. .	
22	80	90	85.0	0.1	Cloudy; thunder; rain.
23	78	84	81.0	. .	Cloudy.
24	70	86	78.0	. .	Fair.
25	76	84	80.0	. .	Cloudy; thunder.
26	76	90	83.0	. .	Fair.
27	76	90	88.0	. .	Fair; clouds; sprinkle.
28	76	86	81.0	0.1	Cloudy; thunder; rain.
29	76	86	81.0	. .	Fair.
30	74	84	79.0	0.5	Cloudy; rain; thunder.
31	74	86	80.0	0.3	Cloudy; rain; thunder.
Means	72.84	86.84	79.84	1.8	Greatest Rise and Fall of temperature in 24 hours.
Max.	80	98	87.0		
Min.	64	74	70.0		
Range	16	24	17.0		
Extreme range 34					

	Sunrise.	3 P. M.
Rise . . .	6	6
Fall . . .	8	12

August, 1857.

DAY.	THERMOMETER. Sunrise.	THERMOMETER. 3 P. M.	THERMOMETER. Mean.	RAIN. Ins.	REMARKS ON THE WEATHER.
1	76	80	78.0	4.0	Cloudy; heavy thunder at night.
2	74	78	76.0	1.0	Cloudy; rain; thunder at night.
3	74	80	77.0	1.5	Cloudy; thunder; rain.
4	74	80	77.0	0.6	Fair; cloudy; thunder; rain.
5	74	87	80.5	1.5	Fair; cloudy; thunder; rain.
6	74	88	81.0	. .	Fair.
7	74	90	82.0	. .	Fair; clouds.
8	76	91	83.5	. .	Fair.
9	75	90	82.5	. .	Clouds; thunder.
10	76	86	81.0	. .	Fair.
11	74	88	81.0	. .	Fair; thunder.
12	74	80	77.0	0.1	Fair; cloudy; mist; rain.
13	80	87	83.5	. .	Fair.
14	77	88	82.5	0.1	Cloudy; rain at night.
15	76	84	80.0	. .	Fog; clouds.
16	74	86	80.0	. .	Fair.
17	74	86	80.0	. .	Fair.
18	74	80	77.0	0.1	Cloudy; rain.
19	74	76	75.0	1.5	Cloudy; thunder; rain.
20	70	78	74.0	1.5	Rain.
21	66	82	74.0	. .	Fair.
22	68	84	76.0	. .	Fair; clouds.
23	72	82	77.0	. .	Clouds.
24	72	84	78.0	1.0	Cloudy; rain.
25	74	80	77.0	0.9	Cloudy; thunder; rain.
26	76	80	78.0	0.9	Cloudy; thunder; rain.
27	76	82	79.0	0.2	Cloudy; thunder; rain.
28	76	86	81.0	. .	Cloudy; fair.
29	68	76	72.0	. .	Fair.
30	64	76	70.0	. .	Fair.
31	. .	. .	. .	. .	
Means	73.53	83.17	78.35	14.9	Greatest Rise and Fall of temperature in 24 hours.
Max.	80	91	83.5		
Min.	64	76	70.0		
Range	16	15	13.5		
Extreme range 27					

	Sunrise.	3 P. M.
Rise . . .	6	7
Fall . . .	8	10

September, 1857.

DAY.	THERMOMETER. Sun-rise.	3 P. M.	Mean.	RAIN. Ins.	REMARKS ON THE WEATHER.
1	66	80	73.0	..	Fair.
2	70	83	76.5	..	Clouds.
3	70	80	75.0	..	Cloudy; fair.
4	72	82	77.0	..	Cloudy.
5	70	86	78.0	..	Fair.
6	70	86	78.0	..	Fair.
7	72	84	78.0	..	Cloudy; fair.
8	74	85	79.5	0.5	Cloudy; thunder; rain.
9	74	84	79.0	..	Fog; thunder; rain.
10	72	82	77.0	..	Cloudy.
11	74	84	79.0	..	Cloudy.
12	72	82	77.0	..	Fair; cloudy.
13	74	80	77.0	0.5	Cloudy; rain.
14	76	82	79.0	0.8	Rain; showery.
15	76	84	80.0	..	Cloudy; fair.
16	72	84	78.0	..	Cloudy.
17	74	84	79.0	..	Fair.
18	74	85	79.5	..	Fair; thunder; rain at night.
19	72	78	75.0	1.4	Rain.
20	62	72	67.0	..	Fair.
21	56	74	65.0	..	Fair.
22	64	72	68.0	..	Fair.
23	54	76	65.0	..	Fair.
24	56	78	67.0	..	Fair.
25	56	79	67.5	..	Fair.
26	56	80	68.0	..	Fair.
27	56	82	69.0	..	Fair.
28	58	82	70.0	..	Fair.
29	61	76	68.5	..	Fair.
30	52	76	64.0	..	Fair.
Means	66.83	80.73	73.78	3.2	
Max.	76	86	80.0		
Min.	52	72	64.0		
Range	24	14	16.0		

Extreme range 34

Greatest Rise and Fall of temperature in 24 hours.

	Sunrise.	3 P. M.
Rise . . .	8	4
Fall . . .	10	7

October, 1857.

DAY.	THERMOMETER. Sun-rise.	3 P. M.	Mean.	RAIN. Ins.	REMARKS ON THE WEATHER.
1	62	74	68.0	..	Cloudy; fair.
2	57	74	65.5	..	Cloudy; rain.
3	56	70	63.0	2.3	Rain.
4	68	74	71.0	0.8	Rain; thunder.
5	70	76	73.0	0.6	Fog; rain.
6	54	74	64.0	0.2	Fair; thunder; rain at night.
7	64	72	68.0	..	Rain; fair.
8	56	74	65.0	..	Fair; cloudy.
9	56	74	65.0	..	Fair; cloudy.
10	60	76	68.0	..	Fair; cloudy.
11	64	76	70.0	0.1	Cloudy; rain.
12	64	74	69.0	..	Fair.
13	60	70	65.0	..	Cloudy; mist; fair.
14	56	72	64.0	..	Fair.
15	52	73	62.5	..	Fair.
16	42	62	52.0	..	Fair.
17	41	62	51.5	..	Fair.
18	52	73	62.5	..	Fair; cloudy.
19	64	64	64.0	..	Cloudy; mist.
20	46	60	53.0	..	Fair.
21	46	54	50.0	..	Cloudy; rain.
22	50	61	55.5	..	Cloudy.
23	56	62	59.0	..	Cloudy; mist.
24	58	66	62.0	..	Cloudy.
25	48	68	58.0	..	Fair.
26	46	62	54.0	0.8	Cloudy; rain at night.
27	54	58	56.0	0.2	Rain.
28	48	60	54.0	..	Fog; fair.
29	46	64	55.0	..	Cloudy.
30	50	64	57.0	0.2	Cloudy; thunder; rain and hail [at night.
31	46	54	50.0	..	Fair.
Means	54.58	67.65	61.11	[illegible]	
Max.	70	76	73.0		
Min.	41	54	50.0		
Range	29	22	23.0		

Extreme range 35

Greatest Rise and Fall of

	Sunrise.	3 P. M.
Rise . . .	12	11
Fall . . .	18	11

November, 1857.

DAY.	THERMOMETER. Sun-rise.	2 P. M.	Mean.	RAIN. Ins.	REMARKS ON THE WEATHER.
1	40	66	53.0	..	Fair.
2	68	70	69.0	0.3	Cloudy; thunder; rain.
3	46	62	54.0	..	Fog; fair.
4	62	62	62.0	0.7	Thunder; rain.
5	68	76	72.0	..	Fair.
6	72	82	77.0	..	Fair.
7	75	70	72.5	1.1	Fair; thunder; rain.
8	46	46	46.0	..	Cloudy.
9	32	50	41.0	..	Fair; killing frost; ice.
10	32	56	44.0	..	Fair.
11	44	58	51.0	..	Cloudy.
12	50	60	55.0	..	Cloudy; rain at night.
13	56	56	56.0	1.2	Rain.
14	46	42	44.0	0.5	Cloudy; mist; sleet; rain.
15	38	39	38.5	1.3	Cloudy; rain.
16	42	47	44.5	..	Cloudy; fair at eve.
17	34	54	44.0	..	Fog; fair.
18	44	60	52.0	..	Fair.
19	46	41	43.5	..	Clouds; wind.
20	27	42	34.5	..	Fair.
21	32	56	44.0	..	Fair.
22	38	58	48.0	..	Fair.
23	48	44	46.0	..	Fair.
24	28	52	40.0	..	Fair.
25	42	44	43.0	0.3	Cloudy; rain.
26	38	52	45.0	..	Fair; cloudy.
27	44	66	55.0	..	Cloudy; rain at night.
28	60	58	59.0	2.8	Rain; thunder.
29	54	59	56.5	..	Fair.
30	42	60	51.0	..	Fair.
Means	46.47	56.27	51.37	8.2	
Max.	75	82	77.0		
Min.	27	39	34.5		
Range	48	43	42.5		

Extreme range 55

Greatest Rise and Fall of temperature in 24 hours.

	Sunrise.	2 P. M.
Rise . . .	28	14
Fall . . .	29	19

December, 1857.

DAY.	THERMOMETER. Sun-rise.	2 P. M.	Mean.	RAIN. Ins.	REMARKS ON THE WEATHER.
1	40	64	52.0	..	Fair.
2	54	64	59.0	..	Cloudy.
3	50	62	56.0	..	Cloudy.
4	54	62	58.0	..	Cloudy; rain at night.
5	60	64	62.0	0.4	Rain.
6	62	68	65.0	..	Cloudy; fair.
7	48	64	56.0	..	Fair.
8	66	72	69.0	..	Cloudy.
9	44	50	47.0	..	Cloudy; wind.
10	34	52	43.0	..	Fair.
11	32	58	45.0	..	Fair.
12	30	58	44.0	..	Fair.
13	32	60	46.0	..	Fair.
14	32	58	45.0	..	Fair; cloudy.
15	42	60	51.0	..	Fair.
16	50	60	55.0	0.1	Cloudy; rain.
17	52	60	56.0	..	Cloudy.
18	40	55	47.5	..	Fair.
19	36	48	42.0	..	Fair; cloudy.
20	40	51	45.5	..	Cloudy; rain at night.
21	18	46	32.0	1.0	Rain.
22	42	44	43.0	..	Cloudy.
23	36	42	39.0	..	Cloudy; rain and snow at night.
24	36	36	36.0	1.8	Snow, large flakes all day—4.5 in.
25	34	37	35.5	..	Fog; cloudy; eaves running.
26	34	42	38.0	..	Fog; cloudy; fair; snow melting.
27	38	52	45.0	..	Cloudy; rain at night.
28	54	54	54.0	1.5	Rain.
29	50	54	52.0	..	Cloudy; mist.
30	48	52	50.0	..	Cloudy; fair.
31	36	60	48.0	..	Fair.
Means	42.71	55.13	48.92	4.8	
Max.	66	72	69.0		
Min.	18	36	32.0		
Range	48	36	37.0		

Extreme range 54

Greatest Rise and Fall of

	Sunrise.	2 P. M.
Rise . . .	24	8
Fall . . .	22	22

January, 1858.

DAY.	THERMOMETER. Sun-rise.	2 P. M.	Mean.	RAIN. Ins.	REMARKS ON THE WEATHER.
1	44	62	53.0	..	Cloudy; fair.
2	37	50	43.5	..	Cloudy.
3	32	46	39.0	..	Fair; cloudy.
4	40	49	44.5	0.3	Fair; cloudy; rain.
5	42	43	42.5	..	Cloudy; fair.
6	32	56	44.0	..	Fair.
7	42	52	47.0	..	Fair.
8	40	48	44.0	..	Cloudy.
9	48	50	49.0	3.3	Cloudy; thunder; rain.
10	60	60	60.0	..	Thunder; rain.
11	44	58	51.0	..	Fair.
12	42	65	53.5	..	Fair.
13	46	52	49.0	..	Cloudy.
14	46	50	48.0	0.8	Cloudy; rain.
15	52	54	53.0	..	Rain; cloudy.
16	34	48	41.0	..	Fair.
17	34	56	45.0	..	Fair.
18	32	58	45.0	..	Fair.
19	36	60	48.0	..	Fair.
20	40	60	50.0	..	Fair.
21	40	63	51.5	..	Fair.
22	38	56	47.0	..	Cloudy; rain at night.
23	50	52	51.0	2.8	Rain.
24	58	64	61.0	1.5	Rain; thunder.
25	50	58	54.0	..	Fair.
26	46	60	53.0	..	Fair.
27	46	58	52.0	..	Cloudy.
28	48	60	54.0	..	Fair.
29	38	52	45.0	..	Fair.
30	37	46	41.5	0.4	Cloudy; rain.
31	41	44	42.5	0.4	Rain.
Means	42.42	54.52	48.47	9.5	
Max.	60	65	61.0		
Min.	32	43	39.0		
Range	28	22	22.0		
Extreme range 33					

Greatest Rise and Fall of temperature in 24 hours.

	Sunrise.	2 P. M.
Rise . . .	12	13
Fall . . .	16	13

February, 1858.

DAY.	THERMOMETER. Sun-rise.	2 P. M.	Mean.	RAIN. Ins.	REMARKS ON THE WEATHER.
1	38	42	40.0	..	Cloudy; rain.
2	36	50	43.0	..	Fair.
3	40	35	37 5	0.8	Cloudy; snow in large flakes, 2
4	34	40	37.0	..	Cloudy. [inches deep.
5	32	44	38.0	..	Fair; cloudy; rain at night.
6	38	46	42.0	0.5	Rain.
7	30	50	40.0	..	Fair.
8	34	58	46.0	..	Cloudy.
9	56	60	58.0	..	Cloudy; wind.
10	32	39	35.5	..	Cloudy.
11	27	36	31.5	..	Cloudy; sleet.
12	34	36	35.0	..	Rain; icicles; rain.
13	38	44	41 0	1.0	Rain.
14	29	56	42.5	..	Fair.
15	42	58	50.0	0.1	Fair; cloudy; thunder; rain.
16	40	52	46.0	..	Fair.
17	34	60	47.0	..	Fair.
18	54	64	59.0	..	Cloudy.
19	38	56	47.0	..	Fair.
20	38	68	53.0	..	Cloudy.
21	64	68	66 0	0.2	Cloudy; rain.
22	27	37	32.0	..	Fair.
23	20	44	32.0	..	Fair.
24	22	44	33.0	..	Fair.
25	30	61	45.5	..	Fair.
26	34	67	50.5	..	Fair.
27	52	72	62.0	..	Fair; cloudy.
28	48	44	46.0	0.1	Rain; wind.
Means	37.18	51.11	44.14	2.7	
Max.	64	72	66.0		
Min.	20	35	31.5		
Range	44	37	34.5		
Extreme range 52					

Greatest Rise and Fall of temperature in 24 hours.

	Sunrise.	2 P. M.
Rise . . .	26	17
Fall . . .	37	31

March, 1858.

DAY.	THERMOMETER. Sun-rise.	2 P. M.	Mean.	RAIN. Ins.	REMARKS ON THE WEATHER.
1	30	42	36.0	..	Fair.
2	24	52	38.0	..	Fair.
3	30	52	41.0	..	Fair.
4	36	64	50.0	..	Cloudy; fair.
5	50	68	59.0	..	Cloudy.
6	60	70	65.0	..	Cloudy; rain at night.
7	42	40	41.0	1.3	Rain.
8	36	50	43.0	..	Fair.
9	32	60	46.0	..	Fair.
10	42	77	59.5	..	Fair.
11	60	70	65.0	..	Cloudy.
12	58	64	61.0	..	Cloudy.
13	54	76	65.0	..	Fair.
14	62	70	66.0	..	Cloudy.
15	66	74	70.0	..	Cloudy.
16	68	70	69.0	3.4	Cloudy; thunder; rain at night.
17	50	66	58.0	..	Fair.
18	50	65	57.5	0.4	Cloudy; thunder; rain.
19	64	76	70.0	..	Cloudy.
20	70	70	70.0	..	Cloudy; thunder; rain.
21	58	62	60.0	..	Fair; cloudy.
22	48	52	50.0	0.3	Fair; cloudy.
23	48	62	55.0	0.6	Cloudy; thunder; rain.
24	46	70	58.0	..	Fair.
25	48	71	59.5	..	Fair.
26	52	74	63.0	..	Fair.
27	56	80	68.0	..	Fair.
28	60	80	70.0	..	Fair.
29	62	73	67.5	0.6	Cloudy; rain at night.
30	58	74	66.0	..	Cloudy.
31	58	70	64.0	..	Cloudy.
Means	50.90	65.93	58.42	6.6	
Max.	70	80	70.0		
Min.	24	40	36.0		
Range	46	40	34.0		
Extreme range 56					

Greatest Rise and Fall of temperature in 24 hours.

	Sunrise.	2 P. M.
Rise . . .	18	17
Fall . . .	18	30

April, 1858.

DAY.	THERMOMETER. Sun-rise.	2 P. M.	Mean.	RAIN. Ins.	REMARKS ON THE WEATHER.
1	54	70	62.0	..	Fair.
2	50	79	64.5	..	Fair.
3	50	82	66.0	..	Fair.
4	58	74	66.0	..	Fair.
5	56	74	65.0	..	Fair.
6	57	81	69.0	..	Fair.
7	62	72	67.0	0.8	Cloudy; thunder; rain at night.
8	58	74	66.0	..	Cloudy; fair.
9	58	74	66.0	..	Cloudy; fair.
10	70	76	73.0	..	Cloudy; thunder; sprinkle.
11	56	62	59.0	..	Cloudy.
12	48	52	50.0	..	Cloudy; thunder; sprinkle.
13	44	51	47.5	..	Fair.
14	42	63	52.5	..	Fair.
15	50	80	65.0	..	Fair.
16	68	85	76.5	..	Cloudy.
17	69	80	74.5	..	Cloudy.
18	68	82	75.0	1.6	Cloudy; thunder; rain at night.
19	64	76	70.0	..	Cloudy.
20	56	62	59.0	..	Cloudy.
21	46	70	58.0	..	Fair.
22	54	80	67.0	..	Fair.
23	52	62	57.0	..	Fair.
24	44	68	56.0	..	Fair.
25	50	76	63.0	0.6	Cloudy; thunder; hail; rain at
26	60	65	62.5	..	Fair. [night.
27	44	65	54.5	..	Fair.
28	50	74	62.0	..	Fair.
29	62	77	69.5	..	Cloudy.
30	68	76	72.0	1.8	Cloudy; thunder; rain at night.
Means	55.60	72.07	63.83	4.8	
Max.	70	85	76.5		
Min.	42	51	47.5		
Range	28	34	29.0		
Extreme range 43					

Greatest Rise and Fall of temperature in 24 hours.

	Sunrise.	2 P. M.
Rise . . .	18	17
Fall . . .	16	18

May, 1858.

DAY.	THERMOMETER. Sun-rise.	THERMOMETER. 3 P. M.	THERMOMETER. Mean.	RAIN. Ins.	REMARKS ON THE WEATHER.
1	64	64	64.0	1.3	Fog; thunder; rain.
2	64	70	67.0	0.5	Cloudy; rain.
3	64	70	67.0	..	Fair.
4	52	68	60.0	..	Fair.
5	54	76	65.0	..	Fair.
6	56	74	65.0	..	Cloudy.
7	60	74	67.0	..	Cloudy.
8	64	66	65.0	0.7	Cloudy; rain.
9	64	70	67.0	..	Cloudy; rain.
10	64	64	64.0	0.5	Cloudy; rain.
11	54	66	60.0	..	Fair.
12	50	76	63.0	..	Fair.
13	60	84	72.0	..	Fair.
14	62	80	71.0	..	Fair.
15	64	80	72.0	..	Fair.
16	64	88	76.0	..	Fair.
17	68	74	71.0	..	Cloudy; thunder; rain at night.
18	64	66	65.0	..	Cloudy.
19	58	64	61.0	..	Cloudy.
20	58	78	68.0	..	Fair.
21	62	80	71.0	..	Fair.
22	66	84	75.0	..	Fair.
23	68	84	76.0	..	Cloudy.
24	76	83	79.5	1.4	Cloudy; thunder; rain.
25	68	82	75.0	..	Rain.
26	64	84	74.0	..	Fair.
27	64	87	75.5	..	Fair.
28	74	85	79.5	0.7	Fair; cl'dy; thunder; r'n at night.
29	70	84	77.0	..	Fair; clouds.
30	74	86	80.0	..	Fair; clouds.
31	76	85	80.5	..	Fair; clouds.
Means	63.55	76.65	70.10	5.1	Greatest Rise and Fall of temperature in 24 hours.
Max.	76	88	80.5		
Min.	50	64	60.0		
Range	26	24	20.5		
Extreme range 38					

	Sunrise.	3 P. M.
Rise . . .	10	10
Fall . . .	12	14

June, 1858.

DAY.	THERMOMETER. Sun-rise.	THERMOMETER. 3 P. M.	THERMOMETER. Mean.	RAIN. Ins.	REMARKS ON THE WEATHER.
1	68	74	71.0	0.1	Cloudy; rain.
2	74	84	79.0	..	Fog; fair.
3	72	86	79.0	..	Fair.
4	74	78	76.0	0.4	Cloudy; rain.
5	68	70	69.0	0.7	Rain.
6	64	78	71.0	..	Fair.
7	65	86	75.5	..	Fair.
8	72	85	78.5	0.2	Fog; cl'dy; thunder; r'n at night.
9	75	84	79.5	..	Cloudy; rain.
10	74	74	74.0	2.5	Rain.
11	70	75	72.5	..	Cloudy.
12	60	70	65.0	..	Fair.
13	58	72	65.0	..	Fair.
14	64	78	71.0	..	Cloudy.
15	64	82	73.0	..	Fair.
16	68	86	77.0	..	Fair.
17	72	82	77.0	0.2	Cloudy; thunder; rain.
18	68	82	75.0	..	Cloudy.
19	68	84	76.0	..	Fair.
20	70	86	78.0	0.2	Fog; cloudy; thunder; rain.
21	72	80	76.0	..	Fog; cloudy; thunder; rain.
22	72	86	79.0	0.2	Fog; cloudy; thunder; rain.
23	72	86	79.0	0.2	Cloudy; thunder; rain.
24	74	84	79.0	..	Cloudy; thunder; rain.
25	74	80	77.0	..	Cloudy.
26	74	84	79.0	0.1	Cloudy; thunder; rain.
27	70	86	78.0	..	Fair.
28	74	90	82.0	..	Clouds.
29	76	90	83.0	..	Fair.
30	76	94	85.0	..	Fair; thunder.
Means	70.07	81.87	75.97	4.8	Greatest Rise and Fall of temperature in 24 hours.
Max.	76	94	85.0		
Min.	58	70	65.0		
Range	18	24	20.0		
Extreme range 36					

	Sunrise.	3 P. M.
Rise . . .	7	10
Fall . . .	10	10

July, 1858.

DAY.	THERMOMETER. Sun-rise.	THERMOMETER. 3 P. M.	THERMOMETER. Mean.	RAIN. Ins.	REMARKS ON THE WEATHER.
1	76	90	83.0	..	Fair.
2	76	90	83.0	..	Fair.
3	76	88	82.0	0.2	Cloudy; thunder; rain at night.
4	78	82	80.0	0.4	Cloudy; thunder; rain.
5	78	84	81.0	0.5	Cloudy; thunder; rain.
6	78	88	83.0	..	Cloudy; fair.
7	78	86	82.0	..	Cloudy; rain; thunder.
8	78	84	81.0	0.3	Cloudy; rain; thunder.
9	74	88	81.0	..	Cloudy; rain; thunder.
10	76	84	80 0	..	Cloudy; thunder.
11	76	80	78.0	0.4	Cloudy; rain; thunder.
12	70	82	76.0	..	Fair.
13	68	80	74.0	..	Fair.
14	70	88	79.0	..	Fair.
15	74	90	82.0	..	Fair.
16	74	90	82.0	..	Fair.
17	74	91	82.5	..	Fair.
18	78	90	84.0	..	Cloudy; thunder.
19	76	92	84.0	..	Fair.
20	76	92	84.0	..	Clouds; thunder.
21	76	94	85.0	..	Clouds; thunder.
22	78	90	84.0	..	Fair.
23	80	94	87.0	..	Fair.
24	76	88	82.0	..	Fair.
25	70	90	80.0	..	Fair.
26	72	90	81.0	..	Fair.
27	74	90	82.0	..	Fair.
28	74	90	82.0	..	Fair.
29	74	91	82.5	..	Fair.
30	76	93	84.5	..	Clouds; fair.
31	76	92	84.0	..	Fair.
Means	75.16	88.42	81.79	1.8	Greatest Rise and Fall of temperature in 24 hours.
Max.	80	94	87.0		
Min.	68	80	74.0		
Range	12	14	13.0		
Extreme range 26					

	Sunrise.	3 P. M.
Rise . . .	4	8
Fall . . .	6	6

August, 1858.

DAY.	THERMOMETER. Sun-rise.	THERMOMETER. 3 P. M.	THERMOMETER. Mean.	RAIN. Ins.	REMARKS ON THE WEATHER.
1	72	92	82.0	..	Fair.
2	74	92	83.0	..	Fair.
3	74	92	83.0	..	Fair.
4	74	94	84.0	..	Fair.
5	72	92	82.0	..	Fair.
6	74	94	84.0	..	Fair.
7	74	92	83.0	1.2	Fair; cloudy; thunder; rain.
8	74	92	83.0	..	Fair.
9	76	92	84.0	..	Fair; clouds; thunder.
10	74	92	83 0	..	Fog; fair.
11	74	94	84.0	..	Fair; clouds; thunder.
12	74	84	79.0	0.4	Cloudy; thunder; rain.
13	74	90	82.0	0.1	Cloudy; thunder; rain.
14	76	90	83.0	..	Fair; cloudy.
15	76	90	83.0	0.1	Fair; clouds; thunder; rain at night.
16	74	88	81.0	..	Clouds.
17	76	90	83.0	0.1	Fair; clouds; thunder; shower at night.
18	72	92	82.0	..	Fair.
19	70	92	81.0	..	Fair.
20	66	90	78.0	..	Fair.
21	68	96	82.0	..	Fair.
22	72	96	84.0	..	Fair.
23	70	94	82.0	..	Fair.
24	67	86	76.5	..	Fair.
25	70	86	78.0	..	Fair.
26	72	96	84.0	..	
27	74	96	85.0	0.1	Fair; clouds; thunder; shower.
28	66	80	73.0	..	Fair.
29	58	74	66.0	..	Fair.
30	64	76	70.0	..	Fair; clouds.
31	56	80	68.0	..	Fair.
Means	71.19	89.81	80.50	2.0	Greatest Rise and Fall of temperature in 24 hours.
Max.	76	96	86.0		
Min.	56	74	66.0		
Range	20	22	19.0		
Extreme range 40					

	Sunrise.	3 P. M.
Rise . . .	6	10
Fall . . .	8	10

September, 1858.

Day.	Thermometer. Sunrise.	3 P. M.	Mean.	Rain. Ins.	Remarks on the Weather.
1	68	84	76.0	0.4	Cloudy; thunder; rain.
2	75	92	83.5	..	Fair.
3	76	68	72.0	1.4	Cloudy; thunder; rain.
4	68	78	73.0	..	Cloudy.
5	66	86	76.0	..	Cloudy; fair.
6	70	90	80.0	..	Fair.
7	74	90	82.0	..	Cloudy; fair.
8	74	86	80.0	..	Cloudy; thunder.
9	74	84	79.0	..	Cloudy.
10	70	82	76.0	..	Fair.
11	62	80	71.0	..	Fair.
12	60	80	70.0	..	Fair. Comet.
13	60	84	72.0	..	Fair.
14	60	82	71.0	..	Fair.
15	62	86	74.0	..	Fair.
16	54	84	69.0	..	Fair.
17	56	85	70.5	..	Fair.
18	64	88	76.0	..	Fair.
19	58	82	70.0	..	Fair.
20	56	84	70.0	..	Fair.
21	58	86	72.0	..	Fair.
22	68	88	78.0	..	Fair.
23	62	88	75.0	..	Fair.
24	62	88	75.0	..	Fair.
25	64	88	76.0	..	Smoky.
26	64	88	76.0	..	Smoky. Comet.
27	64	84	74.0	..	Smoky.
28	64	84	74.0	..	Smoky.
29	64	87	75.5	..	Fair.
30	64	88	76.0	..	
Means	64.70	84.80	74.75	1.8	
Max.	76	92	83.5		
Min.	54	68	69.0		
Range	22	24	14.5		
Extreme range 38					

Greatest Rise and Fall of temperature in 24 hours.

	Sunrise.	3 P. M.
Rise	12	10
Fall	8	24

October, 1858.

Day.	Thermometer. Sunrise.	3 P. M.	Mean.	Rain. Ins.	Remarks on the Weather.
1	64	88	76.0	..	Fair.
2	68	88	78.0	..	Fair.
3	68	87	77.5	..	Fair.
4	70	88	79.0	..	Fair.
5	72	90	81.0	..	Fair.
6	70	90	80.0	..	Smoky; fair.
7	70	90	80.0	..	Fair.
8	40	74	57.0	..	Fair; cloudy.
9	50	68	59.0	0.3	Smoky; cloudy; rain at night.
10	60	64	62.0	1.8	Rain.
11	66	64	65.0	..	Cloudy.
12	52	60	56.0	..	Fog; fair.
13	50	78	64.0	..	Fair.
14	58	72	65.0	..	Fair.
15	58	78	68.0	..	Fair.
16	58	78	68.0	..	Fair.
17	64	82	73.0	..	Fair.
18	66	80	73.0	..	Fair; clouds.
19	66	68	67.0	1.2	Rain.
20	46	64	55.0	..	Fair.
21	48	66	57.0	..	Cloudy; rain; thunder.
22	53	70	61.5	2.4	Rain.
23	58	76	67.0	..	Cloudy.
24	64	72	68.0	..	Cloudy.
25	54	76	65.0	..	Fair.
26	62	73	67.5	..	Cloudy; thunder; rain.
27	64	62	63.0	2.4	Cloudy; thunder; rain at night.
28	57	58	57.5	0.3	Rain.
29	52	66	59.0	..	Fair.
30	54	68	61.0	..	Cloudy; sprinkle; fair.
31	56	62	59.0	1.0	Fair; cloudy; thunder; rain.
Means	59.29	74.19	66.74	9.4	
Max.	72	90	81.0		
Min.	40	58	55.0		
Range	32	32	26.0		
Extreme range 50					

Greatest Rise and Fall of temperature in 24 hours.

	Sunrise.	3 P. M.
Rise	10	18
Fall	30	16

November, 1858.

Day.	Thermometer. Sunrise.	2 P. M.	Mean.	Rain. Ins.	Remarks on the Weather.
1	56	52	54.0	..	Cloudy.
2	50	52	51.0	..	Cloudy.
3	44	53	48.5	..	Cloudy.
4	40	48	44.0	..	Fair; cloudy.
5	44	48	46.0	..	Cloudy.
6	36	60	48.0	0.1	Fair; white frost; shower at night.
7	44	50	47.0	..	Fair; clouds; wind; snow-flakes.
8	36	42	39.0	..	Fair. Vegetation killed; top of ground frozen.
9	38	45	41.5	..	Cloudy; fair.
10	40	56	48.0	..	Cloudy.
11	42	50	46.0	..	Cloudy; fair.
12	36	52	44.0	..	Fair; clouds.
13	32	52	42.0	..	Fair; ice.
14	36	50	43.0	..	Fair; cloudy.
15	46	48	47.0	..	Cloudy.
16	28	44	36.0	..	Fair.
17	24	50	37.0	..	Fair.
18	32	46	39.0	..	Fair.
19	32	42	37.0	..	Fair; sleet; snow at night.
20	32	38	35.0	..	Fair; snow 2.5 inches deep.
21	34	40	37.0	..	Fair; rain.
22	40	40	40.0	0.6	Fair; rain.
23	30	44	37.0	..	Fair; cloudy.
24	26	52	39.0	..	Fair.
25	38	58	48.0	..	Cloudy.
26	52	64	58.0	0.2	Rain.
27	54	66	60.0	..	Cloudy.
28	64	55	59.5	0.6	Cloudy; thunder; rain.
29	36	48	42.0	..	Cloudy.
30	36	51	43.5	..	Fair.
Means	39.27	40.87	44.57	1.5	
Max.	64	66	60.0		
Min.	24	38	35.0		
Range	40	28	25.0		
Extreme range 42					

Greatest Rise and Fall of temperature in 24 hours.

	Sunrise.	2 P. M.
Rise	14	12
Fall	28	10

December, 1858.

Day.	Thermometer. Sunrise.	2 P. M.	Mean.	Rain. Ins.	Remarks on the Weather.
1	38	60	49.0	..	Cloudy.
2	56	64	60.0	..	Cloudy; rain.
3	60	50	55.0	..	Fog; mist; thunder; rain.
4	41	48	44.5	2.0	Rain.
5	37	50	43.5	..	Fair; clouds.
6	38	60	49.0	..	Cloudy.
7	52	46	49.0	0.2	Cl'dy; mist; sleet; thunder; rain.
8	28	40	34.0	..	Fair.
9	24	41	32.5	..	Fair.
10	20	47	33.5	..	Fair.
11	42	52	47.0	..	Cloudy; mist.
12	58	68	63.0	..	Cloudy; mist.
13	64	68	66.0	..	Cloudy.
14	68	62	65.0	0.7	Cloudy; thunder; rain.
15	36	52	44.0	..	Fair.
16	38	51	44.5	..	Cloudy.
17	32	38	35.0	..	Fair.
18	31	38	34.5	..	Fair.
19	44	52	48.0	..	Fair.
20	52	58	55.0	..	Cloudy; mist; rain.
21	38	57	47.5	2.2	Rain.
22	30	60	45.0	..	Fair.
23	46	60	53.0	..	Cloudy.
24	48	52	50.0	..	Cloudy.
25	45	45	45.0	1.6	Cloudy; rain.
26	46	58	52.0	..	Rain.
27	52	58	55.0	..	Rain; mist.
28	48	56	52.0	..	Rain.
29	56	60	58.0	..	Rain; mist.
30	56	57	56.5	..	Fair.
31	34	54	44.0	..	Fair.
Means	43.81	54.26	48.71	6.7	
Max.	68	68	66.0		
Min.	20	38	32.5		
Range	48	30	33.5		
Extreme range 48					

Greatest Rise and Fall of temperature in 24 hours.

	Sunrise.	2 P. M.
Rise	22	20
Fall	32	14

January, 1859.

Day.	Thermometer. Sunrise.	Thermometer. 3 P. M.	Thermometer. Mean.	Rain. Ins.	Remarks on the weather.
1	28	36	32.0	..	Fair.
2	40	56	48.0	..	Cloudy; snow; sleet; fair.
3	30	56	43.0	..	Cloudy; fair.
4	44	57	50.5	..	Fair.
5	56	60	58.0	..	Cloudy; rain at night.
6	56	66	61.0	1.8	Rain.
7	28	35	31.5	..	Fair.
8	36	47	41.5	..	Fair.
9	30	60	45.0	..	Fair.
10	30	56	43.0	..	Clouds.
11	46	49	47.5	..	Rain.
12	46	52	49.0	0.8	Mist; cloudy; rain at night.
13	51	58	54.5	0.5	Rain.
14	42	58	50.0	..	Fair.
15	36	52	44.0	..	Fair.
16	34	57	45.5	..	Fair; clouds.
17	34	50	42.0	..	Fair.
18	27	52	39.5	..	Fair.
19	30	58	44.0	..	Fair.
20	60	65	62.5	0.5	Cloudy; thunder; rain.
21	40	50	45.0	..	Fair.
22	30	34	32.0	..	Fair.
23	18	38	28.0	..	Fair; cl'dy; thunder; r'n at night.
24	20	50	35.0	..	Fair.
25	44	46	45.0	..	Cloudy; mist.
26	43	58	50.5	..	Cloudy; mist.
27	58	68	63.0	0.2	Cloudy; rain.
28	32	60	46.0	..	Fair.
29	40	58	49.0	..	Fair.
30	42	56	49.0	..	Cloudy; fair.
31	34	56	45.0	..	Cloudy.
Means	38.23	53.35	45.79	3.8	
Max.	60	68	63.0		
Min.	18	34	28.0		
Range	42	34	35.0		
Extreme range 50					

Greatest Rise and Fall of temperature in 24 hours.

	Sunrise.	3 P. M.
Rise . . .	30	20
Fall . . .	28	31

February, 1859.

Day.	Thermometer. Sunrise.	Thermometer. 2 P. M.	Thermometer. Mean.	Rain. Ins.	Remarks on the weather.
1	50	56	53.0	..	Rain.
2	52	64	58.0	..	Cloudy; fair.
3	30	50	40.0	..	Fair.
4	32	58	45.0	..	Fair.
5	39	60	49.5	..	Clouds.
6	27	42	34.5	..	Fair.
7	28	54	41.0	..	Fair.
8	56	60	58.0	0.5	Cloudy; thunder; rain.
9	32	47	39.5	..	Cloudy; fair.
10	28	42	35.0	..	Fair.
11	47	64	55.5	..	Cloudy; fair.
12	30	54	42.0	..	Fair.
13	36	56	46.0	..	Cloudy.
14	60	64	63.0	0.7	Cl'dy; sh'r; thunder; r'n at night.
15	64	72	68.0	0.3	Fog; thunder; rain.
16	58	70	64.0	..	Fog; fair.
17	64	78	71.0	0.2	Cloudy; thunder; warm S. wind; rain.
18	66	77	71.5	..	Cloudy; thunder.
19	70	78	74.0	0.2	Cloudy; thunder; rain at night.
20	42	56	49.0	..	Fair.
21	32	60	46.0	..	Fair; cloudy.
22	54	64	59.0	0.3	Cloudy; thunder; rain at night.
23	60	80	70.0	..	Fog; fair; thunder; rain at night.
24	60	78	69.0	..	Cloudy; showers; thunder.
25	..	..	..	..	
26	38	62	50.0	..	Fair.
27	47	76	61.5	..	Cloudy; clouds.
28	54	58	56.0	..	Cloudy; west wind.
Means	46.52	62.22	54.37	[illegible]	
Max.	70	80	74.0		
Min.	27	42	34 5		
Range	43	38	39.5		
Extreme range 53					

Greatest Rise and Fall of temperature in 24 hours.

	Sunrise.	2 P. M.
Rise . . .	28	22
Fall . . .	28	22

March, 1859.

Day.	Thermometer. Sunrise.	Thermometer. 2 P. M.	Thermometer. Mean.	Rain. Ins.	Remarks on the weather.
1	50	58	54.0	..	Cl'dy; fair; thunder; rain at night.
2	62	68	65.0	1.0	Cloudy; thunder; rain.
3	46	62	54.0	..	Fair.
4	40	70	55.0	..	Fair.
5	44	71	57.5	0.5	Fair; thunder; rain at night.
6	60	68	64.0	..	Clouds; thunder; rain.
7	44	50	47.0	..	Cloudy; mist.
8	46	63	54.5	..	Fair.
9	41	68	54.5	..	Fair.
10	57	69	63.0	0.1	Cloudy; thunder; rain at night.
11	44	61	52.5	..	Fair.
12	34	72	53.0	..	Fair.
13	62	64	63.0	2.6	Cloudy; thunder; rain.
14	40	57	48.5	..	Fair.
15	38	65	51.5	..	Fair.
16	40	68	54.0	0.3	Cloudy; thunder; rain at night.
17	56	70	63.0	..	Rain.
18	38	58	48.0	..	Fair.
19	34	70	52.0	..	Fair.
20	58	65	61.5	0.6	Cloudy; rain.
21	64	74	69.0	0.3	Thunder; rain.
22	54	80	67.0	..	Fog; fair.
23	60	68	64.0	0.1	Fair; thunder; rain.
24	62	75	68.5	..	Fog; fair.
25	46	60	53.0	..	Fair.
26	48	68	58.0	0.1	Fair; cloudy; thunder; rain.
27	60	76	68.0	..	Cloudy.
28	68	84	76.0	..	Clouds; fair; high wind from S.
29	44	66	55.0	..	Fair.
30	40	68	54.0	..	Fair.
31	34	68	51.0	..	White frost; fair.
Means	48.84	67.23	58.03	5.6	
Max.	68	84	76.0		
Min.	34	50	47.0		
Range	34	34	29.0		
Extreme range 50					

Greatest Rise and Fall of temperature in 24 hours.

	Sunrise.	2 P. M.
Rise . . .	28	13
Fall . . .	24	18

April, 1859.

Day.	Thermometer. Sunrise.	Thermometer. 2 P. M.	Thermometer. Mean.	Rain. Ins.	Remarks on the weather.
1	50	70	60.0	0.3	Cloudy; thunder; rain at night.
2	64	72	68.0	..	Rain; thunder; cloudy.
3	40	62	51.0	..	Fair; cloudy.
4	34	58	46.0	..	Fair.
5	34	56	45.0	..	Fair.
6	36	68	52 0	..	Fair; clouds; smoky.
7	36	75	55.5	..	Smoky.
8	52	82	67.0	..	Fair.
9	70	88	79.0	..	Cloudy.
10	72	72	72.0	0.5	Cloudy; thunder; rain.
11	64	85	74.5	..	Cloudy; fair.
12	72	76	74.0	0.7	Cloudy; thunder; rain.
13	72	75	73.5	0.3	Cloudy; thunder; rain.
14	42	64	53.0	..	Fair.
15	40	72	56.0	..	Fair.
16	40	58	49.0	..	Fair; high wind from N. W.
17	32	68	50.0	..	Fair; ice.*
18	44	82	63.0	..	Fair.
19	68	82	75.0	..	Fair.
20	60	82	71.0	..	Fair.
21	64	74	69.0	1.8	Cloudy; thunder; showers.
22	48	56	52.0	..	Cloudy; fair; high N. W. wind.
23	36	70	53.0	..	Fair.
24	48	80	64.0	..	Fair; clouds.
25	64	80	72.0	..	Cloudy; thunder.
26	70	82	76.0	..	Fair.
27	56	80	68.0	..	Fair.
28	60	60	60.0	0.8	Cloudy; thunder; rain.
29	60	72	66.0	..	Fair; clouds; high wind from N.
30	54	78	66.0	..	Fair; clouds.
Means	52.73	72.63	62.68	4.4	
Max.	72	88	79.0		
Min.	32	56	45.0		
Range	40	32	34.0		
Extreme range 56					

Greatest Rise and Fall of temperature in 24 hours.

	Sunrise.	2 P. M.
Rise . . .	24	14
Fall . . .	30	20

* April 17. Vegetation killed; fruit all destroyed. Forest leaves, full grown, all black and dead. Peaches, apples, plums, &c., large as birds' eggs, all destroyed.

May, 1859.

DAY.	THERMOMETER. Sun-rise.	3 P. M.	Mean.	RAIN. Ins.	REMARKS ON THE WEATHER.
1	60	80	70.0	..	
2	67	80	73.5	..	
3	64	84	74.0	..	
4	68	83	75.5	..	
5	64	80	72.0	..	
6	66	74	70.0	..	
7	62	81	71.5	..	
8	64	82	73.0	0.1	Fog; thunder; rain at night.
9	64	78	71.0	..	
10	62	86	74.0	..	
11	62	86	74.0	..	
12	64	84	74.0	..	
13	68	88	78.0	..	
14	68	88	78.0	..	
15	70	90	80.0	..	
16	70	88	79.0	..	
17	72	86	79.0	..	Thunder.
18	70	90	80.0	..	
19	68	88	78.0	..	
20	68	90	79.0	0.8	Thunder.
21	62	80	71.0	..	
22	62	80	71.0	..	
23	53	82	67.5	..	
24	62	86	74.0	..	
25	70	86	78.0	..	
26	68	88	78.0	..	
27	56	76	66.0	..	
28	52	78	65.0	..	
29	60	82	71.0	0.2	Thunder.
30	74	86	80.0	..	
31	..	..	..	..	
Means	64.67	83.67	74.17	1.1	
Max.	74	90	80.0		
Min.	52	74	65.0		
Range	22	16	15.0		
Extreme range 38					

Greatest Rise and Fall of temperature in 24 hours.

	Sunrise.	3 P. M.
Rise . . .	14	8
Fall . . .	12	12

June, 1859.

DAY.	THERMOMETER. Sun-rise.	3 P. M.	Mean.	RAIN. Ins.	REMARKS ON THE WEATHER.
1	70	90	80.0	..	Fair; gentle breezes. [at 4 P. M.
2	72	90	81.0	1.6	Fair A. M.; thun'r, hail, r'n, wind
3	70	82	76.0	..	Cl'dy at S. R.; fair; gentle breezes.
4	58	74	66.0	..	Fair at S. R.; slight cl'ds; breezes.
5	58	76	67.0	..	Fair at S. R.; slight cl'ds; breezes.
6	62	80	71.0	..	Cl'ds; thunder; sprinkle at 2; fair
7	62	84	73.0	..	Fair; cl'ds; light breezes. [at eve.
8	62	84	73.0	..	Clouds; distant thunder.
9	70	88	79.0	..	Cloudy; fair; clouds.
10	70	86	78.0	..	Cl'ds; thun'r; sprinkle from S.W.
11	68	80	74.0	..	Cl'ds; thun'r; sprinkle from S.W.
12	68	84	76.0	0.2	Cl'ds; thun'r; sh'r at noon from N.
13	72	82	77.0	0.6	Cl'ds; thun'r; sh'r at 2 from S.W.
14	72	88	80.0	..	Fair; gentle breezes.
15	72	88	80.0	..	Fair; gentle breezes.
16	74	88	81.0	0.2	Cl'y; thun'r; r'n at 12; high wind.
17	75	94	84.5	1.1	Cl'dy; fair; thunder; r'n at night.
18	70	82	76.0	..	Cl'dy; fair; thun'r; high N. wind.
19	74	92	83.0	..	Fog; clouds; fair.
20	76	92	84.0	..	Clouds; thunder; shower at 7 P.M.
21	76	80	78.0	0.8	Thunder; shower at 6 A. M. and 2
22	64	78	71.0	..	[P. M. from N.
23	62	80	71.0	..	Fair.
24	64	84	74.0	..	Fair.
25	66	88	77.0	..	Fair. [P. M. from S.
26	66	90	78.0	..	Fair; cl'ds; thun'r; sprinkle at 5
27	74	90	82.0	..	Fair; clouds.
28	74	90	82.0	..	Fair; clouds.
29	74	80	77.0	0.8	Cloudy; mist A. M.; thunder; rain
30	72	90	81.0	..	Fair; clouds. [at 4 P. M.
					..
Means	68.90	85.13	77.02	5.3	
Max.	76	94	84.5		
Min.	58	74	66.0		
Range	18	20	18.5		
Extreme range 36					

Greatest Rise and Fall of temperature in 24 hours.

	Sunrise.	3 P. M.
Rise . . .	8	10
Fall . . .	12	12

July, 1859.

DAY.	THERMOMETER. Sun-rise.	3 P. M.	Mean.	RAIN. Ins.	REMARKS ON THE WEATHER.
1	74	92	83.0	..	Occasional br'zes; thun'r; spr'kle.
2	74	89	81.5	..	Slight breezes, shifting; thunder.
3	72	92	82.0	..	Slight breezes, shifting; thunder.
4	74	92	83.0	..	Slight breezes, shifting; thunder.
5	66	86	76.0	..	Slight breezes, shifting.
6	70	90	80.0	..	Slight breezes, shifting.
7	64	88	76.0	..	
8	64	90	77.0	..	
9	70	94	82.0	0.1	[at 4 P. M.
10	66	82	74.0	0.1	Fog A. M.; cloudy; thunder; rain
11	66	84	75.0	..	Slight breezes, shifting.
12	68	92	80.0	..	Slight breezes, shifting; thunder.
13	70	94	82.0	..	Slight breezes, shifting; thunder.
14	74	98	86.0	0.8	Heavy shower from 3 to 4 P. M.
15	74	88	81.0	..	Slight shower at 2 P. M.
16	72	92	82.0	..	
17	74	94	84.0	..	
18	76	96	86.0	..	Thunder at intervals.
19	76	98	87.0	..	Thunder at intervals.
20	78	102	90.0	..	Clouds in N. E.; heavy thunder.
21	78	101	89.5	3.8	Tornado from N. W. to S. E.
22	72	82	77.0	..	Thunder; sprinkle of rain at noon.
23	74	92	83.0	..	Thunder.
24	72	92	82.0	..	
25	76	93	84.5	..	Thunder.
26	74	92	83.0	..	Thunder at 6 P. M.
27	76	80	78.0	..	Sprinkle of rain.
28	66	86	76.0	..	
29	64	84	74.0	1.4	
30	64	84	74.0	..	Thunder. [eve.
31	72	85	78.5	0.8	Thunder and rain A. M.; fair at
Means	71.29	90.45	80.87	7.0	
Max.	78	102	90.0		
Min.	64	80	74.0		
Range	14	22	16.0		
Extreme range 38					

Greatest Rise and Fall of temperature in 24 hours.

	Sunrise.	3 P. M.
Rise . . .	8	10
Fall . . .	10	19

August, 1859.

DAY.	THERMOMETER. Sun-rise.	3 P. M.	Mean.	RAIN. Ins.	REMARKS ON THE WEATHER.
1	72	90	81.0	..	Fog A. M.; clouds; thunder.
2	74	90	82.0	..	Cloudy; thunder; shower at noon.
3	72	86	79.0	0.6	Fair; cloudy; thunder; rain.
4	74	86	80.0	0.7	Cloudy; thunder; rain at noon.
5	74	88	81.0	0.2	Cloudy; thunder; rain at 4 P. M.
6	72	90	81.0	..	Fog; mist; clouds; thunder.
7	72	90	81.0	..	Fair.
8	72	88	80.0	..	Fair.
9	72	89	80.5	..	Fog; cloudy; fair at eve.
10	72	94	83.0	..	
11	74	94	84.0	..	Fair.
12	74	95	84.5	..	Fair.
13	74	88	81.0	0.1	Cloudy; thunder; rain at 11 A. M.
14	70	86	78.0	..	Thunder; clouds; sprinkle.
15	75	86	80.5	0.2	Shower, at 4 A. M. and 4 P. M.
16	74	86	80.0	..	Sprinkle at 2 P. M.
17	72	92	82.0	..	Fair; clouds; breeze.
18	72	92	82.0	..	Fair; clouds; breeze.
19	72	92	82.0	..	Thunder; rain at 1.30 P. M.; fair
20	72	90	81.0	..	Fair. [at eve.
21	72	94	83.0	..	Fair.
22	76	85	80.5	..	Rain at sunrise, with thunder; fair
23	70	86	78.0	..	Fog; fair. [at noon.
24	60	86	73.0	..	Fair.
25	64	90	77.0	..	Fair; clouds; hazy.
26	70	90	80.0	..	Fair.
27	74	92	83.0	..	Hazy; clouds.
28	78	94	86.0	..	Thun'r; r'n at 6 A. M.; thun'r and
29	76	82	79.0	..	Cloudy. [lightning at night.
30	64	84	74.0	..	Fog; fair.
31	62	86	74.0	..	Hazy.
Means	71.65	89.06	80.35	1.8	
Max.	78	95	86.0		
Min.	60	82	73.0		
Range	18	13	13.0		
Extreme range 35					

Greatest Rise and Fall of temperature in 24 hours.

	Sunrise.	3 P. M.
Rise . . .	6	6
Fall . . .	12	12

September, 1859.

DAY.	THERMOMETER. Sunrise.	2 P. M.	Mean.	RAIN. Ins.	REMARKS ON THE WEATHER.
1	70	80	75.0	..	Sprinkle at 3 P. M.; thunder.
2	70	83	76.5	0.1	Cloudy; shower; fair; thunder.
3	74	82	78.0	0.5	Cloudy; thunder; showers.
4	72	78	75.0	0.5	Fog; cloudy; thunder; rain.
5	60	66	63.0	..	Cloudy; thunder; rain at 8 A. M.
6	62	74	68.0	..	Cloudy.
7	64	80	72.0	..	Fair.
8	66	86	76.0	..	Fair; clouds.
9	74	90	82.0	..	Light sprinkle at 3 P. M.
10	75	90	82.5	..	Clouds; fair.
11	74	88	81.0	..	Cloudy.
12	70	88	79.0	..	Fog; fair.
13	68	84	76.0	..	Fair.
14	70	86	78.0	0.4	Thunder; rain at night.
15	66	88	77.0	..	
16	66	90	78.0	..	Fair.
17	70	92	81.0	..	Fair.
18	72	82	77.0	0.4	Thunder; showers.
19	64	75	69.5	..	Fair; cloudy.
20	60	70	65.0	..	Fair; cloudy.
21	52	78	65.0	..	
22	52	78	65.0	..	
23	58	80	69.0	..	
24	62	84	73.0	..	
25	64	86	75.0	..	
26	66	77	71.5	0.2	Cloudy; thunder; rain at noon.
27	70	85	77.5	0.4	Thunder; rain at 4 P. M.
28	70	80	75.0	..	Thunder; rain at 10 A. M.
29	72	78	75.0	..	Thunder; rain at 3 P. M.
30	66	68	67.0	1.4	Thunder; rain all day.
Means	66.63	81.53	74.08	3.9	Greatest Rise and Fall of temperature in 24 hours.
Max.	75	92	82.5		
Min.	52	66	63.0		
Range	23	26	19.5		
Extreme range 70					

	Sunrise.	2 P. M.
Rise . . .	8	8
Fall . . .	12	12

October, 1859.

DAY.	THERMOMETER. Sunrise.	2 P. M.	Mean.	RAIN. Ins.	REMARKS ON THE WEATHER.
1	58	74	66.0	..	
2	50	74	62.0	..	
3	47	74	60.5	..	
4	49	76	62.5	..	
5	58	80	69.0	..	
6	58	78	68.0	..	
7	58	78	68.0	..	
8	62	76	69.0	..	
9	44	60	52 0	..	
10	40	74	57.0	..	
11	44	74	59.0	..	
12	54	74	64.0	..	
13	56	82	69.0	..	
14	60	84	72.0	..	
15	62	76	69.0	..	[der.
16	64	75	69.5	1.4	Rain all day, from 2 A. M.; thun-
17	74	84	79.0	0.6	Sh'r at 10; then fair; wind at 2;
18	44	60	52.0	..	[thunder and rain.
19	42	64	53.0	..	
20	46	70	58.0	..	
21	46	66	56.0	..	
22	56	70	63.0	..	
23	52	78	65.0	..	
24	54	80	67.0	..	
25	52	80	66.0	..	
26	54	78	66.0	..	
27	50	64	57.0	..	
28	36	50	43.0	..	First white frost.
29	34	58	46.0	..	White frost.
30	32	54	43.0	..	Killing frost.
31	42	60	51.0	..	
Means	50.90	71.77	61.34	[illegible]	Greatest Rise [illegible] 24 hours.
Max.	74	84	79.0		
Min.	32	50	43.0		
Range	42	34	36 0		
Extreme range 52					

	Sunrise.	2 P. M.
Rise . . .	10	14
Fall . . .	30	24

November, 1859.

DAY.	THERMOMETER. Sunrise.	2 P. M.	Mean.	RAIN. Ins.	REMARKS ON THE WEATHER.
1	34	64	49.0	..	Smoky. Woods on fire.
2	40	74	57.0	..	Smoky.
3	52	74	63.0	..	Smoky.
4	46	76	61.0	..	Smoky.
5	54	78	66.0	..	Smoky.
6	50	74	62.0	..	Smoky.
7	46	74	60.0	..	Smoky.
8	52	74	63.0	..	Smoky.
9	58	74	66.0	..	Smoky.
10	56	74	65.0	..	Fog; mist.
11	67	82	74.5	..	Flying clouds from south.
12	56	40	48.0	..	Cl'dy; mist; cold N. wind; sleet;
13	20	46	33.0	..	Fair; 30° at sunset. [fair.
14	25	56	40.5	..	Smoky.
15	30	58	44.0	..	Smoky; clouds from S. W.
16	52	70	61.0	..	Smoky; clouds from S. W.
17	62	62	62.0	2.5	Thunder and rain.
18	42	56	49.0	..	Fair; strong west wind.
19	34	50	42.0	..	Fair; white frost.
20	52	68	60.0	0.7	Cloudy; thunder; rain.
21	48	60	54.0	..	Fair.
22	45	68	56.5	..	Fair. [sprinkle.
23	57	76	66.5	0.1	Fog; cloudy; thunder at night;
24	66	76	71.0	..	Cloudy; fair; south wind.
25	64	77	70.5	0.3	Cloudy; thunder; showers.
26	62	76	69.0	..	Cloudy; thunder; showers.
27	62	76	69.0	..	Mist; clouds; breezes from S.
28	58	60	59.0	..	Mist; flying clouds from S.
29	45	56	50.5	..	Mist; flying clouds from S.
30	62	74	68.0	..	Mist.
Means	49.90	67.43	58.66	3.6	Greatest Rise and Fall of temperature in 24 hours.
Max.	67	82	74.5		
Min.	20	40	33.0		
Range	47	42	41.5		
Extreme range 62					

	Sunrise.	2 P. M.
Rise . . .	22	18
Fall . . .	36	42

December, 1859.

DAY.	THERMOMETER. Sunrise.	2 P. M.	Mean.	RAIN. Ins.	REMARKS ON THE WEATHER.
1	68	74	71.0	..	Cl'y; r'n at 2 and at night; thun'r.
2	34	26	30.0	2.7	Rain; sleet. Streams swelled.
3	26	32	29.0	..	Sleet; ground covered with snow
4	30	36	33.0	0.2	Cloudy; snow; sleet. [and sleet.
5	36	46	41.0	..	Cloudy; mist; rain.
6	20	14	17.0	..	Cloudy; snow; cleared at night.
7	6	24	15.0	..	Fair; clear and cold all day.
8	14	36	25.0	..	Fair.
9	24	48	36.0	..	Fair.
10	24	54	39.0	..	Fair. } Snow covering ground.
11	36	54	45.0	..	Cloudy. }
12	28	52	40.0	..	Fair. }
13	26	52	39.0	..	Fair. }
14	28	52	40.0	..	Fair. }
15	25	46	35.5	..	Fair.
16	38	44	41.0	0.5	Cloudy; rain.
17	34	50	42.0	..	Fair.
18	39	45	42.0	..	Cloudy; rain at 1 P. M.; snow at
19	34	33	33.5	..	Snow. [night.
20	11	32	21.5	1.0	Fair; snow 6 in. deep. Many sap-
21	10	34	22.0	..	Fair. [lings bent to ground.
22	20	30	25.0	..	Fair.
23	8	34	21.0	..	Fair.
24	20	42	31.0	..	Fair.
25	44	63	53.5	..	Cloudy; snow melting.
26	54	70	62.0	..	Fog; fair; flying clouds from
27	66	70	68.0	0.4	Cloudy; rain. [S. W.
28	64	70	67.0	..	Fog; mist. [noon.
29	48	59	53.5	0.6	Thunder; cold rain from N. till
30	36	44	40.0	..	Cloudy. [2 inches.
31	32	34	33.0	..	Cl'dy; fair; cl'dy; snow at night
Means	[illegible]	[illegible]	[illegible]	5.4	[illegible] temperature in 24 hours.
Max.	68	74	71.0		
Min.	6	14	15.0		
Range	62	60	56.0		
Extreme range 68					

	Sunrise.	2 P. M.
Rise . . .	24	21
Fall . . .	34	48

SUMMARIES

OF THE

METEOROLOGICAL REGISTER, WASHINGTON, ARKANSAS.

SUMMARIES.

I. HIGHEST TEMPERATURE AT SUNRISE.

	Jan.	Feb.	March.	April.	May.	June.	July.	August.	Sept.	Oct.	Nov.	Dec.	Mean.	Year.
1840	60	60	60	68	70	76	74	74	70	74	56	60	66.83	76
1841	58	44	66	68	66	76	75	74	72	70	69	60	66.50	76
1842	64	63	69	67	70	74	76	72	72	64	54	64	67.42	76
1843	59	58	54	70	72	74	74	70	72	67	58	54	65.17	74
1844	65	60	56	68	72	75	76	76	70	70	64	63	67.92	76
1845	66	66	66	70	70	74	74	76	78	66	62	50	68.17	78
1846	58	50	60	70	73	72	76	78	74	66	64	66	67.25	78
1847	64	64	60	70	72	74	74	72	74	70	70	60	68.67	74
1848	64	66	66	62	72.5*	75.5*	78	78	76	68	62	68	69.67	78
1849	66	62	70	70	74	76	76	76	77	74	70	64	71.25	77
1850	62	70	70	70	70	76	76	80	72	76	72	66	71.67	80
1851	62	66	64	68	76	74	76	78	74	72	68	66	70.33	78
1852	66	64	70	74	74	78	76	74	74	78	74	68	72.50	78
1853	56	60	60	70	70	78	76	76	79	68	67	54	67.83	79
1854	68	64	66	72	76	76	76	80	78	74	66	62	71.50	80
1855	64	58	62	68	74	76	78	78	76	66	70	64	69.50	78
1856	48	49	58	78	74	78	80	78	74	72	70	64	68.58	80
1857	60	66	60	66	74	76	80	80	76	70	75	66	70.75	80
1858	60	64	70	70	76	76	80	76	76	72	64	68	71.00	80
1859	60	70	68	72	74	76	78	78	75	74	67	68	71.67	78
Means	61.50	61.20	63.75	69.55	72.47	75.53	76.45	76.20	74.45	70.55	66.10	62.75	69.21	77.65
Max.	68	70	70	78	76	78	80	80	79	78	75	68	72.50	80

II. HIGHEST TEMPERATURE AT 2 OR 3 P. M.

	Jan.	Feb.	March.	April.	May.	June.	July.	August.	Sept.	Oct.	Nov.	Dec.	Mean.	Year.
1840	63	80	80	83	82	92	90	94	91	83	72	72	81.83	94
1841	65	76	75	82	87	92	96	94	88	80	76	67	81.50	96
1842	69	72	84	80	88	90	93	89	92	82	74	70	81.92	93
1843	69	68	70	86	85	90	92	87	88	77	70	62	78.67	92
1844	70	78	74	81	84	88	94	96	93	80	76	70	82.00	96
1845	72	76	80	84	88	89	94	94	89	78	76	60	81.67	94
1846	66	70	76	84	87	92	92	90	92	82	73	72	81.33	92
1847	74	70	75	85	85	88	92	92	88	86	78	72	82.08	92
1848	74	75	83	82	87.6*	91.7*	91	90	88	82	65	74	81.94	91.7
1849	76	78	82	86	87	91	91	94	90	84	80	70	84.08	94
1850	64	78	80	86	90	92	94	101	88	82	78	74	83.91	101
1851	70	76	80	84	88	94	100	102	98	86	80	74	86.00	102
1852	66	78	90	90	90	91	92	92	88	84	72	78	84.25	92
1853	68	76	80	84	86	94	93	96	94	82	78	72	83.58	96
1854	70	74	87	88	86	94	97	96	93	87	76	68	84.67	97
1855	74	77	83	92	92	91	96	96	90	79	80	70	85.00	96
1856	58	74	84	88	94	95	102	99	92	84	72	70	84.33	102
1857	66	78	87	88	88	92	98	91	86	76	82	72	83.67	98
1858	65	72	80	85	88	94	94	96	92	90	66	68	82.50	96
1859	68	80	84	88	90	94	102	95	92	84	82	74	86.18	102
Means	68.35	75.30	80.70	85.30	87.63	91.74	94.65	94.20	90.60	82.40	75.30	70.45	83.05	95.83
Max.	76	80	90	92	94	95	102	102	94	90	82	78	86.18	102

* Interpolation; mean of 19 years.

III. MEAN TEMPERATURE OF WARMEST DAY.

	Jan.	Feb.	March.	April.	May.	June.	July.	August	Sept.	Oct.	Nov.	Dec.	Mean.	Year.
1840	59	67	67	75.5	75	83	85.5	83	75.5	76.5	63	63	72.75	85.5
1841	57.5	58	68	73	76.5	79	84	82	79	73.5	67	62	71.62	84
1842	66.5	67.5	75.5	72	78	80	82	77.5	81	70	64	67	73.42	82
1843	63.5	61	62	76	78.5	82	82	78.5	78	69	62	58	70.87	82
1844	67.5	67	62.5	73.5	78	81.5	84	86	80	75	69	66.5	74.21	86
1845	67	71	71	76.5	76	79.5	83	83.5	83.5	71	71	54	73.92	83.5
1846	61	60	66	72	80	81	83	83	81	73	65	68	72.75	83
1847	68	66.5	65.5	75.5	78	80	81	81	80	73	70	66	73.71	81
1848	68	70.5	73.5	71	78.7*	82.3†	83.5	82	82	72	63	71	74.79	83.5
1849	69	67	75	77	77.5	83	83	85	83.5	79	75	63	76.42	85
1850	62	74	75	75	79	83	84	90	80	79	71	70	76.83	90
1851	65	70	71	73	81	83	87	89.5	85	78	74	70	77.21	89.5
1852	63	68	77.5	82	81	82	83	81	80	79	73	73	76.88	83
1853	59	68	69	76	77	83	84	85	83	72	72	63	74.25	85
1854	67.5	69	76.5	79	78	84	86.5	86	83.5	79.5	66	61	76.38	86.5
1855	67	65	71	78	82	83	86	85.5	82	68	74	67	75.71	86
1856	49	60.5	71	77.5	80	84	91	88	82	75	69	65	74.33	91
1857	63	70.5	72.5	69	79	83	87	83.5	80	73	77	69	75.54	87
1858	61	66	70	76.5	80.5	85	87	85	83.5	81	60	66	75.12	87
1859	63	74	76	79	80	84.5	90	86	82.5	79	74.5	71	78.29	90
Means	63.32	67.02	70.77	75.35	78.68	82.29	84.87	84.05	81.25	74.78	68.97	65.68	74.75	85.52
Max.	69	74	77.5	82	82	85	91	90	85	81	77	73	78.29	91

IV. LOWEST TEMPERATURE AT SUNRISE.

	Jan.	Feb.	March.	April.	May.	June.	July.	August.	Sept.	Oct.	Nov.	Dec.	Mean.	Year.
1840	13	10	31	44	46	56	59	54	43	30	18	24	35.67	10
1841	3	18	28	42	44	52	64	58	44	24	15	21	34.42	3
1842	24	20	32	39	40	54	54	53	48	32	15	15	35.50	15
1843	15	8	6	30	46	50	56	52	52	32	28	26	33.42	6
1844	26	24	29	38	50	60	66	60	36	30	24	16	38.25	16
1845	26	24	25	32	46	60	64	64	54	30	18	—6	36.42	—6
1846	18	23	27	30	44	48	58	58	46	28	20	24	35.33	18
1847	10	16	24	40	42	56	60	56	46	30	16	12	34.00	10
1848	12	24	22	32	47*	56.3*	66	64	52	34	20	20	37.44	12
1849	18	6	34	32	54	60	70	68	55	38	30	10	39.58	6
1850	28	14	28	36	44	56	56	70	52	32	30	12	38.17	12
1851	18	20	28	36	38	62	62	64	43	33	18	12	36.17	12
1852	4	28	28	36	54	54	65	60	52	44	28	25	39.83	4
1853	17	19	30	40	52	58	62	64	50	34	30	22	39.83	17
1854	10	21	32	34	46	62	62	70	60	48	25	20	40.83	10
1855	12	16	20	42	54	54	65	60	53	28	32	10	37.17	10
1856	10	8	26	42	49	58	64	64	42	34	22	20	36.58	8
1857	4	20	22	24	42	54	64	64	52	41	27	18	36.00	4
1858	32	20	24	42	50	58	68	56	54	40	24	20	40.67	20
1859	18	27	34	32	52	58	64	60	52	32	20	6	37.92	6
Means	15.90	18.30	26.50	36.15	47.00	56.32	62.45	60.95	49.30	33.70	23.00	16.35	37.16	9.65
Min.	3	6	6	30	38	48	54	52	36	24	15	—6	33.42	—6

* Interpolation; mean of 19 years.

† Interpolation; mean of 19 years. Mean of the 23d June (one of the eight days observed) was 82.5.

V. LOWEST TEMPERATURE AT 2 OR 3 P. M.

	Jan.	Feb.	March.	April.	May.	June.	July.	August.	Sept.	Oct.	Nov.	Dec.	Mean.	Year.
1840	30	34	42	49	66	76	70	80	68	55	30	29	52.42	29
1841	12	30	32	50	60	64	80	74	58	50	28	30	47.33	12
1842	40	36	40	50	60	70	68	76	68	51	31	34	52.00	31
1843	30	24	24	60	57	60	74	70	60	38	36	40	47.75	24
1844	33	40	38	54	62	76	80	75	52	50	40	31	52.58	31
1845	34	43	44	56	52	76	80	74	70	54	22	26	52.58	22
1846	40	31	48	47	56	70	76	66	65	50	42	38	52.42	31
1847	18	34	32	58	60	76	72	76	70	48	34	36	51.17	18
1848	29	34	36	48	63*	72.4*	76	76	68	56	42	24	52.03	24
1849	34	26	54	52	66	76	76	76	76	50	50	30	55.50	26
1850	40	30	46	48	56	74	80	76	68	50	44	26	53.17	26
1851	36	36	38	58	66	70	84	84	72	62	40	30	56.33	30
1852	21	39	32	36	67	74	76	72	74	54	47	36	52.33	21
1853	32	28	41	54	63	76	76	80	72	50	52	37	55.08	28
1854	25	44	46	60	70	70	76	76	68	60	44	38	56.42	25
1855	32	32	43	58	66	70	76	74	64	48	53	20	53.00	20
1856	26	24	43	64	70	78	75	68	58	57	42	38	53.58	24
1857	23	42	46	39	62	76	74	76	72	54	39	36	53.25	23
1858	43	35	40	51	64	70	80	74	68	58	38	38	54.92	35
1859	34	42	50	56	74	74	80	82	66	50	40	14	55.17	14
Means	30.60	34.20	40.75	52.40	63.00	72.42	76.45	75.25	66.85	52.25	39.70	31.55	52.95	24.70
Min.	12	24	24	36	52	60	68	66	52	38	22	14	47.33	12

VI. MEAN TEMPERATURE OF COLDEST DAY.

	Jan.	Feb.	March.	April.	May.	June.	July.	August	Sept.	Oct.	Nov.	Dec.	Mean.	Year.
1840	22	25	41	47.5	56	66	64.5	68	56.5	43	26.5	27	45.25	22
1841	7.5	25.5	30	48.5	56.5	65	74.5	71	55	37	26.5	27	43.67	7.5
1842	34	28	37	49	53.5	66	66	64.5	59.5	46.5	24	25.5	46.12	24
1843	25.5	21	18	45	53.5	59.5	68	65	58.5	37.5	34.5	35.5	43.46	18
1844	29.5	32.5	39.5	51	59	68	76	69.5	48.5	41	33	28	47.96	28
1845	30.5	35.5	37	49	51	71	72	71.5	62	45	20.5	10	46.25	10
1846	29	27.5	41.5	44	59	63.5	68	66	59	44	33	34	47.37	27.5
1847	18	25	33	54	54	68	69	68	59	42	25	24	44.92	18
1848	23.5	32	32	47	58.1*	67.1*	74	73	61	49	34.5	25	48.06	23.5
1849	29	16	47	45	63	71	75	72	66	44	43	21	49.33	16
1850	35	22	40.5	48	56	68	68	73	64	43	36	20	47.79	20
1851	28	31	37	52	54	72	75	76	57.5	48.5	33	23	48.92	23
1852	12.5	39.5	32	36	63.5	67	71	72	63	53.5	41	33.5	48.71	12.5
1853	24.5	25.5	41	52	57.5	70	69	73	61	45.5	44.5	31	49.54	24.5
1854	18	34.5	47	47	61	66	75	75	68	55.5	38.5	31	51.37	18
1855	22.5	26.5	37	52	61	63	75	72	62.5	39	45	18	47.79	18
1856	20	16	38	56	61	74	75.5	70	52	47	33	31	47.79	16
1857	13.5	33	35	37	59	66.5	70	70	64	50	34.5	32	47.04	13.5
1858	39	31.5	36	47.5	60	65	74	66	69	55	35	32.5	50.87	31.5
1859	28	34.5	47	45	65	66	74	73	63	43	33	18	49.12	18
Means	24.47	28.10	37.32	47.62	58.08	67.13	71.67	70.45	60.45	45.45	33.70	26.35	47.57	19.47
Min.	7.5	16	18	36	51	59.5	64.5	64.5	48.5	37	20.5	10	43.46	7.5

* Interpolation; mean of 19 years.

VII. RANGE OF TEMPERATURE AT SUNRISE.

	Jan.	Feb.	March.	April.	May.	June.	July.	Aug.	Sept.	Oct.	Nov.	Dec.	Mean.	Max.	Min.	Year.*
1840	47	50	29	24	24	20	15	20	27	44	38	36	31.17	50	15	66
1841	55	26	38	26	22	24	11	16	28	46	54	39	32.08	55	11	73
1842	40	43	37	28	30	20	22	19	24	32	39	49	31.92	49	19	61
1843	44	50	48	40	26	24	18	18	20	35	30	28	31.75	50	18	68
1844	39	36	27	30	22	15	10	16	34	40	40	47	29.67	47	10	60
1845	40	42	41	38	24	14	10	12	24	36	44	56	31.75	56	10	84
1846	40	27	33	40	29	24	18	20	28	38	44	42	31.92	44	18	60
1847	54	48	36	30	30	18	14	16	28	40	54	48	34.67	54	14	64
1848	52	42	44	30	25.5†	19.2†	12	14	24	34	42	48	32.22	52	12	66
1849	48	56	36	38	20	16	6	8	22	36	40	54	31.67	56	6	71
1850	34	56	42	34	26	20	20	10	20	44	42	54	33.50	56	10	68
1851	44	46	50	32	33	12	14	14	31	30	50	54	34.17	54	12	66
1852	62	36	42	38	20	24	11	14	22	34	46	43	32.67	62	11	74
1853	39	41	30	30	18	20	14	12	29	34	37	32	28.00	41	12	62
1854	58	43	34	38	30	14	14	10	18	26	41	42	30.67	58	10	70
1855	52	42	42	26	20	22	13	18	23	38	38	54	32.33	54	13	68
1856	38	41	32	36	25	20	16	14	32	38	48	44	32.00	48	14	72
1857	56	46	38	42	32	22	16	16	24	29	48	48	34.75	56	16	76
1858	28	44	46	28	26	18	12	20	22	32	40	48	30.33	48	12	60
1859	42	43	34	40	22	18	14	18	23	42	47	62	33.75	62	14	72
Means	45.60	42.90	37.25	33.40	25.47	19.21	14.00	15.25	25.15	36.85	43.10	46.40	32.05	52.60	12.85	68.05
Max.	62	56	48	42	38	24	22	20	34	46	54	62	34.75	62	..	84
Min.	28	26	27	24	18	12	6	8	18	26	30	28	28.00	..	6	60

VIII. RANGE OF TEMPERATURE AT 2 OR 3 P. M.

	Jan.	Feb.	March.	April.	May.	June.	July.	Aug.	Sept.	Oct.	Nov.	Dec.	Mean.	Max.	Min.	Year.‡
1840	33	46	38	34	16	16	20	14	23	28	42	43	29.42	46	14	65
1841	53	46	43	32	27	28	16	20	30	30	48	37	34.17	53	16	84
1842	29	36	44	30	28	20	25	13	24	31	43	36	29.92	44	13	62
1843	39	44	46	26	28	30	18	17	28	39	34	22	30.92	46	17	68
1844	37	38	36	27	22	12	14	21	41	30	36	39	29.42	41	12	65
1845	38	33	36	28	36	13	14	20	19	24	54	34	29.08	54	13	72
1846	26	39	28	37	31	22	16	24	27	32	31	34	28.92	39	16	61
1847	56	36	43	27	25	12	20	16	18	38	44	36	30.92	56	12	74
1848	45	41	47	34	24.6†	19.3†	15	14	20	26	23	50	29.91	50	14	67
1849	42	52	28	34	21	15	15	18	14	34	30	40	28.58	52	14	68
1850	24	48	34	38	34	18	14	25	20	32	34	48	30.75	48	14	75
1851	34	40	42	26	22	24	16	18	26	24	40	44	29.67	44	16	72
1852	45	39	58	54	23	17	16	20	14	30	25	42	31.92	58	14	71
1853	36	48	39	30	23	18	17	16	22	32	26	35	28.50	48	16	68
1854	45	30	41	28	16	24	21	20	25	27	32	30	28.25	45	16	72
1855	42	45	40	34	26	21	20	22	26	31	27	50	32.00	50	20	76
1856	32	50	41	24	24	17	27	31	34	27	30	32	30.75	50	17	78
1857	43	36	41	40	26	16	24	15	14	22	43	36	30.42	49	14	75
1858	22	37	40	34	24	24	14	22	24	32	28	30	27.58	40	14	61
1859	34	38	34	32	16	20	22	13	26	34	42	60	30.92	60	13	88
Means	37.75	41.10	39.95	32.90	24.63	19.32	18.20	18.95	23.75	30.15	35.60	38.90	30.10	48.65	14.75	72.10
Max.	56	52	58	54	36	30	27	31	41	39	54	60	34.17	60	..	88
Min.	22	30	28	24	16	12	14	13	14	22	23	22	27.58	..	12	61

* This column gives the difference between the highest and lowest observation at sunrise in each year. The range at sunrise, for the whole period of twenty years, was 86°.

† Interpolation; mean of 19 years.

‡ This column gives the difference between the highest and lowest observation at 2 or 3 P. M. in each year. The range at 2 or 3 P. M., for the whole period of twenty years, was 90°.

IX. RANGE OF DAILY MEAN TEMPERATURE.

	Jan.	Feb.	March.	April.	May.	June.	July.	Aug.	Sept.	Oct.	Nov.	Dec.	Mean.	Max.	Min.	Year.*
1840	37	42	26	28	19	17	21	15	19	33.5	36.5	36	27.50	42	15	63.5
1841	50	32.5	38	24.5	20	14	9.5	11	24	36.5	40.5	35	27.96	50	9.5	76.5
1842	32.5	39.5	38.5	23	24.5	14	16	13	21.5	23.5	40	41.5	27.29	41.5	13	58
1843	38	40	44	31	25	22.5	14	13.5	19.5	31.5	27.5	22.5	27.42	44	13.5	64
1844	38	24.5	23	22.5	19	13.5	8	16.5	31.5	34	36	38.5	25.42	38.5	8	58
1845	36.5	35.5	34	27.5	25	8.5	11	12	21.5	26	50.5	44	27.67	50.5	8.5	73.5
1846	32	32.5	24.5	28	21	17.5	15	17	22	29	32	34	25.37	34	15	55.5
1847	50	41.5	32.5	21.5	24	12	12	13	21	31	45	42	28.79	50	12	63
1848	44.5	38.5	41.5	24	20.6†	15.2†	9.5	9	21	23	28.5	46	26.77	46	9	60
1849	40	51	28	32	14.5	12	8	13	17.5	35	32	42	27.09	51	8	69
1850	27	52	34.5	27	23	15	16	17	16	36	35	50	29.04	52	15	70
1851	37	39	34	21	27	11	12	13.5	27.5	29.5	41	47	28.29	47	11	66.5
1852	50.5	28.5	45.5	46	17.5	15	12	9	17	25.5	32	39.5	28.17	50.5	9	70.5
1853	34.5	42.5	28	24	19.5	13	15	12	22	26.5	27.5	32	24.71	42.5	12	60.5
1854	49.5	34.5	29.5	32	17	18	11.5	11	15.5	24	27.5	30	25.00	49.5	11	68.5
1855	44.5	38.5	34	26	21	20	11	13.5	19.5	29	29	49	27.92	49	11	68
1856	29	44.5	33	21.5	19	10	15.5	18	30	28	36	34	26.54	44.5	10	75
1857	49.5	37.5	37.5	32	20	16.5	17	13.5	16	23	42.5	37	28.50	49.5	13.5	73.5
1858	22	34.5	34	29	20.5	20	13	19	14.5	26	25	33.5	24.25	34.5	13	55.5
1859	35	39.5	29	34	15	18.5	16	18	19.5	36	41.5	56	29.42	56	13	72
Means	38.85	38 42	33.45	27.72	20.60	15.16	13.15	13.62	20.80	29.32	35.27	39.47	27.15	46.12	11.50	66.05
Max.	50.5	52	45.5	46	27	22.5	21	19	31.5	36.5	50.5	56	29.42	56	..	76.5
Min.	22	24.5	23	21	14.5	8.5	8	9	14.5	23	25	22.5	24.25	..	8	55.5

X. EXTREME RANGE OF TEMPERATURE.

	Jan.	Feb.	March.	April.	May.	June.	July.	Aug.	Sept.	Oct.	Nov.	Dec.	Mean.	Max.	Min.	Year.‡
1840	50	70	49	39	36	36	31	40	48	53	54	48	46.17	70	31	84
1841	62	58	47	40	43	40	32	36	44	56	61	46	47.08	62	32	93
1842	45	52	52	41	48	36	39	36	44	50	59	55	46.42	59	36	78
1843	54	60	64	56	39	40	36	35	36	45	42	36	45.25	64	35	86
1844	44	54	45	43	34	28	28	36	57	50	52	54	43.75	57	28	80
1845	46	52	55	52	42	29	30	30	35	48	58	66	45.25	66	29	100
1846	48	47	49	54	43	44	34	32	46	54	53	48	46.00	54	32	74
1847	64	54	51	45	43	32	32	36	42	56	62	60	48.08	64	32	82
1848	62	51	61	50	40.6†	35.4†	25	26	36	48	45	54	44.50	62	25	79
1849	58	72	48	54	33	31	21	26	35	46	50	60	44.50	72	21	88
1850	36	64	52	50	46	36	38	31	36	50	48	62	45.75	64	31	89
1851	52	56	52	46	50	32	38	38	55	53	62	62	49.67	62	32	90
1852	62	50	62	54	36	37	27	32	36	40	44	53	44.42	62	27	88
1853	51	57	50	44	34	36	31	32	44	48	48	50	43.75	57	31	79
1854	60	53	55	54	40	32	35	26	33	39	51	48	43.83	60	26	87
1855	62	61	63	50	38	37	31	36	37	51	48	60	47.83	63	31	86
1856	48	66	58	46	45	37	38	35	50	50	50	50	47.75	66	35	94
1857	62	58	65	64	46	38	34	27	34	35	55	54	47.67	65	27	94
1858	33	52	56	43	38	36	26	40	38	50	42	48	41.83	56	26	76
1859	50	53	50	56	38	36	38	35	70	52	62	68	50.67	70	35	96
Means	52.45	57.00	54.20	49.05	40.63	35.42	32.20	33.25	42.80	48.70	52.30	54.10	46.01	62.75	30.10	86.15
Max.	64	72	65	64	50	40	39	40	70	56	62	68	50.67	72	..	100
Min.	33	47	45	39	33	28	21	26	33	35	42	36	41.83	..	21	74

* This column gives the difference between the mean temperature of the warmest and coldest day in each year. The difference between the warmest and coldest day, in the whole period of twenty years, was 83°.5.

† Interpolation; mean of 19 years.

‡ This column gives the difference between the highest and lowest observed temperature in each year. The extreme range of observed temperature, in the whole period of twenty years, was 108°.

XI. GREATEST RISE OF TEMPERATURE FROM SUNRISE OF ONE DAY TO SUNRISE OF THE NEXT DAY.

	Jan.	Feb.	March.	April.	May.	June.	July.	August.	Sept.	Oct.	Nov.	Dec.	Mean.	Year.
1840	29	22	26	16	8	14	6	8	10	18	21	15	16.08	29
1841	20	12	16	17	10	10	5	6	14	30	17	23	15.00	30
1842	20	23	18	18	15	9	6	5	10	8	15	20	13.92	23
1843	20	26	22	16	14	10	14	16	8	13	23	18	16.67	26
1844	23	18	14	8	12	6	8	6	15	12	24	24	14.17	24
1845	28	24	24	22	10	14	4	6	10	20	22	24	17.33	28
1846	18	22	14	14	16	20	14	6	8	12	26	34	17.00	34
1847	28	25	18	10	14	12	6	10	10	20	24	22	16.58	28
1848	22	23	24	18	12.9*	9.7*	10	6	6	20	28	34	17.80	34
1849	24	26	20	18	16	6	6	3	18	17	16	28	16.50	28
1850	18	20	28	16	12	8	12	4	8	14	26	20	15.50	28
1851	20	24	22	26	14	8	6	4	12	26	30	24	18.00	30
1852	20	28	23	22	12	10	6	8	12	12	23	27	16.92	28
1853	16	18	19	14	12	8	6	4	10	24	24	19	14.50	24
1854	28	22	22	14	14	6	8	8	6	12	34	18	16.00	34
1855	22	28	20	16	10	10	10	6	11	15	18	30	16.33	30
1856	21	18	13	16	14	10	6	6	8	16	22	24	14.50	24
1857	24	22	18	20	18	8	6	6	8	12	28	24	16.17	28
1858	12	26	18	18	10	7	4	6	12	10	14	22	13.25	26
1859	30	28	28	24	14	8	8	6	8	10	22	24	17.50	30
Means	22.15	22.75	20.35	17.15	12.89	9.68	7.55	6.50	10.20	16.05	22.85	23.70	15.98	27.20
Max.	30	28	28	26	18	20	14	16	18	30	34	34	18.00	34

XII. GREATEST RISE OF TEMPERATURE FROM 2 OR 3 P. M. OF ONE DAY TO 2 OR 3 P. M. OF THE NEXT DAY.

	Jan.	Feb.	March.	April.	May.	June.	July.	August.	Sept.	Oct.	Nov.	Dec.	Mean.	Year.
1840	16	10	18	16	9	6	8	5	9	10	28	26	13.42	28
1841	19	20	36	26	22	19	5	10	14	12	19	13	17.92	36
1842	13	14	20	19	15	14	11	5	13	11	11	16	13.50	20
1843	20	16	21	12	12	16	9	10	12	15	15	12	14.17	21
1844	17	22	12	12	15	8	6	9	10	20	19	18	14.00	22
1845	10	20	15	14	14	8	6	10	8	10	14	16	12.08	20
1846	11	32	22	16	26	7	10	20	10	10	24	20	17.33	32
1847	17	18	18	16	12	8	12	6	6	12	12	15	12.67	18
1848	16	14	26	18	12.7*	10.3*	6	9	4	12	10	18	13.00	26
1849	30	17	16	14	10	9	12	6	7	17	20	18	14.67	30
1850	18	16	14	14	16	8	10	7	10	10	12	11	12.17	18
1851	18	18	18	10	12	16	12	4	8	8	16	18	13.17	18
1852	14	12	18	34	12	7	10	11	6	8	8	35	14.58	35
1853	16	20	16	22	17	10	8	8	14	12	18	14	14.58	22
1854	26	18	14	12	6	12	8	8	8	12	24	12	13.33	26
1855	15	24	15	21	8	16	10	6	16	20	12	16	14.92	24
1856	17	12	22	16	8	6	8	22	12	12	16	10	13.42	22
1857	22	10	14	20	10	6	6	7	4	11	14	8	11.00	22
1858	13	17	17	17	10	10	8	10	10	18	12	20	13.50	20
1859	20	22	13	14	8	10	10	6	8	14	18	21	13.67	22
Means	17.40	17.60	18.25	17.15	12.74	10.32	8.75	8.95	9.45	12.70	16.10	16.85	13.85	24.10
Max.	30	32	36	34	26	19	12	22	16	20	28	35	17.92	36

* Interpolation; mean of 19 years.

XIII. GREATEST FALL OF TEMPERATURE FROM SUNRISE OF ONE DAY TO SUNRISE OF THE NEXT DAY.

	Jan.	Feb.	March.	April.	May.	June.	July.	August.	Sept.	Oct.	Nov.	Dec.	Mean.	Year.
1840	37	35	21	16	14	10	9	12	13	39	24	20	20.83	39
1841	47	10	28	16	10	10	10	6	10	16	33	36	19.33	47
1842	22	29	19	18	18	7	8	8	14	26	22	22	17.75	29
1843	22	36	24	18	16	16	8	18	14	18	22	22	19.50	36
1844	25	14	22	10	14	9	10	8	17	16	20	20	15.42	25
1845	30	22	20	28	12	8	6	6	8	26	20	25	17.58	30
1846	22	15	18	20	16	22	8	14	12	24	26	36	19.42	36
1847	36	36	19	14	16	10	6	10	20	22	36	30	21.25	36
1848	34	12	23	34	12.8*	11*	9	6	16	20	28	36	20.15	36
1849	34	20	16	12	10	10	4	8	9	27	22	38	17.50	38
1850	20	24	24	18	10	4	20	6	12	20	38	28	18.67	38
1851	38	24	22	18	10	10	12	8	15	19	28	16	18.33	38
1852	26	24	22	20	12	20	6	6	18	12	31	39	19.67	39
1853	39	26	28	25	14	14	6	8	17	17	20	18	19.33	39
1854	57	29	30	22	10	8	6	4	10	18	23	26	20.25	57
1855	32	20	15	10	8	14	9	12	16	20	28	30	17.83	32
1856	20	26	14	16	16	10	8	6	10	26	38	36	18.83	38
1857	34	32	20	40	14	6	8	8	10	18	29	22	20.08	40
1858	16	37	18	16	12	10	6	8	8	30	28	32	18.42	37
1859	28	28	24	30	12	12	10	12	12	30	36	34	22.33	36
Means	30.95	24.95	21.35	20.05	12.84	11.05	8.45	8.70	13.05	22.20	27.60	28.30	19.12	37.30
Max.	57	37	30	40	18	22	20	18	20	39	38	39	22.33	57

XIV. GREATEST FALL OF TEMPERATURE FROM 2 OR 3 P. M. OF ONE DAY TO 2 OR 3 P. M. OF THE NEXT DAY.

	Jan.	Feb.	March.	April.	May.	June.	July.	August.	Sept.	Oct.	Nov.	Dec.	Mean.	Year.
1840	20	21	38	30	14	5	12	12	11	21	26	22	19.33	38
1841	28	26	16	16	16	21	16	11	25	12	26	15	19.00	28
1842	19	19	44	20	21	13	20	9	11	19	19	24	19.83	44
1843	26	34	36	12	19	22	16	10	7	26	20	12	20.00	36
1844	21	26	36	12	18	6	12	14	17	19	30	30	20.08	36
1845	36	14	32	14	16	6	8	7	10	17	28	16	17.00	36
1846	16	34	24	17	14	16	12	12	16	20	16	34	19.25	34
1847	34	26	27	18	14	8	15	12	16	30	22	18	20.00	34
1848	43	16	35	34	15.7*	11.4*	10	8	12	10	17	24	19.67	43
1849	12	20	16	14	13	6	12	14	8	14	20	28	14.75	28
1850	16	20	20	16	17	8	14	10	18	22	30	28	18.25	30
1851	30	34	26	22	10	19	10	10	14	16	22	22	19.58	34
1852	38	23	46	26	19	12	10	8	8	14	16	42	21.83	46
1853	24	32	26	21	19	10	10	10	10	16	14	30	18.50	32
1854	42	16	22	16	10	8	18	11	12	24	18	14	17.58	42
1855	38	27	29	12	14	10	12	21	14	17	14	21	19.08	38
1856	22	22	24	14	14	13	27	18	14	16	24	18	18.83	27
1857	16	28	12	31	24	12	12	10	7	11	19	22	17.00	31
1858	13	31	30	18	14	10	6	10	24	16	10	14	16.33	31
1859	31	22	18	20	12	12	19	12	12	24	42	48	22.67	48
Means	26.25	24.55	27.85	19.15	15.68	11.42	13.55	11.45	13.30	18.20	21.65	24.10	18.93	35.80
Max.	43	34	46	34	24	22	27	21	25	30	42	48	22.67	48

* Interpolation; mean of 19 years. The greatest fall at 3 P. M. during the nine days in which observations were made in June, 1848, was 13; if these figures were inserted, the mean of June would be 11.50.

XV. MEAN TEMPERATURE AT SUNRISE.

	Jan.	Feb.	March.	April.	May.	June.	July.	Aug.	Sept.	Oct.	Nov.	Dec.	Mean.	Max.	Min.	Range.
1840	33.61	39.97	47.58	57.03	60.13	68.52	70.64	65.55	57.70	53.73	38.37	37.94	52.56	70.64	33.61	37.03
1841	33.26	34.04	44.39	53.83	57.19	64.80	69.77	67.45	60.73	49.61	43.23	36.74	51.25	69.77	33.26	36.51
1842	38.13	38.29	53.61	53.00	59.55	66.90	68.09	63.93	62.13	46.35	35.63	35.10	51.73	68.09	35.10	32.99
1843	37.68	32.54	27.77	51.90	58.55	64.77	67.94	60.90	66.70	48.45	44.60	37.06	49.90	67.94	27.77	40.17
1844	38.13	39.10	43.47	59.34	62.64	68.53	72.00	69.52	59.63	49.20	45.57	34.19	53.44	72.00	34.19	37.81
1845	39.00	40.64	44.23	56.47	56.76	67.97	71.29	70.42	67.59	46.29	38.47	28.06	52.27	71.29	28.06	43.23
1846	34.97	34.68	43.48	52.67	59.26	64.33	69.42	68.84	64.53	50.64	43.63	44.06	52.54	69.42	34.68	34.74
1847	31.16	38.29	40.48	55.23	56.32	66.67	69.47	64.81	59.00	48.50	43.50	33.00	50.54	69.47	31.16	38.31
1848	39.90	42.69	45.10	49.20	61.22*	67.90*	71.87	70.71	62.47	52.52	38.53	37.71	53.32	71.87	37.71	34.16
1849	40.03	38.54	53.58	53.10	63.74	69.67	73.93	73.03	65.17	50.45	49.67	39.03	55.83	73.93	38.54	35.39
1850	41.39	43.21	47.30	52.80	58.94	69.80	71.23	74.17	63.80	53.16	43.93	38.07	54.82	74.17	38.07	36.10
1851	36.32	41.78	46.06	51.30	64.22	69.80	70.97	72.84	64.53	50 39	40.83	36.69	53.81	72.84	36.32	36.54
1852	30.77	45.11	51.93	51.87	66.87	65.33	70.65	69.68	64.30	59.71	44.57	43.74	55.38	70.65	30.77	39.88
1853	35.87	40.18	44.23	57.17	62.26	68.10	71.94	72.19	65.20	52.10	48.93	37.33	54.62	72.19	35.87	36.32
1854	34.36	40.04	52.70	53.73	63.23	69.63	73.03	74.84	71.13	58.94	43.50	39.00	56.18	74.84	34.36	40.48
1855	38.71	34.14	42.81	59.07	66.42	67.80	73.20	72.74	70.37	50.55	49.37	36.06	55.11	73.29	34.14	39.15
1856	26.84	35.07	42.71	58.33	60.13	70.73	72.29	71.65	61.73	55.64	40.90	35.03	52.59	72.29	26.84	45.45
1857	30.03	49.93	44.81	45.53	58.77	67.77	72.84	73.53	66.83	54.58	46.47	42.71	54.48	73.53	30.03	43.50
1858	42.42	37.18	50.90	55.60	63.55	70.07	75.16	71.19	64.70	59.29	39.27	43.81	56.09	75.16	37.18	37.98
1859	38.23	46.52	48.84	52.73	64.67	68.90	71.29	71.65	66.63	50.90	49.90	31.70	55.16	71.65	31.70	39.95
Means	36.04	39.60	45.80	53.99	61.22	67.90	71.35	69.98	64.24	52.05	43.44	37.35	53.58	71.75	33.47	38.28
Max.	42.42	49.93	53.61	59.34	66.87	70.73	75.16	74.84	71.13	59.71	49.90	44.06	56.18	75.16	...	45.45
Min.	26.84	32.54	27.77	45.53	56.32	64.33	67.94	60.90	57.70	46.29	35.63	28.06	49.90	...	26.84	32.99
Range	15.58	17.39	25.84	13.81	10.55	6.40	7.22	13.94	13.43	13.42	14.27	16.00	6.28	48.32		12.46

XVI. MEAN TEMPERATURE AT 2 OR 3 P. M.

	Jan.	Feb.	March.	April.	May.	June.	July.	Aug.	Sept.	Oct.	Nov.	Dec.	Mean.	Max.	Min.	Range.
1840	50.61	57.41	66.06	69.43	75.67	83.62	84.42	89.00	78.20	68.03	55.03	48.10	68.80	89.00	48.10	40.90
1841	43.13	50.11	57.77	70.47	76.81	83.07	91.07	85.71	77.17	64.93	57.13	48.55	67.16	91.07	43.13	47.94
1842	54.39	54.71	70.10	71.52	76.26	81.60	86.42	82.93	79.77	68.52	51.57	47.94	68.81	86.42	47.94	38.48
1843	53.74	40.86	42.80	70.97	74.74	81.87	86.00	81.13	80.[illegible]	62.39	55.47	52.06	65.95	86.00	42.80	43.20
1844	49.16	59.86	58.77	71.24	77.84	84.50	89.71	88.03	78.73	67.33	59.60	50.81	69.63	89.71	50.80	38.91
1845	54.16	61.32	60.81	77.37	76.61	85.17	88.61	85.45	79.62	67.58	57.47	43.00	69.76	88.61	43.00	45.61
1846	53.10	49.71	63.00	69.83	79.16	81.63	85.61	82.84	81.20	70.00	60.57	55.79	69.37	85.61	49.71	35.90
1847	43.58	53.07	53.32	74.13	75.93	82.70	85.23	84.55	79.63	71.23	58.67	50.60	67.72	85.23	43.58	41.65
1848	58.94	59.93	62.10	67.73	78.30*	84.29*	84.29	84.65	77.10	73.00	55.23	48.65	69.52	84.65	48.65	36.00
1849	48.65	54.79	71.77	72.97	79.39	85.83	85.00	87.74	82.33	69.77	66.30	49.26	71.15	87.74	48.65	39.09
1850	52.97	54.64	63.63	69.60	73.94	84.20	87.65	92.93	82.17	71.87	59.40	46.55	69.96	92.93	46.55	46.38
1851	56.10	55.18	67.16	70.63	80.77	87.60	92.68	93.21	87.57	74.94	58.00	53.24	73.09	93.21	53.24	39.97
1852	47.19	60.54	70 17	72.10	80.10	83.50	86.58	85.29	80.53	73.84	59.50	56.16	71.29	86.58	47.10	39.39
1853	53.42	54.86	63.35	74.87	77.10	87.17	86.32	90.26	81.77	70.71	67.07	53.27	71.68	90.26	53.27	36.99
1854	50.23	59.36	69.90	73.47	78.97	85.27	90.61	89.22	83.43	74.26	61.85	55.93	72.71	90.61	50.23	40.38
1855	54.55	54.86	62.16	77.57	82.94	83.33	89.13	86.52	83.07	68.35	64.83	50.19	71.46	89.13	50.19	38.94
1856	41.10	53.17	60.65	79.50	82.61	89.20	90.55	90.00	80.03	72.71	60.20	51.32	70.92	90.55	41.10	49.45
1857	43.07	65.07	60.65	64.37	78.52	84.23	86.84	83.17	80.73	67.65	56.27	55 13	69.31	86.84	43.07	43.77
1858	54.52	51.11	65.93	72.07	76.65	81.87	88.42	89.81	84.80	74.19	49.87	53.61	70.24	89.81	49.87	39.94
1859	53.35	62.22	67.23	72.63	83.67	85.13	90.45	89.06	81.53	71.77	67.43	45.16	72.47	90.45	45.16	45.29
Means	50.80	56.09	63.17	72.12	78.30	84.29	87.78	87.07	80.98	70.15	59.07	50.77	70.05	88.72	47.31	41.41
Max.	58.94	65.07	71.77	79.50	83.67	89.20	92.68	93.21	87.57	74.94	67.43	56.16	73.09	93.21	...	49.45
Min.	41.10	49.71	42.80	64.37	73.94	81.60	84.29	81.13	77.10	62.39	49.87	43.00	65.54	...	41.10	35.90
Range	17.84	15.36	28.97	15.13	9.73	7.60	8.39	12.08	10.47	12.55	17.56	13.16	7.55	52.11		13.55

* Interpolation; mean of 19 years.

XVII. MEAN TEMPERATURE OF MONTHS AND YEARS.

	Jan.	Feb.	March.	April.	May.	June.	July.	Aug.	Sept.	Oct.	Nov.	Dec.	Mean.	Max.	Min.	Range.
1840	42.11	48.69	56.82	63.23	67.90	76.07	77.53	77.27	67.95	60.88	46.70	43.02	60.68	77.53	42.11	35.42
1841	38.19	42.07	51.08	62.15	67.00	73.93	80.42	76.58	68.95	57.27	50.18	42.64	59.21	80.42	38.19	42.23
1842	46.26	46.50	61.85	62.26	67.91	74.25	77.26	73.43	70.95	57.44	43.60	41.52	60.27	77.26	41.52	35.74
1843	45.71	41.20	35.28*	61.43	66.64	73.32	76.97	71.02	73.52	55.42	50.03	44.56	57.92	76.97	35.28	41.69
1844	43.65	49.48	51.12	65.29	70.24	76.52	80.85	78.77	69.18	58.27	52.58	42.50	61.54	80.85	42.50	38.35
1845	46.58	50.98	52.52	66.92	66.69	76.57	79.95	77.94	73.60	56.93	47.97	35.53	61.01	79.95	35.53	44.42
1846	44.03	42.20	53.24	61.25	69.21	72.98	77.52	75.84	72.87	60.32	52.10	49.92	60.96	77.52	42.20	35.32
1847	37.37	45.68	46.90	64.68	66.13	74.68	77.35	74.68	69.32	59.87	51.08	41.80	59.13	77.35	37.37	39.98
1848	49.42	51.31	53.60	58.47	69.76†	76.09†	78.08	77.68	69.78	62.76	46.88	43.18	61.42	78.08	43.18	34.90
1849	44.34	46.66	62.68	63.03	71.56	77.75	79.47	80.39	73.75	60.11	57.98	44.15	63.49	80.39	44.15	36.24
1850	47.18	48.93	55.47	61.20	66.44	77.00	79.44	83.55	72.98	62.52	51.67	42.31	62.39	83.55	42.31	41.24
1851	46.21	48.48	56.61	60.97	72.50	78.70	81.82	83.03	76.05	62.06	49.42	44.96	63.45	83.03	44.96	38.07
1852	38.98	52.82	61.05	61.98	73.48	74.42	78.61	77.48	72.42	66.78	52.03	49.95	63.33	78.61	38.98	39.63
1853	44.65	47.52	53.79	66.02	69.68	77.63	79.13	81.23	73.48	61.40	58.00	45.30	63.15	81.23	44.65	36.58
1854	42.29	49.70	61.30	63.60	71.10	77.45	81.82	82.03	77.28	66.60	52.67	47.47	64.44	82.03	42.29	39.74
1855	46.63	44.50	52.48	68.32	74.68	75.57	81.21	79.63	76.72	59.45	57.10	43.13	63.28	81.21	43.13	38.08
1856	33.97	44.12	51.68	68.92	71.37	79.97	81.42	80.82	70.88	64.18	50.55	43.18	61.76	81.42	33.97	47.45
1857	36.55	57.50	55.73	54.95	68.65	76.00	79.84	78.35	73.78	61.11	51.37	48.92	61.90	79.84	36.55	43.29
1858	48.47	44.14	58.42	63.83	70.10	75.97	81.79	80.50	74.75	66.74	44.57	48.71	63.17	81.79	44.14	37.65
1859	45.79	54.37	58.03	62.68	74.17	77.02	80.87	80.35	74.08	61.34	58.66	38.43	63.82	80.87	38.43	42.44
Means	43.42	47.84	54.48	63.06	69.76	76.09	79.57	78.52	72.61	61.10	51.25	44.06	61.81	79.99	40.57	39.42
Max.	49.42	57.50	62.68	68.92	74.68	79.97	81.82	83.55	77.28	66.78	58.66	49.95	64.44	83.55	...	47.45
Min.	33.97	41.20	35.28	54.95	66.13	72.98	76.97	71.02	67.95	55.42	43.60	35.53	57.92	...	33.97	34.90
Range	15.45	16.30	27.40	13.97	8.55	6.99	4.85	12.53	9.33	11.36	15.06	14.42	6.52	49.58		12.55

XVIII. MEAN TEMPERATURE OF THE SEASONS.‡

	At sunrise.				At 2 or 3 P. M.				Day.				Mean of Year, beginning with December.
	Winter.	Spring.	Summer.	Autumn.	Winter.	Spring.	Summer.	Autumn.	Winter.	Spring.	Summer.	Autumn.	
1840	...	54.91	68.24	49.93	...	70.39	85.68	67.09	...	62.65	76.96	58.51	...§
1841	35.08	51.80	67.34	51.19	47.11	68.35	86.62	66.41	41.09	60.08	76.98	58.80	59.24
1842	37.72	55.39	66.31	48.04	52.55	72.63	83.65	66.62	45.13	64.01	74.98	57.33	60.36
1843	35.11	46.07	64.54	53.25	50.51	62.84	83.00	66.06	42.81	54.45	73.77	59.66	57.67
1844	38.10	55.15	70.02	51.47	53.69	69.28	87.41	68.55	45.90	62.22	78.71	60.01	61.71
1845	37.94	52.49	69.89	50.78	55.43	71.60	86.41	68.22	46.69	62.04	78.15	59.50	61.59
1846	32.57	51.80	67.53	52.93	48.60	70.66	83.36	70.59	40.59	61.23	75.45	61.76	59.34
1847	37.84	50.68	66.98	50.33	50.81	67.79	84.16	69.84	44.32	59.24	75.57	60.09	59.64
1848	38.53	...	...	51.17	56.49	...	...	68.44	47.51	...	...	59.81	...§
1849	38.76	56.81	72.21	55.10	50.70	74.71	86.19	72.80	44.73	65.76	79.20	63.95	63.41
1850	41.21	53.01	71.73	53.63	52.29	69.06	88.26	71.15	46.75	61.04	80.00	62.39	62.54
1851	38.72	53.86	71.20	51.92	52.61	72.85	91.16	73.50	45.67	63.36	81.18	62.71	63.23
1852	37.52	56.89	68.55	56.19	53.66	74.12	85.12	71.29	45.59	65.50	76.84	63.74	62.92
1853	39.93	54.55	70.74	55.41	54.81	71.77	87.92	73.18	47.37	63.16	79.33	64.29	63.54
1854	37.24	56.55	72.50	57.86	54.29	74.11	88.37	73.18	45.76	65.33	80.43	65.52	64.26
1855	37.28	56.10	71.28	56.76	55.11	74.22	86.33	72.08	46.20	65.16	78.80	64.42	63.64
1856	32.66	53.72	71.56	52.76	48.15	74.25	89.92	70.98	40.41	63.99	80.74	61.87	61.75
1857	38.33	49.70	71.38	55.96	53.15	69.85	84 75	68.22	45.74	59.78	78.06	62.09	61.42
1858	40.77	56.68	72.14	54.42	53.59	71.55	86.70	69.62	47.18	64.12	79.42	62.02	63.18
1859	42.85	55.41	70.61	55.81	56.39	74.51	88.21	73.58	49.62	64.96	79.41	64.69	64.67
Means	37.80	53.77	69.72	53.24	52.63	71.29	86.48	70.07	45.21	62.53	78.10	61.65	61.89§
Max.	42.85	56.89	72.50	57.86	56.49	74.71	91.16	73.58	49.62	65.76	81 18	65.52	64.67
Min.	32.57	46.07	64.54	48.04	47.11	62.84	83.00	66.06	40.41	54.45	73.77	57.33	57.34
Range	10.28	10.82	7.96	9.82	9.38	11.87	8.16	7.52	9.21	11.31	7.41	8.19	7.33

* March, 1843, was the coldest month in the whole period of twenty years, except January, 1856.

† Interpolation; mean of 19 years.

‡ Winter includes December and the following January and February.

§ If the means for the years 1840 and 1848 be supplied to this column from Table XVII, the general mean will be 61.81—the same as in that table.

XIX. MEAN TEMPERATURE OF EVERY DAY.—January.

	1	2	3	4	5	6	7	8	9	10	11	12	13	14	15
1840	22	29.5	45	42	50	54	47	46	51	51	48	38	43	44	33
1841	26	31	31	35.5	53	53	34.5	33.5	38	41	44.5	40	37	36.5	37.5
1842	39	45	38.5	40	55.5	66.5	60.5	56.5	45.5	45	41	40	42.5	50	42
1843	42	44	33	39.5	50	63	39	29	35.5	37	35	25.5	27.5	39.5	44
1844	49	36.5	35	34	34	42	45	39	43	44	42	57.5	38.5	42.5	49.5
1845	53	62	64	46	54.5	45	40	40	43	43	41	44	58	52	66
1846	57	46	50	41	44	47	41	44	33	29	36.5	36.5	42	46	47
1847	40	34	37	44	41	38	18.5	30	32	23.5	22	29	51	65	68
1848	42	37	50	46.5	60	39.5	45	62	23.5	26	42	54	64	68	65
1849	45	43	46	39	37.5	37	42	38	29.5	29	39	50	51	34	43
1850	35	40	47.5	38	38	42	48	42	42	45	54	50	44	40	49
1851	37	38	40	46	48	56	55	61	48	45	45	48	49	54	64
1852	33	40	44	54	41.5	32	35	52	50	44	32	30.5	18.5	29.5	35
1853	37.5	44	24.5	30.5	38	43	54	58	59	57	53	46	47	41	44
1854	44	49	56.5	52	65	26.5	27	33	36.5	37.5	40.5	37	39	35	54
1855	57	67	61	43	47	60.5	38	36.5	44.5	53	63	66	50	39	43.5
1856	27	38	32.5	39	34.5	41.5	49	28	24.5	22	33	35	40	34	28
1857	41	44	27.5	33	41	41	29	26	30	25	27	25.5	32	37	38
1858	53	43.5	39	44.5	42.5	44	47	44	49	60	51	53.5	49	48	53
1859	32	48	43	50.5	58	61	31.5	41.5	45	43	47.5	49	54.5	50	44
Means	40.57	42.97	42.25	41.90	46.65	46.62	41.30	42.00	40.12	40.00	41.85	42.75	43.87	44.25	47.37
Max.	57	67	64	54	65	66.5	60.5	62	59	60	63	66	64	68	68
Min.	22	29.5	24.5	30.5	34	26.5	18.5	26	23.5	22	22	25.5	18.5	29.5	28
Range	35	37.5	39.5	23.5	31	40	42	36	35.5	38	41	40.5	45.5	38.5	40

	16	17	18	19	20	21	22	23	24	25	26	27	28	29	30	31
1840	30	38	31	29	36.5	48	47	42.5	43	43	45	56.5	59	57.5	29	27
1841	45	7.5	12.5	21.5	30	33.5	33	35	49.5	47	56	57.5	51	46	45	42
1842	42	47.5	51.5	46	34	40	36	38	40	41	43	43	53	59	53	59.5
1843	52	51	58	61	60.5	63.5	61.5	61.5	59	53.5	62	46	38.5	38	36.5	31
1844	37	32	40.5	48.5	59.5	54	67.5	56.5	45.5	46	37.5	39.5	40	29.5	42	46
1845	67	36	30.5	35	39	40	41	41	41	39	47	60	45	45	43	43
1846	50	41	39	40	40	43	42.5	37	41	49	51	52	52	61	49	37.5
1847	36	33.5	40	18	24	22.5	27	42.5	55	64	39	30	33	40	36	45
1848	56	51	46	45	45	48	48	49	55	59	58.5	51	47	50	59	40
1849	38	44	34	35	38	50	38.5	34	61	63	42	35	56	69	69	65
1850	55	55	49	42	58	41	40	49	62	52	58	60	52	40	43	52
1851	56	31	28	32	37.5	50	56	47	44	46	55	58	65	31	31	31
1852	45	54	25	12.5	20.5	30.5	26	33	41	42	43	49	49	59	63	45
1853	44	39.5	39	45	44	38.5	41	45	48	46	41	37.5	44	50	52	53
1854	57	36	42	52	67.5	18	24	30	30	41	64.5	45	34	41.5	45	51
1855	47	49	50	60	61	30	32	47	50	56	35.5	46.5	35	26.5	22.5	28.5
1856	30	39	40.5	42	31	20	28	30	38	39	39	27	29	35	31.5	48
1857	42	36.5	13.5	25	39.5	37	33.5	32	35	40	56	63	46	44	49	44
1858	41	45	45	48	50	51.5	47	51	61	54	53	52	54	45	41.5	42.5
1859	45.5	42	39.5	44	62.5	45	32	28	35	45	50.5	63	46	49	49	45
Means	45.77	40.42	37.72	39.07	43.90	40.20	40.07	41.45	46.70	48.27	48.82	48.57	46.42	45.80	44.45	43.80
Max.	67	55	58	61	67.5	63.5	67.5	61.5	62	64	64.5	63	65	69	69	65
Min.	30	7.5	12.5	12.5	20.5	18	24	28	30	39	35.5	27	29	26.5	22.5	27
Range	37	47.5	45.5	48.5	47	45.5	43.5	33.5	32	25	29	36	36	42.5	46.5	38

XX. MEAN TEMPERATURE OF EVERY DAY.—February.

	1	2	3	4	5	6	7	8	9	10	11	12	13	14
1840	27	25	33	37	51	52	46	46	55	45	42.5	54	60	32
1841	44	42	45	42	47	39	38	37	41	29	25.5	30	30.5	30.5
1842	44	55	60	47.5	40	53.5	39	28	35.5	52	56	44	42	41.5
1843	30.5	39	47	61	38	30	30.5	29.5	41	51	40	51	58	23
1844	65	45	44.5	47	40	38	38	32.5	35	35	39.5	44	55	50.5
1845	56	44	49	35.5	38	36	53	45	47	51	66	69	71	57
1846	37.5	46	48	46	43	44	48	38	36	42	52	49	39	38
1847	45	43	25	37.5	54	60	51	54	55	32	29	38	46	51
1848	38	45	51	45	42	38	41	47	56	63	59	53	49.5	64.5
1849	56	55	36	39	36	45	43	49	40	38	46	39	45.5	39
1850	55	48	30	22	34	51	58	58	46	40	49	44	34	38
1851	36	39	41.5	43.5	47	48	50	65	62	45	38	41	47	60
1852	45	46	51	65.5	66	68	56.5	45	45	48.5	43	45	58	43
1853	61	53	54.5	47	29	25.5	34	37	39	43.5	50.5	57	52	47
1854	56	54.5	34.5	39	48.5	57.5	62	56	40	52	50.5	63.5	69	50
1855	36.5	41	35	44	60	59.5	65	58	43.5	45	47.5	61	49	45.5
1856	46	37	16	19	24	35	34	36	38	49	42.5	47.5	50	48
1857	49	53	66	68	67	69	50	33	34	37	41.5	57	61	67
1858	40	43	37.5	37	38	42	40	46	58	35.5	31.5	35	41	42.5
1859	53	58	40	45	49.5	34.5	41	58	39.5	35	55.5	42	46	63
Means	46.02	45.57	42.22	43.37	44.60	46.27	45.90	44.90	44.32	43.42	45.25	48.20	50.17	46.55
Max.	65	58	66	68	67	69	65	65	62	63	66	69	71	67
Min.	27	25	16	19	24	25.5	30.5	28	34	29	25.5	30	30.5	23
Range	38	33	50	49	43	43.5	34.5	37	28	34	40.5	39	40.5	44

	15	16	17	18	19	20	21	22	23	24	25	26	27	28
1840	34	39	45	52.5	61	55	46.5	56	57	49	50	61	66.5	67
1841	33	42	48.5	47.5	51	38	51	53	58	46.5	45	60	48	46
1842	47.5	40	40.5	59	35	35.5	33.5	41.5	52.5	52.5	51.5	48	59.5	67.5
1843	21	36.5	41	46.5	50	45	45	61	38	42	38.5	49	39.5	31
1844	53	51	49	49.5	54	54	49	50	54	54	52.5	61	67	63.5
1845	42	41	52	55	69	58	55	46	44	46	54	53	50	45
1846	39	45	55	34	33	35	38	47	45	51	32.5	27.5	33	60
1847	56.5	66.5	45	52.5	51	59	37	38	41	51	43	43	35	40
1848	64	65.5	59	68	70.5	65	52	48	42	32	39	44	44	52
1849	28.5	30	30	16	31.5	53	64	65	63	67	61	64	63	64
1850	36	36	44	48	61	66	55	47	41	59	65	69	62	74
1851	34	31	36	47	52	53	46	52	70	52	57	70	46	..
1852	55	48	55	39.5	43.5	54	59	62	61	67	57	..	49	57
1853	48.5	51	47	51.5	43	41	60	47	36	41.5	48	55	68	63
1854	42	35.5	39	44	49.5	51	46	48	47	48	40.5	52	48	59
1855	42	41	44	47	46	42.5	47	56.5	39	34	32	26.5	28	30
1856	58	60.5	41	46	45.5	46	49.5	55.5	49	44	50.5	49.5	55	55.5
1857	63.5	68	70	70.5	64.5	47	48	52	55	67	62	63	68	59
1858	50	46	47	59	47	53	66	32	32	33	45.5	50.5	62	46
1859	68	64	71	71.5	74	49	46	59	70	69	..	50	61.5	56
Means	45.77	46.87	47.95	50.22	51.60	50.00	49.67	50.82	49.72	50.27	49.13	51.89	52.65	54.50
Max.	68	68	71	71.5	74	66	66	65	70	69	65	70	68	74
Min.	21	30	30	16	31.5	35	33.5	32	32	32	32	26.5	28	30
Range	47	38	41	55.5	42.5	31	32.5	33	38	37	33	43.5	40	44

XXI. MEAN TEMPERATURE OF EVERY DAY.—March.

	1	2	3	4	5	6	7	8	9	10	11	12	13	14	15
1840	65	58	61	61	60	62	66	67	67	62	51	51	47.5	59.5	51
1841	49	56	41	57	53	45	43	39	42.5	36.5	34	38	30	54	59
1842	68.5	62	66	63	60	67	52.5	55	70	75.5	67	37	42	51	48
1843	25.5	24.5	31	31	31	32	41	43	53	40.5	34	32	27.5	40	27
1844	55.5	44	44	39.5	40	..	50	60	52	50	55	62	55	59	50
1845	57	66.5	46.5	46	46	57	67	61	46.5	43.5	40.5	45	51	49	42.5
1846	47.5	41.5	47	55	57	64	61	59.5	61	58	50	49	49	55	57
1847	40	41.5	43	43	42	53.5	51	40	42	34	33	37.5	34.5	34	34
1848	37.5	41.5	32	33	39	33	50	51	39.5	46	54	65	47	49	59
1849	63	61	51	59	68	66	65	60	73	72	73.5	64	66	68	64
1850	60	61	47	44	56.5	59	53	59	64	50	51	50	71	72	70
1851	38	43	42	50	61	37	45	46	48	50	57	62	61	61.5	63
1852	62.5	52	58.5	63.5	69	62	62	67	68.5	61.5	66	67	66	62.5	58
1853	49	52	46	46	54.5	48	62	67	41	43	52	51	42.5	43	42
1854	68	67	48	57	54	63	66	67.5	61.5	51	47	52	64	69.5	72
1855	37	48	60	54	61	70	66	71	65	59	65	63	57.5	70.5	50
1856	42	38	45	53	50.5	56	46.5	55	50	42	46	42.5	41	41	49
1857	57	43	52	57	51	39.5	38	44	44	46.5	44	35	38.5	47	47.5
1858	36	38	41	50	59	65	41	43	46	59.5	65	61	65	66	70
1859	54	65	54	55	57.5	64	47	54.5	54.5	63	52.5	53	63	48.5	51.5
Means	50.60	50.17	47.80	50.85	53.50	54.90	53.65	55.47	54.45	52.17	51.87	50.85	50.95	55.00	53.22
Max.	68.5	67	66	63.5	69	70	67	71	73	75.5	73.5	67	71	72	72
Min.	25.5	24.5	31	31	31	32	38	39	39.5	34	33	32	27.5	34	27
Range	43.0	42.5	35	32.5	38	38	29	32	33.5	41.5	40.5	35	43.5	38	45

	16	17	18	19	20	21	22	23	24	25	26	27	28	29	30	31
1840	54	61	63.5	64	46	45	52	60	56	45.5	53	66	67	49	41	49.5
1841	55	48.5	53	60	56	60	59	46	55	65.5	68	65	61	45	49.5	60
1842	50	61	61.5	62	68	67	69	71	73	67	62	64.5	63	65	67	62
1843	18	25.5	36	35	29	38.5	34	26	34	29	..	42	33.5	49	62	54
1844	46	48	51.5	57	55	46	47	42	51	60.5	60	62.5	62	46	41	42
1845	56	64	46	39	37	48	47	48	53	46	51	64	63	70	71	60
1846	51.5	56.5	66	62	51	53	49	61	43.5	43	52.5	57	45	47	50	51
1847	43.5	53.5	64.5	60.5	47	45	54	51	53	41.5	41	48	58	62	63	65.5
1848	59	66	65	70	70	69.5	60	53	59	73.5	57	50	49	55	68	61
1849	63	68	65	65	75	62	54	59	65	58	49.5	47	55	59	61	64
1850	75	75	53	49	51	60	50	41	48	59	52	40.5	42	48	53	..
1851	61	57	60	54	59	67	60	54	52.5	59.5	64.5	68	70	71	68	65
1852	66	32	40	43	45	57.5	55	58	63	72	72.5	68	71	77.5	65	..
1853	49	61.5	54	48	57	60	65	61	61	65	55	49	52	58	64	69
1854	76	76.5	65	48	53	59	69	64	65	54	48	51	60	71	72	..
1855	48.5	40.5	44	49	38	46	42	47	57	50	55	41	41	43.5	43.5	44
1856	47	43	51	49	59	56	53	63	71	69	67	51.5	51.5	57	66	50.5
1857	53	57	54.5	54.5	68	63	70	70	71	67	69	72.5	71	69	67	67
1858	69	58	57.5	70	70	60	50	55	58	59.5	63	68	70	67.5	66	64
1859	54	63	48	52	61.5	69	67	64	68.5	53	58	68	76	55	54	51
Means	54.72	55.77	54.95	54.55	54.77	56.57	55.30	54.70	57.87	56.87	57.79	57.17	58.05	58.22	59.60	57.62
Max.	76	76.5	66	70	75	69.5	70	71	73	73.5	72.5	72.5	76	77.5	72	69
Min.	18	25.5	36	35	29	38.5	34.	26	34	29	41	40.5	33.5	43.5	41	42
Range	58	51.0	30	35	46	31.0	36	45	39	44.5	31.5	32	42.5	34	31	27

XXII. MEAN TEMPERATURE OF EVERY DAY.—April.

	1	2	3	4	5	6	7	8	9	10	11	12	13	14	15
1840	55	58.5	60	67	65	67	65.5	56	60	64	66	52.5	54	65	67.5
1841	63	61	53	55	57	61	65	68	73	71	57	48.5	62	62	58
1842	56.5	65	71	72	64.5	66	65	59	61	69	72	71.5	65	53	59
1843	45	53	55	52	54	54	58.5	69	65	62	71	64.5	60	66	67
1844	51	56	63	67	66	69	70	66	66.5	67	67	68	65	61	67
1845	51	57	60	71	66	53	49	53	53	68	69	69	68	72.5	71
1846	53	61	63	65	63.5	63	59	49	59	63	47.5	44	47.5	53	60
1847	68	73	74.5	72	75.5	68	70	61	64	68	56	61	63	67	54.5
1848	47	50	66	57.5	50	50	54	58.5	63	68	70	71	65	57	54
1849	63	62	64	60	64	75	77	70	69.5	64	68	62	65	55	45
1850	62	64	62	57	52	53	53	59	66	51	50	52	54	62	67
1851	70	68	67	65	55	53	57	48	53	60	69	65	64	55	56
1852	57	59	66	74	51	36	57	57	59	66	66	67	62	68	61.5
1853	71	74	69	53	58	68	67	69.5	61	52	63	68	71	61	53
1854	47	47	58	65	67	64	68	70.5	61	54.5	61	66	71	70.5	56
1855	55	53	55	61	60	58	52	67.5	68	68	61	66	74.5	76.5	73
1856	56	72	65.5	67	57	63	60	65	73	73.5	70	73	76	71.5	83
1857	57.5	48	51	63	51.5	37	55	57.5	50	60	42.5	44.5	49	47.5	53
1858	62	64.5	66	66	65	69	67	66	66	73	59	50	47.5	52.5	65
1859	60	68	51	46	45	52	55.5	67	79	72	74.5	74	73.5	53	56
Means	57.50	60.70	62.00	62.77	59.35	58.95	61.22	61.82	63.50	64.70	62.97	61.87	62.85	61.45	61.32
Max.	71	74	74.5	74	75.5	75	77	70.5	79	73.5	74.5	74	74.5	76.5	83
Min.	45	47	51	46	45	36	49	48	50	51	42.5	44	47.5	47.5	45
Range	26	27	23.5	28	30.5	39	28	22.5	29	22.5	32	30	27	29	38

	16	17	18	19	20	21	22	23	24	25	26	27	28	29	30
1840	69.5	73	50.5	51.5	61	68	71	73.5	75.5	74	64	47.5	60	66	67
1841	65	73	61	57	65.5	61	66	67	69	70	69	53	64	53.5	56
1842	56.5	50	58.5	57	60	64.5	66.5	68	66	49	..	54.5	60.5	55	70
1843	65	59	52.5	58	61.5	60.5	68	69.5	75.5	76	71	62	53	60.5	55
1844	65	55.5	60	60.5	63.5	69	71	..	73.5	72.5	72	70.5	64	62	65
1845	74	70	76.5	71	73	73	76	70	75	58.5	65	73	73	74	75
1846	63	65.5	67	68.5	68	72	68	72	70.5	68	65.5	57	62	60	60
1847	54	59	60.5	64	66.5	69	72	67	54	57	58	62	68	63	71.
1848	54	58	62	51	56	56	67	66	67	47	49	57	65	57	61
1849	49	51	48	54	54	61	69	68	64	63	66	67	67.5	73	73
1850	71	71	69	74	70	75	66	49	48	56	68	74	56	58	67
1851	59	58	68	73	54	56	52	57	55	63	66	65	66	68	64
1852	68	61	58	55	52.5	52	59	66	69	73.5	69	61	57	70	82
1853	61	56	64	66.5	74.5	76	76	75	75	57.5	58.5	66	70	73	73
1854	53	52	57	66	71	73.5	73	74	71	79	79	69	54	51	59
1855	74.5	76.5	78	75	65	67	73.5	73	77	73	74	72	73	73.5	76
1856	77.5	70	66	63	58.5	60.5	70	70.5	73	77	77	70	67	72	70
1857	54	68	52.5	49	58	63	51	53	56.5	62	65	56	63.5	69	61
1858	76.5	74.5	75	70	59	58	67	57	56	63	62.5	54.5	62	69.5	72
1859	49	50	63	75	71	69	52	53	64	72	76	68	60	66	66
Means	62.92	62.55	62.35	62.95	63.12	65.20	66.70	65.71	66.72	65.55	67.08	62.95	63.27	64.70	67.65
Max.	77.5	76.5	78	75	74.5	76	76	75	77	79	79	74	73	74	82
Min.	49	50	48	49	52.5	52	51	49	48	47	49	47.5	53	51	55
Range	28.5	26.5	30	26	22	24	25	26	29	32	30	26.5	20	23	27

XXIII. MEAN TEMPERATURE OF EVERY DAY.—May.

	1	2	3	4	5	6	7	8	9	10	11	12	13	14	15
1840	65	71.5	69	68	69	68	72	66	59	56	60.5	63	65	67	67
1841	61	65	68	71	68	67	64	57	59	68	67	72.5	71	58	56.5
1842	74.5	73	58	54	53.5	56	61.5	70	67	71.5	71.5	72	69	62	64.5
1843	59.5	63	63	65.5	69	68	57.5	53.5	63	62.5	68	74	71	71	75
1844	68	73	71	64	64	68	68	71	71	74	74	74	74	75	75.5
1845	63	51	59	65	59	57	61	61.5	63.5	66	66	70	73	66	62
1846	66	59	63	66	59	73	68	63	68	67	65	72.5	68	66	64
1847	64	56	54	56	57	65	72	66	61.5	69	73	64	64	67	65
1848	68	75	77	..	..	..	..	..	..	..	..	..	..	..	..
1849	76.5	75.5	75	75	73	74	68	69	63	64	70	72	74.5	70.5	68
1850	61.5	60	65	59	56	57	60	66	67	67.5	56	57	57	59	64
1851	54	59	63	63	58	59	60	69	72	78	79	79.5	77	73	75
1852	76	81	77	77	78	67.5	71	73	74	71.5	72	72	71	78	75
1853	69	68	69	68	72.5	71	68	70	67	57.5	66	63.5	69	76	75
1854	61	66	66	67	68	68.5	69.5	70	75	71	68	71	74	72	72
1855	78.5	74	69	67	65	70.5	75	71	61	65	65	67	69	72	73
1856	68.5	71.5	71	79	77	70	69	61	61	65	64	65	69	71	74.5
1857	62.5	61	61.5	59	71	70.5	69.5	74	76	79	77	74.5	76	76.5	72
1858	64	67	67	60	65	65	67	65	67	64	60	63	72	71	72
1859	70	73.5	64	75.5	72	70	71.5	73	71	74	74	74	78	78	80
Means	66.52	67.65	66.97	66.27	66.00	66.58	66.98	66.79	66.63	67.90	68.21	69.50	70.61	69.95	70.00
Max.	78.5	81	77	79	78	74	75	74	76	79	79	79.5	78	78	80
Min.	54	51	54	54	53.5	56	57.5	53.5	59	56	56	57	57	58	56.5
Range	24.5	30	23	25	24.5	18	17.5	20.5	17	23	23	22.5	21	20	23.5

	16	17	18	19	20	21	22	23	24	25	26	27	28	29	30	31
1840	71	72	74	75	68	66	70	74	66	65	65	70	73	71	71	..
1841	60	61.5	65	66	67	70	74	73.5	71.5	69	71	70	71	76.5	66	73
1842	58	66	67	74	75	63.5	71.5	73.5	69.5	69	68.5	69	72.5	75	77	78
1843	70	62	60.5	66	62.5	65.5	64	70	69	77	75.5	78.5	75	61	61	65
1844	75	75	74	75	67	59.5	63.5	71	78	71	71	70	74	65	59	65
1845	61	61	65	69	74	74	76	74	75	68	68	72	74.5	74	70	69
1846	64.5	65	68	72.5	72	72	74	73	71	76	78	80	75	73	71	73
1847	71	63	66	68	70	71	63.5	64	69	60	64	66	72.5	74	76.5	78
1848	..	..	..	..	..	..	..	..	..	..	..	..	..	..	..	..
1849	68	73	69.5	71	72	73	77.5	68	74	76	73	70	68	67	76	74.5
1850	66	71.5	66.5	66	70	71	77	74	76.5	76.5	77.5	76	79	67	65	68
1851	76.5	75	76.5	78	81	80	78	72	69	77	76	78	79	78	78	79
1852	74	67	64	63.5	68	73	76	75	75	72	70.5	75	75	78.5	79.5	78
1853	75.5	76.5	77	67	65.5	69	73	69	65	64	64	65	72	77	76	75
1854	77	71	67	69.5	73	73	67	71.5	74	70	71	75	76	76	78	76
1855	75	80.5	80	80	79	81.5	82	82	82	82	81	81	78.5	77.5	78	73
1856	76	68	63	67	73	80	74.5	77.5	76	76	79	80	71.5	72.5	72	70
1857	62	64.5	59	63	61.5	62	65	66	69.5	70	70	72.5	70	69.5	75.5	68
1858	76	71	65	61	68	71	75	76	79.5	75	74	75.5	79.5	77	80	80.5
1859	79	79	80	78	79	71	71	67.5	74	78	78	66	65	71	80	..
Means	70.29	69.61	68.79	69.92	70.82	70.84	72.24	72.19	72.82	72.19	72.37	73.13	73.74	72.65	73.13	73.12
Max.	79	80.5	80	80	81	81.5	82	82	82	82	81	81	79.5	78.5	80	80.5
Min.	58	61	59	61	61.5	59.5	63.5	64	65	60	64	65	65	61	59	65
Range	21	19.5	21	19	19.5	22	18.5	18	17	22	17	16	14.5	17.5	21	15.5

XXIV. MEAN TEMPERATURE OF EVERY DAY.—June.

	1	2	3	4	5	6	7	8	9	10	11	12	13	14	15
1840	74.5	81	78	72	78	..	71.5	66	69.5	73	74	74.5	74	77	78.5
1841	72	74	75	77	78.5	76	76.5	79	79	79	78.5	72	72	72	69
1842	79	80	80	78.5	77.5	76	75	78.5	73	73.5	69	66	70	66	69
1843	66	69	74.5	74	76	66	72.5	76.5	78	59.5	61	64	73	73	77.5
1844	68	72	74	75.5	76	78	78	76	78	75	77	75	74	76	76.5
1845	72	76	71	75	72	75	76	76	77.5	78.5	78.5	79	79	75	75.5
1846	73	63.5	77	75	65	68	70	70	68	68	70	69	71.5	72	70
1847	76	79	77	72	74	73.5	74.5	77.5	80	73	69	79	79.5	80	73
1848	..	..	..	..	..	..	..	..	..	..	..	..	..	..	..
1849	71	73	75	76	73	77.5	80	83	75	77.5	81	79	79	80	80
1850	68	73	71	75	81	77	78.5	77	77	71	71	73	74	76	77
1851	78	79	79.5	79	80.5	72	78	80	77	74	78	79.5	80	81	82
1852	77	78	78	75	67	67	70	67	68	71	69	74	74.5	76.5	74.5
1853	78.5	80	80	80	79	76	74.5	73	73	75	78	77	77	77	78
1854	77	69.5	70	66	75	76	78	71	69	72	73	74	77	77	75
1855	73	65	63	73	78	79	71	70	72	74.5	68.5	73	76	73	77
1856	74	77	80	81.5	82	82.5	83.5	82.5	80	78	77	81.5	82.5	79	71
1857	66.5	68	69	75	76	79	79	83	83	80	80	79	80	81	76
1858	71	79	79	76	69	71	75.5	78.5	79.5	74	72.5	65	65	71	73
1859	80	81	76	66	67	71	73	73	79	78	74	76	77	80	80
Means	73.40	74.58	75.11	74.82	74.98	74.47	75.53	75.66	75.56	73.92	73.63	74.28	75.53	75.92	75.40
Max.	80	81	80	81.5	82	82.5	83.5	83	83	80	81	81.5	82.5	81	82
Min.	66	63.5	63	66	65	66	70	66	68	59.5	68.5	64	65	66	69
Range	14	17.5	17	15.5	17	16.5	13.5	17	15	20.5	12.5	17.5	17.5	15	13

	16	17	18	19	20	21	22	23	24	25	26	27	28	29	30
1840	74	75	76	77.5	75	76.5	74	75	79	79	80.5	79	80	81	83
1841	76.5	75	75	77.5	77.5	70	74.5	71	66	65	66	70.5	73	74	77
1842	68.5	69.5	76	70	73	77.5	72	72	74	77.5	77.5	78	76	75	80
1843	77.5	82	69.5	77	77	75	78	76.5	70	73	69.5	75	79	80	80
1844	80	77	80	81	81.5	75	73	71	75.5	76	78	80	79.5	79	80
1845	76	75	78	78.5	79.5	79	79	79	79	78	73	78	79	76	74
1846	72	74	77	76	77	73	75	73	77	75	78	76	78	77.5	81
1847	78	77	78	75	73	68	69	70	72	70	77	75	76	73.5	72
1848	..	..	..	..	..	..	..	82.5	75	80	79.5	79.5	78	79	76
1849	78	78	79	77	77	77	80.5	78	77	75	77	79	81	80	79
1850	78	80	78.5	80.5	81	78	79	76	79	82	81	77.5	78	79	83
1851	82	83	77	75	75.5	75	80	80	79	80	81.5	80.5	81	79	75
1852	78	80	77	80	76	80.5	80	82	75	67	67.5	71.5	75	76	80.5
1853	77	79.5	79.5	80	78	81	83	79	70	70	70	79	82	82	83
1854	81	83	82	82	83	79	77.5	75	81	83	84	84	84	83.5	82
1855	79.5	81	80.5	81	76	74.5	80	75	75	74	80.5	83	81	81	79
1856	79	84	83	74	77	80	80	80	80	80	83	81	80	83	83
1857	75	74	70.5	70	73.5	74	71	72	71	77	77	80	82	78.5	80
1858	77	77	75	76	78	76	79	79	79	77	79	78	82	83	85
1859	81	84.5	76	83	84	78	71	71	74	77	78	82	82	77	81
Means	77.27	78.34	77.24	77.42	77.50	76.16	76.61	75.85	75.37	75.77	76.87	78.37	79.32	78.85	79.67
Max.	82	84.5	83	83	84	81	83	82.5	81	83	84	84	84	83.5	85
Min.	68.5	69.5	69.5	70	73	68	69	70	66	65	67.5	70.5	73	73.5	72
Range	13.5	15	13.5	13	11	13	14	12.5	15	18	16.5	13.5	11	10	13

XXV. MEAN TEMPERATURE OF EVERY DAY.—July.

	1	2	3	4	5	6	7	8	9	10	11	12	13	14	15
1840	77	75	64.5	67	73	70	75	75	78	85.5	75	79	80	81	79
1841	79	81	79	81	82	82.5	80	80	79	81	80	80	81	83	83.5
1842	66	67.5	70	70.5	69	76	79.5	80.5	80	82	79.5	79	79.5	78	78
1843	77	74	72	68	72.5	80	79	81	79	76	76	74	76.5	77.5	80
1844	80	78	80	82.5	80	80	80	81.5	82.5	83	81	83	83	78	82
1845	78	76.5	75	78	77	79	78.5	81	81	82	78	81	81	82	82
1846	78	78	80	80	80	80	79	79.5	78	80	78	80	80	79	76
1847	69	71	75	75	74	79	77	79	78	75	78.5	79	78	78	80
1848	80	75.5	76.5	78	80	82	81.5	75	78	76	79	79	80	81.5	83.5
1849	82	80	82	80	75	79	80	83	82.5	81.5	81	81	79	79	79
1850	68	77	83	82	80	81.5	82	81	77	80	83	84	77	80	78.5
1851	75	76	78	81.5	83	83	83	79	84	84	80	83	83	84	86
1852	83	76	71	78	79	78.5	82	82	78.5	80	80	79	81	76.5	79
1853	83	78	79	80	76	77	79	81	79	77	82	81	82	82	83.5
1854	83	83.5	85	83	84	83	83.5	84	75	76.5	76	75	76	75	80
1855	75.5	78	78	81	80	84.5	85	86	84.5	84	82.5	83	85	82	82
1856	83	86	85.5	87.5	91	75.5	76	80	82	84	80.5	76	80	83	83.5
1857	74	76	70	70	71.5	73	75	76	78	78	75	79.5	81	83	85
1858	83	83	82	80	81	83	82	81	81	80	78	76	74	79	82
1859	83	81.5	82	83	76	80	76	77	82	74	75	80	82	86	81
Means	77.82	77.57	77.37	78.30	78.20	79.32	79.75	80.12	79.85	79.97	78.90	79.57	79.95	80.37	81.17
Max.	83	86	85.5	87.5	91	84.5	85	86	84.5	85.5	83	84	85	86	85
Min.	66	67.5	64.5	67	69	70	75	75	75	74	75	74	74	75	76
Range	17	18.5	21	20.5	22	14.5	10	11	9.5	11.5	8	10	11	11	9

	16	17	18	19	20	21	22	23	24	25	26	27	28	29	30	31
1840	81	81	78.5	79	80	78	80	79	77	77.5	79	80	82	80	77	80.5
1841	83	83	80	77	78.5	78	80	80.5	82	81.5	79	80.5	82.5	84	77	74.5
1842	76	77.5	78.5	80.5	82	74	79	77	77.5	79	78.5	79.5	81	80.5	81.5	78
1843	80.5	82	79	81	78	75.5	74.5	75.5	77	78.5	78.5	81	80	80	72	70.5
1844	84	82	81	81	76	76	79	79	80	79	80	82	84	83	82	84
1845	82	81	82	81	82	83	82	82	79.5	80	82.5	81	80.5	81	77	72
1846	73	68	68	69	71	73	79	78	79	79.5	81	83	80	80	77	79
1847	81	80.5	73	77	78.5	77	79	77	79.5	80.5	80	80	78	78	74	..
1848	78.5	75	74	76	76.5	78	76	77	78	77	80	79	81	76	77	76
1849	80	80	76	75	75	82	80	79	80	79.5	78	79	..	81.5	80	75
1850	80	82	78	77	75	79	81	83	80	78	77	75	80.5	81	81	81
1851	85.5	86	84	80	76	76	79	78	85.5	83.5	84	81	82.5	85	87	81
1852	77	76.5	75	76	74	75.5	78	80.5	79	76	80	80.5	81.5	82	82	80
1853	81	81	82	84	81	83	79	80	80	83	74	71	71.5	69	75	79
1854	80	82	85	83	83	83	83	83	85	86.5	82	82	82.5	85.5	84.5	84
1855	86	82	85	84	81	82	77	80	79.5	76	78	75	80	79.5	80	81.5
1856	83.5	84	83.5	81	81	78	78	77	79	80.5	80	79	82	82	84	78
1857	86	87	85	86	85	85	85	81	78	80	83	88	81	81	79	80
1858	82	82.5	84	84	84	85	84	87	82	80	81	82	82	82.5	84.5	84
1859	82	84	86	87	90	89.5	77	83	82	84.5	83	78	76	74	74	78.5
Means	81.10	80.85	79.87	79.92	79.37	79.52	79.47	79.82	79.97	80.00	79.92	79.82	80.45	80.27	79.27	78.78
Max.	86	87	86	87	90	89.5	85	87	85.5	86.5	84	88	84	85.5	87	84
Min.	73	68	68	69	71	73	74.5	75.5	77	76	74	71	71.5	69	72	70.5
Range	13	19	18	18	19	16.5	10.5	11.5	8.5	10.5	10	17	12.5	16.5	15	13.5

XXVI. MEAN TEMPERATURE OF EVERY DAY.—AUGUST.

	1	2	3	4	5	6	7	8	9	10	11	12	13	14	15
1840	79	81	80	82.5	80	82	83	71	68	70.5	70	72	79.5	74	70.5
1841	74	71	73	77	77	79	82	80	80.5	74	78	75.5	74	76	76
1842	69.5	66	64.5	66	67.5	72.5	75.5	75	76	75.5	77	75	76.5	76	74
1843	67	68	66	68	72.5	72.5	74.5	73	76	73.5	78.5	73	77	73	75
1844	84.5	82	82	86	80	79.5	79	83	83	82	81	72	69.5	74	75.5
1845	71.5	74	73	74	75	75	77	73	74	72	76	77.5	78	78	78.5
1846	79.5	79	79	74	72	74	76	77	75	75	66	77	80	77	79
1847	69	70	77.5	79.5	81	75	71	71	72	72.5	74	77.5	79	80	77
1848	74	79	82	81	75	74	75	73	74	75	76.5	77.5	79.5	80	77
1849	77.5	78	79.5	78	79	79.5	80	79	82	78	80.5	83	83.5	84	83
1850	82	81.5	83	83	85	85.5	85	85.5	86.5	85.5	87	90	88.5	89	86
1851	79	80.5	79	76	76	79	82	85	85.5	85	85	86.5	88	89	89.5
1852	78	80	80	79.5	80	78	79	79	77	74	75.5	74	72	76	78
1853	79.5	79	82	82	83	81	82	80	81.5	82	80	81	81	81	81
1854	84.5	85	85	85	85	83.5	79	83	86	86	85.5	85	86	85	86
1855	81	82	82	82.5	82.5	83	82	84	84	84	85	82	80	82	85
1856	79	79	70	81	78	79	82	84	83	82	81	81	81	81	77
1857	78	76	77	77	80.5	81	82	83.5	82.5	81	81	77	83.5	82.5	80
1858	82	83	83	84	82	84	83	83	84	83	84	79	82	83	83
1859	81	82	79	80	81	81	81	80	80.5	83	84	84.5	81	78	80.5
Means	77.48	77.80	77.83	78.80	78.60	78.90	79.50	79.10	79.55	78.68	79.28	79.00	79.98	79.92	79.58
Max.	84.5	85	85	86	85	85.5	85	85.5	86.5	86	87	90	88.5	89	89.5
Min.	67	66	64.5	66	67.5	72.5	71	71	68	70.5	66	72	69.5	73	70.5
Range	17.5	19	20.5	20	17.5	13	14	14.5	18.5	15.5	21	18	19	16	19

	16	17	18	19	20	21	22	23	24	25	26	27	28	29	30	31
1840	72	74	77	74	78	80	81	81	78	78.5	74.5	82	81.5	81	81	79
1841	77	79	81	81.5	76.5	76	77.5	72	72	75	76.5	77.5	78	78	74	75.5
1842	73	74.5	73	74	72	72	74	73	74.5	72.5	75	76	75	77	77.5	77
1843	68	77	74	71.5	71	69	67	67.5	67	70	67	65	70	68	70	72
1844	77	79	80.5	82	82	84	84	77	80	75	75.5	73	72	72	78	78
1845	81	79	81	82	82.5	83.5	83	82	81	81.5	82	80.5	80	76.5	77	77
1846	83	82	82	82	78	78	75	69.5	67	70.5	71	71	75	74.5	77	76
1847	79	79	81	81	75	70	74	74	69	76	74	74	74	68	71	70
1848	78	78	77	76	79	76	75	74	79.5	80.5	80.5	79	79	81	82	81
1849	83	84	83	82.5	82	82.5	82	84	85	84	76	77	74.5	79	77	72
1850	82	85	84	85	85.5	86	85	83	86	83.5	78	74	73	79.5	74	. .
1851	89	89	87	85.5	84.5	83	79	80	82.5	85.5	86	79	79	80	80	80
1852	77.5	76	75	72	77.5	80	79	81	81	79	80	80	75	72	78	79
1853	80.5	80.5	81	84	84	84	85	84.5	83	85	80	76	73	79	81	81.5
1854	81	79	75	78.5	78.5	79	79	79	79	79	79	80	81.5	80	84	82
1855	85.5	76	73	72	75	80	78	74.5	75	75	75	76.5	74	78	80	80
1856	77	84	87.5	87	82.5	84	88	86	83	81	76.5	80	77	80	79	75
1857	80	80	77	75	74	74	76	77	78	77	78	79	81	72	70	. .
1858	81	83	82	81	78	82	84	82	76.5	78	84	85	73	66	70	68
1859	80	82	82	82	81	83	80.5	78	73	77	80	83	86	79	74	74
Means	79.23	80.00	79.65	79.43	78.83	79.30	79.30	77.95	77.50	78.18	77.43	77.38	76.58	76.03	76.73	76.50
Max.	89	89	87.5	87	85.5	86	88	86	86	85.5	86	85	86	81	84	82
Min.	68	74	73	71.5	71	69	67	67.5	67	70	67	65	70	66	70	68
Range	21	15	14.5	15.5	14.5	17	21	18.5	19	15.5	19	20	16	15	14	14

XXVII. MEAN TEMPERATURE OF EVERY DAY.—September.

	1	2	3	4	5	6	7	8	9	10	11	12	13	14	15
1840	72	70	72	65	62	67	74	75.5	75	71	65.5	63	64	66	67
1841	74	77	78	78	71	75.5	79	79	79	72.5	67	69	60.5	65.5	70
1842	77	75	75	75	78	77	81	79.5	79	81	78	78.5	72	68	64.5
1843	77	77	75.5	75	76.5	76	74	77	75	74	76	70	77	74	67
1844	80	78	79.5	80	79	79	76	75	73.5	75.5	76	73	69	72	72
1845	77.5	81	83.5	81	81	80	79.5	80	78	73.5	72	77	78	75.5	68
1846	76	73	74	79	79	76.5	77	76	75.5	78	78.5	79	79.5	81	81
1847	76	75.5	77	76	77	79	80	68	63	59	60.5	65.5	65.5	63	67
1848	78	80	81	81	75	68	68	67	69	71	74	76	79	82	76
1849	71.5	68	71	75	78	75	71	67	69	71	70	70.5	71	80	78.5
1850	65	65	66	73	77	65	70	70	71	72	73	76	77.5	79	80
1851	81	78	80	82	82.5	81	83	85	78	70	78	79	81	81	83
1852	80	77	75	72	71	74	75	75.5	75	75.5	78	68	68	69	72
1853	82	83	82	83	80	79.5	75	71	74.5	72	73	75	75	73	77
1854	81.5	81	78	80	79	79.5	82	81	83.5	83	83	82	82	79	78
1855	76	70	78	79	81	81	78	78	76.5	76	79	81	79.5	79.5	80
1856	71	71	75	77	78	79	79	82	80	81	82	81.5	78	78	75.5
1857	73	76.5	75	77	78	78	78	79.5	79	77	79	77	77	79	80
1858	76	83.5	72	73	76	80	82	80	79	76	71	70	72	71	74
1859	75	76.5	78	75	63	68	72	76	82	82.5	81	79	76	78	77
Means	75.97	75.80	76.27	76.80	76.10	75.90	76.67	76.10	75.72	74.57	74.72	74.50	74.07	74.67	74.37
Max.	82	83.5	83.5	83	82.5	81	83	85	83.5	83	83	82	82	82	83
Min.	65	65	66	65	62	65	68	67	63	59	60.5	63	60.5	63	67
Range	17	18.5	17.5	18	20.5	16	15	18	20.5	24	22.5	19	21.5	19	15

	16	17	18	19	20	21	22	23	24	25	26	27	28	29	30
1840	70	74	66	56.5	62.5	65	62	63	69.5	74	72	68	68	68	71
1841	70	67	67	69.5	74.5	60	59.5	60.5	55	63	70	70	66	63	58.5
1842	61	61	61	64	72.5	72	68	64.5	66	68.5	67	68	67	70	59.5
1843	76	78	77.5	77	76	77	75.5	76	76	71	69	58.5	59	69	69
1844	74	75.5	75.5	74.5	73	64.5	56	58.5	62.5	62	57.5	51	55	48.5	50
1845	67.5	70	71.5	72	71	67	62	67	68	67	69	70	73	74	..
1846	81	81	72	67	66	70	72.5	74	70	66	64.5	61	60	59	59
1847	67	71	71	64.5	61.5	61.5	63	68	69	71	77	78	73	63	69
1848	65	67	67	68	66	62	61.5	61	62	63	63	66.5	66.5	67	63
1849	76	80.5	81.5	83.5	81	75	77	70	66.5	67	74	66	68.5	78	81.5
1850	72	73	74	76	68	69	76	78	79	77	78	77	78	71	64
1851	83	78	77	74	75	75	73	74	78	74.5	72	66	57.5	60	62
1852	73	75	75	74	72	63	66	74	79	75	66	64	72.5	69	70
1853	79	79	78	79.5	71	64	61	61	64	64	67.5	69	69	70	73.5
1854	74	76	73	71	69	68	70	74.5	78	73.5	73	74.5	78	77	76.5
1855	81	82	81	80.5	80.5	79	80	78	79.5	78	74	63	63	67	62.5
1856	77	78	76	70	65	57	64	56	55.5	59	63	65	64	57	52
1857	78	79	79.5	75	67	65	68	65	67	67.5	68	69	70	68.5	64
1858	69	70.5	76	70	70	72	78	75	75	76	76	74	74	75.5	76
1859	78	81	77	69.5	65	65	65	69	73	75	71.5	77.5	75	75	67
Means	73.57	74.82	73.82	71.80	70.32	67.55	67.90	68.35	69.62	69.60	69.60	67.80	67.85	67.47	65.69
Max.	83	82	81.5	83.5	81	79	80	78	79.5	78	78	78	78	78	81.5
Min.	61	61	61	56.5	61.5	57	56	56	55	59	57.5	51	55	48.5	50
Range	22	21	20.5	27	19.5	22	24	22	24.5	19	20.5	27	23	29.5	31.5

XXVIII. MEAN TEMPERATURE OF EVERY DAY.—October.

	1	2	3	4	5	6	7	8	9	10	11	12	13	14	15
1840	72.5	67	47.5	53.5	55	..	65	74	75	76.5	72.5	68	71	69	71
1841	57	55	51	52.5	54	58	62.5	70	73	73.5	72	67	63	53.5	54
1842	62	60.5	62	65	66.5	69	70	64	49.5	51	56.5	61	61	59	53
1843	60.5	63	62.5	58.5	62	67.5	64	57	61	57.5	67	57	49.5	48	50
1844	58	63	60	61	62	63	60	56	57	63	..	57	60	64	57
1845	63	64	64	67	51.5	50	56	58	53	56	47	45	49.5	57	51.5
1846	66	63	65	69	73	73	69	73	70	65	70	67	53	58	59
1847	73	73	69	70.5	70	..	67	63	66	66	65	71	54	52	51
1848	52	52.5	64	70	68.5	68.5	68	66	63	65	65	66	66	70	70
1849	79	63	66	70	71.5	56	56	52	57	64	63.5	64	55	65	65.5
1850	67	70	68	64	65	56	59	63	68	77.5	79	72	64	64	72
1851	63	66	70	71	72	71	71	72	78	75	64	56.5	55	61	55
1852	74	79	78	75	75.5	75	77	73	64	61	62	60	59	61.5	63
1853	72	61	60	61	65	68	70	65.5	68	71	67.5	72	70	68	60
1854	78	78	79.5	63	61	63	64	64	64	69.5	74	77.5	78	79	63
1855	65	63	63	68	58	50	53.5	55	65	64	66	55	55	60	64
1856	55.5	66	72	74	73	73	73	71	69	72	74	75	73	59	48
1857	68	65.5	63	71	73	64	68	65	65	68	70	69	65	64	62.5
1858	76	78	77.5	79	81	80	80	57	59	62	65	56	64	65	68
1859	66	62	60.5	62.5	69	68	68	69	52	57	59	64	69	72	69
Means	66.37	65.62	65.12	66.27	66.32	65.17	66.05	64.37	63.82	65.72	66.27	64.00	61.70	62.45	60.32
Max.	79	79	79.5	79	81	80	80	74	78	77.5	79	77.5	78	79	72
Min.	52	52.5	47.5	52.5	51.5	50	53.5	52	49.5	51	47	55	53	48	48
Range	27	26.5	32	26.5	29.5	30	26.5	22	28.5	26.5	32	22.5	25	31	24

	16	17	18	19	20	21	22	23	24	25	26	27	28	29	30	31
1840	67.5	70	72	65	63	62	52	53	50	43	45.5	50	56	46	48	46
1841	61	57	57	64	52	52	43	40	41.5	37	45	57.5	58	68	67	59.5
1842	57	60	62	52.5	53	53	60	66	63.5	49	46.5	46.5	49	49.5	50.5	52.5
1843	51	50	62	56	65	69	54.5	54.5	65	47.5	38.5	37.5	45	46	45.5	46
1844	65	53.5	46	42	48.5	59	62	70	75	70	68	56	51	41	44	56
1845	45	50	55	64	67	53	47	48	60	59	58	61	61	64	69.5	71
1846	63	49	44	44	49	49	54	59	64	62	67	64	54	52	51	52
1847	60	62	66	59	61	70	60	48	52.5	49	45	42	44	48	53	66
1848	70.5	57	53	53	49	55	62.5	71	66	70	67	72	65	54	57	49
1849	56	50	44	44.5	58.5	60	61	60	61.5	57	56	62	63	65	57.5	60
1850	76	73	62	52.5	52	64	64	65	64	43	44	46	50	58	58	58
1851	58	58.5	60	60	64	59	51	48.5	55	61	52	54	66	67	68	60
1852	66	68	68	66	66	68	69	70	65	65	71	64.5	63	54	56	53.5
1853	63	66	65	65	63	66	55	50.5	45.5	49	63	46.5	48	49.5	51.5	58
1854	67	59	63.5	64	67	67	67	61	55.5	61.5	61	62.5	65	60	64	64
1855	62	63	61	66	64	66.5	49	49	41	39	52.5	63.5	67.5	65	62.5	67
1856	47	49	51	65	67	72	73	75	73.5	58	58	58	54	55	54	52.5
1857	52	51.5	62.5	64	53	50	55.5	59	62	58	54	56	54	55	57	50
1858	68	73	73	67	55	57	61.5	67	68	65	67.5	63	57.5	59	61	59
1859	69.5	79	52	53	58	56	63	65	67	66	66	57	43	46	43	51
Means	61.22	59.92	58.95	58.32	58.75	60.37	58.20	58.97	59.77	55.45	56.27	55.97	55.70	55.10	55.90	56.55
Max.	76	79	73	67	67	72	73	75	75	70	71	72	67.5	68	69.5	71
Min.	45	49	44	42	48.5	50	43	40	41	37	38.5	37.5	43	41	43	46
Range	31	30	29	25	18.5	22	30	35	34	33	32.5	34.5	24.5	27	26.5	25

XXIX. MEAN TEMPERATURE OF EVERY DAY.—November.

	1	2	3	4	5	6	7	8	9	10	11	12	13	14	15
1840	47	51	56	54	62	58	63	49	49	54	54	49	49.5	55	38
1841	53	41	53	47.5	42.5	37.5	50	55.5	67	65.5	65	60.5	52	48	46
1842	56.5	60.5	64	64	64	55	51	53	45	40	46	37	40.5	52	44.5
1843	53	42	47.5	58	50.5	48	48.5	42	61	58	44	38	39.5	47	56
1844	65	69	65	50	55	54	55.5	59	66	64	65	40	33	35	39
1845	71	59	52	53	67	61	52	50	38	39	45	46	45	56	58
1846	53	55	53	60	52.5	45	52	54	65	57.5	56	60	59	46	62
1847	70	68	69	68	61	69	68	70	45	47	42	45.5	63	45	48.5
1848	45	46	62.5	40	41	47	42	49	53	38	54	55	50	54	49.5
1849	59	66.5	68	75	73	66	58	50	54	56	59	59	55	60	62.5
1850	55	69	67	66	71	49	44	48	49	50	44	44	48	51	50
1851	74	56	57	56	53	40	38	49	61	58.5	55	61	48	46	41
1852	62	59	66	72	73	55	49.5	53	49.5	51	62.5	41	46.5	47	44
1853	59	63	53	50	52	56	56	64	47.5	44.5	59	63	51	50	65
1854	63	60.5	60	58.5	43.5	46	60	62	59	62	54	45	40	47	60
1855	69	70	66	74	61	53	52.5	58	57	56	66	60	60	68.5	74
1856	61.5	67.5	69	48	45	52	64	33	35	39	46	47	46	51	55
1857	53	69	54	62	72	77	72.5	46	41	44	51	55	56	44	38.5
1858	54	51	48.5	44	46	48	47	39	41.5	48	46	44	42	43	47
1859	49	57	63	61	66	62	60	63	66	65	74.5	48	33	40.5	44
Means	58.60	59.00	59.67	58.05	57.55	53.92	54.17	52.32	52.47	52.35	54.40	49.90	47.85	49.30	51.12
Max.	74	70	69	75	73	77	72.5	70	67	65.5	74.5	63	63	68.5	74
Min.	45	41	47.5	40	41	37.5	38	33	35	38	42	37	33	35	38
Range	29	29	21.5	35	32	39.5	34.5	37	32	27.5	32.5	26	30	33.5	36

	16	17	18	19	20	21	22	23	24	25	26	27	28	29	30
1840	47	38	36	36	55	57	34	30.5	33.5	26.5	33	41	35	57	53
1841	50.5	60	67	62	64	66.5	48	51	60	44	32	27.5	30.5	26.5	32
1842	50	29.5	25	24	29	36	34.5	36	27.5	41.5	51	39.5	31.5	38	42
1843	60	57	46.5	52.5	54	56	52.5	62	43	46.5	50.5	52.5	56.5	44	34.5
1844	56	50	45	42	44.5	47.5	41	46	42	41.5	52	59	62	65.5	69
1845	59	68	56	48	52	60	38	37.5	45	45	39	30	24	25	20.5
1846	64.5	51	48	40	39	50	45	43	48	35	33	58	62.5	56	60
1847	51	63	49	38	38.5	52	56	49	41.5	38	25	33	39	38.5	42
1848	47	46	37	34.5	40	42.5	48.5	42.5	48.5	63	50	47	36	46	42
1849	68.5	63	48	50	48	61	65	71	57	46	44	43	51	55	48
1850	37	36	45	50	51	47	52	51	51	62	66	65	40	44	48
1851	52	52	54	60	47	45	48	43	34	33	48	52	38	41	42
1852	51	50	41.5	41	49	46	46	43	55.5	48	41	42.5	52.5	61	62
1853	71.5	72	66	68	67	64	56	58	48	50	50	62	65.5	59	50
1854	50	54	46	38.5	51.5	66	58	64	52	44	42	39.5	44	51	59
1855	68	48	45.5	45	55	50	48	51.5	52.5	59.5	51	48.5	51	45	40.5
1856	57	43	38	42	49	50	42	59	55	65	57	48	50	52	50.5
1857	44.5	44	52	43.5	34.5	44	48	46	40	43	45	55	59	56.5	51
1858	36	37	39	37	35	37	40	37	39	48	58	60	59.5	42	43.5
1859	61	62	49	42	60	54	56.5	66.5	71	70.5	69	69	59	50.5	68
Means	54.07	51.17	46.65	44.70	48.15	51.57	47.85	49.37	47.20	47.50	46.82	48.60	47.32	47.67	48.32
Max.	71.5	72	67	68	67	66.5	65	71	71	70.5	69	69	65.5	65.5	69
Min.	36	29.5	25	24	29	36	34	30.5	27.5	26.5	25	27.5	24	25	20.5
Range	35.5	42.5	42	44	38	30.5	31	40.5	43.5	44	44	41.5	41.5	40.5	48.5

XXX. MEAN TEMPERATURE OF EVERY DAY.—December.

	1	2	3	4	5	6	7	8	9	10	11	12	13	14	15
1840	41	40	43	34	36	36.5	51	56	62	61.5	63	42	36.5	53	56
1841	34	43	50	38	41	42.5	45	57.5	62	62	43.5	48	51.5	50.5	54.5
1842	40	52	58	60.5	67	44	49	38	36	35.5	33.5	31	33	29.5	34
1843	37.5	38.5	39	49	37	37	39	40.5	44	47.5	53	38	35.5	46	58
1844	44	47	46.5	61	39	33.5	31	32	34	28	31	42.5	41.5	40	44.5
1845	10	18	21	23	30	33	37.5	44	40	36	36	35	43.5	44	42
1846	67	63	43	43	48	62.5	68	37	35	39	35	37	46	56	55
1847	44.5	38	34	39	42	45	57	47	61	43	43	41	36	33	32
1848	40.5	42	61	67.5	64	40	40	34.5	41	36	28	36	44	51	33
1849	47	39	41	50	56	42	42	51	32.5	27	21	28	35	38	49
1850	63	70	42	37	28	25	20	24.5	36	41	50	55	47	45	52
1851	47	43	36	35	42	49	61	66.5	65	60	44	49	46	41	28
1852	58	58	53	51	57	70.5	45	46	43	41	43	50.5	37	42	44
1853	50	53.5	48	52.5	63	61	47	38	40	43	49	48	44	50	53
1854	61	59	50	40	31	36	43	45	51	54	42	41	. .	45	53
1855	50	51	40	43.5	45	47	55.5	62	47	47	46	60.5	63.5	50	44
1856	59	44.5	32	32	37	33	36	36	45	56	44	46	57	33	40
1857	52	59	56	58	62	65	56	69	47	43	45	44	46	45	51
1858	49	60	55	44.5	43.5	49	49	34	32.5	33.5	47	63	66	65	44
1859	71	30	29	33	41	17	15	25	36	39	45	40	39	40	35.5
Means	48.27	47.42	43.87	44.57	45.47	43.42	44.35	44.17	44.50	43.65	42.10	43.77	44.63	44.85	45.12
Max.	71	70	61	67.5	67	70.5	68	69	65	62	63	63	66	65	58
Min.	10	18	21	23	28	17	15	24.5	32.5	27	21	28	33	29.5	28
Range	61	52	40	44.5	39	53.5	53	44.5	32.5	35	42	35	33	35.5	30

	16	17	18	19	20	21	22	23	24	25	26	27	28	29	30	31
1840	52	39	36	38	40	46	49	44	27	39	47	36	27	39	35	28
1841	41.5	34	33.5	51.5	56.5	41.5	54	31	27	30.5	28.5	29	54.5	34	35.5	36.5
1842	43	37	44.5	46.5	44	41	36.5	25.5	37.5	35.5	47	51	53	38	31	35
1843	54	42	41	45	45	50	45	48	50	50	46	40	40	40.5	53	52.5
1844	30	30	29	36	49	51	44	43	54	66.5	47.5	37.5	45	47	56.5	56
1845	37	49	38	26	18.5	28.5	43	48	45	37.5	24	28	35	48	49	54
1846	56	39	38	37	34	40.5	50	47	60	58.5	60	66	65	59	43	60
1847	32.5	30	34	42	38	24	37	44	43	39.5	33	40	57.5	58	66	. .
1848	39	48	67	71	53	50	25	28.5	36	39	33	37	38	40	37	38.5
1849	54	32	40	63	62	48	46	51.5	52	43	56	60	62	47	28.5	25
1850	55	46	49	50	42	43	46	46	41	42	43	39	38	34	34	28
1851	27	26	23	34	37	36.5	35	34	45	66	47	53	58	70	. .	. .
1852	55	38	49	65.5	73	34	34.5	64	53	50	45.5	67	33.5	39	51	57.5
1853	52	45	41.5	34	31	36	44	39.5	32.5	36	42	48.5	46	43	48	. .
1854	49	48	35	35	32.5	43.5	49.5	56	58.5	57.5	54	53	55.5	45	47	54
1855	50.5	43	35	44	48	67	49	33.5	23	20	20	32.5	39	36	18	26.5
1856	38	41	53	58	31	31.5	33.5	32	40	50.5	65	64	42	49	41	38.5
1857	55	56	47.5	42	45.5	32	43	39	36	35.5	38	45	54	52	50	48
1858	44.5	35	34.5	48	55	47.5	45	53	50	45	52	55	52	58	56.5	44
1859	41	42	42	33.5	23.5	22	25	21	31	53.5	62	68	67	53.5	40	33
Means	45.30	40.00	40.52	45.00	42.82	40.67	41.70	41.42	42.07	44.75	44.52	47.47	47.10	46.50	43.16	42.06
Max.	56	56	67	71	73	67	54	64	60	66.5	65	68	67	70	66	60
Min.	27	26	23	26	18.5	22	25	21	23	20	20	28	27	34	18	25
Range	29	30	44	45	54.5	45	29	43	37	46.5	45	40	40	36	48	35

XXXI. MEAN TEMPERATURE OF EVERY DAY IN THE YEAR.

	Jan.	Feb.	March.	April.	May.	June.	July.	August.	Sept.	Oct.	Nov.	Dec.
1	40.57	46.02	50.60	57.50	66.52	73.40	77.82	77.48	75.97	66.37	58.60	48.27
2	42.97	45.57	50.17	60.70	67.65	74.58	77.57	77.80	75.80	65.62	59.00	47.42
3	42.25	42.22	47.80	62.00	66.97	75.11	77.37	77.83	76.27	65.12	59.67	43.87
4	41.90	43.37	50.85	62.77	66.27	74.82	78.30	78.80	76.80	66.27	58.05	44.57
5	46.65	44.60	53.50	59.35	66.00	74.98	78.20	78.60	76.10	66.32	57.55	45.47
6	46.62	46.27	54.90	58.95	66.58	74.47	79.32	78.90	75.90	65.17	53.92	43.42
7	41.80	45.90	58.65	61.22	66.98	75.68	79.75	79.60	76.67	66.05	54.17	44.35
8	42.00	44.90	55.47	61.82	66.79	75.66	80.12	79.10	76.10	64.37	52.32	44.17
9	40.12	44.32	54.45	63.50	66.63	75.56	79.85	79.55	75.72	63.82	52.47	44.50
10	40.00	43.42	52.17	64.70	67.90	73.92	79.97	78.68	74.57	65.72	52.35	43.65
11	41.85	45.25	51.87	62.97	68.21	73.63	78.90	79.28	74.72	66.27	54.40	42.10
12	42.75	48.20	50.85	61.87	69.50	74.28	79.57	79.00	74.50	64.00	49.90	43.77
13	43.87	50.17	50.95	62.85	70.61	75.53	79.95	79.98	74.07	61.70	47.85	44.63
14	44.25	46.55	55.00	61.45	69.95	75.92	80.37	79.93	74.67	62.45	49.30	44.85
15	47.37	45.77	53.22	61.32	70.00	75.40	81.17	79.58	74.37	60.32	51.12	45.12
16	45.77	46.87	54.72	62.92	70.29	77.27	81.10	79.23	73.57	61.22	54.07	45.30
17	40.42	47.95	55.77	62.55	69.61	78.34	80.85	80.00	74.82	59.92	51.17	40.00
18	37.72	50.22	54.95	62.35	68.79	77.24	79.87	79.65	73.82	58.95	46.65	40.52
19	39.07	51.60	54.55	62.95	69.92	77.42	79.92	79.43	71.80	58.32	44.70	45.00
20	43.90	50.00	54.77	63.12	70.82	77.50	79.37	78.83	70.32	58.75	48.15	42.82
21	40.20	49.67	56.57	65.20	70.84	76.16	79.52	79.30	67.55	60.37	51.57	40.67
22	40.07	50.82	55.30	66.70	72.24	76.61	79.47	79.30	67.90	58.20	47.85	41.70
23	41.45	49.72	54.70	65.71	72.19	75.85	79.82	77.95	68.35	58.97	49.37	41.42
24	46.70	50.27	57.87	66.72	72.82	75.37	79.97	77.50	69.62	59.77	47.20	42.07
25	48.27	49.13	56.87	65.55	72.19	75.77	80.00	78.18	69.60	55.45	47.50	44.75
26	48.82	51.89	57.79	67.08	72.37	76.87	79.92	77.43	69.60	56.27	46.82	44.52
27	48.57	52.65	57.17	62.95	73.13	78.37	79.82	77.38	67.80	55.97	48.60	47.47
28	46.42	54.50	58.05	63.27	73.74	79.32	80.45	76.58	67.85	55.70	47.32	47.10
29	45.80	...	58.22	64.70	72.66	78.85	80.27	76.03	67.47	55.10	47.67	46.50
30	44.45	...	59.60	67.65	73.13	79.67	79.27	76.73	65.69	55.90	48.32	43.16
31	43.80	...	57.62	...	73.12	...	78.78	76.50	...	56.55	...	42.06
Means	43.42	47.78*	54.51	63.08	69.82†	76.11	79.57	78.52	72.60	61.12	51.25	44.04

* If the 29th of February be omitted in computing the means of that month for the leap years in Table XXII, the general mean of February in that table will be 47.78.

† If the three days observed in May, 1848, be omitted in Table XXIII (as they are in Table XVII), the mean of this column will be 69.77.

XXXII. AMOUNT OF RAIN, IN INCHES.

	Jan.	Feb.	March.	April.	May.	June.	July.	Aug.	Sept.	Oct.	Nov.	Dec.	Year.	Max.	Min.	Range.
1840	7.5	14.5	4.2	13.6	5.7	.9	2.5	1.3	2.8	8.0	3.8	2.7	67.5	14.5	.9	13.6
1841	5.0	.4	8.6	5.4	7.2	5.0	1.4	3.0	4.6	8.3	2.6	3.0	54.5	8.6	.4	8.2
1842	3.4	3.7	4.6	4.0	2.1	5.5	1.8	4.1	1.7	2.7	2.7	5.3	41.6	5.5	1.7	3.8
1843	2.9	1.6	5.8	9.2	5.7	3.6	2.7	3.1	7.1	6.8	11.3	3.6	63.4	11.3	1.6	9.7
1844	3.0	3.0	6.8	7.7	4.1	5.4	1.2	1.3	4.6	4.2	2.6	1.6	45.5	7.7	1.2	6.5
1845	7.2	2.8	7.4	5.5	5.1	6.8	2.7	.7	2.1	.8	1.2	4.4	46.7	7.4	.7	6.7
1846	2.7	4.2	3.6	6.9	3.5	4.2	3.5	1.0	1.8	2.8	2.3	4.9	41.4	6.9	1.0	5.9
1847	2.7	6.7	9.6	6.0	3.9	4.0	5.5	7.4	1.5	1.1	5.6	4.3	58.3	9.6	1.1	8.5
1848	3.1	2.7	4.7	5.8	5.4	8.9	6.7	2.2	1.0	2.8	6.9	9.8	60.0	9.8	1.0	8.8
1849	8.9	5.8	5.7	2.7	3.5	3.2	19.5	4.1	1.6	3.3	6.4	5.7	70.4	19.5	1.6	17.9
1850	10.9	5.2	3.5	9.7	4.0	4.0	4.7	7.3	1.2	4.7	5.2	5.3	65.7	10.9	1.2	9.7
1851	1.3	12.7	4.5	2.6	3.9	2.8	2.0	2.7	.6	1.2	3.4	3.8	41.5	12.7	.6	12.1
1852	2.8	8.0	4.8	3.8	3.3	2.9	15.1	11.8	3.9	2.4	7.7	3.0	69.5	15.1	2.4	12.7
1853	1.1	5.6	9.1	4.0	9.7	1.6	7.5	1.1	8.0	2.8	2.5	2.2	55.2	9.7	1.1	8.6
1854	3.6	2.7	5.9	3.1	16.0	3.1	2.3	3.4	8.3	4.0	1.7	5.1	59.2	16.0	1.7	14.3
1855	4.4	2.3	2.0	3.6	2.7	3.6	4.6	4.1	6.2	1.8	8.7	3.6	47.6	8.7	1.8	6.9
1856	6.1	5.5	2.1	3.2	1.0	3.0	4.6	2.1	3.8	4.3	6.7	3.8	46.2	6.7	1.0	5.7
1857	1.7	7.0	1.4	3.4	3.6	1.9	1.8	14.9	3.2	5.2	8.2	4.8	57.1	14.9	1.4	13.5
1858	9.5	2.7	6.6	4.8	5.1	4.8	1.8	2.0	1.8	9.4	1.5	6.7	56.7	9.5	1.5	8.0
1859	3.8	2.2	5.6	4.4	1.1	5.3	7.0	1.8	3.9	2.0	3.6	5.4	46.1	7.0	1.1	5.9
Means	4.58	4.97	5.33	5.47	4.83	4.02	4.94	3.97	3.48	3.93	4.73	4.45	54.70	10.10	1.25	9.35
Max.	10.9	14.5	9.6	13.6	16.0	8.9	19.5	14.9	8.3	9.4	11.3	9.8	70.4	19.5	..	17.9
Min.	1.1	.4	1.4	2.6	1.0	.9	1.2	.7	.6	.8	1.2	1.6	41.4	..	.4	3.8
Range	9.8	14.1	8.2	11.0	15.0	8.0	18.3	14.2	7.7	8.6	10.1	8.2	29.0	19.1		14.1

ERRATA.

Page 10.	February, 1843, mean at sunrise	. . . .	*for* 29.39	*read* 32.54
" "	" " " 2 P. M.	. . . .	" 45.03	" 49.86
" "	" " " of month	. . . .	" 37.21	" 41.20
" "	March, 1843, greatest rise at sunrise	. . . .	" 34	" 22
" 13.	January, 1844, mean at sunrise	. . . .	" 39.40	" 38.13
" "	" " " 2 P. M.	. . . .	" 50.80	" 49.16
" "	" " " of month	. . . .	" 45.10	" 43.65
" 23.	August, 1847, greatest fall at sunrise	. . . .	" 12	" 10
" 28.	January, 1849, amount of rain	. . . .	" 2.7	" 8.9
" 33.	September, 1850, greatest fall at sunrise	. . . .	" 14	" 12
" 34.	March, 1851, greatest fall at sunrise	. . . .	" 24	" 22
" 37.	January, 1852, greatest fall at sunrise	. . . .	" 36	" 26
" 57.	December, 1858, mean at 2 P. M.	. . . .	" 54.26	" 53.61

SMITHSONIAN CONTRIBUTIONS TO KNOWLEDGE.

RESEARCHES

UPON THE

VENOM OF THE RATTLESNAKE:

WITH AN INVESTIGATION OF THE ANATOMY AND PHYSIOLOGY OF THE ORGANS CONCERNED.

BY

S. WEIR MITCHELL, M. D.,

LECTURER ON PHYSIOLOGY IN THE PHILADELPHIA MEDICAL ASSOCIATION.

[ACCEPTED FOR PUBLICATION, JULY, 1860.]

COMMISSION

TO WHICH THIS MEMOIR HAS BEEN REFERRED.

FRANKLIN BACHE, M. D.,
ROBLEY DUNGLISON, M. D.

JOSEPH HENRY,
Secretary S. I.

COLLINS, PRINTER,
PHILADELPHIA.

PREFACE.

IN the following pages are set forth the results of a long and conscientious experimental study of the venom of the Rattlesnake.

During a large part of two years I have given to this work almost all the leisure which could be spared from the everyday exactions of my regular professional duties.

In its progress, I have been constantly aided and encouraged by many friends, principally members of the Academy of Natural Sciences, of Philadelphia; more especially am I in debt to my fellow-members of the Biological Department of the Academy, to Prof. Wm. A. Hammond, and to Mr. Vaux.

My thanks are due to the Smithsonian Institution, without the aid of which I should have been unable to procure the serpents which were essential to my purposes.

The historical references and the Bibliography owe much to the manuscript notes of Prof. John Le Conte, which were collected with much care and labor, that they might be used in a research which he at one time contemplated. Becoming aware of the investigation in which I was engaged, he most liberally placed at my disposal this collection of literary materials.

To Drs. Brinton and Kane I am greatly obliged for intelligent assistance in numerous experimental investigations, for which their ready surgical skill so well fitted them, and I am also in debt to Messrs. Cantrell and Picot, for like aid, which, owing to the nature of the service, was not always free from danger. My thanks are further due to Drs. La Roche and Stillé, to Dr. Fisher, the librarian of the Academy of Natural Sciences, and to Dr. T. H. Bache, the librarian of the College of Physicians, whose assistance in consulting its extensive collection of American journals has been to me of great service.

With the exception of the microscopic delineations, the plates were drawn by Dr. Packard, from my recent dissections, and owe their chief merit to his accurate pencil.

The conclusions arrived at in the pages of this Essay, rest alone upon experimental evidence. That in so varied and so difficult a research, it may be found that I have sometimes been misled, and at others erred in the interpretation of facts, is no doubt to be anticipated. I began this work, however, without preconceived views, and throughout its prosecution I have endeavored to maintain that condition of mind which is wanted in experimentation, and that love of truth which is the parent of rational inferences.[1]

S. WEIR MITCHELL.

1226 Walnut St., Philadelphia.

---

[1] The reader who desires further information in regard to the therapeutics of the subject, and to the relative value of the various antidotes still in repute, is referred to a forthcoming paper, by the author, in the North American Medico-Chirurgical Review, in which the whole subject will be considered from a purely medical point of view. The author takes this occasion to mention the omission in the medical portion of the present essay of the composition of Bibron's antidote. It contains five drachms of bromine, four grains of iodide of potassium, and two grains of corrosive sublimate.

TABLE OF CONTENTS.

CHAPTER IV.

PHYSICAL AND CHEMICAL CHARACTERS OF THE VENOM.

CHAPTER V.

TOXICOLOGY OF THE VENOM OF THE CROTALUS.

CHAPTER VI.

TOXICOLOGICAL ACTION OF THE VENOM UPON WARM-BLOODED ANIMALS.

CHAPTER VII.

ACTION OF VENOM ON THE TISSUES AND FLUIDS.

CHAPTER VIII.

CROTALUS POISONING IN MAN.

LIST OF WOOD-CUTS.

[1] In Fig. 3, p. 9, Description—*d* is described as the spheno-palatine muscle. It should be labelled, Central raphe at the base of the skull.

INTRODUCTION.

POPULAR tradition has long nourished a general aversion to serpents. This dread, fostered by the singular qualities of the snake tribe, has become so familiar an idea to most minds, as to lead to the belief that it is of instinctive origin, and not sown, as it surely is, by the hand of traditional prejudice.

However produced, dread and disgust seem to have had some influence in preventing physicians in this country from investigating the venom of the species of serpents, whose strange peculiarities and fatal powers have most urged them upon their notice. It has thus happened, that with the exception of the Essays of Barton and Brainard, the cis-Atlantic literature of this subject has been confined to scattered notices and incomplete statements of cases, to be found with difficulty in the pages of our numerous medical journals.

Apart from the European and East Indian publications upon snake-bites, we know or have learned but little that is new; and if we except the works of Fontana, Mangili, Bonaparte, and one or two others, in no part of the world has modern science done much to further this inquiry.

Such being the case, I conceive that no excuse is required in presenting the results of investigations upon a subject which has peculiar claims on the attention of our countrymen.

A large part of what is here set forth has some pretension to be regarded as original research; but the subject is so ample, and has presented itself under so many points of view, that I can scarcely regard this paper as more than a re-opening of the matter; and I feel that however full it may be upon some points, it is rather the pledge of future labors than a complete exposition of the subject upon which it treats. For the researches which form the novel part of the following essay, I claim only exactness of detail and honesty of statement. Where the results have appeared to me inconclusive, and where further experimental questioning has not resolved the doubt, I have fairly confessed my inability to settle the matter. This course I have adhered to in every such instance, thinking it better to state the known uncertainty thus created than to run the risk of strewing my path with errors in the garb of seeming truths.

In the following researches I have made use almost altogether of the single species of Rattlesnake, usually known as the *Crotalus durissus.* Of this I have had living specimens from Lake George, and from various localities in the Alleghanies of Pennsylvania and Virginia. In Mr. Cope's Summary at the end of this Essay, the reader will find all the necessary details as to the zoological characters of this serpent.

CHAPTER I.

OBSERVATIONS ON THE HABITS OF THE CROTALUS WHEN IN CAPTIVITY.

During a large part of two years, the period which this research has occupied, I was a portion of each day in the room where the reptiles were kept, and consequently observed with care such of their habits as could be studied while they were in confinement. In regard to these I have a few observations to make, before considering their physiology and toxicology.

It is by no means my intention to give a full account of the habits of the Crotalus, since this would involve a great deal of detail which is to be found elsewhere, and which would be foreign to the general purpose of this essay.

The Rattlesnake of our Northern States, when at liberty, sometimes lives in the company of his fellows, but more frequently alone. I have had, in a single box, from ten to thirty-five snakes, and have never observed the slightest signs of hostility towards one another. Even when several snakes were suddenly dropped upon their fellows, no attempt was made to annoy the new-comers, while the sudden intrusion of a pigeon or a rabbit was met with ready resentment, whenever the snakes were fresh and in vigorous health.

The habits of Rattlesnakes, when in confinement, are singularly inactive. Even in warm weather, when they are least sluggish, they will lie for days together in a knotted mass, occasionally changing their position, and then relapsing into perfect rest. The contrast between this ordinary state of repose, or sluggish movement, and the perilous rapidity of their motion when striking, is most dangerously deceptive. In contrast also with their slow locomotion is the marvellously rapid action of their rattles, which, when annoyed or molested, they will sometimes continue to agitate for hours at a time.

It is the general experience of those who have kept rattlesnakes, that they seldom eat in captivity. I have known a snake to exist for a year without food, and although I have made every effort to tempt my own snakes, I have never seen any one of them disposed to avail itself of food, when placed within its reach. Dumeril states that this is the usual experience in the Garden of Plants, but that at the end of six or eight months they commonly accept food. He also adds that the very young pigeon is the food they are most inclined to eat.

After tempting the snakes with this, as well as with birds, mice, rabbits, etc., and finding the food as often untouched, I finally gave up the attempt, and contented myself with feeding, by force, such of them as seemed feeble and badly nourished. For this purpose, I used milk and insects, which I placed in their throats, while they were properly pinioned. To effect this, the snake was secured, and the lower jaw held in the grasp of a pair of forceps, while a funnel, with a long stem, was thrust down the œsophagus. Into this, insects, such as flies and grasshoppers, were pushed, or milk poured in proper quantity. Yet, even when this precaution of forcible feeding was not employed, the snakes remained healthy, and secreted, as usual, a sufficient amount of venom.

To preserve them, however, in good condition, it is absolutely necessary that they should be frequently supplied with water, especially in hot weather, and when they are about to shed their skins. The free snake is said, in this climate, to shed its cuticle in the month of August. My snakes lost their old integuments at different periods, during the summer. In all cases, the old skin became very dark, as the new one formed beneath it. If, at this time, the snakes were denied access to water, the skin came off in patches. Where water was freely supplied, they entered it eagerly at this period, and not only drank of it, but lay in it for hours together. Under these circumstances, the skin was shed entire—the first gap occurring at the mouth, or near it. Through this opening, the serpent worked its way, and the skin reverting, was turned inside out, as it crawled forth in its new and distinctly-marked outer covering. When the old skin was very loose, the snake's motions were often awkward for a time. It is said to be blind during this period, which is probably true to some extent; since the outer layer of the cornea is shed with the skin, and there must obviously be a time when the old corneal layer lies upon the new formation. It is also said that the fangs are lost at the same time as the skin. In some instances, this was observed to be the case; but whether or not it is a constant occurrence, I am unable to say from personal observation.

It is most probable, as I have elsewhere stated, that not only are the fangs shed when the skin is lost, in summer, but that their loss is a frequent occurrence, like the loss of teeth in certain fish, and takes place at intervals, more or less frequent, certainly oftener than once a year.

A general opinion prevails that, immediately after the loss of the skin, the snakes become most virulent. As they are slothful during the period of change, and strike then with reluctance, if at all, and as the loss of the fang involves, to some extent, the accumulation of poison in the gland cavities, this view may be correct. There is no ground, however, for supposing that the effect of this storing up of the venom would be greater at this period than after a similar amount of accumulation at another time.

After such numerous and long-continued opportunities of observation, it might be supposed that I should be prepared to speak authoritatively, as to the still disputed power of the snake to fascinate small animals. If the power exist at all, it is probable that it would only be made use of when the serpent required its aid to secure food. We have seen that even the most healthy snakes lose their appetite when imprisoned, and beyond this condition, my chances of observation have been limited. Those who are still curious in the matter will find the fullest account of it in the Essay of Dr. B. S. Barton. In despite of the learned and ingenious argument of this author, there are not wanting large numbers, who claim to have witnessed, again and again, the exercise of the power of charming on the part of the Rattlesnake and Black Snake. Dr. Barton, who does not deny that the appearance of fascination has been often observed, explains it by supposing that in these cases the parent bird, alarmed at the near approach of danger to her nest of young, hovers anxiously about the snake, as she would about any other cause of danger, and thus sometimes falls a victim to her maternal anxiety. This theory, Dr. Barton believes sufficient to account for the fluttering and strange movements of the bird, and the arguments with which this view is upheld, are certainly entitled to great respect. While the anxiety and terror of the parent bird would readily attract notice, the real object of the snake, and the true cause of the mother's approach to the very jaws of destruction, would be more than likely to escape the notice of such persons as are usually called upon to observe the supposed fact.

I have seen but one occurrence that might mislead as to the subject of fascination. I have very often put animals, such as birds, pigeons, guinea-pigs, mice, and dogs, into the cage with a Rattlesnake. They commonly exhibited no terror after their recovery from alarm, at being handled and dropped into a box. The smaller birds were usually some time in becoming composed, and fluttered about in the large cage until they were fatigued, when they soon became amusingly familiar with the snakes, and were seldom molested, even when caged with six or eight large *Crotali*. The mice—which were similarly situated—lived on terms of easy intimacy with the snakes, sitting on their heads, moving round on their gliding coils, undisturbed, and unconscious of danger. Larger animals were not so safe, especially if they moved abruptly and rapidly about the snakes. The birds, mice, and larger animals, often manifested an evident curiosity, which prompted them to approach the snake cautiously. Sometimes this was rewarded by a blow, as was sure to be the case, when a dog indulged his inquisitiveness by smelling the snake with his muzzle. Sometimes the snake retreated, and struck only when driven to bay. Usually, the smaller animals indulged their inquisitive instinct unhurt, and were allowed to live for days in the same cage with the dreaded reptiles.[1]

These are the sole facts which I have seen, bearing any relation to the supposed fascinating faculty. They appear to me to lend no strength to the idea of its existence.

There is a popular belief which ascribes to the Rattlesnake a most disagreeable odor, and even naturalists have been led to believe that the serpent owed to this its power to lure and stupefy animals. In this matter, I agree with Barton.[2] I have never perceived that any peculiar odor issued from my snake-box, and as to its ability to injure birds, the facts above stated should suffice to disprove it. As usual, however, this pound of error contains its grain of truth. When a Rattlesnake is roughly handled, especially about the lower half of its length, a very heavy and decided animal odor is left upon the hands of the observer. If the snake be violently treated, causing it to throw itself into abrupt contortions, thin streams of a yellow or dark brown fluid are ejected to the distance of two or three feet. This fluid appears to come from glands alongside of the cloaca. Its odor is extremely disagreeable, and it is irritant when it enters the eye, although not otherwise injurious.

---

[1] It is proper to add, that the curiosity thus exhibited by animals, and especially by mice and dogs, was as active when the snake was not regarding the intruder, as at other times.

[2] Barton, p. 24.

CHAPTER II.

ANATOMY OF THE VENOM APPARATUS.

THE subject of the myology of the Rattlesnake has been considered at length, in several systematic works, and in the monographs referred to at the close of this paper. For the fullest details, it would be necessary to refer the reader to the books in question. Since, however, it is impossible otherwise to convey an accurate idea of the mode in which the fangs are employed, I am forced to describe the parts concerned, and the general mechanism of their motions. It is the more necessary to dwell, at least, briefly, on this matter, because some of the French observers have fallen into error, as regards the action of certain of the muscles concerned in the elevation and depression of the fangs.

I shall first describe, as shortly as possible, the bones involved; then the muscles, and lastly the gland and its duct. Thus prepared, we shall next study the mode in which the blow is given, and the mechanism, through the agency of which the poison is ejaculated.

The heads of the true serpents are so constructed as to admit of a large amount of movement in the component bones. Thus the zygomatic bones which support the lower maxillary bones, are loosely articulated to the mastoid bone, which is itself so mobile as to permit of the greatest possible expansion of the throat. Anteriorly the superior maxillary bones are united, by ligaments only, to the intermaxillaries, and the lower maxillary bones of each side are also so connected anteriorly as to permit of their being widely separated, and of one or the other side of the inferior jaw being drawn down to some distance, without involving a corresponding motion on the part of its fellow. Finally, the superior maxillary bones, the pterygoid and palate bones admit of considerable movement, so that the arches which they form can be widened or narrowed as circumstances may require.

The mobility of these parts is essential to the motions which raise and depress the fang, and to the deglutition of the large animals upon which the snakes are accustomed to prey.

The poison fang, when at rest, projects downwards and backwards into the mouth of the serpent. It is firmly anchylosed in the alveolar process, which crowns the summit of the shortened upper maxillary bone, Fig. 1, *d*, whose peculiar brevity is characteristic of venomous snakes. The superior maxillary bone is of a rather irregular triangular shape, abruptly cut off below to form the alveolar socket. One face of this bone is smooth, and looks inwards and slightly forwards.

A second looks forwards and outwards. This facet is smooth below,[1] but is excavated above into a deep fossa, which in the fresh snake is partially closed by

Fig. 1.

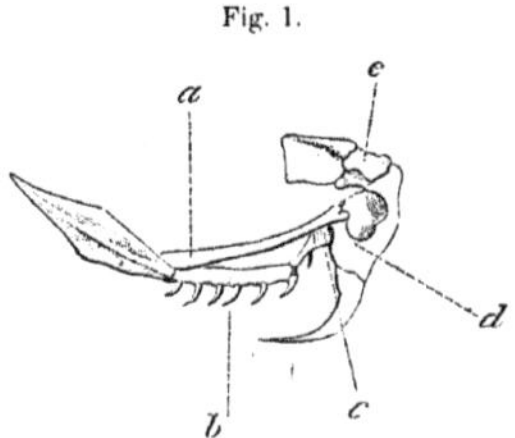

PORTION OF CRANIUM OF CROTALUS.—Right side. Osteology. Bones concerned in the movements of the fang. *a*, external pterygoid bone; *b*, internal pterygoid bone; *c*, palatal bone; *d*, superior maxillary bone; *e*, lachrymal bone.

soft tissues, but is still sufficiently remarkable as lying between the eye and nares. In the dry bone this large fossa opens upwards freely through the base of the bone, and thus separates the two surfaces by which the bone articulates with the ecto-pterygoid and lachrymal bones respectively. Anteriorly, the superior maxillary bone presents a rounded angle, from which diverge the two lateral sides just described. Posteriorly, the superior maxillary exhibits a third face, which is flat only half way down the bone, and terminates in an abrupt edge forming the posterior boundary of the alveolar socket.

Anteriorly, and above, the maxillary bone articulates by a ginglymoid joint with the short triangular lachrymal bone, Fig. 1, *e*, which projects forwards from the anterior external angle of the frontal bone. The articular facet of the maxilla lies at the upper end of its front angle. It moves with great freedom on the concave face of the lachrymal bone, its motion being partially restrained by a short, round, strong ligament, which runs from the posterior and inner edge of the lachrymal bone to be inserted on the back edge of the base of the maxilla, just above the articulation of the ecto-pterygoid bone.

The lachrymal bone has itself some movement on its frontal articulation, and by this the maxilla obtains indirectly an additional extent of forward motion. At the upper edge of the posterior surface of the maxillary bone, it receives the expanded and flattened end of the ecto-pterygoid bone, Fig. 1, *a*. Upon tracing the line of motion, of which this bone is capable, it will be seen that it lies below the lachrymal joint, and that, consequently, when it moves forwards, the fang must rise, as the superior maxillary rocks on the articulating face of the lachrymal bone.

The superior maxillary is indirectly attached to the palate bone, Fig. 1, *c*, and internal pterygoid, Fig. 1, *b*, by virtue of the strong connection of these bones with the ecto-pterygoid. This connection is so close that every free motion of either of

[1] The parts are described as though in sitû.

the two former bones must inevitably affect the latter, and through it again the maxilla and its single tooth.[1]

The motion of the maxillary bone on its lachrymal articulation will, perhaps, be better understood upon reference to the accompanying diagram of the parts.

Fig. 2.

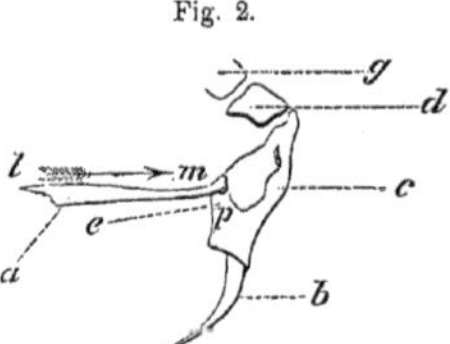

DIAGRAM OF THE BONY PARTS CONCERNED IN RAISING THE FANG.—*a*, pterygoid bone; *l*, *m*, arrow marking its line of motion; *p*, *e*, pterygoideus externus muscle; *g*, frontal bone; *d*, lachrymal bone; *c*, superior maxillary bone; *b*, fang.

The myology of the subject is more complicated; yet even here our purpose will still be answered, if we describe only the muscles concerned, begging the reader to remember that all further details would be misplaced and useless. On reference to Fig. 3, it will be seen that the spheno-pterygoid, *a*, a strong muscle, arises along the raphe at the base of the cranium, and running backwards and outwards, is inserted fan-like upon the pterygoid plate. Acting from the fixed base of the skull upon the movable pterygoid bone, it must draw this bone forward, and, rocking the superior maxillary on its lachrymal joint, erect the fang, Fig. 2, *l*—*m* and arrow.

A second large muscle, the pterygoideus externus, Fig. 3, *b*, arises from the tough aponeurosis covering the zygomatico-mandibular articulation of the lower jaw, and as it runs forward below the poison gland and to its inner side sends a strong layer of white fascial tissue out upon the capsule of the gland. Some of its lower fibres are finally inserted directly into the two lips or edges of the mucous sheath of the tooth fang. A larger part of the muscle is inserted tendinously into an apophysis of the superior maxillary bone exteriorly to the articulation of that bone with the external pterygoid, and a little below it. The mechanical necessities arising from the position of this muscle are easily seen; for when the external pterygoid acts, it will necessarily depress the fang. This movement will be more readily comprehended on reference again to the diagram, Fig. 2, in the text, where *p*—*e* marks the line of action of the force applied by the pterygoid muscle to the superior maxillary bone and to the edges of the vagina dentis, the sheath of the fang. The action of this muscle is probably aided by the spheno-palatine, which arises along the raphe of the base of the skull, above the spheno-pterygoid and thus nearer the skull, and running diagonally outwards and backwards finds

---

[1] These bones rest posteriorly against the articulation of the mandibulæ of the lower jaw with the zygoma; they consequently share, to some extent, in the movements of this joint.

insertion along the inside of the palatal bone. As its fibres cross those of the spheno-pterygoid, its action antagonizes that muscle and aids the purpose of the

Fig. 3

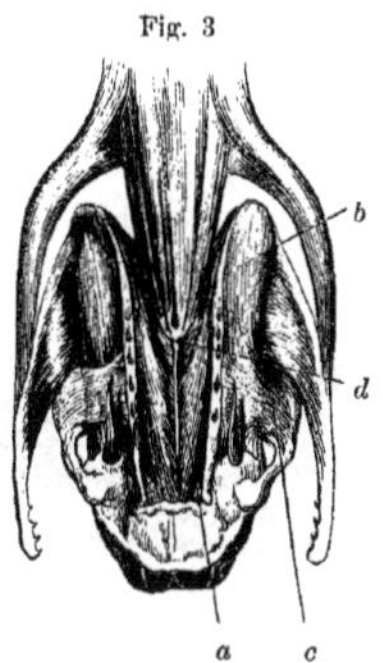

MYOLOGY.—Palatal view of the muscles of the upper jaw and base of the skull. *a*, spheno-pterygoid muscle—the elevation of the fang is caused by its action on the pterygoid and palate bones; *b*, external pterygoid muscle—the retractor of the fang—inserted into the outside of the superior maxillary bone; *c*, fascial sheath of this muscle attached to the capsule of the venom gland; *d*, spheno-palatine muscle.

pterygoideus externus. The connection of the palate bone and the pterygoid bones, which we have already noticed, is essential to this result.

Almost all of the muscles about the head, neck, and jaws of the serpent, take part either in the motions which precede the blow, or those which inflict and follow it. Most of these muscles have functions which are obvious and easily demonstrable; and we shall, therefore, content ourselves with the briefest reference to all but the anterior temporal, which plays a far more important part, and requires a fuller description.

The mouth is opened by muscles, such as the costo-mandibular and the vertebro-mandibular, with the help of a muscular layer analogous to the platysma myoides. The articulation of the jaws is fixed by the double action of the digastricus and cervical angular muscles.

Of the temporal muscles there are three. The anterior temporal, Fig. 4, *a*, functionally the most important, arises from behind the orbit and from the upper

Fig. 4.

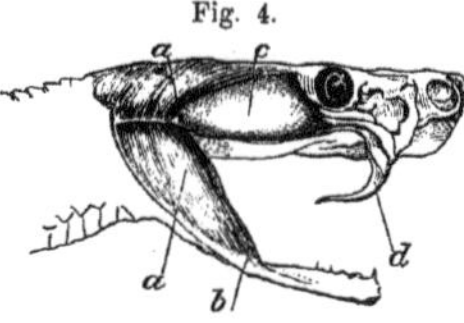

EXHIBITING THE RELATION OF THE TEMPORAL MUSCLES TO THE VENOM GLAND. *a*—*a*, anterior temporal muscle; *b*, its insertion in the lower jaw; *c*, venom gland; *d*, the fang half erected.

2

two-thirds of the firm fascia of the poison gland. Its fibres run backwards over this body and descend between it and the middle temporal muscle. In this course the fibres lie posteriorly to the suspensory ligament, and the outer ones, as they fold about the articular end of the gland, lie in contact with the prolongation of the external lateral articular ligament upon that body. Finally, the muscle winds around the commissure of the lips, and is inserted into the lower jaw some distance in front of the angle of the lips at *b*, Fig. 4.

The middle and posterior temporal muscles, Figs. 4 and 5, arise chiefly from the

Fig. 5.

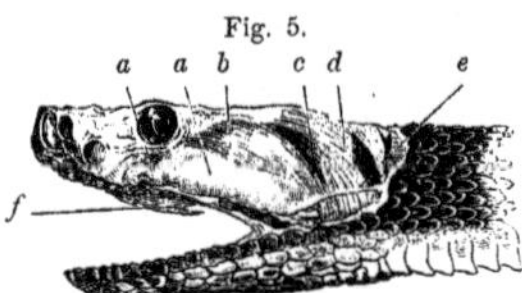

MYOLOGY.—Lateral view. *a*—*a*, gland; *b*, anterior temporal muscle; *c*, posterior temporal muscle; *d*, digastricus muscle; *e*, posterior ligament of the sheath of the gland; *f*, vagina dentis—the fang slightly raised.

temporal fossa and are inserted, one behind the other, into the lower jaw. As these two latter muscles descend nearly vertically, their obvious function is to close the jaws. The use of the anterior temporal is in part also the closure of the jaws, but its more obvious office is to press upon the poison gland, as we shall presently see.

The poison gland of the Crotalus occupies the side of the head, behind the eye, and beneath the anterior temporal muscle, Fig. 5. Its posterior extremity extends three or four lines beyond the commissure of the lips. Its anterior end lies below and just behind the eye. Thus situated, the gland is in relation with the bony surface behind the eye, with the middle temporal muscle, with nerves which emerge under the suspensory ligament, and with the anterior temporal muscle above and behind, where that muscle descends to its insertion. Beneath, the gland is in contact with the external pterygoid muscle, with whose aponeurosis it has peculiar relations. So much of the gland as lies below the anterior temporal and above the line of the lip, is in relation with the skin which is here loosely connected with its fascia by areolar tissue.

The general form of the gland is that of a flattened, almond-shaped oval, the posterior end being somewhat obtuse, and the anterior tapering to the duct, which begins just behind and below the eyeball.

The length of the organ, from the insertion of the articular ligament to the beginning of the duct, was found to be eight-tenths of an inch, in a snake which was four feet long, and weighed two pounds and two ounces. Its breadth was nearly two-tenths of an inch, its thickness about one-eighth to one-tenth of an inch.

The poison-glands of six snakes were carefully weighed, after exhausting them of their contents, during the life of the snakes, and after the ducts and ligaments had been removed. In the following table, the weight of the gland, and the weight and length of the snake are given.

It is proper to mention that almost all of these snakes had been in captivity during periods of from two to eight weeks.

No.	Weight.	Length.	Weight of gland.
1	1 lb. 6 oz.	2 ft. 1 inch	7½ grains
2	4 "	4 ft. 3¼ inches	11½ "
3	3 "	2 ft. 9 "	9 "
4	3 lb. 6 oz.	3 ft. 1½ "	9⅓ "
5	2 lb. 4 oz.	3 ft. ½ "	7¼ "
6	3 lb. 9 oz.	4 ft.	12½ "

It will be seen from this table that very little relation can be established between the size and weight of the snake, and the weight of the gland, beyond the mere fact of the general increase in the size of the organ, with that of the snake.

The poison gland is invested with a double layer of white, and not very yielding fibrous tissue. The two layers of this membrane are united at the base of the gland, and becoming thinner anteriorly, they run off upon the duct, constituting a portion of its thickness. Besides furnishing attachment for the anterior temporal muscle, the outer layer of this capsule gives off three remarkable ligamentous expansions which suspend and confine the gland.

The posterior of these is a narrow, but strong ribbon of fibrous tissue, see Fig. 5, *e*, which runs from the posterior extremity of the gland to the articulation of the jaw, where it appears by its continuation backwards, to constitute one of the external ligaments of that joint.

The second, which we shall term the suspensory ligament, lies behind the gland,

Fig. 6.

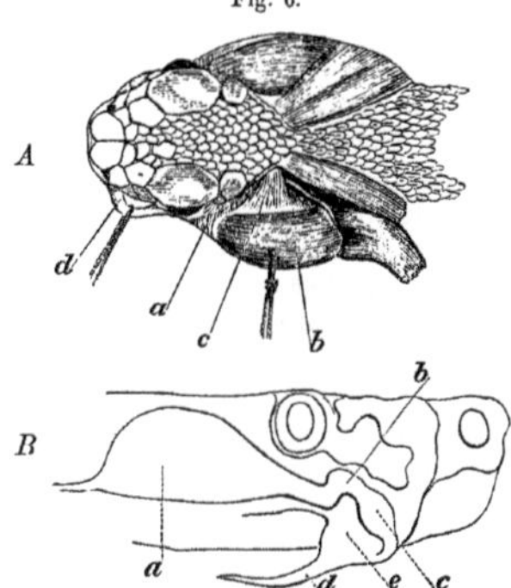

A. The Gland and Temporal Muscles seen from above.—*a*, the gland; *b*, anterior temporal muscle; *c*, suspensory ligament of the gland extended; *d*, duct, drawn from its position.

B. Diagram of Duct and Gland—side view.—*a*, the venom gland; *b*, the duct, at its curve; *c*, the sphincter; *d*, fang; *e*, superior maxillary bone.

Fig. 6 *A*, *c*, a little above its middle line. It arises as a fan-like expansion upon the capsule, and finally narrows to one-third, and is inserted on the bony surface to the inner side of the gland. This ligament is remarkably strong and unyielding; it supports the gland perfectly, and even acts as a passive antagonist to the force exerted by the anterior temporal muscle, while at the same time it shelters the large nerves which emerge beneath it from the skull.

The third attachment of the gland is by means of a fascia, which forms a strong expansion upon the external pterygoid muscle, Fig. 3, *c*, and then runs off laterally, to be inserted upon the outer capsule of the gland. This connection is principally with the lower and anterior portion of the gland. Its object will attract our attention in another place.

Anteriorly, and along its upper edge, the gland is secured by areolar tissue, connecting it with the edges of the temporal fossa, and the posterior edge of the orbit. At the extreme anterior point of the temporal muscle, however, a portion of its proper aponeurosis is gathered into a band, to which run also similar fibres from that part of the capsule of the gland which lies below the muscle. This collection of rather delicate fibres—for in the Crotalus it can scarcely be called a tendon—runs forward above the flexure in the duct, and below the eye, to lose itself on the edge of the fossa, and about the base of the superior maxillary bone. Soubeiran describes in the Viper a tendinous insertion of the anterior temporal, as taking the track here described. I have been unable to discover this insertion in any of my dissections of the Crotalus.

In almost every account of the anatomy of the Crotalus, and in nearly all of the essays upon the effect of its venom, some allusion is made to a sac, or reservoir of poison. Strictly speaking, there is no such organ, and the only provision for the accumulation of venom is to be found in the duct, and its enlargement within the gland.

The duct expands somewhat suddenly, as it enters the gland, and being directed backwards and a little upwards, forms an irregularly-rounded cavity, which runs nearly the whole length of the gland. Into this receptacle, the smaller ducts of the gland empty their contents. From the sides of this cavity there run obliquely upwards, and a little backwards, from five to eight layers of white fibrous tissue, which, lying transversely to the long axis of the gland, separate its secreting portion into lobes, which narrow as they approach the central cavity. The septa here described are finally lost in the capsule of the gland. On their passage outwards, they send off numerous branches and thin sheets of tissue which proceed upwards, for the most part, but also across the lobes, and thus involve the secernent structure in a supporting scaffolding, of the firmest possible character.

The gland so constructed, resembles very strikingly, in section, the appearance of a small testicle. Its color is usually of a pearly or gray-white within, except under certain pathological conditions, when it is full of blood, and presents externally a darkly-mottled look.

The intimate structure of the poison gland resembles very closely that of the typical salivary glands. From the open space at the base of the gland, a number of ducts run up into its substance, and dividing, pass towards the periphery. The direction of these ducts is, for the most part, backwards and upwards. Owing to the strength of the fibrous bands which traverse the gland, and to the extreme softness of the intermediate tissue, I have found great difficulty in tracing the smaller ducts, Fig. 7, *b*. Soubeiran[1] describes them in the Viper, as terminating in minute pouches of amorphous matter. Rymer Jones (article "Reptilia," *Cyclopedia of Anatomy and Physiology*) also speaks of the ducts dividing, to form smaller

Fig. 7.

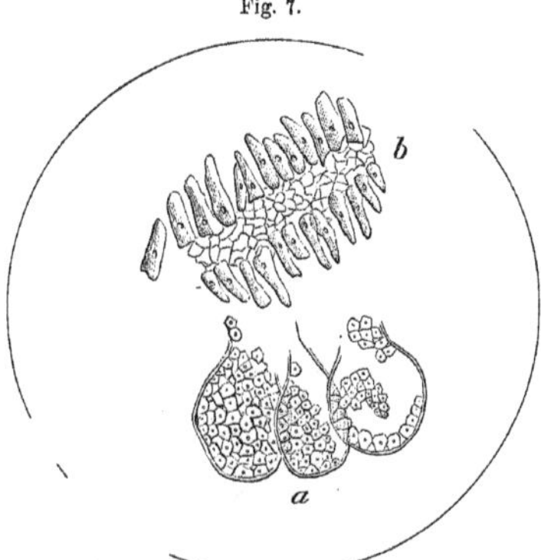

MICROSCOPICAL STRUCTURE OF THE VENOM GLAND.—*a*, secernent cœca; *b*, small ducts.

tubes, on which are finally developed secernent cœca, Fig. 7, *a*, like those of the ordinary salivary glands. In perfectly fresh specimens, these cœca can sometimes be made out. They are lined with pale tessellated and nucleated rounded epithelia, and are commonly filled with amorphous and granular matter, Fig. 7, *a*. The epithelia in question are very easily altered, and in glands kept for a few hours in summer, are scarcely to be recognized. The smaller ducts are lined with a pale and narrow columnar epithelial cell, Fig. 7, *b*. The cavity at the base of the gland, as well as the main duct which connects with the fang, are lined with large pavement-epithelial cells, which possess distinct nuclei, Fig. 8, *a*. This form of epithelia is not usually encountered in this position, in homologous glands, whose ducts are, on the contrary, covered internally with columnar epithelia. Outside of this cellular layer, the poison duct is made up principally of white fibrous tissue, with a small proportion of very fine fibres of yellow elastic tissue. The walls of the duct are provided throughout with an abundant supply of bloodvessels.

Just above the line of the lip, and consequently at the base and outer side of the maxillary bone, the duct, in turning to descend this bone, becomes abruptly larger, for a distance of a line, or a line and a half, Fig. 6 *B*, *c*. Its color at this point is also a little redder than the rest of the duct. Beyond this point, the duct again becomes smaller. If now a probe be introduced into the duct, and its whole

---

[1] J. L. Soubeiran, De la Vipère. Paris, 1855, p. 47.

length divided, it will be observed that the calibre of the canal does not enlarge, until it reaches the gland, and that the appearance of increased size here described, is due to a distinct thickening of the walls of the tube.

Fig. 8.

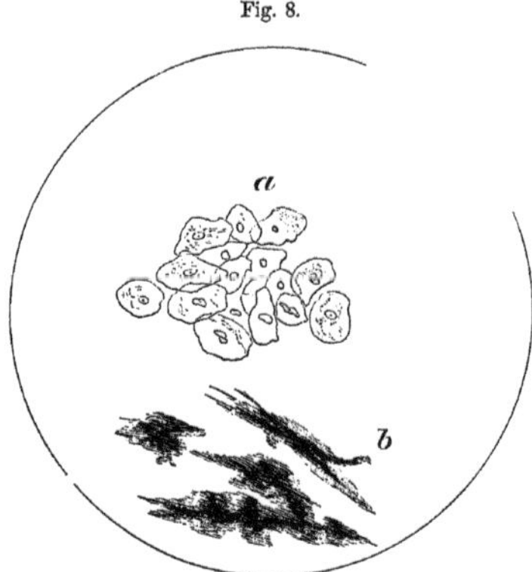

a, Epithelial cells of main duct, and of the receptacle at the base of the gland; *b*, pigment-cells of the duct.

Fig. 9.

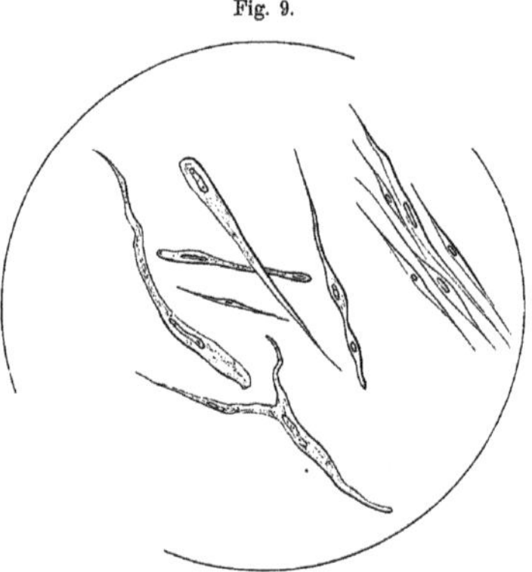

Non-striated Muscular Fibre-cells of the Sphincter of the Duct.

Upon careful examination of the nature of this tissue, I found it to be formed by an increase in the amount of fibrous tissue, and by the addition of a layer of .

elongated fusiform cells, Fig. 9, each having a single nucleus, and sometimes a long, dark nucleolus.

These elements are undoubtedly the characteristic cells of non-striated muscular tissue.[1] Their presence, together with the form and position of this enlargement, enables us to view it as a sphincter placed upon the duct, for the purpose of restraining the wasteful flow of the secretion. This portion of the wall of the duct contains numerous irregular, stellate, pigment-cells, Fig. 8, *b*. So far as I am aware, no author has described this adjunct to the venom apparatus. Of its purpose, however, I have no doubt; and that some such provision does exist, is plain, from the fact that, when in the living Rattlesnake the jaws are separated, and the fangs caught on the edge of a thin cup, and erected, it is usually very difficult to produce a flow of venom. Even when the operator presses upon the glands, the poison is rarely ejected, without the voluntary aid of the snake itself.[2] After death, the remnant of fluid in the gland, although small in amount, is easily forced out along the duct, and through the fang. It is, therefore, very plain, that the snake has the power to restrain the flow of venom, even when the fangs are in such a position as that without the aid of the arrangement we have described, they must inevitably permit of the escape of the poison.

Beyond the sphincter, the duct becomes smaller in calibre, and the walls thinner. To reach the fissure at the base and anterior aspect of the fang-tooth, the duct runs up the posterior edge of the fossette, and winds over the rounded antero-lateral shoulder of the superior maxillary bone to reach its anterior face, where it communicates with the fissure in the fang. The value of the course thus taken by the duct, we shall elsewhere consider.

Another peculiarity in the course of the duct, should, however, claim attention, as it has also a mechanical use. Just below the eye, the duct is abruptly bent, as indicated in Fig. 5.

In its passage from the gland to the tooth, the duct is held in place by a sheet of rather close areolar tissue, which admits of the curves in the tube being straightened, as occasion requires. The part nearest to the gland also receives some of the fibres from the dense fascia which invests the external pterygoid muscle.

The structure of the fang in venomous serpents has been so minutely described by Owen,[3] that a brief synopsis of his views will be all that we shall require. I have carefully examined the fang-tooth by the aid of fine sections, and I have nothing to add to the following excellent description by the author above mentioned.

"To give an idea of the structure of this tooth, we may suppose a simple, slender tooth, like that of a boa-constrictor, to be flattened, and its edges then bent towards each other, and soldered together, so as to form a tube, open at both ends, and inclosing the end of the poison duct. The duct which conveys the poison,

---

[1] Dr. Woodward, who was so kind as to examine these structures, agreed with me as to their nature.

[2] This is only true of the active animal; when insensible from chloroform, the glands are easily emptied by pressure.

[3] Owen on the Skeleton and Teeth, Philada. 1854, p. 257, and Cyclopedia of Anatomy and Physiology, article Teeth.

although it runs through the centre of the tooth, is really on the outside of the tooth. The bending of the dentine beyond it, begins a little beyond the base of the tooth, where the poison duct rests in a slight groove, or longitudinal indentation, on the convex side of the fang; as it proceeds, it sinks deeper into the substance of the tooth, and the sides of the groove meet and coalesce, so that the trace of the inflected fold ceases, in some species, to be perceptible to the naked eye, and the fang appears, as it is commonly described to be, perforated by the duct of the poison gland."

The tooth fang, in the Rattlesnake, has a peculiar double curve. The lower curve is large, and has an anterior convexity; the upper involves only two or three lines of the length of the tooth from the point down, and is nearly straight, or presents a slight concavity anteriorly. The whole length of the fang, from point to base, was $\frac{5}{10}$ of an inch in a snake, four feet two inches long. One-tenth of an inch below the point in this tooth, the poison canal opened on the anterior, or convex surface of the fang. Above this, the fang was solid; as the true pulp cavity terminated some distance lower down. The point of this singular weapon is brittle, but of an exquisite fineness. The tooth thus described, is firmly anchylosed to the submaxillary bone, its base being luted to the portion of bone around its side and anterior aspect. Posteriorly, the bone possesses a hollow, in which is lodged the tooth sac. In the open mouth of this alveolar process, within the mucous membrane, and upon the pterygoid bone, lie one behind and below another, the reserve fangs, each smaller than the one in front, and less and less developed, until the situation of the last which is visible, is marked by a minute papilla alone. I have counted from eight to ten of these on each side. A very good account of their gradual development has been given by W. J. Burnett.[1] The details do not directly concern us here.

When the fang is lost by a natural process, it is replaced within a few days. When violently displaced, several weeks sometimes elapse before the next fang is fixed firmly enough to be useful to the snake.

If the functional fang be lost or shed, the next tooth gradually assumes its position, but of the mode in which the communication is re-established between the poison duct and the fissure of the lower part and front of the new tooth, we have had no correct knowledge until a recent period.

Burnett states, that "the original tooth follicle appears to him to become the poison gland or sac." He then goes on to support this view briefly, still speaking of the poison gland as possibly accompanying the tooth in its forward movement. Dr. Burnett must have made this statement under a misconception, as it is well known there is no poison sac or gland at the base of the fang, or in immediate connection with it.

More recently, the subject of the development of the fangs and the mode in which the fixed fang is replaced, when shed or broken, have been carefully studied by my friend, Dr. Christopher Johnston, of Baltimore, whose skill as an observer,

---

[1] W. J. Burnett, M. D., Boston Nat. Hist. Soc., vol. iv. p. 311–323.

as well as his peculiar knowledge of dental structures, entitle his views to great respect.

At my request, Dr. Johnston has repeated his observations, and most kindly placed them at my disposal. The following statement is in his own language:—

"The study of heads prepared by me, leads me to entertain the following opinion as to the manner in which secondary fangs establish a communication with the poison duct. There appears to me good reason to believe that there is a periodical fall of the venom fangs, quite independent of violence; and this is to be regarded as a physiological circumstance agreeing with what takes place in fishes, as Pike or Gar, and in reptiles, as Iguana, as well as with what occurs in the jaws of Megalosaurus, Hadrosaurus, etc. For I have not observed in the jaws of Crotali of the same species a constant relation between the size of the serpent and of its fangs; and when I couple with the disproportion alluded to, the fact, that at nearly all seasons, reserve fangs and germs are found in *every* degree of advancement or development, I cannot suppose that the almost mature secondaries are awaiting an accident to effect their promotion. We know that in Alligator especially, the secondaries occasion by their development the erosion of the base, and the consequent displacement of their predecessors, and assume positions from which they are to be in turn expelled.

"In Crotalus, the secondary fangs lie in separate capsules at the bottom of the dens in the mucous membrane, where the fangs crouch when not erected. Their pulps are arranged in order upon a gum which lies at the base and to the inner side of the functioning fang; and each developing fang is inclosed in a separate capsule and points directly backwards.

"Now a transverse section of a pulp in any part of its extent, gives a crescentic figure, hardly perceptible as a crescent at the point, evidently lunate with separate horns on either side of the distal aperture of the poison canal, and again a crescent, but with closely approximated cornua, throughout the rest of the crown, where the two longitudinal folds of dentine meet along the median line and are fused together.

"As the growth of the tooth advances, a slight annular enlargement marks its neck, or at least the limit of the crown, and then the two horns of the pulp diverge widely, at the upper part of the base, which is in process of formation, but again approach each other, yet without meeting, as the base goes on to completion. It may here be remarked, that the pulp acquires greater volume at this part of the fang, which is more extended along the posterior edge than in front, and is marked, both internally and externally, with conspicuous longitudinal flutings.

"The dentine of the basal portion in front, necessarily follows the modelling pulp; and as this, by the separation of the anterior lamellæ, leaves an ovoidal hiatus, so the tooth substance investing the matrix shows the free edge of its folds on either side as the margin of a large aperture, the *inlet* of the poison canal. All this occurs while yet the tooth-capsule is entire.

"In this condition the secondary fang remains until the fang in use falls spontaneously or by violence; and the secondaries behind it will be found to exhibit successive inferior stages of development. At length the prime fang is removed, if spontaneously, by the atrophy of the pulp, and, I believe, by erosion of the basal anchylosed portion; if it be broken off by violence, the freedom of the pseudo socket is accomplished by the same means. And now the first tooth of reserve is urged forwards into a recess in the maxillary bone directly adjacent to, and on the *inner side* of the fallen fang; and the requisite advancement is brought about by the developmental vis à tergo of the remaining reserve pulps, and probably also by the traction in front, exerted by the cicatrizing parts. It is evident that the fang emerges from its capsule, and that the point and crown repose in the den, but the base is closely invested with the capsular remains under the form of a periosteal expansion, which is the mediate bond of union between the base and the new and shallow socket of the maxilla.

"As may be perceived, upon examination at this stage, two sockets co-exist in the same jaw. The inner, new one, supporting the recently promoted fang, and the outer, old, and now vacant one, which is fast being disencumbered of the vestiges pertaining to its former resident. In this maxilla, the new fang occupies the innermost part, having the old socket on the outer side, while in the opposite maxilla, the older venom fang may be discovered in its normal situation, leaving the recess to its inner side vacant, for the temporary lodgment of its successor. Or, both fangs being recently fixed to the jaw, the vacuities will both be formed on the outside, and all the reserve fangs will appear to follow backwards and outwards in direct line.

"Now let us look at the situation of the poison duct, and examine into the mode by which it is brought into relation with the fang.

"The venom duct arising from the gland makes a bend upwards, immediately beneath the eye, then advances forwards under the skin, as far as the crotaline fossette, and lying upon the maxilla externally, plunges downwards, and pierces the gum in front of the fang, where it terminates in a papilla, which projects slightly into the proximal aperture of the tooth. In this position, it is maintained by the gum which clasps the base laterally and in front, with considerable firmness, its inferior or distal edge, encompassing the annular enlargement already alluded to. Nor is there any other than a mediate application of the poison papilla against the fang, for as the whole venom canal of each tooth is really upon the outside of the organ, no special membrane lines it which might be continuous with the duct that discharges into the upper aperture.

"Such is the condition of things in an old fang, occupying its normal exterior position. But when the tooth drops out, or is broken, the gum is left entire; or, if its exodus has been forced, the gum escapes with laceration only. In either case, however, the gum remains as a barrier, limiting the progress of the advancing reserve fang; and while the latter is establishing itself provisionally, the gum encircles it, clasps it tenaciously, and brings the poison papilla in apposition with its dental aperture. As time passes, the new fang moves gradually outwards to its permanent seat; the inner maxillary recess is restored, and the first fang of reserve is again discovered on the inner side of its senior, resting with its pulp attachment in the bottom of the recess.

"Thus, the reserve fang has become an adult functioning fang, nor does its pulp relax its hold, until fate or mischance dislodge the now fatally-armed tooth which it animates."

Before leaving this portion of the subject, it is proper to state that the views expressed by my friend Dr. Johnston, as to the want of direct continuity between the duct of the poison gland and the tooth canal, have been recently advocated by Prof. Jeffries Wyman, of Boston. It gives me great pleasure to point out this coincidence of opinion; and while acknowledging Prof. Wyman's priority of claim as established by publication, I must not omit to add that Dr. Johnston's manuscript notes—which I have quoted above—bear the date of Oct. 3d, 1859, since which time they have been in my own possession.[1]

The accompanying diagram, Fig. 10, illustrates our views as to the direction taken by the new fang, in its progress towards the alveolar socket.

It will have been observed that Dr. Johnston states, that the first reserve fang enters the semilunar socket in the maxilla, to the inside of the active fang. Although this is often or usually the case, it is not uncommon to find the two fixed

Fig. 10.

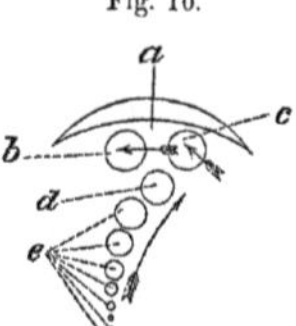

a, Alveolar socket; *b*, functionary fang; *c*, its successor; *d*, the next fang in order of age; *e*, remaining germs.

fangs, unsymmetrically placed, one on the inner, the other on the outer side, of their respective alveolæ, or both on the inner side; or again, both on the outer side of the said socket.

In all other points, my own researches agree with those of Dr. Johnston.

---

[1] May 16th, 1860; Proc. Boston Nat. Hist. Soc.

CHAPTER III.

THE PHYSIOLOGICAL MECHANISM OF THE BITE OF THE CROTALUS.

The preceding details will enable us to understand the following statement of the functions of the various parts described, and to appreciate the mode in which they combine to effect a given purpose.

Of the many authors who have treated of the anatomy and physiology of the Rattlesnake and other venomous serpents, no one has entered fully into the subject of the mechanism of the movements which inflict the bite and inject the poison. Redi, Fontana, Tyson, Ranby, Smith, Home, Duvernoy, Soubeiran, and others, have nearly all in turn contributed something to this subject, but I find nowhere a full and complete account of the part played by the various muscles and of the exact uses of many of the peculiar arrangements of tissue which characterize the poison apparatus. Nothing, in fact, can be more admirable than the mode in which the motions in question are effected, and yet while they interest the physiologist, from the wonderful example they afford of a series of complex acts following one upon another in ordered sequence, to effect a certain end, they are not less interesting to the physician, who may learn from their study how he may be deceived as to the occurrence of poisoned wounds, and how the snake which appears to strike may really fail in its object, even though seeming to have inflicted a wound.

When the Rattlesnake is in repose and unmolested, it sometimes lies at length, sometimes coiled, or wrapped fold on fold in the loops formed by other snakes which may happen to be in the same box. So soon, however, as cause is seen for alarm, the snake extricates itself, if among others, and at once throws its body into the coil so familiar to any one who has seen serpents, whether venomous or not. Sometimes on the edge, more often in the centre of the coil, the tail projects far enough to admit of its vibrating freely, and with singular swiftness.

The head is raised a little above the rest of the body, but not, usually, more than three or four inches, even in large snakes. The neck and upper end of the trunk are not thrown into complete circles, but lie in two or three abrupt curves across the mass of the coiled body. The snake is now in position to strike. While thus at bay, in an attitude of singular grace, the long black tongue is frequently protruded, a common movement among all serpents when irritated. Just before the blow the snake makes a hissing sound, which is caused by the act of expiration, and is due to the passage of air through the narrow glottis. It is louder in certain innocent serpents than in the Crotalus.

The mechanism of the forward cast of the body, which next occurs, is a very simple matter. The muscles which lie upon the convexity of the bendings formed by the upper part of the snake, are suddenly and violently contracted, so as abruptly to straighten the body, and thrust it forward in a direct line. The force resulting from this motion is not very great, as I have often ascertained when a snake has struck the end of a pole which I was holding, nor would it alone suffice to bury the fang in a tough skin, were it not for the acts which follow and aid it. In effecting this forward thrust of the neck and head, the serpent employs only the upper part of its body, and, consequently, is unable, under any circumstances, to strike at a greater distance than one-half its length, while usually its projectile range does not exceed a third of its length. An impression prevails that when the snake lies coiled, its head is raised very high to enable it to strike downwards. It seems, however, to be of no moment, in what direction the danger threatens, since it can, at will, cast itself forwards, downwards, or almost directly upwards.

As the animal comes within reach, of which the snake does not always judge with accuracy, the latter executes the movement just described. At the instant, and while in motion, the jaws are separated widely, and the head is bent somewhat back upon the first cervical bones, so as to bring the point of the fang into a favorable position to penetrate the opposing flesh. Owing to the backward curve of the tooth, this, of necessity involves the opening of the jaws to such an extent, that an observer standing above the snake, can see the white mucous membrane of the mouth, as the blow is given. The peculiar articulation of the lower jaw upon an intermediary bone, in place of upon the body of the skull, greatly facilitates this action. On examining the neck and head, it will also be seen that the head, under the influence of the cervical prolongation of the mass of the spinal muscles, is capable of being bent backwards to no inconsiderable extent. Consentaneously with the forward thrust of the body, and with the opening of the mouth, the spheno-pterygoids act from their firm cranial attachments to draw forward the pterygoid plate, and thus, through its attachment to the maxillary to erect the fang. The function of elevating the fang belongs alone to this muscle, which has no analogue in the other vertebrate animals. I have frequently tested its power to raise the fang, by stimulating it with galvanic or other irritants, after decapitating the snake, and although some French observers seem to have had doubts as to the agencies which effect the elevation and depression of the fang, there does not seem to me to be any reason to doubt the share which the spheno-pterygoid takes in this mechanism. That the mere act of opening the mouth, of necessity raises the weapon, has often been affirmed, but it is only necessary to separate the jaws of a living Crotalus to be convinced that this is not the case, and that even when the mouth is widely opened, the animal has the most perfect control over the movement of the fang, raising or depressing it at will.

As the spheno-pterygoid acts, the submaxillary bone rocks forward upon its lachrymal articulation. When the motion reaches its limit, and is checked by the ligament which I have described, the supporting lachrymal bone, in turn, yields to the power applied through the maxillary bone. These movements elevate a little the muzzle of the snake, so as to give to the face a very singular expression during the act of striking. Their more obvious and important result, is the elevation of the fang, which, rising, thrusts off, from its convexity, the cloak-like vagina-dentis so that it gathers in loose folds at its base.

As the unsheathed tooth penetrates the flesh of the victim, a series of movements occur, which must be contemporaneous, or nearly so. The body of the snake still resting in coil, makes, as it were, an anchor, while the muscles of the neck contracting, draw upon the head so violently, that when a small animal is the prey, it is often dragged back by the effort here described. If now the head and fang remained passive, the pull upon the head would withdraw the fang too soon; but at this moment, the head is probably stayed in its position by the muscles below, or in front of the spine; while the pterygoideus externus and spheno-palatine, acting upon the fang through their respective insertions, into the posterior apophysis of the submaxillary bone, and the inside of the palate bone, draw its point violently backwards, so as to drive it more deeply into the flesh. The muscles alluded to, therefore, antagonize the spheno-pterygoid.

At this instant, occurs a third series of motions, which result in the further deepening of the wound, and in the injection of the poison.

The lower jaw is closed upon the bitten part, or member. Where the surface struck is flat and large, this action will have but slight influence. Where the jaw shuts on a small limb, or member, the consequent effects will be far more likely to prove serious, since the power thus to shut the mouth materially aids the purpose of the blow. The closure of the jaw is effected by the posterior middle, and anterior temporal muscles. The first two tend simply to shut the mouth; the anterior temporal, however, is so folded about the poison gland, that while it draws up the lower jaw, it simultaneously compresses two-thirds of the body of the gland. This force is applied in such a manner as to squeeze the fluids out of the upper and back parts of the gland, and drive them forwards into the duct. The anterior lower angle of the gland, as well as a portion of the duct, is subjected to similar pressure at the same instant, owing to the flat tendinous insertion of a part of the external pterygoid upon the parts in question.

It will thus be observed, that the same muscular acts which deepen the wound, fix the prey, and inject the venom through the duct, and into the tissues penetrated by the tooth.[1] The whole process here described at such length, is the work of an instant, and the serpent's next effort is to disentangle itself from its victim. This step is effected by relaxing the muscles of the neck, so as to leave the head passive, while the continued traction of the muscles of the body pull upon it, and thus withdraw the fang, over which glides the elastic mucous sheath as the

---

[1] It follows from the observations of Dr. Johnston, and Prof. Wyman, that no tissue connection exists between the venom duct and the basal opening in the fang. It becomes necessary, under these circumstances, to explain how the poison is carried from one to the other. Usually the projecting papilla at the end of the duct, is held by the gum in close contact with the fang opening, and when the fang, in rising, thrusts back its mucous cloak, this presses upon the parts at the base of the fang so firmly, as to bring them into perfect apposition. This explanation is given by Prof. Wyman. It does very often happen, however, that a part only, or even none, of the venom enters the fang, but is violently ejected between that weapon and the edges of the vagina dentis.

pterygoid, again acting, depresses the fang, and the serpent recovers its posture of defence.

It happens, not unfrequently, that the teeth of the lower jaw catch in the skin of the bitten animal, and thus prevent the snake from retreating at once. When this takes place, the serpent shakes its head from side to side, with a motion which so nearly resembles the shake a dog gives his prey, that it has been mistaken by at least one observer for an expression of rage. It is really an attempt to escape; nor is it always successful, since a large animal will often drag a snake until the fangs themselves break loose, and are left in, or on, the bitten part.

In considering this portion of our subject, it is well to notice what has been too much overlooked, the fact that, while the snake commonly employs both fangs, it does often inflict but a single wound. When obtaining venom from living snakes, I have been accustomed to allow them to bite upon the inner edge of a cup, and I have observed that on some occasions both fangs were used at once, and that on others only one was active. Or, the fangs were used in succession, an appreciable interval of time intervening. If this occur, when a snake at freedom strikes an object, it is, of course, possible that the animal may escape before the second fang is driven in by the traction of its proper external pterygoid muscle. At all events, it is certain that these facts should receive due appreciation, in estimating the danger of a given bite, and the value of an antidote.

There remains for consideration one muscular motion, which I have observed to accompany the effort to bite, when the snake is held by the back of the neck. It consists in a turning outwards of the points of the fangs, so as to separate them from one another.[1] This divergence of the fang points is disadvantageous, inasmuch as it causes them to enter somewhat obliquely, and frequently throws one fang beyond the part bitten, when that part happens to be small. It has a use with reference to the snake itself, since the fang-points, when thus widely separated, lie outside of the lower jaw, and are thus prevented from wounding it. This purpose is greatly aided by the action of a muscle analogous to the mylo-hyoid, which approximates the anterior extremities of the lower maxillary, or mandibular bones, so as to make narrow the extremity of the jaw. The protection thus obtained is very essential, since the serpent always closes the jaw violently when biting, but does not always succeed in seizing its prey. Whether or not this divergence of the fang-points occurs when the snake bites unrestrainedly, I cannot say; but as I have been very often astonished at the distance between the wounds, where both fangs had taken effect, it is highly probable that it occurs under all circumstances.

We have still left for consideration certain points of minor interest, in connection with the part played by the gland in the train of actions which I have described. This organ, as we have seen, is violently compressed by the anterior temporal muscle, and perhaps by the posterior temporal, as well as indirectly by the external pterygoid. Under the pressure thus applied, the venom passes through the duct, and out of the fang. Now, as it is clear that the temporal muscles must be often used to

---

[1] I could not determine whether this divergence took place when the snake, at freedom, struck an animal.

close the jaws, under circumstances which do not demand the ejection of venom, we must suppose, either that the anterior temporal is, at times, functionally inactive, or else that some provision exists for restraining the flow of poison, when the gland is incidentally compressed during the ordinary movements of the lower jaw, as in gaping (a common action with snakes), deglutition, etc.

The closure of the duct is provided for in two ways, one of which is peculiarly ingenious. The first and most effective of these is the sphincter, which I have already described. The second consists in a peculiar relation between the maxillary bone and the duct. The antero-lateral surface of the bone is somewhat rounded, and the duct being confined at the base of the bone, and also perfectly fixed at its junction with the fang, it happens that when the fang tooth lies flexed in the mouth, the maxillary portion of the duct is stretched over the rounded shoulder of bone upon which it rests, thus flattening, and closing its canal more or less completely.

It is worthy of remark, that the abrupt curve of the duct under the eye, has, also, a mechanical value. First, as an additional means of interrupting the flow of venom, when the fang is not in use, and, second, as a provision for preventing injury to the duct, when, during the action of fixing the fang, the duct is drawn backward by the muscles, and forward by the sudden and momentary flexion of the fang, which occurs at this time. Under these two forces, the bend in the duct is temporarily obliterated.

The power with which the venom is ejected from the tooth, depends somewhat upon the amount contained in the gland and its ducts. When the snake fails to strike the object aimed at, the poison is sometimes projected several feet. In one case which is known to me, it was thrown into the eye of a man standing five or six feet from the snake, when it struck upwards at a stick held above its coil.[1]

---

[1] For an account of many facts in connection with snakes, which are of popular scientific interest, but remote from my present subject, the reader will do well to consult Professor Leconte's paper, Shaw's Zoology, the various Encyclopedia articles, and the memoir of Prof. Dumeril, to which I have already referred.

The great tenacity of life on the part of snakes, is alluded to by several of these authors, and is well known in the form of a very singular popular belief. It is certainly very remarkable in the Rattlesnake, whose reflex motions are admirably retained for some hours after decapitation, and occasionally are seen as late as the 36th hour. At this late period, they consist in wave-like movements, which run from the tail upwards, and are most readily excited by pinching the parts about the cloaca. Immediately after the head has been cut off, the body writhes slowly along the floor, or, if hung up, returns on itself, twining the pendant trunk around the tail. If, when the body is entirely fresh, we seize the tail, the headless trunk frequently returns on itself, in the effort to strike the offending hand. Occasionally, this movement is so perfectly executed, that the bleeding and headless trunk smites the operator's hand before it can be withdrawn. In one or two instances, persons who were ignorant of the possibility of this movement, have been so terrified at the blow which has greeted them, as to faint on the spot. To hold thus the headless snake, has been made a test of firmness in some parts of the West; and few have been found composed enough to retain the tail until the innocent, but ghastly stump, struck the hand. Indeed, any one who may try this little experiment, will discover that it is no easy task to keep a steady grasp upon the tail, even when, in ineffectual efforts, the bleeding neck is thrown towards the irritated parts, but does not fully succeed in reaching it. It is interesting to observe that, while the person whose nerves are thus tried, looks at the snake, he can scarcely ever so control himself as to be unmoved; but, if he close his

The study of the complicated mechanism which we have endeavored to explain, will aid us in understanding several points of interest in connection with the bite of the Rattlesnake.

It must be perfectly apparent that in a sequence of movements so elaborate, it will occasionally happen that, from a failure in some one of the essential motions, the ultimate purpose of the whole will be interfered with. Thus, it sometimes chances that the serpent miscalculates the distance, and fails from this cause. Or, again, when the object aimed at is very near, the initial force of the blow is lost, and the tooth does not enter; no uncommon occurrence, where the animal struck is an old dog, with a tough skin. Again, if the upper jaw be not elevated sufficiently, the fangs are sometimes driven backwards, by the force of the forward impulse, as they touch the part attacked, and the venom is then apt to escape between the tooth and the covering mucous cloak. Upon one occasion, having allowed a small snake to strike a dog, the former became entangled, owing to the hooked teeth of the lower maxillary bone having caught in the skin. Upon examining the snake closely, the dog being held, I found that the convexity of the fangs lay against the skin, on which were thrown one or two drops of venom. On removing the snake, and inspecting the part struck, I could find no fang wound, although the skin was visibly torn by the smaller teeth. I have seen the Rattlesnake strike with great apparent ferocity, a number of times, when I have been unable to discover any fang wound whatsoever; and this has taken place, occasionally, with small animals, such as the rabbit, which must have been seriously affected by even a small amount of venom.

It scarcely ever happens that an animal is bitten, without a part of the injected venom being cast on the skin, near the wound made by the fangs. This wasted material probably escapes from the duct, where it is in apposition with the lower opening of the fang canal, and may be merely that excess of fluid which the fang cannot carry. In some cases, however, it is quite possible that the relations of the fang and the duct are so disturbed, that the venom never enters the tooth at all. It is certainly true, as has been already stated, and as Dr. Wyman has shown, that the fang must be fully erected in order that the duct shall be so firmly held in contact with the fang, as to insure the passage of the venom through this latter organ.

Finally, it sometimes happens, that the blow is given, the fang enters, and from the quick starting of the animal injured, or from some other interrupting cause, it is withdrawn so soon that the larger portion of the poison is thrown harmless upon the surface near the wound. Under these circumstances, the resulting symptoms are, of course, trifling; and how well such an occurrence would be calculated to deceive the observer, who employed an antidote in a like case, can be readily conceived.

---

eyes or look away, the source through which the involuntary start of alarm, or nervousness, is, so to speak, dictated, appears to be cut off, and the intellectual and memorial recognition of the snake's powers is not sufficiently lively to overcome the force of will which is exerted to retain the grasp.

When speaking of the difficulties which surround the study of antidotes to serpent poison, we shall return again to this subject. Here it is sufficient to have pointed out such of the fallacies as are due to a want of exact knowledge of the mechanism concerned in producing the poisoned wound.

The minute details, here given, of the mechanism of the bite, are collected from many sources already mentioned, and are carefully corrected by numerous original observations, dissections, and experimental demonstrations of the mode in which different muscles acted under galvanic stimulus, applied after decollation and removal of the skin. So far as I am aware, it is the only full account of the mode in which the bite is given, and of the parts played by the different organs and tissues concerned.

CHAPTER IV.

THE PHYSICAL AND CHEMICAL CHARACTERS OF THE VENOM.

THE venom, the injection of which is the sole object of the mechanism we have been considering, will now claim our attention. In my own researches, I have felt seriously the want of statements as to the manipulation and mechanical means employed by preceding observers, when handling, and otherwise using, their snakes. For this reason, as well as to place the reader upon the same logical ground with myself, by giving him every known condition and accompaniment of each observation, I have, in all cases, described minutely the whole manual of each experiment. Where these details would have confused the statements of results, I have placed them in the form of notes.

It would have been an easy task to swell this Essay to an imposing bulk, by quoting throughout all the comparative results obtained by those who have experimented on venomous snakes, other than the Crotalus. So full a summary would not be without use and interest; but, since the mass of these researches have but little value, I have contented myself with the briefest relation of the opinions of others, where they did not directly concern the rattlesnake. My main object has been to present, with brevity, my own results, as regards the Crotalus, with such illustration, contrast, and comment, derived from the works of others, as seemed to me essential to this purpose.

Amount of Venom in the Ducts.—The amount of venom contained at any one time in the ducts of the poison gland, varied with the size of the snake, and the period which had elapsed since the last bite. I have again and again collected the venom, and have found that serpents of from three to four feet long rarely threw out more than from two to four drops, after the first ejection had taken place. When perfectly fresh, healthy, and undisturbed for some weeks in summer, the first gush of their venom was sometimes astonishingly large. A snake which had served as a show in Washington, reached me in a box with a glass top, which was firmly fixed by screws. In all probability this snake had been several weeks without using its fangs.[1] It was secured as usual, and the lip of a cup placed in its mouth. It

---

[1] *Manipulation.*—The authors who have written upon serpents, have usually obtained their venom by killing the animal, and compressing the gland (Fontana), or by anæsthetizing it with chloroform (Burnett), and then exerting pressure, until the fluid exuded through the duct. Where snakes are abundant, the first method is perhaps the best, if the head be cut off rapidly and suddenly, without

struck at once with the right fang, but missing the cup, poured a large amount of venom into its own mouth. The left fang struck an instant after, and threw into

---

allowing the snake to bite at any object, and thus exhaust its venom. Where the snakes are not easily replaced, this plan is plainly not economical.

Others have allowed the snake to bite upon soft substances which imbibed the venom readily, and from which it could be removed by water (Bonaparte). The methods which, after long practice, I have found most available, I will detail here, after describing the various means which I have found useful in securing the snakes for experiment, or in removing them from box to box.

In moving snakes, it is customary to employ long-handled tongs, or forceps, which are apt to pinch and otherwise injure them. I have been in the habit of using for this purpose, a bar of wood four feet long, and cut off at the end, so as to present a slightly roughened surface, one and a half inches square. On one side of the end, a piece of soft and pliant leather strap was nailed securely. This strap was then carried across the end of the bar, and through a flat staple upon the side opposite to that on which the strap was fastened. A stout cord, attached to the strap above the staple, was held in the operator's hand. To use this simple instrument, the strap was drawn down, so as to form a loop, which was easily slipped over the head of a snake, and there tightened by drawing on the cord. Where it was desirable merely to secure the venom, the loop was slipped over the head and drawn closely around the neck.

Thus prepared, the snake was placed on the table and retained by an assistant, while the operator obtained the venom. When it was desirable to have an animal bitten without placing it in the cage, the loop was carried to the middle of the snake's body, and it was thus allowed movement enough to enable it to draw back and strike. It is unnecessary to add that during these manipulations, the utmost caution is necessary to avoid accident.

As it is sometimes essential to detain the snake on the table for some time, without being forced to employ a person to guard it, I devised a little apparatus, which, although imperfect, answered my ends well enough. A box, about four inches square, and thirty-six inches long, was divided lengthwise, and arranged with hinges so as to close readily. The two sections were deeply grooved, so that where the sides of the box met, the grooves formed a tube large enough to receive the body of a serpent five feet in length. The large end of the box was fitted with a sliding door which could be secured by a wooden wedge driven in behind it. The lower edge of the door was made concave, and a piece of leather was tacked across the concavity, designed to press on the snake's neck, and secure without injuring it.

To employ this arrangement, the box was closed and the door raised, a cord having been previously run through the central tube. This cord bore on its extremity a loop which was thrown over the tail of the snake, and carried up between three and four inches. To effect this manœuvre, I was usually obliged to hold the snake down with a long stick notched at the end. The serpent being thus noosed, the loop was tightened, and an assistant tilted the box over the cage, and rapidly drew the snake backwards into the tube, while a second person standing in front, guided the snake with a long rod.

As soon as the tail appeared at the small end of the box, it was secured by the assistant, and the looped string which held it was wound around a nail. At this instant, the head sometimes retreated into the box. After waiting a moment, it usually reappeared again, and was then seized with a pair of long forceps, and held while the door was pushed down on the neck, and made fast with the wedge. When the snake was small, it sometimes contrived to turn around in the box before the tail emerged, and thus reverse its desired position. This occurrence twice exposed the operator to great danger. It was finally provided against by the aid of a large cork, which was strung upon the cord, and was used to close the small end of the tube, when the snake was of a size to make it possible for it to turn in the tube. When the snake was thus properly imprisoned, it could be placed on the table and studied to great advantage, while it was still able to bite with sufficient vigor.

At various times I have employed all the methods of procuring venom, which I have enumerated at the commencement of this note. I have finally laid aside all but the plan of stupefying the snake by chloroform. This is accomplished by seizing the snake about the middle with the looped staff, and placing it on the table. An assistant then controls the head and neck, by confining the latter with a notched stick, while with the other hand he slips over the head a glass vessel about two inches wide, and containing at the closed end a sponge soaked in chloroform. The snake breathes for a time with only

the cup fifteen drops of venom. This is the largest quantity which I have ever seen ejected by natural process. In a subsequent attempt, the next day, this serpent, which bit eagerly, threw out only one or two drops from each fang. The snake was fifty-three inches long, and weighed two pounds four ounces.

It is difficult to compare the amount of venom ejected by the Crotalus, with that excreted by the Viper, and the Naja, since, although both Russell[1] and Fontana[2] speak on this point, they seem to have secured the poison from the exsected gland, or, at least, by pressure after death, and they are, moreover, silent as to the length and weight of the animals examined.

Jeter[3] states that the enlarged duct at the base of the poison gland will hold usually about ten drops, when distended with accumulated poison.

In four snakes I filled the duct and gland with water. The injection was made by introducing a small syringe into the duct itself outside of the gland. The fluid was afterwards expressed from the gland, and measured. In place of estimating the fluid by the gross plan of dropping it, I employed the following means: A narrow tube was graduated, so that each division represented a drop of distilled water. The point being drawn to a fine capillary termination, enabled me to collect, by gentle suction, the venom, or other fluid, even when it was spread over a rough surface, or accidentally spilled.

In the accompanying table, I have given the weight and length of the serpents used, and the amount in water-drops which a single gland in each snake was capable of containing.

No. 1.	C. Durissus.	Length[4] 18 inches.	Weight 9½ oz.	Capacity of gland 11 drops.
No. 2.	" "	" 25 "	" 18 "	" " 19 "
No. 3.	" "	" 49½ "	" 3 lbs. 2 oz.	" " 29 "

Color of Venom.—The color of the venom varied from a pale emerald green to orange and straw color. Where the poison had remained a long time in the gland, it was deeper in hue than when its ejection followed rapidly upon its formation.

I have also observed that in some snakes, it was uniformly of a darker color

---

a few inches of lung which lie in front of the stick, but as it becomes more insensible, the pressure of the stick is removed, and the strap of the staff loosened. About twenty minutes are required to complete the process. If it is then found that the lower jaw hangs relaxed when opened, the neck is seized firmly, the fangs caught on a saucer edge, and the glands stripped from behind forwards by pressure with the thumb and forefinger. The venom usually escapes alongside of the fang, from under the mucous cloak. To secure all of the available venom, it is best to wash the fang and the vagina dentis with the aid of a little water, and a pipette; but one objection can be urged against this method. One snake in every four died within from two to five days, and this after apparent recovery from the effects of the chloroform. It is not impossible that too severe a compression of the venom glands may produce rupture of its substance, and consequent blood-poisoning. This, however, is but conjecture; and I have not further examined the subject experimentally.

[1] Russell on the Poison Serpents of India, p. 40.

[2] Fontana on Poisons, Trans. by J. Skinner. Lond. 1787, vol. i. 277—287.

[3] Poisoned Wounds, etc., a Report of a Committee to the Med. Assoc. of Missouri, by A. F. Jeter, M. D., p. 10.

[4] Not inclusive of the rattles.

than in others; but of the cause of this difference I know nothing, nor am I able to associate an increased virulency with any particular hue of the poison.

Fontana[1] describes the color of the venom of the Viper as yellow. Jeter[2] speaks of the Crotalus poison as being more frequently of a greenish tint, though sometimes yellowish. Russell gives no information as to the color of Cobra venom, or that of other East India serpents.

Specific Gravity.—On the subject of the specific gravity of the venom, all authors are silent, usually contenting themselves with the statement that it is heavier than water.

As it is very difficult to collect at any one time enough of the venom to admit of the use of the specific gravity bottle, I was obliged to resort to other means.

Having prepared a solution of sugar in water, of a specific gravity of 1030, I threw into it with a pipette, a drop of pure venom. Finding that it sunk rapidly, I increased the strength of the sugar solution, until the venom was found to float in it midway. This rather coarse means enabled me to estimate the average specific gravity of the clear poison at 1044. The specimen employed came from a snake which had been unmolested for several weeks. To test the matter further, I collected some poison from the same snake on the two following days, obtaining but a drop or two on each occasion. The first of these specimens had a specific weight of 1030. The second was estimated at 1035, so that it is probable that the poison becomes concentrated by long residence in the gland.

The method of examination here employed is, of course, open to criticism, and can furnish only approximate calculations; but, as I know of no other facts in this direction, I do not deem it proper to omit even the imperfect results thus attained.

Physical Characters.—The venom examined by me was always more or less glutinous. In the Viper, it so nearly resembled a gum, that it was described by Fontana as such.[3] That of the Crotalus dries very slowly, and is as adhesive as thick solutions of gum-acacia. When completely desiccated, it resembled dried albumen, and presented itself in thin yellow and transparent layers, traversed by numberless cracks which in the Viper-poison were supposed by Mead to be the edges of crystals peculiar to the secretion.

Whether fluid or dried, the poison of the Crotalus was devoid of taste, and also of smell, unless it had undergone putrefaction, to which, like other albuminoid solutions, it is liable. I have tasted the rattlesnake poison repeatedly, once by design, and several times through accident, when engaged in collecting it by sucking it into a pipette.

I could not perceive that it had the slightest taste or acridity. Mead alone describes the venom of the viper as acrid and caustic to the tongue. Fontana could discern no taste in it, but thought that it benumbed the part on which it was placed. Brainard[4] states that the Crotalus venom has "a peculiar and dis-

---

[1] Fontana on Poisons, VI. p. 12. Skinner's Translation.

[2] Jeter on Poisoned Wounds, p. 20.

[3] Fontana, p. 263, vol. i. Skinner's Transl., where the Abbé examines and disproves this idea.

[4] Brainard, Smithsonian Institution, Annual Report of, for 1854, p. 125.

agreeable odor, and is said to have a pungent taste." No authority is given for the latter statement. Jeter[1] speaks of it as tasteless, but ascribes to it the power to benumb the tongue when a drop is placed on that organ. I can only add that I have never experienced the sensation in question. As respects Prof. Brainard's account of its odor, it is proper to observe that, although, as I have said, the venom was usually free from smell, specimens which had remained a long time in the gland, sometimes had the peculiar animal odor of the snake itself.

Reaction of the Venom.—The subject of the acidity or alkalinity of the venom of the European viper, was very early a matter of keen dispute. Mead and James both asserted that it reddened litmus, and was of a distinctly acid reaction. Mead afterwards disavowed this idea, and agreed with Fontana in calling it neutral. Jussieu, who followed Mead in his earlier view, also agreed with him in recommending the local and general treatment by volatile alkali, in the hope of neutralizing the acid in question. Dr. Brickell,[2] of Savannah, appears to have been the first to examine the reaction of rattlesnake poison. This observer found that the venom was strongly acid, and reddened litmus paper. Dr. Harlan,[3] of Philadelphia, also describes it as invariably acid. Brainard, Barton, Jeter, and others, do not seem to have examined the question.

My own observations on this subject were very numerous, and were directed, not only towards ascertaining whether or not the venom was acid, but also as to the normal reaction of the snake's mouth, when free from venom.

I find in my notes the record of eight observations, in all of which the venom reddened litmus paper more or less distinctly. In a great many unrecorded observations I obtained no other result. It was uniformly acid, and this reaction was common to all specimens of the poison, whether moist or dry, dark colored or pale in tint. One of these specimens was two years old, and, when placed on litmus paper, and touched with a drop of water, it reddened the paper distinctly. I do not think that the venom increases in acidity upon being kept; nor, on the other hand, does the acid of the venom appear to be volatile, since litmus once reddened by it, kept the red hue, until exposed to an alkali, which restored the original blue tint of the test paper. That, finally, the acid was not due to changes which occurred, exterior to the body of the snake, was shown by the constancy of the acid reaction in specimens obtained by allowing the serpent to bite upon test paper folded so thickly as to arrest the fang, and receive the poison directly from it.

The reaction of the mucous membrane of the mouth was almost as consistently alkaline as that of the venom was acid. This observation of course suggested the possibility of neutralization taking place, when the poison accidentally reached the mouth. It was found, indeed, that litmus reddened by the venom became blue again when left in the serpent's jaws; but, although the acid was neutralized,

---

[1] Jeter, p. 20.

[2] Brickell, Med. Depository, conducted by S. L. Mitchill, M. D., and E. Miller, M. D., New York, 1805, second hexade, vol. ii. p. 441.

[3] Harlan, Med. and Phys. Researches, 1835, p. 502.

the poisonous properties of the fluid remained unaltered, as I shall have frequent occasion to demonstrate.

The want of agreement among observers, as to the reaction of viper poison, is such, that the point in question should be re-examined by some competent person. Prince Louis Lucien Bonaparte,[1] to whom we owe a chemical analysis of viper poison, does not appear to have touched the matter, and contents himself with stating that echidnine or viperine, the essential principle, is neutral, making no allusion to an acid, when detailing the other ingredients present.

Decomposition of the Venom.—Like most albuminoid matters, the venom entered into decomposition when long kept in the moist state, but although it then developed vibriones, and even low confervoid growths, and smelt most horribly, it was still poisonous. How long it would retain its virulence under these circumstances, and what extent of putrefactive change might be needed to destroy this quality, I cannot state from my own experience.

Many specimens of venom let fall, on repose, a white sediment, which, in a few cases, was very abundant. The clear poison presented no points of interest when viewed microscopically. When dry, it cracked like dried white of egg, but under no management has it afforded me crystals. My friend Prof. Hammond[2] has been more successful, and has obtained crystals by diluting the venom of the *C. confluentus*, and allowing the mixture to dry slowly, sheltered by a cover-glass. (Fig. 11.) The crystals thus formed, resembled those of ammoniaco-magnesian phosphate, which affect the feathery form of crystallization.

Fig. 11.

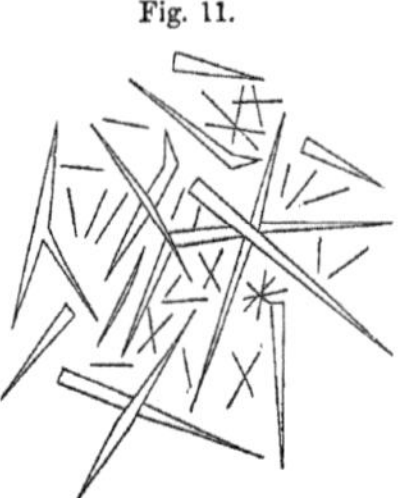

The white deposit was composed chiefly of amorphous, granular matter, with a few pavement epithelial cells, compound granular bodies of oleaginous character, and finally of the peculiar masses known and described as colloid bodies,[3] and in

---

[1] Prince Louis Lucien Bonaparte, Gazetta Toscana, delle Scienze Medico-fisiche, Anno primo, Firenze, 1843. I have been unable to find this memoir, and have been forced to employ Orfila's quotation of his results. Orfila, Tox. Gen., p. 844.

[2] Fig. 11 is taken from Prof. Hammond's drawing, which he kindly put at my disposal.

[3] Wedl, Pathological Histology, Trans. of the Sydenham Society, pp. 38, 264, 271, etc.

appearance so much resembling starch granules, as to have induced me to neglect them at first, and to suppose them to be really that substance, accidentally present. These corpuscular bodies were marked with delicate radiating lines. Iodine stained them of a yellowish-brown. They were doubtless due to some concrete modification of albuminous material.

Occasionally, when the snake had been seriously maltreated, the venom contained more or less blood.

Chemical Examination.—I much regret having been unable to collect the venom of the Crotalus in such amount as would have enabled a competent chemist to make of it an ultimate analysis, to which I believe it has never yet been submitted.

In the following examination, I have contented myself with a qualitative analysis, which, although not so perfect as I could have desired, appears to me to have thrown some light on this novel and curious subject.

The fresh venom of the Crotalus begins to coagulate at 140° F., and is almost solid at 160°. The mode in which I accomplished this observation upon minute amounts of venom, without desiccating it, will be found detailed in the account of the influence of temperature upon the virulency of the venom.[1]

When a drop of the pure poison was thrown upon platinum foil and heated, it boiled, whitened, and at last became charred before it took fire.

When a drop of venom was thrown into cold distilled water, it fell rapidly, and presented a white appearance, which became marked, as it dispersed through the fluid. It finally dissolved in the water, without residue. This phenomenon of the whitening of the venom in water, has also been noticed in regard to fresh white of egg similarly treated.

The pure venom of the Crotalus was subjected to the action of various chemical reagents, either with the primary object of learning how they would affect it, or with the purpose of observing whether or not they altered its power to poison.

Nitric acid threw down from Crotalus venom a dense precipitate. Added in excess, it re-dissolved the larger part of the precipitate, and formed a thin yellowish fluid, in which floated undissolved minute yellow flocculi. Liquor ammoniæ, added in excess, did not re-precipitate the dissolved material.

Chlorohydric acid threw down a dense white precipitate, and, added in excess, completely re-dissolved it, forming a solution colorless, or of a pale yellow, from which ammonia in excess re-precipitated the dissolved substance in opaque white masses.

Sulphuric acid threw down from the venom a white precipitate, which, if the acid were hastily added, or if heated, became yellow or brown.

Acetic acid caused no precipitate from the venom, whether added to it in large or small amount.

Tannic acid produced a dense white precipitate, which proved to be insoluble in water, and in an excess of the acid, but was re-dissolved on the addition of a small amount of ammonia.

---

[1] These observations were amply verified at another time, when larger quantities of venom were used.

Chlorine water caused a dense. precipitate. A solution of iodine and iodide of potassium caused a precipitate which redissolved in an excess of the reagent.[1]

Soda and potassa had no visible effect on the venom.

Ammonia was also without action upon it, as was also lime-water.

Bichloride of mercury gave with the venom a dense white precipitate.

Sulphate of soda produced a dense precipitate, which redissolved on the addition of water in excess. The precipitate was, therefore, soluble in a weak solution of the salt employed.

Sulphate of magnesia, in like manner, caused a precipitate which proved soluble in an excess of water, as in the last observation.

In both cases the precipitate could be reproduced by increasing the amount of the salt present, and again, an added excess of water was competent to redissolve the new precipitate.

Alcohol invariably produced in the venom a heavy, flocculent precipitate, which, when carefully dried, turned of a pale yellow, and was still more or less soluble in water. The latter fact was observed, even when the poison had been kept in alcohol during five weeks. I have also examined the poison found in the ducts of Rattlesnakes, which had remained in alcohol for two years or more. It proved to be very slightly soluble in water. There is in this observation, however, a cause of error; since in snakes which die violent deaths, the whole gland is often filled with blood, so that the coagulated substance in the ducts can, with no certainty, be regarded as venom alone; unless we are informed very fully as to the condition of the organs, when first immersed in the preserving fluid. This question is one of considerable interest, and will engage our attention in another place.

An aqueous solution of the venom was evaporated to dryness. A drop of a solution of sulphate of copper was then added, and the mixture treated with a solution of caustic potassa in excess. In a few minutes it exhibited the violet color characteristic of albuminous matters thus tested.

The venom was next examined for sulphocyanide of potassium, a constituent of human saliva, although with slight expectation of detecting it. Five drops were tested with sulphate of sesquioxide of iron. It produced a heavy white precipitate, but no red color was observed. Seven drops of the venom were evaporated to dryness, and treated with the same salt of iron, but without any appearance of the red hue which indicates the presence of the sulphocyanide mentioned. These examinations were repeated several times on as many specimens of the poison, but always with a negative result. From the small amount of venom employed, they did not entirely satisfy me, and the subject may still repay a fuller examination. At present it is only safe to affirm that the sulphocyanide, if it exist in the venom at all, can only be present in a very minute amount, and can in no way be considered as a causative element, in the production of the symptoms which follow upon the insertion of the venom into the tissues of living animals.[2]

---

[1] Brainard's antidote—Iod. potass. grs. xxx; iodine grs. x; water ℥j.

[2] In the following work by M. Bernard: Leçons sur les Propriétés Physiologiques, et les Altérations Pathologiques des Liquides de l'Organisme, vol. ii. p. 242, he says: "Ainsi on a dit d'abord, que la présence du sulfocyanure de potassium dans la salive, rappelait les glands à venin des serpents vemineux."

Thus far we have only learned, from the preceding details, that the venom of the Crotalus is an acid-fluid, abounding in albuminous matter, and yielding precipitates, or coagula, with certain reagents.

It was highly probable, for various reasons, that the active element of the venom was to be sought in the albuminoid compound just referred to. Accordingly, the greatest attention was paid to this substance, and at every step in the analysis the coagula and filtered solutions were studied toxicologically, as well as chemically.

Prince Charles Lucien Bonaparte has given us the only analysis of a snake venom with which I am acquainted; it is that of the viper. I have been unfortunate in not having had access to the original Essay of this observer, and have been forced to content myself with such analyses of his paper as are to be found in the systematic works on poisons, and in one of M. Bernard's recent volumes.[1] Thus aided, I have partially followed M. Bonaparte's method of analysis; but have found it insufficient for the thorough examination of rattlesnake venom.

The observations and analyses which I have thus introduced, were conducted in the following manner:—

1st. Ten or twelve drops of pure Crotalus venom were secured, as usual. Of this, a minute amount was employed as a toxicological test of the activity of the specimen about to be studied.

2d. The remainder of the venom was mixed with two drachms of cold water, and thoroughly boiled for five or ten minutes. A dense coagulum took place, and settled quickly, leaving above it a pearl-colored fluid, free from sedimentary matter. On shaking the test-tube, so as to mingle the coagulum and the supernatant fluid, and then injecting one-half into the breast tissues of a pigeon, it was found that the mixture proved speedily fatal. Boiling had not destroyed its power.

3d. The remaining half of the mixture (coagulum and fluid), was cast on a small filter, and when the pearly fluid had passed through, the coagulum which remained was carefully washed, drop by drop, with cold water. On the filter was finally left the white coagulum, thoroughly washed; in the filtrate were all the parts of the venom which could be dissolved either in cold or boiling water.

4th. The toxicological test was now introduced, to decide whether the poisoning activity lay in the clot formed by heat, or in the separated fluid. Upon numerous repetitions of this observation, it invariably happened that the coagulum was innocent, and that the pearly supernatant fluid, with the washings of the coagulum, was a deadly poison. The experiments were made as usual, by injecting the venom into the breast or leg tissues of healthy pigeons.

5th. As I was aware that alcohol threw down all of the albuminoid elements of venom, it occurred to me that it might also precipitate from the boiled venom the material which appeared to escape the coagulating influence of the heat. Accordingly, a considerable quantity of venom, about fifteen drops, was boiled, in half an ounce of water. When the coagulum settled, the opalescent supernatant liquid was decanted with care, the coagulum washed on a filter, and the washings mixed with

---

[1] Orfila, Toxicologie Générale, Art. Vipère. Bernard Cl. Leçons sur les Effets des Substances toxiques et médicamenteuses. Paris, 1857, p. 393. Nysten, Dict. de Médecine, Art. Échidnine.

the liquid. To this was now added a small amount of alcohol of 95 per cent. A cloud of a white and granular character was immediately seen at the line where the alcohol and water met. Upon this an ounce and a half of the alcohol was added, when the fluid clouded throughout, and a white precipitate soon settled to the bottom. The supernatant alcohol and water being poured off and carefully evaporated at a temperature of 100° F., was examined toxicologically as usual. The evaporation was, of course, carried nearly to dryness, so as to avoid the risk of killing the bird with alcohol. No poisonous results were observed, except in two cases, where the alcohol originally used proved to have been diluted with water, and to have acted as a partial solvent for the active material. It is necessary, on this account, to employ the strongest alcohol.

6th. The precipitate caused by the alcohol was washed repeatedly with successive portions of that fluid, and allowed to settle. Then the last alcohol used to wash it was removed by pipette, and the precipitate spread on a plate to dry. On testing it toxicologically, it was found to be actively poisonous, giving rise, even when employed in minute amount, to all the local and general phenomena of Crotalus poisoning.

The material thus obtained, was of a pale yellowish tint when dried, and was perfectly neutral in reaction. It dissolved readily enough in water, cold or hot, and its aqueous solutions were troubled by alcohol. Its nitrogenous nature was established by its reaction with Millon's test of nitrate of mercury, and with the cupro-potassa test. As it appeared to me to be the active toxicological element of the venom, I propose to distinguish it by the name of *Crotaline*.

It seemed from the statements of those who quote Prince Bonaparte's method of analysis of viper-poison that he procured the essential principle, which he termed *échidnine*, or *viperine*, in the following manner: The venom was treated with an excess of alcohol, and filtered; the residue on the filter being well washed with fresh portions of alcohol. The alcoholic solution was evaporated to dryness, and found to contain a coloring matter, and a small amount of an undetermined substance, which, of course, was soluble in alcohol. The coagulum was next washed, drop by drop, with cold water, so as to dissolve the échidnine, and leave the "mucosine," become now insoluble from the influence of the alcohol. The échidnine was separated from the aqueous solution by evaporation. In all essential particulars, échidnine and crotaline are alike. Upon repeating and varying M. Bonaparte's method of analysis, I found, however, some discrepancy of results.

Thus, if to the venom of the Crotalus an excess of alcohol be added, a large precipitate occurs. In some instances, all of this precipitate was soluble in water; in other cases, a small proportion remained undissolved, behaving as ov-albumen would do after being coagulated by alcohol. Generally, as I have said, the bulk of the alcohol precipitate was soluble in water. The aqucous solution thus obtained could be coagulated by boiling, so as to throw down a harmless precipitate, and to leave above it a fluid still actively venomous, but representing in its dissolved albuminoid substance but a small part of the nitrogenous precipitate caused by the alcohol in the first instance. In other words, the aqueous solution of the alcoholic precipitate behaved in the presence of heat exactly like the diluted venom itself.

On reviewing these facts, it appears that in Crotalus venom, 1st, alcohol precipitates all the albuminoid material, innocent, as well as poisonous. 2d. That heat throws down from diluted venom the bulk of these albuminous compounds in an insoluble and harmless form, and that the residual water still contains an albuminoid body uncoagulable by heat, but precipitable by alcohol, and of great poisonous activity.

Now, the yield of crotaline from the plan first mentioned, and that of M. Bonaparte, is very different. So much larger is the quantity obtained by the latter means, that I cannot help suspecting that, besides seizing on the active principle, the water also takes up from the alcoholic precipitate a certain quantity of albuminous material which is quite innocent, and can only be coagulated by a heat of 160° and upwards.

Besides the two albuminoid bodies, whose presence in venom I have thus made probable, there is also at times a little nitrogenous matter which behaves like the ordinary egg albumen.

The ether washings of dried venom I found to contain now and then a little oil, which was only to be detected under the microscope. As in M. Bonaparte's analysis, when the alcoholic solution was evaporated, it was found to contain a small quantity of uncrystalline flakes of some unknown body, tinged yellow, and dotted here and there with specks of a deeper hue.

Besides these elements, we have also a small amount of saline constituents, probably chlorides and phosphates of alkalies. The determination of these bodies seemed to be of no great moment in the present case, and I have therefore failed to study them with minute attention.

We have thus far determined that the venom of the Rattlesnake is composed of—

1. An albuminoid body. *Crotaline*, not coagulable by heat of 212°.
2. An albuminoid compound coagulable by a temperature of 212° F.
3. A coloring matter, and an undetermined substance, both soluble in alcohol.
4. A trace of fatty matter.
5. Salts, chlorides, and phosphates.

At this period of our investigation it would be interesting to compare the venom more carefully with the ordinary salivary fluids, a step which is rendered necessary by the fact that De Blainville and others have considered the venom gland as the analogue of the parotid, and the venom as only a peculiar salivary fluid.

Before we carry on such a comparison, it is necessary to state the results of a number of experiments and observations, which, while they aid us in elucidating the present branch of our subject, have also an important bearing upon the question of the true character of the poison of the venom. We shall proceed, therefore, to the statement of the observations in question, and afterwards to the discussion of the claims of the poison gland and its secretion, to the titles of salivary gland and saliva.

If the poison gland is a salivary gland at all, it is, of course, from its anatomical relations a parotid gland, and its secretion is comparable only with the parotid secretion. In the lack of information as to the nature of this saliva in serpents generally, we can only compare the venom with the parotid saliva of the horse, dog, and man, a circumstance which necessarily impairs the interest and value of this particular branch of our subject.

Since the discovery by Leuchs, of the power of saliva to convert boiled starch into grape sugar, observers have been undecided as to whether or not pure parotid saliva possesses this power. The weight of authority at present is undoubtedly against it, but in the absence of any positive decision, I have conceived it necessary to learn whether or not the supposed venom saliva had this faculty.

Experiment.—In three test tubes of the same size, was placed an equal amount of boiled starch-water, in which I had failed to detect the presence of grape sugar. To the first of these were added three drops of pure venom. To the second were added three or four drops of mixed saliva from my own mouth. The third was left without any addition, and all were exposed to a temperature of 78° F.

No. I. Venom and starch-water was examined at intervals, but gave no reaction with the cupro-potassa test until forty-eight hours had elapsed, when sugar was found to be present, but not in large amount.

No. II. Starch-water and saliva contained sugar at the close of half an hour. Within three hours the sugar was present in abundance.

No. III. Starch-water alone exhibited no traces of sugar until forty-eight hours had elapsed, when it was to be detected, although present in no large quantity.

In a second series of experiments, results so nearly similar were obtained, that it is needless to relate them here.

Since it has been asserted by Wright, that acid saliva does not possess the same converting power as the ordinary alkaline fluid, and as the venom saliva was constantly acid, I repeated the experiments with the following modification.

Experiment.—In two test tubes was placed about half an ounce of thin starch-water. To the first were added four drops of venom, which I had rather more than neutralized with potassa.

The second I left without this addition, and exposed them both to a temperature of from 77° to 87° F. At the close of twenty-four hours, neither of them exhibited any traces of sugar, but after twenty-eight hours, sugar was present in the venom tube and not in the other. These experiments were also repeated on subsequent occasions with like results.

I conceive that we have a right to infer that the venom has no peculiar power to convert boiled starch into grape sugar, and is, in this respect, almost absolutely inactive.

My next observations were directed towards ascertaining whether the venom gland, like the ordinary salivary glands, would yield to water its active principles, and so give rise to infusions, in each case, resembling the saliva of the respective glands. Thus, since M. Bernard's researches, it is well known that an infusion of the submaxillary or parotid glands has all the properties of the normal saliva of these organs. According to this author, the solid matters of the various salivas are constantly deposited in the glands, and are rapidly washed out of them by a flow of thin solvent fluid from the bloodvessels, at such times as the secretion may be needed. If, now, the solid matter of the venom be in like manner a constant portion of the bulk of the gland, it was to be presumed that an infusion of the gland tissues would afford a considerable amount of venomous fluid, manufactured, as it were, artificially.

This question divides itself naturally into two queries:—

1st. Is the gland tissue poisonous?

2d. Are infusions of the gland tissue poisonous?

At first sight, nothing seems easier than to answer these questions, by inoculating animals with infusions of the gland, or portions of its tissue. On direct experiment, sources of fallacy at once appeared. The first of these was due to the difficulty of clearing the gland of poison already contained in it, in the form of venom, filling its smaller ducts. Supposing us to have eliminated this element of doubt, and to have ready a gland tissue washed clear of its actual secretions, if we should have in its secernent cells but a small amount of poison, it may not act upon a large animal. On the other hand, if a very small animal be employed, the reagent may prove too delicate a test, and the animal die from a mere trace of the venom remaining in the ducts, or even of the operation required to insert a whole venom gland under its skin.

Experiment.—A large Crotalus, fifty-three inches long, was secured as usual, and four drops of venom obtained from it. It was then replaced in its box, supplied with a bath, and not disturbed during five days, after which an attempt was made to rob it of the poison formed in the interval. It yielded but one drop, although it struck several times at the collecting vessel. Seeing this, and knowing, from previous experience, that it might be retaining its venom, I placed within its jaws a pigeon's thigh, freed from its feathers. The serpent bit fiercely, the animal dying in twenty-nine minutes. A second pigeon having been plucked, so as to expose the breast, the snake was allowed to bite it three times. It died stupefied, at the close of an hour.

A third pigeon was next arranged, so as to be bitten four times about the breast. The snake, by this time, was very unwilling to use its fangs. The pigeon died in two hours and a half. It is clear from these experiments, that in confinement at least, the venom is formed but slowly, and that in the present case the gland was, in all probability, well emptied of its juices. The snake's neck was next severed about two inches below the head, and the glands of both sides rapidly removed.

The ducts were cut away near to the gland, the gland tissue pressed between two slips of board, and finally washed by repeated injections, and subsequent compression, until at length the returning fluid brought away with it no sediment. The whole of one gland was then minced up with twenty-five drops of water, and introduced under the skin of the breast of a pigeon. None of the usual local or general evidences of Crotalus poisoning followed, and within fifty hours the wound looked dry and healthy. After this time, an extensive slough took place above the site of the gland. As the previous signs and appearances did not warrant the idea that any poisoning could have taken place, I made several experiments to learn how far the skin of the pigeon can be separated from subjacent tissues, without endangering its vitality. These observations soon taught me that any foreign tissue which raised the pigeon's skin for a circumference of more than three or four lines, was apt to occasion a slough.

Experiment.—In this experiment, I prepared a large gland, as above described, and inserted it in seven localities about the body, back, and legs of a pigeon. Around two of these, on the back, a little darkening was visible, and one of them sloughed after several days.

Experiment.—A snake thirty inches long was properly secured, a pigeon arranged as usual, and placed within reach. The snake bit it on the neck, where a local discoloration showed itself at once. On further provocation, by pinching its tail, it bit the pigeon several times, until, as I supposed, the venom was exhausted. As the snake had been used to kill a rabbit five days before, I presume the quantity of venom not to have been large, nor, indeed, could it have been so, as the pigeon did not die for forty minutes. The snake's head was next cut off. Placed on a plate, it bit eagerly, but threw out no venom, even when I galvanized the anterior temporal muscle after removing the cuticle.

Both of the venom glands were removed, squeezed thoroughly, divided lengthwise and across, and repeatedly wiped with a soft towel. Twelve drops of water were then added, and both glands hashed up with it, a drop or two being added as it dried. The temperature was that of the air, 75° F. At the close of thirty-five minutes, I carefully removed all the fluid with a pipette, and injected it under the breast-skin, and into the muscles of a pigeon. Five hours later, the bird was well, and the wound quite dry. Eighteen hours after inoculation, it yielded, upon pressure, a little serous fluid, and around the part, infiltrated with the artificial secretion, there was a slight darkening of the skin, whether due to the presence of a small amount of poison, and the consequent extravasation, or to my having wounded small vessels, I am unable to say. Certainly, no other evidences of poison were noted, and the wound healed after a little serous oozing. No slough took place.

Experiment.—The gland tissue employed in the last observation, was dried by frequent wiping, and being minutely divided, was put under the skin of a rabbit's back. The animal had no constitutional disturbance as a consequence, and was sacrificed after five days to another purpose. A small abscess had formed around the foreign tissues, and was making its way outwards. No extravasation was visible.

Experiment.—On another occasion, an infusion of two small glands from a snake twenty-nine and a half inches long, was used upon a rabbit, without effect visible to the eye. The fluid seemed to have been absorbed without local or general injury to the animal.

Experiment.—The whole tissue of the glands just mentioned was finally minced, bruised, dried in bibulous paper, and carefully introduced under the skin of a pigeon's breast, by pushing in a small tube laterally, and through this distributing the crushed gland tissue as the tube was withdrawn. In this way, the inoculation was effected without much separation of the skin from the parts beneath. In despite of this precaution, extensive inflammation ensued, and a large slough of skin took place, the tissues about the wound becoming infiltrated with serum. No local or general symptoms of poisoning were noted, but the bird sank, became thin, refused food, and died at the close of eight days.

It was evident from these experiments that, for some reason, the gland and its infusions were less virulent than had been anticipated. Reflecting upon the great relative size of the gland, and upon the minute amount of secretion elaborated by it, it seemed to me possible that the quantity of gland matter stored up for its production, might also be but small, and that if this were so, the pigeon might not suffice as a test of its existence. The following experiments were the result of this view.

Experiment.—A large snake, weighing four pounds, and measuring three feet eight inches, was secured, and allowed to bite a reed-bird, which died within one minute, exhibiting both local and general symptoms. The snake was then teazed until it struck, and threw out a drop or two of poison from each gland, after which its head was cut off, the ducts divided, and the gland thoroughly emptied by pressure. It was then finely divided as usual, washed, and dried in bibulous paper. Thus prepared, the gland was considered to be free from any poison which might have been already secreted in a fluid form, and was treated with twenty-five drops of water, and kept at a temperature of 90° F. for thirty minutes, during which time it was frequently stirred, and compressed with a small pestle, while the water was renewed as it evaporated. The whole of the fluid was next drawn up into a fine tube, and carefully injected under the skin of the breast of a reed-bird. After four hours and twenty minutes, the bird was seen to be weak, but the local signs were of uncertain value. Twenty-one hours after poisoning, the bird was found dead. Its muscles were firm, the blood dark and loosely coagulated.

Experiment.—The remnant of gland tissue was put under the skin of a reed-bird, one portion being placed in the breast, another in the thigh. This bird died within twenty-one hours, and in it, also, the symptoms of local poisoning were deficient. The blood was even better coagulated than in the last case.

Experiment.—A snake of middle size (about two and a half feet long) was made to employ its glands, and was then decollated, the glands extracted, divided, and washed as usual. Ten drops of water were mixed with the tissue of this gland, and being placed in a test-tube, it was left at a temperature of 85° F. for two hours. The fluid was then drained from the gland, and injected into the thigh of a reed-bird. In two hours and four minutes the bird was becoming weak, and the extravasation of blood—which is the most marked symptom of Crotalus poisoning—was sufficiently distinct. Two hours later, the bird was rocking on its feet, and the extravasation was larger. It died during the following night. On examination, the muscles about the wound were softened, and even decomposing, and the blood was chiefly uncoagulated with an occasional clot of minute size and loose texture.

Experiment.—The remnant of gland used in the last observation was again treated with ten drops of water, which became slightly milky in hue on being agitated, and incorporated with the bruised tissue. After half an hour it was finally drained from the gland, and injected as usual under the breast skin of a reed-bird; proper precaution being always observed to avoid raising the skin too much. Within two hours and ten minutes the bird was weak, and the breast tissues contained a little extravasated blood. One hour and ten minutes later, the local symptoms were unaltered, and the bird weaker. It died during the ensuing night. Its wounds were slightly tinted with effused blood; but the muscles were not softened to the same extent as in the last case, nor were they at all decomposed. The blood of this bird was imperfectly coagulated.

Upon considering the foregoing experiments, it will be seen that all the pigeons escaped but one, that the rabbit was also unhurt, and that the reed-birds all died. These little birds are, however, uncommonly hardy, and, as we shall see in future, do not succumb readily when mechanically injured. Again, when, at this period, I subjected other reed-birds, to the number of ten, to similar wounds, and injected these with water and infusions of fresh muscle, only two out of the ten died. It is difficult, therefore, to avoid the belief that the reed-birds which received in their tissues the minced gland and its infusions, really perished from the rattlesnake poison; a belief which, on the whole, was strengthened by the state of their blood and muscles, and by the local signs which some of them exhibited. It is also to be observed that the reed-bird is remarkably susceptible to Crotalus venom, and will frequently die from a quantity of poison so minute that it would be hard to conceive of its power to destroy life, until we had made the experiment. Thus, while half a drop will often kill a reed-bird in a minute or two, one-eighth of a drop will prove fatal after a lapse of from two to eight hours; so that it is probable that even a smaller quantity would be found sufficient to destroy its existence. Now, as it is possible that quantities so minute may escape any mode of separation, and thus may remain in the gland tissue until the final infusion is formed, or even afterwards, we are not logically called upon to infer from the last series of experiments, that the material for a sudden temporary supply of venom-saliva is stored away in the gland in a semi-solid state. In this respect, therefore, the venom secretion is probably unlike saliva.

Again, unlike saliva, venom is formed slowly, and thence we have some right to infer that those provisions for rapid secretion, which belong to the salivary glands of man or the dog, need not exist in the poison gland of the serpent, and this view is certainly fortified, upon the whole, by the general result of the experiments above detailed.

In despite of what has here been urged, it is still desirable that these experiments should be repeated, with every possible modification; since, as I have endeavored to show, this, like all other portions of our subject, is girt about with such difficulties as may well baffle the most careful.

We have now to ascertain how much right the venom gland has to be regarded as a salivary organ, analogous to the parotid gland.

The argument from anatomy alone would certainly teach us to respect this view as correct, and to consider the poison gland as a true salivary organ. Its position and general structure all favor this idea, just as the appearance and minute anatomy of the pancreas were once believed to authorize us in placing that organ among the salivary bodies, and in giving to it the name of the abdominal salivary gland. But in this case, as in the one before us, the broader light of physiological inquiry has revealed the truth, that anatomical resemblance, even to the minutest details, does not of necessity involve physiological likeness. When, therefore, we turn from the anatomy of the poison gland to examine it under other points of view, we learn that in Crotalus its secretion is constantly acid, and in the Viper neutral, while the saliva of the parotid in all animals yet examined is as unchangeably alkaline. Again, while saliva is a secretion of rapid formation, and appropriated to specific mechanical and chemical purposes within the economy, the venom fluid is slowly elaborated, slowly reproduced when lost, and destined to no end *within* the body which produces it. Lastly, its singular nature as a ferment, poisonous to other animals as well as to its owner, constitutes a distinction, which, with the other points of difference already considered, forbid the physiologist to regard it as, in any true sense, a salivary secretion, or its forming organ as a salivary gland.

Effect of Various Temperatures on the Activity of Venom.—When I contemplated a series of researches upon the antidotes to Crotalus poisoning, I planned and executed a large number of experiments directed towards increasing our knowledge of the influence of physical and chemical agents upon the noxious properties of venom. Some of these researches were modified repetitions of work already done by others, but the majority were novel, and appear to me to cast considerable light upon the subject.

Especially do they clear the ground for more just conceptions of the real value and therapeutic possibilities of antidotes. Without them, also, no fitting idea of the singular energy of this poison could be formed, nor should we be able to conceive of the tenacity with which its powers are preserved in the presence of violent chemical reagents and extremes of heat and cold.

I was well aware that the dried venom retained its potency after two years of climatic changes, and that even the fresh poison, although prone to partial decomposition, might also remain active, after a sojourn of several weeks in an atmosphere of 65° to 70° F.

In the experiments upon the influence of extreme temperatures, I was obliged to resort to the following means:—

First. I established the fact that dilution did not injure the venom; and next, that minute quantities, as one-eighth or one-half of a drop, were fatal to the reed-bird within a few hours, more or less. As it was impossible to use large amounts of venom, owing to the economy with which I was forced to employ it, I arranged a tube of such size, that a marked half inch held one drop of a mixture made by adding four drops of water to one of the venom.

Experiment.—The marked tube was drawn to a capillary point, and a little venom sucked up into it, and so manipulated as to leave in the tube one drop of the mixture, representing one-fifth of a drop of venom. By very gentle suction, this was next drawn two inches up the tube, and the capillary point below, closed in the blowpipe flame.

Thus prepared, the tube was plunged in a freezing mixture, and kept at a temperature 3° to 4° above zero F. At the close of half an hour, the tube was placed in water at 70° F., and when the contents became fluid, the point of the tube was broken off, and the venom ejected into the breast tissues of a reed-bird, which died convulsed in twenty-seven minutes. Two repetitions of this experiment gave no different result.

The same little apparatus was also employed in the following experiments on the effects of heat on the venom. In each case the tube was charged, sealed at one end, and placed in water of the required temperature. In sustaining the standard of heat, it occasionally happened that the temperature rose one or two degrees too high, but this in no way affected the general result or its value. When the higher temperatures were used, the finger was sometimes placed on the open end of the tube, both to prevent the bubble of air below the venom from enlarging in the heat so as to expel the fluid above it, and also for the purpose of limiting evaporation.

The results attained are expressed in the following table:—

TIME OF EXPOSURE IN ALL THE CASES TWENTY OR THIRTY MINUTES.
AMOUNT OF VENOM ONE-FOURTH TO ONE-EIGHTH OF A DROP.

No.	Temperature.	Visible effects on the venom.	Result when injected into the breast of reed-birds.
1	112° F.	None	Killed in 35 minutes. Convulsions and marked local phenomena.
2	120° F.	None	Death in 27 minutes, convulsions, local signs.
3	130° to 134° F.	None	Death in 39 " " " "
4	140° to 142° F.	None	Death in 45 " " " "
5	(½ drop of venom) 148° to 151° F.	Slight coagulation took place.	Death in 43 " " " "
6	180° to 184° F.	Coagulation	Death in 48 " " " "
7	212° F.	Dense coagulation	Death in 2 hours. No convulsions or local signs.
8	212° F.	" "	No malady, except marked feebleness for 2 or 3 hours.
9	212° F.	" "	" " " " " "
10	212° F.	" "	The bird became weak in 20 minutes, and breathed laboriously for a time, but finally recovered. Slight and doubtful local signs.

The results exhibited in the table seemed to show that, while freezing did not alter the powers of the venom, it lost its toxicological vitality at a temperature of 212° F.

Upon re-examining this question at a later date, and with larger quantities of venom, I came to the conclusion that I had been mistaken, and that the most prolonged boiling was inadequate to destroy the virulence of the venom. The error into which I previously fell was due to the following causes:—

I have shown that after boiling, the active portions of the poison were the supernatant fluids, and not the coagulum. Now, when the amount employed was small, and the boiling was conducted in tubes of moderate calibre, the quantity of fluid surrounding the coagulum was in proportion minute. The larger part of it, therefore, clung to the tube, and was practically lost. That which adhered to the precipitate proved insufficient, in most cases, to destroy life, although some of the animals suffered from its use.

In August, 1860, a year after the first examination of this point, I carefully studied it anew. Not less than four drops of venom were employed in each case, and the process of boiling was varied in duration, so that in some cases it was continued for five minutes, in others for half an hour or more. Thus prepared, the coagulum and the supernatant fluid were thrown into the tissues of full-grown pigeons. Of six thus treated, all died with the usual symptoms.

In a second series of experiments, to which I have already alluded (see chemistry of the venom), the coagulum and supernatant fluid were separated by filtration; the coagulum washed, and the two products injected separately into two pigeons. In eight experiments of this kind it was found that the coagulum by heat was always innocent, the fluid as uniformly poisonous. It is unnecessary to relate these cases in detail, but it was further observed that the fatal cases died with the usual rapidity, a fact which permits us to suspect that the venom loses no power by being heated, and that the albuminoid compound, which constituted the coagulum, was not poisonous before its condition was altered by elevation of temperature.

We thus arrive at the conclusion that the venom of the Crotalus is toxically unaltered by freezing or boiling, and of course by the intermediate temperatures to which it may be subjected.

It is not a little curious that the animals which perished from the injection of boiled venom exhibited very trifling local evidences of the action of the poison. I am unable to offer any plausible explanation of this curious deficiency.

Influence of Certain Chemical Agents on the Activity of Venom.—In the following observations upon the influence of chemical agents on the activity of the Crotalus poison, certain necessary precautions were carefully attended to, without which the results attained would have been of but trifling value. Thus, for example, in using strong acids, alkalies, etc., it was necessary to make sure that the caustic action of these substances did not prove fatal to animals as small as the reed-bird. This end was obtained by carefully neutralizing the substances employed, after they had been allowed to affect the venom for a time. Where this could not be done, as with alcohol, etc., the result was checked or tested by experimenting with the substance alone, free from the presence of the venom.

It will be sufficient to give detailed accounts of some of these experiments, and to state merely the results of the remainder; since the precautions employed were similar in all the cases.

Alcohol.—I cannot find that Fontana actually mixed this fluid with venom, and then essayed its powers, with the object of ascertaining to what extent they were modified. Dr. Brainard[1] was probably the first to make this direct observation, not only with alcohol, but also with oil of turpentine, and the solutions of nitrate of silver, ammonia, soda, and potassa. He found that the mixture of these agents with venom did not alter or delay its action, provided the reagents were not of caustic strength.

Experiment.—The venom to be used having been previously tested and found to be potent, two drops of it were treated with twenty-five drops of alcohol. A dense coagulum formed, and at the close of ten minutes the mixture was injected into the breast tissues of a pigeon, which died, with slight local signs of poisoning, at the close of thirty-seven minutes. A check experiment was made at the same time, to learn how much the amount of alcohol used (twenty-five drops) would

[1] Smithsonian Report, 1854, p. 133.

affect the pigeon when injected alone. It appeared to cause slight stupefaction, which passed off rapidly.

Experiment.—About one-third of a drop of venom was treated with a drachm of alcohol. The mixture, which was allowed to evaporate to about seven drops, was placed under the skin of a reed-bird. It died in twelve minutes. When eight drops of alcohol were used alone, the bird was a good deal stupefied for two hours, but no serious result was observable.

Experiment.—About one-half of a drop of venom was mixed with about one drachm of alcohol, and kept four weeks. The precipitate at the bottom was then collected into a pipette, dried, redissolved in water, and thrown under the breast skin of a reed-bird. Slight local evidence of poisoning was visible, but the bird died within nine hours; an unusually long period. A repetition of this experiment gave a more sudden result, the bird dying in two hours.

A great number of observations similar to those just related convinced me that mere mixture with alcohol did not render the venom innocent.

As it appeared from Dr. Brainard's experiments, that in mingling the venom with active reagents, he had used these in a diluted state, I made a number of observations to learn whether or not these agents would affect the potency of the poison when allowed to act on it without previous dilution.

Experiment.—About one-third of a drop of pure venom was put upon a glass slide, and three drops of strong nitric acid were dropped upon it. Coagulation occurred, and in twelve minutes the acid was neutralized with liq. potassæ, and the mixture injected in three places into the breast and thigh of a reed-bird, which died in three hours. The wound was red, and not dark as usual, a fact which may have been owing to the presence of the nitrate of potassa. This observation was repeated twice with like results.

Similar experiments were made with strong sulphuric and muriatic acid, and with ammonia, chlorine-water, iodine, soda, and potassa. None of these agents destroyed the virulence of the venom. It is to be observed that in each case the contact was preserved during several minutes, and that the substances employed were neutralized before making the several injections.[1]

---

[1] When venom was mingled with certain of these agents, such as iodine in solution, tannic acid, etc., and then injected, the constitutional symptoms declared themselves as usual in the pigeons employed, but the local phenomena were more or less wanting. With this latter fact Dr. Brainard has made us acquainted, so far as iodine is concerned.

CHAPTER V.

TOXICOLOGY OF THE VENOM OF THE CROTALUS.

THE strange and subtle poison which we have hitherto considered chemically, will hereafter claim our attention in its relations to animal and vegetable life. In the course of study thus laid down, we shall be called upon to examine, first, its influence upon the lower vegetable existences. Secondly, its power to affect higher vegetable organisms, and the germination of seeds. Thirdly, its activity with relation to the lower animals; and, fourthly, the influence of the venom upon the mammalia, such as the dog, and, finally, man himself.

The subject of the power of serpent venom to destroy vegetable life has attracted the notice of but two, among the many observers who have studied the poison of Indian, European, or American reptiles. Neither of the observers alluded to has investigated the matter very fully, and I have, therefore, endeavored to fill the void thus left, as completely as possible.

Before I proceed to detail my own results, it will be proper to state, briefly, the conclusions at which others have arrived.[1]

Dr. Gilman says: "During the process of robbing several species of serpents (of venom), I inoculated several small, but vigorous and perfectly healthy vegetables with the point of a lancet well charged with venom. The next day they were withered and dead, looking as though they had been scathed with lightning."

The experiments thus described are so very limited, and so wanting in statement of details, that it is difficult to accord to them any great value as scientific evidence. Even in so trifling a matter as this, the sources of error are numerous, and we have a right to demand every possible knowledge as to the temperature and season, the size of the plants, the amount of venom employed, and the effect of wounding similar plants to the same extent, but without the use of the venom.[2]

---

[1] On the Venom of Serpents, B. J. Gilman, A. M. M. D., LL. D., St. Louis Med. and Surg. Journal, 1854, p. 25.

[2] An amusing story, which passed through three persons, reached the Philosophical Transactions (vol. xxxviii. p. 321) in the following form: "Sir Hans Sloan learned from Col. Beverley (Hist. of Va., 2d ed. p. 260) that Col. James Taylor, of Metapony, had stated to him that, having found a Rattlesnake, they cut off his head, with three inches of his body. A green stick, the bark being peeled off, was put to the head. It bit it, when small green streaks were observed to rise up along the stick towards the hand. At this juncture, the Colonel wisely dropped the stick, which, in a quarter of an hour, of its own accord, split into several pieces, and fell asunder from end to end."

The only remaining authority upon this portion of our subject, is Dr. Salisbury.[1]

A large female rattlesnake, without food for a year, died, and on dissection its poison ducts supplied Dr. Salisbury with a small amount of venom. This was used on plants, without having been tested upon animals.

"About fifteen minutes after its removal, four young shoots of the lilac (*Syringa vulgaris*), a small horse-chestnut of one year's growth (*Œsculus hippocastanum*), a corn plant (*Zea mays*), a sun-flower plant (*Helianthus annuus*), and a wild cucumber vine, were severally vaccinated with it. The vaccination was performed by dipping the point of a penknife into the poisonous matter, and then inserting it into the plant, just beneath the inner bark. No visible effect from the poison was perceptible until about sixty hours after it had been inserted. At this time, the leaves above the wound, in each case, began to wilt. The bark in the vicinity of the incision exhibited scarcely a perceptible change; in fact, it would have been difficult to have found the points, had they not been marked when the poison was inserted.

"Ninety-six hours after the operations, nearly all the leaf-blades in each of the plants, above the wounded part, were wilted, and apparently quite dead. On the fifth day, the petioles and bark above the incisions began to lose their freshness, and on the sixth day they were considerably withered. On the tenth day, they began to show slight signs of recovery. On the fifteenth, new but sickly-appearing leaves began to show themselves on the lilacs, and the other plants began to show slight signs of recovery in the same way. Neither of the plants was entirely deprived of life."

Dr. Salisbury afterwards comments upon the fact of the edges and apices of the leaves being the parts first attacked. He also states that the leaves below the points of innoculation were altogether unaffected, while those on the side upon which the venom was inserted were the first to suffer.

These experiments were made in June.

An objection to the want of a precedent test experiment upon animals as to the virulency of the poison used has been above suggested. This objection, it is true, loses some weight in the presence of a positive result. I have mentioned it, however, because it was possible that the secretion of the snake in question might have been altogether harmless, and the apparent results upon the plants only the effect of a mechanical injury to their tissues. This very result occurred to me during the summer of 1859.

A large snake, nearly five feet long, was sent to me from Iowa. It came in a very small, flat box, and was so coiled that it must have been difficult for it to move. When I removed it from its confinement it was sluggish, and was only induced to bite upon being much irritated. During the month of July the snake made no use of the bath in its cage; and, like the rest, took no food, nor did I feed it as I did some of its companions. A week before its death, there is a record on my notes of its having bitten a pigeon, which recovered in spite of a deep wound from

[1] Influence of the Poison of the Northern Rattlesnake (Crotalus durissus) on Plants. By J. H. Salisbury, M. D., N. Y. Journ. of Med., vol. xiii. New Series, 1854, p. 337.

one fang in the thigh. The snake was found dead on the seventh day after this occurrence.

Upon careful dissection, I found that the venom gland and the ducts on the right side, were full of a bloody fluid, with a faint alkaline reaction, and containing an abundance of club-shaped epithelial cells. The gland on the left side was nearly empty; its tissue was stained with blood. As I was curious to learn whether or not the altered poison had lost its power, I collected all the fluid contents of both glands, and their ducts, and inoculated with them the back, breast, and thigh of a pigeon, inserting in all about nine drops. The pigeon was slightly affected after the lapse of an hour, and was disposed to seek a corner and sleep. Four hours later, however, it was seemingly none the worse for the operation. A small oozing of serum took place from one of the wounds in the back, some days afterwards, but the pigeon suffered no permanent injury.

This result was enough to convince me that disease might alter the secretion of the venom glands, as it sometimes does that of the human salivary glands. I have alluded to it here, in order to fortify my criticism upon Dr. Salisbury's experiments. It is further to be observed, that Dr. Salisbury did not make any comparative observations, by wounding in a nearly similar manner, but with a clean weapon, plants of the same species and of equal size.

Beyond the points alluded to, there seems to be no objection to the experiments of Dr. Salisbury. He certainly appears to have been entirely successful in poisoning plants, with Crotalus venom; since, of eight plants injected, each and all seem to have suffered the same changes.

I have been the more willing to quote these results in full, because my own efforts to affect plants in the same way were singularly unfortunate. The point on which our experiments admit of no comparison is in regard to the species of the plant employed. At the season when I made my researches upon plant poisoning, I was unable to obtain the same plants as were used by Dr. Salisbury.

My first experiments upon plant poisoning were incidental to an examination of the power of Crotalus venom to prevent the occurrence of fermentation. After ascertaining, as I have already stated, that the conversion of starch into grape sugar was in no way interfered with when the venom was added to the mixture, I proceeded to ascertain whether or not the vinous fermentation would also take place in its presence.

Accordingly, a small amount of poison having been procured as usual, I found that it was fatal to a reed-bird, and then proceeded to make the following experiment.

Experiment.—Two test tubes of equal size, and capable of holding about one and a half ounces each, were fitted with corks, through which ran glass tubes, long enough to reach to the bottom. At the lower end, the contained tubes were bent at an acute angle, and drawn to a fine orifice. Above the cork they were also bent so as to form a double U-curve external to the test glass. Each of the test glasses was then filled with a solution of sugar in water, twenty grains of sugar being placed in each apparatus. To No. 1 were added a few drops of yeast, and to No. 2 about the same amount of yeast, together with five drops of venom. Both test tubes were next corked with care, so as to exclude any bubbles of air, and the level to which the fluid rose in the tubes having been marked, they were finally placed in an atmosphere of 75° F. Through accident the temperature was allowed to rise to 128° F. It afterwards fell to 80° F., was kept at this during two hours and a half, and was then abandoned to the atmospheric temperature, which varied during the experiment from 69° to 77° F. Experiments previously made, convinced me that the accidental rise of temperature would not be likely to injure the venom. The action of the ferment was unusually slow, but at the end of forty-eight hours both solutions had fermented, the test glasses were half full of carbonic acid gas, and the fluid thus displaced had risen through the tubes and overflowed externally.

Experiment.—On this occasion, I modified the process by leaving the ten drops of yeast in contact with three drops of venom for two hours, at a temperature of 79° F. In all other respects, the experiment resembled that last described. Within thirty-nine hours, both tubes had fermented freely. The remnant solutions within the test-tubes contained an abundance of yeast fungus, and I was, therefore, driven to the conclusion that the venom does not interfere with alcoholic fermentation, nor with the accompanying growth of sporules.

The next observations upon the effect of the venom on the lower vegetable growths, were accidentally introduced to my notice. They appear to me to be still more decisive than those last mentioned.

During the warm weather of August, I had mixed two or three drops of venom with eight or ten of water, and left the mixture in a corked test-tube on my table. It was neglected during two weeks, and when microscopically examined, was found to contain a number of what I took to be the sporules of fungi. During the month of September I repeated this observation upon some diluted poison which had been left in a test-tube during three weeks. In this specimen, I found an abundance of sporules.

As it was possible that the solution of venom might, by decomposing, have lost its virulence, I tested it by inoculating with it the breasts of two reed-birds which died with the usual local and general symptoms within two hours.

In passing to my experiments upon a higher order of plants, I began by using dried venom about two years old, but, as my experiments upon animals will show, of a potency only inferior to that of the freshest material.

Experiment.—During the month of June, 1859, four young shoots of tradescantia, a very succulent and rather tender trailing plant, were selected for experiment. Each of the shoots was split half way through, and about one-third of a grain of dry, pulverized venom was dropped into the opening, which was then allowed to close on the poison. The plants were next well watered, and a drop or two allowed to fall on the line of the incision. Four other shoots, two on the same, and two on other plants, were similarly, or even more mutilated, and in all cases the shoots chosen were from five to seven inches long. During a week, no result was obtained from these experiments. After that period, two of the unvenomed shoots, and one of the poisoned, became sickly, and gradually lost most of their leaves within the ensuing fortnight. So complete a negative result forbade any definite conclusions.

Later in the year, during the month of September, and early in October, I repeated these experiments upon the following plants, viz:—

A young shoot of the common bean, four inches high.

A young dahlia six inches high, and constituting the whole plant.

A long flower, or budding flower-stalk of medicinal colchicum, *C. Autumnale*, about ten inches high.

Three branches of geranium, growing on a large and healthy plant.

A small succulent garden weed, three inches high, of a species unknown to me.

I had no duplicates of the dahlia, bean, and weed mentioned above, which I could wound as a means of comparison, but in the case of the colchicum, I wounded, without poisoning, the remaining flower-stalk, which was rather more fully in bloom, and in the geraniums I wounded, in like manner, three branches, of sizes about equal to those of the stalks which I both wounded and poisoned.

The mode of introducing the venom, which, in these cases was perfectly fresh, and of tried and known potency, I varied in several ways. In the dahlia and colchicum I merely raised the outer bark longitudinally, and with a fine pipette slipped one drop of venom into the opening. I then bent the stalk slightly, so that the divided bark would rise a little from the surface beneath, and thus hold the venom by capillary attraction.

The weed was inoculated by splitting it near to the earth, and inserting a full drop of venom. The geranium branches were each surrounded by a little lip of wax, within which I put from one to two drops of the venom, and then filled the cups with four or five drops of water, having previously punctured the stems, so as to place the incisions below the level of the poisoned water. The water was renewed twice a day, and into one of the geranium branches I introduced, three days later, about one-third of a drop of venom, just above the wax. The cups fell off after four or five days, but neither in the bean, dahlia, colchicum, or geranium, did the leaves die, or the plants in any way suffer, although they were watched daily, during three weeks.

The weed alluded to was an accidental growth in the pot with the geranium. It appeared to droop two days after the poisoning. This was due, I presume, to a very cold night, after which the plants were carried into the house, when the one in question very soon revived. In many successive efforts to poison other plants with venom, I failed in every instance.

It is clear from the foregoing statements, that the venom of the Crotalus is not fatal to the growth of the *lower* orders of vegetable existence; but, unfortunately, no such definite inference can be drawn with regard to plants higher in the scale. My own experience, it is true, would, if considered alone, entitle me to assume the inactivity of Crotalus venom within the tissues of the plants essayed, and this conclusion would gain value, also, from what we know of the mode of its influence upon animals, and from the facts which we have made known as to the power of some forms of vegetative life to defy its influence. But, in the face of strong affirmative results, such as were obtained by Dr. Salisbury, I am unwilling to draw from my own negative experiments the same definite opinion which I should otherwise have felt authorized to base upon them. As I was indisposed to allow the question to remain without further answer, I made a number of experiments upon the ability of seeds to germinate in the venom, hoping to obtain in this manner a more complete solution of my doubts.

Here, owing to the circumstances of the experiment, the result may again be a negative one, and may still be open to all the doubts which encumber negative results.

Experiment.—October 5th, 9 A. M. I placed in each of two short test-tubes eight drops of water, and to one of them added one and a half drops of venom of known activity. On both tubes, upon the surface of each of the fluids, I laid a mesh of cotton wool, and upon it in each vessel fifteen canary seeds. The water in the two tubes was kept always at the same level, by the daily addition of the requisite amount of fluid. On the ninth day, none of the seeds in the venom had germinated, while two in the water were sprouting.

Twenty-one days after the observation began, the venom-tube offered no signs of seed-growth, and smelled very unpleasantly. The germs in the water were nearly half an inch in height.

As the small number of seeds which germinated in the water made it possible that none but incapable seeds might have fallen to the share of the venom-tube, I repeated the experiment without other variation of the circumstances than the substitution of mignionette seed for those last employed, and the use of a bell glass to limit the too rapid evaporation. Twenty seeds were allotted to each vase. This observation began Oct. 15th. On Oct. 24th, none of the seeds in the venom capsule had sprouted, while three of those in the water were in healthy bud, and some a little above the mesh of cotton. One additional test was required to add to these observations all the strength that could be given to them. It was possible that the venom, in decomposing, had lost its potency, and, as detailed previously, I tested it on animals, but still found it actively poisonous. At various times these experiments were again and again repeated, with slight modifications, but with no other result than continual failure to germinate on the part of seeds put in contact with venom.

It appeared probable from these observations, that venom has the power to prevent the germination of the seeds of plants such as those which I have mentioned above.

Action of Venom on Animal Life.—We have now reached a point where we turn from the influence of the venom upon vegetables, to study its power to affect animal existence.

In place of doubtfully deciding as to the cause of death, we are summoned to witness the operations of a substance which sometimes acts with a potency so swift as to defy observation, and which has a power to alter the blood and tissues in a manner, and with a celerity, which is a source of unending wonder, even to one who, by daily repetitions, has become familiar with the changes thus produced.

In the course of study now before us, I shall examine, as fully as possible, the effect of the venom upon cold-blooded animals, including the Crotalus, and upon various classes of warm-blooded animals.

After this general survey of the symptoms and pathology of the acute and chronic forms of venom poisoning, in these various classes of animals, I shall examine separately the influence of the venom upon the muscles, nerves, bloodvessels, and blood itself. This general practical examination will enable us to review the theories hitherto in vogue, and to ascertain, if possible, the proximate mode in which this mysterious substance may be supposed to act.

In following the track here pointed out, I shall relate, at length, the cases, symptoms, etc., observed in a considerable number of animals, and I shall allude, briefly, to a still larger number whose cases it will be needless to state in detail. Although I shall thus record more experiments than have been made by any other observer who has studied the subject of Crotalus poisoning, it will, I fear, be but too plain that the research is one which demands the labors of many, and is, indeed, of such a nature that some of the questions involved in it, can only be settled by persons of greater leisure than myself, and who, at the same time, are so situated as to be able to procure a constant supply of fresh snakes.

It would, perhaps, be more in order to begin this section of our subject by an examination of the relations of serpent venom to the absorbing surfaces. It will, however, prove a convenience, as well as an economy of space, if, in place of this we defer the study of the absorption of venom until we have fully considered its effects on animals; since, in so doing, we shall be obliged to detail many of the facts which bear upon the deferred question.

It will be remembered that, upon page 50 of this Essay, I stated that, on several occasions I had noticed the production of fungi in moist venom, long kept upon my table, in an atmosphere of from 64° to 70° F. I have also observed in the same and in other specimens of venom long kept, and somewhat diluted, that after seven to ten days, the poison acquired an odor of a peculiar and very disgusting character. The production of this animalized and indescribable stench was accompanied by the appearance of vibriones, and, a few days later, of rotiferæ and other minute forms of animalcular life. The occurrence of these little beings in a fluid so deadly, prompted me to learn whether or not it had lost, by decomposition, any part of its specific nature as a poison; for, although I was aware that the cuticles of higher animals opposed a perfect resistance to the passage of the venom, I did not suppose that the delicate organisms here spoken of could, by any possibility, escape its action, when born and developed within it. At all events, this view opened to me a channel for observation of which I had not thought before, and whose value I therefore proceeded to test, as stated on page 52, by determining what power yet remained in the venom which had become the nidus of so much active vitality.

It was my intention to examine, in the next place, the effect of the venom upon leeches, fish, eels, and crustacean animals, but for reasons which it is needless to relate, I was obliged to postpone these observations until some future occasion.

I was the more desirous, however, of making these examinations, because Fontana had already decided that leeches, snails, and slugs, were unaffected by the venom of the viper, and because some of his numerous observations in this direction were open to criticism, from his having failed to observe the animals as long as he should have done after the infliction of the poisoned wound, a precaution which, as I shall show, is absolutely essential when studying the influence of the venom upon cold-blooded animals.

Action of Venom on Frogs.—This industrious and most able writer is also the only one who has recorded the effects of the viper poison on frogs,[1] and, so far as I am aware, no one has repeated these observations. It is to be regretted that he did not state the size of the frogs bitten, since in such facts, or in the fresher state of his snakes, might have been found the reasons why the frogs which were subjected to the Crotalus venom, usually lived so much longer than those upon which the learned Abbé experimented. In the total want of knowledge as to the power of rattlesnake poison over frogs, I shall quote the passage from Fontana, in which he relates the results he obtained when making use of viper poison.

He says, "I procured fifty of the largest and strongest frogs I could meet with. I had each of them bit by a viper, some in the thighs, others in the legs, back, head, etc. Some of them died in less than half an hour, others in an hour, and others again in two, three hours, or somewhat more. There were some again that were not affected, whilst others that did not die became nevertheless swelled. There were, likewise, others among them that fell into a languishing state, their hind legs that had been bit, continuing very weak, and even paralytic. In some of them I contented myself with introducing cautiously into a wound, made with a lancet at the very instant, a drop of venom. These last, however, lived longer than those I had bit; neither of them, however, escaped. I constantly took the precaution to prevent the venom I introduced into the wound being carried out by the blood that flowed from it. Some of these frogs swelled very much, others but little, and others not at all. The wounds of almost all of them were inflamed more or less. There were some, however, that died very suddenly, without the smallest mark of inflammation. A short time after these animals had been either bit, or wounded and venomed, the loss of their muscular force, as well as that of the motion of their extremities, was very evident. When they were set at liberty they no longer leaped, but dragged their legs and bodies along with great difficulty, and could scarcely withdraw their thighs when they were pricked with a needle, of the pain of which they seemed almost insensible. By degrees they became motionless and paralytic in every part of the body, and after continuing a very short time in this state died."

With this exception, and a few further remarks by the same author, we are without information as to the effect of viper venom upon the frog.

Of the effects of Crotalus venom upon the same animal, we know as little, and, so far as I am aware, only a single recorded experiment of this kind is to be found in the writings of American authors;[2] their only observations upon cold-blooded reptiles having been made on the Crotalus itself, or other serpents. We shall now proceed to study the details of the experiments which I have made upon cold-blooded animals.

Upon classifying the cases before us, it will be discovered that they divide them-

---

[1] Fontana on Poisons, Chapter VI. p. 34, vol. i. Translation by J. Skinner, London, 1787.

[2] A single observation by Harlan.

selves naturally and conveniently into two classes, which I shall term acute and chronic, or primary and secondary poisoning.

While in the batrachia the distinction between these two sets of cases is sufficiently clear, it is less well marked than in warm-blooded animals. At the time I was engaged upon this portion of my investigation, the active serpents in my collection were not so large as those which I afterwards received. This may account for the fact that, although I have some records of frogs more or less acutely poisoned, the majority of those bitten lived long enough to exhibit, in a marked manner, the secondary lesions which I shall have occasion hereafter to describe.

The class of cases which I shall term acute, were marked by the negative character of the symptoms. In them the local signs of poisoning were very slight, and the changes in the blood which occurred where life was prolonged after a serious bite, were absent, or but very slightly marked.

Experiment.—A large frog recently caught, was attached to a string and lowered into a cage containing four snakes, none of which were over thirty-six inches long. As I had often observed, no provocation induced them to strike the frog, and, therefore, after many vain efforts, I drew a snake into the snake-tube, and placed the frog in its jaws. The serpent bit with eagerness, and the frog, uttering a cry, leaped from its re-opened jaws to the floor, and for a few moments used its legs so well as to avoid being caught. When at length it was secured, I searched in vain for the fang wound, which must have been very small; I did not discover it until after death, although I was sure that the skin had been penetrated, because a large bubble of air had found entry to the dorsal sub-cuticular sac.

The presence of air in this situation often enabled me to be confident that the fang had pierced the skin. It is occasioned by the attempt on the part of the serpent to withdraw its fang, which, catching, raises the loose skin, and creating a partial vacuum, thus draws air alongside of the fang into the subjacent cavities. A little quivering on the right flank, also, caused me to suspect that as the part bitten. Except in dogs, who shiver so much from mere fright, the local muscular twitchings alluded to are also of some value in calling attention to the part bitten. Two hours after this frog was poisoned, it was dead, having exhibited during the interval occasional convulsive motions of the limbs.

P. M. Dissection.—As soon as all motions, reflex and other, were at an end, the thorax and belly were laid open. The intestines responded to irritants. The heart was beating feebly, but in all of its cavities, and was large and dark. It ceased to pulsate at the close of three hours and ten minutes after the poisoning, and on being opened, was found to contain blood which coagulated perfectly after short exposure. The clot was well formed and firm. The muscles were irritable to all forms of stimulus during eleven hours, and, as I have usually observed, this property lasted longest in the muscles under the chin.[1] Nervous irritability existed until the close of the fourth hour. The seat of the wound was the right flank, into the muscles

---

[1] Brown-Séquard, Bernard, Vulpian, and before them, Fontana, have noted the long retention of irritability by the diaphragm muscles. In the frog, the sub-mental group corresponds in function to these, as I have shown elsewhere.

of which the fangs had entered obliquely, both teeth taking effect. There was more serum than usual in the dorsal sac, through which the weapons passed, and their track was marked by a little darkening of the neighboring muscles.

In twenty-four hours the muscular parts about the bite were almost diffluent, while the rest of the frog had no odor, or any other sign of putrefaction.

Experiment.—A large snake, from which I had in vain attempted to extract venom, was secured in the snake-box as usual. Before releasing it, I placed a small frog, about four or five inches long, in its mouth, so that when it bit, which it did fiercely enough, the fang entered the belly. Slight local quivering of the nearer muscles, and some convulsive extensions of the hind legs, were the only marked signs, and no notable changes in the pupil was perceived until death took place, when it dilated. At the close of sixty-two minutes, neither voluntary or reflex motions could be elicited.

P. M. Section.—The wound exhibited no local evidences of poisoning. The aperture in the skin was small, and but one fang had entered. In passing through, or out of the sub-cuticular abdominal walls, the fang tore these structures, so as to make a distinct opening, through which a little serum from the dorsal sac had passed, and carrying with it a little blood, had found its way into the peritoneal cavity. None of the abdominal viscera were transfixed. The ventricle of the heart beat only for fifteen minutes after it was exposed. The auricles beat feebly for one hour and forty minutes after this period. The nervous irritability was extinct everywhere thirty minutes after voluntary and reflex movement ceased, while the muscular irritability lasted but half an hour longer, and was thus entirely absent when the auricles of the heart were still pulsating. The blood in the heart clotted on exposure.

Experiment.—A small snake was teased until it struck a frog of medium size, and was itself so caught that it hung for a moment, when I drew the frog out by pulling on the string with which I had secured it. Upon inspection, it seemed that the fang had struck upon the spine. On being released, the frog appeared very uneasy, and for ten or twelve minutes was incessantly leaping about in the glass vessel in which it had been placed. At the close of half an hour, the frog became suddenly quiet, and shortly after was attacked with a general quivering of the muscles, followed by the loss of volitional control. Slight reflex acts were still capable of being produced, when the limbs were violently stimulated by mechanical means, but at the close of an hour from the period of poisoning, these also ceased, the eyelids became motionless when touched, and the frog being considered dead, was opened.

P. M. Section.—One fang was found to have entered the spine, and slightly wounded the medulla, which was rather too much injected with blood, but otherwise unaltered in structure. All the remaining viscera were healthy, and the heart was still acting with all its cavities as late as two hours and a half after the poisoning, when the observation stopped for a time. Four hours later, the organ had ceased to pulsate, and was only possessed of a slight localized irritability under stimulus. The blood was well coagulated.

The above quoted instances were the only cases of rapid death which I was called upon to observe in this class of animals. Their discussion will occupy us at another time.

From a large number of instances of death in frogs, from the secondary or chronic action of the venom, I have selected the most interesting, and those which best illustrate the nature of the symptoms.

Experiment.—Temperature 84° F. A very large frog was struck by a snake two and a half feet long, on the back of the pelvis, upon the left side. Twenty-five hours and five minutes after the blow, the frog was re-examined, and found to be inert and sluggish, but still able to move. During the interval, it occupied a glass jar containing a large wetted sponge, and partly open at top. The back of the frog was darker than usual, and presented a fluctuating mass of fluid beneath the skin. The eyes were natural, the respirations occurred now and then, and the lymph-hearts, at the end of the spine were acting as usual. One day later the frog's condition was much as before. On the third day it was motionless, except under excessive stimulus, when it leaped once or twice, or if placed on its back, turned itself over with great difficulty. On the fourth day the swelling on the back diminished somewhat, and the subcuticular sacs of the legs became swollen.

From this time the frog grew weaker, although put in water daily for an hour or two, and every pains taken to preserve it in a healthy state. It died during my absence on the fifth day.

P. M. Section.—The muscles in the track of the fang which had not entered deeply, were dark in color, and underwent extreme decomposition within twenty-four hours, while the rest of the body was not sensibly affected. About the wound, in the dorsal sac, were large quantities of bloody serum, which coagulated feebly upon exposure. The other sacs, wherever examined, were also filled with bloody serum, and a similar fluid was found in the peritoneum and pericardium. Bloody mucus flowed from the mouth and nostrils, and the stomach and mucous surface of the intestines were stained with frequent patches of extravasated blood. The lungs were shrunken, but contained no blood. The heart, which was pale and unirritable, contained only two minute and very pallid clots, adherent to the auricular walls. The muscles of the legs and the flanks responded feebly to galvanism during one hour and thirty minutes after exposure. Those of the forelegs were also irritable, but, singularly enough, the muscles under the jaw had lost their power to act. The muscles were generally pale, owing to the great loss of blood. The sheaths or fascia were stained with blood in nearly every part of the body, and even between the separate muscles and the bone. There was no post-mortem rigor observed.

Experiment.—Temperature 74° F. A large frog was bitten fiercely by a snake three feet long, which thrust one fang deeply into the left thigh. The other fang missed the leg entirely. During the five succeeding hours, the subject was watched by an assistant, who described the wound as exuding bloody serum, while the animal remained in one position, quite motionless. It died during the following night, when unobserved, and was found the next day in a state of rigor, a good deal shrunken, although great pains had been taken to keep it constantly moistened.

P. M. Section.—The bitten leg was greatly swollen, and the muscles beneath were livid with extravasated blood. Everywhere in the injured limb the muscles were deeply stained with blood, and this appearance was not confined to this limb, but existed also in the leg not bitten. About the bite, the muscular structure was almost diffluent, and could be torn with the utmost ease. A slight effusion of blood was found under both forelegs, in the axillary spaces. Elsewhere the organs were healthy. The heart was unirritable, and contained a little thin uncoagulated blood. Nervous irritability was extinct, and that of the muscles absent, except under the chin, where it remained for an hour or more after exposure.

Experiment.—Temperature 74° F. A second frog of large size was bitten twice by the same snake which had just bitten the last one. On each occasion, a single fang entered, the leg and the thigh being thus wounded. From these wounds, a bloody serum continually oozed, until I ceased to observe it. Certainly, a drachm or more of fluid exuded in this manner. On the second day, matters were as before. On the third, the frog was very sluggish. The bitten leg was enormously swollen to the very end of the toes, which, on being held up to the light, were seen to be distended with red serum. The skin of this member was also soaked, in places, with extravasated blood. On the fourth morning, the frog was found to have died during the night.

P. M. Section.—Slight rigor mortis. The bitten leg was literally soaked in blood to the extreme edges of the web, and was everywhere swollen by this local accumulation. The flexors of the thigh were filled with blood, so as to be dark crimson throughout their thickness. A little bloody fluid was present in most of the sub-cuticular sacs. The heart was pale, bloodless, and unirritable. The other organs were normal. The nerves and muscles proved to have lost their power to react under stimulus. The little blood found in the vessels was diffluent. As in some other cases, the fluid of the dorsal lymphatic sac coagulated feebly upon exposure to the air.

Experiment.—Temperature 73° F. A small frog was bitten on the back, below the scapula, by a snake about three feet long, which had already used its fangs once within twenty-four hours. The fang-mark was not visible, but from the presence of air in the dorsal sac, I was convinced that the weapon had entered. The muscles about the bitten part immediately began to quiver, and this motion soon extended to both flanks. The frog became rapidly weak, and within an hour and a half could not turn when laid on its back, and was unable to use its hind legs. At this time the pupils were contracted, the eyes half closed, and the lids of the right organ completely insensible, the left one nearly so. The frog shortly afterwards lost all voluntary power, even in the forelegs, but exhibited slight reflex phenomena up to the fifth hour, when it was apparently dead.

P. M. Section.—The wound passed through the muscles below the scapula, and into the liver and peritoneal cavity, which contained a little bloody fluid. The heart was beating forty-four to the minute, auricles and ventricle acting. Half an hour later the auricles alone were acting, and these were arrested during the ensuing period of ten hours, although carefully protected from desiccation. The nerves everywhere were highly irritable, but this passed away completely within half an hour. The muscular irritability remained good during two hours. Ten hours later, no muscle responded to irritants. The small amount of blood found in the heart was fluid. It is to be remarked that, in some of these cases, nothing was more difficult than to ascertain whether the minute amount of blood present was coagulated or not. Both lungs were gorged with blood, and the intestines were dotted with specks of extravasated blood, although no free blood was found in the intestinal canal.

The cases above quoted illustrate nearly every peculiarity of the effects of the venom upon batrachia, whether affecting them rapidly or slowly.

It is necessary to the completion of this study, that we recount, also, the manner in which the dried venom of the Crotalus acted upon these cold-blooded animals. In one respect its action is undoubtedly peculiar.

I have already alluded, in several instances, to the dried venom of the Crotalus. The specimen used in the following experiments was given to me by Prof. Leidy, who received it from my friend Prof. Wm. A. Hammond. It was obtained in Kansas, in the autumn of 1857, by a process similar to that which I have described on page 28. It had been allowed to dry into thin yellow scales, and was preserved in this condition in a small bottle, not very well secured from the air.

Prof. Christison had already stated that cobra poison, fourteen years old, was still effective. Mangili[1] had ascertained the same of viper poison eighteen months old.

Orfila,[2] in recounting the experiments of the author last named, observes that they proved contradictory of the statements of Fontana,[3] an assertion which is only partially correct, since the learned Abbé distinctly states that viper poison is active after being preserved for several years in the cavity of a dry fang. He adds, moreover, that the powdered and dried venom had been kept by him for several months without loss of its power, and he also adduces Redi's[4] experience to the same effect. At the close of these statements he remarks, however, that the poison may lose its potency by being kept, and that this took place frequently when he attempted to preserve it longer than ten months. As we shall have occasion to see, this is not the only instance where the learned Abbé has been misquoted and misunderstood. Few authors of such merit as Fontana have had so little justice at the hands of those who have followed them, and this remark applies not alone to his work on the Viper, but to his researches on Ticunas, and to other labors, many of the results of which have been assiduously re-discovered by more modern observers.

Experiment. Poisoning by Dried Venom.—Temperature 79° F. A frog of middle size received in the muscles of the back a small quantity of dried venom. An unenvenomed wound of corresponding size was inflicted upon the other side of the spine. On inspection, twenty-one hours after, the frog was found seated and quiet. During half an hour no respiration occurred. Upon touching the eye, the frog breathed once and moved its entire body, after which no further motion could be provoked, and the animal seemed to be dead.

P. M. Section.—On comparison, the two wounds were so much alike, that no dif-

[1] Mangili, Annales de Chimie et de Physique, Février, 1817, from Giornale di Fisica Chimica, etc., vol. ix. p. 458.

[2] Orfila, Traité de Toxicologie, t. ii. p. 852.

[3] Fontana, vol. i. Chapter XXII. p. 65.

[4] Redi, see also Russell, p. 63.

ference could be perceived between them. Not the least sign of swelling, congestion, or inflammation, was visible about either. The heart, which was large and dark, beat fifteen in the minute, all its cavities acting feebly until it was cut out, at the close of half an hour.

The nerves of the legs were irritable for rather over an hour, and the muscular excitability endured but two hours longer, when post-mortem rigor came on. The cardiac blood coagulated very well.

Experiment.—A little dried venom was placed in the muscles of the thigh of a frog. As the wound bled rather freely, a second portion was inserted in the lumbar muscles. The frog died during the ensuing night, within twenty-one hours of the poisoning. When examined, there was not the slightest local sign of the presence of venom, nor was there bloody serum in any of the lymphatic sacs. The nerves and muscles were unexcitable. The heart was at rest, and was not irritable. It contained a little coagulated blood. Other viscera healthy.

Experiment.—A fang recently shed, together with a small quantity of dried venom, was buried in the muscles of the back. After death, the muscles about the imbedded fang were softened, and dotted with points of blood. A little bloody serum was found in the cuticular sac of the wounded thigh. About the spot wounded with the dry venom, there was a little redness, but no softening or extravasation. The remaining symptoms of the case are valueless in this connection.

The chief reason for quoting the above cases here, is to call attention to the almost utter absence of local symptoms when dried venom was used in frogs.

Effect of the Venom upon the Crotalus.—This research resolves itself into two propositions, or rather, questions. First, Can the Crotalus kill its own species? Second, can any individual snake destroy itself?

The first of these queries has been more or less completely answered, as regards certain Indian snakes, the viper of Europe, and our own Crotalus. Russell[1] made a Cobra bite a nooni-paragoodoo near the anus. It died in one hour and a quarter. A little local discoloration existed about the wound, and the lungs were full of blood. A Cobra bit another Cobra, with a negative result. How long it was observed, is not stated.

A Coodum-nagoo bit a Cobra, the two fangs taking effect, the result, as before, being negative. All of these snakes were venomous.

A Coodum-nagoo bit a Tortutta, a harmless serpent, which perished within two hours.

Fontana's[2] experiments on the effect of the venom of the viper upon its own kind, were briefly as follows:—

One viper was bitten by another several times. The wounds swelled a little. It was killed by Fontana after thirty-six hours, and found to have been deeply wounded, the bites being a little inflamed and swollen.

A middle-sized viper received from two large ones six fang wounds. The viper remained agile, and was well at the end of four days. When killed, it was found

---

[1] Russell, p. 56.

[2] Fontana, vol. i. p. 29 *et seq.* Skinner's translation.

to have been bitten through and through. The wounds were somewhat inflamed. Five other vipers thus bitten, did not die. Length of observation not mentioned. Again, a portion of skin having been removed from the backs of four vipers, seven vipers were made to bite them. None of the bitten animals died, and only one of them was at all languid, and had a little swelling about the wound. Three vipers were wounded in the back, and the wound filled with venom. The wounds inflamed, but did not swell. The animals seem to have been killed at the end of several days. A viper was forced to bite itself; it did not die. Another was made to bite on a piece of jagged glass, so that its mouth was wounded as the poison flowed into it. On the seventh day the wounds were healed.

M. Bernard[1] recently repeated Fontana's experiments, and found that a viper which had been both bitten and inoculated artificially with venom, died on the third day. Upon this experiment, M. Bernard criticizes Fontana, as having observed the viper and pigeons together, and having concluded that, because the cold-blooded animal was not affected so soon as the other, that it was incapable of being killed by the venom. As we have seen, however, some of Fontana's experiments were observed during periods of time much greater than that required to destroy the viper observed by M. Bernard. Thus, although Fontana was most probably mistaken in his conclusions, he did not fail in the point criticized, from any glaring neglect of continued observation.

The American authorities upon this matter are brief, but decided. They refer principally to the power of the snake to destroy itself, and to this point, indeed, my own experiments have been directed, since it was plain that if the individual could thus be made to kill itself, there could be no added difficulty in comprehending its ability to kill its fellows.

Besides including the general proposition, the question before us has a specific interest, from the fact that snakes are often accidentally hurt about the mouth, and that abrasions of this cavity must frequently occur. We are, therefore, called upon to say why the snake suffers so little from wounds on which a poison so deadly to other animals must fall from time to time.

Our own writers[2] state almost unanimously that the Crotalus is able to kill itself. Without quoting them in full, it is enough to add that their experiments were commonly made by switching a snake until it turned and struck itself. Death is usually described as following within a few minutes.

At the close of a series of experiments on warm-blooded animals, I made use of some of my largest snakes in the following manner:—

Experiment.—Temperature 65° to 75° F. A small snake about twenty-seven inches long, was caught by the neck, and its tail placed in its mouth. It bit, but did not wound. A portion of skin having been removed from the back, it was

---

[1] Claude Bernard, Leçons sur les Effets des Substances Toxiques, etc., 1857, p. 291.

Dr. Brown-Séquard appears to have made experiments upon the Viper, but I have been unable to find his paper.

[2] Burnett, p. 323.

allowed to bite again, and when the fangs were fixed in the naked muscles, the upper jaw was violently pressed downwards, so as to wound the part deeply.

Upon the sixth day, the wound was covered with a gray exudation, such as is usually found upon the healing surface of the wounds of serpents. This snake died on the fourteenth day. The tissues about the bite were congested, the gall-bladder full, mucus in the stomach, the venom glands dark from effused blood.

Experiment.—A large snake was made to bite himself twice, in a space near the cloac, where the skin had been removed. This serpent also died on the fourteenth day. The wound was apparently healthy, and not to be distinguished from any other wound, except that the muscles about it were a little softened. The blood was uncoagulated, but there was no other visible lesion of any internal organ.

Experiment.—On the same day a large snake, fifty-six inches long, had a small portion of the skin on the back loosened and turned over, so as to make a flap. On this wound was placed about a drop of venom from the snake itself. The poison was finally thrust into a number of superficial cuts made in the muscles on which the drop fell. On the second day, the snake being well to appearance, half a drop of its own venom was put in a superficial wound half way up the back. This wound seemed to excite the snake, which, on being replaced in its box, continued in very rapid and violent motion for some minutes, as though in pain. On the sixth day, both wounds were covered with gray exudation, and beneath, the muscles were soft, but in this, as in other cases, no effusion of blood existed about the wound. The snake was sluggish, and indisposed to bite. It died on the tenth day.

P. M.—There were no visceral lesions, except that one lung contained a little effused blood. The venom glands were dark and congested. The heart blood coagulated firmly, thirty minutes after removal. In all probability this serpent died from some other cause than venom poisoning.

Experiment.—A snake forty-six inches long was secured, and the skin just above the anus removed from a space of about one inch by two. On this, the snake bit itself three times, throwing out a good deal of venom which was thrust deeply into the muscles of the part. On the second day, the wounded muscles were softened, but no blood was effused. The wound had been re-covered with skin, and secured by sutures. At the close of two weeks this snake was healthy, and bit eagerly. The wounds were partially healed.

Experiments.—Three large serpents were made to disgorge their venom, and the poison from each snake was injected under the skin of its back, with the aid of a small syringe and trocar. The snakes, which I will distinguish as numbers one, two, and three, received respectively ten, eight, and seven drops of poison.

No. 1 died in thirty-six hours. The wound was surrounded by softened tissues, but was not stained with blood. The organs generally were normal, except the stomach, which contained bloody mucus. The heart was full of clotted blood.

No. 2 died in sixty-seven hours. The local appearances in this case were much as in the last one, but less extensive. The interior organs were healthy, and the heart contained two loose and soft clots.

No. 3 died during the seventh day. The wound, in this case, penetrated the muscles, which were dark and much softened. The blood in the heart was mostly diffluent, presenting but a single small coagulum of loose structure. The intestines were spotted with ecchymoses, and the peritoneal cavity contained about a drachm of fluid blood.

I may add to these cases the numerous instances in which I have wounded the mouths of snakes, or torn the vagina dentis, while robbing them of poison. On none of these occasions has any serious result followed the injury, even where venom had fallen upon the abraded surfaces in considerable amount.

The above experiments were on the whole so definite in their results, that I did not think it necessary to multiply them. I had very many times injured snakes far more than these were injured by their own fangs, or the preparatory manipulations, and I, therefore, felt at liberty to conclude that the animals employed on these latter occasions really died from the venom. The length of time required for this to occur was curious, and far exceeded in most of them that which was noted in Bernard's case, or in the many instances of which I have been told where rattlesnakes had stricken themselves.

One of the factors in the experiment, and one which has been too much neglected, is the temperature, which in my own cases was very moderate during the day, and fell a good deal lower at night, the observations having been carried on during a cool period in September, 1859. M. Bernard, Russell, and Fontana, give no record of the temperature during their observations. That it is a very important condition in the venom poisoning of the cold-blooded batrachia I have frequently observed, and it is highly probable that in all cold-blooded animals the elevation of temperature carries with it an increase of danger from poisons, and especially from those of a septic nature.

When we examine the pathological effects of the venom in warm-blooded animals, we shall see that, while the general phenomena were essentially the same as in cold-blooded reptiles and batrachia, they were far more rapidly produced. The Crotalus itself was a good illustration of this contrast, and was in other respects exceptional in the mode in which it was affected, since, while the muscles were altered, as in warm-blooded creatures, the blood coagulated better than was usual in them, and the visceral lesions were less severe, and less frequent. On the other hand, while the frog was for its size remarkably unimpressible by Crotalus venom, the phenomena which in it accompanied the examples of slow poisoning, were in no respect different from those developed in the warm-blooded animals. To this subject we shall recur, after studying the effects of the venom upon the higher animals.

CHAPTER VI.

TOXICOLOGICAL ACTION OF THE VENOM UPON WARM-BLOODED ANIMALS.

We shall now enter, without other comment, on the study of the effects of Crotalus venom upon warm-blooded animals.

Of all warm-blooded creatures, birds are most susceptible to the influence of this poison. So sudden, indeed, were its effects in some of them, that when the dose of the venom was large, there was hardly time to observe the resultant phenomena. In larger birds this extreme sensibility to the poison also existed, when the dose was in proportion greater. So minute, however, was the quantity required to kill a small bird, such as the reed-bird, that under certain circumstances these little creatures became very delicate tests of the presence or relative activity of the venom.

Experiment.—A pigeon was lowered into the snake-box, and was struck once, high up on the back, by a snake of middle size, which had just used its fangs. Upon this occasion, both fangs were buried deeply. On being released, the pigeon walked across the table, and seeking a corner, remained at rest, until, at the close of three minutes it fell down, and immediately began to breathe convulsively, now and then gaping, and making efforts to rise. The difficulty in the respiration seemed to be due to the general weakness, which interfered with all the other movements at the same time. The bird became more and more feeble, the breathing more labored, and at the end of the seventh minute the head fell to one side, the breathing ceased, and the bird died without convulsions.

P. M. Section.—Both fang marks were surrounded by circles of extravasated blood, about three lines in breadth. The motor nerves of the wings and legs were irritable nine minutes after death. The muscles remained irritable during twenty-nine minutes, when post-mortem rigor appeared in the legs, and soon became general. The heart beat with all its cavities, four minutes after respiration ceased. Both auricles and ventricles were sensitive to mechanical stimulus nine minutes after death. Two minutes later, the ventricles ceased to respond, but the auricles were more or less irritable fifteen minutes after death. The blood coagulated moderately well. It was very dark, but on exposure became bright red.

Experiment.—Temperature 74° F. A pigeon secured by a string was thrown into a snake-box. Two snakes of middle size, two and a half to three feet long, struck at it as soon as it began to flutter. The pigeon was at once removed and put on the table, where, in two minutes it showed signs of weakness, staggered to and fro, and at last, as usual, sought refuge in a corner. At the sixth minute, its breathing became labored and jerking, and the muscles about the wound were twitching locally. At the sixteenth minute, the breathing was still jerking, but more rapid, the bird crouched as if asleep, the eye natural; the pupil, if changed at all, a little contracted. At the thirty-sixth minute the head fell, the eyes closed, respiration became rare and labored, and the pupils contracted. Cloac temperature 104½° F. At the fortieth minute, the head was bent suddenly forward on the breast, and after three such motions of a convulsive nature, respiration ceased at the forty-second minute.

P. M. Section.—The head was cut off at once, and the blood received in a capsule. It was dark, but became red on exposure, and coagulated firmly, at the close of four minutes. Nervous irritability existed feebly in the sciatic nerves, nine minutes after death. Elsewhere it continued to the twelfth or thirteenth minute, when a probe thrust down the spine occasioned no motion. Ten minutes after death the muscles were everywhere very irritable. Thirty-three minutes after death this property was present only in the thighs and the diaphragm. In both of these localities it was still perceptible fifty-six minutes after death. Ten minutes later, I could not feel sure of its existence. The heart, which was large and dark, ceased to beat ten minutes after respiration stopped, and two minutes later had totally lost all irritability to stimulus. The auricles contained a little dark blood, chiefly uncoagulated, with the exception of two small and soft clots.

Experiment.—A snake four feet long was secured and made to bite a pigeon, which it seized so that one fang entered the knee. This pigeon had recovered from a former bite with the loss of a portion of the pectoral muscles. It was well and active. Upon its being bitten, I threw it from me, but, to my surprise, its wings were motionless, and it fell a dead weight on the table, and did not afterwards breathe or move. Thirty seconds elapsed between the bite and the death.

P. M. Section.—Some little delay occurred, owing to the unexpected nature of the death, and on exposing the heart within three or four minutes, it had ceased to beat, although it responded to stimulus feebly and locally for a few minutes longer. The nerves in the thigh were irritable during twenty-eight minutes. The muscles everywhere lost their irritability within two hours and ten minutes.

Cases of chronic or secondary poisoning were, naturally, rare in birds, and if they survived a few hours, they frequently recovered. The following cases illustrate sufficiently well the chronic form of poisoning.

Experiment.—Temperature 77° F. A large white pigeon was thrown into the snake-box, the inmates of which seemed, for a time, reluctant to use their power. Finally a snake two feet in length bit the pigeon once in the breast, and became so entangled, that bird and serpent rolled over together. On examining the wound, two fang marks were found in the pectoral region, but so much of the venom had been cast upon the neighboring feathers, that I presumed the wound could not be rapidly mortal. Three hours after its infliction, the bird drooped a little and was disposed to sleep. A few hours later this tendency had passed away, but the wound was dark and swollen from effused blood. No signs of active inflammation existed. On pressure, a little serous blood flowed from the wound. Within five days the skin gave way and the parts beneath sloughed to the bones. At the close of this process on the sixth day, the bird died, probably of mere exhaustion and constitutional irritation.

Experiment.—Two pigeons were bitten by a snake which had made frequent and recent use of its fangs. Both birds were purposely exposed in such a way that they were bitten in the thigh. Both were enfeebled by the poison and seemed disposed to sleep. One of them sunk slowly, lower and lower, until its head touched the table, when it rolled on its side. It died without convulsions nearly eleven hours after the bite. The second pigeon, which was also the last bitten, died in violent convulsions with the head thrown backwards, during the eighth hour.

P. M. Section.—In neither of these birds was the blood coagulated, nor did it pass into that state upon exposure. In the pigeon first struck the pericardium was very full of serous blood, but no other organ was altered. In the second pigeon, the lungs, air passages, and mouth were full of blood, the mucous walls of the stomach were deeply congested in spots, and the peritoneal surface of the small intestines was marked with star-like points of extravasated blood.

Experiment.—A pigeon was struck in the back by a small snake, only one fang entering. The bird was placed on the table, where it instantly sought a corner and in ten minutes fell into the usual stupor with jerking, abrupt respiration. This condition seemed to lessen an hour later, but only for a time, and the bird finally sinking down, became weaker and weaker, and died without convulsions at the close of five hours and a half. The pupils gradually contracted before death, and suddenly dilated afterwards.

P. M. Section.—The wound in the back was dark, and a little thin dark blood oozed from it. The tissues around it for an inch or more, were soaked with extravasated blood, which had even passed through between the ribs, so as to stain the tissues behind the intestines and crop. The heart was large and full of perfectly fluid blood. No other lesions were observed, except that the pericordial serum was a little bloody.

My chief reason for recording at length the cases above reported, is to show the great increase in the internal lesions which occurs when the venom is long in killing the animal. Among these changes, it was found, as a general rule, that the blood was most affected, and least coagulable, the longer the death was delayed.

I have not thought it necessary to report in full the whole of the numerous cases of the malady in the pigeon. In some instances, the birds recovered from the immediate effect of the poison to die of the secondary lesions induced by it. In others, the death was sudden and early, and in a third class it was delayed for a few hours. All of these find illustration in the cases already quoted. One point, however, appeared to me to demand further attention.

When a number of any class of animals are poisoned, certain phenomena and lesions occur constantly, others exceptionally; and this is true of what are usually known as diseases, as well as of more easily studied cases of poisoning. To illustrate this, I have selected seven cases of a fatal character in pigeons, none of which have been reported in the foregoing pages. To save space, I have presented them in tabular form, so as to show, at a glance, the variety of symptoms and pathological appearances which may occur. No cases of very early death are admitted into this report.

TABLE OF SYMPTOMS AND LESIONS IN SEVEN CASES OF PIGEONS POISONED BY CROTALUS VENOM.

No.	No. of fang marks.	Locality bitten.	Duration of life from time of bite.	Occurrence of convulsions.	Internal lesions.	State of blood.
1	1	Thigh.	2 hours.	None.	None.	Loosely coagulated.
2	2	Breast.	4 hours and 10 minutes.	None.	Spots of extravasation under the peritoneal surface of the intestines and on the heart.	Chiefly uncoagulated, one small heart clot of loose texture.
3	2 1	Back and Breast.	2 hours and 17 minutes.	Violent.	None.	Coagulated well.
4	2	Breast.	5 hours.	Slight spasms at death.	None.	Coagulated loosely after a few minutes.
5	1	Thigh.	9 hours and 10 minutes.	None.	Bloody serum in pericardium, bloody mucus in lung.	Blood diffluent.
6	2	Back.	3 hours.	Slight at death.	Ecchymosed spots on the heart, abundant yellow serum in pericardium.	Blood diffluent; one small, soft clot in right auricle.
7	1	Leg.	6 hours and 30 minutes.	None.	No visible lesions.	Blood perfectly fluid.

The remaining observations were made upon reed-birds, and were principally incidental to researches upon special points to which I shall have to refer so much at length in another place, that it is needless to duplicate them here. The reed-bird proved so susceptible a test, that one-eighth of a drop of venom sufficed in most cases to destroy it, the length of life in these instances being always in inverse ratio to the amount of poison employed.

Among warm blooded quadrupeds, I have examined the influence of venom on the rabbit, the guinea pig, and the dog. On the first mentioned animal I have made ten observations. Of these, I shall report two at length, the remainder in full tabular form. Upon the guinea pig I have made only four experiments, all of them incidental to special points of research, and not so fully reported in my note book as to enable me to detail at length their symptoms and lesions.

Experiment. Poisoning of Rabbits.—A large white rabbit was lowered into the snake-box, and was instantly struck by a small snake. The wound took effect on the left hind paw. The rabbit was removed and put upon the table, when it rolled over, gasping and slightly convulsed, and was dead in one minute.

P. M.—No lesion was found in any organ. The fore feet twitched for some few minutes after death, and the skin muscles moved to and fro in a singular manner. The heart was beating actively, but feebly, just after death, and continued locally irritable for over an hour and a half. The muscles and motor nerves were perfectly excitable several minutes after death. The blood coagulated firmly and rapidly; a perfect case of acute poisoning.

Experiment.—In this instance the animal was struck once in the back by a large snake already exhausted by frequent use. A few minutes after the bite took place the rabbit was seized with weakness, gritting of the teeth, and rapid respiration. It passed urine and feces, and remained feeble during some hours. From this period the weakness abated somewhat, but the back continued to swell. On the second day the local signs were improving, but the animal had passed a very albuminous urine, and a large amount of blood mixed with feces. The symptoms of general weakness now increased, the hind legs began to drag, the motions were uncertain, and the bloody purging grew worse. The rabbit died on the third day, during my absence.

P. M. Section.—Rigor well developed. The period of death being uncertain, the irritability of the tissues was not tested. The wound was surrounded by half an ounce or more of dark fluid blood. The vessels in the neighborhood were full of a similar fluid, but there was no vascular redness, like that of acute inflammation. The muscles in the track of the bite, which was a double fang mark, were remarkably softened and could be torn with the utmost ease. The brain was highly congested, and there was a good deal of bloody serum in the cavities of that organ. Similar congestion existed in the spinal canal, and at several points the white nervous tissue was stained with small patches of blood. The lungs were healthy. The pericardium was curiously distended with bloody serum. The heart was contracted and contained but little blood, and that dark and diffluent. The intestines were spotted at intervals with ecchymoses four to five lines in diameter and apparently just beneath the serous covering, the cavity of which contained a little bloody serum. The intestines from the œsophagus to the rectum were dotted with ecchymoses and filled, especially the large gut, with blood and mucus. The right kidney was large and absolutely soaked with dark fluid blood. The left kidney was more healthy. The bladder and ureters contained a good deal of bloody urine. How the rabbit lived so long with such a singular complication of serious lesions it is difficult to conceive. In most cases of chronic poisoning, some one or two organs may become the seat of local extravasations, but for extent and character of lesion this case stands alone in my experience.

TABLE OF SYMPTOMS IN EIGHT RABBITS.

No.	Duration of life after bite.	Early local symptoms and place of wound.	General symptoms.	Mode of death.
1	38 minutes.	Slight swelling in fore shoulder.	Prostration and loss of power without loss of sensation or cerebration, jerking respiration, general twitching.	Gradual, without convulsions.
2	5 hours and 4 minutes.	Hind right leg swelled enormously up to the spine.	Prostration, gritting the teeth, local and general twitching, jerking respiration, gradual loss of power, with continued ability to hear, see, &c., until near death.	Gradual, with slight general convulsion; head thrown forwards, feet extended.
3	1 hour and 10 minutes.	Neck; slight swelling, local twitches.	Sudden loss of motor power, gaping, prostration, very quick respiration.	Gradual, no convulsions.
4	27 minutes.	Neck; slight swelling, local twitches.	Sudden prostration.	Violent convulsions.
5	43 minutes.	Right hind leg.	Loss of motor power, prostration, jerking, respiration, general twitching.	Violent convulsions.
6	9 hours.	Left fore paw.	Prostration, gradual loss of motion, gritting the teeth, jerking respiration not so well marked as usual, singular and incessant movement in the skin muscles.	No convulsions; gradual and easy death.
7	12 minutes.	Neck and head; local twitching.	Sudden prostration and loss of motion, respiration quick and labored, not jerking.	Gradual, with slight convulsive motions of the limbs and skin muscles.
8	2 hours and 9 minutes.	Left fore leg.	Symptoms of weakness suddenly developed, 15 minutes after bite; respiration jerking.[1]	Gradual and easy; no convulsions.

[1] In all of the above cases the heart pulse became rapid and feeble.

TABLE OF LESIONS IN THE EIGHT RABBITS MENTIONED ABOVE.

No.	Local appearances.	Heart and lungs.	Abdominal viscera.	Nervous system.	Blood.
1	Small area of extravasated blood.	Heart dark, relaxed, and full of blood, on right side especially.	Healthy.	Slight fulness in the vessels of the brain.	Coagulated pretty well.
2	Extensive effusion of blood, partly clotted, and reaching up the leg to the flank and down to the foot, and soaking the muscles to the bone.	Heart contained a good deal of blood on both sides; a little bloody serum in the pericardium.	The cæcum contained a good deal of dark blood in patches.	The usual vascular fulness only.	One small clot in left ventricle, and elsewhere the blood was fluid.
3	Slight extravasion of blood.	Heart full on both sides.	Intestines dotted with small spots of extravasated blood.	None.	Blood uncoagulated.
4	Slight extravasation.	Heart full on both sides.	None.	None.	Coagulated well.
5	Slight and thin layer of extravasated blood.	Heart as usual, no lesion.	None.	A little bloody serum in the ventricles of the brain.	Loosely coagulated.
6	Part enormously swollen with blood, partly in loose clots when let out by incision at the third hour.	Bloody serum in pericardium and both pleuræ; two extensive extravasations in the right lung; a rare occurrence.	None.	Great vascular fulness.	Blood uncoagulated.
7	Scarcely a trace of any lesion except the fang wound.	No lesion; right side of heart much distended with blood.	None.	None.	Blood perfectly coagulated.
8	Extravasated blood between skin and muscles up to the thigh.	No lesion; heart large and full of blood in all of its cavities.	A few small spots of blood under the peritoneum of the small intestines.	None.	Uncoagulated.

Effect of Crotalus Venom on Dogs.—Thus far we have dealt with animals who were almost inevitably destroyed by the bite of the Crotalus. The canine species are far less liable to die, because their larger size is in itself a protection, as must be evident, when we consider that the poison is active in proportion to the amount injected, and that this will be the same, whether the animal bitten be a bird or a horse. In the following cases, therefore, some will be found to have resulted favorably. On the other hand, the most rapidly fatal termination was consequent upon a number of bites, and took place at the close of twenty minutes. On this point I have a brief explanation to make, before going further.

At the time of my experiments upon dogs, my snakes had been often used and handled, and had taken but little food, although in confinement from two to five weeks. It was not to be expected that, under these circumstances, they should prove as deadly as if they had been fresh, and were biting for the first time during some weeks or months. I have thought proper to make this prefatory statement, because it is well known that very often dogs have been destroyed in one, two, or three minutes after the bite of a fresh animal.

The following experiments were selected from a series, made with the view of establishing a rate of mortality, so as to compare the results with those obtained when a supposed antidote was employed. They were made with care, the snakes employed having been previously left undisturbed during a week.

With the defects which underlie this plan, so far as it has reference to antidotes, we have here nothing to do, and the cases are quoted only on account of their value as such.

Experiment.—A large Spaniel, weighing sixteen and a half pounds, was muzzled, and lowered into the box containing one large snake, which struck it fiercely in the right fore-shoulder, and again, an instant afterwards, a little higher up. Upon a careful removal of the hair, only one fang seemed to have acted in either wound. The blows appeared to be excessively painful at the time, but upon removing the dog at once, he gave no after signs of pain or distress. Within twenty-five minutes he was languid, and remained standing with his head down, as though sick and confused. The local twitching about the wounds was highly marked, but there was no general fremitus, and the respiration was only quickened a little, without being either jerking or laborious. During the ensuing twenty-four hours, the dog refused to eat, but drank at frequent intervals, and passed urine and clay-colored stools. He was able to move about, but preferred to remain at rest.

The wound was not swollen, but when examined with care, a slight hardening of the neighboring tissues could be felt, extending two inches around the wound.

On pressure, a little bloody serum could be forced out of the fang track. This continued to be the case during three days, when pus also flowed out. The local evil was very limited, however, and the animal was so well on the ninth day, that it was used for another purpose.

Experiment.—The dog employed in the last observation was perfectly well, and eating and drinking as usual, when he was bitten in the left fore-shoulder, and in the left hind leg below the knee. Both wounds swelled, that in the shoulder most. The local fremitus was very remarkable, and extended up and down the hind leg, and for some distance around the anterior wound. Although the dog whined at intervals for some hours, and, to appearance, suffered considerably, the parts bitten soon ceased to swell, and but little oozing took place from either wound. No suppuration occurred, and the dog was entirely well within two days.

Experiment.—A black and white mongrel setter, weighing thirty pounds, was lowered into the cage. The only snake in the box struck him repeatedly, but without seeming to cause much pain. Upon looking for the wounds none could be detected, and the snake was, therefore, caught in the loop as usual, and held to the dog again, until it bit eagerly. Still no wound beyond slight abrasions could be found, and on the bitten skin lay adherent a large fang. On inspecting the snake's mouth, I found that both fangs were recent, and not yet anchylosed in their maxillary sockets. The snake's skin was loose, and was shed entire two days later. Two other snakes were next caught and made to bite the hind leg and fore-shoulder of the dog. The latter wound gave great pain, and the swelling extended to the neck and chest. The local trembling was slight. There were no marked general symptoms, except a slight ineffectual effort to vomit, half an hour after being bitten, and some evidence of general feebleness which passed off in five hours. Next day the dog was well and active, eating and drinking as usual. He remained thus for ten days, during which time the wounds grew smaller, and from that in the shoulder oozed a little red serum, and finally some pus, but neither in this or in other cases did the skin slough extensively. I found in most instances only a small orifice leading into an abscess cavity, which was rarely above the size of a large walnut.

Experiment.—A white mongrel, weighing seventeen pounds, was placed in the cage with a large snake. He was struck at once in the left hind thigh, and again by the same serpent about three inches above the first wound. The dog suffered terribly, and during two hours whined and yelled incessantly. Enormous swelling occurred, involving the whole limb up to the pelvic joint. Two hours after being struck the dog was weak, but still kept his feet, and drank almost without ceasing. His respiration was occasionally jerking, his heart as usual rapid but feeble. No local or general fremitus was noted. At the third hour he was again howling frightfully. The weakness was greater than before, and he staggered in his gait, but the other symptoms were unchanged. Four and a half hours after the poisoning, the dog became still weaker, ceased to drink, and finally lay down. The parts wounded were still enlarging. At this time he vomited a little food and mucus, and soon after purged and urinated. From this time he began to mend, and although he howled all the following night, he was able to run about the next day, with only a slight appearance of lameness. The wound discharged blood, and at length bloody pus, and finally pure pus, up to the period of recovery, three weeks later. During the first week of this time, the dog took scarcely any food, and was subject to profuse dysenteric discharges, so that he became remarkably emaciated. From this condition he gradually improved, all the symptoms abated, and at the end of the third week he was as fat as when first injured.

The cases here related are selected from a larger number of a similar nature, all illustrating the more or less grave character of the symptoms, and also the possibility of recovery, even under apparently unfavorable circumstances. The next case, and the last of this kind, I have placed alone, because it has especial value, as showing how exceedingly grave may be the signs of poisoning, and yet how rapid and complete may be the rally and escape.

Experiment.—A small brown terrier was struck twice on the fore leg and shoulder by a large snake, which I held in the loop, as usual. Within ten minutes the dog vomited, urinated, and passed solid feces. All this time he whined a good deal, and finally, at the fifteenth minute, lay down on his side, breathing in jerks, and twitching in almost every muscle. No fremitus could be seen at the wound, owing, perhaps, to the swelling, which was great, and might readily have concealed it from view. An hour after being bitten, the dog had a slight convulsion, and vomited again. Meanwhile I could scarcely feel the heart beat, and the respirations were long and labored. On leaving this animal, late in the evening, and about seven hours after he was hurt, he was lying on the floor, scarcely breathing, and nearly pulseless. He had passed liquid and very dark stools, and some water. Even at this period, his sensorium seemed unaffected, and he felt injuries, heard well, and followed with his eyes the movements about him. To my surprise, when I entered my laboratory the next morning, the dog ran by me and attempted to escape; I caught him with no little difficulty. His wound was like a hump on his side and back, and discharged fluid blood in occasional drops. The floor of the box in which

I had left him contained a good deal of dark, semi-fluid excrement streaked with blood, and he had drunk nearly the third of a bucket of water during the night.

The remaining instances of Crotalus bite in dogs were all fatal, and were selected, like the last series, as being the most illustrative records in my possession. It will be observed, as I have already stated, that no deaths took place so early as to give us perfect specimens of acute poisoning with absence of visceral lesions, and with a perfectly red and coagulable blood. That such cases may occur in the dog, under more favorable experimental conditions, I cannot doubt from what I have already seen in other animals.

Experiment.—A dog of mongrel bull-terrier breed, weighing thirty-one pounds, was lowered into the cage, where he was struck on the outside of the right hind leg in the thigh. He drew up the leg when released, and whined for a few minutes. The wound, which was double, bled a drop or two, and the muscles about it twitched considerably at intervals for an hour, when this symptom was obscured by the swelling. His pulse, which was naturally about 145 and irregular, was, at the fifth minute, 140 and regular, respiration 35. At the fifteenth minute he lay down, much weakened, pulse 160 and feeble, respiration 40. At the twentieth minute the bowels moved loosely, with a gray discharge, and there seemed to be some tenesmus in the rectum. Twenty-fifth minute, pupils so far natural and mobile; he could stand when urged, but lay down again at once, and was much weaker. Forty-fifth minute, pulse 160, respiration 45 and laborious. Fifty-fifth minute, loss of power in the hind legs. Eightieth minute, respiration quick and labored, and so irregular as to make it impossible longer to count the heart pulses. The eyes were natural, and followed my motions; and he wagged his tail when fondled. At this time the observation was temporarily interrupted, and, on its resumption at the third hour, the dog was found dead. He had no foam about his mouth, and probably died quietly.

P. M. Section.—The whole muscular and areolar tissue of the leg and thigh, half way up and down the limb, was dark with infiltrated blood. About the wound the swelling was due to a mass of blood partially coagulated. The extravasated blood extended through the limb, and on the inside it passed half way up the sartorius and adductors, and along the sheath of the vessels to within two inches of the femoral ring. Nearly an inch of the sheath was clear of it, but one-half inch below the ring the tissues were shaded with blood, and the same appearance was seen around the ring itself. From this point the extravasation extended under the peritoneum, into the pelvis, and on to the inner face of the ilium. The color of the tissues thus stained was a brilliant scarlet. The abdominal viscera were healthy, except that the mucous membrane of the lower bowels was somewhat congested. The lungs were sound. The heart was relaxed, the right side full, the left nearly empty. The blood on the right side was a little darker than that on the left; on both sides and everywhere else it was perfectly fluid and free from clots. Placed in a vial, it remained fluid until decomposition ensued. Two hours at least after death, some of the blood globules found in the heart were slightly indented; those taken from the small vessels of the ear were perfectly normal. At the period of examination, the muscular and nervous irritability had entirely departed.

Experiment.—A young dog, weighing nine and a half pounds, of terrier breed, was lowered into a box containing a fresh snake. The snake struck at him twice without effect, once striking to one side of the part aimed at, and the second time miscalculating its distance. The third blow took effect, but I could not ascertain the exact locality wounded. The dog cried out, as though in great pain. Within five minutes he was trembling in every muscle. At the twentieth minute he was so much better that I subjected him to a second bite, which took effect on the neck in front, above the left shoulder. The dog at once lay down, then rose, and passed water and solid feces, and, at the fifth minute from the second bite, fell on his side, and vomited freely. The vomiting was instantly followed by general convulsions, in which the limbs were extended and the head thrown back. Meanwhile, the heart was very feeble, the breathing laborious, and the pupil contracted. The character of the respirations at this time was singular. Eight or ten rapid respirations took place, and then none occurred until twenty seconds had elapsed. The heart-beat, previously 180 to the minute, fell, at the fifteenth minute after the second wound, to 80, and became remarkably feeble. At the seventeenth minute the respiration stopped, and the heart pulse, though so weak as to be counted with difficulty, rose to 156, falling again, at the twenty-fourth minute, to 58, when it became indistinct through weakness. The pupils rapidly dilated.

P. M. Section was delayed twenty-four hours. Post-mortem rigor came on first about the fore legs and neck, and was complete four hours after death. It was so strong as to snap a small cord with which I had drawn the legs of the dog apart. The wound was the seat of an extravasation which had passed over the shoulder and on to the neck. The vessels near it were filled with dark and diffluent blood. The muscles near the wound were softened and readily torn. The heart contained an abundance of blood chiefly fluid, with a number of small clots of very loose structure, in the right side and somewhat less in the left cavities. In the pericardium there was about an ounce and a half of bloody serum. The abdominal organs were healthy, and the peritoneum contained only a little straw-colored serum. The bladder was partially contracted, and held an ounce or two of slightly albuminous urine.

The brain was normally firm, though somewhat congested, and its vessels were distended with fluid blood and a few bubbles of gas. At the side of the long sinus a little blood seemed to have soaked through all the membranes to the bone, but there was no large quantity of blood present at this spot, and no coagulum. It looked like a post-mortem stain.

Experiment.—A white dog, weight nineteen and a half pounds, of unknown or mixed breed, was exposed for a special purpose, to be bitten by several snakes, all of whom had used their fangs or been robbed of venom within four days. The dog was hit at least six times, and perhaps received some wounds which escaped notice. Those found on removing the skin were in the neck and face, fore-shoulders and hind legs. There were absolutely no marked symptoms in this case, except increasing weakness, and consequent vomiting. The bowels also were moved and water was passed. The breathing then became jerking and labored. The fremitus, at first localized in some of the bites, soon became general, until it disappeared before the profound debility, which seemed to affect the entire economy. Three hours after the poisoning the animal died without convulsions. At the moment of the infliction of the wounds, there certainly was great pain, but at no time afterwards was this sensation expressed. Until near death, the cerebral functions appeared to preserve their integrity, so that the dog wagged his tail on being patted, and even followed with his head the motions of the flies which hovered over him. The numerous bites were really the most formidable lesions found after death. Around them, in each case, was an irregular circle of extravasated fluid blood. None of them, however, were much swollen, although the amount of blood spread out in their layers and soaked into the muscles must have been considerable. Except some congestion of the vessels of the brain and its membranes, there was no morbid appearance in any viscus. The right heart was full of fluid blood. The left heart also contained more blood than usual, and its color was a little brighter than that of the other side.

Experiment.—A white mongrel bitch, weighing fifteen pounds, was put in the cage with a large snake, which had not used its fangs for ten days. The snake struck the animal with both fangs just above the eye, and again, after some teasing, on the inside of the thigh high up. This latter wound gave great pain, and the bitch, when lifted from the box, yelled and whined during several minutes. On examination, it was found that only one fang had taken effect in the thigh. Around this was a growing circle of flattened swelling, of which the dark color was easily seen through the skin, which in this place was white and very delicate. During half an hour the animal stood on her feet, her head hanging a little, and blood running so freely from the wound in the thigh, that an ounce or two may have been thus lost within an hour of the period of the bite. At the close of the half hour the bitch suddenly staggered, and fell on her side, then rose and again fell. The heart, which before the poisoning was 154, rose immediately after the bite to 175, stimulated, perhaps, by pain and terror. When the animal fell the pulse was about 160, and irregular and feeble. After this, its force diminished gradually, but the rhythm changed very little until just before death, when it fell rapidly. An hour after the bite, the animal still lay on her side making efforts to vomit. Upon lifting her up she succeeded in vomiting a little mucus. At this time she also passed a loose stool, and soon after lying down again, made water freely. The urine ran over a board on which the dog lay. A little of it drawn up with a pipette, proved to be acid and to contain no albumen. One hour and twenty minutes after the poisoning, the head was suddenly thrown back, the pupils contracted and the limbs extended, although not violently. At the close of this momentary convulsion, the bitch drew a long breath and expired.

P. M. Section.—The wound was a good deal swollen, and contained some loosely-clotted blood, and much more that was quite fluid, and so continued upon removal. The tissues in the track of the fang were only a little softened, but the thigh was literally soaked with blood down to the periosteal membrane, which was darkly stained. The other wound was but little swollen. The brain was apparently healthy. The lungs were normal, the pericardium contained a little bloody serum, the heart was marked over the right ventricle with three star-like spots of ecchymosis, and a little ribbon of extravasated blood ran along each side of several of the smaller coronary veins.

The abdominal organs were healthy, and the intestines the seat of active movement. The extravasation in the thigh extended up through the femoral ring, and over the brim of the pelvis, so that the areolar tissues between the left side of the bladder and the pelvic bones were filled with fluid blood. The heart had ceased to beat when the animal was examined, but it acted for a few seconds when galvanized, and was locally and feebly irritable for half an hour. The muscles were excitable during about the same time, and the diaphragm a little longer. The sciatic nerves responded during thirteen minutes, and the phrenic nerves during twenty-eight minutes.

Experiment.—A small brown dog, weighing twelve pounds, was struck with both fangs by two snakes, one biting him on the muzzle, and one on the side. The wound on the side did not swell, that on the flank formed within two hours a prominent, almost pendulous mass, several inches long and wide. Within ten minutes this animal became feeble and reeled about, as if giddy. At length he lay down on his side, breathing heavily. The muscles about the flank wound twitched a good deal at first, and the general fremitus was well marked within thirty minutes. It passed off after half an hour longer, only recurring at intervals. Meanwhile the dog lay quiet, and although evidently sensible of surrounding objects, seemed in no pain. The heart-beat, which, after the bite, was strong and rapid, became scarcely perceptible to the hand. At the time the dog lay down, he passed urine and solid feces, but did not attempt to vomit. After lying thus for five hours he died quietly.

P. M. Section.—The wound on the flank presented the usual appearance. The skin beyond the bitten nostril was puffy and tumid, the nostrils exuding bloody mucus. All the thoracic organs were normal, the heart as usual, the right side full of fluid blood, with some loose dark clots, the left side almost empty. Elsewhere the organs were healthy, excepting the kidneys, which were full of blood, and presented the appearance of acute congestion. On further inspection, a long thin clot was found in the left ureter, and bloody urine in the bladder below. Brain not examined.

The cases above reported represent so well the character of the pathological lesions in mortal cases of Crotalus bite, that it would be needless to intrude them upon these pages in larger number.

CHAPTER VII.

ACTION OF THE VENOM ON THE TISSUES AND FLUIDS.

In this section, the subject of absorption, hitherto deferred, naturally presents itself at the outset.

The most important of the questions raised in this connection, regards the power of the stomach to absorb the venom of serpents, a question to which Redi[1] gave a negative reply, founded on the experiments of his viper catcher, and upon one of his own on a kid, to which he gave internally the venom of four vipers. Fontana,[2] on the other hand, took the affirmative, owing to a single experiment on a pigeon, down the throat of which he poured nearly thirty drops of venom, killing it thus in six minutes.[3]

Prof. Mangili[4] has since repeated these experiments, and arrived at the conclusion that the venom of the viper is harmless, when taken internally. These results were founded on the most satisfactory data, and leave no room to doubt that the venom is innocuous when thus administered. Before and since his experiments, many observers have been found bold enough to taste, and even to swallow, the venom of serpents. Thus, Mead and his assistants tasted the venom of the viper, Russell[5] *tasted* the poison of the Cobra, but does not seem to have swallowed it, although he has credit in some of the books for having done so.

In our own country, experience upon this matter is limited. Harlan,[6] who gave the venom internally to a single young dog, without effect, and Jeter,[7] who states that when given to fasting cats and dogs, it causes sickness, and is followed by the usual consequences of snake bite, are the only authorities, if we except an extraordinary statement made by Burnett[8] upon the authority of another person, whose

---

[1] Francis Redi, Nobilis Aretini Experimenta. Amstelodami, 1675. Ex. Italico Latinate Donata, p. 14.

Also, Celsus, who says of the venom of snakes, "Non gustu, sed in vulnere nocent;" and Lucan before him, puts into the mouth of Cato "Morsu virus habent, et fatum dente minantur; pocula morte carent." Fontana, vol. ii. p. 323.

[2] Fontana, vol. ii. p. 321.

[3] Fontana had previously arrived at the negative conclusion from experiments upon dogs, who took, however, very small doses. Vol. i. p. 58.

[4] Mangili, quoted in Orfila, Tox. Gén., vol. ii. p. 852, from 'Il Giornale di Fisica Chemica, etc. Vol. ix. p. 458 (1817).

[5] Russell, p. 63.

[6] Harlan, Physiological Researches, p. 501.

[7] Jeter, p. 20.

[8] Burnett, Proc. Boston Soc. of Nat. Hist., vol. iv. p. 323.

imaginative powers must have been of the strongest. Other native authors state that the poison has this or that taste, but do not directly assert that they have acquired such knowledge by personal experiments.

I have already stated that I found the venom tasteless. I did not venture to swallow it, feeling no inclination to repeat the rash acts of the servants of Fontana and Redi.

As regards the question of absorption by a mucous surface, I once saw incidentally made, a rather curious experiment to which I have already referred.

A large Crotalus swallowed a mouthful of its own venom, but, although watched for several weeks, it seemed to have suffered no ill consequences.

From the experiments of Harlan, Mangili, Russell, Davy and others, it seems to be sufficiently proved that the unbroken mucous surface of the mouth has no power to absorb the venom of serpents, and that the stomach also is incapable of admitting this poison to the system in any form possessing noxious properties.

Circumstances interfered to prevent me from extending my experiments on absorption to the length which I contemplated, but I hope to resume them at a future period. I have, however, performed two experiments upon pulmonary absorption, which possess so much interest that it would scarcely be proper to omit them.

Experiment.—A large pigeon was placed between my knees and somewhat compressed so as partially to empty the lungs. At this moment a small tube, well rounded and with an opening on the side near the end, was thrust carefully through the glottis and down into the trachea. As soon as the tube was in place I blew into its upper orifice, thus discharging into the trachea its entire contents, consisting of about two drops of venom with a little water. This manœuvre, suddenly followed by relaxation of the pressure on the respiratory organs of the bird, secured the passage of the venom into the smaller bronchi, and perhaps even into the air-vesicles themselves. A good deal of wheezing and coughing ensued, and within ten minutes the pigeon became drowsy, rocked to and fro, and at the close of thirty-eight minutes fell down. Convulsions followed at the forty-third minute, and terminated in death at the forty-ninth.

P. M. Section.—The heart was still irritable and contained a little loosely clotted blood on both sides. No lesions were visible, except in the lungs, both of which contained large extravasations of dark blood soaked through their tissues to such an extent as to make it impossible to say, whether or not, it was fluid or coagulated.

Experiment.—Another pigeon was treated in the same manner as the one last described, except that the venom used was three weeks old, and amounted to two drops. Death, without precedent convulsions, took place at the close of eight and a half hours. The blood was diffluent in every locality examined, and the left lung contained a large extravasation of dark blood.

The above cases render it probable that the delicate lung tissue offers no permanent barrier to the passage of the venom. There is, however, a possibility of fallacy in these experiments, and it is still desirable that they should be repeated on a larger scale, and on higher animals.

The Wound.—The wound made by the fang sometimes penetrates half an inch, but is oftener more superficial. So far as a fatal result is concerned, it seems to be indifferent, whether the bite takes place about the head and neck, or in the limbs.[1] The local quivering which is so common, seems to depend upon the muscles of the part having been wounded and envenomed, whereas, when the venom enters only the areolar or adipose tissue, this symptom either does not occur at all, or occurs only after a time. The swelling, which in a large majority of cases surrounds the wound, is never inflammatory in the first instance, at least in animals, and especially in those which die, and in which the rapidly increasing loss of tones forbids the presence of such a condition. In some of the animals who recover, secondary inflammation and gangrene, with more or less formation of pus may ensue. The primary swelling, then, is always due to a collection of blood, sometimes partially coagulated, at others perfectly fluid, and apt to leak drop by drop, out of the open fang track, when the opening is large, and the part bitten is highly vascular.

The effusion of blood in such large quantities as sometimes takes place, is explained by the rapidity with which its fibrin undergoes destruction at high temperatures (100° F.), and in the presence of such amounts of venom as are occasionally injected. Under these circumstances the usual arrest of hemorrhage by coagulation of the fibrin of the blood fails to take place, and the incoagulable blood soaks through all the neighboring tissues.

In other instances, as we have seen, the blood about the wound clots, owing either to the relatively small amount of venom present, or to the fact of a sudden and great escape of blood from some vessel of larger size than is usually punctured by the fang. In no case are the clots thus formed of very firm texture.[2]

The veins about the wound are commonly found to be filled with dark and uncoagulable blood, so that the effect here described, is exerted not only upon the effused fluid, but also upon that which is still retained within the vessels.

Effect of the Venom on the Muscles.—The influence of the venom upon the muscles of the wounded part has been already described. It appears to be due to the direct action of the venom upon the sarcous elements.

As I supposed it possible, however, that the mere puncture might be competent to cause protracted local quivering, I punctured exposed muscles, with dry fangs, previously boiled, and then stopped with wax. Slight twitches followed, but no further results were visible. When, on the other hand, I exposed the living muscle and moistened it with venom, the twitching took place as usual, while, when the venom was injected through the fang into the interior of the muscle, the convulsive quivering was yet more active and prolonged. To ascertain whether or not this was due to direct stimulation of the muscular tissue, or to an indirect influence first affecting the nerves of the part, I executed the following experiment:—

---

[1] Unless the mere swelling destroys life, or the poison be deposited near a large vessel.

[2] It is said that the pig is not liable to die from Crotalus bite, and it is well known that it attacks the Rattlesnake with vigor and success. Its comparative immunity may, possibly, be due to the fact that its skin is very thick and tough, and that the large deposit of sub-cuticular adipose tissue is scantily supplied with bloodvessels. Notwithstanding this, I am assured upon competent authority, that when the pig is struck in thin and vascular parts it enjoys no peculiar privilege.

Experiment.—A large frog was poisoned with woorara. This active agent possesses the power to paralyze the motor nerves, and to leave the muscles in a highly irritable state.[1] The animal was thus placed in the same condition as though the whole motor nervous system had been removed by dissection, without serious injury to the remaining parts. It was found that in a frog so prepared, and in which the motor nerves no longer responded to irritants, the muscles still quivered as long as usual when bitten by the snake, so that I felt free to infer that this interesting local phenomenon was in reality due to the direct influence of the venom upon the ultimate sarcous elements.

After a few minutes, or at the utmost, half an hour, these spasmodic movements cease; but without entirely exhausting the irritability of the muscles, which will, sometimes, continue to respond to other stimulants until their structure is more profoundly altered by the continued action of the venom. The quivering often extends to the whole muscular system, but although a frequent, this is not an invariable symptom, and is liable, in dogs, to be confounded with the fremitus of terror, to which they are very subject. It is in them a more common symptom of the poisoning than it is in rabbits, while in birds the general quivering is very rarely met with.

The influence of the venom upon the duration of muscular irritability I have examined in many animals, but especially in frogs. Many of these observations were made in very hot weather, but were finally resumed in the early autumn under more favorable conditions for the preservation of the muscular functions.

Both in the cases of acute and of chronic poisoning, the muscular irritability of the frog was lost earlier than is usual in other modes of death.

Notwithstanding this result, the property in question was perfect at the time of the death, and for a short space afterwards, especially in acute cases, while, in some rare instances, it survived in the chin muscles during twenty-four hours.

The muscular irritability of the warm-blooded animals left them very rapidly, but was often so well marked at, or just after, death, as to forbid us to refer the death to the loss of muscular irritability as the immediate, or even the remote cause.

Rigor Mortis.—The action of the venom did not seem to prevent the occurrence of the strongest rigor mortis. It came on in different animals at varying periods, but, so far as I have observed, was never entirely absent in any case. Even when the blood was perfectly diffluent, this post-mortem phenomenon was noted, *a fact which should utterly forbid us to connect its occurrence with the coagulation of the blood, as was at one time a not uncommon opinion.*

Ultimate Effect of Venom on Muscles.—The final influence of venom upon the muscular structure was extremely curious. In every instance it softened it in proportion to the length of the time during which it remained in contact with it, so that after even a few hours in warm-blooded animals, and after a rather longer time in the frog, the wounded muscle became almost diffluent, and assumed a dark

[1] Cl. Bernard, Leçons sur les effets des substances toxiques et médicamenteuses. Bailliere et fils. Paris, 1857, p. 239 *et seq.*

color and somewhat jelly-like appearance. The structure remained entire until it was pressed upon or stretched, when it lost all regularity, and offered the appearance under the microscope of a minutely granular mass, dotted with larger granules. The altered character of the muscle is illustrated in Fig. 12.

Fig. 12.

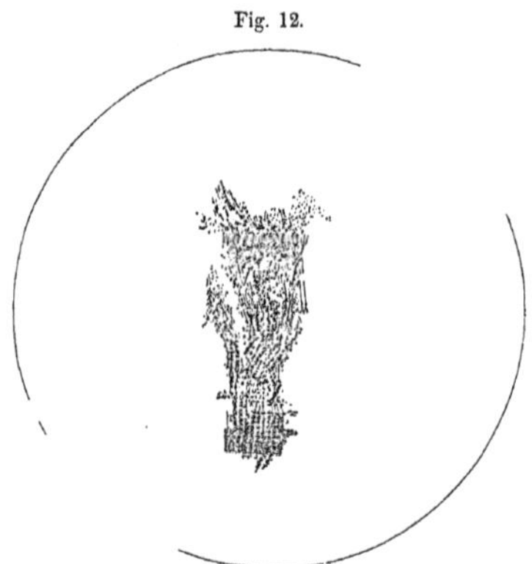

Appearance of muscular fibre when mechanically disturbed after contact with venom.

Effect on the Heart.—Continuing the study of the action of the venom on muscular parts, it remains to examine the extent to which the heart is influenced.

This question is one of extreme interest, and of no less difficulty. It is so important, however, in its bearings upon the causation of death in acute poisoning, that I have spared no pains to investigate it by every means in my power.

My first observations were made by exposing the heart of the frog, and observing it before and after the animal was bitten. Many of these observations failed partially, or entirely, owing to the frogs having survived long enough to pass into the stage of secondary poisoning.

In most of the cases of acute poisoning the rhythm and force of the heart became affected before the respiration was suspended, and the organ continued to pulsate more or less perfectly for some time after all voluntary and reflex motion had ceased.

It is scarcely requisite to detail these observations more fully, since examples may be found in the chapter which treats of the action of the venom on the batrachia. I shall therefore limit myself to stating that, under the influence of Crotalus venom the batrachian heart becomes enfeebled, and acts more slowly; that it continues to act after the limbs have ceased to respond to stimulus by reflex acts, and that it usually stops before the motor nerves lose their vitality.

As the heart of the frog is remarkably independent of the respiratory and other functions, and as, moreover, it will beat longer, when cut out and suspended, than it usually does when subjected in its normal situation to the influence of the venom, it is difficult to avoid the conclusion that it is more or less directly affected by it. It seemed to me equally plain, however, that it was not owing to the arrest of the heart that the animal died. In fact, the heart continued to act after some of the principal nervous functions, such as reflex acts, were over, so that their loss was not due to an arrested circulation.

The study of the effect of venom on the hearts of warm-blooded animals was one of still greater difficulty. This arose from the fact that their functions are more closely related to one another, so that the cessation of respiration necessarily leads to loss of cardiac power, and *vice versâ;* since, however, the determination of the question before us was essential to a proper study of the remedies for venom poisoning, I felt forced to continue my researches in this direction, notwithstanding the obstacles in my path.

As in the frog, I began by a series of simple observations upon the changes in the heart which were apparent to the eye. For this purpose, I opened the chests of rabbits sufficiently to obtain a view of the heart, the action of which was sustained during the experiment by artificial respiration.

Experiment.—Small male rabbit; pulse 280; respiration 120. Struck at 12 o'clock, 32 minutes, in the right flank. The animal fell in two minutes. Artificial respiration was at once used, and, owing to want of caution, the right lung was torn, and the diaphragm ruptured. The chest was then opened. The heart was acting very rapidly, and pretty well up to the thirteenth minute, when its rhythm became disturbed, the right and left cavities acting separately. The respiration was continued, with brief intervals, up to the sixty-third minute, when the auricles alone responded, and the observation terminated.

Experiment.—Small black female rabbit. A string was placed under the trachea. The heart beat too rapidly for numeration. Bitten thrice in the side by a small snake at 6.15 P.M. Fourth minute, pupils contracting. Fifth minute, head falling. Seventh minute, slight general convulsions; respiration feeble and laboring. Tenth minute, slight convulsions; pupils dilated. Twelfth minute, respiration stopped, and a tube being placed in the trachea, regular artificial respiration was accomplished while the chest was opened, and the heart exposed. At first, the heart beat regularly, but not very strongly. At the eighteenth minute, its rhythm became altered, two auricular contractions taking place during each ventricular act. At the twenty-second minute, the organ was acting very feebly, the auricles alone beating, and the respiration was therefore discontinued.

Experiment.—Small male rabbit. In this case, the artificial respiration was made before the natural movement was over, about forty-four minutes after the bite was inflicted. No convulsions were observed. Although the artificial respiration was admirably sustained, the rhythm of the heart became disturbed within twelve minutes, the auricles beating twice as fast as the ventricles. Before this occurred, the heart acted well, except that it did not seem to possess the energy which it usually does under other circumstances.

Experiment.—Large male rabbit. The trachea was prepared as usual, except that a tube of sufficient size was placed in it before the bite, so that no time might be lost.

The animal was struck twice in the left thigh at 4.20 P. M. At the seventh minute it fell, and at the thirtieth minute, the respiration being very feeble, artificial respiration was made, and the chest opened. The heart was acting well, but not perfectly, the same want of completeness in its systole being seen as was noticed in former cases. At the close of the sixtieth minute from the time of the bite, the organ became more markedly feeble, and the ventricles acted but rarely. In this, as in all other like observations, the heart remained irritable to galvanism for a short time after it ceased to pulsate, and locally responsive for a still longer period. It was plain enough from these experiments that the artificial respiration was capable of prolonging the cardiac functions, but not usually for any great length of time. Moreover, the heart was always found beating in animals poisoned, and opened as soon as respiration ceased. Again, its tissues were always alive to stimulus for a short period after its rhythmic movements stopped, so that there was evidently no such complete local paralysis of the muscular structures as is caused by upas-antiar or corroval. When an animal is poisoned with these last-mentioned substances, death begins at the heart; and so complete is the palsy of this organ, that the most violent galvanic stimulus fails to provoke in it the least response, even when applied immediately after it has ceased to pulsate rhythmically.[1]

These views were strengthened by the following experiment: Being aware that the young of warm-blooded animals approximate to the condition of cold-blooded creatures, in regard to the comparative independence of their cardiac and respiratory functions, I exposed several kittens of a week old to be bitten. As soon as respiration ceased their hearts were laid bare, and found to be beating quite actively. Thus, in one case, the kitten was bitten thrice, by as many rather exhausted snakes, between three minutes of six, and eleven minutes after six.

At 6.19 P. M. sensation was gone in the limbs; and at 6.23, all motion ceased, except occasional diaphragmatic acts. At 6.25, the dorsal spine was divided, and no movement took place, the left sciatic remaining perfectly irritable. During this time the heart continued to act regularly, and at 6.44, was still able to respond to stimulus by feeble, but repeated pulses; one stimulation being followed by three or four complete pulsations.

In all human cases of Crotalus poisoning, the general feebleness which follows a severe bite is most notable. As we have seen, there is reason to believe that at least a part of this deadly prostration may be due to an effect on the heart, while on the whole, there is not reason to suppose that its tissues are so paralyzed as to permit us to assert that death begins at the cardiac centre.

As it was possible that I might be deceived as to the appearance of lack of power in the heart, I subjected the matter to more accurate examination. For this purpose, I instituted the following experiments :—

Experiment.—A large brindled dog was properly secured on the table, and his

---

[1] See a paper on new varieties of woorara by Prof. Hammond and the author, Amer. Jour. of the Med. Sci., July, 1859.

right femoral artery laid bare. The brass nozzle of M. Bernard's cardiometer[1] was tied fast in the vessel, and the blood allowed to act on the column of mercury.

At 4 o'clock, 58 minutes, the pulse being 99, and the respiration 21, the constant pressure in the artery was found to be represented by eighty millimetres of the column of mercury, which at every heart beat rose to 115 millimetres.

The following record was then obtained:—

Time.	Constant arterial pressure.	Rising at each heart beat to	Difference.
4.58 to 5.14	80mm	115mm	35mm
	A clot forming, the column ceased to move. The tube was cleansed and replaced at		
5.16,	when again a clot formed, and the artery was tied, and the left carotid laid bare. On inserting the tube in this latter vessel, the record was as follows:—		
5.58	110	145	35
6	"	"	"
6.1	One large snake was allowed to bite the dog's left thigh. The dog struggled, and the muscles about the wound quivered remarkably.		
6.4½	105	120	15
	Respiration perfect as yet. Heart pulse 115, respiration 22.		
6.6	95	115	20
6.7	Pulse beats 120, respiration somewhat laborious.		
6.9	102	120	18
6.10	105	115	10
	A clot having formed, the tube was again removed, cleaned, and replaced.		
6.19	85	105	15
6.20	87	109	22
6.21	85	110	25

At this time a clot formed, and as some blood was lost in replacing the tube, the observation terminated. The artery was tied, and the dog set at liberty. He was very sick for two or three days, but finally recovered, surviving the ligation of two arteries, and the bite of the snake.

Experiment.—A yellow mongrel of middle size was secured as usual. About two ounces of blood were lost while placing the tube in the carotid. At 5 o'clock, 30 minutes, the column rose to 114 millimetres, and at each heart beat to 127 millimetres, so that 13 millimetres represented the heart force.

These figures remaining the same during two minutes, and the respirations being 26, and tranquil, the dog was bitten by three snakes, so as to be the more profoundly affected.

---

[1] The cardiometer consists of a vessel, about three inches high, and of the same diameter. A glass tube, with a scale of millimetre divisions, passes down to the bottom of the vessel, and is open at both ends. A second tube opens through the top of the vessel into its interior, and is provided with a stopcock. To its nozzle is attached a short caoutchouc tube, which is terminated by a brass tube, made to fit the artery selected for trial. The main vessel is now filled with mercury up to 0 of the scale. The caoutchouc tube is next filled with a strong solution of carbonate of soda, and secured in the artery. The stopcock being turned, the mercury rises to a point which marks the height of a column of mercury capable of being sustained by the constant pressure under which the blood circulates in the arteries. At each heart beat, and at each deep expiration, the column rises a little, to fall anew, as the increased pressure thus exerted is removed.

Time.	Constant arterial pressure.	Rising at each heart beat to	Difference.
5.34	94mm	110mm	16mm
5.35	95	110	10
	Pulse 138. The respiration was now laborious, at each expiration the column rising 27mm.		
5.36	93	97	4
	Respiration irregular.		
5.37	92	95	3
5.38½	85	90	5
	Respiration but 12 in the minute.		
5.48	Clots formed, and the tube was replaced.		
5.49½	70	72 or 73	
	The heart pressure was now so slight, that I feared lest a clot might exist in the trunk of the artery, and therefore repeated the observations on the femoral artery, which gave at—		
6.10	50	54	4
	rising in deep expiration to—		
		67	
6.15	35	56	3
	Still doubtful as to the correctness of the observation, I allowed a small jet of blood to escape, and having thus made sure of the absence of clot, replaced the tube, and at once marked at—		
6.21	53	56	3
	The respiration was now labored and slow, the pulse being about 190.		

At 6.23, the artery was cut across, and the dog allowed to bleed to death. Despite the slow and embarrassed breathing, the blood ran red from the divided vessel. It clotted very well in three to five minutes. The effect of the venom on the force of the heart is well seen in the above stated experiments. In them, and in other like observations, the power of the ventricular systole diminished very rapidly soon after the bite, and at the same time, or just afterwards, the general loss of tone was strikingly indicated by the diminution of the independent arterial pressure. In the first case, the animal rallied from the early effect of the venom, and the heart force increased, although not so much as to regain completely its primary power. The cases just stated were selected from a series of seven similar experiments, which I do not think it requisite to quote at length. In all of them the results were the same in kind, although varying somewhat in degree.

In most of these cases, the heart suffered somewhat before respiration was enfeebled or visibly altered. But it was possible that the respiration might be embarrassed, and yet not in so marked a manner as to betray itself to the eye. I thought it likely that by destroying the normal respiratory influence, and sustaining the heart by insufflation, I might be able to place the cardiac organ in a condition which would render it independent of any possible influence from the pulmonary organs.

At first, I attempted to attain this end by cutting both pneumogastric nerves, and thus destroying the main channels through which impressions originating in the lungs are conveyed to the heart. My first experiments failed, owing to my having used young dogs in whom the section of both nerves above the point at which the recurrent laryngeal nerves are given off, never fails to cause asphyxia by collapse of the lips of the larynx. To guard against this result, which, even in older animals, embarrasses the respiration, I placed a tube in the trachea, before dividing the nerve trunks. The respiratory acts became immediately very deep and labored, and, as usual, the heart began to beat with excessive rapidity, but with such feebleness as to raise the mercurial column in the cardiometer only five or six millimetres at each systole. With so feeble a beat it would have been difficult to estimate any such slight increment of feebleness as might at first be produced by the venom. Reluctantly, therefore, this method, which had promised so much, was abandoned. I finally succeeded by resorting to the method detailed in the following cases, which I have chosen for record here, as being sufficiently illustrative of the series to which they belong.

Experiment.—A small black and yellow cur-bitch was secured as usual. The pulse was 140; respiration 29. The trachea was opened, and a tube placed in it. Next, the medulla oblongata was destroyed by pithing, during which about four ounces of blood were lost. Respiration instantly ceased, and the heart-pulse rose to 160. Artificial respiration was now made about forty times in the minute.

The femoral artery was opened, and the cardiometer tube fitted in it, and secured at 5.20 P. M. The constant of arterial pressure was sixty millimetres, the heart beat raising the column from six to twenty millimetres. During three or four minutes these numbers remained about the same, and accordingly a standard of comparison having thus been attained, the dog was bitten twice in three minutes by two snakes of large size. In the next two minutes, the column fluctuated between sixty-seven and seventy-five millimetres, thus giving but eight millimetres to represent the heart force. The change was so notable, that my assistants supposed a clot might be forming, and the tube was therefore removed, cleansed, and replaced. It was perfectly patent, and the artery was unobstructed.

Six minutes after the bite, the constant was forty millimetres, with ten millimetres of rise at each systole. At the eighth minute, the constant was thirty millimetres, the rise fifteen millimetres. This was, however, the maximum, and usually the heart force was but four to five millimetres. The constant was now rapidly falling. The heart beat very irregularly, never raising the mercury above twelve millimetres. There was usually one strong pulsation, and then four feeble ones, of two to four millimetres.

The quivering about the wound continued very remarkable throughout the observation. Upon studying this case, it appeared that the heart and the constant of arterial pressure were both affected very early, but I was not disposed to regard all the ultimate effects as due to the venom. In a case so removed from normal physiological conditions, and so surrounded with causes of depression, it was only possible to draw an inference from the occurrences of the first few minutes after the introduction of a new element—the bite of the snake.

Additional observations, similar to that just recorded, went equally to show that the heart loses power in the first stage of Crotalus poisoning, and that the constant arterial pressure undergoes a rapid and singular diminution. Considerations above stated, would have induced me to question still more rigidly the results of experiments of so complicated a nature, were it not that they are so well supported by all the preceding evidence, and by the numerous records of symptoms in cases of venom poisoning in man.

It is proper to add that in some instances of death, in rabbits, for example, artificial respiration failed almost totally to sustain the cardiac power; but even in these the heart remained irritable to direct stimulus, and there was consequently no such thorough paralysis of the sarcous elements as is seen in some other poisonings.

Action of Venom on the Capillary System.—The experiments on the heart force furnish incidental information as to the absence of capillary irritation from the presence of venom in the circulation.

John Reid, of Edinburgh, has very well shown in his experiments on asphyxia that when black blood, or any other stimulant, enters the capillaries, the arterial pressure increases largely, as is proved by the rise of the mercury in the cardiometer. No such increase of pressure followed the introduction of venom into the system, and we may therefore infer that it exerts no very marked influence of this kind upon the vessels in question.

In frogs, poisoned by venom, the capillary circulation is unaltered, until the heart itself becomes too feeble to sustain it.

When the frog's foot is placed under the microscope, and wetted with venom, no change occurs, because the skin refuses to admit the poison. If we attempt to introduce it into the web through a wound, the mechanical irritation produced by the instrument so affects the local circulation as to baffle the observer completely.

Action of the Venom upon the Intestinal Movements.—The motions of the intestinal canal were unaffected by Crotalus poisoning, and in all cases were as active as after other modes of death.

Action of the Venom upon Ciliary Movement.—In a number of cases of acute and chronic poisoning, I examined the cilia from the mucous membrane of the throat of the frog. Their activity appeared to be undisturbed in both forms of the malady.

Action of the Venom on the Nervous System. Direct Effects of Venom on Nerve Trunks.—The older observers had already shown that the direct contact of venom and nerve matter produced no early local paralysis of the nerve thus treated. I have repeated and modified these experiments, making use of the venom of the Crotalus.

Experiment.—The leg of a frog, prepared as if for use for a galvanoscope, was placed in a wide test-tube, and the long sciatic nerve laid upon a glass slide. Upon applying gentle mechanical or galvanic irritants to the nerve trunk, the muscles of the leg moved freely. A drop of pure venom was then let fall on the nerve, along which it ran by capillary attraction, so as to wet about one-third of an inch of its length. At the close of ten minutes the nerve still reacted well. In a second case treated in the same way, but subjected to rather more of the venom, the nerve acted well after eighteen minutes; and in a third nerve similarly situated, irritability was excellent at the close of thirty-two minutes.

In a second series of experiments, the same conclusion was reached by another route.

Experiment.—A large frog was chosen, and the right sciatic nerve isolated in almost half an inch of its course. A little gutter of wax was slipped under the nerve, and a rather thin solution of venom in water applied to the nerve trunk during five minutes. The wax groove, in which lay the nerve, served to retain the venom in contact with its exterior. At the close of seven minutes the leg still moved with ease, when the frog's body was irritated. The nerve was then incised lengthwise, and a little pure venom dropped within the slit and on the nerve.

A minute amount of moisture being applied to the nerve, with the aid of a camel's hair brush, from time to time, it was found to carry impressions to or from the nerve centres quite well at the end of an hour. On irritating the right foot, both legs were moved freely, and on irritating the unwounded left leg, a like result was observed. When released, the frog leaped about, using both legs with ease and activity. Twenty-four hours later it was still able to use both legs, although the muscles about the wounded part were softened by the venom, a change which had not visibly acted on the nerve trunk. The frog finally recovered. Upon several occasions, as opportunity offered, I repeated these experiments, but without arriving at any other conclusion than that the venom exerted no early action upon the vital properties of nerves to which it was applied.

Action of the Venom upon the Sensory and Motor Nerves, and upon the Nerve Centres.—In the conduct of this portion of my research, I endeavored to ascertain which order of nerves was first affected by the venom. For this purpose,

Experiment.—I tied the left femoral artery of a frog high up, and then had the frog bitten in the back by two snakes. At the seventy-sixth minute all motion, voluntary and reflex, had ceased. On galvanizing the right sciatic nerve, no reflex acts ensued, but the muscles of the right leg moved as freely as those of the other limb, which I had insulated from the effects of the venom by cutting off its circulation. The motor nerves were therefore unaffected. If the sensory nerves and the centres had been also capable of transmitting impressions, and responding to them, there would have been reflex movements produced.

Numerous repetitions of this experiment convinced me that either the sensory nerves had lost their powers, or that the nerve-centres were at fault. This question was set at rest by the following means:—

Experiment.—A frog was poisoned, and as soon as all movement was over except that of the heart, the spine was divided, and a probe thrust up and down. No motion resulted. The irritability of the motor nerves in the sciatic trunk was next tested, and found to be nearly perfect.

The loss of nervous function begins, then, at the centres; and such being the case, we cannot infer logically that the sensory nerves are paralyzed, but only that they have no longer any means of expressing their sensibility, if it still exists.

These experiments were repeated again and again upon warm-blooded animals, in whom the action of the heart proved capable of being sustained for a time by artificial respiration.

Experiment.—A large rabbit, male, was twice struck at 5.10. At 5.20 it fell, and in twenty-eight minutes from the time of the bite, the respiration stopped. Artificial insufflation was then employed, as usual. It seemed to sustain the heart's action pretty well for about twelve minutes. During this time the dorsal spine was cut across; no motion resulted. A probe being thrust up and down the spine, feeble quivering of the nearer spinal muscles took place, but the limbs did not move. On dividing the sciatic nerves, free motion was observed, and the phrenic trunk was likewise irritable.

In another set of cases, the centres and nerve-trunks were galvanized immediately after the natural respiration ceased, and before the heart was quite at rest. Still, the same results were observed, so that it became clear that death took place rather from paralysis of the centres than from loss of function in the efferent nerves.

The duration of irritability in the motor nerves of the frog was observed to be less under venom poisoning than under death by decapitation, for example. It is to be borne in mind, however, that where the heart ceases to beat, or beats too feebly to circulate the blood, the loss of nerve power may be due to this cause alone, as Kölliker has very well demonstrated. Yet, as we have seen, this source of fallacy may be readily eliminated.

Effect of the Venom upon the Calorifacient Functions.—In very acute cases of Crotalus poisoning, death may occur so suddenly as to preclude the possibility of a fall of temperature. The following experiment is a fair type of what occurs in most cases which do not perish within a few minutes.

Experiment.—Temperature of the air 72° F. At eight minutes to five P. M., a very accurate thermometer capable of indicating tenths of degrees[1] was placed in the cloac of a pigeon, and was found to mark 108° F. As the pigeon became tranquil, it fell to 107.5° F. The pigeon was then exposed to the bite of a snake two and a half feet long. Great quivering of the muscles ensued.

At the tenth minute, the temperature was 107.2° F., respiration 31.

The following record was then obtained :—

Time after death.	Temperature.	
14th minute	106.8°	
19th "	105.5	
22d "	105.8	
25th "	104.8	
28th "	104.3	The bulb at this time slipped a little further into the cloac.
31st "	104.4	
34th "	104.4	
37th "	104.2	Respiration 40.
40th "	103.9	Respiration jerking.
43d "	103.5	
46th "	103.3	
49th "	103.1	
52d "	103.	Respiration 52.
55th "	102.5	Slight convulsions.
58th "	101.5	Respiration irregular and slow—12.
61st		Respiration ceased.
62d "	101.3	
63d "	100.9	
66th "	100.	

[1] This instrument was made by J. W. Queen & Co., the well-known opticians, No. 924 Chestnut Street, Philadelphia, to whom I am indebted for much valuable aid in making and altering the numerous instruments which from time to time have been necessary in various physiological researches.

The observation here ended. The heart blood clotted very rapidly, but not very firmly. In addition to these facts, I may observe that in dogs who survived the first action of the venom, and died at the close of twenty-four or thirty-six hours, the temperature of the rectum was found to be a degree or more below the normal standard. On the near approach of death it fell rapidly.

The experiments just related point plainly to the necessity of sustaining the normal temperature of the body in severe cases of Crotalus bite. The value of this precaution in other forms of poisoning has been admirably illustrated by M. Brown-Séquard. All that he has said of narcotic and other depressing agents applies with equal force to the cases before us.[1]

Effect of Venom on the Blood.—The study of the vital fluid in cases of acute or primary poisoning is of a merely negative value. An animal, and especially a warm-blooded animal which dies within a minute or two, or after even a longer time, presents us with none of those profound alterations of the blood which characterize all instances of secondary poisoning. A pigeon, for instance, is stricken, it droops, falls, and dies within thirty seconds, as may happen. Its blood is red, and coagulates perfectly. Its blood-corpuscles are ideally healthy. The tissues and fluids beyond the wound are, pathologically, as they would be after poisoning by opium or woorara. In such a case no physiologist could impute the death to an altered blood, and its positive or negative effects on the essential nutrition and oxygenation of nerve and muscle. The line of difference here between acute or primary, and chronic or secondary poisoning by Crotalus venom, is drawn most definitely, and although every possible variety of modified cases may occur, so as to mingle the two modes of death into one deadly draught, the two sets of fatal cases will still remain characteristically separated, and by no stronger difference than that of the pathology of the blood in the respective instances.

If in the secondary poisonings we examine first the obvious physical characters of the blood, we shall observe that it is very dark in all parts of the body, but somewhat redder in the left than the right heart. Both the color and the accumulation in the veins seem to be due to the apnœa which ushers in the death, as is clear from what I already have said, and from the experiments which I shall presently relate in connection with the question of coagulation.

As I have before stated, the longer the death is delayed, the more apt is the blood to become incoagulable. So diffluent was it in some cases, that I have poured it from glass to glass like water and kept it thus until it decomposed completely. In other cases the heart contained a few loose and very weak clots, and in others again, only rare shreds of coagulum were met with.

What effect has the direct mixture of venom and blood? what becomes of the fibrin in venom poisoning? and what is the cause of the change in the condition of the fibrin? are the material questions which naturally present themselves for answer.

Experiment.—One drop of venom was put on a slide and a drop of blood from a

---

[1] Experimental Researches applied to Physiology and Pathology, by E. Brown-Séquard, M. D., of the Faculty of Paris, etc. etc. N. Y. H. Bailliere, 1853, p. 26 *et seq.*

pigeon's wounded wing allowed to fall upon it. They were instantly mixed. Within three minutes the mass had coagulated firmly, and within ten it was of arterial redness.

Experiment.—One drop of arterial blood from the pigeon was mixed with one of venom. Coagulation took place as usual, but the blood did not darken.

The last experiment was repeated, substituting venous blood, coagulation ensued, and on exposure the blood became of arterial redness.

Experiment.—Two drops of venom were added to one of pigeon's blood. Coagulation took place within four minutes. Pure blood from the pigeon was frequently found to coagulate a little sooner than this. So small a degree of retardation may have been due to the thick and gummy nature of the admixed venom.

As I was anxious to verify these observations, I instituted a number of experiments, some of which are briefly stated in the table below. Simple as the conduct of such experiments may seem, they are liable to fallacies. If, for instance, care be not taken, the blood coagulates before time is allowed to mix it with the venom. Or again, the mechanical process of mingling is carried on too long, and the feeble clots which alone are formed in the case of some animals, may thus be so broken up as to escape notice in the minute amounts of blood we are compelled to employ.

No.	Kind of blood used.	Amount of venom previously mixed with one or two drops of water.	Amount of blood.	Result.
1	Crotalus durissus.	One drop.	About ten drops.	Coagulated within half an hour, clot weak.
2	" "	One-half of a drop.	About twenty drops.	Coagulated in ten minutes.
3	Frog, Rana pipiens.	One-fifth of a drop.	Six drops.	Coagulated well.
	" " "	One-half of a drop.	" "	" "
4	Reed-bird.	One-fifth of a drop.	Five drops.	Clot formed rapidly, and was so loose and weak that it broke up completely and easily during the process of mingling the blood and the venom, and at first led to the belief that none had formed.
5	"	One-fifth of a drop.	" "	Coagulated loosely. All the clots in this blood were of this nature.
6	Dog (a small brown terrier).	One-quarter of a drop.	" "	Coagulated perfectly well.
		One-half of a drop.	" "	" " "
		One-fifteenth of a drop.	" "	" " "
7	Man.	One-fifteenth of a drop.	Seven drops.	" " "

The specimens of blood described in this table were usually set aside after coagulating, and the watch-glasses in which they were placed remained covered with smaller ones during twenty-four hours, the temperature being from 78° to about 82° F. To my surprise, the clots, which were in some instances very firm, became in all more or less altered during this period of time. The blood was darker, the structure of the clots softened and partially or entirely dissolved.

It becomes clear from these results that the mixture of venom and blood does not alter the vital fluid at first in any way which is appreciable to our senses. The blood drawn into venom and rapidly mixed with it in any proportion, clots as firmly as usual. After a time, however, it seems that a catalytic change is induced, the clot softens, and even becomes perfectly redissolved when the amount of mingled venom has been large and the temperature of the air high. This alteration of the formed clot, external to the body, finds its illustration within the system in those cases of chronic poisoning, in which the fibrin of the blood, subjected to long contact with venom, finally loses its power to coagulate. When under ordinary circumstances, in summer weather, blood is protected from desiccation, the clot not unfrequently softens after a few days, or even entirely redissolves. This change, however, is produced by extensive putrefactive alterations in the blood, and is most readily induced in the blood of such persons as are anæmic, or still more rapidly in the blood of some reptiles and fish. The condition of diffluence attained within twenty-four hours, under the influence of the venom, was such as usually requires, in pure blood, several days of warm weather to effect. It is proper to add that in almost all of the specimens of mingled blood and venom the odor made it evident that putrefactive changes had taken place, an inference which was further justified by the evidence which they soon afforded of continued progress in this direction.

Fontana's[1] observations on the subject of the direct action of venom on blood are altogether insufficient and unsatisfactory. He seems to have been of opinion that admixture with venom darkened the blood, and prevented coagulation. In this view he differed from Mead. Dr. Brainard,[2] so far as I am aware, was the first to state that when the animal bitten dies soon, the blood is coagulable, and that when death is delayed, it ceases to exhibit this condition.

The statements of Dr. Brainard in regard to changes effected in the blood-disks by Crotalus, or rather Crotalophorus venom, prepared me to find them more or less altered in my own cases. He seems to have held an opinion, common enough at the date of his paper,[3] namely, that woorara owed its potency to a serpent venom, and that this poison as well as true venom seriously injured the blood-globules, and produced a fatal result by causing their arrest in the capillaries. Fontana, who examined the blood after death from viper bite, and who studied the mixture of blood and venom, states that it prevented coagulation, but that he found the globules unaltered.

The general result of my own experiments on this subject may be very briefly summed up. I have made very many careful examinations of the blood-disks of frogs, birds, dogs, etc., which had been killed by snake bites. In a few rare cases of prolonged secondary poisoning, I found a small proportion of the globules altered and indented on the edge, but in no case were these changes very remarkable. In primary or acute poisoning, I have never been able to detect the least alteration in the blood-cells. It should be needless to add that I examined the cells taken from the heart and from capillaries, and that these observations were made so soon as death took place.

I have also studied the effect on the disks of mixing the venom with blood, but even in these circumstances no notable change took place in the blood-disks within any brief period of time, as half an hour. Whether or not this direct contact would affect them after a longer time, I cannot say, and it is a question which is partially open for further study.

---

[1] Fontana, vol. i. pp. 313 and 384. Skinner's Translation.

[2] Brainard, op. cit.

[3] Essay on a New Method of Treating Serpent Bites, etc., by Daniel Brainard, M. D. Chicago, 1854, pp. 14, and plates.

Dr. Burnett[1] states that direct union of venom and blood causes the disks to lose their tendency to arrange themselves in rows. This observation, also, I am unable to verify entirely. Where the blood and venom were mixed in equal quantities, the nummulation of the disks was very often prevented, but the poison is so glutinous and gum-like that its mechanical properties may be very well supposed to exert some effect on this process, and certainly, so far as I have seen, the presence of venom to the amount of a tenth or twentieth in no way retarded, much less stopped, the union of the globules of freshly-drawn blood.

One other observation was yet to be made to complete the study of the influence of venom upon the various parts of the blood. It was clear that in slow venom poisoning the blood plasma became profoundly altered. As it was possible that the contents of the blood-disks might also undergo a like degradation without of necessity involving changes in the form of these elements, I examined the blood of several guinea-pigs to determine whether, after death from Crotalus bite, the blood would still crystallize. In some of these cases the blood was very feebly clotted, in one only was it perfectly fluid. In all of these, specimens of blood from the heart afforded me, after the usual preparation, beautiful crystals, nor did these differ in form, size, or color, from the characteristic tetrahedrons of the blood of this animal.

In order to complete my study of the blood, I desired to ascertain the rate at which the fibrin disappeared from the vital fluid.

Experiment.—The first observation on this point was made upon a small dog, weighing about ten pounds. A tube was placed in the left carotid artery, that blood might be drawn from time to time. The various portions of blood were received in glasses of like shape, which were labelled and set aside.

At 4.15 minutes P. M., a drachm of blood was drawn from the artery; it coagulated perfectly well in three or four minutes.

At 4.20, at 4.24, and 4.26, the dog was bitten by separate snakes, which had been frequently used within four days. From the second wound ran a little blood, which collected in the hollow of the groin, and coagulated feebly.

At 4.37 about half an ounce of blood was drawn. At 4.36 the dog fell.

At 4.46 I removed about two drachms of blood. Like that removed at 4.37, it clotted perfectly.

At 4.55 respiration ceased, just as a fourth specimen was taken, and at 4.58 all motion was over. The specimen last collected coagulated rather freely.

The wound in the flank was at once laid open, and about two drachms of fluid blood collected from the tissues, which were soaked down to the bones. The heart blood, being drawn into a seventh glass, was still found to be coagulable, but the clot which formed was by no means so perfect as in the blood first drawn.

At the close of twenty-four hours, the temperature being about 78° F., the specimens one, two, and three were unaltered, and had no unpleasant odor; number four was slightly altered, but the blood from the heart was already unpleasant in smell, and that from the wound was quite putrid. At the end of a second period of twenty-four hours, these changes were much more marked.

---

[1] Burnett, op. cit.

Experiment.—In a second case, the dog, which was large and vigorous, survived the bites several hours, and died during my absence. He was bitten by a strong and fresh snake at 5.15, and again by a second at 5.18. At 5.57, blood drawn from the femoral artery was red and perfectly coagulable. At the close of two hours, the blood drawn still clotted well. At this time, as I have said, I ceased to observe him. He was able to walk when I left him, and was drinking eagerly. I do not suppose that he could have died before five or six hours from the time of the bite. Eighteen hours after, I returned to find him dead and rigid. His blood was everywhere dark and fluid.

Experiment.—In another instance during the spring of 1859, a dog was accidentally dropped into my snake-box. He was bitten in a dozen places by as many snakes, and perished in about eighteen minutes. His blood was entirely fluid, and so remained. This was the most rapid case of alteration of the blood with which I have met.

The last observation of this series was one of great interest, owing to the fact that the dog survived very serious visceral lesions and lived during two days with his blood in a condition of complete diffluence.

Experiment.—The dog, a small terrier weighing about fifteen pounds, was intended to make one of a set of observations on the value of Bibron's antidote. For this purpose he was placed in the snake-box, where instantly he was struck twice by a large snake, both wounds being double fang marks, and both being in the right flank. On removing him I observed that from one of the wounds blood was running in a thin stream. After it had run for some time, I caught a few drops in a watch-glass, and found that it coagulated well. Before I thought fit to use the supposed antidote, I was called away. Returning at the end of an hour I found the dog standing with his head pendent, having just vomited glairy mucus. His pulse was quick and feeble, his respiration occasionally panting. The hemorrhage had ceased. Owing to an accident which at this time deprived me of the supply of Bibron's antidote, which I had prepared, I was unable to make further use of the animal in the manner proposed, and not desiring to lose the observation altogether, I utilized the opportunity in the following way:—

One hour and a half after he was bitten I drew a drachm of blood from the jugular vein. It clotted perfectly.

Four and a half hours after the bite a drachm of blood from the same vein coagulated equally well.

Twenty hours from the time of the poisoning, the dog was found lying on his left side, having passed slimy and bloody stools in abundance. At intervals he seemed to suffer much from tenesmus, but was so weak that he stood up with difficulty. His gums were bleeding, a symptom I had seen before, and his eyes were deeply injected. At this time about two or three drachms of blood were drawn. It was very dark, and formed within five minutes a clot of feeble texture.

Twenty-seven hours and a half after the time at which he was bitten, the dog was weaker. His hind legs were twitching, and the dysentery continued. Three drachms of blood were drawn as usual, but no clot formed in this specimen, although it was set aside and carefully watched for some time. While I was collecting the fluid for observation the dog suddenly discharged per anum at least four ounces of dark, grumous blood. At this time I supplied the dog with water, and left him. Fifty-four hours after the bite he was seen again, and found to have drunk freely of water, and to have passed fewer stools. Up to this date he declined all food.

From this time he improved rapidly, and took with eagerness whatever nutriment was offered. On the fourth day his blood again exhibited a clot, although it was very small and of loose texture. I made no further examinations of the blood. The dog lost flesh as he gained strength, and had profuse suppuration from an abscess in the bitten flank. At the close of two weeks he was active and well, except that the wound was still open.

The case last related is doubly valuable, as pointing out even in a single instance the time at which the blood became altered, and also as showing, once more, how profound may be this change, and how perfect the recovery.

The study of envenomed blood has thus far taught us—1st. That in animals which survive the poisoning for a time, the blood is so altered as to render the fibrin incoagulable.

2d. Experiments in and out of the body have given proof that this change is gradual, and that the absence of coagulation is not due to checked formation of fibrin, but to alterations produced by the action of the venom in that fibrin which already exists in the circulating blood.

3. The influence thus exerted is of a putrefactive nature, and imitates in a few hours the ordinary results of days of change. It is probably even more rapid within the body, on account of the higher temperature of the economy.

4th. The altered blood retains its power to absorb gases, and thus to change its own color.

5th. The blood-corpuscles are unaffected in acute poisoning by Crotalus venom, and are rarely and doubtfully altered in the most prolonged cases which result fatally.

6th. The contents of the blood-globules of the guinea-pig can be made to crystallize as is usual after other modes of death.

Altered Relation between the Blood and Tissues.—Among the most constant and most curious lesions in the cases of secondary poisoning are the ecchymoses which are found on and in the viscera of the chest and belly; most frequently affecting the intestinal canal, they may and do occur in any cavity and on any organ. These spots contain blood whose globules are more or less deformed, but still of dimensions not less than usual. As they do not take place until the blood is considerably altered, and as the intra-vascular blood-disks undergo no apparent change, this leakage of the blood into the serous cavities and areolar interspaces is plainly due to the loss of coagulating power in the blood, or to alterations in the vascular tubes, or perhaps to both. Unfortunately, we can but revive anew the unanswered question as to the possibility of the escape of blood-disks through yet unwounded vessels. It is likely, however, that the tissues share in the incipient putrefactive fermentation which characterizes prolonged cases of this poisoning, and are more or less weakened thereby; so that, with a degraded blood, and, of a consequence, with an embarrassed capillary circulation, aided by laboring respiration, we can readily conceive how capillary ruptures may take place, and so give rise to transudations of blood in any portion of the body.

I have grouped together all the visceral lesions, because it seemed to me that, however various the seat of the affection, it was, in all organs and throughout the tissues, alike in its character. In other words, owing to the changes in blood or tissues, or both, extravasations are met with in the lungs, brain, kidneys, serous membranes, intestines, and heart. As a result, we may have functional derangement grafted on the main stem of the malady, and the accompaniments of bloody serum in the affected cavities, bloody mucus in the intestinal canal, and bloody urine in the bladder.

Causation of Death in Acute and Chronic Crotalus Poisoning.—Perhaps scarcely one intelligent medical reader will have followed me thus far without arriving at the conclusion that the venom of the Crotalus, like that of other snakes, is a septic or putrefacient poison of astounding energy. This very obvious view has long been held by toxicologists, and the cases and experiments of this paper assuredly do not weaken it.

The rapid decomposition of the blood, and of the tissues locally acted upon by the venom, leaves no doubt upon the matter, and makes it apparent that an incipient putrefaction of this nature may so affect the blood as to destroy its power to clot, and, perhaps, also to nourish the tissues through which it is urged.

The alterations thus brought about are probably the results of a continued fermentative change, which, begun by a small amount of poison, is gradually made to involve in fatal change the whole mass of the circulating fluids. Like all fermentations, however, the rapidity depends on temperature and on the amount of the primary ferment. In one instance, a dog, struck by eight snakes, died in eighteen minutes, and exhibited an uncoagulable blood. I am aware of no other case of loss of coagulating power so rapid. It was rendered thus by the number of localities from which the ferment attacked the system. On the other hand, the frog, a small animal, receives the same dose of venom as would have entered the tissues of a larger animal, yet it resists the poison most remarkably, by virtue of its powers as a cold-blooded creature, existing at the temperature of the atmosphere itself.

Admitting, then, that the changes effected in the blood may be sufficient to account for the fatal results in chronic cases of poisoning by Crotalus, are we justified in referring to similar causes the sudden deaths which sometimes take place in small, or even larger animals, in whose tissues or fluids we can detect no change whatsoever?

In the present state of this inquiry, the question scarcely admits of a positive answer. It is clear that in acute cases, the symptoms of depression are most marked, and the heart and nerve centres are suddenly and fearfully enfeebled, so that their irritability is lessened, and is finally lost earlier than occurs in other forms of death. If now, we knew of no other property of the poison than this one, we could properly pause here, and regard the venom as having a specific influence on the heart, and on the nervous irritability of some part of the cerebro-spinal centres, such as characterizes certain of the better known poisons, such as corroval, woorara, upas, opium, aconite, etc. Since, however, we are aware that serpent venom, after remaining for a time in the body, has a specific power of attacking at least one element of the blood, and through its degradation, perhaps, of affecting the whole circulating fluid, we are naturally inclined to ask whether this power may not also be invoked to explain even the *ultimate* nature of the *sudden* cases of death from the venom. If, for instance, a pigeon is struck by a snake, and dies in thirty seconds, its tissues normal in appearance and its blood unaltered, have we any logical right to infer that the blood may have been inappreciably, but fatally, altered, so as to be unable to sustain the life of the tissues which it feeds? Is it this possible, but imperceptible, change in the blood which acts to produce those losses of irritability in the nerve-centres which we have been led to regard as the proximate cause of early and rapid death? If such be the case, then *the suddenness of the general change* in the blood must account for the failure of life, because it can be shown that animals whose blood is considerably altered may live for some time, or even survive to renew and refibrinate their vital fluids.

The cause of death in chronic or secondary poisoning may, with propriety, then, be referred to the incipient putrefactive changes which affect the blood, as well as to the continued influence of the agencies which first act to depress the heart's action, and destroy nerve function.

The cause of death in the acute cases, where the result is so sudden that no change is perceptible in the blood in the vessels, is amply explained in the preceding pages. But, while we are able to state where death begins, and in what order the functions succumb, we are still far from knowing why, or precisely how, this or that structure is affected. The proximate causes are open to experimental study, the ultimate reason, as we have seen (page 95), is as yet unknown.

Summing up, then, what we have learned of the acute form of poisoning, we may feel justified in concluding, 1st. That the heart becomes enfeebled shortly after the bite. This is due to direct influence of the venom on this organ, and not to the precedent loss of the respiratory function. Notwithstanding the diminution of cardiac power, the heart is usually in motion after the lungs cease to act, and its tissues remain for a time locally irritable. The paralysis of the heart is, therefore, not so complete as it is under the influence of upas or corroval.

2d. That in warm-blooded animals, artificial respiration lengthens the life of the heart, but does not sustain it so long as when the animal has died by woorara, or decapitation.

3d. That in the frog, the heart-acts continue after respiration has ceased, and sometimes survive until the sensory nerves and the nerve-centres are dead, the motor nerves alone remaining irritable.

4th. That in warm-blooded animals respiration ceases, owing to paralysis of the nerve-centres.

5th. That the sensory nerves, and the centres of nerve power in the medulla spinalis and medulla oblongata, lose their vitality before the efferent or motor nerves become affected.

6th. That the muscular system retains its irritability in the cold-blooded animals, acutely poisoned, for a considerable time after death.

7th. That the first effect of the venom being to depress the vital energy of the heart and nerve-centres, a resort to stimulants is clearly indicated, as the only rational mode of early constitutional treatment.

Analogy between the Symptoms of Crotalus Poisoning and those of Certain Diseases.—I am unwilling to leave this unsatisfactory, but necessary part of my task, without calling attention to the singular likeness between the symptoms and lesions of Crotalus poisoning, and those of certain maladies, such as yellow fever.[1] If for a moment we lose sight of the local injection, and regard only the symptoms which follow, and the tissue changes which ensue, the resemblance becomes still more striking.

In both diseases, for such they are, we have a class of cases in which death seems to occur suddenly and inexplicably, as though caused by an overwhelming dose of the poison. In both diseases, these cases are marked by symptoms of profound prostration, and in both the post-mortem revelations fail to explain the death. I have spoken, as an example, of yellow fever, but similar instances are not wanting in cholera, typhoid, and typhus fevers, and in scarlatina.

A second class of cases, both of Crotalus poisoning and of yellow fever, survive the first shock of the malady, and then begin to exhibit the train of symptoms which terminates in more or less complete degradation of the character of the blood. Varying remarkably among themselves, exhibiting, as it were, preferences for this or that organ, all of these maladies agree in the destruction of the fibrin of the blood which their fatal cases frequently exhibit. In yellow fever, the likeness to venom poisoning is most distinctly preserved, as we trace the symptoms of both diseases to the point where the diffluent blood leaks out into the mucous and serous cavities. The yellowness which characterizes many yellow fever cases, I do not find described as a current symptom of the venom malady, but it is often mentioned as one of the accompaniments of the period of recovery from the bite.[2] It is, indeed, most probable, that if small and repeated doses of venom were introduced at intervals into the body of an animal, a disease might be produced even more nearly resembling the malady in question. In the parallel thus drawn, I have given but the broad outlines of resemblance, nor was it to be expected that the minor details would be alike. From a general and philosophic point of view, this similarity is sufficiently striking to make me hope that the complete control of one such septic poison for experimental use, may enable us in future to throw new light on those septic poisons of disease whose composition we know nothing of, and whose very means of entering the body they destroy, is, as yet, a mystery.

---

[1] This analogy has been noted by S. L. Mitchill, by Magendie, and by Gaspard, who has also called attention to the resemblance between ordinary putrefactive poisoning, such as arises from injection into the blood of decayed animal substances, and the poisoning by venom. Neither in this, or in any other cases of the kind, is the likeness perfect; and while, to use a naturalist's phrase, we recognize these septic maladies as of one genus, we cannot regard them as so nearly allied as to be mere varieties of one species. Yellow fever and putrefactive poisoning both begin, in the mass of cases, with a fever, which is absent in the first stages of venom poisoning; and there are other and wide differences which it is needless to enumerate here. See Gaspard, Journal de Physiologie, tome iv. p. 2 *et seq.*, and tome iii. pp. 81–85 of same Journal. See also La Roche on Yellow Fever, vol. ii. p. 597.

[2] Jaundice, occasionally observed in France as an early symptom of viper bite, has been usually regarded as the jaundice of fear, a cause which certainly cannot be invoked to account for the icterus seen in late stages of the malady caused by the venom.

CHAPTER VIII.

CROTALUS POISONING IN MAN.

The cases of Rattlesnake poisoning in man have been separated from the rest of this paper, owing to the difficulty of grouping the phenomena of human poisoning with those observed in animals. This difficulty arose from the imperfect reports of such cases as have been recorded, and from the fact that, in man, the symptoms were possibly modified, in some instances, by the remedies used, and were thus no longer comparable with such as had been seen to exist in animals submitted to no modifying treatment. Some of these objections would, of course, disappear in a collection of cases so large as to enable us distinctly to separate the essential from the induced, or accidental features of the malady. Unfortunately, although I have collected at least fifty cases of Crotalus bite, the most of these scarcely deserve the name of medical reports, and among the whole number I have been able to select but sixteen which were sufficiently rich in details, to be of the slightest value. The numerous gaps in the accompanying table, show but too well the want of full medical statements of the order and character of the symptoms, even in these select cases, and it is humiliating to observe that, of the four post-mortem examinations of the lesions in this mode of poisoning, but two were made in this country.

If, then, in the table of symptoms in man, and in the following remarks upon them, such a lack of detail is met with as would disgrace the most ordinary report of "an interesting case," the blame must rest where it belongs, with the physicians of our own country, who have failed thus much in their duty as medical observers.

It is impossible to review the whole field of observation upon this important subject, without arriving at the conclusion that whatever may be the degree of virulence in the poison of different venomous snakes, its mode of affecting the system varies but little, whether the bite be inflicted by the Viper, the Copperhead, the Rattlesnake, or the dreaded, but not more deadly, Cobra. Thus, in each case, we have the local poisoning, the constitutional malady, and the possibility of inexplicably rapid death on the one hand, and of a strange zymotic disease upon the other. There may yet remain some room for doubt as to whether the apparent difference in the activity of the venom from various serpents is not due to the quantities formed or stored up in each case, and to unobserved peculiarities in the structure and form of the poison apparatus. However this may be, it is quite certain that two cases of rattlesnake poisoning may sometimes differ as much as either one of them will, from a case of Moccasin or Cobra bite. This fact should make us cautious in asserting distinctions between the mode of action of the venoms of the several poisonous serpents upon evidence of any limited number of facts.

With these brief preliminary remarks, we shall pass to the consideration of the symptoms of Crotalus bite in man. In this review, I shall make use not only of the cases in the accompanying table, but also of the many brief notices of cases which were found unfit for tabular analysis. All that I have to say at present with regard to antidotes and treatment, will be found at the close.

TABLE OF CROTALUS

No.	Reporter.	Sex.	Seat of wounds, *i. e.* fang marks.	Early local symptoms.	Later local symptoms.	Immediate or early constitutional symptoms.	Respiration and circulation.	General later symptoms. Nervous system.
1	Moore	Male	Instep twice bitten	Pain, swelling, hemorrhage from bites	Continued pain, and swelling to the knee	None stated	None stated	Probably none of moment
2	W. Mayrant	Male	Throat	Swelling and pain	Caustics used. Small slough	Sudden and excessive prostration; vomiting; locked-jaw; loss of speech	Feeble fluttering pulse	... ...
3	W. Mayrant	Male	... ...	Pain	... ...	Violent vomiting and prostration	... ...	... ...
4	W. E. Horner	Male	Bend of elbow, two fang marks	There seems to have been none felt (see remarks) except itching	Itching, pain great, swelling	Apparently none	Feeble pulse, respiration easy	Convulsion; mind generally clear up to death
5	H. B. Phillips	Female	Struck twice on foot	... ...	Inguinal glands enlarged; great pain and swelling; mottled skin	Vomiting, depression, and thirst	Feeble, pulse 60; great gen'l swelling; great thirst; loss of speech; tongue swollen	Mind clear
6	Post	Male	Last phalanx of middle finger	Small jet of blood from wound; swelling	Continued swelling up to pectoral muscles, followed by great discoloration	... ...	Pulse 2½ hours after bite 80, not weak; after this it became faster, to 120, and more and more feeble	Excited manner
7	J. Trowbridge	Male, æt. 12 years	Foot near small toe	Swelling and pain	Leg swollen to the groin; great pain and discoloration	Probably none of the usual symptoms, none stated	Pulse rapid 2½ hrs. after bite	... ...
8	Withmire	Male (boy)	Ankle	Pain and swelling	Continued pain and swelling	... ...	... ...	... ...
9	Hammond	Male	Finger	Pain and swelling	Pain and swelling disappeared after use of antidote, and returned in 40 minutes	... ...	... ...	... ...
10	Hammond (Coolidge)	Female æt. 15 years	Finger	Pain, swelling, and discoloration	Pain, swelling, etc., to the elbow	Depression and nausea	... ...	Case too short for the later constitutional symptoms to develop
11	John Louis Xantus. (de Vésey.)	Boy	Leg	Pain, swelling	Increasing pain and swelling	Prostration	... ...	Great prostration
12	Home	Male (the reporter)	Thumb and finger twice bitten, four fang wounds	No immediate swelling	Swelling, pain extending rapidly up the arm, which grew cold and sloughed before death	Incoherence possibly due to drunkenness and alarm	Pulse feeble, throughout 100 to 138	The mind confused at first, became clear; depression, nausea, faint feelings; vomiting on the second day
13	Woodhouse	Male	Finger	Pain, shock, and nausea	Pain, swelling of hand and arm, and axillary glands, vesications over the lymphatics on third day	Nausea	... ...	... ...
14	Harlan	Male	Metacarpal joint of finger, two fang wounds	Bleeding from the punctures; swelling, discoloration	Extensive swelling and pain	Repeated and sudden fainting and pallor	Feeble pulse; difficult respiration; hiccough	Delirium, restlessness, anxiety, insomnia, incessant thirst
15	Atchison	Female æt. 12 years	Instep, two fang punctures	Slight swelling and discoloration	Intense pain shooting up the leg	2½ hours after the bite almost moribund; pulse feeble and wavy; surface cold and perspiring; face swollen; mind wandering; pupils dilated; subject to sensory delusions	Feeble pulse until the stimulus acted	Delusions, etc., passed away under the use of the stimulus
16	Pihorel	Male, adult	Twice bitten on the palm and [illegible] thumb and forefinger on the back of the thumb, the last wound was single	Swelling and discoloration at [illegible] due to the ligature, which was applied 3 or 4 minutes after the bites	No increase of the primary swelling after removal of the ligature	Within 10 minutes pallor, cold sweats, anxious expression, general depression	The physician removed the ligature in consequence of the swelling [illegible] when— The pulse became feeble (50) but rose to 110 before death; noisy respiration	The limbs insensible, repeated syncope, pupils contracted, mind clear
							At the seventh hour there was a swelling of the lip; no general tumefaction; great anxiety; painful and difficult deglutition and respiration.	

POISONING IN MAN.

No.	Secretions and discharges.	State of skin and temperature.	Result of disease.	Duration of disease.	Mode of death.	Local and general consequences if recovery occurred.	Local treatment.	General treatment.	Remarks.
1	... ...	...	Cure	At work in 3 days	...	Limited local suppuration	Ammonia, ligature	Ammonia	Mild case; alludes to 14 cases of snake bite successfully treated with ammonia.
2	... ...	...	Cure	Within 24 hours	...	Small local slough	Caustic	Alcohol and red pepper; 2 quarts of whisky given in one night, and renewed as the pulse fell	Severe case.
3	... ...	...	Cure	In 12 hours	...	... ...	... ...	Whisky one quart in 10 or 12 hours	
4	Dark bilious stool, vomiting	Extremities cold	Death	In about 18 hours, without convulsions	...	... ...	Cups, scarification, etc.	Ammonia, olive oil, no persistent treatment	In this case the man was somewhat intoxicated when bitten.
5	Constant vomiting, loss of speech	...	Cure	Much better in 30 hours, well in 3 weeks	...	... ...	Scarifications, blisters	Carb. ammonia and arsenic	Severe case.
6	None mentioned	...	Death	5½ hours, coma	...	... ...	Suction following on incomplete excision within half an hour, ligature	Carb. ammonia and brandy in as large doses as the patient could be prevailed on to take	
7	... ...	...	Cure	... ...	...	... ...	Frictions, with olive oil	℥ij of olive oil given every half hour	Relates 3 other cases of cure by olive oil, all incompletely told.
8	Nausea and vomiting	...	Recovery	24 hours	...	... ...	Repeated applications of tinct. iodine	None	
9	... ...	...	Recovery	1 hour	...	... ...	None	Bibron's antidote, given twice (dose gtt. x)	No general symptoms occurred.
10	... ...	...	Recovery	Relief in 1 hour	...	Suppuration on back of hand, perhaps from local treatment	Suction, ligature, free incisions, iodine injections	Bibron's antidote, given twice (dose gtt. x)	Expressed distinct relief from the use of the bromine.
11	... ...	...	Recovery	Within 48 hours	...	... ...	... ...	Bibron's antidote, given twice (dose gtt. x)	Effects of 2 doses of bromine said to be immediate and well marked.
12	Vomiting on 2d day, diarrhœa 11th day, and continuously until death	Constant coldness of extremities	Death	Seventeenth day	Asthenia from typhus state	... ...	Ammonia	Chiefly by ammonia and alcoholic stimuli, with such other remedies as the symptoms demanded	A severe case, well reported
13	Nausea and vomiting on movement during five days	...	Recovery	Gradual, the general symptoms passed off on the fifth day, the local results were persistent during some months	...	Slough, exfoliation of last phalanx, anchylosis of first joint of finger	Incision, suction, ligature, ammonia	Took in a few hours one quart of 4th proof brandy and a ½ pint of whisky; intoxication ensued but lasted only four hours	
14	Continual nausea & vomiting, pain & stricture at epigastrium	...	Recovery	Left his bed in a week, depression passed off on the 2d day	...	Suppuration	Ligatures, free excision, ammonia, repeated washing	Camphor, ammonia, opium, and treatment by symptoms	Severe case.
15	Vomiting of bile took place after a dose of carb. ammonia, but did not recur	Cold and perspiring	Recovery	Speedy relief from use of stimulus, and sudden and complete cure within 24 hours	...	Remarkable and entire relief from hooping-cough, under which the patient had suffered	Scarification, cups, local saline bath, sedative fomentations	Free use of stimulants, 80 grains of carb. ammonia, and three pints of brandy in a few hours, without causing intoxication	
16	Involuntary urinary and fecal evacuations, vomiting one hour after bite	Cold and moist	Death	9 hours, some relief followed the severe symptoms caused by removing the ligature, but during the 8th hour respiration and deglutition more and more difficult, pulse imperceptible, and death ensued apparently from syncope; the mind clear to the close	...	Ligature in 3 to 4 minutes, actual cautery within 18 minutes of the bites	... ...	Half ounce of olive oil, a sedative enema, and leeches to the throat, seem to have been the whole treatment	

Sex.—It is needless to state that men are the most frequent subjects of Crotalus bite, owing to the nature of their occupations, which necessarily bring them within reach of the reptile. Children and women are sometimes bitten, and, as may be seen from the table, even young children may recover from the effects of the accident. It is not possible or right to infer from this, that young or weakly persons suffer no more than the strong or fully grown, because we do not know how much venom may have been inserted in each case. Thus, a child struck by an exhausted snake would have a far better chance of escape than a vigorous man bitten by a serpent which had been caged for months. This element is, of course, deficient in calculations upon the prognosis of our ordinary maladies, such as typhoid fever and others, since in them the severity of the resultant symptoms alone informs us as to the probable amount of poison received by the system. In the present instance, it is an important, and usually an attainable factor, in estimating the probabilities of any given case, which it never can be in those modes of septic poisoning which we call diseases, and know only through their symptoms.

The Situation of the Wound.—In almost every reported case, the wound has been upon an extremity. A woodman steps over a log which conceals a snake; a child thrusts an arm into the hollow trunk, where a serpent lies; or, an intoxicated man, ignorant and reckless, puts his hand into a snake cage, or handles a snake which is benumbed with cold, and to appearance harmless. Another not uncommon cause of bite, is due to want of caution in dealing with serpents which have been wounded, or even decapitated. One of the best of the reported cases, that of Dr. Woodhouse, was thus produced.

Local Symptoms.—The pain of the wound made by the snake is usually the earliest symptom, but it is by no means a constant phenomenon in either men or animals. Thus, while one reporter speaks of the sudden and intense pain, another does not mention it at all, or expressly states that the wound was at first disregarded. In most instances, the bite is certainly painful, and when we consider the hooked form of the fangs, the double wound, the injection of a foreign fluid, and the final forcible withdrawal of the teeth, we can feel no surprise that, in most cases, pain is felt, and may wonder that it is not felt in all. Certainly we need not look to the specific nature of the venom, to explain the primary pain here described.

The succeeding local symptoms are almost inevitably swelling, discoloration, and increasing pain. The reader who has followed this Essay thus far, will have no difficulty in explaining at least two of these symptoms. The swelling is due, not to inflammation, but to a large or small collection of effused blood about the wound.

In some loose tissues the amount thus accumulated may be very great, but in other cases the anatomical peculiarities of the part wounded may limit the early extravasation of blood, by confining it under a fascia, of which I have seen repeated examples in animals. The discoloration is to be explained in the same manner.

Hemorrhage from the wound may limit, *for a time*, the last two symptoms. It is, however, a rare occurrence, and depends upon the size of the external opening of the wound inflicted by the fang, and perhaps, also, upon the character of the vessels accidentally encountered by the fang. In one of the dogs whose medical history is recorded in this Essay, the hemorrhage from the fang wounds amounted to several ounces.

In estimating these early local evidences of poisoning in man, as well as the local signs which follow, it is well to remember that in almost every instance the ligature was applied at once, and very tightly. In animals bitten and not subjected to the ligature the swelling occurs, it is true, but forms much more slowly than is usual in the cases of men.

The primary local symptoms thus described increase progressively, so that within a period which varies extremely, the swelling and discoloration extend up the bitten limb, accompanied on their march by pain of the most excruciating character. At this time, and after the first few minutes, the increase in the local symptoms is probably due to the influence of the septic poisoning upon the tissues near the wound, to the irritation thus resulting, and to the direct and indirect effect of the venom upon the local circulation. Thus the extremity becomes larger and more and more discolored until the skin offers every tint of an old bruise. Vesications appear on the surface, the pain lessens, the local temperature early diminished, falls still lower, and unless the poison has ceased to act, or a potent remedy has interfered, gangrene ensues, and the system, already weakened by the effect of the poison upon its own tissues, dies in the effort to separate the mortified and corrupted part.

If, on the other hand, the poison is not present in a dose so large as to insure these fatal effects, or is properly antagonized by medical agents, *the swelling declines, and the pain disappears, with a celerity which every practitioner or reporter has assumed to be evidence of his own skill, or of the utility of his therapeutic means, but which, as we shall have reason to see, is in reality, an essential and most striking feature of the Crotalus malady*, and is either attributable to none of the remedies employed, or to every one of the scores of them which popular credulity has placed like blunt weapons in the too yielding hand of the physician.

It is rather remarkable, that only one reporter, Dr. Woodhouse, has alluded to the occurrence of swelling in the lymphatic glands of the part bitten. His case was in other respects somewhat peculiar, inasmuch as the lymphatic trunks also appear to have been inflamed, which is not a common symptom of Crotalus bite. The venom usually seems to enter the system through the bloodvessels alone, and to sap the life of the parts with which it comes in contact, without of necessity involving the lymph vessels or their glands.

Local Results.—It is not very easy to form a correct estimate of the local consequences in the cases which finally recover. This difficulty will be explained upon glancing over the column of local treatment in the table, when it will be observed that ligatures, the cautery, excision and incision, alone or combined, were resorted to with a freedom dictated by therapeutic despair or the fears of the sufferer and his friends.

It is hence impossible to learn positively how much was due to remedies, how much to disease. It seems, however, to be certain that in many cases slight or extensive local suppurations follow the cure, that in others local gangrene and sphacelus of flesh and bone occur, while in the graver cases, the economy is too seriously deranged to enjoy the power of spontaneously amputating the mass of a limb. The well-known case reported by Sir E. Home (*See* Table of Crotalus Poisoning in Man, Case 12), approached most nearly to the condition last described. In this instance the poison produced great local swelling. When the system began to recover from the primary depressing effects of the venom, it found the bitten arm for the most part dead. Intense inflammation ensued as the patient rallied, but being unequal to the effort of repair, he died before it was accomplished.

In connection with the local signs, it is as well to note that no reporter has described in man the local twitching which is so common in dogs and other animals.

The constitutional symptoms of Crotalus poisoning sometimes declare themselves very early, and if we can believe their reporters, almost immediately after the bite. It is more probable, however, that an interval of several minutes elapses, or that the faintness of terror and pain has been mistaken for the constitutional effects of the venom. In a few instances these symptoms do not announce themselves for twenty or thirty minutes, but aside from these exceptional cases, it seems evident that the general manifestations of the influence of the venom on the system appear with a rapidity which is sufficiently surprising, so that the local symptoms are sometimes overshadowed and forgotten for a time, in the singular phenomena which characterize the systemic disturbance.

The principal constitutional effect of the venom is a general prostration of the most appalling character. Sometimes within a few minutes, sometimes within one or two hours, this condition of profound sedation attains its height. The snake strikes and the faintness comes on while the person injured is endeavoring to kill the reptile. Or, as in another instance, he walks for some time and suddenly finds his limbs giving way beneath him.

I have looked in vain through the reports for any evidence of a primary stimulating power on the part of the poison, but neither in the published cases, or in my own observations, have I met with any early symptoms of excitement which might not with reason be attributed to terror and pain.

The condition of prostration referred to, is accompanied by a variety of phenomena which are in general such as accompany the action of any sudden and violent depressing agency. The patient staggers or falls, cold sweats bathe the surface, nausea and vomiting ensue, the pulse becomes quick, and rapid, and feeble, the expression anxious, and, in a few cases, the mind slightly disturbed.

A patient dying in this condition would probably exhibit no lesion of fluid or solid, and would be an example of acute or primary poisoning, such as sometimes occurs in the early stage of epidemics of cholera or yellow fever. So great, however, is the power of resistance on the part of man, owing, perhaps, in some degree to his bulk, that very early death seems to be a rare incident of venom poisoning, so rare, indeed, that I have met with no reported example of its occurrence.

If death does not intervene, the local symptoms soon begin to play a more important role, and the swelling and discoloration extend up the limb, and pass on to the trunk, so that when the arm has been wounded, half of the chest and back have been seen to be discolored, as though severely bruised.

Meanwhile, the signs of general blood-poisoning develop themselves, and within a few hours, or a day, the face and other parts become swollen and puffy. At the same time, the general weakness remains well marked, as shown by repeated syncope, the heart quick, feeble, and fluttering, and the respiration labored.

In the majority of cases, the slight mental disturbance now passes away, and the mind remains singularly clear to the close, whatever the event may be. In other instances, as in Dr. Harlan's case, delirium, restlessness, and insomnia are present, but in general the nervous symptoms of this and of the earlier stage of the malady are confined to slight incoherence, and to rare sensory delusions.

The state of the secretions and discharges seems to have been thought of so little moment, that in most of the cases they are not even alluded to. For example, the state of the urine is not spoken of in any one instance. The vomiting is so frequent and so enduring a symptom, that it is more constantly referred to; but of the character of the evacuation thus effected, we learn almost nothing. From the fact that in some of the cases the reporter states that it was necessary to give a purgative to complete the cure, we may, perhaps, infer that in the milder cases, at least, no diarrhœa occurred. In two of the fatal cases, diarrhœa came on late in the disease, and in one we are told that the stools were of a dark bilious character, but beyond this we are left in ignorance.

Four fatal cases are found in the table. Of these, the most rapid was that of the medical man, reported by Dr. Post (Table, Case No. 6); the malady ending in death by coma, within five hours and a half. This was the nearest approach to a case of acute or simple primary poisoning, which we have met with in man.

M. Pihorel's case (Table, Case No. 16) died quietly in about nine and a half hours, without loss of intellect, but with a rapidly increasing difficulty of breathing and swallowing.

Dr. Horner's case (Table, Case No. 4) terminated about eighteen hours after the bite was inflicted. One or two hours before death, the patient had a general convulsion, with involuntary evacuation from the bowels, but without any foaming at the mouth. He appears to have regained his senses after this time. Just before he expired, he complained of pain in the colon, said he felt sleepy, closed his eyes, and died quietly without agony, and without convulsions.

In the third of the fatal cases, Sir E. Home's (Table, Case 12), the sufferer rallied from the primary poisoning, and died on the seventeenth day, with well expressed typhous symptoms.

The duration of the various cases, and their mode of recovery or death, is of considerable interest. If we analyze the table of sixteen cases, we shall find that, as I have just stated, the four fatal cases terminated in five and a half hours, nine hours, eighteen hours, and seventeen days respectively. If, again, we analyze these four cases with respect to the question of death from primary or secondary poisoning, we shall discover that Case No. 12 (Home's) survived not only the early effects, but also, to a great extent, the constitutional affection, and perished in the effort to get rid of the gangrenous arm.

On examination, the blood proved to be coagulable. It is probable that the blood had survived the infected condition, and was gradually regaining its normal standard.

Case No. 4 (Horner) seems to have been a fair representative of those instances of Crotalus poisoning which I have termed secondary or chronic. The patient never rallied completely from the depressing effect of the venom, but he was found after death to have a perfectly incoagulable blood.

Case No. 16 (Pihorel) died in nine and a half hours. It seems to have ended before the blood lost its coagulability, so that, although the veins of the bitten arm contained but little clotted blood, large coagula of loose structure were found in the main venous vessels of the trunk, and in the right auricle.

Case No. 6 (Post) was not examined after death. Of the remaining twelve cases of the table, all recovered within variable periods. Where the patient was several days or longer indisposed, the delayed recovery was usually due to the local lesions, rather than to prolonged constitutional malady.

In connection with the history of the amelioration or cure, in almost every case, we are struck by one fact, which is of singular value, because its neglect has led to almost every one of the fallacies attending upon the use of the supposed antidotes which have attained to a local or general notoriety. If the reader will glance at the Table of Crotalus poisoning in man, and at the column headed "Mode of Recovery," he will observe that in almost every case the relief from urgent symptoms was sudden, and the completed cure almost nearly so. If, again, he will look at the column in which are grouped the constitutional symptoms, he will certainly feel some astonishment at their gravity in relation to the character of the convalescence. So extraordinary was this contrast, that within a few hours, or a day in most cases, the patient, whom thè physician regarded as almost moribund, went on horseback to see him, or was able to move about the house, or engage in his ordinary avocations. The general practical inference will at once suggest itself, upon an examination of the numerous and varied remedies employed. It will then be seen that, under the most different systems of treatment, the several cases grew better, or entirely recovered, with equal abruptness. Are we not driven to the absurd conclusion that each and every remedy is equally useful, or to the more logical inference that sudden relief and rapid recovery are peculiarities which belong to those cases of Crotalus bite in which the amount of venom injected has not been so unusually large as to insure a fatal ending?

The bearings of these conclusions upon the study of antidotes require but little comment, and must at once suggest themselves to every thoughtful physician. It is almost needless to add that the reporters have usually assumed the suddenness of the cures to be due in each case to the peculiar therapeutic means employed.

I have already described the local consequences of the bite. The various reports make no mention of constitutional results succeeding recovery. One very curious statement, however, is found in connection with case No. 5 (Phillips). The patient, a female, was suffering when bitten, from a severe attack of hooping-cough, of which she was suddenly and completely cured by the effects of the venom.

P. M. Section.—The three cases of post-mortem examination offer very little, save negative information, as to the character of the lesions.

The Head.—Dr. Horner found the brain of a healthy consistence, but congested so that the cortical substance was of a deep brown tint. A good deal of serum oozed from the cut surfaces. About a drachm of transparent serum was present in each lateral ventricle. The medulla spinalis was healthy; its tunica arachnoidea being somewhat turbid in places, as if from some former cause. The veins of the pia mater and the vertebral veins were full of blood.

M. Pihorel makes a similar report of his case. He found some thickening of the cerebral arachnoid, which was also adherent to the pia mater, but to what extent he does not state. The blood of the sinuses and of the dura mater was fluid. The same condition as to fulness of blood, and the same slight excess of serum in the ventricles and sub-arachnoid spaces, existed in Sir E. Home's case.

Thorax.—Dr. Horner found all the thoracic organs healthy, except that the left ventricle of the heart was described as hypertrophied. The heart was nearly empty, owing to the escape of its fluid when the head was opened.

M. Pihorel found the walls of the trachea and bronchial tubes congested, a spot of distinct inflammation corresponding to the cricoid cartilage. The trachea and bronchiæ were full of a red and frothy mucus. The lungs were healthy and crepitant, but were somewhat congested ("premier degré d'engorgement sanguin"). Two inches below the pharynx the œsophagus was narrowed, but no notable alteration of its tissues could be discovered.

In Sir E. Home's case the lungs were healthy, the anterior fold of the pericardium was dry, resembling a dried bladder. The cavity of this membrane contained half an ounce of serous fluid, frothy from admixture with gases which escaped in bubbles.

Abdomen. Horner's Case.—The peritoneum contained a few ounces of serum. The mucous membrane of the stomach was intensely injected with blood, and most remarkably so in the wrinkles of the mucous membrane. It exhibited neither ecchymosis or softening, and contained the articles prescribed in the morning, with but little gas.

The mucous coat of the small intestines was dotted "with patches of acute inflammation. These spots were of a lively red and very numerous, especially in the jejunum. This latter intestine had its parietes considerably thickened by an infiltration of serum, and was partially filled with a dark bilious matter. The colon was sound but contracted, and contained at its head some hard fecal excrement. The liver was yellow and enlarged, which was attributed to the habits of the patient."

M. Pihorel found all the abdominal organs healthy. Sir E. Home describes the stomach in the case of Soaper as turgid with blood. All the other abdominal organs were healthy. In Pihorel's and Home's cases the blood was more or less coagulated. In Horner's it was everywhere perfectly fluid. Dr. Horner says that the muscles were of a brownish yellow color throughout the body.

The local swelling in Dr. Horner's case was due to serous infiltration; in that of M. Pihorel, but little swelling existed during life after the ligature was removed, and at the post-mortem inspection the tumefaction of the bite between the two metacarpal bones extended only half an inch around it. The bite on the dorsal face of the thumb was not at all swollen. The muscles in these localities were unaltered. Sir E. Home's case presented at the time of death extensive sloughs of skin on the arm and forearm. A large abscess existed on the outside of the arm, elbow, and forearm. The parts in the immediate neighborhood of the bite and in the palm were healthy, except that there was a little extravasated blood in the areolar spaces. The skin still adhered to the biceps flexor muscle in the arm and to the flexor muscles in the forearm, by a dark-colored cellular tissue. Elsewhere in the arm and forearm, the skin and muscles from the axilla down were separated by a dark fluid of an offensive odor, containing sloughs of the dead cellular tissue floating in it. "The muscles had their natural appearance everywhere, except on the surface which was next to the abscess. Beyond the limits of the abscess, blood was extravasated in the cellular membrane, and this appearance was observable on the right side of the back as far as the loins, and on the right side of the chest over the serratus major anticus muscle."

Dr. Horner's case occurred in Philadelphia, in the month of July, and was examined four and a half hours after death. M. Pihorel does not give the exact date of his case. It took place at Rouen, and from various allusions in the text of his report, it is plain that the weather was cold. The examination did not occur until five days after death, but the cold was so great that the body is said to have been in excellent preservation. Sir E. Home's case occurred in London, during the month of October. It was examined sixteen hours after death.

Antidotes.—It might naturally be supposed that the question of antidotes and remedies would be considered fully and experimentally, at the close of this Essay. Such, indeed, was my intention when I began the present investigation, but it soon became clear to me that a just and useful experimental testing of this matter was out of the question until I became thoroughly acquainted with the habits and movements of the Rattlesnake, the precise character of the venom, and its various modes of acting on the system. Portions of this information were to be found scattered through books and journals, but these disjointed studies were incomplete, and it soon grew more and more apparent that a consideration of the entire subject, and a certain familiarity with the powers of the poison must still, of necessity, precede an investigation of antidotes. Impressed with this idea, I have endeavored, in the present paper, to render more easy the still difficult task of examining the therapeutics of Crotalus bite.

It was well said by a distinguished physician, that there are always a great number of medicines for those diseases which are either very easy or very difficult to cure. Such has been the fate of Crotalus poisoning to a remarkable degree, for not only have physicians exhausted their ingenuity in the discovery of antidotes, but the popular medicine of log-cabin, or rough border clearings, has contributed to its strange therapeutics, some twenty or thirty plants which owe their reputation to Indian traditions, and to other, and often accidental, circumstances.

Each one of these remedies has acquired a local credit; has passed from the people to the physicians; has seemed to cure in their hands, as it had done in those of the good wife or herb doctor, and finally, after going the rounds of the daily press and the medical journals, has died a natural death, or received a fatal blow at the bedside of some too deeply injured patient. Accepted upon slight evidence, and thrown aside upon equally feeble proof of inutility, such has been the career of the many and famous antidotes, which in this and other lands have embarrassed the therapeutics of these much-dreaded injuries.

While, however, the larger part of the reputed constitutional remedies are mere sudorifics, or entirely inert, the local therapeutics of Crotalus bite have been always of the most decisive and potent character. Without entering into the history of these means, I desire to assign to them their proper place in the treatment, and also to define the real limits of their utility. We shall, therefore, discuss them in turn, and for this purpose shall divide them into, 1st, Those which remove the poison and the poisoned part, as excision, amputation.

2d. Those which partially remove the venom, and more or less detain it in the wounded part. In this class, we have a variety of agents acting in ways as various, as

Scarifications.	Suctions.
Ligature.	Caustics.

3d. Those agents which, being injected *into* the wound, or wounded part, are supposed to destroy the venom, or to render it innocuous, as injections of iodine.

4th. Local applications of various substances, as alcohol, ammonia, indigo olive oil, etc.

Class 1*st.* Excision, the only local means which proposes to remove at once and entirely the poison and the poisoned part has been occasionally resorted to. Dr. Harlan, Case 14 of the Table, used it freely. In another instance, in France, even amputation of a finger was promptly and successfully resorted to in a case of Crotalus bite.

Excision and amputation are more or less usefully available, as the resort to them is more or less early, and their utility is also increased when a ligature has been so applied as to arrest the local circulation, immediately after the bite. In the French case, the instant ablation of the part was perfectly successful; in Dr. Harlan's case the malady was extremely grave *after* the operation, and we have, indeed, no means of saying whether or not it proved useful. It seems likely that in so severe a case, the removal by excision of any part of the poison might favorably determine the issue of the almost balanced chances. Necessarily, excision would be unavailable where the fang had buried itself deeply in a part like the neck.

Where the snake has been long confined without using its venom,[1] so that the amount injected has probably been great, and where the part bitten is a small extremity, excision, or, rather, amputation, would be justifiable. Where, on account of the serpent being at large, we cannot judge as to the quantity of poison stored up in its ducts, and where excision would affect important parts, it is certainly better to accept for the patient the ordinary prognostic chances of the poisoning, under a less heroic local treatment. Above all, is it to be remembered that, while it may be good practice to amputate a finger within a few moments of the bite, the value of the operation lessens as we recede from this period, because the poison exerts its power so rapidly, that its effects soon pass beyond the reach of any justifiable operation, and excision then could do only what other and safer means might effect.

---

[1] It is curious that the fatal cases found in the journals were nearly all occasioned by the bite of snakes which, during long imprisonment, had accumulated a large amount of venom.

Class 2d of local means acts in ways so various as to make it necessary to consider these separately.

Scarifications.—It is not easy to see how mere incisions could be of much value, unless made expressly so as to cut off the wound from the system, by destroying for a time its vascular connection with the centres. Where ablation or excision is no longer justified, incisions may be made into the part, and so directed as to traverse the line of the fang wounds.

Suction. Cups.—Suction by the mouth is an ancient practice, and one which is supposed to be effectual. It is not probable that the narrow fang-track would allow of the return of the poison under any suctorial power of which the lips are capable, unless the wound were unusually large. Where a previous incision has been carried deeply through the bitten part, it is possible that suction may remove some of the venom, but as Dr. Pennock has shown, it is more likely that the cups and suction merely delay the constitutional poisoning, by retarding the local circulation and the subsequent distribution of the venom. Either may be thus of value, as Barry proved in regard to cups, but neither can do more than afford time for the administration of general and more permanent local means. Cups are available only in certain localities; suction by the lips may be used on the small extremities, in advance of all other means.

Ligatures.—The first resource in serpent bite has been to tie a ligature around the limb. Of course, there are localities in which this cannot be done, and where only cups can be used. The value of the ligature has been repeatedly tested, not only in this, but in other modes of poisoning, and it is perfectly clear that a ligature tightly applied above the wound will, for a time, secure the system from the consequences of the venom inoculation. But this is all which it can do. Time is obtained for the use of other means, both local and general, and then a period arrives when the swelling and interrupted circulation threaten the bitten member with gangrene, and at last the physician reluctantly loosens the band which quarantined the deadly material, and the system passes rapidly under its influence. Allowing the ligature—as we must do—to be of the utmost value for a time, can we not derive from its use yet further advantages, without subjecting our patients to the sudden influx of the poison when the guarding band is loosened? Two precautions will probably insure the requisite end. Let the cord be loosened for a few minutes at a time, and at intervals, with a constant eye to the constitutional symptoms, and let the delay secured by the ligature be used not only to apply local means, but to administer general remedies. This method, which I shall term the *intermittent ligature*, seems to have been first employed by the well known naturalist, Prof. Holbrook, of Charleston, South Carolina, in conjunction with Dr. Ogier. Their experiments, which were numerous and satisfactory, have never been published.

The precautions in the use of the ligature which I have just recommended have been advocated singly, or together, by several more recent authors, and especially by Drs. Alexander and Jeter.

Several writers have recognized the danger of suddenly removing the ligature, and it would be easy to criticize some of the reports of treatment in which the above precautions have been neglected, and where the sudden prostration which ensued was most appalling.

Dr. Alexander relates a singular, but instructive case, in which the ligature was retained for sixteen hours. Meanwhile, the parts below were swollen and vesicating, but the system remained unaffected, and readily passed under the influence of stimulants. Either during the profound intoxication which ensued, or soon after, at all events, sixteen hours from the time of the bite, the ligature was removed. The swelling at once passed the line of the ligating cord, and advanced up the leg to the body. The patient died in two hours after the release of the previously isolated poison. Instructed by this sad case, the reporter directs that the ligature should be merely relaxed, and the pulse kept up with stimulants as required, and that the cord should be tightened or loosened as the symptoms direct. This plan is so clearly recommended by common sense, that it is needless to dwell upon it further.

Unfortunately, the ligature can be used only when the bite is on an extremity. In other cases, cups may be similarly employed, but even these are not always available, as where the nose is the part bitten, and moreover, they are not always at hand.

Caustics.—These agents are supposed to be useful, not only by destroying the tissues, and so unfitting them for absorption, but also by chemically acting on the venom itself. So far as they do act on the tissues, they are beneficial, when fully applied along or through previous incisions. As to their power to alter the venom, it is clear that the actual cautery does do this effectually, but, as we have seen, potassa, soda, ammonia, and the undiluted mineral acids do not affect its toxic potency. Except, then, as they alter the tissues, it were better to reject them, and to depend upon the actual cautery alone, where such means is deemed of value.

Class 3d.—Dr. Brainard, some time ago, directed attention to the injection of an iodized solution of iodine, as a means of destroying the activity of Crotalus venom. His process is as follows: Ten grains of iodine and thirty grains of iodide of potassium are dissolved in one ounce of water. The bitten part is first cupped, or a ligature is applied on the limb, until the tissues are swollen with serum sufficiently to enable the injection to be diffused through the distended areolar spaces. The sharp point of a trocar, or injecting-tube, is then pushed laterally into the bitten part, and the injection effected by pressing down the piston of the syringe, while the exhaustion of the cup is still carried on. Apart from the antidotal value of this ingenious method, it is clear that the necessary apparatus is not easily procurable in time to be of use. Moreover, Dr. Brainard adds that, to render it effectual, we must be provided with cups of various curves adapted to fit the surfaces of the body and limbs. Dr. Brainard states that the iodine does not act as a caustic. M. Reynose, in an admirable paper, has examined the statements of Dr. Brainard, and especially with reference to the action of iodine as an antidote to woorara. He arrived at the conclusion that the iodine was a caustic, and that its value was due to this fact, a conclusion in which his experiments did not entirely justify him.

The question of the reality of the influence of the iodine upon the active qualities of Crotalus venom still rests upon rather insecure ground. It certainly seems to have been successful in pigeons, but the fallacies which surround these researches are numerous and baffling, and the experimentum crucis of mixing the iodine with the venom before innoculating with it, was not made by Dr. Brainard. To set the matter at rest, I have recently made a number of experiments. It was apparent that if animals previously bitten could be saved by subsequent injections of iodine into the part, they should run no risk when a mixture of venom and the iodine solution was thrown into their tissues. On pursuing this method, I observed, as Dr. Brainard had done, that the local symptoms were slight, or did not appear at all, but whereas his cases recovered, mine died despite the absence of local phenomena. The explanation of this latter fact, as well as the full details of numerous observations upon the use of reputed constitutional antidotes, I shall set forth at length in a future essay. At present I can only add that iodine as a local antidote has uniformly failed in my hands, although every means was taken to give it a fair trial. It is proper to state here that Dr. Brainard made use, not of the Crotalus, but of the *Crotalophorus tergeminus*, or prairie Rattlesnake of the west. As yet, Dr. Brainard's antidote has never been employed upon the body of man, except by Dr. Coolidge, who unfortunately used the Bibron treatment at the same time.

Class 4th.—Consists of various substances which have been applied to the skin on and about the wound, or placed in contact with the raw surfaces of the incisions or excisions. Among them are warm and cold water, ammonia, alcohol, olive oil, etc. My own experiments, and the observations of others, justify us in rejecting them altogether, so far at least as they are supposed to exert specific power.

Although, as I have already said, I consider this essay as but a preparation for the full experimental examination of the treatment of serpent bite, I do not wish to conclude without some comment upon the constitutional remedies which I have necessarily been called upon to survey and judge in the course of my researches. A host of these may be dismissed with a word, but before I criticize those of greater pretension, it will be proper to make some statements regarding the misconceptions which have crept into this part of the subject.

If, as I have elsewhere urged, we could dismiss from view the mode in which the virus enters the body, and were called upon to consider only the resultant malady, we would as little have dreamed of specifics or real antidotes, as we now do in yellow fever, or ordinary putrefactive poisoning. We should at least have confessed that such belonged only to the hopes of therapeutics, and not to its attained realities. Such, however, is the tangible and visible nature of the poison that we have been continually seduced into the idea that we must possess some available and directly efficient means of actually neutralizing its power, when once in the system itself.

Apart, then, from the question of local antidotes, which is altogether a different matter, what probability is there that we really possess specific general remedies? Even here, the knowledge that our local means, however active, and with all our power to place them in direct contact with the venom, are but too ineffectual, should at least have taught us to receive with wise mistrust every account of constitutional antidotes.

Antidotes considered with reference to the system at large, are of only two kinds. Those which meet the poison in the vessels of the economy, and then and there *chemically alter it*, so as to destroy its potency, and those which, like most of our medicines, are absorbed, circulate, and *counteract the effects of the poison*. Thus a sedative may counteract a stimulant, and vice versa, and each would, in this sense, be for the other a physiological antidote, but would in nowise correspond with the popular conception of an antidote.

The remedies which still hold repute as antidotes are few in number. They are ammonia, olive oil, arsenic (as the Tanjore pill), Bibron's antidote (Bromine), and alcoholic stimuli.

The pretensions of ammonia in this connection have been long since settled by the experiments of Fontana on Vipers, and of Brainard on *Crotalophorus*. I have also tested its supposed utility in cases of animals poisoned by Crotalus venom, and it will answer our present purpose to add that it failed almost uniformly. Notwithstanding the continued faith still reposed in it by some, and the cures attributed to its use, I am convinced that it has no powers which alcohol does not enjoy to a superior degree, and I feel equally sure that its exhibition should never be allowed to supplant the use of other and better stimulants. That it has no value as a chemical antidote, the experiments elsewhere related in this paper sufficiently prove, if proof were wanting.

Olive oil is another remedy which has been gravely urged and has received the support of numerous successful cases. What these are worth, or with what allowance they should be entertained, has, I trust, been set in clear light by the general argument which I have founded on all the cases which I have analyzed. After the experiments of Fontana on its use in Viper poisoning, it is strange that the most confident should have dared to employ it again.

Arsenic, unlike olive oil, certainly does not belong to the class of expectant remedies. Its use in snake-bites comes from the East, where as the "Tanjore pill" it attained great celebrity.

This well-known medicine is composed of arsenious acid, three East Indian roots, two of which are purgative, and one an acro-narcotic, mixed with pepper and the juice of the wild cotton plant. Two of the pills, containing each three-fourths of a grain of the arsenic, are given at once, and one at the close of an hour, a rather formidable dose of so active a medicine. Russell (p. 65), who examined this remedy, was not satisfied with it, nor am I aware that it has retained its celebrity, or that any one has used it in Rattlesnake bite.

Bibron's antidote is a more novel remedy, of the value of which I am not fully prepared to judge. Its history is rather curious. Mr. Xantus obtained it in the first place from Prince Paul, of Wurtemberg, the well-known traveller and naturalist. This gentleman stated that it had been invented and employed by Prof. Bibron, of Paris, but neither Mr. Kantus or Dr. Hammond has been able to find any printed account of it, nor have I been more successful. The chief evidence in its favor rests upon a considerable number of experiments made by Dr. Hammond and Mr. Kantus, and upon three cases reported by the same observers. Mr. Kantus states one fact which I have been thus far unable to verify, namely, that dogs which were under the influence of the antidote, were for some time incapable of being affected by Rattlesnake bites. This experimenter states that after seventeen experiments, in which three dogs were at different times bitten by seventeen different serpents, he met with no case in which the antidote failed. These results are not stated with sufficient precision as to the condition of the snake, the number of fang-marks, or the place of the bite, but they are still sufficiently interesting to awaken further research.

Dr. Hammond was not so fortunate as Mr. Xantus. He experimented with the antidote on a wolf which was apparently saved by the use of the bromine after being once bitten, but upon another occasion, having been thrice bitten, died suddenly, exhibiting, however, some evidence of having been aided by the remedy. A dog severely injured by snake-bite was successfully treated by Dr. Hammond with the bromine antidote.

One of the cases of man in which Dr. Coolidge (Dr. Hammond's Report) used this antidote, was also treated with local injection of iodine, and must, therefore, be laid aside. The patient expressed herself relieved by the use of the antidote.

The case directly reported by Dr. Hammond also seemed to experience great assistance from the antidote, so that even the local symptoms were promptly relieved by its use. No local means seem to have been employed, and the case is thus unusually free from complication.

Mr. Kantus' case was said to have been almost hopeless when the bromine was employed. The worst symptoms rapidly subsided when the antidote was given, although but two doses were used. Were it not for our knowledge of the natural history of the malady, and of the strange suddenness with which cases almost moribund rapidly amend, we could not fail to be greatly impressed with the evidence thus furnished. As it is, perceiving no obvious adaptation of means to ends, we can only await the issues of a larger and more general experience to determine the question.

My own experiments upon the use of this antidote were made on sixteen dogs, and were conducted with scrupulous care. It does not suit my present purpose to enter into the details; it will suffice to state that their results were nearly negative. Of eight dogs bitten and treated with the antidote, two died; while of eight bitten, and not so treated, three died.

The last of the reputed antidotes which we shall criticize is alcoholic stimulus. In one form or another this has been employed in India and in this country, and no single remedy is so much in repute along our borders or in our Rattlesnake regions. Perhaps the evidence in its favor is not much better than that which exists for some other means, but its real strength, in the lack of proper and numerous reports, lies in its obvious adaptation to the wants of those who seek its aid. Moreover, the experiments on the state of the heart and nervous system of animals, in the first stage of the Crotalus malady, clearly indicate a condition of things which is to be met alone by the use of supporting agents, and these the most rapid and effective which we can command.

When, too, we consider the state of a person bitten, and constitutionally affected, we perceive at once that we have to deal with a degree of prostration which instantly suggests the free use of stimulus. When this is given, and is successful in raising the pulse, the result is commonly a rapid and easy cure, but the amount of alcoholic fluids necessary to secure even partial intoxication is scarcely credible. Quarts of brandy have been thus taken by delicate females and mere children without injury, and almost without effect. This alone is, to some extent, evidence in favor of the remedial means under discussion.

It is very plain, then, that in the state of profound sedation, or, rather, prostration, which ushers in the general malady, stimulants are distinctly indicated. It is also clear that the means thus pointed out is a physiological antidote, a counteractive agent, and is to be used to an effect and with certain precautions.

When, therefore, a person has been bitten, it would be proper slightly to intoxicate him, then to loosen the previously applied ligature or cup, and watching the pulse, and relaxing or tightening the ligating cord to control thus the inlet of the poison, with the aid of the stimulus destroy its effects in detail. Finally, the stimulus should be most cautiously and by degrees abandoned, with continued regard to the state of the system.

There is a popular, I might almost have said a medical belief, that the condition of perfect protection is complete intoxication. Two or three authors, as Jeter, Alexander, and others, protest against this idea, and with every appearance of right on their side.

Profound drunkenness is a condition of sedation and not of excitement, and yet the whole object of using alcohol in snake-bites has been among rational men to stimulate and not to lull or depress the system. In fact, it is well known that persons who were at the time "dead drunk," or nearly so, have been bitten by Rattlesnakes, and have obtained thereby no immunity from the effects of the bite. Dr. Brainard, who is opposed to the use of stimulus in Crotalus bite, thinks the evidence in its favor insufficient, and thus sums up his argument against its utility:—

"When mixed with alcohol, the venom is rapidly fatal, if inoculated." This opinion is correct, but has no value as in opposition to the constitutional use of stimuli, because they are not to be regarded as chemical antidotes, and their direct reaction with the venom becomes, therefore, a matter of indifference.

Dr. Brainard also urges that when venom is injected into the tissues, or introduced into the stomachs of birds or small animals bitten, it only hastens death.

This, he adds, is not conclusive, because alcohol is a poison to birds and other small animals. The authority for these statements I have been unable to find. It is not Fontana, and I cannot discover in Dr. Brainard's papers that the conclusion here stated is based upon his own experiments. If true, it would have little value, the real point in question being whether stimulation is useful in cases of Crotalus bite. To determine this, we should intoxicate animals and then inoculate them with known amounts of venom, or first inoculate and then give the stimulant. Moreover, we should resort to as large animals as can easily be managed; the venom being so fatal to all small animals, and especially to birds, as to give but little time for remedies. Again, in small animals, and particularly in birds, it is not always easy to ascertain and govern the degree of stimulation which may be present or desirable.

The last argument against stimulants used by Dr. Brainard, is the fact that intoxicated persons have died from Crotalus bite. He states that he has authentic information as to four such cases. Now it is plain, as I have urged, that deep drunkenness is not the condition which we desire, and it is most probable that a person who was in this state would be overcome by the venom with more than common facility, as indeed may be inferred from Dr. Brainard's statement. If, however, the cases which he refers to were only somewhat intoxicated when bitten, it would be very requisite to know whether or not any means were taken to sustain the stimulation, without which the primary state of excitement would very soon disappear before the terrible depression caused by the poison.

The remaining instance of death from a bite given to an intoxicated man is the case of Adam Lake, reported by Dr. Horner. The particulars are as follows: The patient was in the habit of drinking daily from half a pint to one pint of alcoholic liquors, and, as was seen at the autopsy, was constitutionally the worse for this habit. When somewhat intoxicated, he was bitten at the bend of the arm, both fangs entering. Some time, I presume at least two or three hours, passed by before he sought aid, and during this period so little effect was produced that he paid no attention to the wound until the itching annoyed him. From this time he was under treatment, the arm rapidly swelling and becoming painful. Now, Crotalus poison may produce but slight local effects, but when it is in such amount as finally to kill, it does not long delay the exhibition of its influence on the system. Yet in this person, who did afterwards die, some time evidently elapsed without any constitutional expression of poisoning. Was this reprieve due to the partial intoxication of the sufferer? Whatever answer we may give, it is quite clear that this was no case to quote against the use of stimulants, since, in addition to what I have urged, we learn yet further that with the exception of a little ammonia and two half-ounce doses of sp. vin. dilut., used late in the malady, he took no stimulants, and that no regular effort was made to sustain or renew the primary stimulation, which, at first, had so guarded his system.

It sometimes happens that the physician finds it impossible to produce stimulation in the presence of so potent a sedative as the venom. When this is the case, it is possible that absorption does not occur with sufficient rapidity, or at all events, that cases may occur, where it is necessary to stimulate fully and suddenly.

Under these circumstances I would recommend *inhalation of the fumes of warm alcohol, or even of ether if used with caution.*

While advocating the employment of stimuli as rational therapeutic means of meeting a most obvious indication, it is proper to admit that cases have been and will be encountered, in which the dose of venom has been so great, that no remedy is of any avail. Such, however, must be rare, and it is on the whole more than probable that the danger from the bite of the Rattlesnake has been over-estimated, and that in a large majority of cases the patient would recover, even if unassisted by any remedy.

Where stimulants are of any use, the patient commonly recovers without further difficulty. In some cases, however, which attain to the stage of alteration in the blood, we have to deal with conditions which are also present in other cases of putrefactive poisoning, but for which we have no remedies of well determined power. Possibly, tonics, astringents, and continued stimulation might be of some value in supporting the strength until the blood recovers its normal condition.

In the foregoing brief indication of my views as to the proper treatment of Crotalus bite, I have endeavored to make it plain that in the absence of any certain specific, this malady should be treated as the symptoms dictate, and that no other guide can be safely or conscientiously followed in the present condition of the therapeutics of this mode of poisoning.

It would be improper to close these pages without repeating that I have given my views as to treatment, in the briefest and most condensed manner, and that every criticism of the treatment advised by others, and every remedial method recommended by myself, rests upon the authority of experiments which I shall detail at length on a future occasion.

I sincerely trust that the publication of this essay may induce the physicians of this country to study more zealously, and record more exactly, every case of snake poisoning which may fall under their notice, since, without such aid, it is impossible for the most ardent student to do justice to the subject, and since it is only by a large accumulation of experience, that any fair appreciation of the true value of remedies can be attained.

APPENDIX A.

AN ENUMERATION OF THE GENERA AND SPECIES OF RATTLESNAKES, WITH SYNONYMY AND REFERENCES.

By E. D. COPE.

I.

THAT large assemblage of serpents, known as the Viperidæ of Bonaparte, Viperina of Gray, or Solenoglyphes of Duméril, exhibits the most perfect degree of development of those points of structure which distinguish all venomous serpents from those that are innocuous. Of the subgroups of genera and species contained in this "family," or "suborder," none is more truly representative than that denominated by the authors just mentioned, Crotalina, Crotalidæ, and Crotaliens respectively, and which is characterized by the possession of a deep pit in the maxillary region, in front and below the level of the eye. Preëminent among the Crotalina for size, strength, and power of inflicting injury, are those species in which the tail terminates in a jointed corneous appendage, termed the rattle, from which their name of Rattlesnakes is derived. These serpents exhibit two types of form, which are distinguished by the following characters:—

Anterior part of the top of the head covered by small scales. CAUDISONA.
Anterior part of the top of the head covered by nine plates, symmetrically arranged. CROTALUS.

In the following pages will be given an enumeration of the species of these two genera, under their correct names, with a description of the *Caudisona horrida*, the species which has been the subject of Dr. Mitchell's experiments.

II.

CAUDISONA LAURENTI.

1768. Caudisona: LAURENTI, Specimen Synopsis Reptilium, p. 92.
1789. Crotalus: LACÉPÈDE, Histoire Naturelle des Serpens, II, 130. Nec Linnæi.
1802. " DAUDIN, Histoire Naturelle des Reptiles, V, 297.
1817. " CUVIER, Règne Animal, II, 77.
1830. " WAGLER, Naturlich. Syst. der Amphibien, p. 176.
1837. " SCHLEGEL, Essai sur le Physionomie des Serpens, II, 555.
1842. " GRAY, Zoological Miscellany, p. 51.
1843. " FITZINGER, Systema Reptilium, p. 29.
1849. " GRAY, Catal. Brit. Museum, p. 19.
1853. " BAIRD et GIRARD, Catal. Serp. Smiths. Inst., p. 1.

1854. Crotalus: DUMÉRIL, Erp. Générale, VII, 1453.
1830. Uropsophus: WAGLER, Natur. Syst. der Amph., p. 176.
1842. " GRAY, Zool. Misc., p. 51.
1843. " FITZINGER, Syst. Rept., p. 29.
1849. " GRAY, Cat. Brit. Mus., p. 19.
1843. Urocrotalon: FITZINGER, Systema Reptilium, p. 29.

Caudisona durissa.

1768. Caudisona durissa: LAURENTI, Spec. Syn. Rept., p. 93. Exclus. cit. Catesb. et Habitat.
1766. Crotalus durissus: LINNÆUS, Syst. Nat. Edit., XII, I, 372. Citatio prima; [*Amoen. Acad.*, I, 500, 1748. *Crotalophorus durissus, descriptio prima*, p. 501, *nec secunda*]. Citatio tertia falsa; [*Seba* II, 95, f. 2, *Caud. terrifica delineatur*].
1788. " " var. γ. GMELIN, Linn. Syst. Nat., I, 1081.
1789. " " LACÉPÈDE, Hist. Nat. Serp., II, 423, Excl. cit. Laurenti. Nec "Le Durissus," tab. xviii, f. 3, p. 390, ubi C. *horrida* (hujus enumerationis) delineatur.
1790. " " BONNATERRE, Ophiologie, p. 2.
1817. " " CUVIER, Règne Animal, II, 78.
1820. " " MERREM, Syst. Amphib., p. 156. Homonyma accuraté enumerata.
1830. " " GRIFFITH, Cuv. Règne Animal, IX, 267.
1853. " " LE CONTE, Proc. Acad. Nat. Sci. Philada., 1853, 416.
1859. " " COPE, Proc. A. N. S., p. 337. Exclus. homon. *C. cascavella* Wagl. et spec. "No. 3."
1802. " horridus: DAUDIN, Hist. Nat. Rept., V, 311. Exclus. cit. Linn. Laurenti, Lacépède.
" " WAGLER, Nat. Syst. Amph., p. 176. Exclus. homon. *C. cascavella* Wagl.
1837. " " SCHLEGEL, Essai, II, 561. Exclus. cit. Laurenti, Wagler, Neuwied.
1854. " " DUMÉRIL, BIBRON, VII, 1472. Exclus. cit. Linn. Wagl. (in Spix Serp. Braz.), Neuw. ?Gray.

Icones—?Seba, tab. xlv, 4. ?Bonnat, tab. iii, f. 1. Daudin, V, 69, I. ?Schlegel, Essai, tab. xx, xii, xiii, xiv. ?Dum. Bibr., lxxxiv, bis, 2. ??Cuv. Règne Animal (Edit. Audouin, Blanch. etc.), pl. xxxii. Dict. Sci. Nat. Cloquet, Poiss. et Rept., t. xxiv.

Habitat.—In Guiana, ?Mexico.

Caudisona terrifica.

1768. Caudisona terrifica: LAURENTI, Spec. Syn. Rept., p. 93.
1789. Crotalus boiquira: LACÉPÈDE, Hist. Nat. Serp., II, 130, 390. Excl. fig. 1, tab. XVIII, et cit. Kalm.
1802. " simus: DAUDIN, Hist. Rept., V, 321.
1824. " cascavella: WAGLER, Spix Serp. Braz., 60.
1825. " horridus "Daud:" NEUW. Naturgeschichte Brazil., p. 435.
1849. " " ?GRAY, Catalogue Brit. Mus., p. 20. Exclus. cit. Linn. Daudin, Schlegel; et homonym. *horridus, adamanteus, rhombifer, Oregonus.*
1827. " durissus: BOIE, Isis von Oken, p. 562.

Icon.—Seba, xcv, f. 1. Spix Serp. Braz., xxiv. Neuwied Naturgeschichte Braz., tab.?

Habitat.—In Brasilia, Guiana.

Caudisona Loeflingii.

1833. Crotalus Loeflingii: HUMBOLDT, in Humboldt et Bonpland, Recueil d'Observ. de Zoologie et Anat. Comp., p. 6.

Habitat.—In Venezuela.

Caudisona adamantea.

1799. Crotalus adamanteus: PAL. DE BEAUVOIS, Trans. Am. Phil. Soc., IV, 368.
1842. " " HOLBROOK, N. Am. Herp., III, 17.
1853. " " BAIRD et GIRARD, Catal. Serp. Smiths. Inst., p. 3.
1853. " " LE CONTE, South. Med. and Surg. Journ., IX, 664.
1790. " ?horridus: BONNAT. Ophiologie, p. 1. Excl. cit. Linn. Mus. Ad. Fried. et Tab.
"1801. " rhombifer: LATREILLE, Hist. Rept., III, 197."
1802. " " DAUDIN, Hist. Rept., V, 525.
1854. " " DUMÉRIL, BIBRON, Erp. Gen., VII, 1471.
1802. " durissus: SHAW, Gen. Zool., III, 333.
1853. " terrificus: LE CONTE, Proc. Acad. Nat. Sci. Philada., VI, 419. Exclus. homon. *Caudisona terrifica* Laur., p. 418.
1859. " " COPE, Loc. cit., p. 337. Exclus. homon. *terrifica* Laur.
1842. ? Crotalus Oregonus: HOLBROOK, N. Am. Herp., III, 21.
1853. " " BAIRD et GIRARD, Cat. Serp., p. 145.

Icones.—? Shaw, Gen. Zool., III, t. lxxxix. Daudin, Hist. Rept., V, pl. lx, figs. 22, 23. Holbrook, N. Amer. Herp., III, t. ii. U. S. Pacific R. R. Rept. Reptiles, tab. xxiv, f. 2.

Habitat.—In "United States" orientalibus circa oram Maris Mexicani et "South Carolina," in America Septentrionali.

Caudisona atrox.

1853. Crotalus atrox: BAIRD et GIRARD, Catal. Serp. Smiths. Inst., p. 5.
1859. " " BAIRD, U. S. and Mex. Boundary Surv. Reptiles, p. 14. U. S. Pacific R. R. Rept., X. Whipple's Rept., p. 39.

Icones.—U. S. and Pac. R. R. Rept. Reptiles, t. xxiv, f. 3. U. S. and Mex. Boundary Survey, Reptiles, t. i.

Habitat.—In Texas.

Caudisona lucifer.

1852. Crotalus lucifer: BAIRD et GIRARD, Proc. Acad. Nat. Sci. Philada., p. 177, et (1853), Catalogue, p. 6.
1858. " " GIRARD, Herpetology U. S. Expl. Exped., p. 187.
1859. " " BAIRD, U. S. Pacif. R. R. Report, X, Williamson's Report, p. 10.
1859. " " COOPER et SUCKLEY, Nat. Hist. Wash. Terr., p. 295.

Icones.—U. S. Pac. R. R. Surv. Rept. Reptiles, Williamson's Rept. Reptiles, tab. xi. Girard, Herp. U. S. Ex. Exp., tab. xv, figs. 1–6.

Habitat.—In Oregon, California.

Caudisona Le Contei.

1852. Crotalus Le Contei: HALLOWELL, Proc. Acad. Nat. Sci. Philad., VI, 180.
1853. " " " Rept. Exped. Zuni and Colorado Rivs. Sitgreaves, p. 139.
1859. " " " U. S. Pac. R. R. Rept., X, Williamson's Rept., p. 18.
1853. " confluentus: "Say," BAIRD et GIRARD, Catal. Serp. Smiths. Inst., p. 8. Exclus. homon. *C. confluentus* Say.
1859. " " BAIRD, U. S. and P. R. R. Surv. Rept., Whipple's Rept., p. 40. U. S. and Mex. Bound. Surv. Reptiles, p. 14.
1859. " " COOPER et SUCKLEY, Nat. Hist. Wash. Ter., p. 295.

Icones.—Sitgreave's Exped. Colorado and Zuni, tab. xviii (icon pej.). U. S. Pac. R. R. Surv. Rept. Reptiles, tab. xxiv, fig. 4. Ibid. Williamson's Rept. Reptiles, tab. iii. Cooper and Suckley, Nat. Hist. Wash. Terr., tab. xii.

Habitat.—In Nebraska usque ad "Rocky Mountains," Texas et "New Mexico."

Caudisona confluenta.

1823. Crotalus confluentus: SAY, Long's Exped. Rocky Mts., II, 48.
Icon.—Nulla.
Habitat.—"Red River," circa fontes.

Caudisona tigris.

1859. Crotalus tigris: KENNICOTT, U. S. et Mex. Boundary Surv., II, Reptiles, p. 14.
Icon.—Loc. cit., tab. iv.
Habitat.—In Eremis Gila et Colorado, "New Mexico."

Caudisona lugubris.

1860. Crotalus lugubris: JAN, Rev. et Mag. de Zoologie, p. 156.
Icon.—Jan Prodrome d'un Iconogr. Descr. Ophid., tab. E, f. 4.
Habitat.—In Mexico.

Caudisona horrida.

1766. Crotalus horridus: LINNÆUS, Syst. Nat. Ed. XII, I, 572. Primó cit. Mus. Ad. Fr., I, 39, ubi "Frons tecta squamis obtusissimis, palpebræ superiores planæ magnæ" legatur. Porro Catesby Carol. Hist. (*A*) et Amoenitat. Acad. (*B*) citantur. (*A. "Vipera caudisona americana," et "V. c. a. minor" describuntur*, pp. 41, 42; *sed "V. c. a. minor caput scutis magnis instructum habet."*[1]) (*B. In. Amoen. Acad.*, II, 139. *C. durissa* (*hujus enumerationis*) (*Amoen. Acad.*, I, 500) *citatur! et "Virginianis rattlesnake" denominatur!*) Secundo cit. Seba, 95, f. 1, ubi *C. terrifica* delineatur!!

1802. " " SHAW, Gen. Zool., III, 317.
1817. " " CUVIER, Règne Animal, II, 78.
1830. " " GRAY, Synopsis Rept., p. 78.
?1830. " " GUERIN, Iconogr. R. Anim., tab. n. 23, f. 2.
1831. " " GRIFFITH, Cuv. Règne Animal, IX, 267.
1853. " " LE CONTE, Proc. Acad. Nat. Sci. Philada., VI, 417.
1859. " " COPE, Proc. Acad. Philada., p. 338.
"1801. " durissus: LATREILLE, Hist. Rept., III, 190."
1802. " " DAUDIN, Hist. Rept., V, 304. Exclus. cit. Linn. Laurenti, Lacép.
1825. " " HARLAN, Journ. Acad. Nat. Sci. Philada., p. 368. Exclus. cit. Linn. Laur. Ibid. Med. and Phys. Res., p. 132.
1837. " " SCHLEGEL, Essai sur le Phys. Serp., II, 365. Exclus. descrip. color., p. 366, et homon. *Uropsophus triseriatus* Wagl. et *Crot. confluentus* Say.
1839. " " STORER, Report, Rept. Mass., p. 233.
1842. " " HOLBROOK, N. Am. Herp., III, 9. Exclus. cit. Linn.
1842. " " DE KAY, Zoology of New York, pt. III, 55. Exclus. cit. Linn. Say.
1853. " " LE CONTE, Southern Med. and Surg. Journ., p. 663.
1853. " " BAIRD et GIRARD, Catal. Serp. Smiths. Inst., p. 1. Exclus. cit. Linn.
1854. " " BAIRD, Serpents of New York, p. 9. Exclus. cit. Linn.
1854. " " DUMÉRIL et BIBRON, Erp. Gen., VII, 1465. Exclus. cit. Linn. Latreille, Wagler.
1859. " " BAIRD, U. S. Pac. R. R. Expl. Surv., X. Whipple's Rept. Reptiles, p. 39. Exclus. cit. Linn.
1859. " " ?JAN, Rev. et Mag. de Zool., p. 153.

[1] Linnaeus Syst. Nat., in *C. miliarii* diagnosi.

"1801. Crotalus atricaudatus: LATREILLE, Hist. Rept., III, 209."
1827. " " ?BOIE, Isis von Oken, p. 562.
1830. " " ?WAGLER, Nat. Syst. Amphib., p. 177.
1842. " " GRAY, Zool. Miscell., p. 51.
1843. Urocrotalon durissus: FITZINGER, Syst. Rept., p. 29.
1849. Uropsophus durissus: GRAY, Catal. Brit. Mus., p. 19. Exclus. cit. Linn. et homon. *confluentus* Say, *rhombifer* Latr., *triseriatus* Wiegm. Wagl. Gray.
1826. ? Crotalus Catesbaei Hempr.: FITZINGER, Neue Class, p. 63, fide Gray.
1851. ? Urocrotalon Catesbyanum Fitz.: DIESING, Syst. Hélminth., II, 431.

Icones.—Catesby, Hist. Car., II, tab. xlii. Lacépède, Serp., II, tab. xviii, f 3. Shaw. Zool. III, t. lxxxviii. Daudin, V, t. lxviii. Guerin, Iconogr. R. Animal, t. xxiii, f. 2. Schlegel, Essai, xx, f. 15, 16. Dict. Univ. Hist. Nat. Atlas, II, t. xiii. f. 1. Dum. Bibr. Erp. Gen. Atlas, t. lxxxiv, bis. fig. 1. Holbrook, N. Am. Herp., III, t. i. De Kay, Zool. New York, pt. III, Atlas, fig. 19. Baird, Serp. New York, t. i, f. 1. U. S. Pac. R. R. Expl. Rep. X, Reptiles, t. xxiv, fig. 1.

Habitat.—In "United States" orientalibus, usque ad "The Plains."

This species may be distinguished by the following peculiarities:—

Upon the top of the extremity of the muzzle there are two subtriangular shields (prefrontals) in contact with each other. A large oval shield covers the region over each eye (superciliary). These shields are in contact anteriorly upon each side with a smaller one, which is in contact anteriorly with the prefrontal, and forms upon each side, the external shield of a cross series (post-frontals) immediately behind the prefrontals, which is usually composed of five plates. The remaining part of the upper surface of the head is covered with small subtuberculous scales.

The shields bounding the upper lip (superior labials) are from twelve to fourteen in number, the fourth or fifth the largest; those bounding the lower lip (inferior labials) thirteen to fifteen. Three rows of scales separate the eye from the superior labials. Two plates in front of the eye (preoculars), the lower usually reaching the pit in the side of the face; the upper larger, and separated from the hinder of the two plates between which the nostril is pierced (nasals), by two or more small plates (loreals). The scales of the body are in twenty-three or twenty-five longitudinal rows, all keeled, the row on each side next the shields of the abdomen (gastrostega) faintly.

The ground color above varies from bright yellowish tawny or fulvous to black brown; beneath from whitish yellow to black gray. A light line extends from the superciliary plate to the angle of the mouth, behind which is a dark band or blotch. Upon each side of the medial dorsal line there are two series of brown or black spots. The spots of the upper or medial series are larger, rhomboid, running obliquely upwards and backwards. They are frequently confluent across the middle line of the back anteriorly; *always* upon the posterior half of the body. The spots of the lower series encroach slightly upon the gastrostega, and posteriorly, unite with those of the middle series, to form zigzag cross bands. Anteriorly they sometimes alternate with the central series, or rather become confluent with an indefinite alternating series, and joining the extremities of the former, enclose the ground color, which thus forms a series of light spots. Of these transverse bands or rows of spots there are twenty-one, more or less, from the head to the anus. In southwestern specimens, a narrow rufous band frequently extends along the median dorsal line throughout the whole length. Tail nearly always entirely black.

This species is found from Maine to Kansas, and from Louisiana to Florida.

Caudisona molossus.

1853. Crotalus molossus: BAIRD et GIRARD, Catal. Rept. Smiths. Inst., p. 10.
1859. " " BAIRD, U. S. et Mex. Bound. Surv. Reptiles, p. 14.
1854. " ornatus: HALLOWELL, Proc. A. N. S. Philada., VII, 192, etc.
1859. " " " U. S. Pac. R. R. Expl. Rept., Parke's Rept. Reptiles, p. 23.

Icones.—U. S. Pac. R. R. Rept. Reptiles, xxiv, f. 5. Ibid., Parke's Rept., tab. ii. U. S. and Mex. Bound. Surv., tab. iii.

Habitat.—In "New Mexico."

Caudisona lepida.

1860. Caudisona lepida: KENNICOTT, MSS.

Icon.—Nulla.

Habitat.—In Texas australi.

Caudisona cerastes.

1854. Crotalus cerastes: HALLOWELL, Proc. Acad. Nat. Sci. Philada., p. 95.
1859. " " " U. S. Pac. R. R. Expl. Rept. Williamson's Rep. Rept., p. 17.
1859. " " BAIRD, U. S. and Mex. Bound. Surv. Reptiles, p. 14.

Icon.—U. S. et Mex. Bound. Surv., pl. iii.

Habitat.—In Eremis Colorado et Gila.

CROTALUS LINNÆUS.

1766. Crotalus: LINNÆUS, Syst. Nat. Ed., XII, 372.
1788. " GMELIN, Syst. Nat., I, 1080.
1790. " BONNATERRE, Ophiologie, p. 1.
1820. " MERREM, Tent. Syst. Amphib., p. 156.
1827. " BOIE, Isis, p. 562.
1825. Crotalophorus: GRAY, Ann. Philosophy, p. 205.
1849. " " Cat. Brit. Mus., p. 17.
1842. " HOLBROOK, N. Amer. Herp., III, 25.
1853. " BAIRD et GIRARD, Cat. Serp. Smiths. Inst., p. 11.
1826. Caudisona: FITZINGER, Neue Class. Rept., p. 63.
1830. " WAGLER, Nat. Syst. Amphib., p. 176.
1832. " BONAPARTE, Saggio, p. 24.
1842. " GRAY, Zool. Misc., p. 51.
1843. " FITZINGER, Syst. Rept., p. 29.

Crotalus miliarius.

1766. Crotalus miliarius: LINNÆUS, Syst. Nat. Ed., XII, v. I, 372.
1788. " " GMELIN, Linn. S. N., I, 1080.
1789. " " [illegible] Hist. Serp., II, 401.
1790. " " BONNATERRE, Ophiol., p. 1.

1802. Crotalus miliarius: SHAW, III, 336.
1802. " " DAUDIN, Hist. Rept., V. 328.
1817. " " CUVIER, Règne Animal, II, 79.
1820. " " MERREM, Syst. Amphib., p. 156.
1827. " " BOIE, Isis, p. 562.
1837. " " SCHLEGEL, Essai, II, 569. Exclus. bomon. *C. tergeminus* Say.
1854. " " DUMÉRIL, BIBRON, Erp. Gen., VII, 1477.
1825. Crotalophorus miliarius: GRAY, Ann. Philos., p. 205.
1830. " " " in Griff. Regne Anim., p. 78.
1842. " " HOLBROOK, N. Am. Herp., p. 25.
1849. " " GRAY, Catalogue Brit. Mus., p. 17.
1853. " " BAIRD et GIRARD, Cat. Serp. Smiths. Inst., p. 11.
1859. " " BAIRD, U. S. Pac. R. R. Expl. Rep., X. Whipple's Rept., p. 40.
1826. Caudisona miliaria: FITZINGER, Neue Class., p. 63.
1830. " " WAGLER, Nat. Syst. Amph., p. 176.
1842. " " GRAY, Zool. Misc., p. 51.
1843. " " FITZINGER, Syst. Rept., p. 29.

Icones.—Catesby, Hist. Car., II, t. xlii. ?Bonnaterre, Ophiologie, t. i, f. 1. Schlegel, Essai, t. xv, f. 17, 18. Holbrook, N. Am. Herp., III, t. iv. Dum. Bibr. Erp. Gen., lxxxiv, bis. f. 5. U. S. Pac. R. R. Surv. Rept., X, Reptiles, t. xxiv, f.

Habitat.—In "United States" circa oram maris Mexicani, "South Carolina," et Arkansas.

Crotalus Edwardsii.

1853. Crotalophorus Edwardsii: BAIRD et GIRARD, Catal., p. 15.
1854. " " DUMÉRIL, BIBRON, Erp. Gen., VII, 1483.
1859. " " BAIRD, U. S. and Mex. Bound. Surv., p. 15.

Icones.—U. S. Pac. R. R. Expl. Rept., X, Reptiles, tab. xxiv, fig. 8. U. S. and Mex. Bound. Surv., t. v, f. 1.

Habitat.—In Texas.

Crotalus tergeminus.

1823. Crotalus tergeminus: SAY, Long's Exped. Rocky Mts., I, 499.
1824. " " BOIE, Isis, p. 270.
1827. " " HARLAN, Journ. Acad. Nat. Sci., V, 372.
1827. " " BOIE, Isis, p. 563.
1854. " " DUMÉRIL, BIBRON, VII, 1479.
1830. Crotalophorus tergeminus: GRAY, Synops. Rept., p. 78.
1842. " " HOLBROOK, N. Amer. Herp., III, p. 29.
1849. " " GRAY, Cat. Brit. Mus., p. 18.
1856. " " BAIRD et GIRARD, Catal., p. 14.
1842. " Kirtlandii: HOLBROOK, N. Am. Herp., III, 31.
1849. " " GRAY, Cat. Brit. Mus., p. 18.
1853. " " BAIRD et GIRARD, Catal., p. 16.
1854. " massasauga "Kirtland:" BAIRD, Serpents of New York, p. 11.
1850. " ? AGASSIZ, Lake Superior, p. 381.
1830. Caudisona tergeminus: WAGLER, Nat. Syst. Amph., p. 176.

Icones.—Holbr. N. Am. Herp., III, f. 5, 6, Agassiz, Lake Superior, t. vi, f. 8. Baird, Serp. New York, t. i, f. 2. Ibid. U. S. Pac. R. R. Expl. Rep., X, Rept., t. xxv, figs. 9, 11.

Habitat.—In "Indian Territory," Nebraska, usque ad Michigan et Ohio.

III.

The descriptions of the following supposed species do not coincide with those of any species known to modern naturalists:—

Crotalus dryinus: LINNÆUS, Syst. Nat., I, 372 (1766). Quoted by Gmelin, Lacépède, Bonnaterre, Daudin, Merrem.

Crotalus horridus: BODDAERT, Nova Acta, VII, 16 (1783). Quoted by Gmelin, Le Conte.

The following names refer to species which I cannot identify with, or distinguish from known species either on account of want of specimens, imperfect descriptions, or references which cannot be unravelled.

Crotalus adamanteus: JAN, Rev. et Mag. Zool., 1859, p. 153.

Crotalus atricaudatus: MERREM, Syst. Amphib., 157.

Crotalus cumanensis: HUMBOLDT, Humb. et Bonpl. Recueil d'Observ., p. 6 (1833).

Crotalus durissus: BODDAERT, l. c. Merrem, l. c.

" " var. *a* GMELIN, Syst. Nat., I, 1081 (1788).

Crotalus exalbidus: BODDAERT, l. c.

Crotalus horridus: JAN, Rev. et Mag. Zool., 1859, 153.

Crotalus rhombifer: MERREM, l. c.

Caudisona orientalis: LAURENTI, Synops., p. 94 (1768). = *Crotalus strepitans* Daud., V, 318 (1802). "Said to be Boa canina." Gray, Synopsis Rept., p. 78.

Caudisona Gronovii: LAURENTI, l. c. Perhaps Lachesis mutus, Daud.

Uropsophus triseriatus: WAGLER, Nat. Syst. Amph., p. 176 (1830). Gray, Cat. Brit. Mus., p. 116. Perhaps Caudisona lucifer. Prof. Jan. Iconogr. descr. Ophid., p. 29, places this species in Crotalus (*Crotalophorus*)!

Crotalophorus consors: BAIRD and GIRARD, l. c. Baird, U. S. and Mex. Bound. Surv. Reptiles, p. 15. Ibid. U. S. Pac. R. R. Expl. Rep., X, Repl., pl. xxiv, f. 7.

The following supposed species, according to Boie, Isis, 1827, 562, is *Tropidonotus quincunciatus* with a crepitaculum of a Rattlesnake attached:—

Crotalus tessellatus: HERMANN, Observat. Zool., p. 271 (1804).

The following species are not Rattlesnakes:—

Crotalus mutus: LINNÆUS, l. c. p. 373 et Gmelin, is *Lachesis mutus*, Daud.

Crotalus piscivorus: LACÉPÈDE, l. c. p. 424 (1789) = *C. aquaticus*, Bonnat. l. c. p. 3 (1790), is *Ancistrodon piscivorus*, nobis.

APPENDIX B.

BIBLIOGRAPHY.[1]

ABBATIUS (BALDUS ANGELUS). De Admirabili Viperæ natura et de mirificis ejus facultatibus liber. Ragusæ, 1587–91, in 4.
Anatomical description principally of the organs of Generation. [S.]

ACRELL (JOH. GUST.). De morsura Serpentum. (Linnæi Amœnit acad., VI., 97. 1762, in 8.)
An excellent dissertation on the bite of venomous Serpents. [S.]

ALBERTUS MAGNUS. Opus animalium. In fol. 1651.
Reports certain erroneous opinions as to the viper, and denies its cohabitation with the Lamprey. [S.]

ALDOVRANDUS (ULYSSES). Serpentum et Draconum historia, libr. 11. Francforti, in fol. 1640.
Gives descriptions of the viper, etc., with figures. [S.]

ALESSANDRINI. Ricerche sulle glandoli salivali dei Serpenti a denti solcati o veleniferi confrontate con quelle proprie delle specie non velenate di Schlegel. (Journ. polygr. de Vérone, fasc. XXVIII, 47, 1832.) [S.]

ALEXANDER. Medica commentaria. Edinburgh, II, decad. IV, B., 45. [S.]
On the employment of L'eau de Luce as a remedy. [S.]

ALEXANDER, J. B. Alcohol as an antidote. St. Louis Med. and Surg. Journal, XIII, 116, 1855.

ALOS, (JOH.) Dissertatio de Viperis. In 4, 1664.
Treats of medicines made from the flesh of the viper. [S.]

AMATUS LUSITANUS. Curationum medicarum centuriæ. Cent. I. cur. I, fol. 20. Cent. III, cur. 14, fol. 230. [S.]

ANDRIEUX. Coup d'œil sur les accidents causés par la morsure des serpents venimeux, énumération des différents moyens employés pour les combattre. Journ. des Conn. Méd. et Pharm., 181. 1849.
On the action of Mikania Guaco in snake bites. [S.]

ANEL. Art de sucer les playes sans se servir de la bouche d'un homme. Amsterdam, 1707. [S.]

ANGELINI (BERNARDINO). Del morasso a Vipera chersea rinvenuto sul territorio Veronese. (Bibl. Ital., VII, 451.) [S.]

ANSELMIER (VICTOR). Dissertation sur les indications du cautère actuel dans les plaies virulentes et envenimées. (Thèses de Paris, No. CXXIX), 1854.
Reports two successful cases of persons bitten by vipers; the actual cautery the best mode of local treatment. [S.]

ARETÆUS. De causis et signis acutorum morborum. (Ed. Haller), libr. II, cap. II, 100, in 8, 1772.
Speaks of the effect of the bite of the Dipsade and of the employment of theriac as a remedy for the bite of the viper (136). [S.]

ATCHISON, T. A. Alcohol as an antidote to the venom of the Crotalus. Southern Journal of the Med. and Phys. Sciences, I, p. 47, 1853.

ATWELL (JOSEPH). Observations concerning a man and a woman bitten by a viper. (Philos. Trans. No. CCCCLXIV, 275, 1736.) [S.]
Reports good results from the employment of oil in viper bites. [S.]

AUDOUX. Observations communiquées à M. Ma-

[1] As a general rule, the authorities upon the natural history of serpents are not included in the list. For those especially concerning the Rattlesnake, see Mr. Cope's "Genera and Species," p. 119. The works given by Soubeiran in his excellent Bibliography are marked in mine with the letter [S].

sars de Cazeles. (Jour. de Méd., XXXII, 442.)

Reports a case of viper bite treated by applications of the bruised head of the viper, together with theriac and a vinous decoction of the flesh of the viper and of the bark of the ash tree. Recovery in three days. [S.]

AUZOUX (L. I. I.). Dissertation sur la Vipère. (Thèses de Paris, No. CLXII), 1822.

This work gives a general statement of knowledge relative to the viper. [S.]

AVICENNE. Canon Medicinæ ex Gerardi Cremonensis versione. In fol. II, libr. IV, fen. 6, tract 3, Venetiis, 1608. De regimine morsionis universali. Et de effugatione venenosorum et de curatione morsicationis Serpentum et speciebus eorum.

Treats of the venom of the viper and of the treatment of snake-bites. [S.]

BAJON. Mémoire pour servir à l'histoire de Cayenne. Maladies de Cayenne, I, 352–355.

States that the juice of the Tayove (*Caladium sagittæfolium*) and sugar, are useful in snake-bites. [S.]

BARICELLI. Falsum viperam in coitu masculum occidere, ipsumque a catulis in partu necari. Hortulus genialis Bononiæ, in 12mo, 1617. [S.]

BARSTOW. Account of the singular effects from the bite of a Rattlesnake. Philadelphia Med. Museum, III, 61.

The milk of a woman bitten by a rattlesnake, said to have caused the death of her child, as well as of two puppies and three lambs employed to draw off the milk.

BARTON (B. S.). On the supposed powers of Fascination in serpents. [O.] Pamphlet, Phila., 1814. Also, the same in American Phil. Trans., III, 1793. Also, General Observations on the Rattlesnake. Am. Phil. Trans., IV, 1799.

BARTRAM. On the teeth of the Crotalus. Engl. Phil. Trans., abrd. IX, 60, 1793.

BAUDERON, BRICE. Pharmocopée diusée en deux liures, p. 860, in 4, Lion, 1640. [S.]

BAUQUIER (DE SAINT AMBROIX). Observation d'une morsure de vipère. Journ. de Sci. Méd., XXVIII, 377, 1827. [S.]

BAUREGARD. Anc. Journ. de Méd., VI, 233, 1757.

A case of viper bite treated successfully with the juice of ash leaves, and poultices of the same, as local treatment. [S.]

BECK. Medical Jurisprudence, II, 537.

BÉRARD. Gazette de Santé, No. 16, 1788.

Advises frictions with olive oil in viper bites. [S.]

BERNARD (CLAUDE). Leçons sur les effets des substances toxiques et médicamenteuses, Paris, 1857, p. 388 et seq.

Brief account of viper venom. Experiments to prove the power of the viper to destroy its own kind.

BERNINCK (A.). Dissertatio serpentem sistens Præs. S. F. Freuzel. In 4to. Wittebergæ, 1665. [S.]

BERTIN (J. E.). Ergo specificum viperæ morsus antidotum alcali volatile. Paris, 149, in 4. Haller, dissert., p. vi, No. 218. [S.]

BEST (J. CH.). Dissertation sur la morsure de la vipère fer-de-lance. Thèses de Paris, No. 106, 1823.

Treats of the cause of death, and thinks that fright has a great deal to do with the production and intensity of the symptoms. [S.]

BLAINVILLE. Observations on Crotalus Poisoning. Bull. de la Société Philomatique, Paris, 1825, p. 210. [S.]

BOAG (W.). General observations on the bites of E. Indian serpents. Asiatic Researches, VI, 103, 1801.

BOCHART (SAMUEL). Hierozoicon, sive de animalibus scripturæ recensuit suis notis, L. F. C. Rosenmuller, in 4, III, pars ii, lib. iii, 1793–96.

Gives the etymology of the word viper, proves that it was known to the Hebrews, and cites many oriental authorities, &c., which make mention of the animal in question.

BONAPARTE (LUCIEN). Gaz. Tosc. delle sc. medicofis, p. 169, 1843.

Analysis of viper venom, the only one on record.

BOSC (L. A. G). Vipère Nov. Dict. d'histoire Nat. Déterville, XXXVI, 82, 1819.

Natural history of the viper, with discussions as to its habits. [S.]

BOUÉ (J. F.). Dissertation sur la morsure de la vipère. Thèses de Paris, No. 69, 1823.

Advances cases to prove the gravity of the malady of the viper bite. [S]

BOURDELOT (PIERRE MICHON). Recherches et observation sur les vipères. Paris, in 12mo., also in English, Philos. Trans., VI, 3013, 1671. [S.]

BOYLE (ROBERT). De utilitate philosophiæ experimentalis. Pars II, Exercitat, II, par 34. Lindaviæ, 1 in 4to, 1692.

Reports cures from using a hot iron, which was brought as near to the wound as it could be borne by the patient. [S.]

Brainard (David, M. D.). On the nature and cure of the bite of serpents, and the wounds of poisoned arrows. Smithsonian Reports, 1854, p. 123.

Describes woorara, and considers that it owes its poisoning power to a venom. Advocates the use of iodine as an antidote to be injected into and about the track of the wounds made by serpents or by poisoned arrows.

Brainard (David). Essay on a new method of treating serpent bites and other poisoned wounds. 8vo. pamphlet, Chicago, 1854.

Much the same as the last paper (vide *supra*), with new observations on the phenomena of crotalophorous poisoning.

Brainard and Green. Comptes Rendus de l'Académie des Sciences, p. 811, 1853.

Contains details of observations on the use of iodine in woorara poisoning and in snake-bites.

Breintnal (C.). Engl. Philosophical Trans. abrd., X, 229.

Reports his own case of Crotalus bite.

Brickell. New York Medical Repository, VIII, 441, 1805.

Gives his own experiments upon the reaction of Rattlesnake venom.

Brogiano (Domenico). De Veneno Animantium naturali et adquisito, p. 38, 4to.

An extremely interesting dissertation on the effects of viper venom upon the economy of man.

Brotonne (De). Ergo specificum viperæ morsus antidotum alcali volatile. Paris, 1778. [S.]

Bulletin de Thérapeutique, XXXI, 70, 1846.

Case of viper bite successfully treated by ammonia. [S.]

Burnett (W. I.). Proc. Boston Nat. Hist. Society, IV, 311, 323.

On the succession of the fangs in Crotalus, describes his mode of procuring the venom by chloroforming the snake and then pressing on the glands. Also observation of the effect produced by mingling the venom with blood.

Burton (William). Letter concerning the Viper Catchers, and their Remedy for the Bite of a Viper. (Engl. Phil. Trans., No. 443, 1734.)

Reports experiments tried on a man to show the utility of olive oil in viper bites. [S.]

Camerarus (Elias). Dissertationes Epistolico physico medicæ. Tubingen, 1712, m. 2.

He seeks to prove that the viper is not equally venomous in all localities, and cites facts to support this opinion. [S.]

Cantor. London Zoological Trans., II, 304.

On Pelagic snakes. Action of their venom on the tortoise, etc.

Cardose. Des effets d'une piqûre faite par la dent d'une vipère morte. Annales de la Soc. de Méd. pratique de Montpellier, serie II, I, 179. [S.]

Carminati (B.). Saggi di osservazioni sui veneno della vipera. Opusc. scelti, I, 58, 1778. [S.]

Catesby. Natural History of Carolina; also cited by Mortimer, Engl. Phil. Trans., 1738, p. 8.

Advises the actual cautery as a remedy in snake-bites. Early natural history of the Rattlesnake, etc.

Cauro. Exposition du moyen curatif des accidents produits par la morsure de l'Arraignée 13 guttata ou Theridion mal mignatte du départment de la Corse, suivi de quelques réflexions sur le mode d'agir de son venin et de celui de la vipère, in 4to. Thèses de Paris, No. 128, 1833.

Proposes a secret remedy, camphor and opium, which he describes as useful in spider bites, and which, therefore, he presumes would be valuable in those of the viper. [S.]

Caventou. Relation de quelques nouvelles expériences faites par M. Desaulx, avec le venin de la vipère. Archives Général de Médecine, série I, XIII, 518. [S.]

Cayal. Rage communiquée par la morsure d'un chien, essais de traitement par l'arsenic, l'hydrogène sulphuré et par le venin de la vipère, mort 70 heures après l'invasion des premiers symptômes; nécropsie. Révue Méd., III, 387, 1831. [S.]

Cazentre (de Bordeaux). Notice sur les propriétés thérapeutiques de *cèdron*. (Journ. des Conn. Médico-Chirurg., 1850.)

States that the *cedron* is an infallible remedy in serpent bites. [S.]

Celsus. De re medica; de medicamentis, lib. V, cap. XXVII, § 3, Lyon, 1856, in 8.

Prefers the suction of poisoned wounds to the ligature, to cups, or to incisions. [S.]

Chabert (Jean-Louis). Du Huaco et de ses vertus médicinales in 8, 1853.

Reports marvellous effects of *mikania guaco* in serpent bites, even of the most terrible kind. [S.]

Charas (Moïse). Nouvelles expériences sur la vipère ou l'on verra vne description exacte de tovtes ses parties, la sovree de son venin; ses divers effets et les remèdes exquis que les artistes peuvent tirer de la vipère tant pour la guérison de ses morsures que pour celle de plusieurs autres maladies. Paris, in 8, 1669. [S.]

CHARAS (MOÏSE). Svite des novvelles expériences svr la vipère, in 8, 1772–90. [S.]

CHEVALLIER (TH.). Lettre sur l'efficacité de l'arsenic sur la morsure des serpents. Sedillot Recueil périod de la Soc. de Méd. de Paris. III, 409. [S.]

CHRISTISON (R.). Treatise on Poisons. 1st Am. from 4th Edin. ed., Phila. 1845, p. 484.

CLARKE (R. W.). Attempt to cure Elephantiasis and Leprosy by the Bite of a Rattlesnake. Lancet, I, 1838 and 1839, 443.

Singular case resulting fatally.

COL DE VILLARS (ÉLIE). Cours de chirurgie dicté aux écoles de médecine de Paris, III. Traité des plaies, ch. vi, p. 177, 1746.

Gives a short description of the symptoms and treatment of viper bites, insists on the necessity of internal treatment, owing to the fact that a part of the venom always enters the blood. [S.]

COLBATCH (J.). Cure of the Bite of a Viper. London, 1698, 8vo. [S.]

COLLENUTIUS (PANDOLPH). Libellus de Vipera Venet, 1506. [S.]

COOPER (SAMUEL). Surgical Dictionary, 1828, p. 274.

Describes the viper, his teeth and his bite, and the mode of treatment. [S.]

COSTE. Sur les effets de l'eau de Luce dans la morsure de la vipère. (Journ. de Méd., XXXIII, 524, 1770.)

Reports a cure by the use of fomentations of camphorated alcohol and theriac, followed by scarifications, and the application of eau de Luce on the wound. [S.]

COSTER. Prophylactique du venin de la vipère. (Clin. des Hôpit., III, No. 43, 1828.) [S.]

CRÜGER (DANIEL). De morsu Viperarum. (Eph. Germ. Acad. Nat. Cur., IV, obs. LXV, 143, 1686.)

Treatment of a case of viper bite according to ancient methods, attributes great value to the *sperma ranarum*. [S.]

DAVY (JOHN). On Snake Stones. Asiatic Researches, XIII, 317, in 4to.

Gives analyses of the stones whose application to the wound is supposed in the east to effect a cure of snake-bites.

DAVY (JOHN). On the poison of three of the poisonous snakes of Ceylon. Davy's Physiological and Anatomical Researches, I. 113, London, 1839; and also the author's account of the interior of Ceylon, London, 1821.

A highly valuable and interesting detail of experiments on venom poisoning.

DECERFS (J. P. E.). Essai sur la morsure des serpents venimeux de la France. Thèses de Paris, No. 27, 1807.

Contains nothing novel except the opinion that the viper bite is not mortal in man, even when no treatment has been employed. [S.]

DELACOUX. Amputation complète de la jambe gauche produite par une ligature circulaire permanente de ce membre. Acad. de Méd. Séances des 30 Juillet et 20 Août, 1833. Arch. Gén. de Méd., 2e sér. II, 587 et 592. [S.]

The ligature of the limb was used after a viper bite; no absorption of venom took place, but the leg became gangrenous, and was finally amputated. A case in which the remedy was probably worse than the disease. [S.]

DELPECH. Précis élémentaire des maladies réputées chirurgicales, II, 135 et 136, in 8vo., 1815. [S.]

Thinks that the viper bite is rarely dangerous. [S.]

DEMATHIIS. Moyen de guérir l'hydrophobie. Anc. Journ. de Méd., LXI, 365, Mém. de la Soc. de Méd., p. 210, 1783.

This author treated a dog supposed to be mad by allowing him to be bitten numerous times by a viper. The dog died in four hours. The author supposes that if the bites had been fewer the dog would have been cured; and infers that the venom is a specific against hydrophobic rage! [S.]

DEMEURE. Journ. de la Soc. Gall. de Méd. homœopathique, V, No. 6, 397, Oct. 1854.

Gives the case of a person bitten by a viper. The symptoms seem to have been of an unusual nature. The cure is attributed to the fact that some of the venom from the bite in the thumb having been absorbed in homœopathic amount, the patient was thus protected from the effects of the remaining poison. [S.]

DELILLE. Indication de Thérapeutique directe des morsures les plus vénéneuses. Journ. de Physiologie Exp. et Pathol., VII, 113.

DESBOIS (de Rochefort). Cours élémentaire de Matière Médicale, II, 280, 1789.

Thinks that the effects of the venom of the viper are due to the animal being enraged, and that it acts on the nervous system, producing a tendency to putrefaction. Advises sudorifics, ammonia, and eau de Luce.

DESMOULINS. Mémoires sur le système nerveux et

l'appareil lacrymal des serpents à sonnettes, de Trigonocéphales et de quelques autres serpents. Journ. de Phys., IV, 264, 1824.
Treats of the venom gland of serpents, and desires to prove that it is only an adjunct of the lachrymal apparatus. [S.]

De Vesey (Louis) Xantus. Cases.—Experiments with Bibron's Antidote. Am. Journ. of the Med. Sci., No. LXX, p. 375, 1858.

Dezeimeris. Dict. de Médecine, XXX, 822.
Contains nothing new. Gives an incomplete bibliography.

Drake. On the use of ammonia in cases of serpent bites. West. Journ. Med. & Phys. Sci., I, 60.

Dubébat. Mort spontanée produite par la morsure d'une seule vipère. Bull. de Thér., X, 198, 1836.
Case of a woman analogous to that reported by Dr. Lugeal. [S.]

Dudley (Paul). Account of the Rattlesnake. Phil. Trans. abrd., VII, 409–410, 1722.
On the rattles, on fascination, etc.

Dugès (Alfred). Sur les Vipères Aspis et Pelias. Mém. de la Soc. de Biologie, II, 115. Gaz. Méd., p. 270, 1850.
Corrects certain errors in regard to the French vipers; gives details of their habits, etc. [S.]

Dugès (Alfred). Note sur le redressement des crochets dans les Thanatophides. Ann. des Sc. Nat., 3e sér. XVII, 57, au pl., 1852.
Gives a new explanation of the mechanism concerned in elevating the fangs. [S.]

Duméril (Constant) et Bibron (E.). Erpétologie Générale, VI et VII, 1844. At VII, part II, 1399, Natural History and Anatomy of Serpents; reports case of M. Duméril, bitten by a viper in 1851.

Duméril (Auguste). Note historique sur la ménagerie des reptiles du muséum. Mém. du Muséum, VII, 273.
Contains a large amount of information on the habits of snakes, their food, change of skin, etc.

Dumont. Vide Aug. Duméril, p. 276.
On the use of *cedron* as an antidote and prophylactic.

Duncan. On E. Indian Snake-Bites, strychnia as a remedy in. Lancet, I, 507.

Dusourd. Effets remarquables de l'huile d'olive employée à l'intérieur et à l'extérieur dans les cas de morsure de vipère. Bull. de Thérapeut., XXVII, 489, 1849.
Approves of the internal use of olive oil in snake-bites. [S.]

Dutertre (Jean Baptiste). Hist. Générale des Antilles habitées par les Français, in 4to, 1667, 1671. [S.]

Duvernoy (G. L.). Caractères anatomiques pour distinguer les serpents venimeux. Ann. des Sci. Nat., XXVI, 113, 1830, XXX, 5, 1832.
Gives, amongst numerous other matters, details of the anatomy of the head of the viper; also accounts of experiments upon the poisoning power of venom long kept in alcohol.

Énaux et Chaussier. Méthode de traiter les morsures des animaux enragés et de la vipère, in 12mo., p. 101, 1785.
Advises cauterization. [S.]

Encyclopædia. See article Serpents, in the British, Edinburgh, and Rees' Encyclop.

Erndte (Christ. Henr.). Iter Anglicanum et Batanum, 1714, in 8vo. [S.]

Ettmuller (M.). Dissertation de Morsu Viperæ, præs. S. R. Sulzberger, Leipzig, 1665, 1685, in 4to. [S.]

Fodéré. Médecine Légale, IV, 11 et 12.
Cites many cases observed in the hospital at Martinique, which died from the bites of the vipers of the marshes of Bos.

Fontana (Félix). Ricerche filosofiche sopra il veleno della vipera, in 4to, II, Lucca, 1767. Translated into French in 1781, 4to, II, and into English, by Skinner, in 1787, II, 8vo.
This latter is the edition referred to in the foregoing essay.

Foucher (d'Opsonville). Essai philosophique sur les mœurs de divers animaux étrangers, 1783, p. 26, in 8vo. [S.]

Franzius (Wolfgang). Historia animalium in qua plerumque animalium præcipuæ proprietates in gratiam studiosorum, theologiæ et ministrorum verbi ad usum ἱκονολογικόν breviter accomodantur, in 18vo, Amster., 1665, pars IV, cap. iii, de vipera.
Dwells on the reproduction of the viper, on the consequences of its bite, and on the remedies; but especially on the viper, theologically considered. [S.]

Freiskarn (Faulens). Dissertatio de veneno Viperarum, in 8vo, 1782. [S.]

Gaignepain. Dissertation sur les effets du venin de la vipère. Thèses de Paris, No. 24, 1807.
Contains nothing novel. [S.]

Gale (B.). Crotalus bite cured by salt. Engl. Phil. Trans. abrd., XII, 224, 1765.

GALEN. Opera, XII, Ed. Kuhn, Lipsiæ, 1826, pp. 311–316.
Speaks of various venomous serpents, and of the use of viper flesh in elephantiasis. [S.]

GASPARD (B.). Observations sur la morsure de la vipère. Journ. de Physiol. Expt. et Pathol. de Magendie, I, 248, 1831.
Reports a case of a woman who was cured of a tertian by the bite of a viper.

GASPARD (B.). On putrefactive poisoning. Journ. de Phys. Exp. et Pathol., VII, 7 et seq.

Gazette Salutaire de Bouillon, 1787. Hufeland Neues Annalen, I, 405.
Of the use of ammonia locally and interiorly as an antidote. [S.]

Gazette de Santé du 5 Novembre, 1822.
States that dogs may be saved from the effects of viper bite by the application of a cataplasm of the fresh stems of the helleborus niger. [S.]

GEOFFROY et HUMAULD. Mémoire dans lequel on examine si l'huile d'olive est un spécifique contre la morsure des vipères. Mém. de l'Acad. des Sci., 1737, p. 183.
Concludes that olive oil is not a remedy in these cases, or at least that it is a doubtful one. [S.]

GERDY (P. N.). Traité des pansements proprement dits, 2e édit. p. 152, 1839.
Case of viper bite treated by ammonia. Plan of treatment. [S.]

GIADOROU (VINCENT). Observations médico-pratiques sur l'efficacité de *l'Inula squarrosa* contre la morsure de la vipère. Ann. Univ. de Médic., 1837; Gaz. Médic., p. 424, 1837. [S.]

GILMAN. Soda as an antidote in the bite of the Crotalus. Southern Med. and Surg. Journ., N. S., X, 706.

GILMAN (J.). Action of Crotalus Venom on Plants. St. Louis Med. and Surg. Journ., XII, 25, 1854.
Contains, also, notes on other minor matters connected with serpents.

GOCKEL (EBERHR). De peste et venenis, in 8vo, 1669, cap. xiv, p. m. 59.

GOESLING (I. A.) De spissitudine sanguinis multis in morbis temere accusata. Gutt., 1747.
Affirms that the popular opinion as to viper venom greatly thickening the blood is not correct.

GOODYEAR (AARON). Death from snake-bite at Aleppo. Engl. Phil. Trans. abrd., II, 816–817.

GOUPIL. Sur la vipère de Fontainebleau et sur les effets de sa morsure. Bull. de la Soc. de la Fac. de Méd. Cah., 5 Mai, 1809. [S.]

GRAY (E. W.). Observations on the amphibia of Linnæus, and especially on the means of distinguishing venomous serpents from those which are not so. Engl. Phil. Trans. at large, LXXIX, 21, 1789.

GRAY (J. B.). Observations on Vipers. Proc. Zool. Soc., 1834, p. 101.

GRAY (J. B.). Venomous Water Snakes. Proc. Zool. Soc., 1837, p. 135.

GREVIN. Deux liures de venins auxquels il est complétement discouru des Bestes venimeuses, thériaques, poisons et contre poisons. In 4to, Anvers, 1618, chap. x, p. 72.
Translations from Nicander in regard to the bite of the viper, etc. [S.]

GRIMM (J. F. C.). Historia symptomatum a morsu Aspidis productorum et medelæ. Nova Act. Acad. Cur., III, 64, 1767. [S.]

GRIVE (LOUIS DE LA). Antiparalèlle des Vipères romaines et berbes candiotes. Lion, 1632, p. 77. [S.]

GRUÈRE (J. B. VICTOR). Des venins et des animaux venimeux. Thèses de Paris, No. 9, 1854. [S.]
Gives an analysis of the memoir of Prince Lucien Bonaparte.

GUBLER (AD.). Mémoire sur l'ictère qui accompagne quelquefois les éruptions syphilitiques précoces. Mém. de la Soc. de Biol., V, 263, 1853.
Contains incidental remarks on the icterus consecutive to the bites of serpents.

GULDEN (KLEE). Bald. Timoeus A. Opera Libr. vii, cas. XVIII, p. 323; libr. v. Epist. XVI, p. m. 824, in 4to.
Cases of viper bite. [S.]

GURISCH (MARTIN). Consideratio physico-medico-forensis de saliva humana qua ejus natura et usus insimulque morsus brutorum et hominis, rabies et hydrophobia, demorsurum delecta et defensio, etc. Lipsiæ, 1729, p. 181, de morsu vipèrarum. [S.]

GUYON. Leçons diverses, II, 527.
Describes the treatment of the bite of the viper by saliva. [S.]

HAFENREFERUS (SAM.). De cutis affectibus, in 8vo. Tubingen, 1630, libr. iii, cap. viii, p. 461.
Relates certain facts in regard to the bite of the viper. [S.]

HALL. Expts. on Crotalus venom. Engl. Phil. Trans. abrd., VII, 412, 1727.

HAMMOND (W. A.). On the use of Bibron's Antidote. Am. Journ. of the Med. Sci., No. LXIX, p. 94, 1858.

HANNEMANN (JOS. LUD.). Dissert. de viperæ morsu Miscell. Nat. Cur. Dec. II, An. VIII, p. 203, 1689. [S.]

HANNOVER, Nützliche Sammlungen, p. 1365, 1756.
Advocates the use of olive oil in viper bites. [S.]

HARDER (J. J.). De viperarum morsu dissertatio. Ept. Germ. Acad. Nat. Cur. Dec. II, An. VI, p. 229, 1685.
Relates experiments made to test the truth of Redis' statements. [S.]

HARLAN (R.). Medical and Physical Researches, p. 490, Phila., 1835.
Experiments with Crotalus on animals, antidotes, etc.

HARLAN (R.). A case of Crotalus bite in man. The North Am. Med. and Surg. Journ., Phila., 1831, XI, 227.
Interesting case—recovery.

HARRIS. Asclepias as an antidote in venom poisoning. South. Med. and Surg. Journ., N. S., XI, 414.

HARTMANN (G. L.). Précis sur l'histoire naturelle des Vipera Berus, Coluber natrix et Anguis Fragilis, lu à la Soc. d'hist. nat. de Saint-Gall., 1819. Neue Alpina, I, 169.
Advises as treatment suction, the ligature, and cauterization.

HEEREY (O. C.). Use of Bibron's Antidote. Am. Journ. Med. Sci., 1859, No. LXXVI, p. 574.
Reports a case of its use.

HELMONT (VAN). Ontus Medicinæ. Amsterdam, Elzevir, 1548, in 4, p. 177.
Disputes the opinion that the virulence of viper venom is due to the animal being angry. [S.]

HEMPRIEZ. De absorptione et secretione venenosa, 1822. [S.]

HERING (CONSTANTINE). The Effects of Snake Poison. Allentown, Pa., and Leipzig, 8vo, 1837. Translated into English in 1844, in the Brit. Quart. Journ. of Homœopathy.
A collection of wild absurdities in regard to the analysis of venom, and to its use in hydrophobia, etc.

HERODOTUS. Histoire, Libr. III, cap. 109.
Speaks of the viper and its mode of propagating. [S.]

HERRAN. Graine du *Cêdron* employée dans l'Amérique tropicale comme remède contre la morsure des serpents. Journ. de Pharm., 3e série, XVIII, 296, 1850.
Thinks the seed of the *Simaba Cedron* an infallible remedy. [S.]

HODIERNA (JOH. BAPT.). De dente viperæ virulento epistola, 1651. [S.]

HOFFMANN (FRIED.). Disputatio de saliva et ejus usu medico, in 4to, 1678, cap. V, p. 18. [S.]

HOME (SIR E.). Case of a man bitten by a Crotalus, with additional cases of E. Indian serpent bites. Engl. Phil. Trans. at large, 1810, p. 75.

HORNER (WM.). Death from Crotalus bite—post mortem examination. Am. Journ. of Med. Sci., VIII, 397, 1831.
An interesting case.

HUBBLE. *Prenanthes Altissima* as an antidote. N. Am. Med. and Surg. Journ., I, 447, 1826, from N. Y. Med. and Phys. Journ., Jan. 1826.

IRELAND (J. P.). Treatment of snake-bites, cases, etc. Med.-Chir. Trans., II, 394.
East Indian snakes—arsenic as a remedy.

JAGERSCHMIDT. De morb. Serpentarum: Miscell. Nat. Curioso Acad. Dec. II, An. 2, p. 240.

JETER (A. F.). Poisoned wounds, their distinctive features, and classification, with remarks on the classes; and a special treatise on the nature and treatment of the wounds resulting from the bites of venomous reptiles. Being a report of a committee to the Med. Assoc. of Missouri, 1854.
Contains many points of interest, and a number of experiments.

JOMARD. Comptes Rendus de l'Acad. des Sci., XXXI, 141, 150, vide Herran. [S.]

Journal Encyclopédique, VI, 297, 1772.
External and internal use of olive oil in snake bites. [S.]

Journal de Méd. pratique de Hufeland, Analysé dans. Bibl. Médic., LXXIV, 125, 1821. [S.]
Reports two cases of viper bite, illustrating the proper and the improper mode of treatment.

JUSSIEU (BERNARD DE). Sur les effets de l'eau de Luce contre la morsure des vipères. Mém. de l'Acad. Roy. des Sci., p. 54, 1747.
Case of a student bitten in the hand. Cure. [S.]

KALM. Travels in America (Hist. Caudisonæ). 1753, II, 490.

KIRKER. Épreuve de la pierre de serpent faites à Vienne par ordre de S. M. I. Journ. litt. de Nazari, 1668; Collect. Academ. part. étr., VII.
Reports favorable results. [S.]

KNOX. On the mode of growth, reproduction and structure of the poison fangs in serpents. Memoirs of the Wernerian Nat. Hist. Soc., V, part ii., 411, 1826, pl.

KOSTER. Voyage au Brésil, II, 247.
Permanent effects of Crotalus bite renewed at the full and wane of the moon.

KRUZENSTEIN. Dissertatio de oleorum ex vegetabilibus expressorum salutariusu medico. Hafn, 1773. [S.]

KUTZCHIN (J. C.). Dissertatio inauguralis medica de viperarum usu medico. Præs. J. Juncker Hake., Magd. 1744. [S.]

LANTIER (ÉTIENNE). Dissertation sur la morsure de la vipère et celle des animaux enragés. Thèses de Strasbourg, 19 Fruct. An. XI, 1803.
An incomplete abridgment of Fontana's views. Contains no novelty. [S.]

LANGONI. De venenis, cap. 33 et 61, 1509. [S.]

LAPRE. Symptômes d'une morsure de Vipère décrits par un médecin qui a failli en être victime. Union. Med., Sept. 1850. [S.]

LAURENTI (J. N.). Synopsis Reptilium emendata, cum experimentatis circa venena et antidota Serpentum Austriacorum. Viennæ, in 8vo. 1768.

LE BRUN. Observations sur l'usage des alcalis volatils contre la morsure de la Vipère, qui tendent à prouver que tous les alcalis volatils tirés des animaux peuvent, ainsi que l'eau de Luce, guérir les personnes mordues par les Vipères. Journ. de Méd., XVIII, 150, 1763.
Four cases of viper bite terminating favorably—three of the number being infants. [S.]

LE CONTE (J.). On the Venomous Serpents of Georgia. Southern Med. and Surg. Journ., IX, 1853, 645.
A very interesting collection of observations, new and old, on the natural history, habits, and poison of the Georgia serpents.

LEMERY (NICOLAS). Traité universel des drogues simple, p. 812 in 4to., 1598.
Gives the symptoms of the bite, the mode in which the venom is supposed to act, and the treatment.

LIMPERANI (G. PAOLO). Relazione di una Vipera che ha partorito i viperini per bocca—(in Vallisneri, op. Med. fis., III, 1733.) [S.]

LINDELIUS (JOH. H.). Dissertatio de Vipera ejusque morsu, in 4to., 1690.
Attributes the action of the venom to the anger of the animal, and denies that there is any difference in danger between the bite of the male and female viper. [S.]

LINNÆUS (CAROLUS). *Coluber Smolandiæ.* Act. Holm, Coll. Acad. part étr., XI, 91, 1772.
Insists upon the dangerous character of the bite of this serpent, which is the *Vipera Chersea.* [S.]

LUGEOL. La morsure d'une seule Vipère peut entrainer la mort. Bull. de Thér., XXV, 211, 1766.

MANGILI (GIACOMO). Sul. Veleno della Vipera. Paris, 1809. Bibl. Med., XXXI, 428, 1811.
Shows that the young viper may be killed by venom. States that the viper cannot raise its fangs during the first few days of its existence. Of the effects of ammonia given internally for the cure of viper bites.

MANGILI (GIACOMO). Discours sur le venin de la Vipère. Giorn. di fisica chemica, IX, 458, 1817. Ann. de Chimie et de Physique, IV, 159.
Contains experiments to show that the venom of the viper is harmless when taken internally.

MANZINI (NICOLAS B. L.). Histoire de l'inoculation Préservative de la Fièvre Jaune. Paris, 8vo. 1858.
The active element of the substance used in Cuba supposed to be the venom of a Crotalus. The description of the phenomena of the inoculation are very curious. The *likeness* between yellow fever and the Crotalus malady is remarked upon at length, but the essential differences are not sufficiently noted.

MARTIN. Recueil périodique d'observations de Médecine, IV, 412, 1756. [S.]

MASARS DE CASELES. Vide AUDOUX. [S.]

MAYER (C. A.) Exercitatio historico-medica de Viperarum usu medico. Altdorf, 1727. [S.]

MAYERNE (SIR THEO. DE). Engl. Phil. Tr. abrd., II, 817–818.
Marrubium a remedy in viper bite.

MAYRANT (WM.). Cases of Rattlesnake bites. Alcoholic stimulants as remedies. Amer. Med. Recorder, VI, 1823, 619.

MEAD (RICHARD). Mechanical account of Poisons. 4to. London, 1673.
Contains Mead's well-known theories and observations upon viper venom.

MECKEL (J. FRÉD.). Sur les glandes de la tête des Serpents. Arch. für Anat. und Phys., I, 1. [S.]

MENTZELIUS (CHRÉTIEN). Observation sur les Vipères d'Italie. Eph. Nat. Cur. germ. dec. II, Ann. 2, obs. vii. Collect. Academ. III, 535, 1755.

Observations on the habits of the viper, and the arrangement of its teeth. [S.]

MESUÉ. Opera, in f. Venetiis, 1762, p. 107, 109. 354, 393.

Gives brief account of numerous medicines used in cases of viper bites. [S.]

METAXA (LOUIS). Monographie des Serpents de Rome et de ses environs. In 4to., 1823. Bull. de Férussac, I, 184, 1824.

Describes the organs which secrete and conduct the venom; also, the nature of this fluid, its effects, and the remedies employed. [S.]

MILLER (A. G.). Ammonia as an antidote in Rattlesnake bite. Boston Med. and Surg. Journ., VIII, 1833, 240.

MIQUEL. Morsures de Vipère, moyen de prévenir l'absorption du virus après la cautérization de la plaie, et de combattre l'engorgement consécutif du membre. Bull. de Thér., XXXV, 283, 1848.

Described by Soubeiran as an interesting and suggestive essay. [S.]

MONGIARDINI. Essai d'expériences sur le mode d'action du venin de la Vipère dans l'économie animale. Analys. Bibl. Médic., XVI, 257, 1807.

Endeavors to prove that the venom of the viper does not cause death by cardiac paralysis, and does not attack only the muscular irritability. [S.]

MONTI. Opusc. Scelti., I. Weigel Bibl. Ital., III, 207.

States that he found useful the topical application of earth moistened with urine. [S.]

MOORE (J.). Ammonia as an antidote in the bite of the Rattlesnake. Am. Journ. of the Med. Sci., I, 341, 1827.

Reports cases.

MORGAGNI (J. B.). Recherches Anatomique sur le siége et les causes des maladies. Trad. Desormeaux et Destouet, IX, Lett. 59, ch. 294, p. 390, 1824 (1761).

Interesting study of the viper bite, &c., from a therapeutical point of view. [S.]

MORO. Journ. de Leroux, XXXIX, 278.

Used carbonate of ammonia with good effect internally. [S.]

MORTIMER (CROMWELL). Case of Wm. Oliver, who allowed himself to be bitten by Vipers, using olive oil locally as a cure. Engl. Phil. Tr. abrd., IX, 61 et seq., 1736. See BURTON and ATWELL.

MOSELEY. Tropical Diseases, etc., p. 34.

Jaundice a secondary consequence of snakebites.

MOTTE (LA). Chirurgie, Observ., 314.

Advises the use of theriac and spirit of wine internally and externally. [S.]

MULLER. De glandularum secernentium structura penitiori, in fol., 1830, VI, fig. 1, 50.

Structure of the venom gland in snakes.

NICANDER. Les Œuvres de Nicandre médecin et pöete grec, traduites en vers françals. Ensemble devx hures des venins, auxquels li est amplement discouru des Bestes venimeuses, thériaques, poisons et contre poisons par Jaques Gréuin in 4. Anvers, 1617. [S.]

ORFILA. Traité de Toxicologie, 5th Ed. Paris, 1852, pp. 840 et seq.

A good summary of the present state of knowledge in regard to venomous serpents.

OWEN (R.). Cyclopædia of Anat. and Phys. Ed. Todd. Articles: Teeth and Reptilia.

PARÉ (AMBROISE). Œuvres, cap. 22, p. 577, in fol. Paris, 1633.

Bite of the viper. Reports his own case. [S.]

PATTERSON (WILLIAMS). Four voyages into the Hottentot country and into Caffraria, in 4to., 1791.

Advises the use of the Tanjore pill, and failing this, Madeira wine strengthened with brandy, and given in full doses.

PAULET. Observations sur le Vipère de Fontainebleau, et sur les moyens de remédier à sa morsure, in 8vo., 1805.

Report many fatal cases of viper bite, and tends to exaggerate its gravity.

PAULUS (ÆGINETA). Opera, lib. v, p. 8, in fol., 1532.

Extols the use of garlic and of wine in these cases, etc. [S.]

PERONI. Lettera su un caso di morso d'una Vipera instantaneamente fatale, con reflessioni su tale avvenimento. Giorn. della Soc. Med.-Chir. di Parma, XIV, 209.

PHILLIPS (H. B.). Case of Rattlesnake bite. Am. Journ. of the Med. Sci., VIII, 546, 1831.

Use of arsenic (see IRELAND), favorable result.

PIHOREL. Observations sur la morsure d'un ser-

pent a sonnettes. Journ. de Phys. expér. et path. de Magendie, VIII, 97. Paris, 1827.
The well-known case of Drake.

PIHOREL. Note sur l'appareil secrétaire du venin chez les serpentes a sonnettes. J. de Phys. et Path. Exp. de Magendie, VII, 109.

PLATT (THOMAS). Letter from Florence concerning some experiments there made upon Vipers. Engl. Phil. Trans., VII, No. 87, 5060, 1762.

POLETTA (GIOV. BAT.) Sul morso della Vipera. Mem. dell' imper. reg. instit. di Lombardia, II, parte ii, 1, 1821.
Failure to cure canine madness by the bite of the viper. [S.]

POST. Case of Rattlesnake bite ending fatally. Buffalo Med. Journ. and Monthly Rev., IV, 1848, 115.

POUTEAU. Œuvres posthumes, III, 73, 1783, in 8vo. [S.]
Contains observations on the use of olive oil in viper bites, and reports many cases of serious symptoms resulting from these injuries. [S.]

PRAVAZ. Moyens mécanique propres à prévenir l'absorption du virus. Acad. de Méd., Sept. 1828; Arch. Gén. de Méd., 7e série, XVIII, 309, 1828. [S.]
Proposes the use of cups which admit at the same time of lotions being employed. Cauterizes by electricity; gives experiments on animals. [S.]

PRINA. Observation sur un empoisonnement par la morsure d'une Vipère, traité avec succès par des ablutions d'eau froide. Gaz. de Santé, 5 Juillet, 1824.
An exaggerated statement of a case. [S.]

PURPLE. Cedron as a remedy in snake-bites. N. Y. Journ. of Med., N. S., XIII. 173.

PUZIN (J. B.). Observations raisonnées sur quelques faits de médecine pratique. Thése de Paris, No. 84, p. 54, 1809.
A case of viper-bite tending to show that it may be mortal in cold weather, and that the cessation of the symptoms is not a certain sign of cure. Thinks that the venom acts like a ferment.

QUENAT (HENRY). Des animaux venimeux de la France, p. 21, in 8, 1835.
A highly colored statement of the symptoms of a case of viper bite. [S.]

RAFFENEAU (DELILLE). Indications de Thérapeutique directe des morsures les plus vénéneuses. Journ. de Phys., etc., de Magendie, VII, 110, 1827.
Advises the use of incisions and the cautery in viper bites. [S.]

RAMSAY (D). Case of snake-bite treated by ammonia. The Med. and Phys. Journ., London, 1804, XI, 332.

RANBY. On the Teeth of the Rattlesnake, and experiments on the action of the venom upon animals. Engl. Phil. Trans. abrd., VII, 416, 1727.

RAYGER (C.). De lapide serpentis pileati contra Viperarum morsum antidotum. Misc. germ. Acad. Nat. Cur., Dec. 1, ann. 4 et 5, p. 2, 1673–74. [S.]

RAZOMOWSKI. Histoire Naturelle du Jorat, I, 118. [S.]

REDI (FRANÇOIS). Observationes de Viperis scriptæ literis ad gener. dominum Laurentium Magalotti in 18. Amsterd., 1675. Misc. Med. Acad. Nat. Cur., I, 305, 1672. Collect. Acad., III, 27, 1755. [S.]
Gives his own experiments, and refutes the prevalent errors as to the viper.

REDI (FRANÇOIS). Experimenta circa res diversas naturales, speciatim illas quæ ex Indiis adfertuntur, in 18, p. 4, Amst., 1675.
On the inutility of snake stones. [S.]

REDI (FRANÇAIS). Epistolæ ad aliquas oppositiones factas in suas observationes circa Viperas, scriptæ ed. D. Alex. Morus et D. Abb. Bourdelot, in 18. Amst., 1675. Collect. Acad., III, 85, 1755.
Refutes certain views put forth by Charas. [S.]

RENEALMUS (PAULUS). Observationes, in 8vo. Paris, 1606. [S.]

REYNOSO. Experimental criticism upon Brainard's views as to Iodine as an antidote in poisoning by woorara. Comptes Rend., XXXIX, 67, and XL, 118, 825, 1153.

RICHARD (ACHILLE). Observations sur la morsure de la Vipère commune, *Vipera Berus*. Noue. Journ. de Méd.-Chir. et Pharm., VIII, 279, 1820. [S.]
Reports three very serious cases of viper bite. [S.]

RIDOLFI (CAMILLO). Sur l'inutilite de la ligature dans la morsure de la Vipère. Ann. Univ. de Méd., 1834. Gaz. Méd., II, 280, 1834.

RIVERIUS. Observationes, Cent. IV, No. 96.
Proposes the use of garlic internally and externally, and also local treatment by scarifications. [S.]

ROBERT. Cas de morsure de Vipère observé et traité à l'Hôtel Dieu. Bull. de Thér., VII, 307, 1834.
Reports very severe cases treated successfully by ammonia, mercurial frictions, scarifications, ipecacuanha, leeches, etc.

ROBINEAU (DESVOIDY). Viviparité de la Vipère rouge. Compte Rend. de l'Acad. des Sci., 21 Oct. 1829; Journ. de Ch. Médic., V, 639, 1829. [S.]
States that it is more dangerous than the gray viper; thinks nitrate of silver useful in these cases, and cups and ammonia valueless. [S.]

ROCHEFORT. Histoire Nat. des Antilles, I, 294. Lyon, 1667. [S.]

RONEAU (J. B.). Observations sur la morsure de la Vipère. Thèses de Paris, No. 121, 1828.
Reports fatal cases, and others of great severity. [S.]

ROSE (DE). Remède contre la morsure de la Vipère. Fil. Sebez, de 1846; Gaz. Méd. p. 562, 1846.
States that he used with success a cataplasm of the *Trifolium lupinella.* [S.]

ROUSSEAU (EMMANUEL). Des serpents venimeux en général, et de la Vipère en particulier. Gaz. de Santé à l'usage des gens du monde.
Three cases of viper bite. [S.]

ROUX. Hist. de la Soc. Roy. de Méd., ad. 1782 et '83, II, 212, 18—.
Used the ligature, oil "septiques" (sic), and the cautery in viper bites. [S.]

RUDOLPHI (respondente Saïffert). Dissertatio sistens spicilegium adenalogiæ, in 4to. Berlin, 1825. [S.]

RUEZ. Recherches sur les empoisonnements pratiqué par les nègres à la Martinique. Annales d'hygiène publique. Paris, 1844, XXXII, 383.

SABAL (A. M.). Experiments with Bibron's antidote. Savannah Journal of Medicine, Sept. 1858; Amer. Journal of the Med. Sci., Oct. 1858, p. 575.

SAGE. Expériences propre à faire connaitre que l'alcali volatil est le remède le plus efficaces dans les asphyxies, avec des remarques sur les effets avantageux qu'il produit dans la morsures de la Vipère, la rage, etc. Paris, 1777, in 8vo. [S.]

SALISBURY (J. H.). Action of venom on plants. N. Y. Journ. of Med., XIII, 337, 1854.

SAUVAGES (FR. BOISSIER). De venenatis Galliæ animalibus. Montpellier, in 4, 1764. [S.]

SAVA. Introduction d'une Vipère dans l'estomac d'un enfant, Filiat Sebez. Gaz. Méd., p. 743, 1843. [S.]

SAVARY. Lettres sur l'Égypte, p. 62, 1788–89.

SAY. Herpetology, etc. etc. Silliman's Journal, I, 259.

SCHLEGEL. Untersuch der Speïcheldrusen bei den schlangen suit gefurchten Tahnen. Nov. Act. Leop. XIV, 143, 1828; Bull. de Ferussac, XVIII, 462, No. 310.
On the structure of the venom gland and fangs. [S.]

SCHLEGEL. Materiallen für die Stahtarzneikunde, IV, Samml., No. 16.
Treatment of snake-bite by the internal and external use of caustic potassa. [S.]

SCHUCHMANN (CHRISTIAN). Sur les effets d'une morsure de Vipère. Eph. Germ. Acad. Nat. Cur., Dec. 11, Ann. VII, Obs. 140, 1688; Collect. Acad. VII, 661, 1766.
Cure by the use of theriac and mithridate with moderate heat, as local treatment, and finally with scarifications. [S.]

SCHULZE (J. H.). Dissertatio de viperarum in medicina usu. Altdorf, 1727. [S.]

SCOUTETTEN. Morsure de la Vipère en France près Metz, suivie d'accidents très grave. Trans. Mèdic., II, 92, 1830.
A case treated at first by bleeding, without good results, and finally treated successfully with large doses of quinine. [S.]

SCRIBONIUS (LARGUS), (in Matthiale Commentaires).
Extols the use of οξυτοριφυλλον (*oxalis*), which must be gathered before sunrise, and by the left hand. [S.]

SEMMEDUS (JOH. CVR.). Pvgillvs rervm Indicarvm qvo comprehenditvr historia variorvm simplicivm ex India orientali, America, alliisqve orbis terrarum partibvs allatorvm, cvra, Abrahami Vateri, in 4. Wittemb., 1572, p. 24 et 53.
Snake stone and "racine de mungo" useful in viper bites. [S.]

SEVERINO (MARC. AUREL.). Vipera Pithya seu de Viperæ natura, veneno, etc., in 4to, 1651.
Account of the viper—of his bite, and of the remedies for it. [S.]

SHAW. General Zoology. London, O, III, 368.
Contains general information as to the natural history and habits of venomous serpents, etc.

SIGAUD. Du Climat et des Maladies du Brésil, p. 394. Use of the venom of the Crotalus in tubercular lepra, with remarks on the effects of the venom of other serpents, p. 431.

SIMMONDS. Sur les propriétés médicale du *guaco*. Journ. de Pharm., 3e série, XX, 357, 1851.

SLOANE (SIR H.). Engl. Philos. Trans., abrd., IX, 53, 1733.
Droll snake story, etc.

SMITH (TH.). Structure of the Fang. Engl. Phil. Trans. at large, CVIII, 471, pl. xxii, 1818.

SONNINI (DE MANONCOUR). Observations sur les Serpents de la Guyane, et sur l'efficacité de l'eau de Luce pour en guérir. Journ. de Physique, VIII, 469, 1776.
Reports cases of snake-bite. [S.]

SONNANI. Expériences faites sur l'hydrophobie avec le venin de la Vipère. Bull de Thér. XII, 294, 1837.
This singular treatment failed. [S.]

SOUBEIRAN (J. L.). De la Vipère de son venin et de sa morsure. O. Paris, 1855.
A well written essay. The Bibliography is excellent, except as regards the Crotalus.

SOUCHAY (ABBÉ). Discours sur les Psylles Hist. de l'Acad. roy. des inscript. et belles-lettres, VII, 273, 1733.
Gives a history of the Psyllæ, and concludes that their power to cure snake-bites was due only to the suction which they employed. [S.]

SPIELMANN. Dissert. de animalibus nocivis Alsatiæ. Argent. 1768. [S.]

SPONTONUS (J. B.). Conachiduelogia seu discussus de pulvere viperino. Romæ, 1648, in 4to. [S.]

SPRENGEL (CONRAD J.). Some observations upon the viper. Engl. Phil. Trans. at large, XXXII, 296, 1722. [S.]

STORR (TH. CONTR. CHRIST.) De curis Viperinis, in fol., 1768. [S.]

STUPANAS. Dissert. Viperæ et venenorum correctio. Basil, 1640. [S.]

TACHENIUS. Extrait d'une lettre contenant une expérience faite à Venise de la vertu d'une pierre qui guérit la morsure des serpents. Coll. Acad. I, 262; Journ. des Savants, 1668. [S.]

TAVERNIER. Remarques touchant la pierre de serpent. Coll. Acad., I, 275, 1755; Journ. des Savants, 1668.
Describes the properties of these stones, states where they are found, and gives receipt for making artificial snake stones. [S.]

TAYLOR. Effect of Pennyroyal on Crotalus. Engl. Phil. Trans. at large, II, 373, 811, 1665.
This plant said to be fatal to the rattlesnake.

TIEDEMANN (FR.). Ueber Speicheldrusen der Schlangen Mém. de l'Acad. de Munich, p. 25, pl. ii, 1813.

TIXIER. Morsure des serpents venimeux, Vipère, morsure de Crotale. Rapport gén. des Trav. de la Soc. des Sci. Méd. de Gannat, in 8, p. 25, 1854, par M. Gilliot.
General remarks on the habits of the viper, etc. [S.]

TOWGOOD (J.). Dissertatio de Vipera. Lugd-Bat., in 4, 1718. [S.]

TRACY (J. G.). *Uvularia grandiflora* an antidote to the bite of the Crotalus. Trans. Albany Instit., I, 32.

TROWBRIDGE. Olive oil an antidote to the bite of the Rattlesnake. Buffalo Med. Journ. and Rev., IV, 203, 1848.
Reports successful cases.

TRUDAINE (DE MONTIGNY). Lettre à M. Le Marquis de Chesnaie, contenant une observation sur la guérison d'une morsure de Vipère, opérée par l'alcali volatil. Journ. de Méd., XXIV, 162, 1766.
Case of a girl, aged twelve, cured in six hours. [S.]

TYSON. Anatomy of the Crotalus, etc. Engl. Phil. Trans. abrd., II, 797, 1683.

VALLISNERI. Risposta in cui dimostra, come nascano naturalmente i viperini et come le Vipere e gli altri animali si fecondino, spiegando come sia quel raro caso accaduto, e levando molti errori antichi, alla suddetta serpe, ed a' serpentelli spettanti. Opere fisico-mediche, III, 285, 1733.
Opposes Limperani's views (vide L.), and states that he found good results from the use of spirits of hartshorn in snake-bites. [S.]

VAN LIER. Traité des Serpents et des Vipères qu'on trouve dans le pays de Drenthe, auquel on a ajouté quelques remarques et quelques particularités relatives à ces espèces de serpents et à d'autres, p. 84, in 4. Amsterdam, 1781 (fig.). [S.]

VARGAS (DON PEDRO FIRMIN DE). Semanario de agricultura y artes dirigido á los párrocos, IV, 397. Madrid, 1798.
Observations on the use of *mikania guaco* [S.]

VATER (A.). Dissert. de olei olivarum efficacia et virtute adversus morsum animalium venenatorum, casu singulari confirmata. Wittemb., in 4to, 1751. [S.]

VATER (A.). Dissertatio de antidoto novo ad-

versus viperarum morsus præstantissimo in Anglia detecto. Wittemb., in 4, 1736.
Extols the use of olive oil. [S.]

VESLINGIUS. Observationes de viperæ anatome et generatione. Observ. Anat., a Th. Bartbolino editæ, II, 36, in 4, 1740.
Points out with accuracy the seat, etc., of the fang teeth. [S.]

VEYRINES (C. DE). Dissertation sur la morsure de la Vipère et sur son traitement. Thèse, 15 Mars, 1817.
Reports cases, and describes the pathology of snake-bites. [S.]

VIREY. Plantes usitées contre les morsures des serpents venimeux; extrait du travail de Moreau de Jonnès sur le trigonocephalus. Journ. de Pharm. et de Chim., III, 143, 1817.
States that the Euphorbias are the most successful remedies. [S.]

VIREY. Sur l'aspic rougeâtre ou Vipère des environs de Paris. Journ. de Pharm. et de Chim., XIII, 333, 1827. [S.]

VOIGT (M. GODOFREDUS). De congressu et partu viperarum, in 12, 1698. [S.]

WAGNER (FRÉD. AUG.). Observations sur les mœurs de la Vipère commune. Journ. der Practisch. Heilkunde, p. 3; Bull. des Sci. Nat., XXI, 322, 1829.
States that the viper bite is not fatal to vipers. [S.]

WALKER (E. M.). Experiments with Bibron's Antidote. Am. Journ. of Med. Sci., Oct. 1858, p. 568.
Reports an interesting case in man bitten by the *Trigonocephalus piscivorus*. Took whiskey and 20-drop doses of Bibron's antidote; nearly the whole hand sloughed; amputation and cure. Thinks the recovery due to the antidote.

WEGER. Cas de morsure de Vipère, trachéotomie, guerison. Wochenschrift für die Gesammte Heilkundt Casper's, 1839; Gaz. Méd., VII, 632, 1839. [S.]

WHITMIRE (J.). Iodine an antidote to snake-bites. Northwest. Med. and Surg. Journ., Chicago and Indianapolis, I, New Series (V of the whole series), 396.

WILLIAMS (J). Seven cases of E. Indian serpent bites, treated with ammonia. Asiatic Researches, II, 323.

WILLIAMS (STEPHEN). Letter concerning the Viper Catchers, and the efficacy of olive oil in curing the bite of Vipers. Engl. Phil. Trans. at large, p. 27, 1737.

WILLIAMS (S. W.). The *Viola Ovata* as a remedy in Crotalus bite. Am. Journ. of the Med. Sci., XIII, 310, 1833.

WILLIS (G.). On the bite of the Viper. Assoc. Med. Journ., No. 83, 1854.

WOLFF (WEICHEL). De Paulo a Vipera demorso, in 4to, 1710.

WOODHOUSE. Case of Crotalus bite, reported by the patient. Sitgreave's Expedition to the Colorado and Zuni Rivers, 1851–52; also in Buffalo Med. Journ. and Rev., VIII, 72, 1853.
A well described case of some severity.

WYDER (J. F.). Essai sur l'histoire naturelle des serpents de la Suisse. Lausanne, in 8vo, 1823.
Reports cases of viper bite collected by Drs. Schwartz and Lantz. [S.]

XANTUS. *See* DE VESEY.

INDEX.

V.

W.

X.

Y.

Lightning Source UK Ltd.
Milton Keynes UK
UKHW021033191218
334260UK00012B/1088/P